P9-AFI-917

DeGowin & DeGowin's

Bedside

DIAGNOSTIC EXAMINATION

Contributors:

PETER R. JOCHIMSEN, M.D., F.A.C.S.

Professor of Surgery,
University of Iowa College of
Medicine, Iowa City

and

ERNEST O. THEILEN, M.D., F.A.C.P.

Professor of Internal Medicine,
University of Iowa College of
Medicine, Iowa City

DeGowin & DeGowin's

Bedside

DIAGNOSTIC EXAMINATION

FIFTH EDITION

Revised by

RICHARD L. DEGOWIN, M.D., F.A.C.P.

Professor of Internal Medicine, University of Iowa College of Medicine, Iowa City

Macmillan Publishing Company
NEW YORK

Collier Macmillan Canada, Inc.
TORONTO

Collier Macmillan Publishers
LONDON

Printed in the United States of America

Macmillan Publishing Company
866 Third Avenue, New York, New York 10022

Collier Macmillan Canada, Inc.

Collier Macmillan Publishers • London

Library of Congress Cataloging-in-Publication Data

DeGowin, Elmer Louis, 1901–
DeGowin & DeGowin's bedside diagnostic examination.

Rev. ed of: Bedside diagnostic examination/Elmer L. DeGowin, Richard L. DeGowin. 4th ed. c1981.
Bibliography: p.
Includes index.
1. Physical diagnosis. 2. Diagnosis. I. DeGowin, Richard L. II. Jochimsen, Peter R. III. Theilen, Ernest O. IV. Title. V. Title: Bedside diagnostic examination.
RC76.D45 1987 616.07′54 86–33212
ISBN 0–02–328080–8

Printing: 5 6 7 8 Year: 1 2 3 4 5

Dedicated to the late Elmer L. DeGowin, M.D., M.A.C.P.

Preface to the Fifth Edition

Since the publication of the fourth edition, remarkable changes have occurred in the practice of medicine. Many more physicians have entered an increasingly competitive practice, in a system with strong pressures to reduce the costs of highly technologic medical care and in which rapid diagnosis and treatment yielding near-perfect results are expected. These developments have made the office and bedside diagnostic examination even more critical in establishing good rapport with patients, as well as in quickly evaluating their complaints, selecting appropriate laboratory and imaging studies, and making rational decisions regarding their need for hospitalization and therapy.

Computerized tomography and magnetic resonance imaging have joined ultrasonography in revolutionizing diagnostic imaging, thus requiring that this textbook inform the student and physician about how and when these new modalities may extend their examinations to assist in accurate diagnosis. New syndromes, like AIDS, toxic shock, and Lyme disease, have been described in the interim and now appear in this fifth edition. Système International units for laboratory values were introduced in all American Medical Association publications in July 1986 and are included with conventional units in Chapter 11. Students opening this book for the first time, however, should not feel intimidated by its 1000-plus pages of tightly organized information. Rather, they should be reassured by their instructors that it is not possible to memorize the contents by the end of their second year in medical school. Initially, they will wish to concentrate on how to elicit and interpret symptoms and signs. Later, as house officers and seasoned practitioners, this portable companion should remind the physician of symptoms and signs to seek and diseases to consider in formulating a differential diagnosis of the problems confronting him in the office and hospital.

Twenty years ago, a friend predicted the evolution of a totally automated diagnostic examination that would render obsolete the history and physical examination. He envisioned the reclining patient conveyed on a belt through a series of devices designed to image and sense the body's structure and function. The ill person would receive a computer printout of the diagnoses and recommended treatments at the end of his short journey. With contributions from the manned space program and other sources, the technology to realize this fantasy has probably been at hand for several years. You, my tolerant reader, can undoubtedly offer more reasons to explain why this has not occurred than I can. Indeed, it is surprising how many recent papers in the general medical literature stress the need for teachers of clinical medicine to accompany students and residents to the bedside, where they can observe and help improve the trainee's skills in taking a history and performing a physical examination.

The popularity of the earlier editions among medical students, physicians, physician assistants, and nurses in North America and among their counterparts abroad (who have used translations into French, German, Italian, Greek, and Spanish) has encouraged me to retain the original format and update the material within that structure. The late Elmer L. DeGowin, senior author of the fourth edition, would be the first to disclaim the beauty of his artwork for the book. His intent was to present line drawings like he might sketch for a student after demonstrating a physical sign in a patient. He thought that photographs could not depict concepts as well, and fine art would distract the reader from the points we wished to make. For these reasons, and to contain the cost, I have retained my father's simple, but clinically accurate, illustrations with slight modifications.

After reviewing and suggesting changes for Chapter 6 ("The Thorax and Cardiovascular System") for the fourth edition, Ernest O. Theilen, M.D., F.A.C.P., has taken the responsibility for revising that chapter in this fifth edition. As Professor of Medicine at the University of Iowa, he regularly attends patients and teaches on the Coronary Care Unit, the Cardiology Inpatient and Consultation Services, and the Outclinic. His broad interests in undergraduate and postgraduate medical education include his service as Governor of the Iowa Chapter of the American College of Physicians. Moreover, he was my father's physician and is frequently consulted by members of our faculty for their personal medical care; he is a doctor's doctor. Peter R. Jochimsen, M.D., F.A.C.S., joins us as a contributor, revising the section on examination of the breast, Chapter 7 ("The Abdomen and Rectosigmoid"), and Chapter 8 ("The Genitalia"). It has been my pleasure to work with this fine surgeon in the mutual care of our patients who require both medical and surgical therapy. Dr. Jochimsen serves as Professor and Vice-Chairman of the Department of Surgery at Iowa and is Associate Director for Clinical Programs in the University of Iowa Cancer Center. Other interests and responsibilities include service on the Executive Committee of the National Surgical Adjuvant Breast and Bowel Project and president of the Iowa Academy of Surgery.

I am especially grateful for the thoughtful review and recommendations of other chapters by my colleagues: Lee A. Harker, M.D., F.A.C.S., Professor of Otolaryngology and Head and Neck Surgery—Chapter 5 ("The Head and Neck"); Joseph D. Brown, M.D., F.A.C.P., Associate Professor of Medicine—the section on the thyroid gland; Joseph A. Buckwalter, M.D., F.A.C.S., Professor of Orthopaedic Surgery—Chapter 9 ("The Spine and Extremities"); and Harold P. Adams, M.D., F.A.C.P., Professor of Neurology—Chapter 10 ("The Neuropsychiatric Examination"). All of these teachers have major clinical responsibilities and vigorously participate in programs of undergraduate and postgraduate education.

Joan C. Zulch, Vice-President of Macmillan Publishing Company, has personally edited and guided publication of these five editions during the last 25 years. She has concerned herself not only with the overall objective, but also with all of the small but critical details of the book and its production. I wish to thank her and her staff at Macmillan for their successful work in producing an attractive, durable, and functional book within the means of students, house officers, and other health care professionals.

Finally, I thank those who have taken the time to write recommendations for revisions, and I encourage the readers of this book to let me know how subsequent editions can be improved.

RICHARD L. DEGOWIN, M.D., F.A.C.P.

Iowa City, Iowa

Contents

[including key symptoms and signs]

DeGowin & DeGowin's *Bedside* DIAGNOSTIC EXAMINATION

Diagnostic Reasoning

Disease Names—Indices to the Medical Literature

For several thousand years physicians have recorded their observations and clinical trials about patients. In the accumulated facts they have discerned disordered patterns of bodily structure, function, and mentation. Some patterns of features recur with such frequency as to suggest a common cause; the disorder with these features is called a *disease* and is given a specific name. Wulff has aptly called a disease "a vehicle of clinical experience." Other clusters of attributes, less closely related to a single cause, but known by a combination of features, are called *syndromes.* In the medical literature clinical facts are collected under the names of diseases and syndromes, so the names serve as "catchwords" leading to definitions, descriptions, causations (etiology), courses (prognosis), diagnostic features, and treatments.

The Two Meanings of Diagnosis

The name of the patient's disease is *the diagnosis.* In English, the word *diagnosis,* meaning the patient's disease, may or may not be preceded by the article *a* or *the.* When diagnosis means a *search for clues,* the noun diagnosis is always used *without the article,* but a better style is *diagnostic process* or *procedure.*

Triage—The Prelude to Diagnosis

Triage (tre-ahzh') (*Fr.* "sorting"): the sorting out and classification of casualities of war or other disaster, to determine priority of need and place of treatment [*Dorland's Illustrated Medical Dictionary, 26th ed.* 1981, Philadelphia, W. B. Saunders Co.]

Although the French term *triage* is usually applied to military or civil *mass* casualties, the same diagnostic process is used informally with *every* individual patient in civil medicine. In the latter case, there are usually two stages of decision-making: one by nonprofessionals and the other by professionals.

Nonprofessional Triage. Someone must make the initial decision that the patient needs medical attention. This conclusion may be made by the patient, or a relative, friend, or a bystander, none of whom usually has medical training. But the average adult in civil life can judge when a person is sick. He will have been sick himself in the past and will have seen sick persons. Sometimes he will make correct diagnoses, as acute respiratory infections, some febrile diseases, pregnancy, burns, malpositioned limb fractures, compound fractures, lacerations, exanthemata, and hemorrhage. If a precise diagnosis is not made, he will at least be able to judge the *severity* and *urgency* of the situation. This is done by registering subtle signs, as facial expressions of *pain* or *dyspnea, pallor* or *cyanosis* of the skin, and the appearance of *weakness*. These conclusions temper the arrangements for getting the patient to the site of medical attention.

Professional Triage. The site of contact between patient and physician may be in the field where first aid is rendered, the patient's home, in the physician's office, in the emergency room of a hospital or clinic, in a hospital intensive care unit. Before meeting the physician, the patient may meet with intermediaries with various degrees of medical sophistication: physician's assistants, ambulance drivers, or attendants, hospital orderlies, physician's secretaries, receptionists, social workers, nurses; all may lend assistance in expediting the patient's course through diagnostic procedures; all may form conclusions about the diagnosis and conduct the patient accordingly. When the physician has made a more thorough examination, the diagnosis is either made or enough information obtained to direct the patient to an appropriate medical specialist for further examination and treatment. In each case, each person meeting the patient judges the degree of disability and urgency.

The Diagnostic Examination

Intelligent medical care depends upon the physician's knowledge of the patient's abnormalities of function, structure, and mentation—best combined in a diagnosis. Each recognizable disease in the corpus of medicine must *a priori* possess distinguishing features that may serve as *clues*. So the physician embarks upon two parallel courses: (1) a search for clues, leading to (2) the generation and selection of hypotheses.

Course of Clue-Search/Hypothesis-Selection. The dual courses begin about simultaneously with the first contact between patient and doctor. The *age* calls to mind a list of diseases common to the patient's contemporaries, and another list is excluded by age. The *duration of illness* tells the doctor much: e.g., diseases lasting more than three years are unlikely to be cancer. *Race* is important in some diseases, e.g., sickle-cell anemia is not found in Northern European whites. *Sex-linked* diseases are obvious for some structural abnormalities. Diseases such as hemophilia are rarely encountered in females.

Processing of Clues. During the progress of the clue-search, each emerging clue is scrutinized closely before being accepted. If it be a symptom, its accuracy is questioned as to the reliability of the observer; is the observer acceptable or does he/she permit observations to be highly colored by emotions or a desire to malinger? Is the observer's memory adequate? What importance does the patient attach to the symptoms? Is it regarded fearfully or with relative unconcern? If the clue be a sign, is it within normal limits or is it highly significant? Is it constantly present or does it vary with bodily motions? With laboratory findings, one must constantly suspect the mixing of specimens. Are the reports in accord with what else you know about the patient? Was there opportunity for the adulteration of specimens? What is the reputation for accuracy of the laboratory? If the clue was found in the x-ray films, was it present in previous films? Was there proper identification of the patient in taking the films? Were the films read by competent persons?

Clue-Search in Four Compartments. The examiner carries on the dual clue-search/hypothesis selection sequentially in four compartments. The boundaries of these compartments are determined by the physical contacts of the patient with the physician, nurses, and technicians: (1) *History-taking* where clues are *symptoms* (abnormalities perceived by the patient's own senses); (2) *physical examination* where the *physical signs* are clues (abnormalities perceived by the physician's senses); (3) *laboratory examination* where the clues are findings from cytologic and chemical tests of tissues, body fluids, and excreta; (4) *special anatomic and physiologic examinations* where the clues appear on x-ray films, computed tomographic (CT) or magnetic resonance image (MRI) scans, ultrasonograms, and electrical measurements, such as ECG, EMG, or EEG. The examiner searches in each compartment, using the same general procedure in each. A clue is uncovered and verified. It prompts the examiner's recall of a list of diseases and syndromes all having the one clue in common. The examiner maintains an *imaginary slate* upon which the names of the diseases are inscribed that are considered as hypotheses for the diagnosis. As each name is slated, its other attributes are matched with those already slated to determine whether prior entries should be dropped, or whether the new entrant has attributes suggesting other hypotheses for the slate.

Studies have shown that the average clinician carries coincidentally four or five diseases on the slate; but a total of 13 or 15 will have appeared on the slate at some time or other during the examination.

Decision on Hypotheses. This process has attracted much attention from physicians, mathematicians, and psychologists writing on the topics of medical decision-making, medical logic, or clinical problem-solving. Although several methods of problem-solving have been considered, *branching* and *matching* are most commonly used.

Branching Hypotheses. Most clinicians follow a clue-search that leads from one hypothesis to another. A clue calls to mind a disease with a similar attribute; the other attributes of the new entry are considered, and they introduce other diseases for consideration. The hypotheses are entered on the examiner's imaginary slate, revised, and reviewed, and the attributes of the new entry may introduce for consideration other diseases.

Matching Hypotheses. The attributes found in the patient are matched with those of the hypothetic disease on the imaginary slate. The best match is selected as *the diagnosis* of the patient. For example, suppose the examination of the patient (*pt*) yields attributes or clues *a, d, e, k,* and *n;* we may designate the patient as (*pt*)*adekn*. From memory or references in this book under the heads *Clinical Occurrence* the examiner enters upon his slate a list of diseases having the same attribute *a*. The diseases on the list can be designated as *V, W, X, Y,* and *Z*. In matching one finds the diseases have the following attributes in common with the patient: *(V)abcde* has *ade* in common; *(W)acefg* has *ae* in common; *(X)adfij* has *ad* in common; *(Y)afhkl* has *ak* in common; *(Z)aekgn* has *aekn* in common. Without any other considerations, this last would be eligible as *the diagnosis.*

[We have described the diagnostic process from our own introspections after reviewing the following references: A. R. Feinstein: *Clinical Judgment,* 1967, Baltimore, Williams & Wilkins Co. E. A. Murphy: *The Logic of Medicine,* 1976, Baltimore, The Johns Hopkins Press. H. R. Wulff: *Rational Diagnosis and Treatment,* 2nd ed., 1981, St. Louis, C.V. Mosby Co. A. S. Elstein, L. S. Shulman, and S. A. Sprafka: *Medical Problem Solving,* 1978, Cambridge, Mass., Harvard University Press. J. M. Harris: The Hazards of Bedside Bayes, *J.A.M.A.,* **246:**2602–05, 1981. F. M. Wolf, L. D. Gruppen, and J. E. Billi: Differential Diagnosis and the Competing-Hypotheses Heuristic, *J.A.M.A.,* **253:**2858–62, 1985. P. Cutler: *Problem Solving in Clinical Medicine, From Data to Diagnosis,* Williams and Wilkins Co., Baltimore, 1985.] We have avoided the attempted applications of mathematics to diagnosis because we are not convinced that the approach has contributed practical results. We decry the obfuscation in discussions of this subject by the unnecessary displacement of familiar and time-tested terms with such jargon as *iatrotropic symptoms* = chief complaints; *criterial subject* = experienced clinician; *uncriterial subject* = inexperienced person; the redundant *data base* = data; *lanthanic disease* = asymptomatic disease; *cue-hypothesis matrix* = ?

Decisions Based on Probability. As far as we know, the mathematics applied to decision-making in medicine has been focused on the determination of the most probable for a diagnosis. If the examiner followed that principle rigidly, a rare disease would never be diagnosed. Considerable time is devoted to the physician's education to learn about diseases that may never be encountered in his/her practice; nevertheless the physician has the responsibility of taking care of patients with rare diseases.

Use of Computers. There are several special areas in which computers have proved valuable in the diagnostic examination. One of these areas is in the rapid communication of laboratory results and radiologic interpretations to office and nursing-station computer terminals and printers. Another is in the comprehensive search of the medical literature by computers to evaluate clues found during an examination. Today, computer searches are frequently made in most hospital libraries and in the offices and homes of an increasing number of physicians.

Proposals for the use of computers in other areas, however, have not enjoyed the same acceptance. Obviously, the fully computerized chart, promised in the 1960s, has not accommodated the needs of an actively growing hard-copy record that constantly and immediately receives new data from nurses, physicians, receptionists, dieticians, social workers, technicians, and others as it joins the patient's odyssey from clinic to radiology department to laboratory and elsewhere. More recent proposals for the use of computers include history taking and construction of a differential diagnosis. In the former, you are asked to picture a patient seated comfortably before an interactive computer terminal, stylus in hand, answering questions flashed on a screen by user-friendly software. Introducing this practice will hardly mollify dissatisfied patients whose most frequent complaint is, "The doctor did not listen to me or appear interested in my problem." Second, a certain level of training and understanding, not required in a verbal interview, is necessary.

The computer display of a list of diseases in rank order of probability as a cause of a diagnostic clue may reassure physicians who fear they will forget an item. Such a list would be valuable in solving complex problems of differential diagnosis, but its use by an experienced clinician would probably be too infrequent to encourage dependence upon such a system for most problems. Undoubtedly, technologic progress will provide physicians with new opportunities for computer assistance in the diagnostic examination. Satisfactory answers to a few basic questions should precede the adoption of a computer-assisted system: Who developed the program and with which data? How frequently will it be updated and by whom? Will it save time? Is it portable? Are there enough constantly operative computer terminals available to make it accessible when needed? How will access to confidential information be controlled? Will it alienate my patients? Is it easy for me and my patient to learn and use? How expensive is it?

Modifications of Hypothesis Selection

"Snap" Diagnoses. With certain diseases the clinician gives one glance at the patient and renders the diagnosis, when not enough time has elapsed to permit the complicated processes we have just described. The German word for this is *Augenblick* [= movement of the eye]. From another approach, the German *Gestalt* [= form] expresses the psychologic concept of the process. It depends upon recalling an entire image as a unit. Some disorders are favorite subjects for this method: myxedema, Marfan's disease, acromegaly. Apparently dermatologists recognize many skin lesions in this fashion. Other local disorders are hernias, Dupuytren's contracture, Peyronie's syndrome, compound fractures.

Specialist's Diagnoses. The foregoing discussions of the diagnostic process have built-in hidden biases. Actually this complex process deals primarily with the problems of chronic and relatively obscure diseases commonly assigned to the fields of internal medicine and pediatrics. The majority of patients seen by most physicians escape the necessity for such a process. Although the principles of diagnosis hold for all patients, wide deviations from the described details are induced by the patient's condition and the medical or surgical specialty involved. Many conditions requiring minor surgery need few or no symptoms to make a diagnosis; the situation is obvious by noting the anatomic derangement or taking x-ray films. The dermatologist can make many diagnoses without hearing any symptoms. On the other hand, the psychiatrist leans heavily upon the history given by friends, relatives, and attendants, or from dialogue with the patient. It follows that the scope and length of the history vary greatly among medical specialties.

Tests of the Diagnosis

In choosing a diagnosis from several hypotheses, the matching of the patient's attributes with those of the hypothetic disease may not be entirely conclusive; so several criteria may be added for further confirmation and adjustment to the patient's situation.

Parsimony. The diagnosis has a higher probability of being correct if one disease is accepted to explain the entire cluster of clues, rather than trying to account for the findings by supposing a coincidence of several diseases. However, the older persons get, the more often they may acquire two or more coincident disorders, especially in the category of degenerative diseases.

Chronology. It is possible to have a perfect match of attributes between patient and disease, but the hypothesis is incorrect because the timing of onset and course are incorrect.

Degree of Sickness. Not infrequently an inexperienced person will diagnose the patient's condition as an upper respiratory infection when a more experienced clinician will look at the patient and make a diagnosis of pneumonia, explaining that the patient looked "too sick" for the first condition. This perception of degree of sickness is valid and diagnostically useful, but it is difficult to explain or describe.

Prognosis. If two hypotheses seem equally probable and neither can be immediately proved, temporarily select the one with the better prognosis for the benefit of the patient and the family.

Therapeutic Tests. If there is a choice of diagnosis between a fatal disease and one with successful therapy, try a *therapeutic test.* Although experience shows that these are often inconclusive or difficult to interpret, they are better than nothing.

Selection of Diagnostic Tests. Experienced clinicians select diagnostic tests indicated by clues from the history and the physical examination. They have repeatedly learned that routine testing or uncritical testing for remote diagnostic possibilities frequently yields questionably abnormal results requiring explanation by more testing. This "cascade effect" heightens the patient's anxiety, is hazardous and expensive, and delays treatment [J. W. Mold and H. F. Stein: The Cascade Effect in the Clinical Care of Patients, *N. Engl. J. Med.,* **314:**512–14, 1986.]

Rare Diseases. Some physicians, especially the inexpert, have a tendency to diagnose rare diseases with suspicious frequency. It is well to recall that rare diseases occur rarely.

Deferred Diagnoses

When a suitable match for the patient's clues cannot be found, or the patient lacks any distinctive clues at the time, the physician can proceed with the following supplementary steps:

1. Repeat the History-Taking and the Physical Examination. This tests the patient's memory; it may prove to have been faulty, or more recall may have been stimulated by the first trial. Talk to more relatives and attendants to confirm or deny the original story and to add details. Carefully repeat the physical examination for signs that were overlooked the first time. Repeat examination often uncovers cardiac murmurs.

2. Repeat Laboratory Tests. The specimens may have been mixed on the initial occasion, or an error in the first test may be uncovered.

3. Deferral of Diagnosis. Carefully explain the situation to secure his/her confidence so that a return examination may be made when new symptoms or signs may have appeared, or extended chronicity shall have given more perspective to the case. Mark the record "Diagnosis Deferred"; do not let the Record Room rules or the insurance company force a premature diagnosis.

Varieties of Medical Examinations

There are at least seven varieties of medical examinations that differ from one another in their purposes, their stereotyped procedures, and their diagnostic tests.

1. Examination of Young Schoolchildren. The examination usually emphasizes tests of vision and hearing, sometimes coordination, and a search for birth defects.

2. Examination of Athletes. The examiner stresses tests of cardiopulmonary function and muscle performance. Other systems affecting stamina are tested.

3. Examination for Military Service. This resembles the examination for athletes but adds testing of the special senses and the psyche.

4. Examination for Life Insurance. The routine is generally established by the insurance company; it usually consists of a simple history form, an abbreviated physical examination, and a few laboratory tests, to exclude the presence of chronic diseases that affect longevity.

5. Periodic Health Examination. For infants, the physician searches for birth defects; he measures growth and development. In persons over 45 years old, annual examinations seek to detect the early onset of degenerative diseases, or to find diabetes mellitus, pulmonary tuberculosis, or cancer of the lung. Hypertension is also sought.

6. Industrial Examinations. Specialized procedures detect the hazards of particular industries: testing for lead and carbon monoxide in the blood, seeking signs of pneumoconiosis or tuberculosis in radiograms of the lungs, the measurement of radiation of workers exposed to x-rays or radioisotopes.

All six of these examinations are special stereotyped routines upon persons presumed to be well and therefore *having no symptoms as clues* to disease. Recommendations based on yield and cost are periodically revised by various professional groups. [Medical Evaluations of Healthy Persons, *J.A.M.A.*, **249**1626–33, 1983.] The lack of symptoms imposes a set of conditions far different from those surrounding a diagnostic examination.

7. Diagnostic Examination. This procedure is much less routinized, more searching, has symptoms as clues, and starts with the problem of *finding a disease that is causing discomfort or dysfunction.*

Certainty of the Diagnosis

When *the diagnosis* is established for a patient, how certain can one be of its correctness? Unfortunately there is no accepted scale of *degrees of certainty* whereby the examiner can express the extent to which he has proved his diagnosis. The term *the diagnosis* is applied, on the one hand, to a fracture of the tibia where the fracture line can readily be seen in the x-ray film with perfect accuracy. On the other hand, the same term is applied to a diagnosis of rheumatoid arthritis, a situation often with much less certainty, where the clinical appearance is supported by such nonspecific tests as x-ray examinations, tests of rheumatoid arthritis factor, etc. Many types of neoplasia can be diagnosed with great accuracy in biopsy specimens, but diseased lymph nodes occasionally are the subjects of great uncertainty to pathologists.

Although a meticulous physician may qualify his diagnosis by the word *probable* or a question mark, these modifiers often get dropped when the record has passed through several transcriptions. These important adjectives and adverbs are impatiently discarded by operators of computers, lawyers, insurance adjustors, and medical librarians. Other statements of uncertainty in use are *preliminary diagnosis, diagnostic impression, tentative diagnosis, working diagnosis, provisional diagnosis,* and *probable diagnosis.*

Another attempt at grading diagnoses is encountered in some hospitals and in some insurance forms that call for a *primary diagnosis* and a *secondary diagnosis.* On the face of it this seems rational, but the absurdity appears when the same records are graded by different specialists. The primary diagnosis is often quite different from the view of the internist, the surgeon, the orthopedist, or the otolaryngologist. Each selects the disease pertaining to his own specialty.

Part I: Symptoms and Signs

(Chaps. 2–10)

This part presents the classic approach to diagnosis, evolved over two thousand years, in which the diagnostic clues to diseases are sought as *symptoms* (abnormalities perceived by the patient's own senses and conveyed to the physician during history-taking), and *physical signs* (abnormalities perceived by the physician's senses and found by him in the physical examination).

The symptoms and signs are set in boldface italic type as paragraph heads, with or without preceding modifiers. To emphasize relative importance, certain symptoms and signs are distinguished by preceding keystone symbols (▼) and the words "Key Symptom" or "Key Sign." These are the authors' choices for clues most likely to lead the search to a finite number of disease entities as diagnostic hypotheses. Most of the key symptoms commonly occur as chief complaints.

Most of the physical signs are placed in order as they are encountered by the physician who conducts the physical examination from head to foot of the patient.

2
The Medical History

The Patient's Medical Record

The patient's medical record is a written document containing (1) the medical history, (2) the findings from the physical examination, (3) the reports of laboratory tests, (4) the findings and conclusions from special examinations, (5) the findings and diagnoses of consultants, (6) the diagnoses of the responsible physician, (7) notes on treatment, including medication, surgical operations, radiation, physical therapy, and (8) progress notes by physicians, nurses, and others.

Purposes. The varied purposes of the patient's medical record may be classified as follows:

Medical Purposes

1. To assist the physician in making diagnoses
2. To assist physicians, nurses, and others in the care and treatment of the patient
3. To serve as a record for teaching medicine and for clinical research

Legal Purposes

4. To document insurance claims for the patient
5. To serve as legal proof in cases of malpractice, claims for injury or compensation, cases of poisoning, cases of homicide

Usually the physician composes the patient's record with his attention focused upon the *medical purposes* of making diagnoses, caring for the patient, and teaching medicine and furthering research. After the illness, sometimes years later, the medical record may be consulted to fulfill the *legal purposes* in support of claims and the demonstration of facts in litigation.

In these contingencies, the physician belatedly discovers omissions and inaccuracies. To prevent late recriminations, certain rules should be rigidly observed when the record is composed.

Physician's Signature. Each sheet and briefer entry composed by the physician for the medical record should be accompanied by his *signature* and the *date of signing*, as proof of authorship. In the hospital record, the physician's initials are inadequate; his *complete signature* should be employed; it should be *written* and *legible*. All dates should include the *month, day of the month,* and *year*. In teaching hospitals, where many persons contribute to the record, the entries of medical students and nurses should be accompanied by their signatures, affixed with suitable abbreviations indicating their status in the medical organization.

Custody of the Record. The record may repose in the physician's locked office files, or it may be in the custody of the hospital where the patient received medical care. The contents of the medical record must be guarded against the scrutiny of unauthorized persons; the recorded facts are *privileged communication* under the law; they cannot be revealed to another person without the written consent of the patient. In some states, privileged communication does not extend to nurses, unless they are the specific agents of the physician, or unless the information is given in their presence in line of duty. Generally, it is undesirable that the patient should read his own record; he may misinterpret the contents and suffer unnecessary anguish. The medical record should be composed with the constant realization that at some future time it may become a legal document; the date and authorship of each entry may be important. The record should not contain flippant or derogatory remarks about the patient or colleagues that would give embarrassment when read in court.

Taking the Medical History

Definition of the Medical History. The medical history is an account of the events in the patient's life that have relevance to his mental and physical health. Much more than the patient's unprompted narrative, it is a specialized literary form in which the physician composes and writes an account based upon facts, supplied by the patient or other informants, offered spontaneously or secured by skillful probing. Items are accepted for the record only after rigorous evaluation by the physician, who employs his knowledge of the natural history of diseases to secure pertinent details and establish the sequence of events.

Scope of the History. When a patient consults his physician for a dermatitis, the necessary diagnostic history is very brief, possibly only a few sentences. For a man brought into the hospital with a fractured tibia, a long diagnostic history is unnecessary, and even inhumane. In contrast, a chronic obscure disease may require a long careful history, perhaps repeated and expanded, with supplements from time to time as the results of further studies open new vistas of diagnostic possibilities. Writings on history taking always discuss the *extended history,* which is complicated and demands maximal skill. But it would be folly to insist on an extended history for every patient; in many conditions, it is unnecessary; the physician could care for only a few patients in a day. The experienced physician adjusts to the patient's problems. Whether the history is sufficient for the individual case will plague the clinician during his entire professional career.

Interrogation in History Taking. To learn the art of history taking is probably more difficult than acquiring skill in physical examination. Beginning students, and even experienced clinicians, often slight the interview to indulge in the motor activity of palpation, percussion, and auscultation. This appears to be a response to a primitive instinct; even young infants seem to prefer palpating a newfound object to looking at it. For this reason and others, it seems easier to teach students the mechanisms of physical examination first and the techniques of history taking later, after they have acquired more knowledge of the symptoms and signs of diseases.

We believe that extensive written instructions about interrogation of the patient are unprofitable; the student can only learn to pose questions by actually interviewing patients. But no one can take a meaningful medical history unless his memory is well stocked with lists of diseases that can be recalled by catchwords of symptoms and signs. When a disease name thus comes to mind, it should recall a cluster of symptoms and signs, and chronologic data about which to ask the patient. When the student has acquired an intellectual capital of disease names associated with their symptoms and signs, he can face the patient confidently without embarrassment and readily improvise methods of interrogation.

Diagnostic history taking has the triple quest of (1) searching for symptoms, (2) eliciting accurate quantitative descriptions, and (3) securing precise chronologies of events.

CONDUCTING THE INTERVIEW. ***Arrangement.*** **This description deals with the taking of an *extended history* in the physician's office: the patient is in no acute distress, time limitations are not urgent, and the disease is relatively obscure. Circumstances often vary greatly from these stipulations. The conversation should not be overheard by others, although the presence of the patient's spouse or a relative is often helpful in confirming the narrative and supplementing the patient's observations. We prefer to limit a single interview to the patient and one other informant; more informants waste time in their disagreements on details that outweigh the slight extra yield of information.**

Physician's Manner. **Present to the patient the appearance of being *unhurried, interested,* and *sympathetic,* to obtain his confidence and rapport. In no way should you express adverse moral judgment on his actions. Permit him to begin his story in his own way; listen for a short time before gradually injecting questions to guide the interview. Gently but firmly keep the discussion centered upon the patient's problems. By all means, avoid discussing your own health, even when he invites you. One of us knew a resident who violated this injunction on a women's ward. On rounds each morning the patients interrupted our interviews with them by anxiously inquiring about the health of "poor Dr. X." Incidentally Dr. X's health needed no attention.**

Writing. **Write sparingly while the patient talks. After you have recorded some routine data on vital statistics, sit back and listen to the narrative for a while, interjecting only a few questions. Avoid writing the patient's narrative verbatim; it is too lengthy and poorly organized. After obtaining the present illness, take time to write it down. Then write the past history as it is elicited by your questions.**

Use of Language. **From the beginning, gauge the patient's understanding of the language; words may have different meanings for both of you. Put your questions in simple nontechnical words. Even lay words may be misunderstood; the English vocabulary is vast and formidable to the scholar. Excluding your scientific and medical vocabulary, you may be able to use 100,000 words, while the adult with average education gets along with 30,000 to 60,000 [Mario Pei: *The Story of English.* J. B. Lippincott Co., Philadelphia, 1952]. So the patient may not know half the words you may use in English. Patients often leave the interview with the fear they have presented their symptoms poorly because they have answered questions they did not understand.**

Patient's Motivation. **The use of the history to secure diagnostic clues depends on the tacit assumption, frequently forgotten, that the patient's description of his symptoms is *truthful,* because his sole motive is to assist the physician in treatment. As far as possible, this assumption must be confirmed by excluding other motives that might prompt misrepresentation of the facts. Many patients, entirely truthful, present symptoms that are baffling until the physician learns their resemblance to those of a friend or relative who has died of cancer and the patient fears the same fate. The physician must ascertain whether the patient is contemplating a lawsuit for damages, claiming workman's compensation, or applying for war veteran's benefits. The narcotic addict presents symptoms calculated to obtain drugs. Lacking discernible motives, a few patients fabricate medical histories that defy the psychiatrist's attempts to explain (Münchausen's syndrome).**

Sequence of Components in the Medical History

The parts of the medical history follow a standardized sequence, differing only in small details from one institution to another. The following is employed for adult patients in the Department of Internal Medicine at the University of Iowa. A different order is usually preferred by pediatricians, who set the birth history and the past history ahead of the present illness.

I. Identification and vital statistics
II. Informant, his relation to the patient
III. Chief complaints
IV. Present illness
V. Past history
  A. General health
  B. Infectious diseases
  C. Operations and injuries
  D. Previous hospitalizations
  E. System review (inventory of systems)
    1. Integument
    2. Lymph nodes
    3. Bones, joints, and muscles
    4. Hematopoietic system
    5. Endocrine system
    6. Allergic and immunologic history
    7. Head

8. Eyes
9. Ears
10. Nose
11. Mouth
12. Throat
13. Neck
14. Breasts
15. Respiratory system
16. Cardiovascular system
17. Gastrointestinal system
18. Genitourinary system
19. Nervous system
20. Psychiatric history

VI. Social history
VIII. Family history

1. Identification and Vital Statistics

Data under this heading are frequently recorded by the physician's receptionist or the hospital registration clerk. During the history taking, the physician should check with the patient the accuracy of all prerecorded items.

Patient's Name. Insist upon recording the *complete name,* including the family name and *all* given names. Strangely, some men object violently to using their given names when they usually employ their initials. The family name should be placed *first,* followed by a comma and all given names. Be meticulous to obtain the correct spelling. Any file of considerable size contains the records of several patients with identical or closely similar names. Fatal errors have occurred when two patients with the same name have been under treatment in the hospital simultaneously; so each patient is given a unique hospital number that should be used for identification before a treatment is instituted. With a married woman, use her *own given names* after the family name of her husband; after these place her husband's given names in parentheses, as *Brown, Mary Elizabeth (Mrs. Edward Charles).* The arrangement is necessary because she may sign her name as *Mrs. Edward C. Brown* in correspondence about her case. She can be distinguished from other Mary Browns with differing middle names. By her husband's name, she may be isolated from other Mary Elizabeth Browns.

Sex. Usually, this is obvious. In cases of intersex, the problem of sex may be difficult to establish accurately, but it is sufficient to give the sex the patient has assumed.

Residence. The address should be recorded as completely as possible to facilitate efficient mailing of correspondence; occasionally it is used to distinguish identity between two patients with the same name.

Birth Date and Age. The patient's statement of the *birth date* should be recorded, in addition to the *stated age.* The birth date is required for some insurance claims. Comparison of it with the stated age on subsequent hospital visits may disclose discrepancies, reflecting on the patient's veracity or memory. The birth date may help distinguish between patients with the same name.

Place of Birth. The information may be useful in assessing social or nationalistic incidence of disease. The examiner may gain some insight into the probability of the patient's understanding the nuances of the English language in giving a history.

Nationality and Race. The correct classification may require considerable knowledge of geography, history, and anthropology. The patient may not be able to give a satisfactory answer. It may be helpful to learn the nationality and race of the parents before accepting the patient's statement. The race is of some importance in diagnosis; sickle-cell anemia occurs almost exclusively in Blacks, while erythroblastosis fetalis is rare in that race. The absence of a beard in a full-blooded American Indian man should not lead the examiner in pursuit of an endocrine disorder.

Marriage Status. Under this heading, note whether the patient is single, married, divorced, a widow or a widower. More details may be included in the genitourinary or social history.

Occupation. Precise knowledge of the patient's work sheds light on social status, physical exertion, psychologic trauma, exposure to noxious agents, and a variety of other conditions that may cause disease. Do not accept the patient's categorization of an occupation without detailed questioning about what he actually does. The manual laborer may have little physical exertion; he may be exposed to heavy metal poisons or silica dust; ask the patient whether his coworkers recognize some disease connected with their surroundings. Some diseases produce symptoms years after exposure; so tabulate *past occupations* as well as current work. Women often give their occupation as "housewife," neglecting to mention additional part-time or full-time employment, unless asked about it. A "housewife" on the farm may or may not do hard manual labor in the field.

II. The Informant

Record the sources of the history, whether from the patient or others. In either case, record your judgment of the accuracy and credibility of the informant's answers. Errors are frequent in judging orientation from a casual conversation. A person who converses normally may, on direct questioning, be unable to tell the day of the week, the month, or the year; or he may not even know the name of the city he is in.

Interpreters. When the patient does not speak your language, be cautious about interpreters who are not medically trained. A frequent experience with a lay interpreter resembles the following. You ask, "Does the patient have any pain?" The interpreter engages the patient in animated conversation in a foreign tongue; it proceeds for three or four minutes, much longer than a simple question should take. You think surely he will provide you with a detailed story. Finally, the interpreter turns back to you and says, "No, he doesn't have any pain." If you could have followed this mysterious exchange, you would have found that the interpreter had embraced the opportunity to apply his concepts of medicine to history taking; he had stated all sorts of questions that you did not propose. You cannot evaluate the answers unless you know what questions they responded to. Your only recourse is to ask short questions and firmly insist that the resulting conversation is not longer than you judge necessary for your question.

III. Chief Complaints (CC)

The history of symptoms begins with the *chief complaints*, abbreviated CC. These should consist of a list of one or more symptoms causing major discomfort. The complaints are usually tabulated, each on a separate line, followed by the approximate duration in time units; they are written as words or phrases, not as complete sentences. Complaints are not diagnoses by the physician or the patient. It is customary to advise stating the chief complaints in the patient's own words; we have been unable to understand the merit of this requirement. Occasionally, the patient is so uneducated that his complaints are obscenities that he cannot translate into polite speech. More often, his words are so ambiguous as to be useless without interrogation. We advise translating the terms into precise medical language.

The purpose of isolating certain symptoms as chief complaints is twofold. They often serve as important clues with which to begin making a differential diagnosis; the details of these symptoms should always be sought out. The other purpose is to present a prominent list that serves to remind the physician that these symptoms brought the patient for treatment; they require therapy or an explanation of why therapy is not given. This would seem obvious, but occasionally, the physician finds an interesting disease, entirely unrelated to the chief complaints; the medically attractive condition receives all the attention, and the chief complaints are ignored.

In eliciting the chief complaints, do not press the patient for them too early in the interview. He will be better able to select them after he has told some of his story; you may have to help identify them. Occasionally, when a patient is asked for his symptoms, he or she produces a piece of paper upon which are written a list of notes. The French label this *la maladie du petit papier*. Formerly considered a sign of psychoneurosis, many doctors now encourage their patients to keep track of symptoms, signs, temperature, blood pressure, weight, blood sugars, blood counts, etc., for a more accurate evaluation of their progress. [J. F. Burnum: La Maladie Du Petit Papier, Is writing a list of symptoms a sign of an emotional disorder? *N. Engl. J. Med.*, **313**:690–1, 1985.]

IV. Present Illness (PI)

This part is the heart of the diagnostic history. It should be written as a lucid, succinct, chronologic narrative with complete sentences in good English. The patient's symptoms should be accurately described; insist upon symptoms from the patient and do not accept diagnoses instead. When a symptom is mentioned that suggests several conditions, accompany it with statements about the absence of concomitant symptoms that you have obtained by direct questioning. For example, when the patient has had attacks of pain in the right upper abdominal quadrant, the description should include the fact that icterus was not present, the urine was not dark-colored, no pruritus was experienced, the pain did not radiate to the right scapula (all signs and symptoms of acute cholecystitis).

Ideally, the section on the present illness should be brief, so that it is easily read and digested by the author and subsequent readers. This objective is obtained only if the diagnosis is relatively simple and easily made. When the condition continues to be obscure during the history taking, the writer includes more details, because he is uncertain what is pertinent and hopes that the information ultimately will be useful. The perfect history can be written only after the diagnosis is known; such a history cannot serve as a diagnostic procedure. One test of the completeness of a history is whether it conveys a clear picture of the patient's sufferings amid his own surroundings, how the illness affected him and his family, how it interfered with his work, how his finances were affected.

Procedure. Start the patient's narrative by saying, "Tell me about your problem," or "Give me your story." Don't ask him, "What is the matter with you?" or "What is troubling you?" because he is likely to respond, "That's what I came here to find out." For a while, listen to his story without interruption with questions or writing. After the general outline becomes apparent, interject questions designed to establish the nature of the symptoms, the medication, the chronology, the disability. Ask also about symptoms not mentioned that are prompted by your search for diagnostic clues. Then pause and write down the present illness.

Searching for Diagnostic Clues. The chief purpose of the history is to furnish clues for diagnosis. As the narrative unfolds, the physician subjects each emerging symptom to the first three of the diagnostic four-step series (p. 3): (1) the accumulation of facts (obtaining the history), (2) evaluation of the facts (testing the credibility of symptoms, seeking more details of time and quantity), (3) preparation of hypotheses. Having formed a list of hypotheses, he interrogates the patient about other symptoms specific for diseases on his list, either to support or to discard the hypothesis. For example, when the patient complains of pain in the chest, the physician inquires whether it is related to respiratory movements. A positive answer prompts questions about inflamed muscles, fractured ribs, and pleurisy. When the patient denies exacerbation of pain by thoracic movement, he is asked for an association with exertion and distribution of pain resembling that of angina pectoris. Admitting to such a distribution, he is then asked about onset of pain in the horizontal position, as in hiatus hernia. Thus each step in the narrative induces another run through the four-step sequence that results in a frequent shift in the hypothetic list.

Nature of the Symptoms. The patient's description of symptoms must be subjected to *clarification* and *quantification*. *Clarification.* Question him until sufficient details are obtained to categorize the symptom in medical terms. Do not accept vague complaints such as "I don't feel well"; ascertain whether he is weak in one or more muscle groups, whether he has lassitude, malaise, or myalgia. When he says he is dizzy, inquire whether he merely feels weak and unstable or his surroundings seem to whirl about, as in vertigo. Determine whether dyspnea occurs at rest or with exertion. When he complains of swelling of the ankles, inquire whether a dent is left in the skin after pressure, as in pitting edema. Ascertain whether pain is sharp, lancinating, burning, or dull like a toothache. *Quantification.* Highly important to the evaluation of symptoms is to *measure* them. Avoid recording a symptom without a statement of quantity. A woman may tell you that she has a "terrible pain," but it attains different significance when she admits on questioning that it has never interfered with her work or other activities. Although pain cannot be measured, severity can be judged by how it affects the patient. Exertional dyspnea can be assessed by the amount of exertion required to produce it; how many stairs can be climbed, how far the patient can walk on the level. Neither you nor your reader can interpret what a "heavy smoker" is. Heavy is a value judgment, whose meaning varies from one to another; but a record of smoking 20 cigarettes a day is a measure everyone can understand. Don't label a patient as an "alcoholic"; put down the volume of whiskey he drinks in a stated time. When the patient has hemoptysis, have him estimate the amount of blood lost in household measures, such as teaspoonfuls, cupfuls, or quarts. Blood-streaked sputum suggests minor lesions of the mucosa, while loss of 100 mL of blood from the respiratory tract indicates more serious disease.

The amount of sputum raised should always be recorded; the volume serves as an important consideration in differential diagnosis.

Chronology. The duration of a symptom and its appearance time in the course of disease are frequently significant for diagnosis. When the disease is chronic and the course complicated, the patient may disclaim his ability to place events in chronologic sequence. A work chart may be sketched that will assist him in clarifying the details. On a piece of paper, the physician draws a series of steps, with their horizontal dimensions representing duration in approximate time units, such as days, weeks, months, or years. After labeling the time units, the physician indicates on the chart the few dates supplied by the patient. Seeing the chart, the patient can frequently recall further details and indicate the occurrence of symptoms on the time scale. The doses and times of medication can also be graphed.

IVa. Current Activity

We recommend this subject be added to the conventional Present Illness in a separate paragraph with its own subhead. Frequently notes of the patient's activities are insufficient or absent from contemporary records. The physician needs this information to substantiate the patient's claim for insurance. Furthermore, a detailed picture of the patient's average day often sheds surprising light on the patient's reaction to illness or the severity of the disease. Special attention should be given to the occupation. Do not be mislead by categories. When a woman says she is a housewife, ascertain the number of rooms in the house; how many persons she cares for; whether she has assistance with her work; whether she takes a nap during the day. If she is on a farm, how much fieldwork does she perform? For both sexes on the farm, what contacts with poisonous chemicals do they have and how much exposure? For some unknown reason, many women give their occupation as housewife but never volunteer that they are also employed in a factory full time. With factory workers of either sex, ascertain whether other workers in the same plant or department have symptoms similar to those of the patient. Determine how much anxiety and tension accompany the job, the attitudes of superiors, the degree of fatigue from work.

IVb. Current Medication

We suggest the addition of this topic to the Present Illness, as a separate paragraph with its own subhead. It should record a list of all drugs being taken, their names, doses, and effects, if known. When the patient brings the pharmacist's containers, the specific data may be on the labels. If the labels are noncommittal, tablets, pills, capsules, and suppositories may be identified by comparing them with the colored pictures in a current *Physicians' Desk Reference* (PDR). If the drugs are not shown in the book, inquire by telephone from the patient's pharmacist who issued the drug. A notation of past medications may be pertinent and should be as explicit as possible. This isolated summary of medications will facilitate future references to the record in deciding whether there has been drug toxicity, and the drugs that should be selected for current treatment.

V. Past History (PH)

Ordinarily the items in the past history have no great diagnostic value. If they provide clues for the diagnosis, the facts should be interpolated in the present illness. Otherwise the data are of some statistical value, or their significance may be appreciated after future developments in the patient's condition. New associations of disease may be introduced to enhance the value of the past history.

a. General Health

The patient's health during his lifetime, before the present illness, is sometimes revealing. *Body weight:* present, maximum, and minimum, with dates of each. *Previous physical examinations:* dates and findings. *Admissions to the armed services:* dates, geographic locations on foreign soil. *Insurance examinations:* dates when accepted or rejected.

b. Infectious Disease

Dates and complications of measles, German measles, mumps, whooping cough, chickenpox, smallpox, diphtheria, typhoid fever, malaria, hepatitis, scarlet fever, rheumatic fever, chorea, influenza, pneumonia, pleurisy, tuberculosis, bronchitis, tonsillitis, venereal diseases, and others. Give dates of chemotherapy and antibiotic treatment with any reactions to drugs.

c. *Operations and Injuries*

Give dates and nature of injuries, operations, and operative diagnoses.

d. *Previous Hospitalization*

Give accounts of each, with dates and names of hospitals and their locations. If the hospital records are available, summarize the dates and diagnoses for each admission.

e. *System Review (Inventory of Systems)*

This is an outline for careful review of the history by inquiring for salient symptoms associated with each system or anatomic region. Primarily, it is a search for symptoms that may have escaped the taking of the present illness. These symptoms should be memorized and their diagnostic significance learned. In practice, the answers are not written down except when positive. After the physician has fully mastered the outline, we suggest that he ask the questions while examining the part of the body to which they pertain. In taking the present illness, when one of the symptoms emerges, the associated symptoms in this outline should be inquired about.

1. Integument: Skin. Color, pigmentation, temperature, moisture, eruptions, pruritus, scaling, bruising, bleeding. *Hair.* Color, texture, abnormal loss or growth, distribution. *Nails.* Color changes, brittleness, ridging, pitting, curvature.

2. Lymph Nodes. Enlargement, pain, suppuration, draining sinuses, location.

3. Bones, Joints, and Muscles. Fractures, dislocations, sprains, arthritis, myositis, pain, swelling, stiffness, migratory distribution, degree of disability, muscular weakness, wasting, or atrophy. Night cramps.

4. Hematopoietic System. Anemia (type, therapy, and response), lymphadenopathy, bleeding (spontaneous, traumatic, familial).

5. Endocrine System. History of growth, body configuration, and weight. Size of hands, feet, and head, especially changes during adulthood. Hair distribution. Skin pigmentation. Weakness. Goiter, exophthalmos, dryness of skin and hair, intolerance to heat or cold, tremor. Polyphagia, polydipsia, polyuria, glycosuria. Secondary sex characteristics, impotence, sterility, treatment.

6. Allergic and Immunologic History. Dermatitis, urticaria, angioneurotic edema, eczema, hay fever, vasomotor rhinitis, asthma, migraine, vernal conjunctivitis. Seasonal incidence of the foregoing. Known sensitivity to pollens, foods, danders, or drugs. Previous skin tests and their results. Results of tuberculin tests and others. Desensitization, serum injections, vaccinations, and immunizations.

7. Head. Headaches, migraine, trauma, vertigo, syncope, convulsive seizures.

8. Eyes. Visual loss or color blindness, diplopia, hemianopsia, trauma, inflammation, glasses (date of refraction).

9. Ears. Deafness, tinnitus, vertigo, discharge from the ears, pain, mastoiditis, operations.

10. Nose. Coryza, rhinitis, sinusitis, discharge, obstruction, epistaxis.

11. Mouth. Soreness of mouth or tongue, symptoms referable to teeth.

12. Throat. Hoarseness, sore throats, tonsillitis, voice changes.

13. Neck. Swelling, suppurative lesions, enlargement of lymph nodes, goiter, stiffness, and limitation of motion.

14. Breasts. Development, lactation, trauma, lumps, pains, discharge from nipples, gynecomastia, changes in nipples.

15. Respiratory System. Pain, shortness of breath, wheezing, dyspnea, nocturnal dyspnea, orthopnea, cough, sputum, hemoptysis, night sweats, pleurisy, bronchitis, tuberculosis (history of contacts), pneumonia, asthma, other respiratory infections.

16. Cardiovascular System. Palpitation, tachycardia, irregularities of rhythm, pain in the chest, exertional dyspnea, paroxysmal nocturnal dyspnea, orthopnea, cough, cyanosis, ascites, edema. Intermittent claudication, cold extremities, phlebitis, postural or permanent skin color changes. Hypertension, rheumatic fever, chorea, syphilis, diphtheria. Drugs such as digitalis, quinidine, nitroglycerin, diuretics, and other medications.

17. Gastrointestinal System. Appetite, changes in weight, dysphagia, nausea, eructations, flatulence, abdominal pain or colic, vomiting, hematemesis, jaundice (pain, fever, intensity, duration, color of urine and stools), stools (color, frequency, consistency, odor, gas, cathartics), hemorrhoids. Change in bowel habits.

18. Genitourinary System. Color of urine, polyuria, oliguria, nocturia, dysuria, hematuria, pyuria, urinary retention, urinary frequency, incontinence, pain or colic, passage of stones or gravel. *Menstrual History.* Age of onset, frequency of periods, regularity, duration, amount of flow, leukorrhea, dysmenorrhea, date of last normal and preceding periods, date and character of menopause, postmenopausal bleeding. *Pregnancies.* Number, abortions, miscarriages, stillbirths, chronologic sequence, complications of pregnancy. *Venereal history.* Chancre, bubo, penile discharge. Treatment of venereal diseases.

19. Nervous System: Cranial Nerves. Disturbances of smell (1st); visual disturbances (2nd, 3rd, 4th, 6th); orofacial paresthesias and difficulty in chewing (5th); facial weakness and taste disturbances (7th); disturbances in hearing and equilibrium (8th); difficulties in speech, swallowing, and taste (9th, 10th, 12th); limitation in motion of neck (11th). *Motor System.* Paralyses, atrophy, involuntary movements, convulsions, gait, incoordination. *Sensory System.* Pain, lightning pain, girdle pain, paresthesia, hypesthesia, anesthesia. *Autonomic System.* Control of urination and defecation, sweating, erythema, cyanosis, pallor, reaction to heat and cold.

20. Mental Status. Describe reactions to and influence of parents, siblings, spouse, children, friends and associates, sexual adjustments, success and failures, illnesses. Lability of mood. Hallucinations. Grandiose ideas. Nervous breakdowns. Sleep disturbances.

VI. Social History (SH)

Birthplace and Places of Residence. Marital History. Duration of marriages and causes for termination. Age, status, and health of spouse and children. *Social and Economic Status.* Standard of living, extent of education, special financial problems. *Habits.* Diet. Use of drugs, tobacco, alcohol, sedatives, other medications.

VII. Family History (FH)

Parents. Age and health or age at death and causes.

Siblings. Age and health or cause of death. Exposure to tuberculosis, syphilis, leprosy. History of hypertension, heart disease, kidney disease, arthritis, gout, allergy, obesity, anemia, diabetes, endocrine disorders, hemophilia or other bleeding diseases, jaundice, cancer, migraine, nervous or muscular disorders, mental or emotional disturbances, alcoholism, epilepsy.

VIII. Customary Summaries and Notes

Case Summaries. After writing the history and physical findings, the physician usually appends some type of summary, its style and purpose often dictated by hospital standards. Frequently it is an abstract of the significant items in the history and the physical findings. He may discuss a brief differential diagnosis. Usually the note ends with the writer's initial diagnoses, variously labeled as *impression, diagnostic impression, tentative diagnosis, provisional diagnosis,* or *working diagnosis.* He may add suggestions for further diagnostic procedures and tests, and indicate the course of treatment.

Progress Notes. While the patient is still in the hospital, or being treated in the office, his various physicians, and sometimes students, nurses, and technicians, write *progress notes* at appropriate intervals. Each note should commence with a date (including the year), and the time of day, preferably in the military style (e.g., *1330 hour* = *1:30* P.M.). The notes are usually brief and include statements on the current condition of the patient, changes in symptoms and signs, response to therapy, suggestions for further management. Diagnoses may be ventured or changed. The *full* and *legible* name of the writer should be appended. This should be followed by a solidus and an abbreviation indicating hospital rank, as *John Doe/*M_3 (junior medical student), or *Richard Roe/*R_2 (second-year resident, *Jane Doe/*N_3 or *RN* (student nurse or graduate), *John Doe/S* (staff).

Off-Service Note. Some hospital services require a note in the chart by the intern or resident as he leaves the service and turns over the care of the patient to his successor. Usually a brief résumé of the case is recorded, stating the diagnosis, the treatment, and response; he may add suggestions for continuing treatment.

Discharge Summary. As the patient leaves the hospital, the physician should enter a final note containing an abstract of the case, elaborate or brief, with the diagnosis and the treatment given in the hospital and prescribed for home use. He notes information and instructions given to the patient and his attendants.

Weed's System for Summaries and Notes

Weed has proposed a system of recording case summaries and progress notes that commits to writing in orderly fashion much of the reasoning used in the differential diagnosis and also provides the means for tracing clinical problems as the patient's medical record expands [Lawrence L. Weed: *Medical Records, Medical Education, and Patient Care: The Problem-Oriented Record as a Basic Tool.* Press of Case Western Reserve University, Cleveland, 1969, and Year Book Medical Publishers, Chicago, 1970]. The system entails the addition of three distinct components to the patient's record. In essence, it provides for making written lists of the problems that the physician usually attempts to carry in his memory.

Working Problem List. After recording the conventional history and physical examination, the writer analyzes the available facts of chronology, symptoms, signs, and laboratory findings. He formulates a written list of all the problems the patient presents, *assigning a number to each one.* This numbered item is repeated throughout the ensuing notes until it is canceled out by a written statement of the reason for its elimination. The problem may be a symptom, a sign, a laboratory finding, or a complex of several items that experience has taught are associated with disease. A previously diagnosed disease, or one under consideration for diagnosis, may be listed as a problem. In the listing, the title of the numbered problem is followed by subtitles: (a) *plans* for elucidation of diagnoses, (b) *therapy* to be given, (c) *education* of the patient and his attendants at home. In addition, a separate page in the record is reserved for listing the numbered titles of problems with notes and dates indicating the disposal of each.

Numbered Problems in Progress Notes. In the Weed system the progress notes have special structure. Notes are made whenever necessary. In most cases the *title of the note* is a numbered problem previously introduced. Each note has four subheads, the initials of whose title make the mnemonic *SOAP.* This stands for *Subjective Data* (symptoms): changes in symptoms; their appearance and disappearance; their response to therapy. *Objective Data* (physical signs and laboratory findings): changes in signs and findings, spontaneously or in response to therapy, or revealed by further examination. *Assessments:* analyses, impressions, interpretations. *Plans:* diagnostic, therapeutic, instructions to the patient and attendants. When a problem is resolved by inclusion in another diagnosis, or by cure, or by disappearance, a dated progress note in the flow sheet heralds the fact.

Critique of Weed's System. The clinical reader will realize that this system is ponderous and time-consuming; so its advantages must outweigh its disadvantages before it becomes attractive. When carefully followed, it can provide good insight into the quality of the diagnosis and treatment of patients. Thus it reflects the capabilities of the physicians caring for the patient. The system is attractive for those who seek to evaluate the work of medical students, house officers, and senior staff being subjected to *peer review.* In a hospital where large numbers of interns and residents rapidly change assignments, records with this system greatly facilitate the succession of various physicians caring for the patient. When the patients have multiple chronic diseases and many hospital admissions that produce fat medical records, the system of numbered problems greatly assists their care.

The disadvantages of the system are mainly *added paper work* for those who write hospital records and the *increased reading time* for everyone dealing with patients. Most of the enthusiastic testimonials to the system have been published by senior academic staff persons who can delegate most of the actual writing to house staff. Paper work detracts from bedside care. One would hesitate to require the system for all patients; it probably should be reserved for those few with chronic diseases and multiple hospital admissions. Most of these patients would be found on the services of internal medicine and pediatrics. Another disadvantage we have observed concerns a tendency by some students to persist in listing related problems separately without realizing that they represent manifestations of one disease appropriately stated as a single diagnosis.

Symptoms

The word *symptom* is derived from the Greek, meaning anything that has befallen one. In this sense, every happening in the medical history is a symptom. But in diagnostication a symptom is usually considered to be an abnormal sensation *perceived by the patient,* as contrasted with a physical sign that can be seen, felt, or heard *by the examiner.* The items previously listed in the outline of the medical history can be classified as (1) sensations that can never be observed by the examiner, (2) abnormalities noted by the patient at some past time so they cannot be confirmed by the physical examination, (3) events in the past, not readily verifiable, such as former diagnoses or treatments. Diagnostic evaluation of a symptom is simple when the patient says, "I've found a lump in my arm" (symptom), and the examiner can palpate a mass (physical sign). But when the patient complains of pain in the chest and no physical signs can be detected, much more information about the nature of the pain is required before the symptom can serve as a diagnostic clue.

Events that involve the patient *before* the physician first examines him may be recorded in the *medical history.* But subsequent events, while the patient is under medical care, belong in the medical records under such categories as *physician's and nurses' progress notes, medications, physician's orders, radiation therapy, physiotherapy, consultant's notes, descriptions of surgical operations.*

Diagnostic Attributes of Pain

Pain is a prime symptom; it often prompts the patient to seek medical care, it directs attention to a specific anatomic region that is the site of tissue injury. Diagnostic clues can be obtained by further questioning the patient about the *attributes of pain* (use the initials PQRST as a mnemonic, although not necessarily in that order):

Provocative-Palliative Factors. Association of pain with bodily movement often localizes inflammation of a specific tissue known to be displaced by such a motion. If the point is sufficiently accessible, the location may be confirmed by pressure to elicit *tenderness.* Pain associated with respiratory motions may indicate a lesion in the thoracic wall or the parietal pleura. Flexion of the spine may cause pain in the region of an injured intervertebral joint. The relief of chest pain by nitroglycerin points strongly to angina pectoris as the cause. Sharp pain at the site of an unsuspected neoplasm may occur within minutes after the ingestion of alcohol.

Quality. Three qualities of pain are recognized: (1) *bright, pricking,* often described as sharp, cutting, knifelike, lightning-like, (2) *burning,* also reported as hot or stinging, and (3) *deep, aching,* variously called boring, pounding, sore, heavy, constricting, gnawing. Physiologically, *superficial pain* includes types 1 and 2 (pricking and burning); the origin is accurately localized; it may be associated with paresthesias, itching, tickling, or hyperalgesia. Type 3, *deep pain,* is more diffuse and difficult to localize; it persists longer and includes the qualities of throbbing, cramping, depending upon the cause.

Region. Pain is usually confined to one or more anatomic regions that the patient can point to. Since each region comprises a separate group of tissues and organs, the diagnostic significance of pain is conveniently discussed in this book in the chapters dealing with the examination of each region.

Severity. Precise measurements of the intensity of pain are impractical for a clinical examination, but meaningful approximations can be obtained from the patient's descriptions and the examiner's observations. The patient is asked to liken the severity of the pain to some common experience such as a toothache, menstrual cramps, labor pains, or a sore throat. Intense pain is usually accompanied by physiologic signs perceptible to the examiner and often noted by the patient, such as facial expressions, bodily postures (protecting a limb by holding it, flexion of the thighs upon the belly for severe abdominal pain), reduced bodily activity, sweating, pallor, dilatation of the pupils, elevation of the blood pressure and acceleration of the heart rate, retching and vomiting.

Tests with a stimulus of measured intensity prove that individuals have remarkably similar thresholds for pain. But clinical observation teaches that persons vary greatly in their reactions to pain depending upon their emotional and social backgrounds. Our society permits women more emotional expression than men. Superimposed *fear* may aggravate the pain. Persons who have never endured sickness seem more sensitive to pain than those who are more accustomed to it.

Temporal Characteristics. Total duration of the pain often indicates the course of the disease. The duration of a single sensation may be *short,* described as throbbing, boring, cramping, shooting, or aching. Shooting pain usually results from irritation of a nerve trunk. Displacement of inflamed tissues surrounding a pulsating artery causes throbbing pain. *Remissions* are usual in the pain of organic disease; *constant pain* for many days is usually psychoneurotic. *Seasonal pain* is frequently experienced in peptic ulcer, especially occurring in the spring and fall of the year. *Daytime pain* is common to many conditions in which motions or muscle spasm intensifies it; *nighttime pain* is likely to result when muscle spasm relaxes its protection of tender tissues.

3

Methods in the Physical Examination

In performing the physical examination the clinician employs most of the classical five senses of sight, hearing, touch, smell, and taste; the last has been supplanted in modern times by laboratory tests. Four chief methods bring his senses to bear upon the examination of the patient: inspection, palpation, percussion, and auscultation; smelling is occasionally useful. Using the same senses as the layman, the experienced physician assigns special meanings to his perceptions as the result of practice and his knowledge of normal and abnormal anatomy and physiology. When he recognizes the abnormal in the physical examination, he utilizes the facts of pathology to make a diagnosis. Slight mechanical skill is required for palpation and percussion. The major effort in becoming a diagnostician consists in acquiring the intellectual background to make his perceptions meaningful—in short, *he must practice and study.*

During our current era of high technology, the resurgence of concern for the proper performance of the physical examination may surprise the casual observer [N. P. Wray and J. A. Friedland: Detection and Correction of House Staff Error in Physical Diagnosis, *J.A.M.A.*, **249:**1035–37, 1983; and J. E. Johnson and J. L. Carpenter: Medical House Staff Performance in Physical Examination, *Arch. Intern. Med.*, **146:**937–41, 1986.]. We believe, however, that this renewed interest stems from several realizations emanating from recent experience: (1) routine ordering of laboratory tests and x-rays unguided by clues discovered from the history and physical examination is expensive and yields results of questionable value [T. G. Tape and A. I. Mushlin: The Utility of Routine Chest Radiographs, *Ann. Intern. Med.,* **104:**663–70, 1986.], (2) interpretation of results from blood tests, imaging procedures, and even biopsy material may be misleading, if not erroneous, without information supplied by the doctor's diagnostic examination, and (3) a person may withhold his trust from the physician who appears so little interested in his patient's symptoms that he fails to examine him.

Inspection

Inspection is seeking physical signs by observing the patient. Of the several methods of examination, inspection is the least mechanical and the hardest to learn, but it yields the most physical signs. More diagnoses are probably made by inspection than by all other methods combined. The method is the most difficult to learn because no systematic approach can encompass the variety of signs. More than any other method, inspection depends entirely upon the knowledge of the observer; we tend to see things that have meaning for us. This fact has been epitomized in such maxims as "We see what's behind the eyes" (Wintrobe), "The examination does not wait the removal of the shirt" (Waring), *"Was man weiss, man sieht"* (Goethe: What one knows, one sees). The layman looks at a person and concludes that there is something "peculiar" about him; the physician gives one glance and diagnoses acromegaly. From his study of disease, he can dissect the "peculiarity" and recognize the diagnostic components, such as the enlarged supraorbital ridges, the widely spaced teeth, the macroglossia, the buffalo hump, the huge hands and feet. Practice is required to learn inspection. Watch a Japanese person distinguish among the ideographs in his printed language and compare it with your unpracticed efforts.

Despite its importance as a method of examination, inspection is frequently slighted. This is probably attributable to the complete absence of motor activity. In learning about his surroundings, the infant does not trust his eyes, he must finger the objects also; apparently palpation is more satisfying than inspection. The adult seems to retain this preference; even experienced clinicians have to restrain consciously their impulses to palpate before adequate inspection has been made.

General Inspection. The initial act of physical examination is the inspection of the body as a whole. Most clinicians believe that composite pictures of disease, although composed of many signs, strike them at a glance; they attempt to teach others to perceive likewise. The Germans seem to recognize this concept when they refer to *Augenblick* diagnoses (literally, "a blink of the eye"). Although difficult to prove, we question the validity of this concept. The focus of attention is sharp, as demonstrated by a classic example in psychology. In the days when pocket watches were common and often had the *6* on the dial replaced by a second hand, the lecturing professor told his audience that they had looked at their watches thousands of times but many could not recall whether they had *6s* on their dials. Whereat many took surreptitious glances at their timepieces. After the watches had been pocketed, he asked if they knew what time it was; many could not tell. It seems probable that the *Augenblick* is a series of events; some salient sign is noted that suggests the composite picture; then other components are sought. Accordingly, we have laid no stress upon such recognition, believing that it comes only with long practice on details.

In looking at the patient as a whole, many facts are noted about motor activity, body build, outstanding anatomic malformation, behavior, speech, nutrition, appearance of illness (a complex defying description).

Local Inspection. Focusing observation on a single anatomic region yields hundreds of physical signs. Since only signs perceived by inspection can be illustrated, the myriads of pictures used in books on surgical diagnosis hint the importance of the method in that field. The dermatologist relies almost entirely on the appearance of skin lesions to make a diagnosis.

Usage more or less confines the term *inspection* to observation with the unaided eyes. Actually, visual signs are the chief or only rewards in the use of the ophthalmoscope, slit lamp, gonioscope, otoscope, nasoscope, laryngoscope, bronchoscope, gastroscope, thoracoscope, peritoneoscope, cystoscope, anoscope, and sigmoidoscope. The pathologist uses the microscope; the radiologist inspects the fluoroscopic screen and photographic films.

Palpation

The usual definition of palpation is the act of feeling by the sense of touch. But this is too limited; when the physician lays his hands upon the patient, he perceives physical signs by his tactile sense, his temperature sense, his kinesthetic sense of position and vibration. As in inspection, all normal persons possess these senses, but practice and special intellectual background in medicine enable the physician to extract meanings that escape the layman. If the reader doubts the influence of practice on palpation, let him observe a blind person reading a book printed in braille, then close his eyes and attempt to distinguish between two braille letters by touching them. Or, let him identify a pocketful of United States coins by touch, then test himself similarly with British coins.

Sensitive Parts of the Hand: Tactile Sense. The tips of the fingers are most sensitive for fine tactile discrimination. *Temperature Sense.* Use the dorsa of the hands or fingers; the skin is much thinner than elsewhere on the hand. *Vibratory Sense.* Palpate with the palmar aspects of the metacarpophalangeal joints, rather than with the fingertips, to perceive vibrations such as thrills or the precordial cardiac thrust. Prove the superiority for yourself by touching first the fingertip, then the palmar base of your finger, with a vibrating tuning fork. *Sense of Position and Consistency.* Use the grasping fingers, so you perceive with sensations from your joints and muscles.

Structures Examined by Palpation. Palpation is employed on every part of the body accessible to the examining fingers: all external structures, all structures accessible through the body orifices, the bones, the joints, the muscles, the tendon sheaths, the ligaments, the superficial arteries, thrombosed or thickened veins, superficial nerves, salivary ducts, spermatic cord, solid abdominal viscera, solid contents of hollow viscera, accumulations of body fluids, pus, or blood.

Qualities Elicited by Palpation: Texture. The skin and hair. *Moisture.* The skin and mucosa. *Skin Temperature.* At various levels of the body. *Masses.* The size, shape, consistency, motility, pulsation (expansile or transmitted) (p. 506). *Precordial Cardiac Thrust* (p. 343). *Crepitus.* In bones (p. 314), joints (p. 651), tendon sheaths (p. 701), pleura (p. 345), subcutaneous tissue (p. 501). *Tenderness.* In all accessible tissues. *Thrills.* Over the heart (p. 345) and blood vessels (p. 403). *Vocal Fremitus* (p. 296).

Special Methods of Palpation: Light Palpation (p. 498). *Deep Palpation* (p. 504). *Ballottement* (p. 505). *Fluctuation* (p. 656). *Fluid Wave* (p. 485).

Percussion

In physical diagnosis, percussion is the method of examination in which the surface of the body is struck to emit sounds that vary in quality according to the density of the underlying tissues.

Methods of Percussion. Bimanual, Mediate, or Indirect. In this method the left middle finger is laid upon the body surface to serve as a *pleximeter;* it is struck a sharp blow with the tip of the right middle finger, the *plexor* (see full discussion, pp. 300*ff.*). *Immediate or Direct.* The body surface is struck directly with one or more fingers of a hand. A special type is *Hoover's damped percussion,* described on pp. 300*ff.*

Sonorous Percussion. This term is applied to any method of percussion when its *purpose* is to ascertain the density of the tissue by the sound emitted when struck. Various densities emit sounds given special names. The percussion notes may be arranged in sequence according to the density that produces them, from least to most dense: *tympany, hyperresonance, resonance, impaired resonance, dullness, flatness.* Certain steps in the scale may be defined by their occurrence in normal tissues. Tympany is the sound emitted by percussing the air-filled stomach; resonance is produced by striking the air-filled lungs; flatness results from percussing the thigh. In general the *pitch* or *frequency* of the sounds progresses through the series from lowest for tympany to highest for flatness; the *duration* of the sound ranges in the series from long to short (see pp. 298*ff.*). Some clinicians have trained themselves to feel changes in resonance as well as to perceive them as sound.

Sonorous percussion is employed to ascertain the density of the lungs, the pleural space, the pleural layers, and the hollow viscera of the abdomen.

Definitive Percussion. Where two structures in apposition have greatly contrasting densities, as demonstrated by their percussion notes, mapping of the area of greater density furnishes a concept of the size of the structure or the extent of its border.

Any method of percussion used for this *purpose* is termed *definitive percussion.* The technique is discussed on pp. 300*ff.*

Definitive percussion is commonly employed to ascertain the location of the lung bases, the width of the lung apices, the height of fluid in the pleural cavity, the width of the mediastinum, the size of the heart, the outline of dense masses in the lungs, the size and shape of the liver and spleen, the size of a distended gallbladder and urinary bladder, the level of ascitic fluid.

Auscultation

Although auscultation might literally imply the act of hearing to obtain physical signs, usage restricts it almost solely to hearing through the stethoscope. There is no formal term for hearing the patient speak, cough, groan, or shriek, although all these sounds furnish diagnostic clues.

The scope of auscultation is expanding with the increase of knowledge gained from phonocardiography and newer diagnostic studies. It is probable that more physicians are extending their routines of examination as progress in vascular surgery makes lesions remediable. The skull can be auscultated for the bruit of an arteriovenous fistula. The vessels of the neck are examined for murmurs in the thyroid, carotid, and subclavian arteries, and venous hums. From the lungs the stethoscope conveys breath sounds, whispers, and voice, as well as rales and friction rubs. Crepitus can be heard in joints, tendon sheaths, muscles, fractured bones, and in subcutaneous emphysema. The heart makes its various valve sounds with their splitting, murmurs, rhythm disturbances, pericardial rubs and knocks. Auscultation of the abdomen reveals bowel sounds, murmurs from aneurysms and stenotic arteries, especially the renal. The stethoscope is applied to the scrotum to detect bowel sounds in a scrotal hernia.

As every musician knows, the ear can be trained to recognize sounds more accurately. Each person learns to recognize the voices of many associates by patterns of pitch and overtones.

Smelling

Although some physicians seem to regard the diagnostic use of the nose as indelicate, odors may provide valuable and immediate clues. *Breath:* Odors on the breath from acetone, alcohol, and some poisons may lead quickly to a diagnosis (p. 148). *Sputum:* Foul-smelling sputum suggests bronchiectasis or lung abscess. *Vomitus:* The gastric contents may emit the odors of alcohol, phenol, or other poisons, or the sour smell of fermenting food retained overlong. A fecal odor from the vomitus indicates violent prolonged vomiting from peritonitis or intestinal obstruction. *Feces:* Particularly foul-smelling stools are common in pancreatic insufficiency. *Urine:* An ammoniacal odor in the urine may result from fermentation within the bladder. *Pus:* A nauseatingly sweet odor, like the smell of rotting apples, is strong evidence that pus is coming from a region of gas gangrene. The fecal odor of pus is imparted by the growth of proteolytic bacteria from the gut (not of *Escherichia coli*). Some proteolytic bacteria in abscesses produce an odor likened to overripe Camembert cheese.

Clinical Measurements

This category includes measurements easily made on the patient in the office or at the bedside.

Height and Weight

Accurate measurements of the height and weight are essential during the initial diagnostic examination and may prove extremely valuable with subsequent encounters in the office or hospital, so they should be obtained routinely. A physician uses the data in a variety of ways. He evaluates the nutritional status of the pregnant woman, the normality of the child's growth, the fluid balance of the ambulatory and bedridden patient. He checks the metabolism and appetite as influenced by mental status, thyroid function, recovery from childbirth, surgery, illness, the progress of cancer and the effects of drugs.

It is convenient to measure the height with a rod attached to the office scales. The patient should stand shoeless and the units should be recorded in centimeters for the physician and in inches for the patient who requests it.

The patient can be weighed with or without clothes, but the circumstances should be recorded with the observed values expressed in kilograms and converted into pounds, if desired.

Body Temperature

In English-speaking countries the usual scales on the clinical thermometers are either Fahrenheit or centigrade. Conveniently remembered clinical equivalents are 104.0° F = 40.0° C; 98.6° F = 37.0° C; 95.0° F = 35.0° C. Despite the designation "half-minute" or "two-minute" on clinical thermometers, maximum readings may require five minutes of contact with body surfaces.

Diurnal Variation of Body Temperature. Persons working in the daytime and sleeping at night register the minimum temperature at 3:00 to 4:00 A.M., whence it rises slowly to a maximum between 8:00 and 10:00 P.M. The pattern is reversed in night workers, but transition from one pattern to the other requires several days for adjustment.

Simultaneous Temperatures in Various Regions. Body heat is produced by chemical reactions in cell metabolism; so a temperature gradient extends from a maximum in the liver to a minimum on the skin surface. Customarily, the body temperature is measured in the rectum, the mouth, the axilla, or the groin. Of these sites, the rectal temperature is about 0.5° to 0.7° F (0.27° to 0.38° C) higher than the oral or groin reading; the axillary temperature is about 1.0° F (0.55° C) less than the oral value.

Normal Body Temperature. Ignore or curse the traditional red line at 98.6° F (37.0° C); it is meaningless; frequently it misleads the patient, occasionally a physician. Modern statistical practice would require a normal range for both maximum and minimum at each hour of the 24-hour day, each point determined by two standard deviations on either side of the mean. A clinical shortcut is to regard as probably in the febrile range a maximum *oral* temperature above 99.5° F (37.5° C) and a rectal temperature exceeding 100.5° F (38.0° C). The minimum normal temperature is more difficult to define; the oral temperature often dips to 96.0° F (35.0° C) or 95.0° F (35.0° C) during sleep.

Causes of Fever. Increased body temperature results from excessive production of heat or interference with heat dissipation. *Impaired Heat Loss.* Climatic temperatures exceeding that of the normal body, moderately hot weather for a person with congenital absence of sweat glands, congestive cardiac failure, heat stroke from failure of the heat-dissipating apparatus. *Increased Heat Production.* Exercise. Thyrotoxicosis. Tissue injury from trauma, thrombophlebitis, myocardial infarction, meningeal hemorrhage. Specific infections. Localized infections. Localized accumulations of pus. Neoplasm. Hematologic disorders, such as hemolysis, leukemia, lymphoma, severe pernicious anemia. Gout and porphyria. Collagen disease. Pleurisy with effusion. Drugs. Polymer-fume fever. Familial Mediterranean fever and etiocholanolone fever. Pemphigus and bullous dermatoses. Sarcoidosis. Catecholamines from pheochromocytoma, hypothalamic disturbances, endogenous pyrogens, and gonadal steroids.

Physical Signs of Fever. Usually the skin is *warm* and flushed; but absence of these signs does not exclude fever. Occasionally the skin temperature may be subnormal or normal while the interior, measured by the rectal temperature, may be excessively warm. *Tachycardia* usually accompanies fever; the increase in the pulse rate is proportionate to the temperature elevation. In infectious fevers, the thermostatic mechanism operates at a higher control level; in rapid transition from normal to a higher control level, shivering from involuntary muscle contractions produces more heat to raise the temperature to the higher level; clinically, these are called *chills* or *rigors.* In fever, the patient usually feels more comfortable in a *warm* environment. *Night sweats* may accompany an elevated temperature at night, but they also occur in patients debilitated from disease and in normal children.

Febrile Temperature Patterns. The pattern of fluctuations on the temperature chart may serve as a diagnostic clue. Many patterns have been defined. ***Continued Fever.*** A fever with a diurnal variation of 1° to 1.5° F (0.55° to 0.82° C). ***Remittent Fever.*** A fever with a diurnal variation of more than 2° F (1.1° C), but with no normal readings. ***Quotidian Fever.*** A fever recurring daily, usually associated with a double infection of *Plasmodium vivax;* also seen in hepatic abscess or acute cholangitis. ***Intermittent Fever.*** Episodes of fever separated by days of normal temperature. Examples: *tertian fever* from *Plasmodium vivax* in which paroxysms of malaria are separated by an intervening normal day; *quartan fever* in which paroxysms from *Plasmodium malariae* occur with two intervening normal days; *intermittent hepatic fever* (Charcot's hepatic fever) in which chills and fever occur at irregular intervals, marking the intermittent impaction of a gallstone and cholangitis. ***Relapsing Fever.*** Bouts of fever occurring every five to seven days from infection with spirochetes of the group *Borrelia.* ***Pel-Epstein Fever.*** Occurring in Hodgkin's disease, bouts of several days of continuous or remittent fever followed by afebrile remissions lasting an irregular number of days.

Factitious Fever. This is usually encountered in hospitalized patients attempting to malinger, although the motives are often obscure. The situation is usually suspected (1) when a series of high temperatures are recorded to form an atypical pattern of fluctuation, or (2) when a recorded high temperature is unaccompanied by warm skin, tachycardia, and other signs of fever. The patient may have surreptitiously dipped the thermometer in warm water, placed it in contact with a heat source, or heated the bulb by friction with bedclothes or even the mucous membranes of the mouth. Occasionally one thermometer is exchanged for another; the substitution may be detected by checking the serial numbers on the tubes given and returned.

Diagnostic Imaging

With progress in nuclear physics, biochemistry, engineering, and computer technology during this century, the development of diagnostic medical imaging has become a remarkable extension of the physical examination and has brought unanticipated benefits to the patient. Physicians, privileged to practice in nations with advanced economic development, may order special examinations using sophisticated instruments that exploit differences in tissue densities and metabolism to diagnose precisely many conditions that previously had remained obscure until observed at surgery or during postmortem examination.

Many of the procedures, however, are expensive and expose the patient to radiation, so their critical selection should be justified by information derived from the physician's diagnostic examination. Special examinations are undertaken with *conventional radiography* with and without contrast materials introduced into the gastrointestinal and genitourinary tracts, the cardiovascular and lymphatic systems, other organs and body cavities; *ultrasound or echography; scintillation scanning* with radionuclides; *computed tomography* (*CT*) and *magnetic resonance imaging* (*MRI*).

Since this book deals with the physician's personal diagnostic examination in the office or at the bedside, discussions of the details of diagnostic imaging techniques are inappropriate here. Although we will indicate when special diagnostic imaging examinations are helpful, we recognize that the field is moving very rapidly. We must rely, therefore, on the initiative of the reader to update our attempts to list the usefulness of these special examinations in the diagnosis of certain diseases.

Routine or Basic Physical Examination

Within practical limits there is no such thing as a routine physical examination. Like history taking, the diagnostic physical examination is a probing here and there for clues; the details of the hunt vary as prompted by the symptoms in the history, the physical signs, and the laboratory findings in each case. Emphasis on parts of the examination varies with the patient; the heart and circulation will be examined more carefully and thoroughly in a patient with exertional dyspnea than in one who has just sustained a fractured femur.

Nevertheless, either unconsciously or after careful consideration, every physician adopts or acquires certain habits of examination. He develops a routine or basic examination that he follows with most patients, until meaningful clues are encountered that concentrate his attention upon an anatomic site or some physiologic problem, to which he devotes more probing. So his procedures not only differ from those of his colleagues but are not exactly repetitive with each of his own patients.

Robert S. Hillman and his students at the University of Washington studied the components of screening examinations employed by various family physicians and internists in their community. They found the duration of examinations varied widely from 2 to 45 minutes, with wide variation in the components emphasized. We are indebted to them for making their findings available. Such a study was badly needed.

It would be impractical to describe a routine for everyone to follow exactly. There are many possible plans of action, each with its advantages and disadvantages; none is perfect. We have chosen to present a routine incorporating the ideas of two physicians who had different medical training and backgrounds. These procedures may serve as points of departure in developing one's own habits. Both experiences recognized certain facts: (1) A routine or basic examination not only discovers diagnostic signs but also reassures the patient. (2) The patient should be examined from head to foot. (3) Many physical signs are recognized and evaluated during the history taking. (4) A routine or basic examination can be performed in 15 minutes. (5) Evaluation of clues consumes additional time. (6) Fumbling with instruments and the accommodations in the examining room consumes much time. (7) Changing the position of the examiner or patient consumes additional time. (8) In some circumstances, a routine or basic examination is inappropriate; a regional or special examination may be indicated.

Routine Examination in the Office

This example of a screening examination is designed to be performed with the patient in only four positions and requiring approximately 15 minutes.

Required Equipment. Oto-ophthalmoscope, sphygmomanometer, stethoscope, tongue blades, reflex hammer, visual testing chart, rubber or plastic gloves with lubricant for rectal and vaginal examinations, reagent for occult blood test.

Phase A. Clues Detected While History Taking: NERVOUS SYSTEM: auditory acuity, intelligence, memory, mood, speech, gait, involuntary movements, other cranial nerve dysfunctions. RESPIRATORY SYSTEM: rate and rhythm of respiratory cycle, vital capacity, cough, hoarseness.

Phase B. Patient Draped and Sitting (Physician Facing). The patient undresses in private and drapes himself while the physician washes his hands. The draped patient sits on the end of the examining table. The examining instruments are ranged on a table within reach of the physician. GENERAL APPEARANCE: description. SKIN AND NAILS: texture, temperature, color, local lesions. Head: configuration. EYES: visual acuity (with test chart), conjunctivae, sclerae, extraocular movements, visual fields by confrontation, pupillary reaction to light and accommodation, funduscopic examination of lens, disks, retinal vessels (with ophthalmoscope). EARS: auditory acuity (with watch or whisper), otoscopic examination, nasal inspection. MOUTH: note control of lips and jaws; oral examination of lips, teeth, saliva, ducts, tongue, tonsils, pharynx, uvula during phonation. NECK AND AXILLAE: inspect thyroid gland and configuration of the neck and breasts; palpate cervical and clavicular lymph nodes; palpate axillary and epitrochlear nodes. LIMBS AND HANDS: note musculature and coordination of shoulders, arms, and hands; palpate both radial pulses; examine palms and nails; elicit deep tendon reflexes (biceps, triceps, knee, and ankle) with reflex hammer.

Phase C. Patient Draped and Sitting (Physician to Right and Back): THYROID AND TRACHEA: inspect and palpate. SPINE: inspect and palpate; percuss. THORAX: duration of the respiratory phase; palpate and percuss lung fields and diaphragm; auscultate the lungs and heart.

Phase D. Patient Draped and Supine (Physician to Right): BLOOD PRESSURE: on right arm with patient reclining. NECK VEINS: observe fullness and pulsations; note presence of orthopnea. CHEST AND PRECORDIUM: inspect and examine each breast and axilla for masses, ulcerations or secretions; palpate for character and location of impulses; percuss left apical border and sternum; auscultate at 5 valve areas; count heart rate and note rhythm; auscultate carotid arteries. ABDOMEN AND INGUINAL REGIONS: auscultate for bruits and bowel sounds and friction rubs; inspect for hernias while the patient performs Valsalva's maneuver; percuss liver and spleen; palpate superficially and deeply the liver, spleen, inguinal nodes, aorta, inguinal and femoral arteries. LEGS AND FEET: inspect skin, muscles, joints, and look for edema; palpate dorsalis pedis and posterior tibial pulses; elicit plantar reflexes.

Phase E. Patient Draped and Supine, Knees and Hips Flexed (Physician at Foot): GENITALIA: inspect and palpate. RECTUM: digital examination of rectum and prostate gland, test stool on glove for occult blood; pelvic examination in women (with aide's assistance).

As stated previously, the preceding routine is simply a recommendation. We encourage those students unable to learn how to examine a patient from the right side to try the left [S. Akgün and J. M. Raskin: Left (Sided Examination) May Be Right, Too!, *N. Engl. J. Med.*, **314:**994, 1986.].

4

The Skin

The skin covers the entire body, protecting the underlying tissues from injury, infection, and dehydration. It supports the peripheral nerve endings. It plays an important part in the temperature regulation of the body by radiation, conduction, and convection of heat and the emission of sweat. Morphologically, the three chief layers of the skin are the epidermis, the dermis, and the subcutaneous tissue.

Epidermis (Cuticle) (Fig. 4-1). This is the most superficial layer. It is subdivided into two important strata. ***Horny Layer (stratum corneum).*** This consists of several layers of dead keratinized cells that normally separate and drop off (desquamation). ***Stratum Mucosum.*** Underlying the horny layer, this

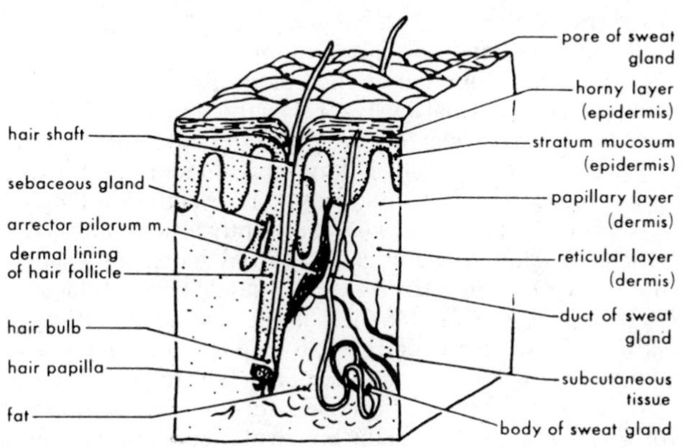

Fig. 4-1. Principal structures of the skin.

stratum is constituted of living cells deriving their nutriment from the underlying tissues because the epidermis is avascular. The mucosum cells contain *melanin,* a brown or black pigment whose concentration is determined by heredity, exposure to sunlight and other irritants, and hormonal control. The mucosum layer contains a network of *furrows* or *rhomboid lines,* visible with the unaided eye through the horny layer; on relaxed surfaces the furrows are narrow, over joints they are widened.

Dermis (Cutis, Corium, True Skin): ***Papillary Layer.*** The superficial aspect is thrown into a series of papillae into which the epidermis is molded. ***Reticular Layer.*** This consists of dense connective tissue that contains blood vessels, lymphatics, nerves, and considerable elastic tissue. Its deeper portion is the site of collagenous bundles mixed with yellow elastic fibers; between the meshes are sweat glands, sebaceous glands, hair follicles, and fat cells. The reticular layer merges with the deeper and looser subcutaneous layer. The dermis is especially thick over the palms and soles; it is extremely thin over the eyelids, scrotum, and penis. In general, the dermis is thicker over dorsal and lateral surfaces than over ventral and medial aspects. The dermal appendages are the nails, hairs, sweat and sebaceous glands.

Nails. These are described on p. 688.

Hairs. The skin is covered with hairs, except on the palms, soles, dorsa of the distal phalanges, glans penis, inner surface of the prepuce, and the labia minora. The *hair follicle* is a long tubular invagination of the epidermis and dermis penetrating the chief dermal level and even the subcutaneous tissue. At its blind end a *hair papilla* protrudes into the lumen of the follicle. The *hair shaft* is long and slender; in a straight hair its cross section is round or oval; a curled hair is flattened. The shaft consists of a *medulla,* frequently absent, and a *cortex* whose cells contain pigment in colored hairs, air spaces in white hairs. Outside is the *cuticle* of a single layer of flat scales. The proximal end of the shaft is the *root,* terminating in a hollow *bulb* that fits over the hair papilla; the root is softer and lighter in color than the shaft. The hair follicle penetrates the dermis obliquely; on the side forming an obtuse angle with the surface of the skin, an involuntary muscle bundle, the *arrector pili,* extends from near the hair bulb to the superficial dermis; so its contraction pulls the hair to a perpendicular position.

Sebaceous Glands. A group of specialized cells in the dermal lining of the hair follicle secretes sebum through a duct that empties into the follicle near its distal end; one or more sebaceous glands are associated with each follicle.

Sweat Glands. The *body* consists of a coiled tube nesting in the subcutaneous tissue; a more or less straight duct leads from this to the epidermis, emerging on the skin surface in a funnel-shaped opening or *pore.* Modified sweat glands are ceruminal glands, ciliary glands, circumanal glands, and mammary glands.

Examination of the Skin

In taking the history, the clinician seeks (1) the symptoms attributed to the skin lesions; (2) the chronology of appearance, change, and disappearance of the lesions; (3) the conditions of exposure, injury, or medication that may have induced or altered the disease.

In the physical examination, inspection is the chief procedure, supplemented by palpation to detect nodularity and infiltration. Three categories of observations should be made in sequence: first, the anatomic distribution of the lesions; second, the configuration of groups of lesions, if any; third, the morphology of the individual lesions. The purpose of this chapter is to define the descriptive terms and the physical signs of skin lesions, so that the physician may construct a good description with which to consult the textbooks on dermatology for a diagnosis.

Anatomic Distribution of Lesions

Many skin diseases have characteristic anatomic patterns that depend upon special skin features of the region or the exposure to noxious agents permitted by the clothing, ornaments, or occupational contact, medication, or other circumstances. A few examples follow.

Rosacea is limited to the face; acne involves the face, shoulders, and upper trunk. Lesions resulting from exposure to light, such as lupus erythematosus, porphyria, pellagra, occur on the forehead, cheeks, tops of ears, the neck (but sparing the submental region), the dorsa of the hands and forearms, and the lateral arms. A bandlike distribution suggests herpes zoster, except where some object of clothing has obviously had contact. Linear arrangement suggests poison ivy. Lesions limited to the legs are erythema nodosum and stasis dermatitis. Cutaneous moniliasis occurs in the moist folds behind the ears, under the breasts, in the axillae, in the umbilicus, along the inguinal and pudendal regions, in the gluteal folds, and in the perianal region.

Group Configuration of Lesions

Some skin lesions are grouped in more or less distinctive configurations; these patterns must be sought when the skin is examined.

Annular, Arciform, and Polycyclic Grouping. The individual lesions are arranged in circles, arcs, or irregular combinations of the two. This pattern is distinctive of some drug eruptions, erythema multiforme, urticaria, psoriasis, and a few others.

Serpiginous Grouping. The lesions occur in wavy lines (serpiginous means "creeping"). Typical are the nodular lesions of late syphilis.

Iris Grouping. A pattern like a bull's-eye occurs as an encircled round spot. It is characteristic of erythema multiforme.

Irregular Grouping. Groups with no distinct patterns, except that of irregular collections, occur in such diseases as urticaria and insect bites.

Zosteriform Grouping. Lesions occur in broad bands, often in the area of a nerve distribution. This is always the case with herpes zoster; often it is seen in diseases such as metastatic breast carcinoma.

Linear Grouping. This is typified by lymphangitis and contact dermatitis due to poison ivy.

Retiform Grouping. The lesions form a network. Examples are erythema ab igne, livedo reticularis, and x-ray dermatitis.

Morphology of Individual Lesions

After noting the anatomic distribution and the group configuration, the clinician should examine carefully several individual lesions to describe their attributes. A magnifying glass may assist. The lesions should be palpated to distinguish papules, nodules, plaques, and infiltration. Viewing the skin through a compressing glass microscope slide discloses deep lesions obscured by erythema.

Diffuse Cutaneous Color Changes. *Erythema* is typified by scarlet fever, scarlatiniform drug eruptions, polycythemia, porphyria, pellagra, lupus erythematosus, first-degree burns. *Transitory erythema* occurs in blushing and in some cases of metastatic carcinoid. *Depigmentation* is usually either vitiligo, tinea versicolor, or albinism. *Brownish pigmentation* is often seen in Addison's disease, hemochromatosis, porphyria, arsenic poisoning, atabrine medication, systemic scleroderma, local irritation from burning or scratching. *Gray-blue coloration* occurs in argyria, deposition of gold or bismuth salts, hemochromatosis, sulfhemoglobinemia, methemoglobinemia. A *yellow color* is produced by deposition of bile pigments, carotenemia, or atabrine dye.

Macules (Fig. 4-2A). These are localized changes in the skin color. The areas may be small or large; they occur in many shapes and colors. Macules are not palpable. The lesions may be associated with desquamation or scaling. They are exemplified in rubeola, rubella, secondary syphilis, rose spots of typhoid fever, drug eruptions, petechiae, purpura, first-degree burns, systemic lupus erythematosus, pityriasis rosea, vitiligo.

Maculopapules. These are slightly elevated macules. Common diseases with this lesion are pityriasis rosea, erythema multiforme, fixed drug eruptions, and the exanthemas.

Papules (Fig. 4-2B). The lesions are solid and elevated; they are defined as less than 5 mm in diameter. Their borders

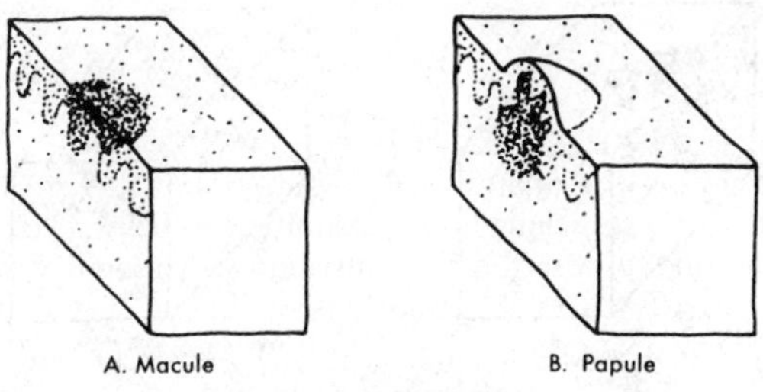

Fig. 4-2. Skin lesions.

and tops may assume various forms. *Pointed* or *acuminate* lesions occur in insect bites, acne, and the physiologic gooseflesh. *Flat-topped* lesions are exemplified by psoriasis, atopic eczema, condyloma latum. *Round* or *irregular* lesions are seen in senile angiomas, eczematous dermatitis, and papular secondary syphilis. *Filiform* lesions are illustrated by condyloma acuminatum. *Pedunculate* lesions are typified by neurofibromas.

Plaques. Since papules have a diameter of less than 5 mm, any elevated area of greater size is a plaque, usually formed from confluent papules. *Red scaling plaques* are seen in psoriasis, pityriasis rosea, discoid lupus erythematosus (with atrophy). Xanthomas are *yellow;* the lesions of seborrheic warts are *brown;* plantar warts are *keratotic;* atopic dermatitis is *lichenified.*

Nodules (Fig. 4-3A). The lesions are solid and elevated; they are distinguished from papules by extending deeper into the dermis or even the subcutaneous tissue. They are usually greater than 5 mm in diameter. The depth may be inferred by palpation; when below the dermis, the skin slides over them; lesions within the dermis move with the skin. Typical nodules are gummas, lymphoma cutis, xanthomas, gouty tophi, and erythema nodosum.

Wheals (Fig. 4-3B). Caused by edema of the skin, these areas are circumscribed, irregular, and relatively transient. Their color varies from red to pale, depending upon the amount of fluid in the skin. Examples are urticaria and insect bites.

Fever, Urticaria, Arthralgia After Foreign Protein Injection: ***Serum Sickness.*** This belongs to the group of necrotizing vasculitides

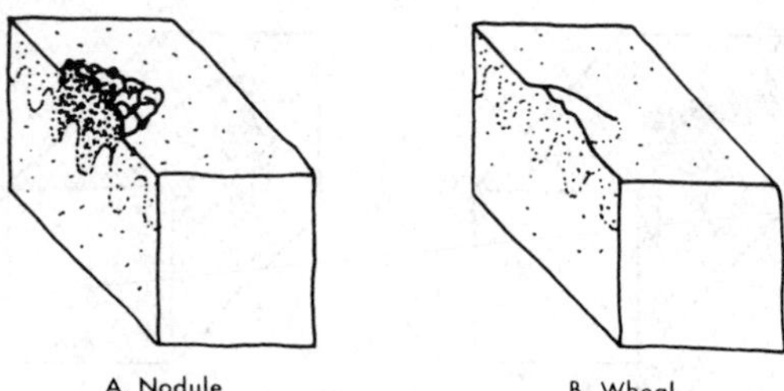

Fig. 4-3. Skin lesions.

[*see* p. 465 for classification and pathophysiology]. *Age and Sex:* no limitations. *Antigens:* originally, from the injection of horse serum therapeutically; more recently, the injection of penicillin has been the most common cause, although a variety of proteins can cause it. *Course:* A few days after injection of protein, onset is attended by *headache, pruritus,* and *wheal formation* at site of injection. The urticaria spreads, and large areas of skin may become *edematous.* An *erythematous rash* accompanies. *Pains in muscles* and *joints* may be severe; *nausea and vomiting* may occur. Generalized *lymphadenopathy* is frequent. The *blood counts are not significantly abnormal. Response to Therapy and Prognosis:* The symptoms and signs promptly respond to corticosteroids and the course is self-limited.

Vesicles (Fig. 4-4A). An accumulation of fluid between the upper layers of the skin produces an elevation covered by a translucent epithelium that is easily punctured to release the fluid. By definition, their diameter is limited to less than 5 mm. *Umbilicated* vesicles are usually the result of viral infections. Examples of vesicles are found in acute eczematous dermatitis, second-degree burns, varicella, and variola.

Bullae. Accumulations of fluid between the layers of the skin, larger than 5 mm in diameter, are bullae. They are typified by some lesions in contact dermatitis, second-degree burns, bullous impetigo, and pemphigus.

Pustules (Fig. 4-4A). Vesicles or bullae that become filled with pus and tiny abscesses in the skin are termed pustules. Through the translucent skin covering, their contents appear milky, orange, yellow, or green, depending somewhat upon the infecting organisms. Pustules frequently arise from hair

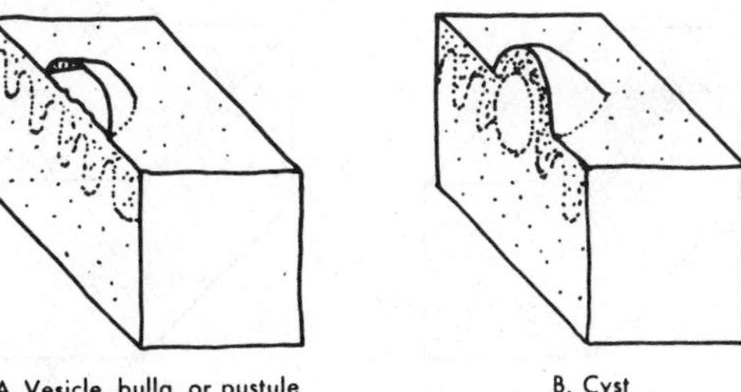

Fig. 4-4. Skin lesions.

follicles or sweat glands. Typical lesions are seen in acne, furuncles, variola, bromide and iodide eruptions.

Cysts (Fig. 4-4B). Elevated lesions containing fluid or viscous material appear as papules or nodules. The distinction is made by puncturing to examine their contents and depth. Typical are sebaceous and epidermal cysts.

Vegetations (Fig. 4-5A). Elevated irregular growths are called vegetations. When their covering is keratotic or dried, they are *verrucous,* as in verruca vulgaris (common wart) and seborrheic keratosis. When covered by normal epidermis, they are *papillomatous,* as in condyloma acuminatum.

Hyperkeratosis. Keratotic cells are piled up to produce elevations. Calluses are the most common. Arsenic produces punctate keratoses of the palms and soles.

Secondary or Consecutive: ***Scales*** (Fig. 4-5B). Thin plates of dried cornified epithelium cling to the epidermis, partly separated. These are exemplified in psoriasis and exfoliative dermatitis. Smaller scales are constant features of the individual lesions in pityriasis rosea and seborrheic dermatitis.

Secondary or Consecutive: ***Lichenification*** (Fig. 4-6A). Repeated rubbing of the skin produces hyperplasia of all layers. This appears as a dry plaque in which the normal skin furrows or rhomboid lines are accentuated. These are typified in atopic dermatitis and lichen simplex chronicus.

Secondary or Consecutive: ***Crusts*** (Fig. 4-6B). A plate of dried serum, blood, pus, or sebum forms upon the surface of any vesicular or pustular lesion when it ruptures. The honey-colored crusts of impetigo are typical.

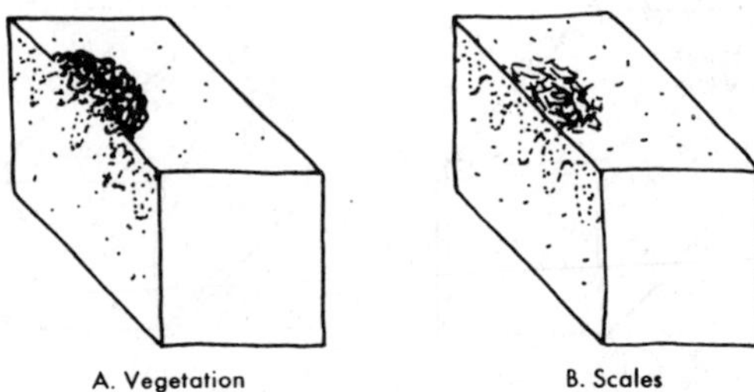

Fig. 4-5. Skin lesions.

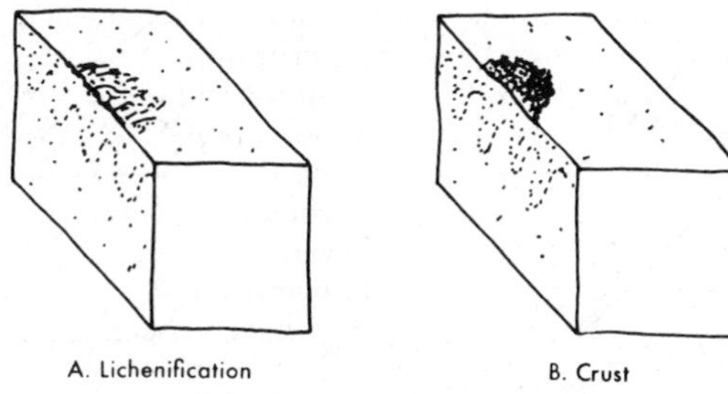

Fig. 4-6. Skin lesions.

Secondary or Consecutive: ***Atrophy*** (Fig. 4-7A). The skin is thinned, as noted by the lack of resilience and loss of skin furrows or rhomboid lines. This is typified in senile atrophy, discoid lupus erythematosus, and insulin lipodystrophy.

Secondary or Consecutive: ***Sclerosis.*** An area of skin is indurated from underlying interstitial inflammation. Examples are keloid, stasis dermatitis, scleroderma.

Secondary or Consecutive: ***Erosions*** (Fig. 4-7B). The moist surface uncovered by the rupture of vesicles or bullae or by laceration from rubbing is termed an erosion.

Secondary or Consecutive: ***Fissures*** (Fig. 4-8A). A cleavage of the epidermis extending into the dermis is a fissure. Commonly it occurs from trauma to thickened, dry, inelastic skin.

Secondary or Consecutive: ***Ulcers*** (Fig. 4-8B). A depressed lesion results from loss of epidermis and the papillary layer of the dermis. Examples are traumatic ulcers, burns, stasis ulcers.

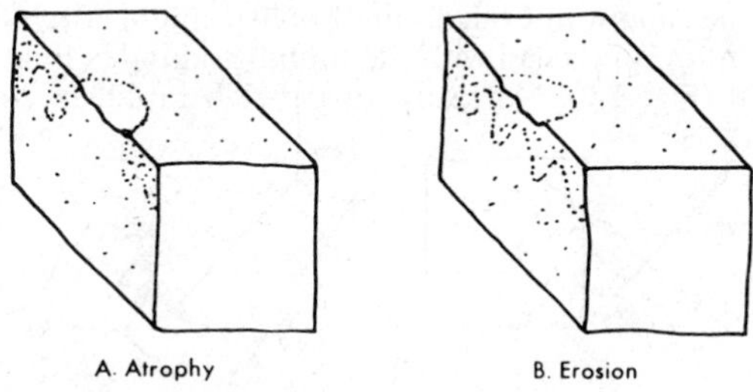

Fig. 4-7. Skin lesions.

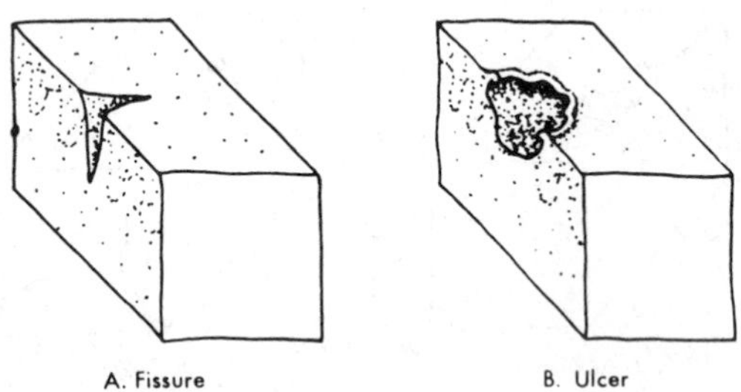

Fig. 4-8. Skin lesions.

Secondary or Consecutive: ***Gangrene.*** Extensive destruction of the skin may leave many dead cells that become blackened.

Changes in the Hair. The quantity of hair may vary. An excessive growth is termed *hypertrichosis* or *hirsutism.* This may occur locally over a nevus or generally as in carcinoma of the adrenal, Cushing's syndrome, testicular tumors, and acromegaly. The presence of less hair than normal is *hypotrichosis,* as in some congenital ectodermal defects. *Alopecia* is the loss of hair in either congenital or acquired conditions. Some examples are physiologic baldness in the male, alopecia areata, hypothyroidism, thallium intoxication, scleroderma. *Graying of the hair* (canities) may be from aging or albinism; it may be acquired in pernicious anemia or from chloroquine therapy. Localized graying occurs in vitiliginous lesions.

Skin Turgor. The turgor of the skin is reduced in general dehydration, senile cutaneous atrophy, rapid loss of body tissue in weight reduction, and pseudoxanthoma elasticum. Loss of skin turgor and longitudinal furrowing of the tongue (p. 154) should be sought in evaluation of dehydration. The skin over the sternum is pinched with the thumb and index finger, then released (Fig. 4-9). Normally, turgid skin rapidly resumes its

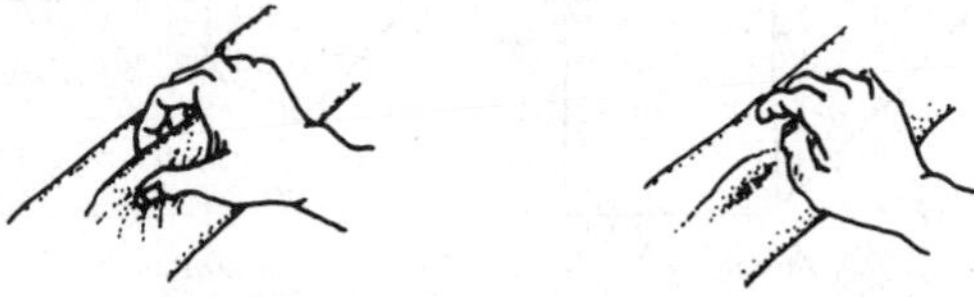

Fig. 4-9. Testing for skin turgor.

customary shape. Loss of turgor is indicated by persistence of the fold for a time after pinching.

Diffuse Skin Colorations in Caucasians*

In human beings the color of the normal skin results from a blend of four pigments: melanin (brown), carotene (yellow), oxyhemoglobin (red), and reduced hemoglobin (bluish-red). Except in albinos, the amount of melanin is the determinant of the normal skin color.

Pathophysiology of Melanin Coloring. Cells in the dermis called *melanocytes* manufacture the enzyme *tyrosinase, which converts ingested tyrosine to the pigment melanin* via stages forming dopa and indoles. The melanin granules (organelles called *melanosomes*) migrate outward through the epidermis to become associated with *keratocytes* in the epidermis and hair. Each individual has dual melanin deposits: one producing a *constitutive* skin color in which the amount of pigment is determined by genetic inheritance, and a deposit for a *facultative* skin color in which an additional amount of pigment waxes or wanes in response to the hormone supply and the character of external stimuli such as untraviolet light.

Inherent Diffuse Brown Skin: ***Normal Melanin Pigmentation.*** This is the constitutive skin color inherited by genes for race and family. The diagnostic importance is to distinguish it from acquired disorders. In racial pigmentation, the Black has the greatest melanin density, and lesser amounts occur in order from American Indians, Indonesians, Orientals (Chinese and Japanese); with the Caucasians having the least. But there is also variation among the ethnic groups of the same race. For example, in the Caucasians the natives of India are almost black; the inhabitants of the Mediterranean region are darker than the Northern Europeans, although the Prussians are also

* WARNING: Most English descriptions of skin lesions refer to disorders in white patients; but neither writers nor readers seem to recognize this limitation. As an intern in Cleveland City Hospital many years ago, E.L.D. was privileged to make rounds with an internationally famous dermatologist from Central Europe. When the Herr Professor was conducted into a ward occupied by black patients, he was nonplussed. He had never before seen a Black, and he failed to recognize common skin lesions, so much did they differ from those of Caucasians.

dark. In many Caucasian families dark complexions are inherited by some members, not by others. *Distinction:* The inheritance of skin color can usually be established by questioning the patient or his acquaintances about the origin and appearance of his relatives. The question of race should be raised; in the United States many white persons have had an American Indian ancestor.

▼ *Key Sign: Acquired Diffuse Brown Skin:* ***Melanism.*** By this term is meant a darkening of the skin color from augmented production of melanin in the facultative pigment deposits. The brown color is diffuse, with accentuation in palmar creases; recent scars; pressure points at elbow, knee, and knuckles. Pigmentation appears in the oral mucosa (this is abnormal when found in Caucasians). *Pathophysiology:* The mechanisms are not well-known except that melanin production is stimulated by adrenocorticotropic hormone and melanocyte-stimulating hormone, active in Addison's disease and some endocrine and nonendocrine neoplasms. The administration of vitamin B_{12} will abolish the excessive pigmentation in patients with pernicious anemia or folic acid deficiency. *Distinction:* The history of a definite onset establishes the pigmentation as acquired. Its presence should prompt an intensive search for serious organic disorders among the following.

Clinical Occurrence. [adapted from F. R. Greipp: Hyperpigmentation Syndromes (Diffuse Hypermelanosis), *Arch. Intern. Med.*, **138:**356–57, 1978]: *skin* (scleroderma); *neck* (Graves' disease, myxedema); *colon* (Whipple's disease); *adrenals* (Addison's disease); *liver* (cirrhosis, hemochromatosis); *spleen* (Felty's syndrome); *genitalia* (Heller-Nelson syndrome); *blood* (pernicious anemia, folic acid deficiency); neoplastic diseases; *nutrition* (malnutrition, starvation); *metabolic* (porphyria); *drugs and poisons* (busulfan, arsenicals, dibromomannitol).

— *Acquired Diffuse Brown Skin:* ***Hemosiderin (Hemochromatosis).*** The actual color may be bronze, blue-gray, brown, or black, accentuated in the flexor folds, the nipples, recent scars, and in parts exposed to the sun. The pigment may be a mixture of hemosiderin and melanin. Only a skin biopsy can prove the presence of hemosiderin by the blue-staining of the iron with potassium ferrocyanate. Skin color may antedate the hepatic cirrhosis and diabetes mellitus by several years.

— *Acquired Diffuse Blue-Gray Skin:* ***Silver (Argyria).*** Silver salts from ingestion or intranasal absorption may be deposited in the skin to produce a blue-gray or slate color, accented in the areas exposed to sunlight. The mucosa and nail lunulae may be deposit sites. The pigmentation may appear years after exposure.

— *Acquired Spotted Blue-Gray Skin:* ***Arsenic.*** The ingestion of arsenic, therapeutically or as chronic poisoning, produces a diffuse gray background with superimposed dark macules, 2 to 10 mm in diameter. This is often accompanied by punctate hyperkeratoses of the palms and soles. The skin manifestations may appear from one to ten years after ingestion of the chemical.

— *Inherent Blue-Gray Skins:* ***Alkaptonuria (Ochronosis).*** This is an inherited metabolic error lacking the oxidase of homogentisic acid, with consequent deposition of black polymers of homogentisic acid in the connective tissues and in the urine. The black accumulations shine through the skin producing a faint blue-gray color to the skin especially over the pinnae, the tip of the nose, and in the sclerae. The blackened extensor tendons of the hands may shine through the skin. Often a dark butterfly pattern will appear on the face; the axillae and genitalia will be pigmented.

— *Acquired Blue-Gray Skin:* ***Gold (Chrysoderma).*** Occasionally the parenteral administration of gold salts in the treatment of arthritis will cause a blue-gray pigmentation of the periocular skin and the regions exposed to the sun.

— *Acquired Diffuse Yellow Skin:* ***Jaundice (Icterus, Bilirubinemia).*** *See* full discussion under Jaundice, p. 479.

— *Acquired Diffuse Yellow Skin:* ***Carotenemia.*** Excessive deposition of carotene appears as yellowness of the skin especially on the forehead, the nasolabial folds, behind the ears, in the palms and soles. *Pathophysiology.* The carotene surplus occurs (1) from excessive ingestion of the pigment in oranges, mangos, apricots, carrots, and all green vegetables or (2) when the liver fails to metabolize the carotene in myxedema and diabetes mellitus. *Distinction:* When the diagnosis is in doubt an elevated serum concentration of carotene should confirm.

— *Acquired Diffuse Yellow Skin:* ***Quinacrine (Atabrine), Dinitrophenol, Tetryl.*** The ingestion of quinacrine, an antimalarial supressant and a therapeutic agent for discoid lupus erythematosus and polymorphous light eruptions, produces a greenish-yellow skin. A similar discoloration occurs from contact with dinitrophenol and tetryl, both used in the manufacture of explosives.

5

The Head and Neck

In clinical medicine no less than six specialties focus on the head and neck: neurology, neurosurgery, ophthalmology, otorhinolaryngology, plastic surgery, and dentistry. A detailed examination has evolved for each specialty, assisted by appropriate instruments. The physician who examines the entire patient employs these methods and instruments to the extent of demonstrating (1) the signs of generalized disease and (2) local lesions requiring the care of the specialist. Presentation of the entire corpus of diagnosis in these specialties is beyond the scope of this book or the competence of the authors. Instead, we shall describe appropriate examinations that can be made with the resources available to the general physician. Traumatic disorders are omitted from consideration.

Symptoms from the Head

▼ *Key Symptom:* ***Headache.*** The term *headache* is usually reserved for pain perceived more than momentarily in the cranial vault, the orbits, and the nape of the neck; pain elsewhere in the face is not included. The common *extracranial* cause of headache is sustained contraction of the muscles of the neck and shoulders. *Intracranial* headaches are produced by (1) dilatation and distention of cerebral arteries, or (2) traction, displacement, or inflammation of cerebral vessels, sensitive portions of the meninges, cranial and upper cervical nerves. Usually the diagnosis of the type of headache must be made from the symptoms; physical signs are often absent or nonspecific.

CLINICAL EXAMINATION FOR HEADACHE. **In taking the history, inquire carefully for the attributes of pain (PQRST):** ***provocative*** **and**

***palliative factors*, such as position of the head and body, coughing, straining, emotional tension; *quality*, whether burning, aching, deep or superficial, throbbing or continuous; *region* of the head involved; *severity* of the pain; and *timing*. The last includes the duration of the history and the periodicity of symptoms. Seek *associated symptoms:* nausea and vomiting, constipation or diarrhea, diuresis, rhinorrhea; *visual disturbances*, such as photophobia, scotomata, tearing, diplopia; *cerebral symptoms*, such as aura, paresthesias, anesthesias, motor paralysis, vertigo, mood, sleep disturbances.**

Inspect the skin and scalp for *bulges* and areas of *erythema*. With deep pressure palpate the bones of the cranium and face for *tenderness* and *irregularities* of contour. Especially, pinch the muscles in the nape of the neck and the upper borders of the Trapezii for unusual *tenderness*. Palpate the carotid and temporal arteries for *pulsations* and *tenderness*. Examine the eyes for *pupillary irregularities, conjunctival injection, abnormal extraocular motion;* use the confrontation test (p. 81) to detect gross defects in the visual fields; look with the ophthalmoscope for *choked disk* and *retinal hemorrhages*. With the stethoscope auscultate the cranium for *bruits*. Make a routine neurologic examination with special attention to the cranial nerves and the deep tendon reflexes.

Muscular Contraction Headaches. Sustained contractions of the muscles of the neck, head, and shoulders cause fatigue and *pain*. The principal physical finding is *tender muscles*. Injection of the tender muscles with isotonic saline can be shown to intensify the headache; injections of procaine relieve it.

— *Muscular:* ***Muscle Tension Headaches* (*Primary*).** *Epitome: chronic intermittent headaches in the occiput, with tenderness in the neck and Trapezii.* Usually the pain has recurred irregularly for many years, without periodicity. The sensation is described as mild or moderate discomfort, vicelike, a heavy feeling, a sense of pressure, a tight band, cramping, aching, or soreness; it is *unvarying* rather than throbbing. The pain is *not augmented* by coughing, straining at stool, or shaking the head. It usually begins in the occiput and extends upward to the parietal regions and down the nape of the neck to the shoulders. It may last for a few hours, with intensification near the day's end; or it may persist for many days, waxing and waning throughout. The onset of an episode is often related to emotional tension or to activity of an occupation. The pain is *relieved* by external support of the head, the application of hot packs or massage to the neck, salicylates or tranquilizers. *Physical Signs. Tender-*

ness in the upper border of the Trapezii and the intrinsic muscles of the neck. *Distinction.* The symptoms and signs diagnose the primary types. But intracranial disorders cause a secondary type that must be excluded by appropriate tests, whenever the history suggests an unusual exacerbation. Muscle contraction headaches are the only type *not intensified* by coughing or straining at stools; they are also the only type *ameliorated* by shaking the head.

— *Muscular:* ***Muscle Tension Headaches (Secondary).*** *Epitome: acute or chronic headaches in the occiput with tender muscles in the neck and shoulders, associated with intracranial lesions.* The quality, location, and severity of the pain and muscle tenderness resemble those of the primary type. But muscle tension is secondary to other types of pain in the head from intracranial disorders. For example, the muscle tension in migraine may not subside when the more severe migrainous pain has been relieved by drugs.

Clinical Occurrence. All intracranial disorders that cause headache.

Vascular Headaches. This term is applied to a variety of entities produced by reversible segmental arterial constriction and dilatation; so vascular headaches are all characterized by their *intermittence* and the *throbbing pain.* The components of the group are distinguished by differences in cause, temporal sequences, and the location of the affected blood vessels.

— *Vascular:* ***Migraine*** (Migram, Hemicrania, Sick Headache). *Epitome: an inheritable disorder with periodic unilateral headache preceded by an aura of transient ischemia in some part of the central nervous system.* An estimated 10% of the population have some migrainous manifestations. The disorder is inherited as a recessive gene with a penetrance of 70%. Members of a family are likely to exhibit the same pattern of symptoms. Women are more frequently affected than men, though boys are more frequently affected in childhood. Patients with migraine have a higher-than-normal incidence of allergy and Raynaud's phenomenon. Commonly patients of either sex experience the onset in adolescence; symptoms often subside in the fifth decade of life. But the onset may be delayed until the fifties. The attacks may occur a few times a year or as often as every few weeks. Often migraine is coincident with some phase of the menstrual cycle. The clinical picture of paroxysms varies so much among individuals that the experience of a single patient is not representative of most; some patterns have received special names. The paroxysm of migraine has four phases. ***The Prodome.*** An attack is often triggered by a period of intense activity associated with anxiety, tension, or rage with stifled expression of resentment. A day or so before the attack, the patient may feel *depressed,* or he may feel a sense of unusual well-being; occasionally *hunger* (bulimia) is noted. Body water is retained with resultant gain in weight. The attack may begin any time of the day or night, frequently on awaking. ***The Aura.*** Although great individual variations occur, each patient tends to repeat his own pattern of aura in successive attacks. Migrainous phenomena are typically *unilateral,* but occasionally they involve both sides; the side may vary in different paroxysms. *Visual Disturbances:* A *scintillating scotoma,* involving one or both eyes, presents as black and white wavy lines, like the shimmering made by heat waves rising from an asphalt pavement; sometimes there are flashing lights. Or a *fortification spectrum* may be exhibited, with zigzag colored patterns with dark centers moving across the visual field. *Variant—Ophthalmic Migraine:* The scotomata may be succeeded by momentary blindness, *anopsia,* in the entire field, or in the lower or upper quadrants; or the pattern may be *bitemporal* or *homonymous hemianopsia. Variant—Ophthalmoplegic Migraine:* Transient unilateral paralysis of the 3rd cranial nerve (oculomotor) produces lateral deviation and palpebral ptosis. This occurs in young girls. *Variant—Dysphasic Migraine:* Unilateral paresthesias or anesthesias may occur in the face, the arm, or the foot. When the right side is involved, expressive dysphasia and homonymous hemianopsia may be added. *Variant—Basilar Artery Migraine:* The scotomata and anesthesias of the face and limbs are bilateral and vertigo or cranial nerve palsies may be present from brainstem nuclear ischemia. The transition from aura to headache may be accompanied by momentary *loss of consciousness or light sleep. Variant—Hemiplegic Migraine:* This is spectacular but rare. The paralysis is most likely to occur in migrainous patients experiencing paresthesias. The right side is more often involved. The patient complains of numbness or "woodenness" of the ipsilateral limbs. Although weakness may be the complaint, it is often revealed only during an attack when the examiner finds exaggeration of the deep tendon reflexes and Babinski's sign. The paralysis lasts for a few minutes to 2 or 3 days; usually there is no permanent damage. Many neurologists are reluctant to make such a diagnosis without excluding more permanent cerebral disorders by arteriography, computed tomography, EEG, and brain scans, or by prolonged observation of the patient. The diagnosis is on a more secure basis when there are other cases of hemiplegic migraine in the family. *The aura usually lasts from 10 to 40 minutes.* **The Headache.** An occasional patient may have a typical aura without succeeding headache. But usually, as the aura diminishes, *unilateral headache* appears on the side opposite any unilateral visual or somatosensory symptoms. The pain may start above one orbit and spread over the entire side of the head to the occiput and neck; or it may begin in the back of the head and move forward. Rarely, the site of pain is below the eye, in front of the ear, behind the mandibular angle, in the nape of the neck, or in the shoulders. For about one hour the pain spreads and intensifies to a severe *throbbing, boring, aching* headache. The pain is often *augmented in the reclining position,* lessened when sitting or standing. Shaking the head, coughing, or straining at stool *intensifies* the pain. Usually the pain is not relieved by mild analgesics, but ergot may abolish it. Although the pain may be severe, usually it *does not disrupt sleep.* In rare instances, a headache equivalent is *mental confusion, excitement,* or *delirium. Associated Symptoms:* Nausea and vomiting often accompany the headache. Frequently the threshold for external sensory stimuli is lowered, so there are *photophobia,* an annoyance from loud sounds (*hyperacusis*), annoyance from odors (*hyperosmia*). *Physical Signs During Headache:* The patient may be prostrated to the point of *stupor,* with cold limbs and pale skin; in others the attacks are relatively mild. Often the *conjunctiva is injected* on the affected side. *Unilateral hyperesthesia* of the face and scalp may be found. On the side of the headache, the superficial temporal artery is often distended and its pulsation augmented. Occlusion of the carotid artery on the affected side with digital compression will temporarily abolish the headache. The retained body fluid may rapidly be lost by *spontaneous diuresis. The duration of the paroxysm is from 1 hour to 3 days.* **The Recovery.** When an attack concludes overnight, the patient usually awakens with headache and experiences a sense of buoyancy and well-being. He may have lost several pounds of body water from vomiting and diuresis. ***Pathophysiology.*** The mechanism of triggering the migrainous paroxysm is unknown. Apparently the manifestations of the aura are caused by segmented arterial constriction; vasoconstriction of the retinal vessels may be directly observed, and the EEG gives indirect evidence of similar activity within the cerebrum. The aura is abolished by certain vasodilator drugs. The headache results from dilatation chiefly of the extracranial and dural branches of the external carotid artery, plus the elaboration of some substance that lowers the pain threshold. *Distinction.* The diagnosis is easy in a long-established case with relatively typical symptoms. When the onset is recent and the symptoms unusual, other intracranial disorders must be excluded. Ophthalmoplegic migraine can be closely simulated by a leaking aneurysm in the circle of Willis. Although hemiplegia has been described as a migrainous phenomenon, most authors are inclined to consider other, more serious causes. Migraine headaches are frequently ameliorated by the *erect* position; in other intracranial disorders the patient seeks the horizontal to relieve the pain. *Whenever the symptoms of the aura persist after the headache has subsided, search for another intracranial disorder is imperative.*

— *Vascular:* ***Atypical Migraine*** (Sick Headache, Headache Qualified by Tropical, Summer, Monday, Weekend, Premenstrual, Menstrual). This is a variant of migraine in which the aura may be absent or rudimentary; the headache may be unilateral or bilateral; the periodicity may be related to occupation, environment, or menses.

— *Vascular:* ***Cluster Headaches*** (Histamine Headache, Histamine Cephalgia, Erythroprosopalgia, Migrainous Neuralgia, Petrosal Neuralgia). *Epitome: brief, severe, unilateral headaches, several times a day or week for several weeks, with long intermissions between clusters.* The principal name emphasizes the occurrence of the headaches in clusters of several times a day or week for several weeks, followed by long and irregular remissions. A single paroxysm lasts from 15 to 45 minutes; there is *no antecedent aura.* The headache is *unilateral, severe, boring,* and *throbbing.* It recurs consistently on the same side. It is usually maximal just inferior to the medial canthus of the orbit, but may occur in the temple, or in the side of the face, and it may spread to the neck and shoulder. *Flushing* of the skin, *lacrimation, congestion* of the nostril *rhinorrhea,* and *dilatation* of the temporal artery may occur on the affected side. *Pathophysiology.* The headache is produced by dilatation of branches of the internal carotid artery, especially those supplying the meninges innervated by the trigeminial nerve. Although the syndrome can be simulated by the injection of histamine into the internal carotid artery, there is no conclusive evidence that this substance is concerned in the natural disorder. The administration of ergot derivatives relieves the headache as in migraine.

— *Vascular:* ***Hypertensive Headache.*** In patients with mild hypertension the incidence of headache and the types are no different than in normotensive persons. But in half the patients with severe hypertension without encephalopathy many headaches occur. According to Wolff, some of these headaches are the muscular contraction type, whereas others are vascular. The occurrence of the vascular type is not associated with periods of highest peripheral blood pressure; they may be more pronounced when pressures are relatively low. The vascular headaches are often occipital, although other regions may be involved; they are not necessarily unilateral; they have no antecedent aura. *Pathophysiology.* The evidence points to segmental dilatation of branches of the external carotid artery. Digital compression abolishes the headache when applied to the external carotid, frontal, supraorbital, postauricular, or occipital arteries. Ergotamine tartrate, whose principal dilating effect is on the external carotid, reduces the intensity of the headaches, even while it increases the peripheral arterial tension.

— *Vascular:* ***Headache from Fever.*** Many febrile illnesses are associated with headache. The location varies; the pain may be slight or severe, throbbing or steady. Evidence suggests that distention of the cranial arteries is the cause of the pain.

— *Vascular:* ***Temporal Arteritis.*** Epitome: persistent throbbing headache with tender arteries of the head, often visual disturbances. The disease is named for the principal accessible vessel involved, although frequently the occipital artery and less often the carotid and others are affected. In many cases a concomitant segmental inflammation of the retinal and ophthalmic arteries causes visual disturbances. This is one of the group of necrotizing vasculitides (cf. p. 465 for classification). The disease is heralded by severe *headache, persistent* and *throbbing.* Jaw claudication is frequent. The pain is located in the region of the involved superficial cranial artery; when an intracranial vessel is affected, the pain cannot be accurately localized. The disease is *unilateral* or *bilateral;* it lasts from 3 months to more than 3 years. It is often associated with polymyalgia rheumatica. ***Physical Signs.*** The inflamed artery feels *hard* and *nodular;* it is *tender* and *pulsating,* even though it may contain a thrombus. The overlying skin is often *red* and *swollen.* Systemic manifestations seem disproportionately severe for the local lesion; there are *profound weakness, malaise,* and *prostration. Fever* is often present. Some *mental symptoms* are common; there may be disorientation. In half the cases one or both eyes are involved. *Vision* is often impaired; *ophthalmoplegia* may occur, temporarily or permanently. The retina may appear normal, or one may see *closure* of retinal vessels, *choked disk,* or *cotton-wool patches.* ***Laboratory Findings.*** Moderate leukocytosis and normocytic anemia; accelerated erythrocyte sedimentation rate; occasionally hypergammaglobulinemia. ***Pathophysiology.*** The cause is unknown. Histologic examination shows patchy medial necrosis of arterial segments, with diffuse mononuclear infiltration and giant cells throughout the vessel walls. Thromboses are frequent. The *carotid artery* may be involved (p. 205).

Distinction. The condition may be attributed to a benign headache *unless* the cranial arteries are palpated and tenderness is discovered. When intracranial arteries are involved first, the ocular disturbances are usually attributed to other causes until accessible vessels show signs.

Traction, Displacement, Inflammation Causing Intracranial Headaches. The pain-sensitive structures within the cranium are the dura and its arteries at the base of the brain, the cerebral arteries in the same region, the great venous sinuses, and certain nerves (5th, 9th, and 10th cranial, and the upper 3 cervical). The greater portion of the dura and cranium is insensitive. Wolff lists the mechanisms producing headaches from intracranial disorders: (1) *traction* on the superficial cerebral veins leading to the venous sinuses and *displacement* of the sinuses themselves, (2) *traction* on the middle meningeal arteries, (3) *traction* on the basilar arteries and their branches, (4) *distention* and *dilatation* of the intracranial arteries, (5) *inflammation* near any pain-sensitive region, (6) *direct pressure* or *traction* by tumors on cranial and cervical nerves. The resulting headaches may be *throbbing* when arteries are involved; otherwise the *pain is steady*. Headaches are often *intensified* by movements of the head, certain postures, rapid changes in the pressure of the cerebrospinal fluid.

— *Traction-Displacement:* ***Brain Tumor.*** *Epitome: constant or paroxysmal headaches, with progressive increasing frequency and duration, changing from customary individual headache pattern.* Although the word *tumor* literally means a mass of any kind, in this context it refers to a neoplasm. *Headache* is often the first indication. At first, the pain is usually in paroxysms, lasting a few seconds to 3 hours, for weeks or months. But there is *progressive increase* in frequency and duration of paroxysms; in the late stages the pain is continuous. A paroxysm is often started by *abrupt change in position*. The pain is *deep, aching*, usually *steady;* throbbing pain occurs when cerebral vessels are involved. *Nausea* and *vomiting* may accompany it, or occur during the pain-free periods. Occasionally, *major seizures* occur. The headache is usually *intensified* in the *erect position,* so reclining is preferred. The pain may be anywhere in the cranium. *Occipital pain* is often caused by subtentorial tumors. *Unilateral pain* localizes the side of the tumor in 90% of cases. The headache may be mild or excruciating; often it is relieved by analgesics; it seldom interferes with sleep. *Physical Signs.* These vary with the location of the tumor and the affected modalities. Localization may be assisted by the nature of the headache and the focal changes in muscle strength and tendon reflexes. *Special Examinations.* Ophthalmoscopic examination for *choked disk;* lumbar puncture for *increased fluid pressure* and the presence of *blood* or *increased protein* in the spinal fluid; mapping of visual fields for *defects;* x-ray films of the skull for osseous *erosion* and *displacement* of the *pineal body;* EEG; scintigrams of the skull with radioisotopes; arteriography, but especially CT and MRI scans. *Distinction.* All other types of headache must be distinguished by the symptoms, the neurologic findings, and the results of the special tests. Brain tumor should be suspected whenever the onset is recent, or a recent change in the customary headache pattern has occurred, or when an apparent aura of migraine persists after the headache subsides.

— *Traction-Displacement:* ***Brain Abscess.*** *Epitome: symptoms and signs of brain tumor coincident with or after infection in the ears,* *paranasal sinuses, or lungs.* A localized region in the brain substance becomes infected and encapsulated, enclosing liquefied brain and pus. To the diagnostician, the condition presents the symptoms and signs of a compact mass (the so-called space-occupying mass), as a sequel of primary infection elsewhere in the body. Frequently the infection has been in the middle ear, the mastoid cells, the paranasal sinuses, or the lungs; rarely, an osteomyelitis or other source is incriminated. When the presence of the primary infection has not been recognized, or proper significance has not been attached to it, the distinction from brain tumor may not be evident until a CT or MRI scan is performed. The course, the attributes of the headache, and the localizing signs are similar to those of brain tumor. *Distinction.* Aside from the history, abscess may be distinguished from brain tumor by finding pleocytosis (25–300 cells per cu mm) and elevated protein content (75–300 mg per 100 mL) in the spinal fluid.

— *Traction-Displacement:* ***Subdural Hematoma.*** *Epitome: symptoms and signs of expanding intracranial mass with a time lapse after head trauma.* After a severe head injury, the immediate accumulation of blood in the subdural space is anticipated and offers no diagnostic difficulty. But minor trauma to the head may be followed by a *latent period* of days, weeks, or months before the onset of headaches. The progression, timing, and attributes of the pain are similar to those of a brain tumor with relatively rapid expansion. Early, no physical signs are present; later, localizing signs of an expanding intracranial lesion are evident. Or frequent episodes of drowsiness, mental confusion, or coma may appear. The cerebrospinal fluid may be *xanthochromic,* or it may contain small amounts of *blood.* Frequently x-ray films of the skull show a shift of the pineal body. The diagnosis is confirmed by CT or MRI scanning.

— *Traction-Displacement:* ***Cerebral Hemorrhage.*** *Epitome: sudden generalized headache succeeded by cerebral disturbances varying with the site of hemorrhage.* In about half the patients the onset is heralded by *sudden severe generalized headache,* followed by clinical evidence of motor or sensory involvement of the brain. Frequently the patient *vomits once.* Often there is *nuchal rigidity.* Cerebral *seizures* or *coma* may supervene. The sequence of events and the neurologic manifestations vary with the side of hemorrhage and its volume. *Putamen:* a sensation of intracranial *discomfort* is followed in 30 minutes by *dysphagia, hemiplegia,* and sometimes *anesthesias. Thalamus: hemiplegia* and *hemianesthesias* with *dysphasia, homonymous hemianopsia,* and *extraocular paralyses* are common. *Cerebellum:* slowly developing, with *repeated vomiting, occipital headaches, vertigo,* paralysis of conjugate lateral gaze and other ocular disorders. *Subarachnoid:* excruciating generalized headaches with *nuchal rigidity,* prompt *coma,* and often death. If there is recovery from the coma, the mental confusion and other neurologic disturbances persist for weeks. *Pons:* prompt unconsciousness and death within a few hours. ***Pathophysiology.*** The mechanism of arterial rupture in hypertension is unknown. The site is usually intracerebral, rarely subarachnoid. Subarachnoid hemorrhage usually results from rupture of a saccular aneurysm (berry aneurysm) of the circle of Willis; often there is repeated leakage, in contrast to the rupture of an artery from hypertension. Rupture of a berry aneurysm is the most frequent cause of subarachnoid hemorrhage in the adolescent and young adult. ***Laboratory Finding.*** Leukocytosis; grossly bloody spinal fluid, often under increased pressure, or xanthochromia.

Clinical Occurrence. Hypertension. Vascular diseases: traumatic, inflammatory, saccular or mycotic aneurysms, angiomas, erosion from neoplasm. Cerebral infarction, embolism, thrombosis. Hemorrhage disorders and coagulation defects.

— ***Inflammatory: Bacterial Meningitis.*** *Epitome: acute generalized headache, throbbing or constant, accompanied by fever and stiff neck.* Headache is a prominent early symptom of meningitis. Although many febrile illnesses are accompanied by some degree of head pain, the *headache* of meningitis is *especially severe;* it is either steady or throbbing. Since the meninges are inflamed, the headache is *intensified* by sudden movements of the head. The headache may be accompanied by or supplanted by *drowsiness* or *coma.* Signs of meningeal irritation are *nuchal rigidity, Kernig's sign,* and *Brudzinski's sign* (p. 823). *When headache is associated with stiff neck, a lumbar puncture is indicated.* In meningitis, the cerebrospinal fluid is under increased pressure and shows pleocytosis; organisms may be seen directly through the microscope or cultured from the fluid.

— *Traction-Displacement:* ***Lumbar Puncture Headache.*** A few hours or days after a lumbar puncture has been performed, the patient may develop *full deep headache, constant* or *throbbing,* usually bifrontal or suboccipital. Moderate *stiffness* of the neck may occur. The pain is *intensified* by the erect position, shaking the head, or bilateral compression of the jugular veins. It is *lessened* by the horizontal posture and flexion or extension of the neck. ***Pathophysiology.*** The pain is caused by traction on the supporting structures when the volume of the cerebrospinal fluid is diminished. The fluid is lost by seepage through the puncture hole in the dura.

— *Localized Headache:* ***Paranasal Sinusitis.*** The pain may be *throbbing* or *steady.* Acute inflammation of the maxillary sinuses usually causes *pain* and *tenderness* over the maxilla and aching of the upper molars on the involved side. In acute ethmoid sinusitis, the pain is frequently localized between or behind the eyes. Frontal sinusitis causes pain over the frontal area; sphenoid sinusitis may refer pain to the vertex, occiput, or bitemporal regions. Acute sinusitis pain is characteristically exacerbated by bending over, straining, lifting or anything that suddenly increases cerebrospinal fluid pressure. There is no pain associated with chronic infection of the paranasal sinuses. The diagnosis of acute or chronic sinusitis is confirmed by the chronicity of the disease and the radiographic findings.

— *Localized Headache:* ***Eyestrain.*** Disorders of refraction or accommodation may cause pain in the *orbits* that radiates toward the *occipital region,* following the distribution of the ophthalmic branch of the trigeminal nerve. The pain usually occurs when the eyes have been used intensively for some time, but the pain does not subside immediately with eye rest. The pain is attributed to sustained contraction of intraocular and extraocular muscles. When present, the pain from glaucoma is a *sharp ache* that is most intense around the *orbital rim.*

▼ *Key Symptom:* ***Pain in the Face.*** Although facial pain is usually well localized so that it indicates the anatomic structure involved, the cause may prove to be a major diagnostic problem, so some disorders should be listed and considered: *Nerves:* trigeminal neuralgia, postherpetic neuralgia. *Blood vessels:* temporal arteritis, cavernous sinus thrombosis. *Teeth:* periapical abscess, periodontitis, unerupted teeth. *Bones:* sinusitis, osteomyelitis. *Joints:* temporomandibular arthritis. *Salivary glands:* parotitis.

— *Facial Pain:* ***Trigeminal Neuralgia*** (Tic Douloureux). The patients experiences periodic pain, always unilateral, initially limited to one division of the trigeminal nerve (5th cranial). During an episode the pain is dull and continuous until some slight stimulus provokes a paroxysm of "hot" lancinating pain, accompanied by flushing and lacrimation on the affected side. The intense pain causes grimacing that prompts the French term *tic.* Each patient has his special adequate stimulus, a light touch, a draft, or a tickling of the skin in a *trigger area.* The 2nd or maxillary division of the trigeminal is most commonly involved; so the pain is in the maxilla, the upper teeth and lip, and the lower eyelid (p. 782). Uncommonly the 3rd or mandibular division is involved, with the pain distributed in the lower teeth and lip, the oral portion of the tongue, and the external acoustic meatus. The 1st or ophthalmic branch is rarely affected. *Diagnosis.* The symptoms are the only indication; there are no motor or sensory changes. Usually an underlying cause is not found, but a local neoplasm should be sought. The initial stages of herpes zoster may suggest tic douloureux, but the distinction is made when herpetic vesicles appear on the skin or mucosa. Among other causes, this has been ascribed to digoxin intoxication [J. L. Bernat and J. K. Sullivan: Trigeminal Neuralgia from Digoxin Intoxication, *J.A.M.A.,* **241**:164, 1979].

The Eyes

The bony orbits are quadrilateral pyramids with bases facing anteriorly and apices pointing backward and medially; their medial sides are parallel, while their lateral walls form an angle of 90° (Fig. 5-1). The *orbital roof* is formed by faces of the frontal and sphenoid bones. Portions of the maxilla, lacrimal, and sphenoid bones constitute the *medial wall;* the front of this wall contains the *lacrimal groove* for the lacrimal sac. The *lateral wall* is composed of the zygomatic and palatine bones. At the apex is the *optic foramen* that transmits the optic (2nd) nerve and the ophthalmic artery. The *superior orbital fissure* is posterior between the roof and the lateral wall; it carries the middle meningeal artery, the ophthalmic vein, and four cranial

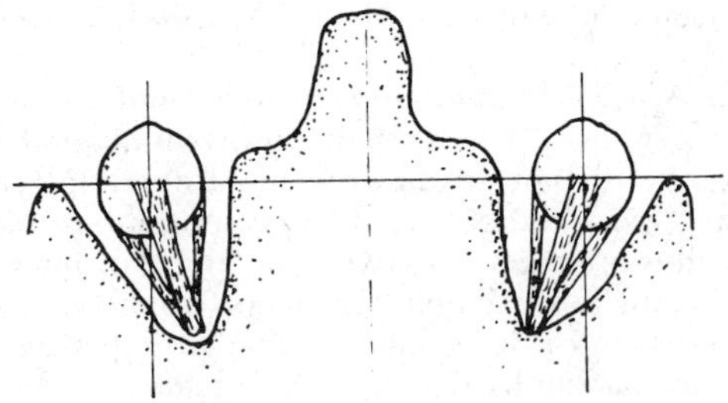

Fig. 5-1. Biorbital relationships. *Diagrammatic horizontal section through the orbits. The medial walls are parallel. When the eyes are in the primary position, the parallel optic axes are also parallel with the medial orbital walls. Since the orbital apices and the origins of the ocular muscles are medial to the optic axes in the primary position, the lateral rectus muscles are longer than the medial; the superior and inferior recti pull medially.*

nerves: the oculomotor (3rd), the trochlear (4th), the ophthalmic division of the trigeminal (5th), and the abducens (6th).

Extraocular Movements

Consider the eyeball as a terrestrial globe with the *optic axis* passing from the midpoint of the cornea, as the north pole, to the back of the eye, as the south pole. Imagine a series of meridians between the poles, all cut by an equator. The globe is suspended at the front of the orbit (the base of the pyramid) by fascia that prevents translation—i.e., movements of all parts of the globe simultaneously in the same direction. Instead, rotation occurs about three axes intersecting perpendicularly at a point 15.4 mm back of the cornea, the *center of rotation.* The vertical axis through the equatorial plane permits *abduction* and *adduction;* rotation about the horizontal axis through the equator produces *elevation* and *depression;* rotation of the uppermost meridian about the optic axis toward the nose is *intorsion;* its movement away from the nose is *extorsion.* Six muscles actuate these motions. The four recti originate in a fibrous ring around the optic foramen in the orbital apex (Fig. 5-2); these muscles insert slightly anterior to the global equator, 90° apart, so the *superior* and *inferior recti* attach in the vertical meridian, while

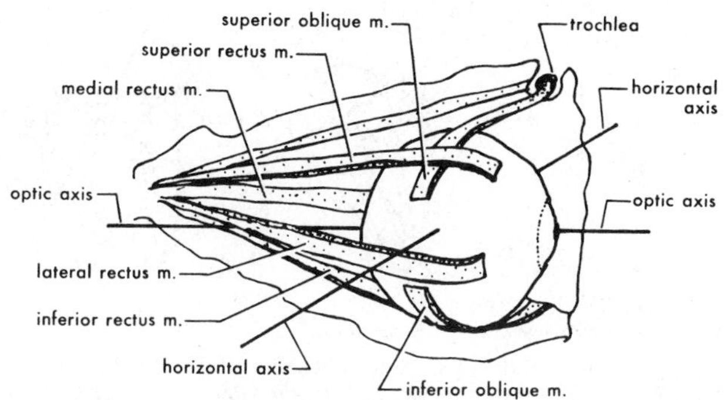

Fig. 5-2. Detail of the ocular muscles. *Diagram of the right orbit as viewed through the lateral wall.*

the *lateral* (external) and *medial* (internal) *recti* oppose on the horizontal meridian. The *superior oblique muscle* inserts behind the equator in the upper lateral quadrant of the posterior global aspect; it passes medially, under the superior rectus, forward and upward to send its tendon through the *trochlea,* a fibrous pulley in the nasal side of the anterior orbit; thence the tendon bends backward to its origin above those of the four recti at the optic foramen, so its physiologic point of action is at the pulley. The *inferior oblique muscle* inserts in the lower lateral quadrant near the superior oblique; it runs medially between the inferior rectus and the orbital floor, passing anteriorly to its origin near the lacrimal groove. The superior oblique is supplied by the *trochlear (4th) nerve;* the *abducens (6th)* nerve innervates the lateral rectus; the other three recti and the inferior oblique are served by the *oculomotor (3rd) nerve.* Some find the mnemonic LR_6SO_4 useful, where *LR* stands for lateral rectus and *SO* indicates superior oblique.

In the primary position, the globes are suspended with their two optic axes horizontal and parallel to the midsagittal plane of the skull. Since the muscles pull toward the apex, the lateral recti are longer than the medial recti; the superior and inferior recti do not pull exactly in the direction of the optic axes. Fig. 5-3A indicates the global movements imparted by the six muscles when the eye is in the primary position. Contraction of the medial rectus, with relaxation of its antagonistic lateral

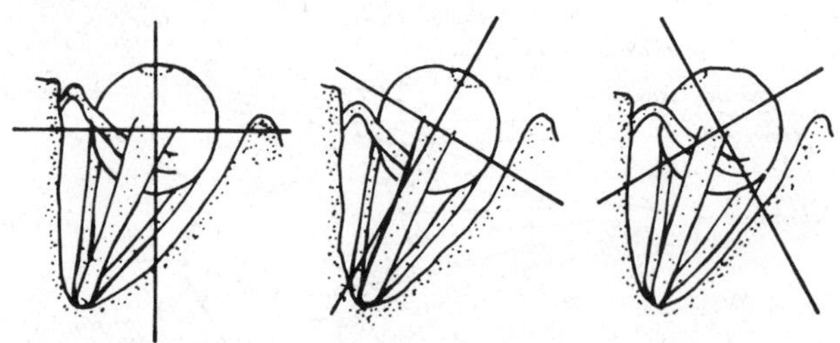

Fig. 5-3. Position of the globe determines the effects of the ocular muscles. *In all positions of the right globe, the lateral rectus produces abduction, the medial rectus causes adduction. When the optic axis is in the primary position* **A,** *the superior rectus elevates and intorts, the inferior oblique elevates and extorts, the inferior rectus depresses and extorts, the superior oblique depresses and intorts. When the globe is abducted so the optic axis coincides with the pull of the superior and inferior recti* **B,** *these muscles produce elevation or depression without extorsion or intorsion. When adduction causes the optic axis to coincide with the pull of the oblique muscles along the equator* **C,** *these muscles produce elevation and depression without intorsion or extorsion.*

rectus, produces *adduction;* pull by the lateral rectus and relaxation of the medial rectus result in *abduction.* With contraction of the superior rectus, the globe *elevates* and *intorts,* because the angular pull produces some rotation about the optic axis. Similarly, the pull of the inferior rectus causes *depression* and *extorsion.* The superior oblique assists the inferior rectus to *depress,* but the oblique also *intorts* to counter *extorsion* by the inferior rectus. The inferior oblique assists the superior rectus in *elevation,* but its *extorsion* counters the *intorting* action of the superior rectus. Deviation from the primary position changes the relative effects of various muscles. When the eye is *abducted* (Fig. 5-3B), a position may be attained where the direction of pull of the superior and inferior recti coincides with the optic axis to produce *pure elevation* or *depression.* As in Fig. 5-3C, *adduction* can attain a position where the oblique muscles pull along the equator to produce *pure intorsion* or *extorsion.* Convergence is accomplished by contraction of the two medial recti.

Ocular Symptoms

▼ *Key Symptoms:* ***Pain in the Eye.*** Some of the more common causes of pain in the eye are the following:

Clinical Occurrence: *Visible lesions:* foreign body, entropion conjunctivitis, sty (hordeolum), chalazion, corneal ulcer, interstitial keratitis, iritis, iridocyclitis, glaucoma, herpes, conjunctiva calcification, and band keratopathy.
Without visible lesions but with blindness: retrobulbar neuritis.
Pain without visible lesion or blindness: eyestrain.
Pain from febrile illness.
Pain from sinusitis: ethmoiditis, sphenoiditis, frontal sinusitis.
Endocrine eye lesion of thyrotoxicosis.

▼ *Key Symptom:* ***Lacrimation.*** Lacrimation usually refers to any condition resulting in tears, although strict usage indicates an overproduction, while *epiphoria* means an overflow from any cause. The various conditions causing the disorder are:

Clinical Occurrence: *Increased secretion of tears:* weeping from emotion, irritaiton from foreign body, corneal ulcer, conjunctivitis, coryza, measles, hay fever, iodism, bromidism, arsenical poisoning. *Obstruction of the lacrimal ducts:* congenital, cicatrix, edema of the eyelids, lacrimal calculus, dacryocystitis. *Separation of the puncta from the globe:* facial paralysis, loss of muscle tone in the aged, chronic marginal blepharitis, ectropion, proptosis from any cause.

Examination of Extraocular Movement

REMOTE EXAMINATION OF THE EYES. **From a distance, note the increased or diminished width of the *palpebral fissures,* whether unilateral or bilateral. Note *protrusion* or *recession* of one or both globes by inspecting the eyes from the front; if in doubt, look at the profile; finally, look downward over the patient's forehead and the superior edges of the orbits.**

Test for *lid lag,* holding your finger or a penlight as a target in the midline above eye level, about 20 inches (50 cm) away (Fig. 5-4); move the target rapidly downward in the midline, watching for the appearance of white sclera between the iris and the upper lid margin. Test the *extraocular movements* by moving the target at eye level from one side to the other, noting failure of the eyes to follow; similarly, test by moving the target from upper right to lower left, and upper left to lower right. Finally, test *convergence* by holding the target in the midline and at eye level, about 20 inches (50 cm) from the face, gradually moving the target toward the bridge of

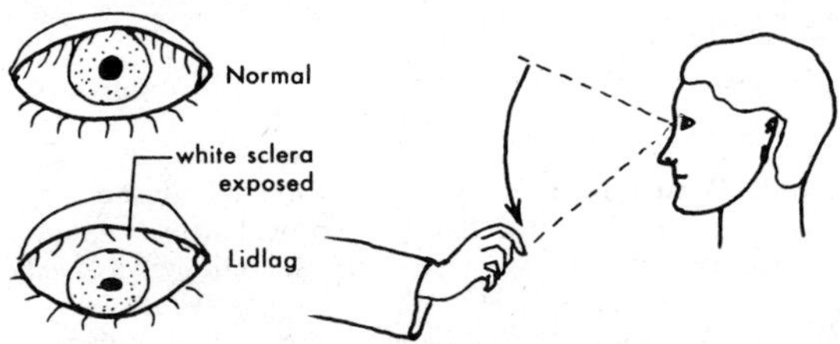

Fig. 5-4. Test for lid lag. *A target, such as a lighted penlight or a flicking finger, is held before the midline of the patient above the eye level; as the target is moved downward, the patient's upper lid is observed for its ability to follow the iris in its downward movement. A lag is indicated by white sclera appearing between lid and limbus.*

the patient's nose; note the near point at which convergence fails (normally 2 to 3 inches, or 50 to 75 mm).

Test for gross defects in the *visual fields* by the confrontation method (Fig. 5-5). Have the patient cover his left eye with his hand. Place your face in front of the patient's at the same eye level, with your nose about 40 inches (1 meter) from the unmasked eye. Ask the patient to fix constantly on your eye. Close your own left eye; fix your right on the patient's unmasked eye. Hold your right hand off to the side in the midplane between your faces. With flicking finger or penlight for a target, bring it slowly toward the midline between you. Ask the patient to indicate when the target first appears and compare with your own experience. Test vertical and oblique runs also. Test nasal field with left hand. Test the second eye similarly.

Widened Palpebral Fissures: ***Lid Spasm*** (Dalrymple's Sign). When the eyes are in the primary position, the upper lid covers the limbus, but a white scleral strip usually shows between the limbus and the lower lid. Widening of the palpebral fissure uncovers the upper border of the limbus to expose white sclera superiorly. A few normal persons seem to have widened palpebral fissures, but the acquired type is usually distinguished when the patient's acquaintances have commented on "the change in the eyes." Fissures may be widened by retraction of the lids or by protrusion of the eyeballs. When there is no actual proptosis, widened fissures produce the optical illusion of global protrusion. The presence of *lid lag* (von Graefe's sign) indicates lid spasm, even when the eyes do not show widened fissures in the primary position. Lid spasm occurs

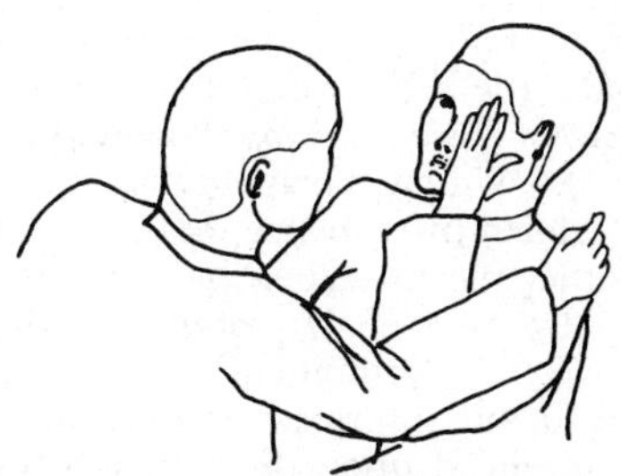

Fig. 5-5. Confrontation test of visual fields. *The patient covers his left eye with his hand. The examiner places his right eye directly in front of the patient's open eye, at a distance of approximately 40 inches (1 meter). The patient fixes on the examiner's right eye. The examiner imagines a line of sight extending between the patient's open eye and his own eye; the two can be termed the opposing eyes. He imagines radii that are perpendicular to the line of sight and center at a point equidistant between the two opposing eyes. A target on any point of such a radius will be equidistant between the opposing eyes at all locations. As a target he uses a flicking finger or a penlight; he moves it slowly along a radius from the periphery toward the center until the patient signifies that he can see it. Simultaneously the examiner checks his view of the target. Many different radii are tested until the entire field has been explored. This method discloses gross defects in the visual fields.*

in thyrotoxicosis; the mechanism is uncertain, but it is usually attributed to sympathetic stimulation. Usually bilateral, occasionally one fissure is much wider than the other.

Widened Palpebral Fissures: ***Lid Lag*** (von Graefe's Sign). In the absence of wide palpebral fissures, the sign must be sought to establish the presence of lid spasm. Have the patient's eyes fixed on the finger or penlight as a target, about 20 inches (50 cm) from the eyes, in the midline above eye level. As the target moves downward, a white scleral strip is uncovered between the upper lid and the limbus, widening with further depression of the globes. The sign is suggestive of thyrotoxicosis.

Other Lid Signs in Thyrotoxicosis. *Stellwag's sign:* infrequent blinking. *Rosenbach's sign:* tremor of the closed eyelids. *Mean's sign:* global lag during elevation. *Griffith's sign:* lag of the lower lids during elevation of the globes. *Boston's sign:* jerking of the lagging lid. *Joffroy's sign:* absence of forehead wrinkling with upward gaze, the head being tilted down.

Widened Palpebral Fissures: ***Exophthalmos*** (Exophthalmus, Ocular Proptosis). Widened palpebral fissures present an optical illusion of global prominence, but actual proptosis must be proved by other means. When proptosis is unilateral, the problem is usually resolved by comparing the two eyes. If both eyes seem equally prominent, the facial profile should be inspected for further impressions (Fig. 5-6). Looking downward over the forehead upon the eyes will sometimes assist in judgment. Accurate measurement of the distance between the anterior surface of the cornea and the outer edge of the bony orbit can be made with an exophthalmometer of the Hertel type. But this instrument, though simple and relatively inexpensive, is usually possessed only by an ophthalmologist, and its use requires some practice. Even with accurate measurements, a judgment of normality must be rendered because individual variation is great, and there are familial and racial trends toward proptosis. The best evidence of pathologic exophthalmos lies in a series of accurate measurements of the patient showing anterior progression. Acquired *bilateral* exophthalmos is most commonly associated with thyrotoxicosis. In thyrotoxicosis the proptosis often occurs after the metabolic imbalance has been controlled by thyroidectomy or radioiodine therapy; it may even occur during myxedema. The proptosis is usually permanent, or at least it persists for many years after other signs of active disease have subsided. Other accompanying but transient signs may be *palpebral edema* and *periorbital swelling.* At onset, the thyrotoxic proptosis may be *unilateral,* and it may precede other constitutional signs and symptoms of the disease. When first encountered, *unilateral* proptosis should suggest also an orbital tumor or inflammation within

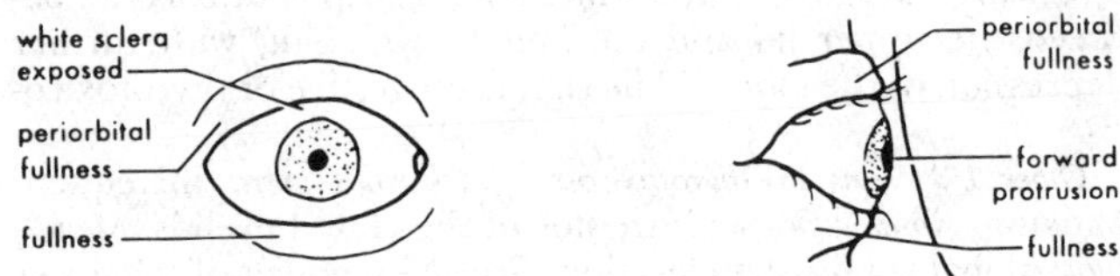

Fig. 5-6. Exophthalmos (exophthalmus, proptosis).

the orbit. When the globe is *displaced medially*, disease of the lacrimal gland should be suspected; *upward displacement* suggests disease in the maxillary sinus; *lateral displacement* can occur from a lesion in the ethmoid or sphenoid sinus. X-ray examination of the orbit frequently furnishes clues, especially when tomography or pneumotomography is employed. Ultrasonic examination is often definitive. The cause may be inferred from evidence of disease elsewhere in the body. In the absence of clues, surgical exploration may be necessary.

Clinical Occurrence: UNILATERAL EXOPHTHALMOS: mucocele, orbital cellulitis and abscess, thrombosis of the cavernous sinus, orbital periostitis, thyrotoxicosis, myxedema, orbital fracture, hemangioma, meningocele, encephalocele, gumma, orbital neoplasm, tubercle of the orbit, arteriovenous aneurysm, granuloma from aspergillosis, histiocytosis (Hand-Schüller-Christian disease).

BILATERAL EXOPHTHALMOS: thyrotoxicosis, myxedema, acromegaly, thrombosis of the cavernous sinus, empyema of the nasal accessory sinuses, lymphoma, leukemia, oxycephaly, leontiasis ossium, histiocytosis (Hand Schüller-Christian disease and Letterer-Siwe disease), and hyperpituitarism.

***Narrowed Palpebral Fissures:* Enophthalmos.** The globe is recessed in the orbit. When the condition is *bilateral*, it is usually caused by loss of fat in the orbits during inanition, dehydration, or congenital microphthalmos. The causes of *unilateral enophthalmos* are trauma or inflammation. Enophthalmos is described as an integral sign of *Horner's syndrome*, although measurements long ago proved this an error; the accompanying droop of the eyelid merely produces an optical illusion of recession of the globe.

***Failure of Lid Closure:* Paralysis of Orbicularis Muscle.** The facial (7th) nerve supplies the Orbicularis oculi muscle. Disorder of this nerve, as in Bell's palsy, causes partial or complete paralysis of the orbicularis. When complete, both upper and lower lids remain retracted so the eye is unprotected and tears drain onto the face. *Bell's phenomenon* occurs: the globes elevate during attempted closure of the lids. Failure of lid closure is also present in severe grades of exophthalmos or lid spasm from sympathetic stimulation.

***Failure of Lid Opening:* Ptosis of the Lid.** The congenital form is usually bilateral from paralysis of the Levator palpebrae superioris. The acquired condition is usually a result of disease of the oculomotor (3rd) nerve; so paralysis of other eye muscles may accompany. Supranuclear lesions, such as encephalitis, may produce it. Paralysis of the superior cervical sympathetic nerve causes *Horner's syndrome,* marked by ptosis, miosis, and anhydrosis on the affected side. In this condition, the ptosis is not complete, distinguishing it from paralysis of the levator muscle.

***Repetitive Jerky Movements:* Nystagmus.** Under many conditions of fixation the eyes may drift slowly to the right to be corrected by a quick movement back to the original position. This is termed *nystagmus to the left,* named after the direction of the quick component. The pattern of the nystagmus may be *horizontal, vertical, rotatory,* or *mixed.* When both eyes participate, the nystagmus is *associated;* movement of only one eye is *dissociated.* Less than 40 jerks per minute is considered *slow;* more than 100 jerks is *fast.* Amplitudes of less than 1 mm are *fine;* more than 3 mm are *coarse.* **End-Position Nystagmus.** The correctional jerks occur only with fixation far to the side; so nystagmus is always in the direction of fixation (Fig. 5-7A). There are several varieties; *Fixation nystagmus* occurs in many normal persons when required to fix to one side or the other; it is horizontal or horizontal-rotatory, moderate to coarse. *Labyrinthine end-position nystagmus* usually occurs in disease of the semicircular canals; it is horizontal-rotatory and is initiated by fixation in the end position, but it persists from some time after the primary position has been resumed. *Muscle-paretic nystagmus* presents as a dissociated movement of an eye with a paretic muscle, when fixation is directed to the paralyzed side; the muscle attempts to renew its position with new impulses. *Gaze-paretic nystagmus* appears in paralysis of conjugate

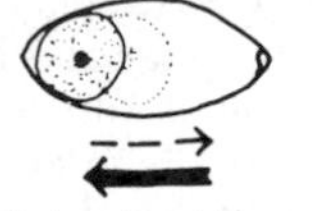

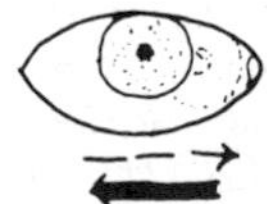

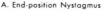

A. End-position Nystagmus B. Nystagmus in Primary Position

Fig. 5-7. Nystagmus. *A slow drift of the eyes away from the position of fixation (indicated by the broken arrow) is corrected by a quick movement back (solid arrow). The direction of the nystagmus is named from the quick component. Nystagmus from the primary position is more likely to be of serious import than that from the end position.*

movements. Both eyes show more nystagmus to one end position than to the other. *Primary Position Nystagmus.* This occurs with fixation in the primary position or at a point away from the direction of the quick component (Fig. 5-7B). *Peripheral labyrinthine nystagmus* is horizontal-rotatory, with medium frequency and amplitude, commonly seen in Ménière's syndrome, benign paroxysmal positional vertigo, viral or bacterial labyrinthitis, perilymphatic or labyrinthine fistula, and vestibular neuronitis. *Central nystagmus* may be horizontal, rotatory, vertical, or mixed, usually in the direction of the diseased side. Commonly it is found in multiple sclerosis, encephalitis, brain tumors, and transient or permanent vascular insufficiency states involving the vestibular nuclei or the medial longitudinal bundle. Vertical nystagmus usually indicates a lesion in the midbrain. *Ocular nystagmus* is characterized by unsystematic wandering movements with various frequencies and amplitudes, in persons who have poor vision from birth.

TEST FOR STRABISMUS (HETEROTROPIA). **Determine whether the patient has useful vision in each eye.* Ask the patient to fixate on an object at the end of the room or at your penlight held about 13 inches (33 cm) away from him. First cover his left eye with your right hand (Fig. 5-8). Watch the uncovered right eye to see if it moves to take up fixation. Uncover the left eye and allow him to look with both eyes. Then cover the right eye and watch the uncovered left to see if it moves to fixation. If there is fixation movement, the patient has heterotropia (strabismus, squint). To determine if the heterotropia is paralytic or nonparalytic, ask him to follow your penlight in the six cardinal directions of gaze (both eyes look to right, right and up, left and up, left, left and down, right and down). If the eyes move equally without restriction, the deviation is nonparalytic. If one eye overshoots and the other fails to look the entire distance in one or more directions, the deviation is paralytic. When**

* Omitting this step may lead to embarrassment of the physician. The patient hugely enjoys the doctor's painstaking attempts to determine the type of heterotropia in an eye with limited movement, only to discover belatedly that it is a prosthesis (glass or plastic)! As one of a group of house officers, one of us helped to confront a distinguished clinician with a brilliantly jaundiced patient lying in bed with one eye yellow, the other chalky white. It required several suspenseful minutes under our amused gaze before the victim finally thought of the only cause of a white sclera in a jaundiced patient.

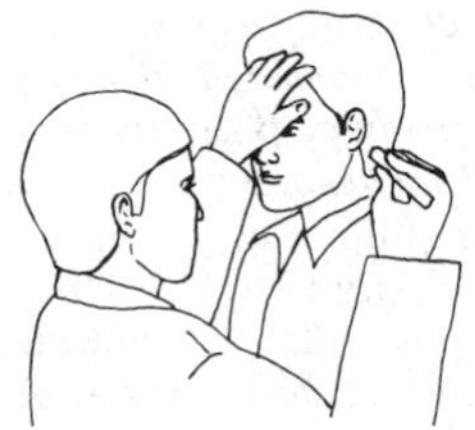

Fig. 5-8. Testing for strabismus.

fixation movements are absent in the cover-uncover test, try the alternate cover test. Cover the eyes alternately and watch the uncovered eye. If there is fixation movement, the eye has heterophoria.

Constant Squint Angle: ***Comitant Strabismus or Squint*** (Nonparalytic Heterophoria) (Fig. 5-9A). The word *comitant,* when applied to strabismus, indicates that the *squint angle* between the two optic axes remains constant in all positions assumed by the globes, no matter which eye fixates. Neither eye has limited motion. Since comitant strabismus occurs in the very young, children learn to suppress the image from one eye and do not have diplopia. The muscles are normal; the disorder probably results from abnormal innervation in the nuclei of the cranial nerves, since the squint angle disappears during general anesthesia. In most cases, the optic axes converge, when the condition is termed *comitant convergent strabismus* or *esotropia.* When hypermetropia causes excessive convergence, the condition is called *accommodative squint.* Occasionally, the optic axes diverge and the term is *comitant divergent strabismus* or *exotropia.*

Varying Squint Angle: ***Noncomitant Strabismus or Squint.*** Paralytic Heterotropia. The squint angle changes with the direction of fixation. This is caused by paralysis of one or more eye muscles. Certain generalizations apply to paralysis of any eye muscle. The squint angle is greatest when the unaffected eye is fixed on the field of action of the paralyzed muscle. The squint is augmented when fixation is made with the paralyzed muscle, *secondary deviation.* When paralysis is acquired during maturity, diplopia occurs at the onset, frequently accompanied by vertigo. In contradistinction to comitant strabismus, the motions of the paralyzed eye are limited. The head is held

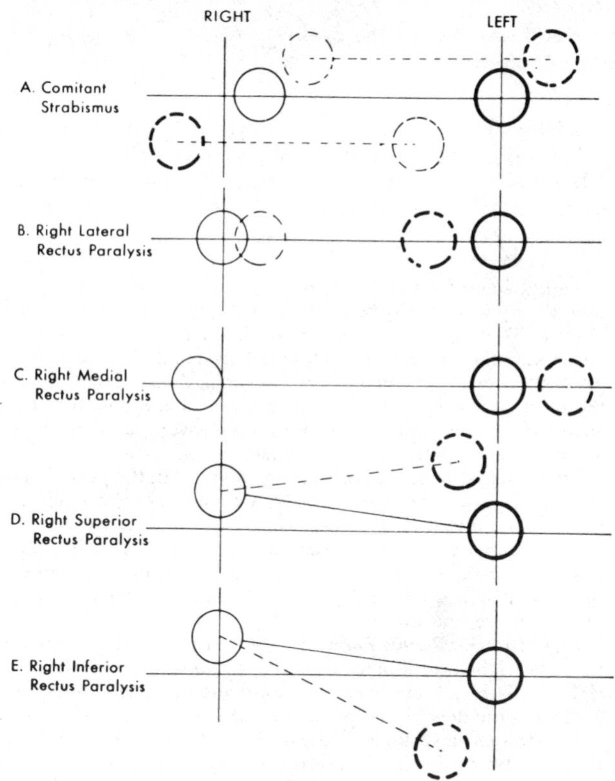

Fig. 5-9. Strabismus (squint). *These terms refer to disorders in which the optic axes are not parallel. The diagrams illustrate positions of the patient's eyes as they appear to the observer. The unbroken circles connected by the unbroken lines show pairs in the primary position with the normal or fixing eye represented in heavier lines. Pairs with broken lines are in secondary positions with the heavier lines for the fixing eye.* **A.** Comitant strabismus. *The squint angle between the two optic axes is constant in all positions regardless of which eye fixates.* **B.** Right lateral rectus paralysis. *Inability of right eye to move laterally.* **C.** Right medial rectus paralysis. *Right eye is lateral in the primary position; it fails to move medially.* **D.** Right superior rectus paralysis. *Right eye slightly elevated in primary position and fails to move farther upward.* **E.** Right inferior rectus paralysis. *Right eye elevated slightly in primary position; it cannot move downward.*

toward the field of the paralyzed eye to avoid diplopia. In the following consideration, only paralyses of the right eye will be employed as examples to avoid confusion. In the figures, only the deficient movements of the eye are illustrated; all others are normal.

Right Lateral Rectus Paralysis (Fig. 5-9B). In the primary position, the optic axes may be parallel, or the right eye may converge slightly. The right eye cannot move laterally. The lateral rectus muscles are the most frequent site of isolated paralysis. The abducens (6th) nerve may be damaged in infectious diseases, periostitis of the orbit, fracture of the petrous portion of the temporal bone, aneurysm of the carotid artery within the cavernous sinus, lesions of the posterior pons near the midline.

Right Medial Rectus Paralysis (Fig. 5-9C). In the primary position, the right eye deviates laterally; it cannot move medially. The head is turned to the left to avoid diplopia.

Right Superior Rectus Paralysis (Fig. 5-9D). In the primary position, the right eye deviates downward; it cannot move upward to the right. The squint angle and the diplopia increase with fixation of the left eye upward to the right.

Right Inferior Rectus Paralysis (Fig. 5-9E). In the primary position, the right eye deviates upward; it cannot move down to the right. With the left eye fixed downward and to the right, the squint angle and the degree of diplopia increase.

Right Superior Oblique Paralysis (Fig. 5-10A). Most characteristic is the tilt of the head toward the left shoulder to compensate for the pronounced extorsion. The assumed position results in the normal intorsion of the left eye; so the torsional diplopia is corrected. If the head is tilted to the right side, the right eye rotates upward. In the primary position, the right eye deviates upward; movement is limited down and to the left. The squint angle is increased when the left eye is fixed downward and to the left.

Right Inferior Oblique Paralysis (Fig. 5-10B). In the primary position, the right eye deviates downward; its movement is limited upward and to the left. The squint angle increases when the left eye is fixed upward to the left.

Varying Squint Angle: ***The Ophthalmoplegias.*** Paralysis of two or more ocular muscles is termed *ophthalmoplegia.* Since only the oculomotor (3rd) nerve supplies more than a single muscle, *partial* ophthalmophegia must be attributed to malfunctioning of that nerve. *Unilateral total ophthalmoplegia* can be caused only by involvement of all nerves in the superior orbital fissure or

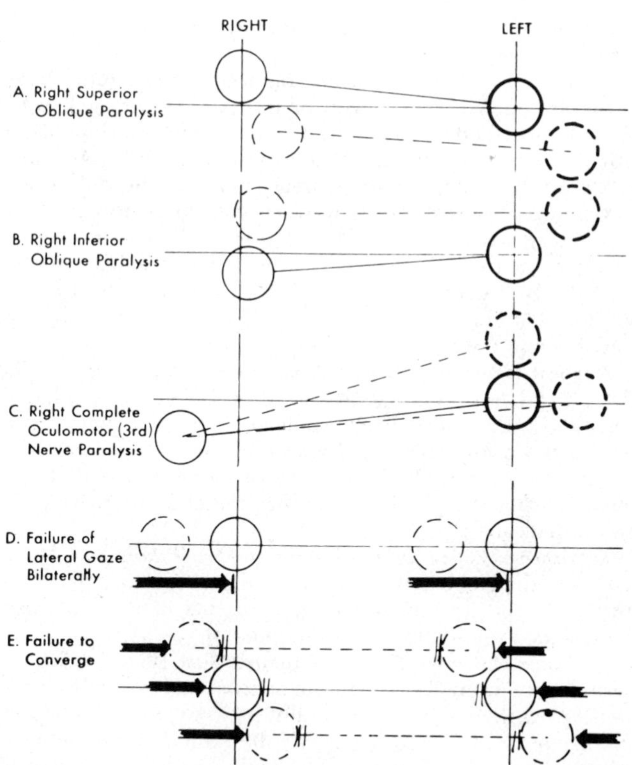

Fig. 5-10. Strabismus, disorders of lateral gaze and convergence. *Diagrams constructed as in Fig. 5-9.* **A.** Right superior oblique paralysis. *In primary position right eye slightly elevated; can only be slightly depressed.* **B.** Right inferior oblique paralysis. *Right eye slightly depressed in primary position; it can be elevated only slightly.* **C.** Right complete oculomotor nerve paralysis. *Right eye fixed in depressed and lateral position.* **D.** Failure of lateral gaze. *Both eyes cannot be moved beyond the median to the left (or right, as the case may be).* **E.** Failure of convergence. *In no position can the two eyes converge.*

the cavernous sinus; a bilateral lesion could result only from a focus in the base of the brain.

Varying Squint Angle: ***Complete Right Oculomotor (3rd) Nerve Paralysis*** (Fig. 5-10C). This produces paralysis of the levator, the superior, medial, and inferior recti, and the inferior oblique muscles. Only the superior oblique and the lateral rectus muscles are functioning. In the primary position, the right eye is deviated downward and outward to the right. Motion to the left and upward is absent. The squint angle and the degree of diplopia are increased when the left eye is fixed to the left. Ptosis is present in the right eye from paralysis of the levator. The most frequent cause of 3rd nerve paralysis is an aneurysm in the circle of Willis.

Transient Weakness of Ocular Muscles: ***Myasthenia Gravis.*** The levator and, to a lesser extent, the other ocular muscles characteristically show normal reactions after rest, but they fatigue as the day progresses so ptosis and other muscle paralyses occur. Ptosis is quickly dispelled by the administration of neostigmine, but the paralyses of other muscles do not respond so dramatically.

Restriction of Motion: ***Orbital Tumors and Exophthalmos.*** Movements of the globe may be restricted in all directions by orbital tumor or the increase in orbital contents in thyrotoxicosis. Ultrasonic examination will differentiate.

Conjugate Movement: ***Failure of Lateral Gaze*** (Fig. 5-10D). A disturbance in the frontopontine pathway will cause this disorder. When the lesion is in the right pathway, there is constant conjugate deviation to the right; the patient turns his head to the left to fixate in front. The optic axes are parallel in all positions; so there is no diplopia. Neither eye can move to the left of the midline. The condition is distinguished from combined paralysis of the left lateral rectus and the right medial rectus by the retention of convergence. In partial failure of lateral gaze, the patient can *will* his gaze to go to the left, but he cannot fix it; so there is bilateral nystagmus to the left.

Conjugate Movement: ***Failure of Vertical Gaze.*** Assumed to be a disorder of the frontopontine pathway, the exact mechanism is unknown. Most frequent is the inability to gaze upward. The eyes cannot move above the horizontal, so the patient tilts the head backward. There is no diplopia. When failure is incomplete, there is slight upward movement with upward nystagmus. Combined bilateral paralyses of the superior recti and the inferior obliques (muscles innervated by the 3rd nerves) produce similar findings, but the frontopontine lesion is distinguished by retention of the normal *Bell's phenomenon* (reflex elevation of the globes when the lids close). This reflex is mediated by fibers between the nuclei of the 3rd nerve and the 7th in the medial longitudinal bundle; the 3rd nerve supplies the superior rectus and the inferior oblique, the 7th nerve serves the orbicularis. Persistence of the reflex proves the intactness of both nuclei, so the lesion must be supranuclear. Rarely, upward failure is combined with downward failure, or failure of downward gaze may be present alone.

Disjunctive Movement: ***Failure of Convergence*** (Fig. 5-10E). A lesion in the frontopontine pathway is responsible. All movements are normal except convergence. Normal abduction of both globes to right and left proves the medial recti to be normal.

Visual Fields

Bilateral Visual Field Defects: ***Hemianopsia*** (Hemianopia). By definition, hemianopsia is bilateral, caused by a lesion in the optic chiasm, the optic tracts, or the brain. The diagram in Fig. 5-11 shows that fibers from the right side of the brain supply the right side of each retina, projected as the left halves of both visual fields. The left brain serves both left retinae. The right *optic tract* carries all fibers to that side of the brain. At the *optic chiasm* the tract fibers divide, part going into the right *optic nerve* to supply the right half of the right retina; the other part crosses the chiasm to supply the right half of the left retina. *Homonymous Hemianopsia:* The same side of each field contains a defect (Fig. 5-12A). A left homonymous hemianopsia can be caused by a lesion in the right optic tract or the right brain; the image projected by the eye reverses the side of the field. With a tract lesion, the pupillary reflex is lost; the pupil reacts when the lesion is in the brain. *Crossed Hemianopsia:* Symmetric sides of both retinae are deficient, so the lesion is either *bitemporal* or *binasal.* A lesion of the decussating fibers in the chiasm causes bitemporal hemianopsia (Fig. 5-12B), by injuring the fibers to both nasal retinae. The lesion at this site is commonly a tumor of the pituitary gland that enlarges from below, so the temporal sides of both fields are

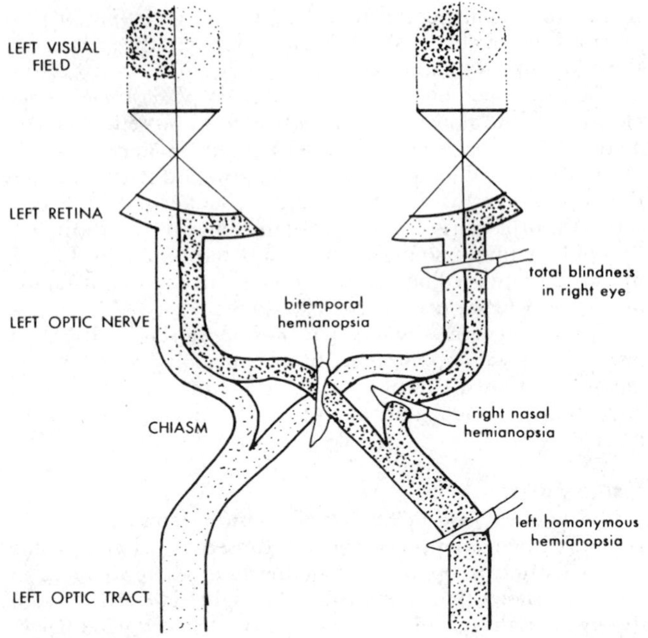

Fig. 5-11. Neural pathways from brain to retina. *The cutting knives indicate points of lesions and the resulting visual defects.*

first affected, the *temporal cut.* Binasal hemianopsia is uncommon because it involves injury of both lateral halves of the optic nerves or optic tracts. When only a quadrant of each field is lost, it is termed *quadrant hemianopsia.* Brain tumor is the most frequent cause.

Bilateral Field Defects: ***Glaucoma.*** Concentric contraction of both visual fields (Fig. 5-12C) is a late manifestation of glaucoma from destruction of the retinae by increased intraocular pressure.

Single Field Defects: ***Lesions of Optic Nerve or Retina.*** Destruction of an optic nerve produces blindness in the eye. Optic neuritis may produce smaller field defects. Destructive lesions of the retina also result in unilateral field defects.

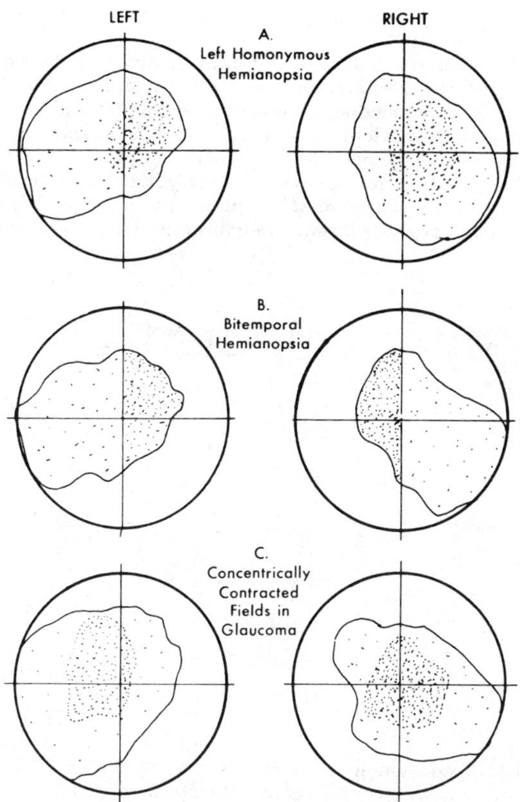

Fig. 5-12. Pathologic visual fields. *The normal visual field areas are enclosed by the heavy black lines that include both kinds of stippling. The areas of heavy stippling indicate portions of the fields that are visible in the pathologic condition; the portions of the normal fields not seen are indicated by light stippling.*

CLOSE EXTERNAL EXAMINATION OF THE EYE. *Eyelids.* **Look for *swelling* about the lids, above, below, and near the canthi. Note *inversion* or *eversion* of the lids. Examine the lid margins for scaling, excess or sparsity of secretions, purulent exudate, papules, or pustules. Look for lashes turned inward (trichiasis). Press on the lacrimal**

sac; if fluid can be expressed through the punctum, the tear duct is obstructed.

Bulbar Conjunctiva and Sclera. **Gently retract the lids with the thumb and forefinger; note the *color* of the sclera, whether white, blue, yellow, or hemorrhagic. Look for pigment deposits and judge whether normal for complexion and race. Look for vascular engorgement. Distinguish the normal pinguecula from ptyergium.**

Palpebral Conjunctiva. **Evert the lower lid (Fig. 5-13A) by placing the thumb tip on the loose skin beneath the margin, sliding the skin down and pressing it gently into the orbit. Look for congestion,**

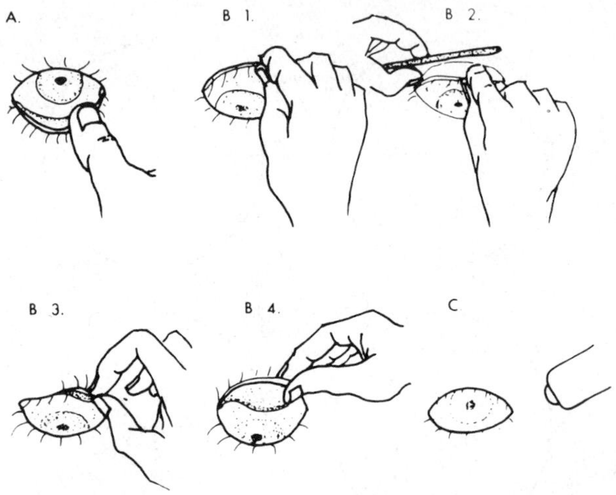

Fig. 5-13. Examination of the eyelids. **A.** Eversion of the lower lid. *This is readily accomplished with the thumb or index finger pressing on the soft tissue below the lid and pulling it downward.* **B.** Eversion of the upper lid. *Tell the patient to look downward and proceed with four steps: (1) With the right thumb and forefinger grasp a few cilia of the upper lid and pull the lid away from the globe; (2) lay a matchstick or applicator along the crease made by the superior edge of the tarsal plate and the soft adjacent tissue; (3) quickly fold the lid over the applicator so the tarsal plate turns over and its upper edge faces downward; (4) replace the right thumb and finger by the corresponding left ones to hold the lid.* **C.** Testing pupillary reaction to light. *Shine the rays from a penlight or other source into the pupil from the side so the macula is not directly stimulated and the patient cannot fix on the light and confuse reaction to light with that of accommodation.*

pustules, and other lesions. If indicated, evert the upper lid (Fig. 5-13B). For this manipulation, either face the patient or stand behind him while he is sitting, so his head rests against your body. Ask him to *keep both eyes open and look downward* to prevent elevation that reflexly accompanies closure of the lids. Grasp some eyelashes of the upper lid between your thumb and forefinger, pull the lid gently *downward* and *away from* the globe. With the tip of your left forefinger or the side of an applicator press against the upper lid just above the superior edge of the tarsal plate, using this pressure point as a fulcrum. Then pull the eyelid quickly upward so that tarsal plate turns on the fulcrum, its lower edge becomes uppermost, and the lid is everted. After the lid has been everted (to the astonishment of the patient) hold the lid with the left fingers, freeing the right hand for other acts. The normal position is regained merely by having the patient glance upward.

Cornea. Shine light from a window or a penlight *obliquely* on the cornea to note scars, abrasions, or ulcers. Abrasions are readily demonstrated by placing one or two drops of 2% aqueous solution of fluorescein in the fornix, closing the lids for a minute to permit staining, then washing away the excess with isotonic saline or boric acid solution. Corneal abrasions stain green. The cornea may also be examined with a lens.

Iris and Lens. Note the *color* of the iris, whether it appears distinct or muddy. Look for *new vessels* and *deposits.* Note the size, shape, and equality of the pupils. Test *pupillary reaction to light* by having the patient fix on an object over 10 feet (3 meters) distant and shining a penlight into the retina *from the side* (Fig. 5-13C), so the patient does not fixate on the light and thus use his accommodation. Test *pupillary reaction to accommodation* by having him fix on a finger that is gradually brought closer to his nose. Shine the penlight obliquely through the lens to discover deposits on the surface and opacities in the matrix such as cataracts.

The Eyelids

The area between the opened upper and lower eyelids is the *palpebral fissure* (Fig. 5-14); the two angles of the slit are the *external* (temporal) and the *internal* (nasal) *canthi.* In the internal canthus is a small protuberance of modified skin, the *caruncle;* nearby is a tissue fold, the *plica semilunaris.* Near the inner canthus on an elevation of the lid margin is the *punctum,* the entrance to the *canaliculus* draining into the lacrimal duct; each lid possesses a punctum. The upper eyelid extends upward from the fissure to the superior edge of the bony orbit, merging with dense tissue bound to the periosteum. The skin overlying

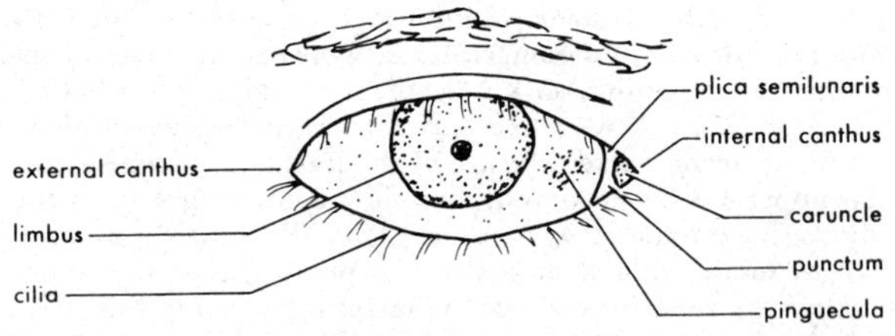

Fig. 5-14. External details of the normal right eye.

the eyelids is the thinnest in the body, so it is readily moved and picked up. When elevated, the upper eyelid invaginates between the eyeball and the upper border of the orbit; the *lower lid* is shorter and does not fold in. From the fissure the lower lid extends downward to the dense tissue and periosteum of the lower outer orbital margin. Edema fluid in the lids is sharply limited by these attachments to the orbit. Both lids are lined with *palpebral conjunctiva;* in their substance they carry the circular fibers of the *Orbicularis oculi muscle,* supplied by the facial (7th) nerve. The upper lid also contains the vertical tendons of the *Levator palpebrae superioris muscle,* originating in the optic foramen, inserting in the tarsal plate, and innervated by the oculomotor (3rd) nerve. The lids are stiffened by tarsal plates, transverse dense plaques of elastic and connective tissue, forming the free halves of both lids; the upper tarsus is much larger than the lower. Both tarsi are adherent posteriorly to the palpebral conjuctiva and contain many *meibomian glands* that run perpendicularly to the palpebral margins and empty through pinpoint openings in the lid margins. At the skin border of the lid margins is a double row of *cilia* or *eyelashes* with their hair follicles. The hairs are deeply pigmented and curve outward from the skin surface.

Medial Canthus Fold: Epicanthus. In one or both eyes, the epicanthus is a semicircular fold of skin that lies vertically over the upper and lower lid so the medial canthus is partially covered. It is present in about one fifth of newborn Caucasian children, but it disappears by the age of 10 years in all but 3%. The epicanthus must be distinguished from the *mongolian fold* that originates in the upper lid and partially or completely overhangs the superior tarsus; this is horizontal while the epicanthus is vertical. The mongolian fold is a normal characteristic of Asian races and some individuals of other races. Epicanthus should not be confused with *esotropia,* in which there is excessive deviation of the visual axis toward the other eye. Four ocular signs of *Down's syndrome* (mongolism) are (1) a higher-than-normal incidence (10% compared with 3%) of *epicanthic fold persisting* after the age of 10 years, (2) a higher-than-normal incidence (72% compared with 14%) of unilateral or bilateral *slanting eyes* in which the lateral canthus is elevated more than 2 mm above the medial canthus when a transparent rule is placed across the bridge of the nose level with the medial canthus, (3) a higher-than-normal incidence (69% compared with 12%) of *Brushfield spots,* accumulations of lighter-colored tissues in the concentric band of the outer third of the iris, (4) a higher-than-normal incidence of *hypoplasia of the iris,* showing as darker discolorations of the iris.

***Shortened Palpebral Fissures:* Fetal Alcohol Syndrome.** The combination of *shortened palpebral fissures, shortened nose* with *epicanthic folds* and *anteverted nostrils, hypoplastic upper lip* with *thinned vermilion* and *flattened or absent philtrum* [vertical groove from nasal septum downward to vermilion], together with mental retardation, have been recognized as the characteristic stigmata of an individual born of an alcoholic mother. [S. K. Clarren and D. W. Smith: *N. Engl. J. Med.,* **298:**1063–67, 1978].

***Lid Inversion:* Entropion.** *Spastic entropion* occurs only in the lower lid and is caused by increased tone of the orbicularis oculi, usually from inflammation of an eye with scanty tarsal plate or poor tissue tone. The lid turns in only when forcibly closed (Fig. 5-15A). *Cicatricial entropion* occurs in either lid by contracture of scar tissue, as in trachoma. Entropion from any cause may be accompanied by *blepharospasm* from irritation of the inverted eyelashes.

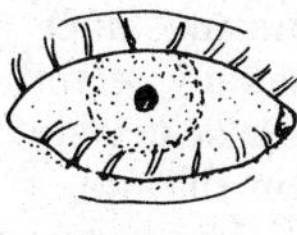

A. Entropion

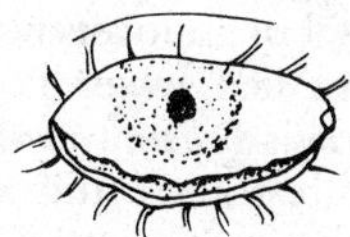

B. Ectropion

Fig. 5-15. Pathologic inversion and eversion of the eyelids.

Lid Eversion: ***Ectropion.*** The lid turns outward (Fig. 5-15B). Both lids may be affected by *spastic* or *cicatricial ectropion,* but the *paralytic* type involves only the lower lid. The spastic type is encountered in severe protrusion of the globe from staphyloma or palpebral edema. Senile atrophy of tissues sometimes results in ectropion rather than entropion.

Lid Redness: ***Local Active Hyperemia.*** Generalized reddening of the lids is nonspecific. Hyperemia of the nasal half of the upper lid suggests inflammation of the frontal sinus. Disease of the lacrimal sac sometimes causes reddening of the adjacent portion of the lower lid. Hyperemia of the temporal side of the upper lid should suggest dacryoadenitis. The lid is frequently red in the region of a sty.

Lid Cyanosis: ***Local Passive Hyperemia.*** Blueness of the eyelid occurs from thrombosis of the orbital veins, orbital tumors, and arteriovenous aneurysms of the orbit.

Lid Hemorrhage: ***Palpebral Hematoma.*** Trauma to the lids may result in extravasation of blood into the surrounding tissue, colloquially known as a "black eye." Palpebral hematoma can occur from nasal fracture. The appearance of hematoma many hours after skull trauma suggests skull fracture; the greater the time interval, the more remote the fracture site. Fractures of the posterior skull may produce hematoma of the lid several days later.

Lid Swelling: ***Palpebral Edema.*** *Inflammatory edema* from local infections is readily distinguished by the signs of inflammation: rubor, thermor, and dolor. *Noninflammatory edema* of the eyelids is frequent in acute nephritis, uncommon in chronic nephritis and cardiac failure (Fig. 5-16A). It occurs early in the course of both myxedema and thyrotoxic exophthalmos. Palpebral edema is frequent in trichinosis. Angioneurotic edema frequently involves the lids. Contact dermatitis is often a baffling cause of palpebral edema until the physician learns that a patient may be able to tolerate contact with an allergen on the hands, but innocently transfers the substance to the soft tissue of the lids, where the swelling readily occurs.

Lid Plaques—Yellow: ***Xanthelasma.*** Raised yellow plaques, painless and nonpruritic, may occur on the upper and lower lids near the inner canthi (Fig. 5-16B). They grow slowly and may disappear spontaneously. The lesion is a form of xanthoma frequently associated with hypercholesterolemia.

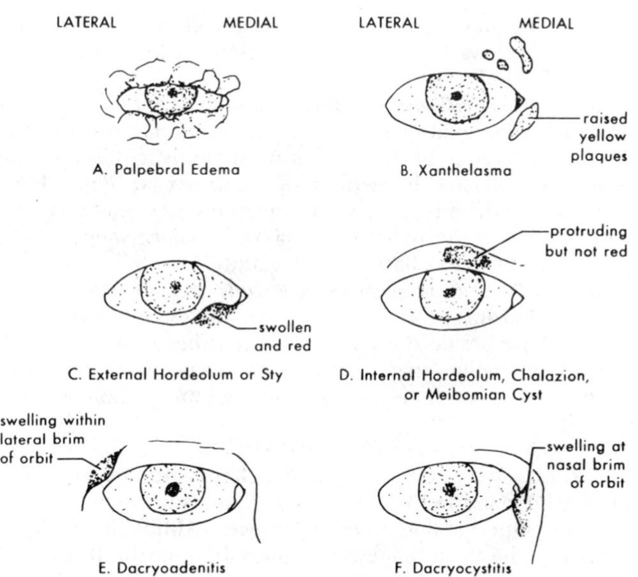

Fig. 5-16. Lesions of the external eye.

Lid Scaling and Redness: ***Marginal Blepharitis.*** *Squamous blepharitis* is a seborrheic inflammation of the lid margins that produces greasy flakes of dried secretion on the eyelashes and reddening of the lid margins. When ulceration of the lid margin occurs, it is termed *ulcerative blepharitis. Angular blepharitis* is a specific disease caused by the diplococcus of Morax-Axenfeld in which the margins near the temporal canthi are inflamed.

Lid Pustule: ***External Hordeolum*** (Sty). When a sebaceous gland near the hair follicle of a cilium becomes inflamed, a pustule forms on the lid margin (Fig. 5-16C). It may be surrounded by hyperemia and swelling. Many rupture and heal spontaneously.

Lid Protrusion: ***Internal Hordeolum, Chalazion, and Meibomian Cyst.*** Acute inflammation of a meibomian gland is termed an *internal hordeolum* or *internal sty* (Fig. 5-16D). A granuloma of the gland is known as a *chalazion* or *meibomian cyst.* These affections of internal sebaceous glands produce localized swelling that frequently causes a protrusion of the lid. Eversion of the lid shows hyperemia and perhaps a localized cyst or enlarged gland.

Lacrimal Gland Inflammation: ***Dacryoadenitis.*** Acute inflammation of the lacrimal gland causes pain and tenderness within the temporal edge of the orbit; it must be distinguished from orbital cellulitis and hordeolum of the upper lid (Fig. 5-16E). The chronic form is painless; it sometimes occurs as a component of *Mikulicz's syndrome,* along with enlargement of the parotid and submaxillary salivary glands.

Lacrimal Duct Inflammation: ***Dacryocystitis.*** Obstruction of the nasolacrimal duct produces acute inflammation with tenderness and swelling beside the nose, near the inner canthus (Fig. 5-16F). The swelling may extend to the eyelid. Its site anterior to the eyelid distinguishes it for hordeolum of the lower lid.

The Conjunctiva

The *palpebral conjuctiva* joins the skin at the anterior edge of the lid margins. It follows the inner surface of the lids into the superior and inferior fornices. Although firmly attached to the tarsal plates, it is quite loose in the fornices to permit movement of the globe. At the fornices the membrane is reflected anteriorly to cover the sclera where it becomes the *bulbar conjunctiva.* The larger episcleral vessels are normally visible through the transparent bulbar conjunctiva; they may be moved by sliding the conjunctiva over the sclera. At the limbus the conjunctiva is firmly attached to the sclera and continues as the epithelium of the *cornea.* The superficial vessels of the bulbar conjunctiva run radially in tortuous courses (Fig. 5-17A); their visible portions lie in the *periphery* of the sclera. The deeper vessels are not individually visible; they radiate *near the limbus.* A raised yellow plaque, the *pinguecula,* normally occurs on each side of the limbus in the horizontal plane, the larger is nasally; their size increases with age. With the exception of the pinguecula, some visible peripheral vessels, and a few patches of pigment, the sclera is normally white.

Subconjunctival Hemorrhage. Bleeding under the conjunctiva is obvious (Fig. 5-17B). Bleeding may be induced by coughing, sneezing, weight lifting, or defecation; frequently, the cause is not apparent. The extravasation is harmless unless

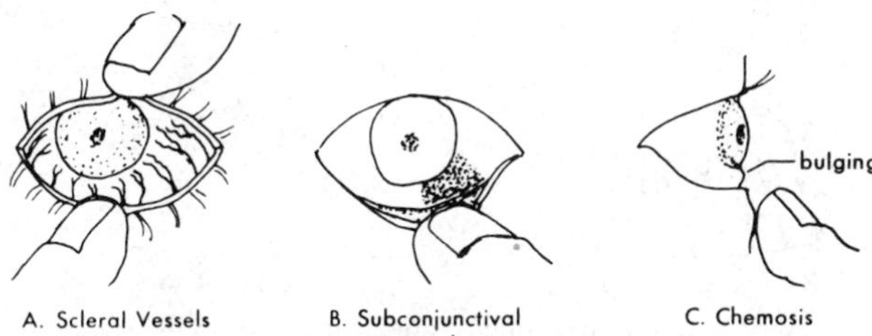

Fig. 5-17. Vascular disorders of the external eye. **A.** Scleral vessels. *These are the most prominent vessels to be seen.* **B.** Subconjunctival hemorrhages. *Bright red superficial blotches show through the sclera. They appear suddenly and painlessly.* **C.** Chemosis. *This is edema of the conjunctiva that may be demonstrated by pressing the lower lid against the globe producing a bulge in the boggy global conjunctiva above the point of compression.*

an excessive amount of blood lifts the conjunctiva so draining is required.

Conjunctival Edema: Chemosis. Usually associated with edema of the lids, the conjunctiva is swollen and transparent. The edema may be demonstrated by looking at the globe in profile while pressing the lower lid against the bulbar conjunctiva; the edge of the lid pushes up a wave of edematous bulbar conjunctiva (Fig. 5-17C). It is frequent in the endocrine eye lesions of thyrotoxicosis.

Global Hyperemia and Congestion. Hyperemia of the global vessels reveals the circulation of the bulbar conjunctiva and iris. The conjunctival vessels are readily visible as radii with tortuous branches, running from the fornices toward the center of the cornea (Fig. 5-18A). The vessels of the iris are deeper; they begin at the limbus and run in straight radii toward the pupil. Even when congested, the individual vessels cannot be seen, but their dilatation produces a pink band surrounding the limbus, the *ciliary flush* (Fig. 5-18B). Suffusion in the conjunctiva blanches with pressure; the ciliary flush does not blanch.

Conjunctival New Growth: Pterygium. As described elsewhere, the *pinguecula* is a normal, slightly raised fatty structure under the conjunctiva in the horizontal meridian, between canthus

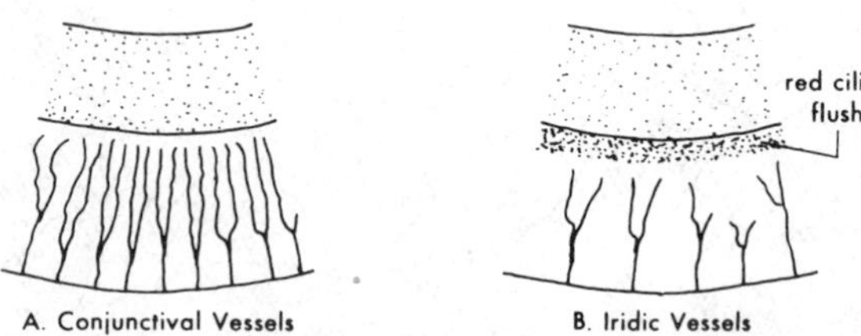

Fig. 5-18. Hyperemia and congestion of the globe. *The scleral vessels are superficial, coursing radially from the periphery to the limbus in tortuous branches, as in* **A.** *The vessels of the iris are deeper; when congested, individual vessels are not visible, but they produce a pink or red band around the limbus—the ciliary flush in* **B.**

and limbus, usually on the nasal side. Chronic inflammation from wind and dust is thought to stimulate the growth of the pinguecula to extend a vascular membrane over the limbus toward the center of the cornea (Fig. 5-19A), called a *pterygium.* Usually, it is bilateral; vision may be obstructed. The structure is distinguished by being in firm contact with the bulbar surface and being limited strictly to the horizontal meridian; a *pseudopterygium* is a band of scar tissue that may extend in any direction and adhere only partially to the bulbar conjunctiva, so a probe may be passed beneath it.

Pigmented Pingueculae: ***Gaucher's Disease.*** Brownish pigmentation of the pingueculae occurs as one of the few physical signs of Gaucher's disease; the other signs are hepatosplenomegaly and pigmentation of the skin.

Hyperemic Conjunctiva: ***Conjunctival Calcification in Calcium-Phosphorus Disorders*** *Conjunctival Lesions.* The segments from limbus to canthus at 7 to 10 o'clock and at 2 to 5 o'clock show (a) *hyperemic reddening,* (b) *calcified plaques,* and (c) *pingueculae.* The eyes are *painful* or feel *gritty.* The affected areas contain calcium deposits, visible to the unaided eye or through the slit lamp. The lesions occur when the serum *calcium-phosphorus produce* (calcium in mg × phosphorus in mg) exceeds 70 in patients with renal disease. Occasionally the lesions have been described in hypercalcemia from renal failure or sarcoidosis. *Corneal Lesions.* These are called *band keratopathy.* White material is visible in the limbal arcs at 2 to 5 o'clock and 7 to 10 o'clock. The slit lamp reveals calcium deposits. Band keratopathy has

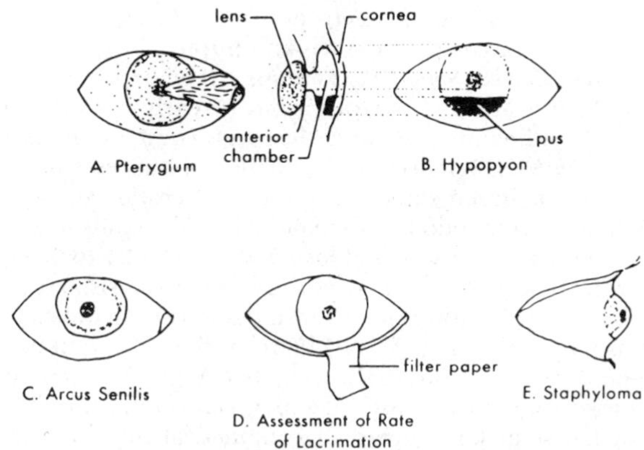

Fig. 5-19. Lesions of the cornea and iris. **A.** Pterygium. *Abnormal growth of the pinguecula appears as a raised, subconjunctival fatty structure, growing in a horizontal band toward a position over the pupil. The lesions are usually bilateral and eventually may obstruct vision.* **B.** Hypopyon. *A result of iritis may be a collection of pus in the lowest part of the anterior chamber between cornea and the iris.* **C.** Arcus senilis. *A gray opaque circular band in the cornea, separated from the limbus by a narrow clear zone. The lesion is bilateral. Early it is arcuate; later it forms a complete circle.* **D.** Assessment of lacrimation. *A fold of filter paper is hung over the lower lid. Nonwetting of the paper for 15 minutes indicates keratoconjunctivitis sicca.* **E.** Staphyloma. *Anterior protrusion of the cornea or sclera.*

been reported in disorders with hypercalcemia and in some patients with renal disease having conjunctival calcification.

Granuloma in Conjunctiva: ***Sarcoidosis.*** Several workers have reported that noncaseating granulomata are often found in the conjunctivae of patients with sarcoidosis; these were proved by biopsy.

The Cornea

The cornea is a convex tissue of five transparent layers that joins the sclera at the limbus. Its surface is highly reflecting so inspection with oblique lighting reveals small imperfections. Normally, it is avascular. Its diameter is about 12 mm, and its radius of curvature is slightly smaller than that of the globe, so it protrudes somewhat from the surface of the globe. Through it may be seen the iris and pupil.

Lusterless Cornea: ***Superficial Keratitis.*** The expert recognizes many forms. Most are characterized by early *lackluster* of the corneal epithelium with underlying grayness of the stroma. A *ciliary flush* is often present. Instillation of fluorescein demonstrates by its green stain that there is ulceration or denuded epithelium. Disruption of the epithelium demands urgent expert therapy, because visual loss can occur in 24 to 36 hours. A corneal ulcer is extremely *painful,* causes miosis and photophobia. Accumulation of pus in the anterior chamber of the eye is a *hypopyon* (Fig. 5-19B), perceived as a gray fluid level in the lowest portion of the chamber angle between cornea and iris. Among the causes of superficial keratitis are infected epithelial scratches, spread of conjunctival infection, herpes simplex and zoster, corneal exposure from muscle paralysis or proptosis, injury to the trigeminal (5th) nerve, tuberculosis.

Tearless Cornea: ***Keratocunjunctivitis Sicca*** (Sjögren's Syndrome). The conjunctival inflammation results from *lack of tears,* demonstrated by *Schirmer's test.* The triad of *Sjögren's syndrome* consists of keratoconjunctivitis sicca, xerostomia (lack of salivary secretion), and rheumatoid arthritis; the presence of two of the three is diagnostic. In the triad, rheumatoid arthritis may be supplanted by lupus erythematosus, scleroderma, or polyarteritis nodosa. The plasma of patients with the syndrome often shows multiple autoimmune stigmata, such as the rheumatoid factor, antinuclear antibodies, complement-fixing antibodies for various tissues and organs. Sometimes the syndrome is followed by large cell lymphoma.

SCHIRMER'S TEST FOR LACK OF TEARS **(Fig. 5-19D). A slip of filter paper is folded over the lower eyelid. When it remains unwetted for 15 minutes, the diagnosis of keratoconjunctivitis sicca is confirmed.**

Cloudy Cornea: ***Interstitial Keratitis.*** The prototype occurs in congenital syphilis in which interstitial keratitis, deafness, and notched teeth constitute *Hutchinson's triad.* During the early stages of inflammation, between the fifth and fifteenth years of age, a faint opacity begins in the central zone of the cornea, together with a faint ciliary flush. Usually, there are pain and lacrimation. Later the cornea becomes diffusely clouded, so the iris may be obscured. Blood vessels grow into the cornea. After the acute stage, there is more or less permanent corneal opacity. Acquired syphilis and tuberculosis occasionally cause this lesion.

Peripheral Corneal Opacity: ***Arcus Senilis.*** A gray band of opacity in the cornea, 1.0 to 1.5 mm wide, is separated from the limbus by a narrow clear zone (Fig. 5-19C). The lesion is bilateral. It is present in some degree in most persons beyond 60 years of age. An arcus before 40 years is often a sign of hyperlipidemia. The term *arcus* comes from the early stage when only a segment of the circumference is involved; later the circle is completed. Regarded as a degenerative change, it has little clinical significance.

Peripheral Corneal Opacity: ***Kayser-Fleischer Ring.*** A circular band of golden brown pigment, 2 mm wide, is apparent on the posterior corneal surface, near the limbus. It is characteristic of hepatolenticular degeneration (Wilson's disease). Extreme hyperbilirubinemia (20 mg/dL) in a patient with normal copper metabolism, however, produced corneal rings independently diagnosed as *Kayser-Fleischer rings* by two ophthalmologists using slitlamp examination [L. M. Weinberg, T. A. Brasitus, and J. H. Lefkowitch: Fluctuating Kayser-Fleischer-like Rings in a Jaundiced Patient, *Arch. Intern. Med.*, **141:**246–47, 1981].

Central Corneal Opacity: ***Trauma.*** This is usually the result of trauma or infection. It also occurs in three quarters of the cases of dysostosis multiplex (Hurler's syndrome).

Dots in the Cornea: ***Fanconi's Syndrome.*** Crystals of cystine are deposited throughout the stroma with no accompanying inflammatory reaction.

The Sclera

Beneath the bulbar conjunctiva, the ocular globe is covered by a tough dense fibrous coat, the *sclera.* It is china white except for spots of brown melanin, varying in number with the individual's complexion and his race. The sclera is pierced by the *scleral foramen,* for the optic nerve, the long ciliary arteries and nerves, the short ciliary nerves, and the venae vorticosae. The tendons of the ocular muscles attach to the sclera with reinforced bands from the capsule.

Yellow Sclera: **Fat, Icterus, or Atabrine.** Commonly deposits of fat beneath the sclera show through the membrane and impart a yellow color to the periphery, leaving the perilimbal area relatively white. The lipochrome is more obvious in elderly persons with thinning membranes and in patients with anemia where the lipochrome is not obscured by the normal concentration of hemoglobin in the blood vessels. In *jaundice,* bilirubin infiltrates all body tissues and fluids; it colors the sclera *evenly.* The conjunctiva of the fornices is usually yellower because thicker. The dye *Atabrine* has been widely employed as an antimalarial drug; in dark-complexioned persons it produces a harmless yellowing of the sclera, skin, and mucous membranes. A distinctive feature is said to be that Atabrine produces more intense coloration near the limbus than in the remainder of the sclera.

Blue Sclera: **Osteogenesis Imperfecta.** The blue color results from thinning of the sclera so the choroid shows through. This finding is distinctive in *osteogenesis imperfecta.*

Brown Sclera: **Melanin or Homogentisic Acid.** Patches of melanin are commonly seen in the sclera of many person of dark complexions, especially in Blacks. In *alkaptonuria* homogentisic acid may color the sclera near the attachments of the ocular muscles upon the globe. Wedge-shaped areas of brown extend their apices toward the limbus.

Scleral Protrusion: **Staphyloma.** Injury to the sclera or increased intraocular pressure forces protrusion in the region of the cornea, forming an *anterior staphyloma* with characteristic profile (Fig. 5-19E). A *posterior staphyloma* cannot be seen by external inspection.

Scleral Ulcers: **Scleritis.** *Suppurative scleritis* is rare; it is usually metastatic from pyogenic inflammation elsewhere in the body. Tuberculosis, sarcoidosis, and syphilis cause a *granulomatous scleritis* in which is found localized elevation of the sclera with nodule formation. Focal necrosis of the sclera occurs as a reaction to collagen disease elsewhere in the body, as in rheumatoid arthritis. The condition is termed *scleromalacia perforans.* There is little inflammatory reaction about the ulcers.

Uveal Tract Inflammation: **Iritis, Iridocyclitis, and Uveitis.** Inflammation may involve only the iris, *iritis,* or extend to the ciliary body, *iridocyclitis;* when the choroid is also involved, the condition is termed *uveitis.* Iridic inflammation is characterized by ciliary flush and miosis, accompanied by deep pain and lacrimation. The iris becomes adherent to the anterior lenticular surface forming *posterior synechiae,* manifest by irregularities in the pupil. Cast-off cells sediment in the anterior chamber of the eye to form a sterile *hypopyon* (Fig. 5-19B). If there is involvement of the ciliary body and choroid, deposits of yellow or white dots of aggregated cells occur on the posterior surface of the cornea, *keratic precipitates* (KP). Inflammation of the uveal tract may be caused by trauma, infection, allergy, sarcoid, rheumatoid spondylitis.

The Iris and the Pupil

The *pupil* is a circular hole surrounded by loose pigmented stroma, the *iris,* which is arranged as an optical diaphragm with a variable opening. The iris contains irregular holes, called *iris crypts.* Embedded in the central part of the iris is the *Sphincter pupillae;* more peripheral is a radial muscle, the *Dilator pupillae.*

Pupillary Reaction: The Normal. The *Sphincter pupillae* is a circular muscle embedded in the iris near the pupillary margin. It is innervated by parasympathetic fibers from the Edinger-Westphal nucleus near the oculomotor (3rd) nerve nucleus (Fig. 5-20). The fibers enter the orbit in the 3rd nerve and accompany its motor branch to the inferior oblique muscle, whence the parasympathetic fibers synapse in the ciliary ganglion; from there, other fibers enter the eye through the short ciliary nerves. The *Dilator pupillae* is arranged radically in the peripheral two thirds of the iris. It receives sympathetic fibers, arising in the cortex, descending to the hypothalamus to Budge's ciliospinal center; new fibers go to the cervical sympathetic chain and ascend to the superior cervical ganglion to synapse with fibers

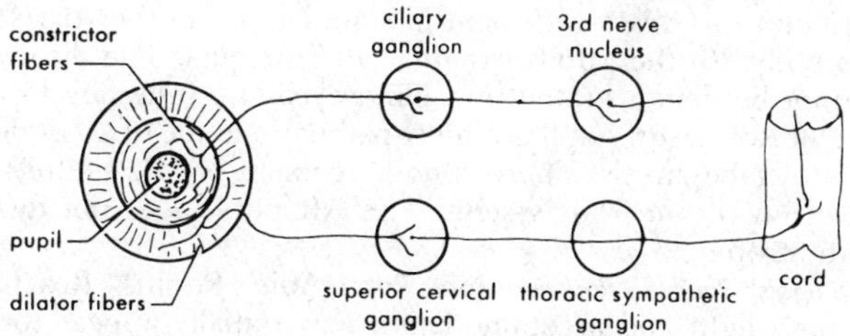

Fig. 5-20. Innervation of the pupillary muscles.

that run to the carotid plexus, and thence to the first division of the trigeminal (5th) nerve into the eye. Thus the sphincter contracts the pupil through *parasympathetic* stimulation; the dilator widens the pupil by sympathetic stimuli. The size of the pupils frequently fluctuate from changes in tone; exaggerated wavering is termed *hippus,* but it is of little clinical significance. Patients with Cheyne-Stokes respiration may have pupils that dilate during the phase of hyperventilation and contract during the periods of apnea. *Mydriasis* is dilatation; *miosis* is pupillary constriction. Bright light causes constriction, accompanied by a consensual reaction in the unexposed eye. In older persons, the pupils may react sluggishly to light; the reaction is hastened after several stimulations. *Near-point contraction* is incorrectly termed *reaction to accommodation,* because it involves convergence. Miosis occurs when the eye is fixed on a near object, say 20 mm away.

Unequal Pupils: ***Anisocoria.*** Inequality between the diameters of the two pupils can be without clinical significance; but a greater disparity in size, from *miosis* of one, suggests iritis, paralysis of the cervical sympathetics, or the use of a miotic drug (as pilocarpin). *Dilatation* of a single pupil can be caused by a mydriatic drug (as atropine), paralysis of the 3rd nerve, increased intraocular pressure in one eye. Inequality may occur congenitally or with luetic meningitis, tabes dorsalis, trigeminal neuralgia, carotid or aortic aneurysm, unilateral intracranial mass, glaucoma, or Adie's pupils. The examiner should beware of the artificial eye.

Sluggish Pupillary Reaction: ***Argyll Robertson Pupil.*** The classic signs are (1) weak or absent contraction to light, (2) contraction to light not improving with dark adaptation, (3) normal or exaggerated contraction to accommodation, (4) miotic pupils, (5) failure to dilate with painful stimulation in other parts of the body, (6) the pupils irregular and unequal. The disorder cannot be demonstrated in a blind eye. The fully developed Argyll Robertson pupil is almost pathognomonic of tabes dorsalis or taboparesis. There is no agreement on the site of the lesion in the nervous system. The AR pupil does not dilate with atropine.

Sluggish Pupillary Reaction: ***Tonic Pupil*** (Adie's Pupil). Reaction to both light and accommodation may initially appear to be lost. Closer observation shows both to be present but extremely sluggish, with a prolonged latent period. The condition may be unilateral. It is frequently encountered in young persons with widened pupils, in contrast to the requisite miosis in the AR pupil. Whatever the degree of reaction in the AR pupil, its reaction is prompt. The tonic pupil dilates with atropine; the AR pupil does not.

Without Reaction: ***Pupillary Paralysis*** (Ophthalmoplegia Internal). The pupil lacks the ability to constrict from either light or accommodation. It is generally dilated, never miotic.

Clinical Occurrence. Luetic meningitis, vasculitis, virus encephalitis, diphtheria or tetanus toxin, lead poisoning, midbrain lesions, bilateral 3rd nerve involvement. Adie's pupils, iris dysfunction from trauma, topical mydriatics, benztropine mesylate (Cogentin).

Unilateral Miosis: ***Miosis of Horner's Syndrome.*** This is caused by a lesion of the sympathetic pathway and is accompanied by ptosis and anhydrosis on the affected side.

The Lens

The anterior and posterior surfaces of the lens are convex; the junction of the two curved surfaces is the *equator*. The lens is suspended behind the iris by a tough membrane, the *zonula ciliaris* (zonule of Zinn), that extends from the entire lenticular equator to the *ciliary body* on the choroid (Fig. 5-21). When the eye is at rest and thus suited for distant vision, the ciliary muscle is relaxed so the pull of the zonula ciliaries *diminishes* the anteroposterior dimension. During accommodation, the ciliary muscle contracts, permitting the lens to thicken in response to its normal elasticity. Normally, the lens is highly transparent; changes in its protein produce opacity.

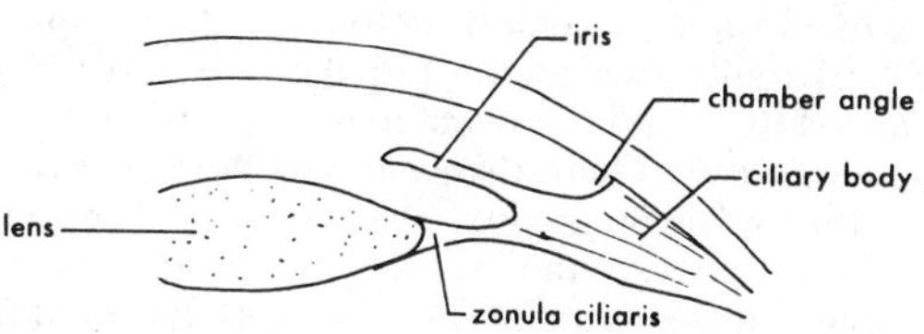

Fig. 5-21. Arrangement of the lens and ciliary body. *Cross-sectional diagram.*

Lenticular Opacity: **Cataract.** Since nearly all adults have some opacity of the lenses, a clinical definition of cataract implies a degree of clouding that interferes with vision. Some cataracts can be readily seen by shining a light beam obliquely through the lens (focal illumination), or by inspection through the ophthalmoscope with + 10 diopter magnification (direct illumination); others can be identified only with the slit lamp. Centrally placed cataracts can be seen without pupillary dilatation; those in the periphery can be visualized only after employment of a mydriatic. This discussion is limited to the types detectable without mydriatics or the slit lamp. *Anterior Polar Cataract.* A small white plaque can be seen in the center of the pupil. It either is congenital or occurs after corneal ulceration. *Nuclear Cataract.* A diffuse pigmentation occurs in the central portion of the lens. Ophthalmoscopic illumination shows a black reflection instead of the normal red retinal reflex. *Cortical Cataract.* Wedge-shaped opacities, arranged radially in the periphery, appear gray with the penlight, black against the red retinal reflex through the ophthalmoscope. Projections extend toward the center of the pupil, so oblique lighting shows them as gray bands. *Secondary Cataract.* Occurring after incomplete removal of the lenticular capsule, this type shows as dense folds of tissue and clusters of clear vesicles. *Complicated Cataract.* Associated with uveal disease or retinal detachment, opacities with rainbow colors extend toward the center as radii. *Diabetic Cataract.* Older diabetics have an increased tendency to develop nuclear or cortical cataracts with no distinctive character. Juvenile diabetics acquire a distinctive *snowflake cataract* containing chalky white deposits; the entire lens subsequently becomes milkly.

Lenticular Displacement: **Subluxation and Dislocation.** Rupture of the zonula ciliaris (zonule of Zinn) permits the lens to move from its fixed position behind the pupil. Slight displacement, with the lens still back to the pupillary aperture, is termed *subluxation* (Fig. 5-22B); it is manifested by tremulousness of the iris, *iridodonesis,* when the eye moves horizontally. Viewed through the ophthalmoscope, the equator of the lens may show as a dark curved line crossing the pupillary aperture; a double image of the retina may be seen with different magnifications, one through the lens, another without. When the lens is displaced completely from the aperture, the condition is

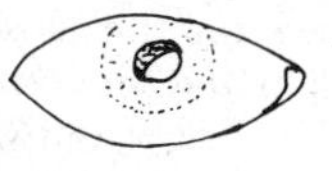

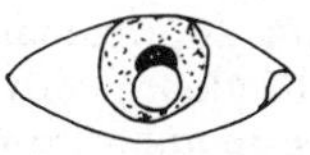

Fig. 5-22. Displacement of the lens. *When the lens is displaced but still remains behind the pupillary aperture, the condition is called subluxation.* **A.** Dislodgment posteriorly. **B.** Anterior chamber subluxation.

called *dislocation.* The lens is readily seen when it emerges into the anterior chamber (Fig. 5-22A); if it falls into the posterior chamber, special methods of visualizing it are required. Lenticular displacement is usually caused by trauma. Nontraumatic dislocation occurs in Marfan's disease and homocystinuria.

Intraocular Pressure Changes. Palpation may disclose gross disturbances in the tension of the eyeball (Fig. 5-23A). Place the

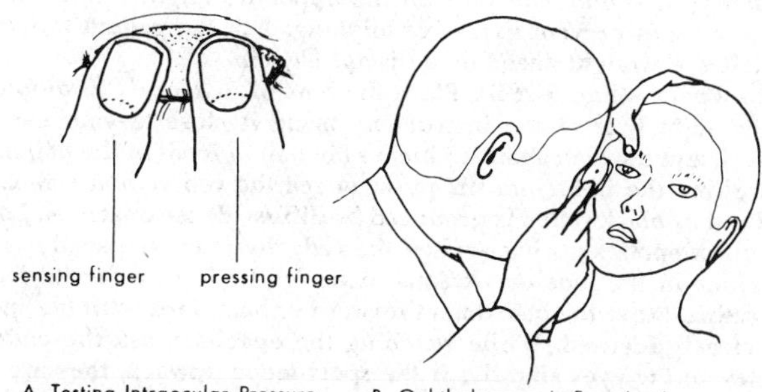

Fig. 5-23. Palpation and inspection of the eye. **A.** Digital testing of intraocular pressure. **B.** Ophthalmoscopic examination. *The media are inspected with a + 8 or + 10 lens, held about 12 inches (30 cm) from the patient's eye. Spots in the globe may be localized by moving the light source to determine whether the spots move in the same or in opposite directions. Inspection of the fundus is performed with the sight hole of the instrument about 3 inches (8 cm) from the patient's eye. The physician's right eye examines the patient's right; his left is employed for the patient's left, so the physician's nose parallels the patient's cheek. The examiner's right forefinger changes the lenses; his left hand rests upon the head of the patient with the thumb gently retracting and holding the upper lid to prevent excessive blinking.*

tips of both approximated forefingers on the closed upper lid; press the globe gently with one finger and sense the amount of pressure required to move the other finger outward. With practice, or by comparison with a normal eye, some judgment of tension is frequently possible. *Increased tension* occurs in glaucoma; *decreased tension* means extreme dehydration. Accurate assessment is made by measurement of pressure with the tonometer.

METHOD OF OPHTHALMOSCOPIC EXAMINATION. **The use of the ophthalmoscope requires practice, so the reader cannot hope to obtain meaningful information on the first attempt. This discussion can only serve to recall what the reader should have learned from supervised practice. Face the patient so that your right eye looks into his right; later, your left eye should examine his left. Examination of the right eye without dilating the pupils will be described. Grasp the instrument with your right hand, your forefinger on the milled disk of lenses. Rest your left hand on the patient's forehead so that your thumb can pull up the upper lid slightly to uncover the pupil and prevent excessive blinking. Ask the patient to fixate his left eye straight ahead on a distant object.**

The Media **(Fig. 5-23B). Place the lens of + 8 or + 10 diopters in the sight hole of the instrument, bring it close to your eye or glasses, and move to about 12 inches (30 cm) in front of the patient's eye. Shine the light into his pupil to see the red retinal reflex. A dull red or black reflex is produced by diffuse dense opacities. Look for black spots showing against the red; these are the shadows of opacities in the lens or vitreous made by the light reflected from the retina. Move the instrument forward or backward until the spots are clearly focused. While watching the opacities, ask the patient to elevate the eyes slightly; if the spots move upward, they are on the cornea or anterior part of the lens; little movement occurs when the location is near the lenticular center; downward movement indicates a location in the posterior lens or in the vitreous. Vitreous opacities appear more distinct when viewed obliquely with the white optic disk as a background.**

The Fundus **(Fig. 5-23B). When the media appears sufficiently clear, hold the instrument about 3 inches (8 cm) from the patient's eye, and run the gamut of lenses in the sight hole from + 10 to − 5, to find the optimal magnification for a distinct view of the retina. The selection will be governed by the refractive error and the degree of accommodation in both patient and examiner. In the absence of both factors, the best view should be obtained when the** sight hole is turned to zero. Minus lenses are required to correct for involuntary accommodation. When a cataract has been extracted, about + 10 is needed for correction. High astigmatism cannot be corrected with the spherical lenses of the instrument; the fundi should then be examined through the patient's glasses. When the correct setting for the instrument is found, move the sight hole closer to the patient's eye, resting your forehead firmly against your left thumb that is over the patient's brow. After studying Fig. 5-24A, examine the following regions. *Optic Disk Region.* Note the shape and color of the optic disk. The shape is round or oval vertically. Most of the disk is red-orange, the color imparted by the nerve fibers. The *physiologic cup* is a pale area in the temporal side of the disk, devoid of nerve fibers so it forms a depression whose base is the nonvascular lamina cribrosa. The size and shape of the cup vary greatly in normal eyes. In the disk, the site of ingress and egress of vessels, called the vessel funnel, also lacks nerve fibers, so it is pale and white. The borders of the disk may emerge gradually into the surrounding retina, or they may be sharply demarcated by a white *scleral ring.* Outside the ring, on the temporal side, a crescent of pigment may occur. *Retinal Vessels.* The arteries are bright red with a central white *reflex stripe.* Note the width of the reflex stripe. Normally the veins are about one quarter wider than the arteries; they are darker red and lack a stripe. The pattern of branching vessels shows great individual variation. As they emerge from the disk, the afferent vessels are true arteries; branches beyond the second bifurcation are arterioles that usually originate about one disk-diameter away from the disk margin. Look for sheathing of the arteries. Note the veins carefully at the arteriovenous crossings for nicking, deviation, humping, tapering, or banking. Veins normally pulsate; arteries in the retina do not.

Macular Region. The macula is in the horizontal plane of the disk and from two to three disk-diameters to the temporal side of its margin. Examination of the macula is usually fleeting because illumination of this region produces discomfort. The macula appears as a small darker red area in the retina, set apart from visible vessels. In its center appears a small darker spot, the *fovea centralis,* whose center gives off a speck of reflected light.

Undifferentiated Retina. The amount of pigmentation corresponds to the patient's complexion and race. The retina is thinner in the nasal periphery and therefore paler. Note areas of *white* or *pigment* from scarring. Look for *hemorrhages* and *exudates.* Express the size of areas in terms of disk-diameters. Measure depression or elevations by the diopters of correction required in the sight hole to focus on an arterial reflex in the area.

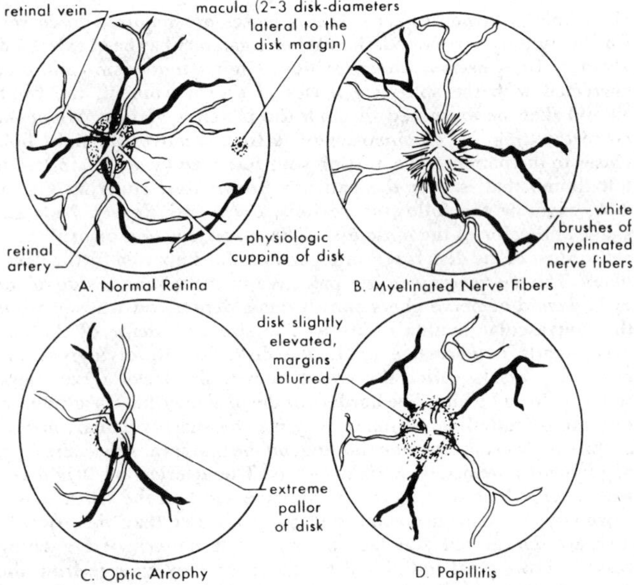

Fig. 5-24. Retinal abnormalities I. **A.** Normal retina. *The background of the retina is red-orange; it contains a variable amount of black pigments, depending on race and complexion. Diverging blood vessels emerge from the optic disk to spread over the retina, usually in pairs of an artery and a vein. The veins are solid, dark red, and they may pulsate normally. The arteries are brighter red, contain central white stripes, and are pulseless. The width of an artery is usually about four fifths that of the adjacent vein. The optic disk is lighter red, with sharp borders, often outlined by a strip of black pigment in the adjacent retina. The physiologic cup is white or pale yellow. The macula lies in the horizontal plane of the disk and from two to three disk-diameters to the temporal side. The macular area is pale red with a central white or shining dot.* **B.** Myelinated nerve fibers. *White brushes of myelinated nerves emerge from the disk, obscuring segments of vessels and disk margins. Despite the spectacular appearance the condition is normal.* **C.** Optic atrophy. *The disk is chalk-white with sharply defined borders. The blood vessels are normal.* **D.** Papillitis. *The disk is hyperemic and its borders are blurred. Focusing shows the disk to be elevated above the retinal background. The appearance alone cannot be distinguished from papilledema, but visual deficit accompanies papillitis from the anterior optic neuritis.*

Proliferation About the Disk: ***Myelinated Nerve Fibers*** (Fig. 5-24B). Semiopaque white patches emerge from the borders of the optic disk and spread into one or two quadrants of the retina. The retinal borders appear frayed and the underlying vessels are partially or completely obscured. The tyro may think he is viewing a serious lesion, when actually it is a normal variation. Usually myelination of the optic nerve fibers ends at the lamina cribrosa; infrequently myelin sheaths are retained by some nerve fibers until they reach well into the retina, causing the picture just described. They are of no clinical significance.

Disk Pallor: ***Optic Atrophy*** (Fig. 5-24C). In primary optic *atrophy* the disk is white, the borders sharply defined, the physiologic cup and lamina cribrosa visible. The blood vessels are normal. The primary type occurs in tabes dorsalis and taboparesis, and in conditions causing compression of the optic nerve without increased intracranial pressure. The lesion is also present in about 5% of the patients with pernicious anemia. Secondary *optic atrophy* also shows pallor of the disk, but the disk margin is indistinct, the lamina cribrosa is obscured, and the physiologic cup is not visible. The emerging vessels may be surrounded by perivascular lymph sheathing, seen as white lines. Pigmented or gray patches in the retina attest to previous hemorrhages or exudates. These findings indicate the presence of increased intracranial pressure that produced the optic atrophy. The common cause is brain tumor. In *optic atrophy from chorioretinitis* the disk may have a yellow cast, and the surrounding retina may contain hemorrhages, areas of atrophy, and pigment.

Disk Edema: ***Papillitis*** (Fig. 5-24D). When an optic neuritis involves the global portion of the optic nerve, *papillitis* is produced with loss of vision. When other portions of the nerve are involved, no retinal sign results. Papillitis causes edema of the disk that is indistinguishable from papilledema; but visual loss occurs in optic neuritis, not with papilledema. The disk is hyperemic and its margins blurred. The disk surface is elevated above the surrounding retina, demonstrated by finding that a + 1 or +2 lens correction is required to focus the surface of the disk. Edema of the disk usually does not produce loss of vision until late. Some causes of optic neuritis are local inflammation, such as uveitis and retinitis, sympathetic ophthalmia, multiple sclerosis, meningitis, sinusitis; infectious diseases, such as syphilis, tuberculosis, influenza, measles, malaria, mumps, and pneumonia; metabolic conditions, pregnancy, and intoxications, such as from methyl alcohol.

Disk Edema: ***Papilledema*** (Choked Disk) (Fig. 5-25A). Increased intracranial pressure causes the cerebrospinal fluid in the optic nerve sheath to compress the central vein of the retina, so return of blood from the eye is obstructed. In contrast to papillitis, the optic nerve is seldom functionally disturbed, so vision is unimpaired. Early papilledema causes blurring of the upper and lower nasal disk margins; later, the physiologic cup is obscured and the lamina cribrosa becomes indistinct. Blurring then extends to diverging vessels; veins become distended and pulseless. The disk surface may elevate 1 to 7 diopters. The emerging vessels can be seen to bend sharply as they pass over the edge of the elevated disk. Edema of the retina in the macular region throws the retina into traction folds, seen as white lines radiating from the macula, the *star figure* (Fig. 5-25B). High degrees of hyperopia cause a similar appearance in the disk, termed *pseudoneuritis;* the disk looks edematous, but the veins are not engorged: hemorrhages and exudates are absent. The principal causes

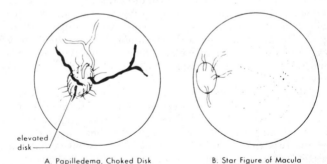

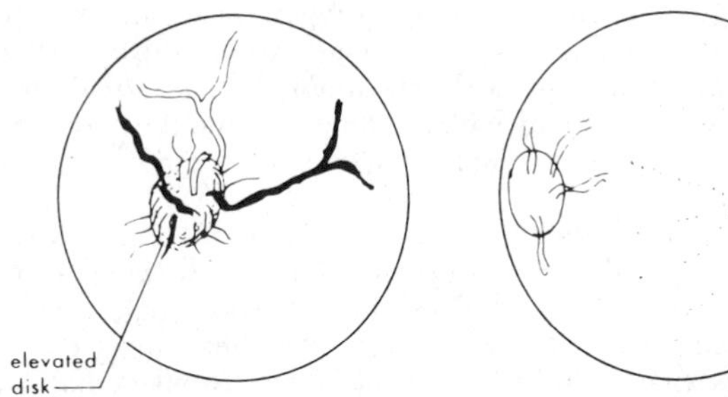

Fig. 5-25. Retinal abnormalities II. **A.** Papilledema (choked disk). *The disk surface is elevated, the nasal borders blurred. The vessels curve downward over the borders. The veins are distended and pulseless. Both arteries and veins in the disk may be obscured by the swollen structure.* **B.** Star figure of the macula. *Edema throws the retina into traction folds that radiate from the macula as white lines.*

of choked disk are brain tumor as well as hydrocephalus from any cause; but occasionally hypertensive, arteriosclerotic, or leukemic retinopathy, subarachnoid hemorrhage, meningitis, salicylate poisoning may be causative. Rarely, papilledema occurs in polycythemia and macroglobulinemia. Unilateral papilledema has been reported in benign intracranial hypertension (Pseudotumor Cerebri) [N. A. Sher, J. Wirtschafter, S. K. Shapiro, C. See, and I. Shapiro: Unilateral Papilledema in 'Benign' Intracranial Hypertension (Pseudotumor Cerebri), *J.A.M.A.*, **250:**2346–47, 1983).].

Drüsen bodies [German plural for "granules"] are granular deposits in the optic disk. The distinctions between early papilledema and drüsen bodies are reported as follows: drüsen cause obvious elevation of the disk, this is slight or absent in early papilledema; drüsen are pink or yellow, the surface of papilledema is hyperemic; drüsen cause the nerve fiber layer to glisten and often show a halo of feathery reflections, the layer in papilledema is dull; drüsen are in the disk center with frequent anomalous trifurcation of vessels, in papilledema the vessels are not deformed but show absence of venous pulsation and the light reflexes are dulled.

Retinal Vessels: ***Venous Engorgement.*** Distention of the retinal veins suggests polycythemia vera, congenital heart disease, leukemia, diabetes, and macroglobulinemia.

Retinal Vessels: ***Hemorrhages.*** The shape of a retinal hemorrhage frequently reveals its source. A very large and deep hemorrhage in the choriocapillaris produces a dark elevated area in the retina that looks like a melanotic tumor (Fig. 5-26). A smaller, more superficial hemorrhage appears as a round red spot, with blurred margins, called a *blot hemorrhage. Microaneurysms* are also round red spots, but their borders are distinct, they are not reabsorbed like hemorrhages, and they may occur in clusters about vascular sprigs. *Flame-shaped hemorrhages* occur in the nerve layers of the retina; they are red and striated. In the *subhyaloid* or *preretinal hemorrhage,* a pool of blood accumulates between the retina and the hyaloid membrane to form a turned-up half-moon with the straight upper side being a fluid level. These lesions sometimes organize slowly to form arcuate strands of white near blood vessels, a condition called *retinitis proliferans.* A small hemorrhagic spot with a central white area is called *Roth's spot;* it occurs in subacute bacterial

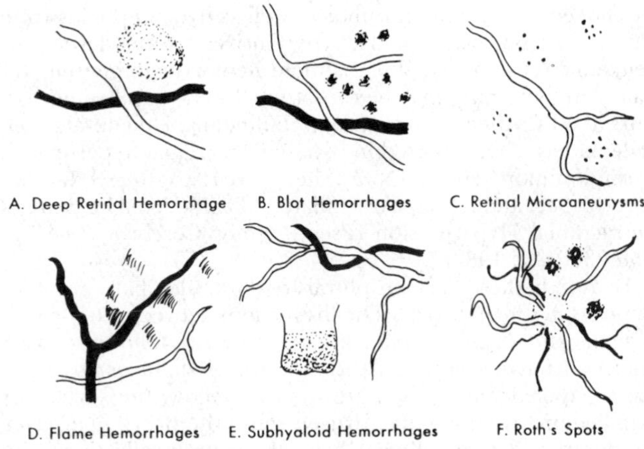

Fig. 5-26. Hemorrhages and similar objects in the retina.

endocarditis and leukemia. Some of the numerous conditions producing retinal hemorrhages are hypertension, diabetes mellitus, choked disk, occlusion of retinal veins, subacute bacterial endocarditis, systemic lupus erythematosus, pulseless disease (Takayasu's disease), macroglobulinemia, leukemia, polycythemia, sickle-cell disease, sarcoidosis.

Retinal Vessels: ***Arterial Occlusion.*** The central artery of the retina may be completely occluded, usually from thrombosis, rarely from embolism. Early the retina is very pale, because of ischemic edema; the arteries are extremely narrowed, the smaller ones invisible (Fig. 5-27A). Although the veins are full, they are pulseless. Pressure on the eyeball induces no pulsation in either artery or vein, proving the lack of circulation. Retinal edema around the macula causes a pallor, and by contrast the macula appears as a *cherry-red spot;* this disappears within a few weeks with subsidence of the edema. Occlusion of a branch artery causes findings limited to its area of supply. The common causes of arterial occlusion are vascular disease, syphilis, rheumatic fever, hepatitis, and temporal arteritis. Rarely, it is a complication of systemic lupus erythematosus, sickle-cell disease, cryoglobulinemia, or thromboangiitis obliterans.

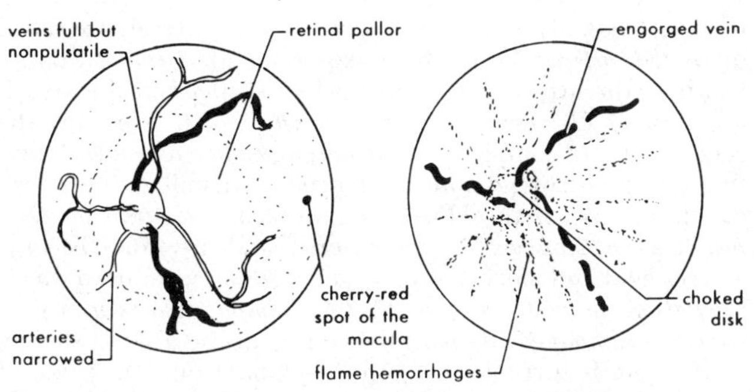

Fig. 5-27. Retinal vascular occlusions. **A.** Occlusion of the retinal artery. *The retinal background is white; the arteries are much narrowed. The veins are pulseless. Pressure on the globe produces pulsation in neither artery nor vein. After 36 hours, a cherry-red spot appears at the macula. Occlusion of a single arterial branch produces findings limited to the supplied area.* **B.** Occlusion of the retinal vein. *The affected veins are engorged and tortuous. Variform hemorrhages occur near the veins. Edema of the disk is present. Involvement limited to a venous branch produces findings in the drained area.*

Retinal Vessels: ***Venous Occlusion.*** Thrombosis of the central retinal vein is accompanied by engorgement and tortuosity of all visible veins (Fig. 5-27B). Variform hemorrhages appear throughout the retina. Occlusion of a branch of the central vein produces findings limited to the area of its drainage. Venous occlusion is often the result of atherosclerosis, but other causes are diabetes, periphlebitis from tuberculosis, polycythemia, multiple myeloma, macroglobulinemia, and leukemia. In sickle-cell disease, multiple venous thromboses may be accompanied by neovascularization.

Retinal Vessels: ***Arteriolar Sclerosis.*** The progress of the disease can be viewed through the ophthalmoscope, although the retinal changes do not necessarily parallel the changes elsewhere in the body, as the disease is notoriously spotty in its distribution. *Arterial Stripe.* Normally, the retinal arteries contain a central white stripe from the light reflection off the curved blood column. Increase in mural thickness causes widening of the stripe and brightening of the reflex. In moderate disease, the walls look like burnished copper and the vessels are called *copper-wire arteries.* When the disease is far advanced, the entire width of the artery reflects as a white stripe, and the vessels are termed *silver-wire arteries.* ***Vessel Sheaths.*** Normally the vessel walls are completely transparent, hence invisible. Mural thickening with lipoid infiltration produces a milky white streak on either side of the blood column, called *pipestem sheating.* ***Arteriovenous Crossings.*** As the arteries and arterioles become less resilient and more dense, certain signs are produced where they cross the veins (Fig. 5-28). *Concealment of the vein* or *arteriovenous nicking* occurs with thickening of the arterial sheath, so the vein is invisible for a short segment on either side of the overlying artery. *Deflection of the vein* is produced by the stiffened artery pushing the vein to assume a crossing at 90° where the normal angle of the two vessels is acute. *Tapering of the veins* results when the artery compresses the vein at the crossing. When dilatation occurs at the end of the vein segment, it is called *banking.* When the vein overlying the artery is uplifted by the latter, it is called *humping.*

The degree of involvement of the retinal vessels by the arteriolar sclerotic process has been variously scored. The following is a modification of Schleie's classification [W. M. Kirkendall and M. L. Armstrong: Vascular Changes in the Eye of

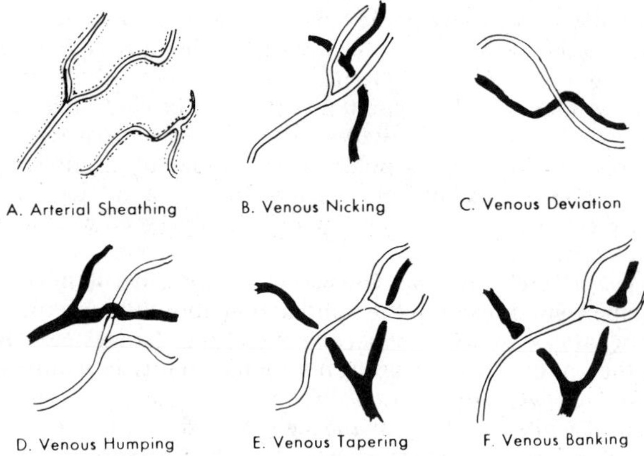

Fig. 5-28. Retinal signs of arteriolar sclerosis.

the Treated and Untreated Patient with Hypertension, *Am. J. Cardiol.*, **9:**663, 1962]:

Grades of Retinal Arteriolar Sclerosis

Grade 1. Thickening of vessels with slight depression of veins at arteriolar-venular crossings.

Grade 2. Definite AV crossing changes and moderate local sclerosis.

Grade 3. Venule beneath the arteriole is invisible; severe local sclerosis and segmentation.

Grade 4. To the preceding signs are added venous obstruction and arteriolar obliteration.

Retinal Vessels: ***Hypertensive Retinopathy.*** Arterial hypertension produces distinctive retinal signs that often coexist with the signs of arteriolar sclerosis. The signs attributed to hypertension may also be graded, using the classification of Kirkendall and Armstrong (*loc. cit.*):

Grades of Retinal Hypertension

Grade 1. Narrowing in terminal branches of vessels.

Grade 2. General narrowing of vessels with severe local constriction.

Grade 3. To the preceding signs are added striate hemorrhages and soft exudates.

Grade 4. *Papilledema is added to the preceding signs.*

For example, the appearance of a retina may be classified as "grade 3 arteriolosclerosis, grade 4 hypertension."

Retinal Vessels: ***Arteriovenous Aneurysms.*** Abnormal communications between arteries and veins have been noted in the lungs and other organs of patients with hereditary hemorrhagic telangiectasia. A single case has been reported in which the abnormal connection was found in the retinal vessels [E. L. Forker and W. B. Bean: Retinal Arteriovenous Aneurysm in Hereditary Hemorrhagic Telangiectasia, *Arch. Intern. Med.*, **111:**778, 1964]. An arteriovenous junction was seen with dilatation of the distal segment of the vein.

Retinal Spots: ***Cotton-Wool Patches.*** Gray to white areas with ill-defined fluffy borders occur in disarray around the posterior pole of the retina. The appearance is caused by thickening and swelling of the terminal retinal nerve fibers. They are often accompanied by red dots, representing microaneurysms, that subsequently rupture to produce striate hemorrhages [Kirkendall and Armstrong: *loc. cit.*].

Clinical Occurrence. Hypertension, lupus erythematosus, dermatomyositis, occlusion of central retinal vein, papilledema from any cause.

Retinal Spots: ***Hard Exudates.*** In contradistinction to the superficial cotton-wool patches, these are small white spots with *sharply defined edges.* They are exudates deeper than the retinal vessels. The cause is probably deposition of fatty or hyaloid-colloid material in old deep hemorrhages [Kirkendall and Armstrong: *loc. cit.*].

Retinal Spots: ***Pigmented Spots.*** The sites of old hemorrhages are marked by groups of pigmented spots over retinal vessels.

White or Yellow Spots in Retinal Arteries: ***Deposits of Talc.*** These are seen in the retinae of drug addicts who have injected ground-up tablets of methylphenidate into their own veins. The granules seem to be harmless in the eye but the associated granules trapped in lung capillaries would be harmful [H. Schatz and M. Drake: quoted in *Med. World News,* Jan. 8, 1979, p. 30].

Macular Region: ***Senile Degeneration.*** Although vision is much reduced, the only visible sign may be a few spots of pigment near the macula and blurring of the macular borders. In other cases, hemorrhages, patches of retinal atrophy, and pigmented areas may be seen.

Macular Region: ***Diabetic Retinopathy.*** In diabetes, the macular region is especially involved. Around the macula occur *microaneurysms,* sharply defined small red spots, to be distinguished from blot hemorrhages with blurred borders (Fig. 5-26). Microaneurysms around the macula are pathognomonic of diabetes. In advanced cases of the disease, the picture is embellished by white or yellow waxy exudates with distinct borders that are often serrated. The exudates gradually coalesce to form a broken circle around the macular region. The signs of atherosclerosis and hypertension are sometimes superimposed.

White Macular Region: ***Tay-Sachs Disease.*** Inherited in Jewish families, the disease is characterized by a white macular region containing a cherry-red spot in the fovea. Late complications are flaccid paralyses of the limbs.

Pigmentary Degeneration of the Retina. Inherited singly, or as a component of several syndromes, the disorder is manifest by diminution in the caliber of the retinal vessels and pigmentation of the retina (Fig. 5-29A). Spidery strands of pigmented spots form a girdle about the global equator. Later, most of the retina is infiltrated with pigment. Night blindness is the earliest symptom; later, all types of vision are greatly impaired. The condition may occur in the *Laurence-Moon-Biedl syndrome,* which includes obesity, polydactylism, hypogenitalism, and mental retardation.

Angioid Streaks in the Retina. Broad lines of pigment radiate from the optic disk, branching in the manner of blood vessels (Fig. 5-29B). They probably represent degeneration of elastic tissue. They occur in Paget's disease and pseudoxanthoma elasticum.

Retinal Detachment. The earliest sign is elevation of a retinal area so it is out of focus with the surrounding structure. The arteries and veins in the separated membrane appear almost black (Fig. 5-30). When widely separated, the retinal sheet is gray and frequently folded. Underlying inflammation may produce areas of choroiditis and vitreous opacities. A torn edge may be encountered, often shaped like a horseshoe. The cause of detachment is often undetermined (idiopathic); post-retinal hemorrhage or tumor may produce it. The retinal detachment can be detected by ultrasonic examination when the lens is

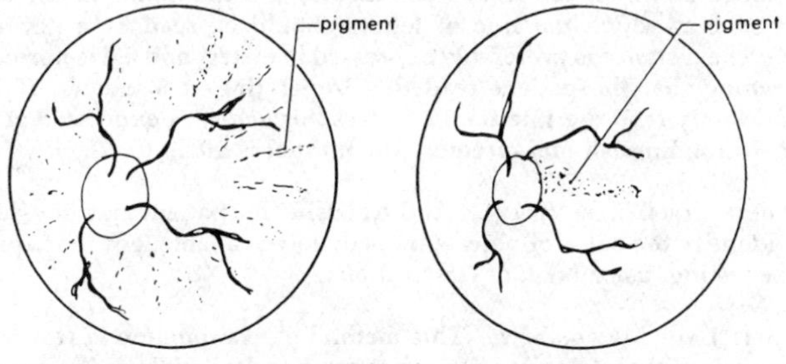

Fig. 5-29. Retinal pigmentation.

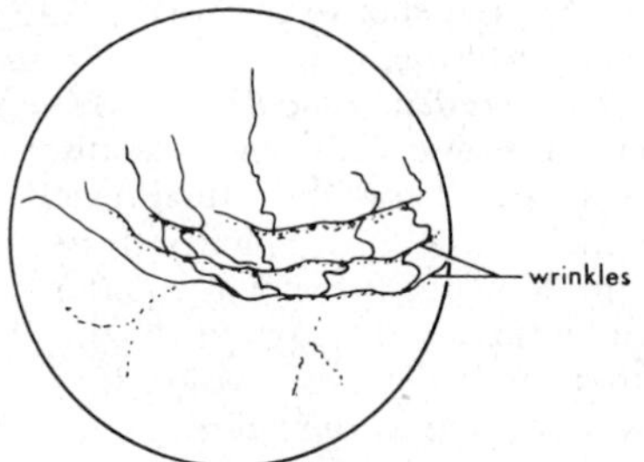

Fig. 5-30. Retinal detachment.

opaque. The examination may distinguish between post-retinal hemorrhage and tumor.

Bedside Tests for Visual Acuity. **Gross tests for visual acuity can be made without special equipment. Test a single eye at a time. Show the patient a newspaper or magazine, testing first with the fine print. If this is not perceived, show the larger letters. When he fails on large letters, hold several fingers up 3 feet (1 meter) away and ask him to count them. If he cannot count them, determine whether he can see movements of the hand. Failing this, flash a light beam into the eye, asking him to indicate when it appears. Test whether he can perceive the direction of the light source.**

When gross visual acuity is fair, more accurate tests can be made in the office with the standard *Swellen charts, provided* the illumination is adequate and sufficient distance from the charts is available. Express the reading in terms of a fraction with the numerator the distance at which the test is conducted, and the denominator the distance at which the line of letters should be read by a normal eye. The distance is preferably expressed in meters and 6/6 is normal, meaning that the patient read the proper line at 6 meters. If he could only read the line for 12 meters, his acuity is expressed at 6/12. In the English measurement the normal is 20/20 (feet).

Tests for Color Vision. **At the bedside the patient may be asked to identify the color of objects immediately available. For more precise testing, use a book of *Ishihara plates*.**

Slit Lamp Microscopy. **This method of examination is reserved for the ophthalmologist with experience and special equipment. A powerful light is focused in a narrow slit upon the various layers of the cornea, the anterior chamber, the lens, and the anterior third** of the vitreous chamber while the objects are examined through a corneal microscope. Accurate inspection of opacities and minute foci of inflammation can be made. Disturbances in protein aggregates can often be detected that are diagnostic of generalized disease.

TRIAGE FOR PATIENTS WITH RED EYE. **[discussion based upon published interview with J. Trobe: The Emergent Eye, *Emergency Med.*, 25–44 (Sept.) 1978].** BENIGN DISORDERS **[for the care of the generalist]: conjunctivitis (except fulminant gonococcal and chlamydial), external hordeolum (sty), and blepharitis—all having conjunctival injection, but no elevated intraocular pressure, corneal haze, visual disturbances, pain, or photophobia.** SERIOUS DISORDERS **(for the urgent care of the ophthalmologist): acute keratitis, acute glaucoma, acute iridocyclitis—all having conjunctival injection, ciliary flush, corneal haze (glaucoma and keratitis), increased intraocular pressure and shallow anterior chamber (glaucoma), all with blurred vision, ocular pain, and photophobia.**

TRIAGE FOR SUDDEN VISUAL LOSS **[for the urgent care of ophthalmologist]: *Monocular:* retinal detachment, vitreous hemorrhage, retinal artery occlusion, compression on optic nerve, temporal arteritis. *Binocular Transient Blindness:* amaurosis fugax (for 5 to 15 minutes, from cerebrovascular insufficiency).**

The Nose

The external nose is a triangular pyramid with one side adjoining the face (Fig. 5-31). The upper angle of the facial side is the *root,* connected with the forehead. The two lateral sides join in the midline to form the *dorsum nasi;* its superior

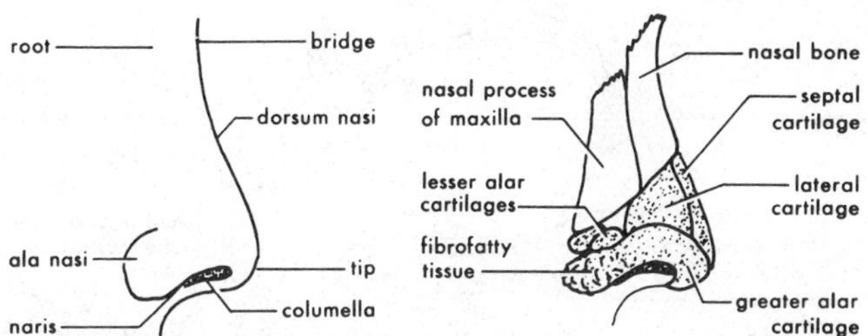

Fig. 5-31. The external nose. *Diagrams show the topographic features and the skeleton. Note that the proximal half of the nose is bone and the stippled distal half is cartilage.*

portion is the *bridge* of the nose. The free angle or apex forms the *tip* of the nose. The triangular base is pierced on either side by an elliptic orifice, the *naris* (plural *nares*), separated in the midline by the *columella* that continued internally with the *nasal septum.* Lining the margins of the nares, stiff hairs, the *vibrissae,* prevent inhalation of foreign objects. The proximal part of each lateral nasal surface ends below in a rounded eminence, the *ala nasi* (plural, *alae nasi*).

The upper third of the lateral nasal wall is supported medially by the nasal bone, laterally by the frontal process of the maxilla. Sustaining the lower two thirds is a framework consisting of the lateral cartilage, the greater alar cartilage, and several lesser alar cartilages. Also part bone and part cartilage, the nasal septum is formed proximally by the lamina perpendicularis of the ethmoid bone and, distally, by the quadrilateral septal cartilage.

The nasal septum divides the internal nose into symmetric air passages. Each passage begins anteriorly at the naris (Fig. 5-32), widens into a *vestibule,* thence it passes into a high narrow chamber that communicates posteriorly with the nasopharynx by an oval orifice, the *choana.* Normally the septal surface of the chamber is planar. But the lateral surface is thrown into convolutions by three horizontal parallel bony plates, each curling downward, the *superior, middle,* and *inferior conchae* or *turbinates.* Under each turbinate is a groove, the *superior, middle,*

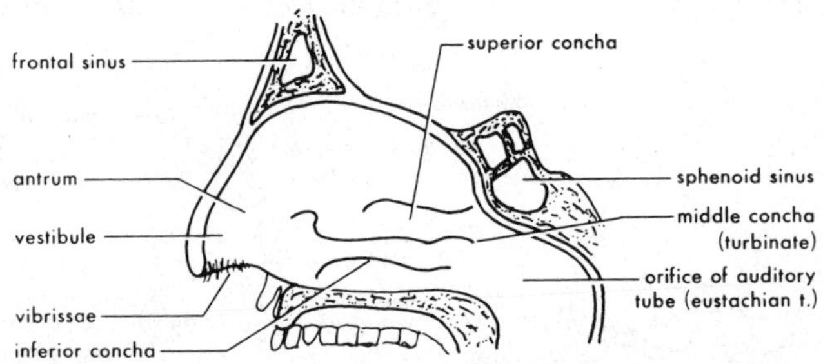

Fig. 5-32. Lateral nasal wall. *Parasagittal section shows the superior, middle, and inferior conchae; under each is its corresponding meatus. Posterior to the inferior meatus is the orifice of the auditory (eustachian) tube.*

and *inferior meatus*. Above and posterior to the superior turbinate is the opening of the *sphenoid sinus*. The superior meatus contains the orifices of the *posterior ethmoid cells*. The middle meatus receives drainage from the *maxillary sinus*, the *frontal sinus*, and the *anterior ethmoid cells*. The inferior meatus contains the orifice of the *nasolacrimal duct*. Just behind and lateral to the choana at the level of the middle meatus, the *auditory tube* (eustachian) opens into the nasopharynx. The mucous membranes of the inferior turbinate are very vascular and semierectile, so this structure is affected most by vasoconstrictor drugs.

The endings of the *olfactory (1st) nerve* are located high in the nasal chamber, above the superior turbinate. Lesions of this nerve may produce loss of smell, *anosmia*, which is invariably accompanied by a perceived change in the taste of food, which seems flat and unpalatable. A vascular network on the portion of the nasal septum, called *Kiesselbach's plexus*, is noteworthy because it is the site of most nosebleeds.

ROUTINE NASAL EXAMINATION. **Inspect the contour of the nose for asymmetry and abnormalities of profile. Test the patency of each naris by closing the other with digital compression, while the patient inhales with the mouth closed. With the thumb, push the soft nasal tip upward, while a lighted penlight in the other hand closes one naris (Fig. 5-33A); through the open naris, view the transilluminated septum for deviations, perforations, and masses. Palpate the cheeks and supraorbital ridges for tenderness over the maxillary and frontal sinuses. If no significant abnormalities have been encountered thus far, no further examination of the nose is required.**

DETAILED NASAL EXAMINATION. **The history or the findings from the routine examination may prompt a more thorough search with special methods and instruments. *Using the Nasal Speculum:* Examine the nasal chambers anteriorly by retracting the nares with the speculum and illuminating with head mirror or penlight. For either naris, hold the handles of the speculum in the left hand (Fig. 5-33B); insert the closed blades about 1 cm into the vestibule; open the blades, *anteroposteriorly* with the left forefinger pressing the ala nasi against the anterior blade to anchor it, thus avoiding painful pressure on the septum. The right hand is free to tilt the patient's head when the head mirror is used or to hold the penlight. Since only a small area can be viewed in a single position of the speculum, explore the region by changing the direction of the speculum and the position of the patient's head. Examine the *vestibule* for folliculitis and fis-**

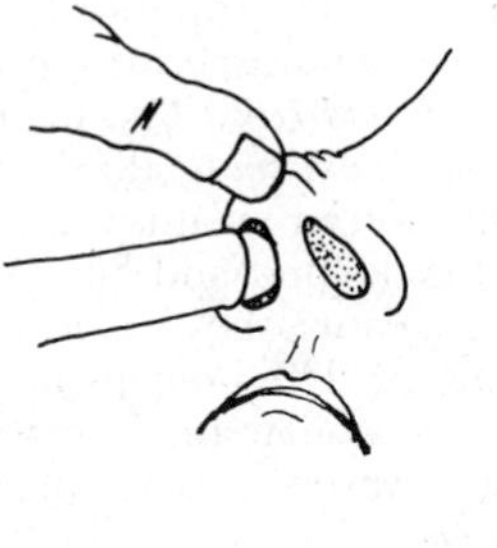

A. Transillumination of Nasal Septum

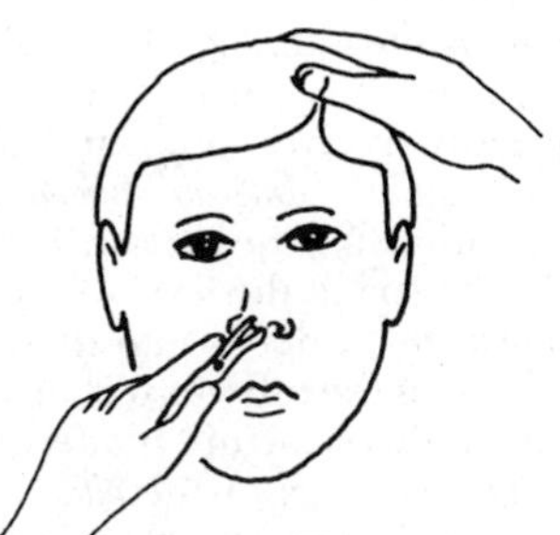

B. Speculum Examination of Nose

Fig. 5-33. Examination of the nasal septum and nares. **A.** Transillumination of the nasal septum. *Shine a light into one nasal cavity so the brightness of the septum illuminates the other nasal passage. This serves for the routine examination of the septum and the contralateral air passage.* **B.** Speculum examination of the nose. *Grasp the handles of the speculum between left thumb and long and ring fingers so the index finger rests along the upper handle and blade. Insert the blades into the naris, one blade above the other, to spread the naris anteroposteriorly so painful contact with the septum is avoided. Press the wall of the naris to the blade with the index finger. With your right hand, hold the patient's head in the desired position or perform other maneuvers in the handling of instruments.*

sures. Note the color of the *mucosa* and any swelling. Inspect the nasal septum for deviations, ulcers, or hemorrhages. Then, direct your attention to the lateral chamber wall. Locate the *inferior turbinate* to note swelling, increased redness, pallor, or blueness. Identify the *middle turbinate* and its underlying *meatus*. Look particularly in the middle meatus for purulent discharge from frontal, maxillary, and anterior ethmoid sinuses. *Using the Postnasal Mirror* (Fig. 5-34A): A head mirror is required for illumination. Use a No. 0 (small) postnasal mirror, warming it by immersion in warm water or by the flame from an alcohol lamp; test its temperature by touching its back to your hand. Secure a tongue blade in your left hand; insert it obliquely onto the tongue from the right side of the mouth; depress the tongue deeply. Reassure the patient that he can breathe through his nose while the mouth is open. Grasp the handle of the mirror in your right hand, like a pencil; steady your hand by bracing your fingers against the patient's cheek. Insert the mirror from the left side of the mouth (opposite the tongue blade), behind the uvula

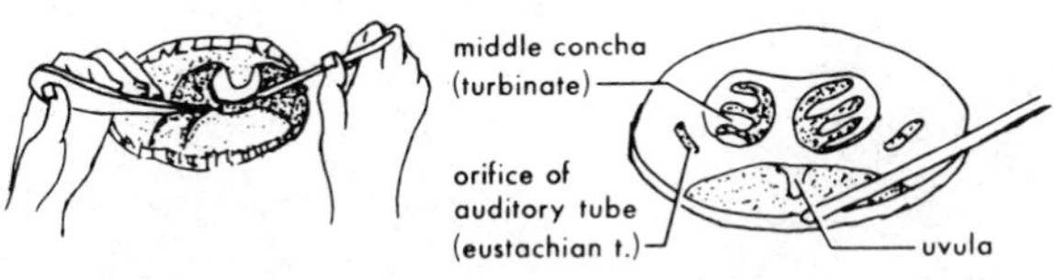

Fig. 5-34. Examination of the posterior nose. **A.** Examination with the postnasal mirror. *Grasp the end of a tongue blade in the left hand so the thumb pushes upward from beneath, while the index finger and long finger press downward on the middle of the blade. Have the tongue tip placed behind the lower incisors. Depress the tongue by inserting the blade from the right corner of the mouth to rest upon the midpoint of the lingual dorsum; press the arched tongue downward and forward by depressing the middle of the blade with the two fingers and the upward push of the thumb serving as a fulcrum at the end. Steady the left hand by pressing the ring and little fingers against the patient's cheek. With the right hand grasp the handle of the mirror (no. 0, small) like a pencil. Warm the mirror by immersion in warm water or heating in an alcohol flame; some hold it against an electric lamp. Test the temperature of the mirror by touching its back to your wrist. Have the patient breathe steadily through the nose with the mouth opened. Then insert the mirror from the left side of the mouth, with mirror upright, avoiding contact with tongue, palate, and uvula. Focus the light from a head mirror upon the nasal mirror and view the various parts of the choana.* **B.** View of the choana in postnasal mirror. *Note the three conchae (turbinates) with their corresponding meatus beneath; view the orifices of the auditory (eustachian) tubes. In the drawing, all deep spaces are heavily stippled.*

and near to the posterior pharyngeal wall. Turn the mirror upward, focus the light upon it, and adjust it to view the various parts of the choana (Fig. 5-34B). Locate the posterior end of the *vomer*, always found in the midline. Identify the *middle meatus;* pus draining from this region posteriorly comes only from the maxillary sinus. The *inferior meatus* is not well visualized posteriorly. The orifices of the *auditory tubes* (eustachian) are behind and lateral to the middle meatus. The orifice appears pale or yellow and is about 5 mm in diameter. The tubes are closed except during swallowing or yawning. Look for masses of pharyngeal tonsil (adenoids), hanging from the roof into the fossa of the tubal orifice. Look for areas of inflammation, exudate, polyps, and neoplasms in the nasopharynx, the uvula, or the soft palate. *Transillumination of the Maxillary Sinuses* (Fig. 5-35):

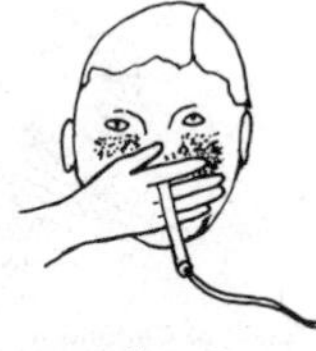

A. Maxillary Sinuses

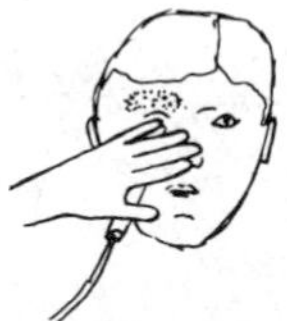

B. Frontal Sinuses

Fig. 5-35. Transillumination of the nasal sinuses. *Use a specially insulated electric lamp on a cord in a darkened room. For the maxillary sinuses, insert the tip of the lamp in the patient's mouth and have him close the lips tightly around it. Occlude the light transmitted from the oral cavity by covering the mouth with your hand. In the clear maxillary sinus, the light will be visible in the stippled areas of the cheeks. For the frontal sinuses, point the light upward from the floor of the supraorbital ridge. Cover the light from the orbit with your hand. The light in the clear frontal sinus will appear in the stippled area over the eyebrow.*

In a darkened room, place a special light in the patient's mouth and have the lips closed tightly about it. Put your hand over the mouth to shield the light coming from the buccal cavity. Usually, the two maxillary sinuses and the orbits are illuminated. Most significant is when one maxillary sinus lights up and the other is clouded. *Transillumination of the Frontal Sinuses:* Use the same arrangements, but place the light under the nasal half of the supraorbital ridge; with your hand, shield the orbit up to the eyebrow. Look for a bright area in the forehead.

External Nasal Deformities: **Congenital.** Disturbances in development of the nose are myriad, but they are so obvious as to pose little problem in diagnosis. Perhaps the most common is *cleft nose* (Fig. 5-36B). The physician should recognize nasal deformities as sources of extreme psychologic trauma that can be alleviated by modern rhinoplasty.

External Nasal Deformities: **Acquired.** Trauma, infection, and neoplasm produce classic types of acquired deformities. *Saddle nose* is distinguished by the sunken bridge (Fig. 5-36C), which most commonly results from loss of cartilage secondary to septal hematoma or abscess. Rarely it can follow relapsing polychondritis or either congenital or acquired syphilis. *Skewed nose* (the term is not in general use), with a curved or oblique dorsum nasi, results from the fracture. *Rhinophima* is a bulbous enlarge-

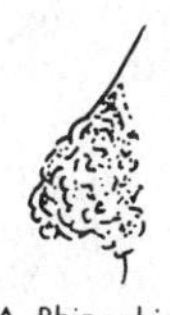
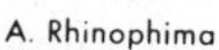

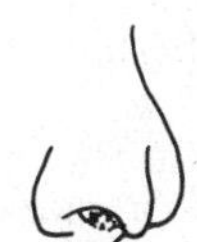

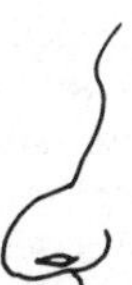

Fig. 5-36. External nasal deformities. **A.** *Rhinophima causes a bulbous enlargement of the distal two thirds of the nose; numerous sebaceous adenomas produce a dull, rough, reddened surface.* **B.** *Cleft nose is a congenital defect from incomplete fusion at the tip and dorsum.* **C.** *Saddle nose results from sinking of the dorsum with relative prominence of the lower third. It may be caused by disease or trauma.*

ment of the distal two thirds of the nose from multiple sebaceous adenomas of the skin (Fig. 5-36A). The mass of tissue is nodular, covered by erythematous skin. These deformities are remediable by plastic surgery.

Nasal Vestibule: ***Folliculitis.*** Mild inflammation around the hair follicles is evident on inspection.

Nasal Vestibule: ***Furunculosis.*** A small superficial abscess forms in the skin or mucous membrane (Fig. 5-37A). The area becomes tender, swollen, and reddened. Swelling may involve the nasal tip, alae nasi, and upper lip. *Avoid* instrumentation or other trauma to pyogenic lesions within the triangle anterior to a line from the corners of the mouth to the glabella, because infection may spread directly to the cavernous sinus.

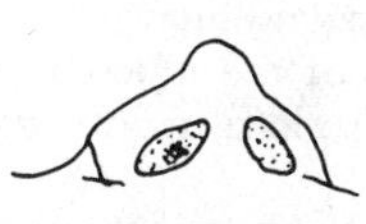

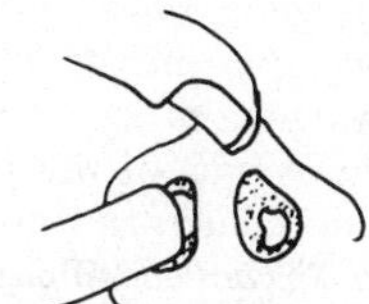

Fig. 5-37. Lesions in the nasal vestibule. **A.** Furuncle. *Easily seen from the exterior, the lesion is typical of all furuncles, except that it is in an extremely painful location. Avoid trauma that might spread infection to the cavernous sinus.* **B.** Perforation of nasal septum. *Transillumination of the septum discloses a hole resulting from operation or ulceration.*

Nasal Vestibule: ***Fissure.*** Often fissures develop at the mucocutaneous junction. They become overlaid with crusts that cover tender surfaces.

Nasal Septum: ***Deviation.*** In the adult, the nasal septum is seldom precisely a midline structure. The cartilaginous and bony septum may deviate as a hump, a spur, or a shelf, to encroach upon one nasal chamber, occasionally causing obstruction. *Columnar dislocation* of the septum may occur.

Nasal Septum: ***Perforation.*** A hole in the nasal septum is commonly caused by chronic infection with repeated trauma in picking off crusts, or as a result of nasal surgery. Formerly attributed to tuberculosis or syphilis, these causes are now quite rare. Perforation is readily demonstrated by looking in one naris while a light is shown in the other (Fig. 5-37B). The cartilaginous portion is usually involved.

Nasal Septum: ***Hematoma.*** Trauma results in a subperichondrial collection of blood on one or both sides of the nasal septum. This is evident as a violaceous, compressible, obstructive mass that will result in a saddle nose if bilateral and not treated appropriately by incision and drainage.

Nasal Septum: ***Abscess.*** The septum swells into both nasal chambers, and the overlying membranes become edematous. Infection of a septal hematoma invariably results in loss of cartilage and must be immediately incised, drained, and treated with appropriate antibiotics. There is risk of progression through the angular veins to produce cavernous sinus thrombosis.

Bilateral Rhinorrhea: ***Acute Rhinitis.*** Beginning with a watery discharge (*rhinorrhea*) and sneezing, the nasal secretion ultimately becomes purulent. Fever and malaise may accompany. Nasal obstruction occurs from edema of the mucosa. A sore throat is not part of the picture. Severe local pain suggests a complication, such as sinusitis.

Bilateral Rhinorrhea: ***Allergic Rhinitis.*** Itching of the nose and eyes, rhinorrhea, and lacrimation are accompanied by sneezing. Headache is common. The membranes are typically pale, swollen, and edematous; occasionally they are dull red or purplish. The appearance is closely simulated by rhinitis medicametosa from excessive use of vasoconstricting drugs. Microscopic examination of stained secretions should be made. When more than 4% of the polymorphonuclear leukocytes are eosinophilic, an allergic cause should be suspected. Allergic rhinitis may be seasonal or perennial; recurrence during the pollen seasons suggests hay fever. Symptoms that occur near animals or other objects may have an allergic basis.

Bilateral Rhinorrhea: ***Nonallergic Vasomotor Rhinitis.*** Symptoms identical to those seen in allergic rhinitis occur in individuals in whom no allergic reaction can be demonstrated. Symptoms are frequently exacerbated by smoke, fumes, and rapid changes in temperature and humidity. The membranes are pale and boggy.

Dry Nasal Mucosa: ***Atrophic Rhinitis.*** The patient complains of nasal discomfort or "stuffiness." The membranes appear dry, smooth, and shiny; they are studded with crusts. A foul odor (*ozena*) may be present. The cause is unknown.

Unilateral Nasal Discharge: ***Choanal Atresia.*** A congenitally closed orifice is occasionally encountered, usually in infants, demonstrated by obstruction when an attempt is made to pass a catheter from the external naris to the nasopharynx.

Unilateral Nasal Discharge: ***Foreign Body.*** Children frequently put objects into the nose that remain for long periods and produce foul, purulent discharge.

Unilateral Nasal Discharge: ***Neoplasm.*** Often carcinoma produces a bloody discharge, in distinction to the brisk bleeding of epistaxis.

Unilateral Nasal Discharge: ***Cerebrospinal Rhinorrhea.*** A unilateral discharge of clear spinal fluid may occur after head injury or surgery. The fluid may be blood-tinged, but is readily distinguished from a brisk nosebleed. Compression of the jugular vein increases the flow. Spinal fluid also gives a positive test for sugar with Benedict's solution.

Facial Pain: ***Acute Suppurative Sinusitis.*** Severe pain in the face, occurring with signs and symptoms of an acute upper respiratory infection, suggests complicating acute suppurative sinusitis. Involvement of the *maxillary sinus* causes dull throbbing pain in the cheek and in *several* of the upper teeth on that side. Thumb pressure discloses localized tenderness in the maxilla. *Frontal sinusitis* produces pain in the forehead above the supraorbital ridge; pressure in this region elicits tenderness. Edema of the eyelids on the affected side is infrequent. The pain of *ethmoid sinusitis* is medial to the eye and seems deep in the head or orbit; there is no localizing tenderness, although palpebral edema is common. *Sphenoid sinusitis* generates pain, either behind the eye, in the occiput, or in the vertex of the skull; no tenderness is produced. Pain in the teeth with maxillary sinusitis must be distinguished from an inflammation about a tooth; in the latter case, only one tooth is painful and may be tender when tapped with a probe. In sinusitis, examination of the affected side with a nasal speculum discloses reddened edematous mucosa and swollen turbinates. When the mucosa is shrunk by the application of a cotton pledget soaked with 3% ephedrine in saline solution, a purulent discharge may be seen; the drug may also be applied as a spray. During the first two days, the discharge may be tinged with blood. With shrinkage, pus in the posterior middle meatus may be seen in the nasopharyngeal mirror. Transillumination may reveal an opaque maxillary or frontal sinus; x-ray films may show clouding of the sinus or even a fluid level.

Protracted Purulent Discharge: **Chronic Suppurative Sinusitis.** When a purulent nasal discharge persists for more than three weeks, *subacute* or *chronic sinusitis* should be suspected. Pain over the sinuses is not a prominent symptom, and tenderness is frequently absent. Examination of the shrunken membranes may disclose the source of the pus. Transillumination of the sinuses and x-ray films may assist in localization. Clouding of the maxillary sinus in the x-ray film, without a fluid level, may require maxillary antral puncture to distinguish between thickened membrane and pus.

Sinusitis and Periorbital Edema: **Periorbital Abscess.** In suppurative ethmoid sinusitis, pus may extend through the lateral wall of the sinus to form an abscess between the ethmoid plate and the periosteum lining the orbit. This is accompanied by some increase in fever, pain on movement of the eye, and edema between the inner canthus and the bridge of the nose. The edematous region is tender and may extend to involve most of both lids. The pus may push the ocular globe slightly downward and laterally. No chemosis is present. Surgical drainage is essential.

Sinusitis and Periorbital Edema: **Orbital Abscess.** A periorbital abscess may extend to produce a diffuse cellulitis of the orbital tissue. Invasion may be heralded by a chill, high fever, and dull pain in the eye. The eyelids become edematous, particularly near the inner canthus. Chemosis develops. Ultimately, the eye becomes fixed. The patient appears very ill and requires the immediate care of a surgical specialist.

Sinusitis and Ocular Palsies: **Cavernous Sinus Thrombosis.** This is the most feared complication of nasal infections; the mortality is still near 50%. Usually infection spreads from the nose through the angular vein to the cavernous sinus, where septic thrombosis occurs. The catastrophe is revealed by sudden chills and high fever. The patient is prostrated and may rapidly become comatose. He complains of pain deep in the eyes. Early, there is *selective* ocular palsy (Fig. 5-38A), involving one of the nerves in the cavernous sinus, either the oculomotor (3rd) nerve, the trochlear (4th) nerve, or the abducens (6th) nerve. Both eyes are involved fairly early with immobilization of the globes, periorbital edema, and chemosis. Death may occur within two or three days. *Distinction.* Selective ocular palsy occurs early in cavernous sinus thrombosis, whereas orbital abscess produces complete immobilization of the globe gradually, without preliminary disorder of a single nerve. Bilaterality strongly suggests cavernous sinus thrombosis.

Intranasal Masses: **Polyps.** Nasal polyps are overgrowths of mucosa that may be either sessile or pedunculated. Developing from recurrent episodes of mucosal edema, they are frequently seen in long-standing allergic rhinitis. Polyps are commonly multiple, most frequently protruding from the middle meatus to present as smooth, pale, spheric masses of mucosa (Fig. 5-

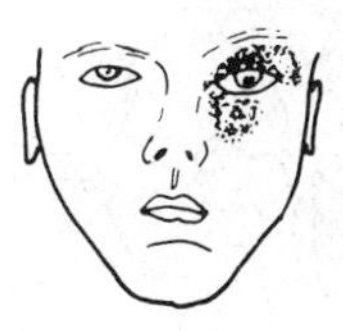

A. Cavernous Sinus Thrombosis

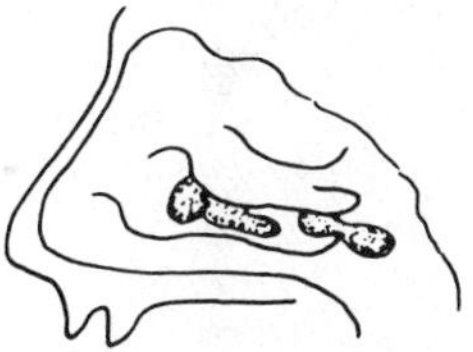

B. Nasal Polyps

Fig. 5-38. Lesions about the nose. **A.** Cavernous sinus thrombosis. *Early there is paralysis of a single ocular muscle, with the development of edema and proptosis* (*shown*). *Later, the globe becomes immobilized and the other eye becomes involved. The diagnosis and treatment of this disorder are an emergency.* **B.** Nasal polyps. *The parasagittal section shows the lateral wall with three polyps emerging from the middle meatus.*

38B); they are quite mobile and insensitive to the probe, which distinguishes them from swollen turbinates. Polyps may enlarge to obstruct the air passages; they frequently recur after removal.

Intranasal Masses: **Mucocele and Pyocele.** Permanent obstruction of the orifices of the frontal or ethmoid sinuses causes accumulation of mucus normally secreted by their lining membranes. A resulting sac or *mucocele* slowly enlarges; the pent-up mucus exerts pressure on the surrounding structures and erodes bone, thus behaving like a neoplasm. A sac from either site eventually erodes through the floor of the frontal sinus or the lateral ethmoid wall to produce a *painless swelling* beneath the supraorbital ridge, medial to the ocular globe (Fig. 5-39). The mass feels rubbery and slightly compressible. The globe is pushed downward and laterally, causing diplopia; proptosis may also occur. Upward and medial motions of the eye are restricted. Intranasal examination may be negative, or the results of ancient surgery may be seen. Occasionally, a previous skull fracture is the cause. An infected mucocele is termed a *pyocele*. *Distinction.* Swelling from the mucocele occurs *above* the inner canthus; dacryocystitis forms a swelling *below* the canthus.

Intranasal Masses: **Neoplasm.** Benign papillomas are often found in the vestibule. Slow-growing benign neoplasms of the

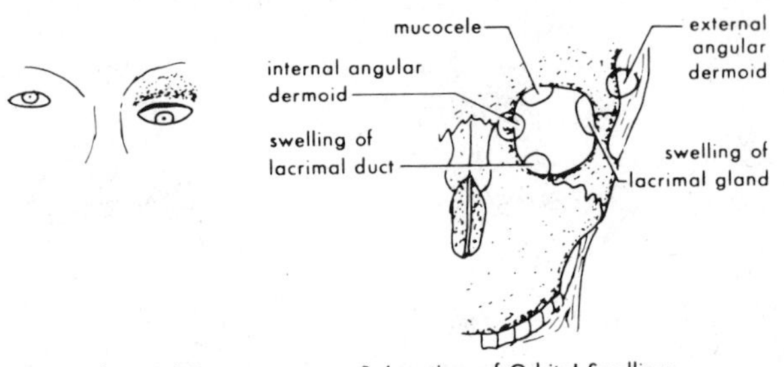

Fig. 5-39. Tumors about the orbit. **A.** Mucocele of frontal sinus. *An example of a mucocele, this occurring in the floor of the supraorbital ridge and presenting medially. It may push the globe downward and cause proptosis. It is painless. It must be distinguished from other swellings about the orbit by knowledge of their exact locations as shown in* **B.**

sinuses are usually osteomas or chondromas. They grow slowly and cause no symptoms until air passages or a sinus orifice is obstructed. X-ray films of the skull frequently lead to the diagnosis. Carcinomas of the sinuses cause obstruction, blood-stained discharge, and constant boring pain. They invade bone; in the orbit, they may cause ocular disturbances; in the antral floor, their presence may be announced by loosening of the teeth, maladjustment of a denture, or bulging and softness of the hard palate.

Nasal Necrosis Without Systemic Disease: ***Midline Granuloma.*** This is a progressive destructive disease that erodes the nose, the paranasal sinuses, the palate, the orbits, and the face, penetrating soft tissues, bone, and cartilage. The cause is unknown, although hypersensitivity is suspected. *Pathophysiology:* the inflammation is attended with granulomatous formation that is often hard to find in biopsies. *Age and Sex:* most common in 5th or 6th decades, with slight preference for women. *Signs:* indolent ulceration and mutilation suggest the diagnosis. *Biopsy:* usually confirms the nature of the disease. *Prognosis and Response to Therapy:* the disease progresses despite surgical débridement. Response to therapy with corticosteroids is questionable. Local radiotherapy may slow the process. *Distinction:* in contrast with Wegener's granulomatosis, this disease does not show systemic involvement.

Chronic Nasal Erosion with Systemic Disease: ***Wegener's Granulomatosis*** (Necrotizing Respiratory G., Rhinogenic Polyarteritis, Arteritis-Pulmonary-Nephropathy Syndrome, Klinger's Disease). This is one of the segmental necrotizing vasculitides (*see* p. 465 for pathophysiology and classification). *Involved Vessels:* small arteries and veins are the sites of granulomatous inflammation. The process may involve the upper and lower respiratory tract, the kidneys, and the small vessels of other systems. *Age and Sex:* mostly the 4th and 5th decades, either sex. *Symptoms and Signs:* these arise from erosion of the nose (with a resulting *saddle deformity*), palate, nasopharynx. *Lungs: invariably affected* with infiltrates, nodules, and cavitations. *Kidneys:* Glomerulitis. *Distinction:* the diagnosis is made by the entire picture, together with biopsies showing typical pathologic lesions. *Prognosis and therapeutic response:* progressive to death unless given cyclophosphamide which produces long-term remissions.

▼ *Key Sign:* ***Epistaxis (Nosebleed).*** Nosebleed may be a spontaneous and trivial occurrence, or it may be a sign of serious local or generalized disease. Some of the causes are listed:

Clinical Occurrence: LOCAL CAUSES: *Forceful expiration:* coughing, sneezing. *Injuries:* nose picking, fractures, lacerations, foreign bodies. *Ulcerations:* adenoid growth, malignant polyp, nasopharyngeal fibroma, angioma, malignant disease. *Varicosities:* multiple hereditary telangiectasia, portal cirrhosis of the liver. *Acute infections:* rhinitis, diphtheria, scarlet fever, influenza, pertussis, psittacosis, typhoid fever, Rocky Mountain spotted fever, erysipelas.

GENERALIZED CAUSES: *Physiologic: exertion. Arterial hypertension:* essential hypertension, coarctation of the aorta. *Venous hypertension:* pulmonary emphysema, cardiac failure, superior vena caval obstruction. *Blood coagulation disorders:* hemophilia and Christmas disease, pernicious anemia, thrombocytopenia, scurvy, leukemia, hypoprothrombinemia from hepatic disease or salicylism. *Infections:* typhoid fever, scarlet fever, influenza, measles, infectious mononucleosis (glandular fever), rheumatic fever. *Changes in atmospheric pressure:* mountain climbing, caisson disease, flying. *Vasomotor:* rhinitis sicca. Uremia.

NASAL EXAMINATION FOR EPISTAXIS. **Hemorrhage from the external nares is obvious, but bleeding from the choana must be distinguished from hemoptysis and even hematemesis. In any case, the first problem is to ascertain the bleeding site and judge whether trauma or some predisposing disease is present. In the anterior nose, the most common site of bleeding is from Kiesselbach's plexus, a vascular network in the anterior nasal septum. Posteriorly, hemorrhage occurs frequently at the back third of the inferior meatus; vessels in the region are large and belong to the external carotid artery system. In some cases, there are multiple oozing points in the mucosa. If he is able, seat the patient in a chair and be seated in front of him. Cover both of you to catch the blood. Remove the clots by suction; or lacking equipment, have the patient clear the nose by blowing it. Inspect the anterior nasal chambers, especially the septum. If hemorrhage is so profuse as to obscure the site, advance the sucker tip backward in small increments, clearing the blood at each step, until a point is reached where the passage immediately fills after clearing; this is the bleeding site. Blood-tinged fluid should suggest that the discharge is cerebrospinal fluid. Consult the textbooks for method of arresting hemorrhage.**

Nasal Trauma: ***Septal Hematoma.*** Even slight trauma to the nose may produce bleeding under the mucoperichondrium, usually causing bilateral hematomas. Breathing through the mouth is necessary because of nasal obstruction. The columella may be widened; the nasal tip pales from stretching of the skin. Pressure on the anterior ethmoidal nerve by the hematoma may cause anesthesia of the tip. Long-standing hematomas interfere with the blood supply of the septum causing slow necrosis of the cartilage.

Nasal Trauma: ***Fracture.*** Usually nasal fractures are simple or comminuted, seldom are they compound. A blow from the side displaces both nasal bones to the opposite side, producing an S-shaped curve in the dorsum nasi. The septum may also be fractured along with the nasal bones, or it may be affected when the nasal bones are left intact. Frontal blows depress the nasal bones. Palpation along the inferior border of the orbit may disclose an irregularity that indicates concomitant fracture of the maxilla, with displacement of a fragment downward into the sinus. Backward displacement of the maxilla is indicated by malocclusion of the teeth. Fracture of the zygoma leaves a flattening in that part of the face.

The Mouth

Surrounding the mouth is the *Orbicularis oris,* a complicated circular band of muscle innervated by the facial (7th) nerve; its contraction closes and protrudes the lips. Each lip is anchored to its adjacent gum by a fold of mucosa, the *labial frenulum.*

▼ *Key Symptoms:* ***Dysphagia.*** A disorder in swallowing is termed *dysphagia.* The patient experiences a *sense of obstruction* at a definite level when fluid or a bolus of food is swallowed. Neurogenic dysphagia may be accompanied by *regurgitation through the nose.* Some varieties of dysphagia may cause localized *pain;* others are painless. Deglutition involves muscles in both the oropharynx and the esophagus. Pain from the oropharynx is accurately localized in the neck; but esophageal pain is dispersed in the thoracic six-dermatome band, so it presents as pain in the chest (pp. 227–51).

Clinical Occurrence: OROPHARYNX. *Painful dysphagia from intrinsic lesions* (diagnosed by inspection of the mouth): glossitis, tonsillitis, stomatitis, pharyngitis, laryngitis, lingual ulcer, carcinoma, pemphigus, erythema multiforme, Ludwig's angina, mumps, bee-sting of the tongue, angioneurotic edema, sometimes Plummer-Vinson syndrome. *Painful dysphagia from extrinsic lesions* (diagnosed by palpation of the neck): cervical adenitis, subacute thyroiditis (p. 212), carotid arteritis (p. 205), infected thyroglossal cysts or sinuses, pharyngeal cysts or sinuses, carotid body tumor (p. 225), spur in cervical spine. *Painful dysphagia from general conditions:* rabies, tetanus, Plummer-Vinson syndrome. *Painless dysphagia from intrinsic lesions* (diagnosed from inspection of the mouth): cleft palate, flexion of the neck from cervical osteoporosis, xerostomia in Sjögren's syndrome, and Mg deficiency. *Painless dysphagia from neurogenic lesions:* globus hystericus, postdiphtheritic paralysis, bulbar paralysis, myasthenia gravis, hepatolenticular degeneration (Wilson's disease), paresis, paralysis agitans, botulism, poisoning (lead, alcohol, fluoride).

ESOPHAGUS. *Painful dysphagia from intrinsic lesions:* (*see* Pain in the Chest, pp. 227–51): foreign body, carcinoma, esophagitis, diverticulum, hiatal hernia. *Painless dysphagia from intrinsic lesions:* congenital stricture, adult acquired stricture, scleroderma, dermatomyositis; xerostomia in Sjögren's syndrome, amyloidosis, and thyrotoxicosis. *Painless dysphagia from extrinsic lesions:* aortic aneurysm, dysphagia lusoria (pp. 245 and 250), vertebral spurs from osteoarthritis, enlarged left cardiac atrium.

TEST FOR ESOPHAGEAL OBSTRUCTION **(contributed by Michael P. Corder, M.D.).** Face the patient and supply him with a glass of drinking water. Place the chestpiece of your stethoscope over the patient's abdominal left upper quadrant. Measure the time elapsing between swallowing and the murmur produced by the bolus passing the cardia. Normally it should range from 7 to 10 seconds.

INSPECTION AND PALPATION OF THE MOUTH. **Face the patient, with both of you seated at the same level. Hold the tongue blade in the left hand and a penlight in the right. If a head mirror is used, your right hand is free to hold a nasal or laryngeal mirror. *Lips:* Look for cleft lip and other congenital and acquired defects. Have the patient attempt to whistle, to reveal paralysis from facial (7th) nerve lesions. Note the color of the lips, evidence of angular stomatitis, rhagades, ulcers, granulomas, neoplasms. Inspect the inner surface of the lips by retracting them with a tongue blade while the teeth are approximated. *Teeth:* Note absence of one or more teeth, presence of caries, discoloration, fillings, bridges. Notice abnormal dental shape, such as notching. Tap each tooth with a probe for tenderness. *Gums:* Look for retraction of the gingival margins, pus in the margins, inflammation of the gums, spongy or bleeding gums, lead or bismuth lines, localized gingival swelling. *Breath:* Smell the breath for acetone, ammonia, or fetor. *Tongue:* Have the patient protrude his tongue; assess its size; look for deviation from the midline, restricted protrusion. Examine the coat of the tongue for color, thick-**

ness, and adhesiveness. Look for abnormalities on the dorsal surface. Describe local lesions and palpate them with gloved fingers. Palpate the accessible portions of a tongue that is painful, or has restricted motion, for deep-seated masses. In palpation, have the tongue *inside* the teeth to relax the muscle tension. Have the patient raise the tip to the roof of the mouth; inspect the undersurface, including frenulum and carunculae sublingualis. Palpate the region of the sublingual salivary glands and the submaxillary ducts for calculi. To *depress the tongue,* have the patient place the tip *behind* the lower incisors and breathe gently but steadily (Fig. 5-40A). Hold the blade in your left hand with the middle finger *over* its midpoint and the thumb *pushing upward* on the nearer end of the blade; place the flat of the farther end about midway back on the tongue; pull *down* on the middle of the blade and push *up* with the thumb to depress the tongue and pull its root forward. Pressing the tongue farther back causes gagging; pressing anteriorly permits posterior bulging. To secure optimal view may require several placements of the blade transversely at the midpoint. Test for vagal (10th) nerve paralysis by noting whether the uvula is drawn upward in the midline when the patient says "e-e-e." *Buccal Mucosa:* Retract the cheek with the tongue blade. Look for melanin deposits, vesicles, Koplik's spots, ulcers, neoplasms. Examine the orifices of the parotid duct, opposite the upper 2nd molar. *Tonsils:* Look for hyperplasia, ulcers, membrane, masses, and small submerged tonsils.

Oral Cavity

The oral cavity is a short tunnel with an arching roof of hard and soft palate, with walls of the cheeks and lateral teeth,

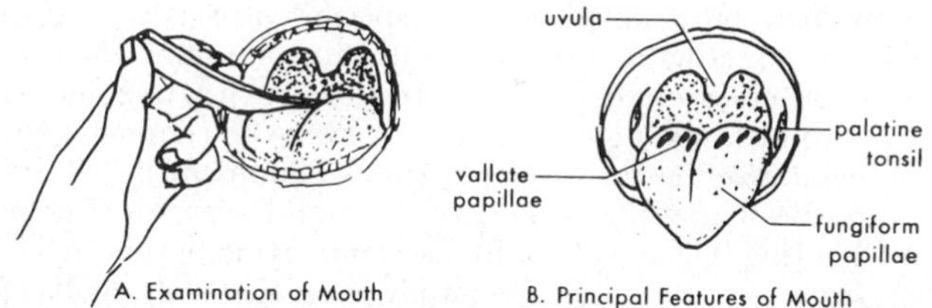

Fig. 5-40. Examination of the oral cavity. **A.** Procedure. *Grasp the tongue blade so the thumb pushes the end upward as a fulcrum while the fingers depress the middle of the blade. The free tip is placed flatly upon the midpoint of the arched tongue when the tip of the tongue is behind the lower incisors. The tongue is pressed downward and forward.* **B.** *Principal anatomic features seen in the oral cavity.*

and with the floor formed by the tongue (Fig. 5-40B). As double portals of the tunnel, the lips and teeth are separated by a shallow *vestibule.* The tunnel's exit is the *isthmus faucium* between the faucial pillars; it opens into a vertical passage, the *oropharynx,* continuous above with the *nasopharynx.*

The anterior two thirds of the roof is formed by the *hard palate,* comprising maxilla and palatine bone covered by mucosa with a median raphe. The *soft palate* continues the roof posteriorly as a fold of mucosa and muscle, hanging free and forming a curtain in the isthmus faucium. From the midline of its free border is suspended the conical or bulbous *uvula.* Laterally, the border of the soft palate splits into two vertical folds, the *pillars of the fauces.* Between the anterior and posterior pillars lies the *palatine tonsil,* a mass of lymphoid tissue containing deep *crypts* or clefts. Similar lymphoid tissue lies in the base of the tongue, the *lingual tonsil.*

Labial Deformity: **Cleft Lip.** In the embryo, incomplete fusion of the frontonasal process with the two maxillary processes leaves a persistent *cleft* in one or both sides of the upper lip. This is incorrectly termed *harelip,* since the rabbit has a midline cleft. Cleft lip is sometimes accompanied by *cleft palate* (see p. 164).

Labial Enlargement. The lips may appear large in cretinism, myxedema, and acromegaly.

Labial Vesicles: **Herpes Simplex** (Cold Sores, Fever Blisters). Groups of vesicles containing clear fluid are surrounded by areas of erythema. Frequently they occur on the lips. The lesions may burn or smart. The specific virus is carried by many adults; it lights up a local inflammation only when the carrier develops another infectious disease, such as pneumonia, cerebrospinal meningitis, malaria, or even the common cold.

Inflamed Labial Corners: **Cheilosis** (Angular Stomatitis). Ulceration of the skin at the corners of the mouth leads to crusting and fissuring (Fig. 5-41A). Often accompanying profuse salivation from any cause, it is specifically associated with riboflavin deficiency or ill-fitting dentures. The entire labial surface may be inflamed from overexposure to sunlight, *actinic cheilosis.*

Local Labial Inflammation: **Carbuncle.** Painful localized swelling, with erythema and increased skin warmth, suggest early cellulitis or carbuncle. When it occurs on the upper lip, this lesion may be exceedingly dangerous, because the venous

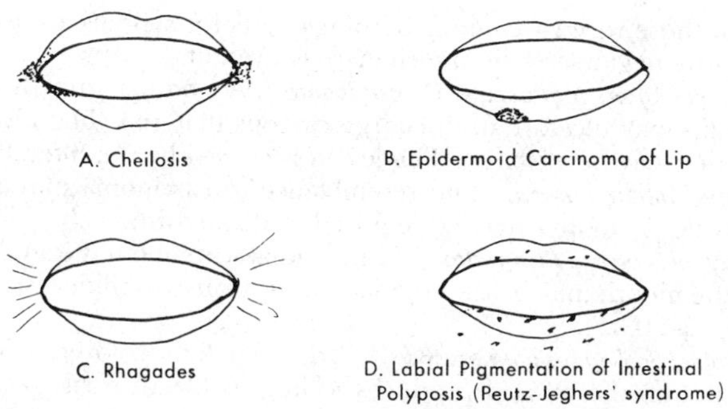

Fig. 5-41. A few lesions of the lips. **A.** Cheilosis. *Maculopapular and vesicular lesions are grouped at the corners of the mouth, on the skin and the mucocutaneous junction.* **B.** Epidermoid carcinoma of lip. *Notice the sharply demarcated elevated edges with the ulcerating base, typically located at the mucocutaneous junction.* **C.** Rhagades. *Linear scars radiating from the lips, especially from the corners of the mouth. These are scars of syphilitic lesions.* **D.** Signs of Peutz-Jeghers' syndrome. *These are blue or black patches of pigmentation in skin or mucosa.*

drainage is into the cavernous sinus, where thrombosis may occur.

Labial Ulcer: ***Epidermoid Carcinoma.*** Early, the lesion is indurated and discoid; later, it becomes warty and crusted, forming a shallow ulcer that slowly extends. The ulcerated border is elevated, sometimes pearly (Fig. 5-41B). The regional lymph nodes are usually involved late; involvement of lymph nodes is less common when the lesion is warty and nonulcerating. More frequent in the male, in 95% of the cases the lesion is on the lower lip. Any ulcer more than two weeks old should be suspected.

Labial Ulcer: ***Chancre.*** The lip is the most common extragenital site of the primary syphilitic lesion; usually the upper lip is involved. The lesion is discoid, without sharply defined borders. Palpation with the *gloved* fingers reveals a plaque that can be moved over the underlying tissues. The lesion soon ulcerates to exude a clear fluid, teeming with *Treponema pallidum,* when examined in the dark-field microscope. The regional lymph nodes are early involved; they feel large and softer than those with carcinoma. Serologic tests for syphilis are frequently negative while the chancre is present.

Labial Ulcer: ***Molluscum Contagiosum.*** A nodular growth in the lip may ulcerate to discharge caseous material. The ulcer border may be elevated. The lesion is caused by the filterable virus *Molitar hominis.* The resemblance to carcinoma may be striking, so biopsy may be required to distinguish.

Labial Scarring: ***Rhagades.*** White radial scars about the angles of the mouth may be the stigmata of previous syphilitic lesions (Fig..5-41C).

Labial Scaling Lesion: ***Keratosis.*** A dry, flat, light-colored lesion occurs on the lip and produces scaling. It bleeds easily when traumatized. It is a precancerous growth.

Labial Pigmentation: ***Intestinal Polyposis*** (Peutz-Jeghers' Syndrome). Multiple pigmented brown to black spots on the lips may resemble freckles, but they are suspect on the mucosa where freckles are uncommon (Fig. 5-41D). The lesions strongly suggest a mendelian-dominant syndrome associated with intestinal polyposis. Their presence may furnish the clue for the cause of gastrointestinal hemorrhage.

The Teeth

Set in the maxilla and mandible, an upper and lower semicircle of teeth approximate at their contact surfaces. The *gums* of tough fibrous tissue and mucosa cover the bony dental ridges and necks of the teeth. The gum borders are called the *gingival margins.*

The child develops 20 *deciduous teeth:* from the midline on either side, uppers and lowers, they are two *incisors,* one *canine,* and a *first* and *second molar.* Gradually, these teeth are lost, to be replaced by *permanent teeth* and the addition of a *first* and *second premolar* or *bicuspid,* and a *third molar,* making a total of 32. The eruption times of various teeth are approximately as follows:

	Deciduous	*Permanent*
1st molars	15–21 months	6 years
Central incisors	6–9 months	7 years
Lateral incisors	15–21 months	8 years
1st premolars	—	9 years

2nd premolars	—	10 years
Canines	16–20 months	11–12 years
2nd molars	20–24 months	12–13 years
3rd molars	—	17–25 years

Absent Teeth: ***Loss or Developmental Failure.*** The absence of teeth should be noted in the record. An insufficient number may seriously impair nutrition.

Absent Tooth with Swelling: ***Odontoma.*** Failure of eruption of a tooth may be caused by a tumor arising from the genetic layers and subsequently produces an unexplained swelling.

Beveled Teeth: ***Worn Teeth.*** The biting surfaces may be worn down by continuous chewing on hard substances, such as a pipe stem.

Widened Interdental Spaces. This may occur congenitally or it may be acquired when the jaw enlarges in a person developing acromegaly.

Eroded Teeth: ***Caries.*** Usually the presence of cavities in the teeth is obvious. Occasionally a postnasal mirror is required to see them.

Darkened Tooth: ***Devitalized Tooth*** (Dead Tooth). When the pulp of the tooth is no longer viable, the enamel appears less white than its companions. The tooth becomes insensitive to cold, as tested by the application of ice.

Pigmented Teeth: ***Fluoride Pits.*** This is a harmless condition found in persons who have ingested large amounts of fluorides in the water.

Notched Teeth: ***Hutchinson's Teeth.*** The *permanent* upper central incisors are misshapen (Fig. 5-42A). They are peg-topped, resembling the frustum of a cone; smaller than normal, their tips are notched. They result from congenital syphilis interfering with the development of the permanent teeth. Notching is one component of *Hutchinson's triad,* together with interstitial keratitis and labyrinthine deafness.

▼ *Key Sign:* ***Bleeding Gums.*** A wide variety of local and general disorders produce bleeding of the gums that prompts the patient to consult physician or dentist.

Clinical Occurrence: LOCAL CAUSES. *Traumatic:* tooth brushing, lacerations, dental caries, tartar on the teeth. *Infections:* pyorrhea alveolaris, actinomycosis, stomatitis (aphthous, ulcerative, Vincent's

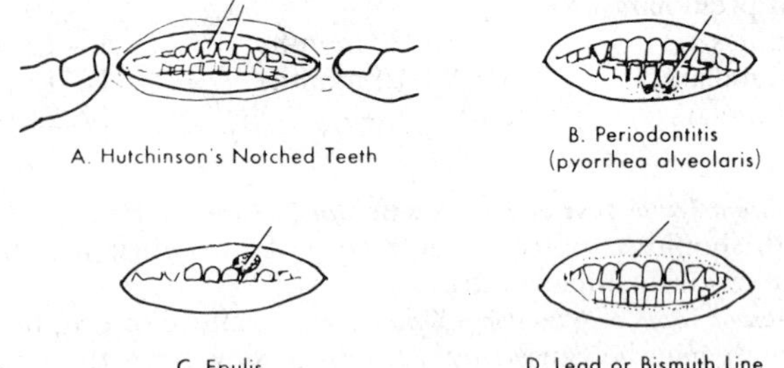

Fig. 5-42. Dental abnormalities. **A.** Hutchinson's notched teeth. *These are stigmas of congenital syphilis. They occur only in the permanent teeth and only the two upper central incisors are involved. The affected teeth are smaller than normal, tapered, and their cutting edges are notched.* **B.** Periodontitis (pyorrhea alveolaris). *In the drawing some of the lower teeth are involved; the gums are retracted and pus is exuding from behind the gingival margins.* **C.** Epulis. *A fibrous tumor arises from the periosteum and emerges from between the teeth. It is sessile, lighter in color than the gums.* **D.** Lead or bismuth line in the gums. *A thin blue line in the gums, about 1 mm from the gingival margin, is visible only when there is also pyorrhea. The metallic deposit appears as a solid line to the unaided eye; with a lens the line is seen to be a series of dots.*

stomatitis), tuberculous gingivitis. *Skin eruptions:* erythema herpetiformis, pemphigus. *Neoplastic:* papilloma of gums, epulis, myeloma, epithelioma.

General Causes. Scurvy, Syphilis. *Blood dyscrasias:* thrombocytopenia from any cause, leukemias, Hodgkin's disease, immune deficiency states, aplastic anemia, hemophilia, Christmas disease. *Metal poisoning:* phosphorus, lead, arsenic, mercury.

Tender Teeth: ***Periapical Abscess*** (Gum Boil). A cause of toothache, abscess in an alveolus may be suspected when the pain is accentuated by tapping the tooth with a tongue blade or probe. Tender swelling occurs in the adjacent gum; a sinus tract may form to drain the pus.

Retracted Gums: ***Recession of the Gums.*** In older persons, the gingival margins may recede to expose the rough lusterless cementum, proximal to the enamel border.

Purulent Gums: ***Periodonitis*** (Pyorrhea Alveolaris). Pockets formed between the teeth and receding gums may become infected and exude pus (Fig. 5-24B). The gingival borders are reddened; pressing the gums against the teeth may express the pus. Anaerobic organisms predominate.

Inflamed Gums: ***Vincent's Stomatitis*** (Trench Mouth, Necrotizing Ulcerative Stomatitis). Inflammation of the gums and adjoining mucosa is attributed to a symbiotic infection with *Borrelia vincentii* and *Fusobacterium plauti-vincenti.* The infection may remain localized in the gums, or it may extend dangerously to involve all pharyngeal structures including bone. On the mucosa, it produces punched-out ulcers, covered with gray-yellow membrane that sometimes must be distinguished from diphtheria by stained smears and bacteriologic culture.

Swollen Gums: ***Scurvy*** (Scorbutus). The gums are deep red or purple; they become swollen, tender, and spongy, so they bleed easily. This is part of the bleeding tendency, along with subperiosteal hemorrhages, that results from ascorbic acid deficiency in scurvy. Purpura may also be present.

Swollen Gums: ***Gingival Hyperplasia.*** The volume of the gums increases so they may overshadow the teeth. Several drugs occasionally induce the condition, notably diphenylhydantoin (Dilantin), the cause for which is unknown. A similar appearance is seen in leukemia, from infiltration with leukocytes, so the dentist first sees the patient.

Mass in Gums: ***Epulis.*** A fibrous tumor of the gum, it arises from the alveolar periosteum and emerges between the teeth as a nodular mass (Fig. 5-42C). It appears as a nontender sessile mass, lighter in color than the gum; rarely, it is pedunculated. A similar tumor, but bright red, is a *fibroangiomatous epulis.*

Mass in Gums: ***Granuloma.*** A mass may occur in the gums spontaneously, or it may result from an ill-fitting denture. It is firm, pink, and nontender; it my break down to form an ulcer.

Blue Gums: ***Lead and Bismuth Lines.*** With chronic exposure to lead (occupational) or bismuth (therapeutic), the heavy metals may be deposited in the gums, forming a blue line about 1 mm from the gingival margin (Fig. 5-42D). Inserting a corner of white paper behind the gingival border aids in seeing the line. A view through a magnifying lens shows the line to be composed of small discrete dots. The deposit does not occur when the teeth are absent, because the lead sulfide is formed only in the presence of bacterial infection.

The Pharynx

▼ *Key Sign:* ***Odor of the Breath.*** Detection of certain odors on the breath is a quick and important diagnostic procedure. Even in man, the olfactory sense is incredibly acute, although many persons profess the inability to smell, or they seem disinterested in trying. Apparently, there is great individual variation in olfactory acuteness. Description of odors is meaningless; the examiner must first smell the properly identified substance before he can recognize it. A foul odor on the breath, *fetor oris,* is common in dental or tonsillar infections, atrophic rhinitis, putrefaction of food in the stomach from pyloric obstruction, infected sputum from bronchiectasis or lung abscess. *Acetone* can be detected on the breath, even when its presence in the urine cannot be shown by usual chemical tests; its presence indicates ketonemia in diabetic or starvation acidosis. In some patients with uremia, *ammonia* is detected on the breath. A curious *musty odor* occasionally is smelled in patients with severe liver disease. *Hydrocyanic acid* is said to impart the odor of bitter almond to the breath of patients who have ingested it. When a person has inhaled *artificial illuminating gas,* the odor is detectable in the exhaled air (natural gas is odorless). *Alcohol* on the breath indicates that the person has been imbibing, but trauma or the ingestion of drugs should not be excluded in explaining the patient's symptoms and signs. Unaccountably, a few patients in coma have no alcoholic odor on the breath when the aspirated gastric contents reek of alcohol. The odor of *paraldehyde,* given as a drug, should be recognized so it will not be confused with other odors. The breath of the chronic alcoholic may reek of acetaldehyde instead of alcohol. When *garlic* is eaten, the methyl mercaptan causing its odor is excreted in the lungs for more than 24 hours. The odor of *chloroform* on the breath can result from use of that anesthetic, or from poisoning with *methylchloroform, used in industry as a substitute for carbon tetrachloride.*

▼ *Key Sign:* **Trismus (Lockjaw).** Trismus is the forceful apposition of the jaws from *spasm* of the masticatory muscles, so failure of the mouth to open from local lesions is not included. The sign is often associated with tetanus, but it has many other causes. The cause is usually found by diagnosing the general condition, but local lesions are more difficult to discover.

Clinical Occurrence: LOCAL DISORDERS. Impacted 3rd molar, arthritis of the temporomandibular joint, trigeminal neuralgia (tic douloureux), scleroderma or dermatomyositis of the face.
DISORDERS WITH WIDESPREAD MUSCLE SPASM. Trichinosis, rabies, tetany, tetanus, strychnine poisoning, typhoid fever, cholera, septicemia. CEREBRAL DISORDERS. Encephalitis, epilepsy (transient), catalepsy, hysteria, malingering.

Etiologic Diagnosis of Acute Pharyngitis. Between 1892, when diphtheria antitoxin was discovered, and 1935, when sulfonamide drugs were introduced to therapeutics, the chief diagnostic problem was to distinguish between diphtheria and nondiphtheritic pharyngitis, for which there was no specific treatment. During this period, the many hospitals in the United States for contagious diseases afforded facilities for physicians to acquire great skill in distinguishing clinically the various pharyngitides. With the advent of sulfonamides and antibiotics, the practical implications of diagnosis changed considerably. Now, the chief problem is to distinguish between bacterial pharyngitis and viral infections for which there is still no specific therapy. But many physicians seem to have abdicated clinical diagnosis in favor of reports from the bacteriologic laboratory. With the current emphasis on testing organisms for antibiotic sensitivity, we have seen house officers confront patients with fever of unknown origin, culture a normal-looking pharynx, and administer antibiotics to which the isolated organisms were found to be sensitive. Accordingly, it seems necessary to recommend the implications of Koch's postulates: acute pharyngitis is the visible bodily reaction to the invasion of microorganisms; without such reaction, there is no disease to treat, regardless of the organisms lying around. In acute pharyngitis, the competent physician will make a diagnosis of the *disease* from the history and physical findings. Should he decide the cause is probably bacterial, he will culture the throat. If treatment is urgently needed, he may elect to begin antibiotic therapy before the bacteriologic report is received; if the pharyngitis appears to be viral, he will probably delay giving antibiotics pending the report on the throat cultures.

Acute Pharyngitis: ***Influenzal Type.*** The patient usually complains of malaise, myalgia, and often of a moderately sore throat and rhinorrhea. Inspection of the oral cavity discloses only swelling of lymphoid tissue in the mucosa of the posterior oropharyngeal wall, as elevated oval islands (Fig. 5-43). The mucosa may be dull red and the faucial pillars slightly edematous. This appearance is often encountered in the mild local epidemics resembling influenza that are attributed to a virus, but never proved. Lymphoid hyperplasia is also present in heavy smokers. This pharyngitis is *not* diphtheria, *not* streptococcal or staphylococcal, unless proved by some means other than throat cultures.

Acute Pharyngitis: ***Streptococcal or Staphylococcal Follicular Pharyngitis.*** The onset is often sudden, pain in the throat is *severe;* the temperature may rise to 103° F (39.5° C) or higher. The pharyngeal mucosa is bright red, swollen, and edematous, especially in the fauces and uvula; it is studded with white or yellow follicles. When the tonsils are present, they are swollen and stippled with more than their quota of follicles. Tender, swollen cervical lymph nodes are common. The picture just described may be caused by either the streptococcus or the staphylococcus. Common before the mysterious decline of *typical* scarlet fever, but still occasionally encountered, is the extremely painful throat with few follicles but brilliant red mucosa in the oropharynx, which extends forward to end abruptly near the

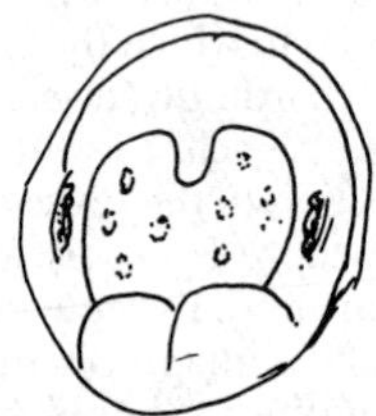

Fig. 5-43. Granular pharyngitis in viral infections. *In the mucosa of the oropharynx islands of lymphoid tissue are elevated. The membranes are only slightly reddened; seldom is there any edema or exudate.*

back of the soft palate and fauces, as if red paint had been applied. This is certainly streptococcal until proved otherwise.

Acute Pharyngitis: ***Pharyngeal Diphtheria.*** The fauces first become dull red and a patch of white membrane appears on the tonsil; in the absence of tonsils, the membrane forms elsewhere. The pharyngeal mucosa becomes reddened, swollen, and edematous. Lifted with tongue blade, the membrane tenaciously holds to the mucosa; when separated, it discloses a bleeding surface. The membrane extends rapidly to involve other structures, while turning gray or yellow. The cervical lymph nodes are enlarged and tender, and the patient appears quite ill with severe constitutional symptoms. The throat is not nearly as sore as follicular pharyngitis. A membrane limited to a tonsil must be distinguished from Vincent's angina (acute necrotizing ulcerative stomatitis); in the latter, the membrane does not extend beyond the tonsil, it is not so tenacious, it is not accompanied by severe constitutional symptoms. A membrane in the pharynx requires quick culturing on media appropriate for the diphtheria bacillus.

Acute Pharyngitis: ***Vincent's Angina*** (Necrotizing Ulcerative Stomatitis). Usually limited to the gums, occasionally, this disease becomes more aggressive and involves the tonsil to form a membrane resembling that of diphtheria. The disease is more locally destructive than diphtheria; an entire tonsil may slough. The membrane covering the ulcer is gray, but more friable than the diphtheritic variety. It rarely overspreads the faucial pillars.

Acute Pharyngitis: ***Infectious Mononucleosis.*** The pharyngitis frequently brings the patient to the physician, but the throat findings do not usually distinguish it from other nonspecific mild infections. Occasionally tonsillar infection produces impressive erythema and exudate, making distinction from streptococcal infection difficult. Disproportionately great enlargement of the cervical lymph nodes may suggest generalized disease, prompting the physician to search for axillary and inguinal lymphadenopathy and splenomegaly. The stained blood smear should be examined for the typical large lymphocytes. Serial tests of the blood serum should be done for a rising titer of anti-sheep-cell (heterophil) antibody over a period of several weeks.

The Tongue

The tongue lies within the horseshoe curve of the mandible, so its dorsal surface forms the floor of the oral cavity. The *tip* or *apex* is thin and narrow, resting against the lingual surface of the lower incisors. Posteriorly and inferiorly is the *root,* composed of muscle masses and their bony attachments. The common word *tongue-shaped* applies only to the visible tip and dorsal surface of the human tongue; like an iceberg, the greater bulk is submerged and is neither thin nor sinuous. Dissection discloses masses of *extrinsic muscles* extending between the symphysis mentis of the mandible, the hyoid bone, and the styloid process of the temporal bone; they cause protrusion and retraction of its tip, convex and concave curving of the dorsum, movements of its root upward and downward. The *intrinsic muscles* alter the length, the width, and the curvature of the dorsal surface. The lingual muscles are innervated by the hypoglossal (12th) nerve.

The tongue is free at its tip, the dorsum, the anteroinferior surface, and the sides (Fig. 5-44A). A midline fold of mucosa underneath, the *lingual frenulum,* attaches the tongue to the floor of the mouth and the lingual surface of the lower gum.

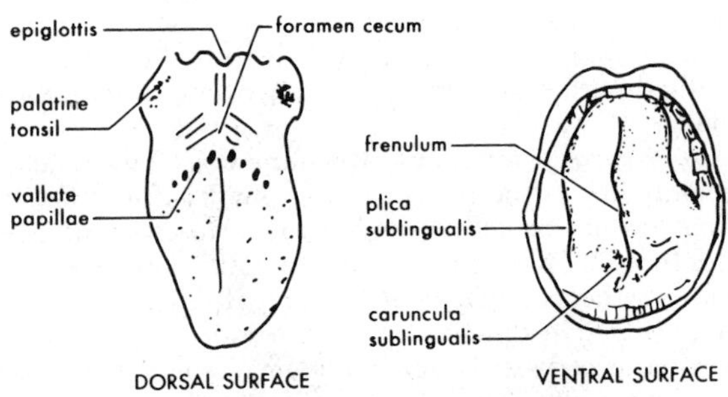

Fig. 5-44. Surfaces of the tongue. *The dorsal surface is depicted from the tip of the epiglottis, showing relations with the palatine tonsils. The ventral surface is viewed from the outside of the mouth. The caruncula sublingualis is at the base of the frenulum; it contains the orifices of the ducts of the submaxillary salivary glands. In the plica sublingualis are some orifices of the sublingual salivary glands.*

Near its base, the frenulum swells to form twin eminences, the *caruncula sublingualis,* each surmounted by the orifice of the submaxillary duct (Wharton's). Running from the caruncu-lae laterally and posteriorly around the base of the tongue is a ridge of mucosa, the *plica sublingualis,* punctured at intervals by orifices of minor ducts from the sublingual gland, lying deep to the ridges.

The dorsum of the tongue extends from its tip to the epiglottis. The *median sulcus* bisects the dorsum from tip to the posterior third, where it ends in the depressed *foramen cecum,* the closure site of the embryonal thyroglossal duct. A *sulcus terminalis* extends forward and lateral from either side of the foramen cecum to form a V with its apex posterior. Slightly anterior and parallel is another V formed by a row of eight to twelve *papillae vallatae.* The vallate papillae are round discrete eminences with concentric fossae. The anterior two thirds of the dorsum linguae is textured like velvet by the protrusion of microscopic *papillae filiformes* that catch desquamated cells, bacteria, and particles of food that form the coating of the normal tongue. Scattered among the filiform papillae, at the apex and sides of the tongue, are the less numerous *papillae fungiformes.* They are readily seen with the unaided eye as large, raised, rounded, and deeper red. Microscopic taste buds are numerous in the vallate and fungiform papillae on the sides and back part of the tongue, in the soft palate and the posterior surface of the epiglottis. The sensory root of the facial (7th) nerve, through the chorda tympani, supplies the taste buds in the anterior two thirds of the tongue. The posterior third is served by the glossopharyngeal (9th) nerve.

▼ *Key Symptom:* ***Thirst.*** The mechanism of thirst is unknown and its diagnostic significance is often uncertain. But the sudden development of thirst is a reliable indication of *dehydration* when it appears with hemorrhage, traumatic shock, the polyuria of diabetes insipidus, and some cases of severe electrolyte or fluid imbalance. It cannot be relied upon to indicate hyponatremia or hypokalemia.

▼ *Key Symptom:* ***Soreness of Tongue or Mouth.*** Pain or tenderness in the tongue or mouth causes such discomfort that it is frequently the presenting symptom for a number of disorders that require a differential diagnosis.

Clinical Occurrence: BURNING TONGUE WITH NO LESIONS: tobacco smoking, early glossitis from all causes, menopausal symptom, heavy metal poisoning.

PAIN IN THE TONGUE FROM DEEP LESIONS: calculus in duct of submaxillary or sublingual gland, foreign body, myositis of lingual muscles, trichinosis, periostitis of hyoid bone, neoplasm of lingual muscles.

PAIN FROM LOCALIZED SUPERFICIAL LESIONS: biting the tongue, trauma to lingual frenulum, dental ulcer, injury from mouth gag while under anesthesia, foreign body such as fish bone, epithelioma or carcinoma, ranula, tuberculous ulcer, herpes. Vincent's stomatitis, leukoplakia, candida.

PAIN FROM GENERALIZED DISEASE: pellagra, riboflavin deficiency, scurvy, atrophic glossitis, leukemia, erythematous disorders, collagen diseases, lichen planus, scarlet fever, heavy metal poisoning, diphenylhydantoin (Dilantin) medication, uremia, antiobiotic sensitivity.

PAIN FROM IRRADIATION: Therapeutic irradiation for head and neck malignancy causes temporary or permanent loss of saliva production. Within two to four weeks of the beginning of treatment and lasting six or more weeks, patients experience increasing dryness and generalized soreness of the mouth and throat.

Dry Tongue Without Longitudinal Furrows. The lingual surface may be dry from mouth-breathing or lack of saliva (xerostomia) in Sjögren's syndrome and irradiation. But the volume of the tongue remains normal, so no longitudinal furrows develop.

Dry Tongue with Longitudinal Furrows. This is the most reliable physical sign of *general dehydration*. Longitudinal furrows develop in the lingual surface from reduction of volume of the tongue. In adults, this occurs regularly with a deficit of 3 liters of extracellular fluid. This degree of dehydration is always accompanied by *loss of skin turgor,* but the latter also occurs in senile cutaneous atrophy or recent loss of body tissue.

Lingual Enlargement. The tongue is enlarged in Down's syndrome, cretinism, and adult myxedema. It increases in size during the development of acromegaly and amyloidosis. Transient swelling occurs with glossitis, stomatitis, and cellulitis of the neck. Occlusions of the lymphatics by carcinoma and obstruction of the superior vena cava often produce enlargement. Transiently, it may be the site of angioneurotic edema, hematoma, or abscess.

Lingual Tremor. A fine tremor of the tongue is often present in thyrotoxicosis. A coarser tremor is frequently seen in nervous persons; it also occurs in alcoholism, paresis, and drug addiction. It may be the accompaniment of debilitating disease of any sort.

Limited Lingual Protrusion: ***Shortened Frenulum*** (Tongue-Tie). A congenitally short frenulum linguae not only limits protrusion, but the patient is unable to place the tip in the roof of the mouth.

Limited Lingual Protrusion: ***Carcinoma.*** Infiltration of the lingual muscles with neoplasm may limit protrusion of the tongue. The history assists in the diagnosis because this is an acquired disability. Inspection usually reveals an ulcerated whitish lesion that is hard on palpation compared with the surrounding muscle. A firm nontender nodule in the base of the tongue may not be visually impressive, but it can represent squamous carcinoma. Palpation of the tongue discloses the buried neoplasm.

Lingual Deviation: ***Paralysis of the Hypoglossal (12th) Nerve.*** During protrusion, the tongue deviates toward the paralyzed atrophic side, because normal movement depends on the balanced action of the bilateral muscle groups (Fig. 5-45). The two halves of the tongue are grossly of unequal size because of the muscle atrophy induced by the paralysis. The condition can be distinguished from carcinoma because it has no palpable mass.

Lingual Deviation: ***Unilateral Carcinoma.*** A neoplasm on one side may hinder contraction of the muscles on that side. Palpation discloses the mass.

Lingual Fissures: ***Congenital Furrows*** (Scrotal Tongue). The median sulcus is deepened, the dorsal surface is interrupted by deep *transverse* furrows (Fig. 5-46A). This is a harmless condition, frequently inherited. It must be distinguished from the *longitudinal* furrowing in syphilitic glossitis.

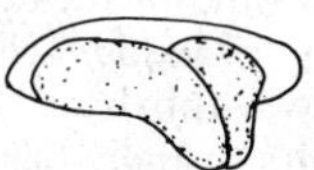

Fig. 5-45. Paralysis of the left side of the tongue. *Protrusion of the tongue depends upon tensing the two lateral muscle bundles; paralysis of one bundle causes the tongue to deviate to the paralyzed side.*

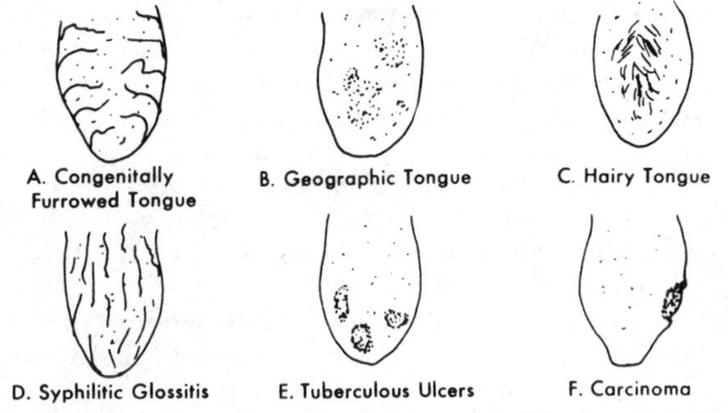

Fig. 5-46. Patterns on the lingual surface. **A.** *The congenitally furrowed tongue contains deep transverse furrows that are not inflamed. This must be distinguished from the furrows of syphilitic glossitis that are chiefly longitudinal.* **B.** *Geographic tongue contains irregular patches of denuded epithelium that show red against the normal coat. The patches heal in a few days and are succeeded by new ones in other areas.* **C.** *Hairy tongue appears to support a patch of black hairs that are actually overgrowths of mold hyphae in the coating; they appear especially during antibiotic treatment.* **D.** *The furrows of syphilitic glossitis are mainly longitudinal and deeper than the congenital type.* **E.** *Tuberculous ulcers are indolent lesions without much surrounding inflammation.* **F.** *A typical location of carcinoma of the tongue is on the lateral edge. The lesion ulcerates and produces elevated borders.*

Lingual Fissures: ***Syphilitic Glossitis.*** The fissures are mainly *longitudinal,* and the intervening epithelium is desquamated (Fig. 5-46D).

Lingual Coat: ***Geographic Tongue*** (Migratory Glossitis, Glossitis Areata Exfoliativa). The normal lingual coating is studied with circular areas of bright red denuded epithelium, surrounded by rings of light yellow piled-up cells (Fig. 5-46B). The pattern changes within a few days; the denuded areas are restored to normal, and new territory is involved. This is a harmless condition of unknown cause.

Lingual Coat: ***Hairy Tongue*** (Furry Tongue, Black Tongue). The distal two thirds of the dorsum looks as if it were growing short hairs, usually black (Fig. 5-46C). The appearance is imparted by hyperplasia of the filiform papillae entangled with an overgrowth of mycelial threads of *Aspergillus niger* or *Candida albicans.* The condition is symptomless. Occasionally the color is green, either from the fungus or because the patient is chewing gum containing chlorophyll. Formerly, the finding was restricted to debilitated patients; now it often appears during treatment with antibiotics that inhibit the growth of normal bacteria and permit overgrowth of fungi.

Smooth Tongue: ***Atrophic Glossitis.*** The patient may complain of dryness of the tongue; intermittent burning, and paresthesias of taste. The tongue becomes smaller, its surface *slick* and *glistening*, mucosa thinned. The color may be *pink* or *red*, depending upon the hemoglobin concentration in the blood and the amount of local inflammation. In the advanced stages there are considerable pain and swelling. The color is red or blue-red with atrophied hyperemic papillae that appear as *small punctate red dots*. *Laboratory Findings:* Hypochlorhydria or achlorhydria, macrocytic megaloblastic anemia (except in iron deficiency). *Distinction:* The diagnosis is confirmed by therapeutic tests.

Clinical Occurrence. *Deficiency of* B_{12}: pernicious anemia, postgastrectomy syndrome, blind intestinal loop, extreme vegetarian diets, infestation with fish tapeworm (*Diphyllobothrium latum*). *Folic acid deficiency:* megaloblastic anemia of pregnancy, megaloblastic anemia refractory to B_{12} administration, megaloblastic anemia in hepatic cirrhosis. Iron deficiency anemia. Idiopathic gastritis. Mixed B-complex deficiency. Unknown causes.

Red Tongue: ***Nonspecific Glossitis.*** Localized infections of the pharynx may also involve the tongue, producing redness and swelling. The tongue may burn and feel tender.

Red Tongue: ***Strawberry Tongue*** (Raspberry Tongue). Notably in scarlet fever, occasionally in other diseases involving a toxin, the lingual papillae become swollen and reddened. According to Osler, some writers gave the name *strawberry tongue* to the stage in which the inflamed and hyperplastic papillae show through the white coat. Later, the epithelium desquamates, carrying away the coat and leaving a fiery red denuded surface surmounted by hyperplastic papillae; this has also been termed a strawberry tongue, but others prefer the more accurately descriptive term *raspberry tongue*. During the desquamated period, the sense of taste is diminished.

Red Tongue: ***Pellagrous Glossitis.*** In the early stages, the patient complains of burning tongue when in contact with hot or spicy foods, but no signs are visible. Later, the burning is constant; diarrhea, mental confusion, and dermatitis may appear (the 3 Ds, if one calls the mental disorder *delirium*). The tongue becomes reddened at the tip and borders; later the erythema spreads and the tongue swells. The surface is denuded to present a fiery-red mucosa with ulcerations and indentations from the teeth. During remission, the lingual surface is pallid and atrophied. A therapeutic test confirms the diagnosis; the oral administration of 100 mg of niacin will cause disappearance of the erythema and burning within 24 to 48 hours.

Magenta Cobblestone Tongue: ***Riboflavin Deficiency.*** Burning of the tongue is relatively mild; more discomfort is caused by the lesions of the lips and eyes. Swollen hyperemic fungiform and filiform papillae produce rows of reddened elevations that suggest the name *cobblestone tongue.* Edema at the bases of the papillae modifies the color to magenta, in contrast to the fiery red of the pellagrous tongue in which the epithelium is denuded. Associated with the lingual lesions, and often without them, are the *cheilosis* and *angular stomatitis.* The first sign of these is a painless gray papule at one or both corners of the mouth. The papule enlarges and ulcerates to produce indolent fissures with piled-up yellow crusts, leaving permanent scars. Similar lesions may occur at the ocular canthi and the nasolabial folds; the sebaceous glands in the nose become hyperplastic. Superficial keratitis and conjunctival injection are common.

Smooth Burning Tongue: ***Menopausal Glossitis.*** Intense burning of the tongue and slight atrophy of the lingual mucosa often occur at the menopause. They are ascribed to the same mechanism that causes senile vaginitis. The symptoms and signs are improved when estrogens are administered.

White Lingual Patches: ***Leukoplakia.*** In the early stages, one or more areas on the dorsal surface are affected by obliteration of the papillae with thin white lesions that are wrinkled and sometimes pearly (Fig. 5-47A). Early lesions coalesce; as they persist and enlarge they become chalk white and thick and are palpable as a more firm nodule than the compliant adjacent mucosa. They often occur at the site of chronic irritation from ill-fitting dentures or a snuff smokeless tobacco. They are precancerous, and biopsy is indicated to ascertain whether invasion has occurred.

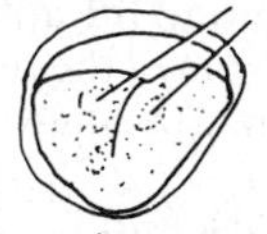

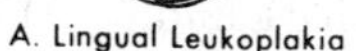

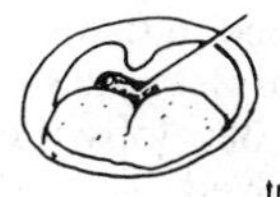

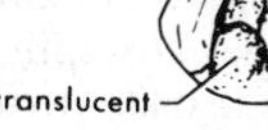

Fig. 5-47. Lesions of the tongue. **A.** Lingual leukoplakia. *In the early stages, the areas are thin and white, often wrinkled or pearly; they obliterate the papillae. Later, the lesions coalesce, thicken, and become chalk-white. In advanced stages, they look like dried cracked white paint.* **B.** Lingual thyroid. *A round, smooth, red mass at the base of the tongue, near the foramen cecum, may be a lingual thyroid arising from the remnants of the thyroglossal duct. Consider the possibility before attempting biopsy.* **C.** Ranula. *This is a translucent cyst of a sublingual or submaxillary salivary gland. It is readily distinguished by its location. The extent may be palpated in the root of the tongue.*

White Lingual Patches: ***Lichen Planus.*** The lesions are thin, bluish white spiderweb lines that may resemble leukoplakia. Circumscribed areas of flattened papules on the flexor surfaces of the wrists and the middle of the shins strengthen the diagnosis of lichen planus.

EXAMINATION OF A LINGUAL ULCER. **Dry off the ulcer by pressing it gently with a cotton sponge. Then inspect it carefully. Palpate the surrounding and underlying tissue with *gloved* fingers (you may be dealing with a chancre). Remember that the pain from lingual lesions may be referred to the ear.**

Lingual Ulcer: ***Aphthous Ulcer*** (Canker Sore). A few small vesicles appear in crops on the tip and sides of the tongue, and on the labial and buccal mucosa. When viewed, the vesicular covering has usually been wiped off, so the lesion appears as a painful, small, round ulcer with white floor and yellow margins, surrounded by a narrow erythematous areola. The cause is variously ascribed to herpes simplex, to food allergy, or to emotional stress.

Chronic Oral Ulcerations: ***Behçet's Syndrome*** (see p. 893).

Lingual Ulcer: ***Chancre.*** A syphilitic primary lesion on the tongue is rare; it usually occurs on the tip. Starting as a small pustule, the top soon ruptures to form an ulcer. When examined with the *gloved* finger, its base is indurated, feeling like a small button embedded in tissue. In contrast to the aphthous ulcer, it is not very painful. Painless enlargement of the regional lymph nodes promptly develops; the submental or submaxillary nodes are usually involved.

Lingual Ulcer: ***Mucous Patches*** (Condyloma Latum). This is the common lesion of secondary syphilis, occurring on the tongue, the buccal and labial mucosa, regardless of the site of the primary lesion in the body. The patches are round or oval, 5 to 10 mm in diameter, slightly raised, and covered by gray membrane. They may ulcerate slightly. Palpated with *gloved* fingers, they feel indurated. They are painless. Regional lymphadenopathy occurs.

Lingual Ulcer: ***Gumma.*** Beginning as a painless nodule in the anterior two thirds of the tongue, the lesion occurs in the dorsal *midline,* whereas carcinoma is usually on the side, base, or ventral surface. When the mass ulcerates, it forms a *punched-out area* with *little induration;* carcinoma forms an ulcer with rolled-up margins and much induration. A syphilitic serologic reaction does not prove the diagnosis of gumma because carcinoma might exist coincidentally with syphilis.

Lingual Ulcer: ***Dental Ulcer.*** Always on the sides or undersurface of the tongue, the ulcer results from irritation of a projecting tooth or an ill-fitting denture. Frequently, the ulcer is *elongated* from trauma; its base is sloughing, its borders erythematous. The ulcer margin may be elevated and surrounded by induration, suggesting carcinoma. Removal of the irritating surface should result in a trend toward healing in a few weeks. Lacking improvement, biopsy is indicated.

Lingual Ulcer: ***Tuberculosis.*** A rare lingual lesion, it is nearly always associated with pulmonary tuberculosis. One or more nodules occur on the *tip* of the tongue or on its anterior sides (Fig. 5-46E). Characteristically, the lesions are *extremely painful.* Later, the nodules ulcerate, forming bases with gray membranes; the margins may overhang slightly. An x-ray film of the chest should be taken to search for pulmonary lesions. Biopsy may be necessary.

Lingual Ulcer: ***Carcinoma.*** The sites of predilection for carcinoma are the sides, the base, and the undersurface of the tongue (Fig. 5-46F). The disease usually appears as an ulcer with *rolled and everted margins,* viewed best when dried. Palpation of the region discloses a discrete firm mass with some surrounding induration. It is not tender unless ulcerated. Inspection and palpation are the keys for establishing the diagnosis, although pain from the ulcer while drinking acidic or alcoholic beverages should arouse suspicion. If no lesions are visible, yet the patient complains of lingual discomfort or dysphagia, or if the tongue does not readily protrude, *palpate the root* of the tongue. *Also feel* the submental, submandibular, and deep cervical lymph nodes.

Posterior Lingual Mass: ***Lingual Thyroid.*** Since aberrant thyroid tissue can occur anywhere in the course of the thyroglossal duct, always consider the possibility that a mass near the foramen cecum may be lingual thyroid (Fig. 5-47B). A lingual goiter is sessile, moderately firm, and nontender; it does not ulcerate. Before attempting to biopsy such a mass, have its uptake of radioiodine tested. It may be the only thyroid tissue in the body.

Sublingual Mass: ***Ranula.*** Hippocrates used the Greek word for "little frog" to describe this lesion, because it looks like a frog's belly. This is a cyst of the sublingual or submaxillary salivary gland, caused by obstruction of the duct. When the tongue is raised, a *translucent* mass is seen beside the frenulum linguae (Fig. 5-47C). The swelling may extend to the other side behind the frenulum. Transillumination of the mass may show the submaxillary (Wharton's) duct traversing the upper part of the cyst. With one forefinger in the mouth and the other outside in the submandibular region, palpate to determine the extension of the mass to the submaxillary gland.

Sublingual Mass: ***Dermoid Cyst.*** This is an *opaque* cyst; when superficial, it may be seen to be white. It may occur behind the frenulum or beside it (Fig. 5-49A). Bimanual palpation in the floor of the mouth and outside in the submandibular region will assist in demonstrating fluctuation and in assessing the size of the mass.

PALPATION OF THE ROOF OF THE TONGUE. **If the patient gags readily, spray the throat with a topical anesthetic: otherwise, proceed without anesthesia. Put the right hand in a rubber glove. Have the patient open his mouth wide (Fig. 5-48). From the outside, with your left fingers push a fold of the patient's right cheek between his teeth, to avoid having your fingers bitten. Insert your gloved right forefinger to the back of the mouth, and palpate the root of the tongue and the valleculae, and the tonsillar fossae.**

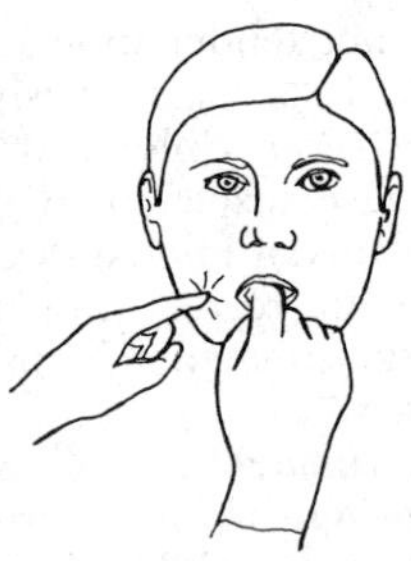

Fig. 5-48. Palpation of the roof of the tonuge. *Insert the gloved index finger into the mouth to feel the posterior portion of the tongue. To avoid being bitten, use the other index finger to press the patient's cheek between his teeth so he bites it if he attempts to close his jaws.*

Sublingual Mass: ***Carcinoma.*** In the floor of the mouth, the patient soon discovers a carcinoma because it is more sensitive to food and beverages contacting it. Ulceration exposes afferent pain fiber endings, and tongue motion may also cause discomfort. Secondary infection is common. It may begin as a leukoplakic area, but ulceration and a palpably discrete mass strongly suggest carcinoma. Extension to the mandible with loss of mobility of the mass occurs early, as do metastases to submental or anterior jugular lymph nodes.

Buccal Pigmentation: ***Addison's Disease*** (Chronic Adrenal Insufficiency). Small patches of pigment in the buccal mucosa are common in Blacks and other darkly pigmented races. In Caucasians, however, dappled brown pigment in the lining of the cheek *strongly suggests.* Addison's disease, or the intestinal polyposis of Peutz-Jehgers.

Buccal Mass: ***Retention Cyst.*** A mucous gland anywhere in the buccal surface may be obstructed to produce a *blue-domed translucent* cyst.

Buccal Ulcer: ***Aphthous Ulcer.*** This is similar to those of the tongue (p. 159).

Buccal White Spots: ***Mucosal Sebaceous Cysts*** (Fordyce's Spots). These appear in the mucosa of the lips, cheeks, and tongue as isolated white or yellow spots, less than a millimeter in diameter, sometimes slightly raised. They are painless and harmless. Often a bit of white sebum may be expressed from the lesion.

Buccal White Spots: ***Koplik's Spots in Measles.*** One or two days before the appearance of the exanthem in measles (morbilli), small white spots appear opposite the molars and sometimes elsewhere on the buccal mucosa (Fig. 5-49B). Each is surrounded by a narrow red areola. They are pathognomonic of measles and forecast the appearance of the rash.

Reddened Parotid Duct Orifice: ***Mumps.*** The orifice of the parotid (Stensen's) duct, in the buccal mucosa opposite the upper 2nd molar, may become reddened in mumps or acute parotitis from other causes.

Bony Palatine Protuberance: ***Torus.*** Often, as an anatomic variation, a bony knob or ridge occurs in the midline of the hard palate (Fig. 5-49C). It has no clinical significance.

Palatine Mass: ***Carcinoma.*** The epithelium of the hard and soft palate can be the site of carcinoma with typical findings, noted elsewhere.

Palatine Mass: ***Mixed Tumor of Ectopic Salivary Gland.*** This occurs in the soft or hard palate. Unless noticed accidentally, it is silent until ulceration causes pain. It may invade the base of the skull.

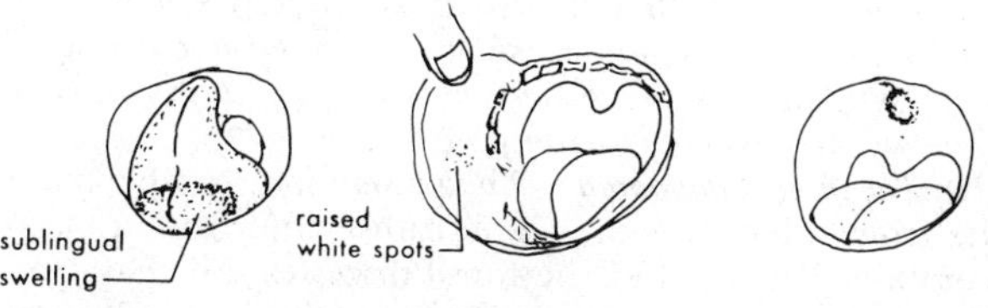

Fig. 5-49. Various lesions of the oral cavity. **A.** Sublingual dermoid cyst. *An opaque fluctuant mass, this often appears white through the mucosa. It occurs either behind or beside the frenulum of the tongue.* **B.** Koplik's spots in measles. *Small white spots form on the buccal mucosa opposite the molars. They antedate the exanthem of measles (morbilli) by 1 or 2 days, so they are the earliest diagnostic sign of the disease.* **C.** Torus palantinus. *A bony protuberance in the midline of the roof of the hard palate; it is a harmless variant in development.*

Arched Palate. There are many causes for high-arched palate. The condition has become associated with arachnodactyly and Turner's syndrome, so these possibilities should be considered.

Cleft Palate. A midline opening in the hard palate is a congenital failure of fusion of the maxillary processes. It is usually associated with cleft lip (p. 142) but also occurs in isolation. Its severity varies from a complete cleft of the entire soft and hard palate, including the alveolar ridge, to a partial cleft of the soft palate alone. A submucous cleft in which only the underlying muscle is deficient is suggested by a bifid uvula.

Palatine Perforation. Tertiary syphilis is a common cause of a hole in the hard palate, but the deformity can result from radiation therapy or from postoperative breakdown after surgical repair of cleft palate.

Tonsillar Enlargement: ***Hyperplasia.*** The normal adult tonsils seldom protrude beyond the faucial pillars; they are larger in children, shrinking when puberty is attained. For adequate examination, take a tongue blade in each hand; depress the tongue with one and retract the anterior faucial pillar laterally with the other, to disclose the anterior tonsillar surface. Normally, the color of the tonsil matches the surrounding mucosa; its surface is interrupted with deep clefts or crypts that may contain white or yellow debris whose presence is not a sign of infection. Hyperplasia is usually attributed to chronic infection, but it may be associated with obesity or thyrotoxicosis. Hyperplasia is usually bilateral.

Tonsillar Ulcer: ***Carcinoma.*** The patient may complain of earache from referred pain. The breath is foul from a bleeding ulceration. Palpation of the tonsil discloses the characteristic induration.

Tonsillar Swelling: ***Peritonsillar Abscess*** (Quinsy). The affected side of the pharynx is very painful. Opening the mouth is always limited and may be difficult because of muscle spasm, *trismus.* When the abscess is *anterior,* between the tonsil and the anterior faucial pillar, the anterior bulging is easily seen: the swelling also displaces the uvula to the opposite side (Fig. 5-50A). The adjacent soft palate is edematous and bulging. In the less common *posterior* abscess, the tonsil is pushed forward and much of the swelling is hidden from direct vision. Earache is a distinguishing feature. Surgical drainage is necessary.

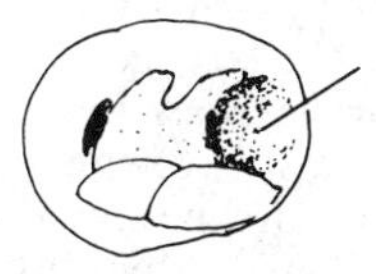

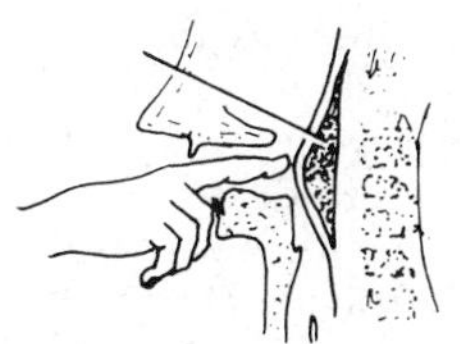

Fig. 5-50. Various lesions of the oral cavity. **A.** Peritonsillar abscess (quinsy). *Usually the abscess occurs between the palatine tonsil and the anterior faucial pillar, so the swelling pushes the tonsil medially, displacing the uvula to the opposite side. Much edema surrounds the swelling. When the abscess is posterior to the tonsil, the tonsil is pushed forward, and earache accompanies the sore throat.* **B.** Palpation of a retropharyngeal abscess. *The sagittal section shows the relation of the abscess to the palpating finger. The finger feels a boggy indentable mass as it presses against the anterior surfaces of the vertebral bodies.*

Posttonsillar Swelling: ***Retropharyngeal Abscess.*** An accumulation of pus occurs in the space between the pharynx and the prevertebral fascia. If the swelling is in the oropharynx, it may be seen directly through the mouth with the tongue depressed as an anterior swelling of the posterior pharyngeal wall. In the nasopharynx, or opposite the larynx, it is never directly visible. The condition should be suggested when nose breathing is impaired (usually attributed to adenoids) or in laryngeal respiratory distress or difficulty in swallowing. The abscess is only demonstrated by *palpation* (Fig. 5-50B). The palpating finger can feel the unilateral swelling that is soft and indentable. It usually occurs in children less than five years, and urgent surgical drainage is necessary because of the risk of airway obstruction by the expanding mass.

Edema of the Uvula. When one encounters edema of the uvula together with bronchitis, asthma, and rhinopharyngitis, one should suspect the patient of recent heavy smoking of hashish. More commonly, localized edema of the uvula represents angioneurotic edema from a topical allergic reaction.

The Larynx

The larynx is immediately behind and below the oral cavity, so in many persons the epiglottic tip is directly visible through the mouth. Since the larynx is on the *anterior* wall of the pharynx with the sloping plane of its rim facing *posteriorly,* it is viewed in the laryngeal mirror held *behind* it. The laryngeal apparatus may be considered a series of three parallel rings, held together by ligaments. Above is the arched *hyoid bone,* opening posteriorly. Suspended from it by ligaments, the arched *thyroid cartilage* also opens posteriorly. The ligaments from the thyroid cartilage uphold the *cricoid cartilage,* a complete ring affixed to the tracheal rings below. Although these structures are practically subcutaneous and palpable in the neck, their openings are posterior and well protected.

The essential mechanism of the larynx depends upon the shape, position, and action of the two *arytenoid cartilages* (Fig. 5-51). Each is a three-sided pyramid with a triangular base. The base is slightly concave to glide on a convex joint surface on the posterior rim of the cricoid cartilage, the *cricoarytenoid joint,* surrounded by a capsule. The two pyramids stand erect on either side of the midline of the cricoid. Appropriate muscles pull on the various faces of the pyramids, causing their bases to rotate in the joints. The apex of each pyramid is surmounted by a horizontal crescent of small cartilages and ligaments, pointing medially toward its opposite and curving anteriorly. From the curve of each crescent, a tough fibroelastic band, the *true vocal cord* (vocal fold), extends forward to the midline of the thyroid cartilage. The two vocal cords thus form an opening into the trachea, the *rima glottidis.* When open, the rima is an isosceles triangle, with apex anterior beneath the epiglottis, and base posterior, formed by the tissue bridge between the two arytenoid crescents. Rotation of the arytenoids brings the legs of the triangle together posteriorly to approximate the cords over their entire length.

Lateral, parallel to, and above the true cords is a pair of tissue folds, the *false vocal cords* (ventricular folds). A membrane covers the epiglottis and continues around posteriorly to envelop the crescents of the arytenoids, forming the *aryepiglottic folds.* Since the larynx protrudes slightly from the anterior pharyngeal wall, several pockets are formed: two *valleculae* between the epiglottis and the base of the tongue; two *piriform sinuses,* one on either side of the cricoid. Most of the intrinsic muscles of the larynx are supplied by fibers of the recurrent laryngeal nerve, a branch of the vagus (10th) nerve.

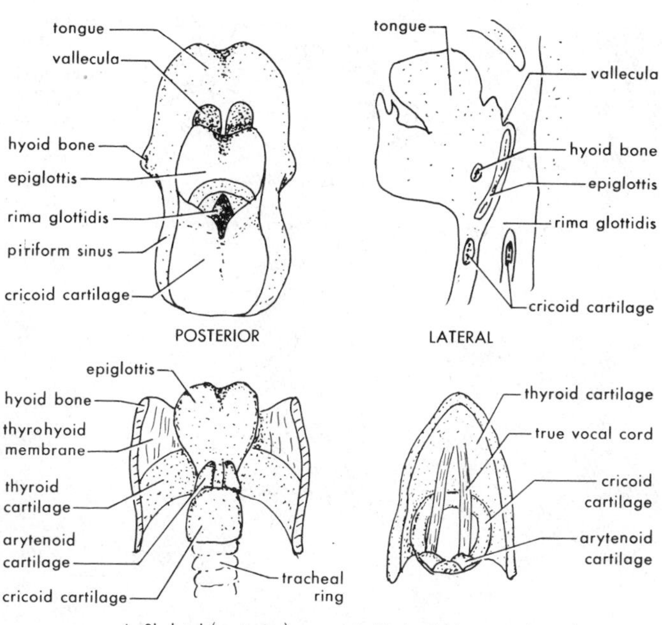

Fig. 5-51. Anatomy of the larynx. *In reviewing the various anatomic facts, it is important to realize that the larynx faces posteriorly so it is seen by inserting the mirror in a position back of the plane of the vocal cords. The arytenoid cartilages are little pyramids that are perched upon the cricoid cartilage to which they are connected by true joints that become the site of joint disease. Notice that the movement of the pyramidal cricoid cartilages is by twisting their bases to vary the tension on the vocal cords.*

MIRROR LARYNGOSCOPY. **Seat the patient in a chair with a clear 150-watt electric lamp immediately behind his head and to his right. Reflect this light with your head mirror, because both your hands must be free. Have the patient sit quite erect with the chin somewhat forward, both feet on the floor, knees together. Seat yourself in front of him with your knees outside his. Explain exactly what you are about to do and have him concentrate on breathing softly and regularly *through the mouth* (Fig. 5-52A). Have the tongue protruded maximally over the lower teeth; with your left hand, wrap a piece**

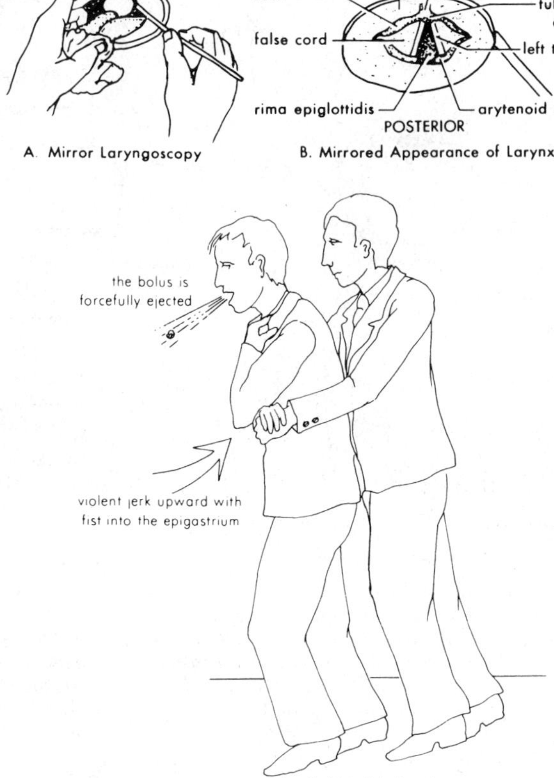

Fig. 5-52. Mirror laryngoscopy. **A.** Method of laryngoscopy. *Have the patient breathe regularly through the mouth. Wrap the protruding tongue with gauze and grasp it with your left thumb and long finger, steadying the hand with the index finger against the patient's cheek. With your right hand grasp the handle of the laryngeal mirror (no. 5, large) like a pencil. After the mirror has been warmed by immersion in warm water or heated in an alcohol flame, touch the back of the mirror to your wrist to ascertain that the temperature is tolerable. Then insert the mirror carefully into the left side of the patient's mouth,*

of gauze over the tongue, grasp the wrapped portion with thumb and middle finger, bracing your hand against his upper teeth with the forefinger; pull the tongue gently to his right side. With thumb and forefinger of your right hand, grasp a No. 5 (large) laryngeal mirror at the midpoint of its handle. Heat the mirror over an alcohol flame or in warm water to avoid subsequent steaming over, test the temperature by touching the mirror back to your left wrist. Holding the handle like a pencil, bracing your hand against his cheek by your fourth and fifth fingers, insert the mirror in his mouth from his left side, with the face of the mirror downward and parallel to the tongue surface. Move it posteriorly until its back rests against the anterior surface of the uvula. Press the uvula and soft palate steadily upward; avoid touching the back of the tongue to prevent gagging. Have the patient breathe steadily while you inspect the larynx. While still viewing the vocal cords, ask the patient to say "e-e-e" or "he-e-e" in a high-pitched voice. Sing along with him in the desired pitch and for the proper duration. When looking in the mirror, remember that upward is anterior, downward is posterior. Examine the *vallate papillae*, the *lingual tonsils*, the *valleculae*, the *epiglottis* (Fig. 5-52B). Then look at the *false cords*, the *true vocal cords*, the *arytenoids*, the *piriform sinuses*. Finally, observe the true vocal cords during *quiet respiration* when the rima is tent-shaped. *During phonation*, watch the cords meet in the midline.

▼ *Key Sign:* ***Hoarseness.*** More than all other signs, hoarseness focuses attention directly upon the larynx. A multitude of disorders exhibit this sign.

Clinical Occurrence: RECENT ONSET. *Overuse:* shouting, cheering. *Infections:* upper respiratory infections, diphtheria, smallpox, measles. *Drugs:* atropine-like drugs (dryness), strychnine (laryngeal spasm), aspiration of aspirin (chemical burn), potassium iodide

---

steadying your hand by resting the ring and little fingers against his cheek. Face the mirror downward and edge it over the arched tongue, gently pushing the uvula and soft palate backward and upward. Focus the light from your head mirror onto the laryngeal mirror and have the patient repeat after you "e-e-e" or "he-e-e"; you set the example for the timing and the high pitch. **B.** Appearance of the larynx in the mirror. *This is the appearance with the cords abducted.* **C.** Heimlich maneuver for choking on food. *From the subject's back encircle his waist with your arms. Grasp your fist with the other hand and give it a sudden forceful jerk that thrusts the fist upward into the subject's epigastrium. Repeat, until the obstructing bolus is forcefully expelled from the throat.*

(edema of cords), uremia (edema of cords). Angioneurotic edema. Insect bites (edema). Foreign body. *Laryngeal spasm:* croup, tetany, tetanus, tabetic crisis. *Burns:* inhalation of irritant gases, swallowing of hot or caustic liquids. *Onset of all chronic conditions.*

CHRONIC COURSE. *Occupational overuse:* in clergymen, orators, singers, teachers. Foreign body. *Lack of mucus:* Sjögren's disease (keratoconjunctivitis sicca). *Chronic inflammation of cords:* nonspecific chronic laryngitis, alcoholism, gout, tobacco smoking. *Edema of cords:* myxedema, chronic nephritis. *Surface lesions of cords:* keratosis, pachyderma, herpes, leukoplakia, pemphigus. *Ulcers of cords:* tuberculosis, syphilis, leprosy, lupus, typhoid fever, trauma, contact ulcer. *Neoplasm of cords:* vocal nodules, sessile or pedunculated polyp, vocal process granuloma, vallecula cyst, leukoplakia, carcinoma-in-situ, epidermoid carcinoma, papilloma, angioma. *Innervation of cords:* compression of recurrent laryngeal nerve by aortic aneurysm, large left atrium of the heart, mediastinal neoplasm, mediastinal lymphadenopathy, retrosternal goiter; severance of nerve in thyroidectomy. *Weakness of cord muscles:* debilitating diseases, severe anemia, myasthenia gravis, myxedema, thyrotoxicosis, normal aging process. *Laryngeal bones and cartilages:* perichondritis of cricoid or arytenoids, ankylosis of cricoarytenoid joints (rheumatoid arthritis, syphilis). *Compression of larynx:* retropharyngeal abscess, caries of cervical vertebrae, neoplasm of pharynx, large goiters, actinomycosis of neck. X-ray radiation of neck region.

EMERGENCY: Choking ("The Cafe Coronary")

Making this diagnosis calls for instant treatment. Even physicians fail to recognize and treat the condition in time to save life. *Immediate Diagnosis:* **Usually during a meal, the victim *rises suddenly* with a *look of panic or anguish*, often *with hand to throat*, unable to speak or breathe; he often rushes from the room, with face rapidly changing from *pale* to *blue*. He then *collapses*. This behavior is presumptive evidence of *choking* (in contrast, myocardial infarction permits speech and breathing), and there is *less than 5 minutes before death* in which to perform:**

HEIMLICH'S MANEUVER. ***With the victim standing:*** **Stand behind him and *wrap your arms around his waist*. With your other hand *grasp your fist* and place its thumb side against the victim's abdomen between his navel and rib cage. *Press your fist deep into the abdomen* with a *quick upward thrust*. Repeat several times, if necessary. [The maneuver has also been successful with drowning persons.] Although Heimlich objected that it required too much time to slap the back between the scapulae four times before initiating his maneuver, cur-**

rent basic rescue teaching recommends this approach. After an adult has aspirated a bolus during inspiration, Heimlich calculated that his maneuver can forcefully expel about 940 cc of residual and tidal air at an average pressure of 31 mm Hg, enough to cause the bolus to pop out [Heimlich, H. J.: A Life-Saving Maneuver to Prevent Food-Choking. *J.A.M.A.*, 234:398–401, 1975].

Laryngeal Malfunction: ***Laryngeal Dyspnea.*** Shortness of breath is not necessarily diagnostic of laryngeal obstruction, since it occurs in a variety of other conditions, discussed on p. 281. In laryngeal disease, the occurrence of dyspnea is a mark of an advanced degree of obstruction, lesser degrees having been heralded by hoarseness. In laryngeal dyspnea, the harder the attempt to inhale, the greater becomes the obstruction, because the inrushing air forces the cords to approximate. Exhalation is unopposed. So quiet breathing is more efficient.

Laryngeal Malfunction: ***Stridor.*** Inhalation is accompanied by a high-pitched sound that has the same pitch and intensity throughout the entire inspiratory effort. Its presence indicates a high degree of laryngeal obstruction, and it is almost always accompanied by significant dyspnea. It may be caused by mass lesions, such as carcinoma, which restrict vocal cord mobility or reduce the size of the glottic aperture, or by bilateral vocal cord paralysis, which limit the effective glottic opening.

Acute Laryngitis. The most common cause of hoarseness, acute laryngitis is often accompanied by an unproductive cough producing pain or a burning dryness in the throat. Through the mirror, the true cords are reddened, their edges rounded by swelling. Erythema of the other laryngeal membranes is present; edema of the larynx is common. A white membrane in the larynx suggests infection with either the streptococcus or the diphtheria bacillus.

Clinical Occurrence. Acute upper respiratory infections, including diphtheria and streptococcal sore throat. Overuse of the larynx. Foreign body in the larynx. Inflammation from the inhalation of hot gases or the aspiration of hot or caustic fluids.

Laryngeal Edema. The usual signs of laryngeal obstruction are present, ranging through hoarseness, dyspnea, and stridor. Inspection through the mirror is diagnostic. Glistening swollen mucosa may be seen on the vocal cords, the arytenoid promi-

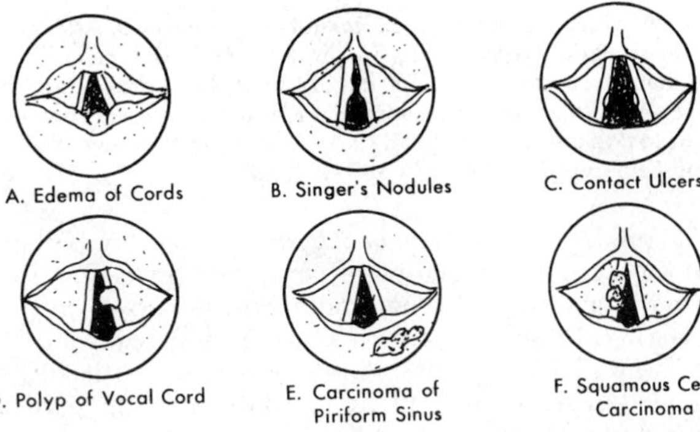

Fig. 5-53. Appearance of laryngeal lesions in the mirror. **A.** *In laryngeal edema the mucosa is swollen and glistening on the vocal cords, arytenoid prominences, and epiglottis.* **B.** *Singer's nodules appear as apposing swellings on the free margins of the vocal cords at a distance one third posteriorly in their extent.* **C.** *Contact ulcers appose on the free margins of the cords at their junctions with the arytenoid cartilages.* **D.** *Laryngeal polyp on the free margin of the left cord.* **E.** *Laryngeal carcinoma in the left piriform sinus.* **F.** *Squamous cell carcinoma along the anterior half of the right cord.*

nences, and the epiglottis (Fig. 5-53A). The membranes may not be reddened, depending on the cause.

Clinical Occurrence. An accompaniment of acute laryngitis and its causes. Lymphatic obstruction by neoplasm or abscess. Trauma to the larynx from instrumentation. Radiation. Angioneurotic edema. Myxedema.

Laryngeal Contact Ulcer. Apposing ulcers occur on the free edges of both vocal cords at their junctions with the arytenoid cartilages (Fig. 5-53C). The irregular borders of the ulcers cause hoarseness. They usually result from trauma of overuse or from instrumentation, as intubation or direct laryngoscopy. Granulation tissue may develop on one or both ulcers and become sizeable enough to cause airway embarrassment.

Chronic Laryngitis. Hoarseness and unproductive cough are usually present. Pain is negligible. The true cords may appear dull and thickened, or edematous and polypoid. Frequently, the false cords are similarly affected.

Clinical Occurrence. Chronic overuse of the cords. Tobacco smoking. Injudicious use of cords in alcoholics. Syphilis. Far-advanced pulmonary tuberculosis.

Laryngeal Leukoplakia. A superficial nonulcerative white membrane appears on one or both vocal cords. Hoarseness may occur, but pain is absent. The condition results from chronic irritation, such as tobacco smoking and may proceed to carcinoma-in-situ or invasive epidermoid carcinoma.

Laryngeal Spasm: ***Croup.*** The term is applied to any laryngeal disorder accompanied by a hoarse brassy cough and dyspnea, usually in children. *Inflammatory croup* is actually acute laryngitis. The cords may appear normal and edema may be greatest in the subepiglottic region. The onset of an attack should warn the physician of the danger of asphyxia. In *spasmodic croup* (laryngismus stridulus), the child is awakened with a barking cough, dyspnea, and stridor. Cyanosis from air hunger is frequent. Recovery is sudden and complete. Viewed in the mirror, the larynx looks normal. The cause of the condition is unknown.

Immobile Vocal Cord: ***Laryngeal Paralysis.*** In *unilateral cord paralysis,* the affected cord may be immobilized near the midline or slightly more laterally in the paramedian position. In the latter case, vocal cord approximation is poor and the voice is husky (Fig. 5-54A). During phonation, a mirror view shows the normal cord crossing the midline to meet the abducted immobile cord. In *bilateral cord paralysis,* the cords are usually fixed near the *midline,* so the voice is normal but dyspnea is extreme and inspiratory stridor pronounced with strenuous exertion (Fig. 5-54B).

Clinical Occurrence. Recurrent laryngeal nerve injury from thyroidectomy (either or both sides). Aneurysm of the aortic arch (left side). Mitral stenosis with enlarged left atrium (left side). Mediastinal tumor (either or both sides).

Immobile Vocal Cord: ***Ankylosis of Cricoarytenoid Joint.*** Hoarseness and voice weakness are common, as in laryngeal paralysis. The mirrored view shows limited or absent motion of the true cords, also resembling paralysis. The *passive mobility test* distinguishes ankylosis from paralysis: with direct laryngoscopy, forceps are used to move the arytenoid cartilages. Arytenoid arthritis should be considered in any patient with rheumatoid arthritis

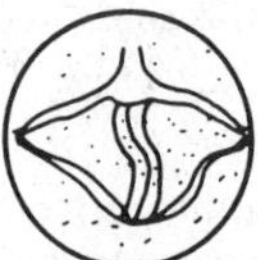

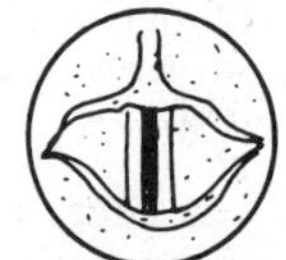

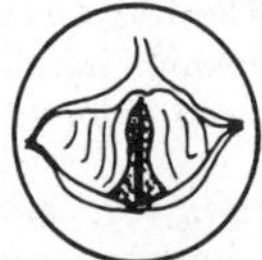

Fig. 5-54. Malfunctions of the vocal cords. **A.** Left abduction paralysis. *In attempting adduction the right cord crosses the midline to meet its immobile mate.* **B.** Bilateral abduction paralysis. *This is the most common condition when both sides are involved; the cords remain nearly in apposition but cannot be abducted.* **C.** Dysphonia plicae ventricularis. *This occurs sporadically between intervals of normal function. During malfunction, the false cords move over the true cords, instead of remaining passive; this causes the voice to break.*

and hoarseness. If the joints are not completely immobilized, *crepitus* over the larynx may be heard with the stethoscope. A traumatic arthritis may be induced by contact with a feeding tube. The condition may be so insidious that dyspnea is not recognized; patients have died from respiratory acidosis.

Hysterical Aphonia. Each of the organic conditions causing aphonia are readily diagnosed by inspection of the larynx. But even before laryngeal examination, hysterical aphonia may be distinguished by demonstrating that the patient can make a *sharp normal cough.* When viewed through the mirror, the cords are morphologically normal. On attempted phonation, the cords promptly approximate, but quickly diverge; or the arytenoids approximate while the free edges of the cords bow outward.

Dysphonia Plicae Ventricularis. Intermittent or chronic hoarseness results when the *false* vocal cords close over the true cords, instead of remaining passive during phonation. A single examination of the cords may disclose no abnormality; subsequent examinations eventually coincide with an occasion when the false cords are seen to close partially or completely over the true cords (Fig. 5-54C). When this occurs, the voice breaks, as in a boy whose "voice is changing." The false cords may also be active when the true cords are separated by tumor, cricoarytenoid arthritis, voice abuse, or emotional instability.

Polypoid Corditis. The entire free margins of the true cords are loose and sagging. Hoarseness results from imperfect approximation of the edematous cords. Causal factors include voice strain, irritation from alcohol and tobacco, and upper respiratory allergy or infection.

Laryngeal Nodes: ***Vocal Nodules*** (Singer's Nodules). With voice overuse, apposing nodules may be seen on the free margins of the true cords at the junction of the anterior one third and the posterior two thirds (Fig. 5-53B). Initially, the lesions may appear red; fibrosis later turns them white. Their size varies from 1 to 3 mm.

Laryngeal Masses: ***Neoplasm.*** Tumors in the larynx may be benign or malignant, pedunculated or sessile, localized or infiltrative. Infiltrative lesions are recognized as malignant; localized masses must be biopsied for diagnosis (Fig. 5-53E and F).

Disorders of Speech. Deviations in speech may be considered in several categories. *Articulation:* This is the production of sounds and their combinations into syllables. *Dyslalia* is impaired articulation from structural defects or from hearing loss. Disorders of the central nervous system produce *dysarthria.* *Rhythm:* This deals with the timing and sequence of syllables. Faltering or interruptions in speech are termed *stuttering* or *stammering.* *Voice:* This concerns phonation, resonation, pitch, quality, and volume. *Dysphonia* is the disturbance in pitch, quality, and volume. *Hypernasality* and *hyponasality* refer to nasal resonance. *Symbolization:* The inability to associate meaning with words is usually termed *dysphasia* or *aphasia.*

The Salivary Glands

Parotid Gland: This is the largest of the salivary glands. Normally, it is *not* palpable as a distinct structure, but its location and extent must be known to diagnose parotid enlargement (Fig. 5-55). A *superficial portion* lies subcutaneously and extends from the zygomatic arch superiorly to the angle of the mandible inferiorly and from the external auditory canal posteriorly to the midportion of the masseter muscle anteriorly. A tail portion wraps around the angle and horizontal ramus of the mandible in the upper neck, and a *deep lobe* extends from the tail medial to the stylomandibular ligament and styloid muscles. The *parotid (Stensen's) duct* is about 5 cm long and runs forward

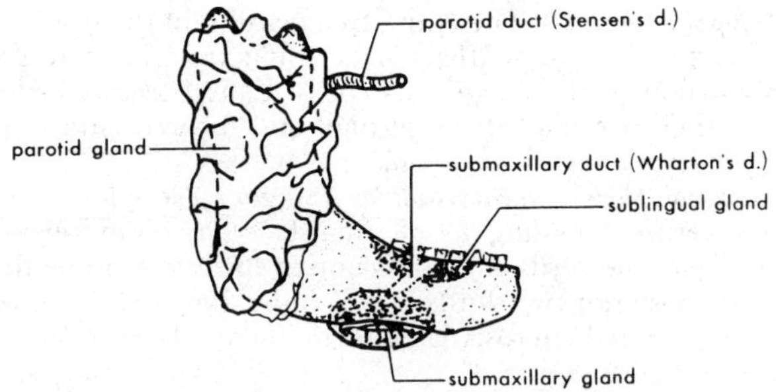

Fig. 5-55. Anatomic relations of the salivary glands to the mandible. *Note that the parotid gland lies on the lateral surface of the mandibular ramus, curling behind its posterior margin. The submaxillary gland is on the medial surface of the mandible with its lower margin protruding below the bone. The sublingual gland is behind the medial mandibular surface near its superior margin. Using the jaw for a landmark, the glands can be located accurately by palpation.*

horizontally, about one fingerbreadth below the zygomatic arch, in a line drawn from the inferior border of the concha of the ear to the commissure of the lips. In its course, it lies on the superficial surface of the masseter muscle; upon reaching the muscle's anterior border, it pierces the buccinator muscle to emerge on the buccal mucosa, with its orifice in a papilla opposite the upper 2nd molar tooth. The normal duct is thick enough to be felt when rolled against the masseter, tensed by clenching the teeth.

Submaxillary Gland: About the size of a walnut, the gland lies medial to the inner surface of the mandible; its lower portion can be palpated from beneath the inferior mandibular border, somewhat anterior to the angle of the jaw. Bimanual palpation with a gloved finger in the floor of the mouth and the opposite hand on the corresponding skin reveals a characteristic sensation from the finely lobulated glandular architecture. The *submaxillary* (*Wharton's*) *duct* is about 5 cm long; it courses upward and forward to the floor of the mouth, where its orifice is crowned by the caruncula sublingualis, beside the lingual frenulum.

Sublinugal Gland: Smallest of the glands, it lies beneath the floor of the mouth, near the symphysis mentis. It empties through several short ducts, some with orifices in the plica sublingualis, some entering the submaxillary duct.

EXAMINATION OF THE SALIVARY GLANDS. *Parotid Gland:* **See whether the facial swelling has the distribution of the parotid gland; especially, whether there is swelling (a) in front of the tragus of the external ear, (b) in front of the auricular lobule, (c) behind the ear, pushing the pinna outward. Have the patient clench his teeth to tense the masseter muscle; palpate the swelling against the hardened muscle to determine extent, consistency, and tenderness of the mass. When fullness is present anterior to the tragus, ascertain whether it is continuous with the inferior mass, as in parotid swelling, or is discontinuous, as in swelling of a preauricular lymph node. Feel for swelling behind the mandibular ramus, always present in parotid enlargement. Inspect the orifice of the parotid duct, opposite the upper 2nd molar; while watching the orifice, press the cheek swelling to observe pus from the duct. Palpate the parotid duct externally for calculus; with gloved finger, feel the region of the orifice and the region posterior to it in a horizontal line, for calculus or other mass. The location of the parotid duct on the cheek is one fingerbreadth below the zygomatic arch, on a line between the inferior border of the concha of the ear and the commissure of the lips. Have the patient clench his teeth and feel the duct against the hardened masseter muscle.**

Submaxillary Gland: **Note a swelling under the mandible and slightly anterior to the angle of the jaw. When no mass is present, but there is a history of a mass appearing after meals, have the patient sip some lemon juice and watch for the development of a swelling. Under such a test, the appearance of a mass or the enlarging of a preexisting swelling is diagnostic of ductal obstruction. Also, in the test, compare the appearance of the ductal orifice with its homologue. Using bimanual palpation, with gloved finger in the floor of the mouth, feel for calculus or a mass; look for the drainage of pus when the mass is pressed in the submandibular triangle. Test both orifices for the secretion of saliva: place dry cotton under the tongue and let the patient sip lemon juice; then remove the swab and watch for salivary flow from each orifice.**

▼ *Key Sign:* ***Ptyalism*** **(*Salivation*).** Ptyalism implies an excessive production of saliva, but it is frequently extended to any condition in which saliva seems overabundant, from rapid secretion, inability to swallow, production of saliva that is more viscid (and more difficult to swallow), or failure of the lips to withhold it.

Clinical Occurrence: OVERPRODUCTION OF SALIVA. *Drugs:* mercury, copper, arsenic, antimony, iodide, bromide, potassium chlorate, pilocarpine, aconite, cantharides. *Stomatitis:* aphthous ulcers, septic ulcers, suppurative lesions, pyorrhea alveolaris, chemical burns. *Specific oral infections:* variola, diphtheria, syphilis, tuberculosis. *Single oral lesions:* alveolar abscess, epulis, salivary calculus.

DIFFICULTY IN SWALLOWING SALIVA. *Infections:* tonsillitis, quinsy, mumps, retropharyngeal abscess, chancre. *Granulomas:* gumma, actinomycosis. *Bone lesions:* fractures, dislocation of the jaw, ankylosis of the temporomandibular joint, sarcoma of the jaw. *Neoplasms:* epithelioma, carcinoma. *Neurologic disorders:* bulbar paralysis, pseudobulbar paralysis, bilateral facial nerve palsy, myasthenia gravis, palsy of the hypoglossal nerve, diphtheritic palsy, paralysis agitans, rabies, botulism. *Inflammation:* radiation therapy.

REFLEX SALIVATION: Gastric dilatation, gastric ulcer or carcinoma, acute gastritis, pancreatitis, hepatic disease.

CEREBRAL DISORDERS. mental deficiency, hysteria.

Lack of Saliva: ***Xerostomia.*** Dryness of the mouth is caused by mouth breathing, obstruction of the salivary gland ducts as demonstrated by sialography, or Sjögren's syndrome. An indication of Sjögren's syndrome has been called the *sourball sign,* when the dryness of the mouth was indicated by the patient sucking on sour candies to relieve oral discomfort [G. E. Ehrich: Sour-Ball Sign of Sjögren's Syndrome, *J.A.M.A.,* **194:**167, 1965].

Painful Parotid Swelling: ***Acute Nonsuppurative Parotitis.*** The parotid region is the site of brawny induration, causing swelling in front of the tragus, back of the mandibular ramus, and behind the pinna pushing it outward. The skin temperature is elevated; there is exquisite pain or tenderness. The pain is accentuated by opening the mouth or chewing, because of the nearness of the gland to the temporomandibular joint. The ductal orifice may be reddened, occasionally with a discharge of pus. One or both sides may be involved. There is moderate fever with *leukopenia.*

Clinical Occurrence. Mumps is the usual cause; occasionally bacterial infection is responsible. Allergy to iodine can cause the same symptoms.

▼ *Painful Parotid Swelling:* ***Acute Supportive Parotitis.*** The gland is swollen, tender, and painful. Local inflammation is accompanied by high fever and *leukocytosis.* The ductal orifices discharge pus. Multiple abscesses may form, although fluctuation may be difficult to detect. Induration and pitting edema are often present.

Clinical Occurrence. Usually the cause is bacterial infection in a patient previously debilitated by other disease or irradiation therapy.

Painless Parotid Swelling: ***Chronic Suppurative Parotitis.*** Repeated episodes of ductal obstruction may produce chronic inflammation in the gland without fever or pain.

Painless Bilateral Parotid Swelling. The phenomenon is associated with a great diversity of conditions: its mechanism is unknown.

Clinical Occurrence. *Malnutrition:* alcoholic cirrhosis of the liver, kwashiorkor, cardiospasm, pellagra, vitamin A deficiency. *Drugs or poisons:* iodine, mercury, lead, thiouracil, isoproterenol, sulfisoxazole. *Endocrine:* pregnancy and lactation, diabetes mellitus, thyrotoxicosis, stress. Allergy and autoimmunity. Obesity. *Neoplasia:* lymphocytic leukemia, lymphoma. *Others:* Sjögren's syndrome, sarcoidosis, ingestion of excessive amounts of starch, bilateral fatty atrophy of the parotid glands.

Parotid Tumors: ***Pleomorphic Adenoma*** (Mixed Parotid Tumor). Characteristically, this neoplasm arises as a firm, painless, nontender nodule, slightly above and in front of the mandibular angle. Less commonly, the site is just anterior to the tragus. It may remain benign for years, growing very slowly. Rarely, it suddenly becomes malignant with rapid growth and metastasis. When confined to the typical sites, the physical examination is diagnostic.

Parotid Tumors: ***Other Neoplasms.*** Neoplasia of the parotid may be either benign or malignant. The second most common benign neoplasm is the *Warthin's tumor* (papillary cystadenoma lymphomatosum), which most commonly occurs in the tail of the parotid in older men and is bilateral more often than any other salivary gland tumor. Malignancy is suggested by pain and tenderness, rapid tumor growth, paralysis of a branch of the facial nerve, and fixation to the skin or underlying tissues. Histologic diagnosis is necessary because biologic behavior of the several tumor types requires different techniques for management.

Salivary Calculus. ***Sialolithiasis.*** In about 85% of patients with salivary calculi, the stone is in the submaxillary gland or duct. Frequently, the symptoms are pathognomonic: submandibular swelling, with or without pain, occurs suddenly while eating and subsides within two hours. The sequence may be invariable for several years. Occasionally, the gland becomes infected or the duct obstructed. In stone of the parotid duct, glandular swelling may persist for several days after onset. In all three glands, calculi are disclosed by palpation quite commonly. About 80% of the calculi are calcified, so they can be demonstrated in x-ray films without contrast media. Intraoral dental radiograms are excellent for demonstrating the calculi because they can minimize the density of the mandible by positioning the film properly. An impalpable stone, without calcium, must be detected by sialography with radiopaque media.

Diseases of the Submaxillary and Sublingual Glands. These glands are subject to the same diseases as the parotid, with slight variations. Rarely, mumps involves the submaxillary gland without affecting the parotid, although it is more common to have the submaxillary involved secondary to the parotid in mumps. Ranula involving the sublingual or submaxillary gland is described on p. 161.

SIALOGRAPHY. **Cannulation of the salivary ducts and the injection of radiopaque media for x-ray examination is a valuable adjunct in diagnosis. It assists in the demonstration of calculi, strictures, and fistulas. Masses can be localized within or without the glands. Evidence can be obtained for the diagnosis of Mikulicz's disease and Sjögren's syndrome. Neoplasms can sometimes be distinguished from inflammatory disease.**

The Ears

The pinna, or auricula, and the external acoustic meatus compose the *external ear;* the *middle ear* consists of the tympanic membrane and the tympanic cavity with its three ossicles. The *internal ear,* or labyrinth, is the organ of hearing; it is not accessible to direct examination.

▼ *Key Symptom:* ***Earache.*** Although the cause of acute pain in the ear is usually readily discovered, chronic earache may offer considerable challenge in diagnosis.

Clinical Occurrence: AURICLE: trauma, hematoma, frostbite, burn, epithelioma, perichondritis, gout, eczema, impetigo, insect bites, rodent ulcer (carcinoma), herpes zoster.

MEATUS: external otitis, carbuncle, meatitis, eczema, hard cerumen, foreign body, injury, epithelioma, rodent ulcer, insect invasion, herpes zoster, trigeminal neuralgia of the mandibular division of the 5th nerve.

MIDDLE EAR: acute otitis media, acute mastoiditis, malignant disease.

REFERRED PAIN (through 5th, 9th, 10th cranial nerves and 2nd and 3rd cervical nerves): unerupted lower 3rd molar, carious teeth, arthritis of temporomandibular joint, tonsillitis, carcinoma or sarcoma of pharynx, ulcer of epiglottis or larynx, cervical lymphadenitis, subacute thyroiditis, trigeminal neuralgia.

▼ *Key Symptom:* ***Tinnitus.*** Ringing in the ears or tinnitus is sufficiently distressing that it serves as a chief complaint in bringing the patient to the physician.

Clinical Occurrence: OUTER EAR: cerumen, foreign body, polyp in the external acoustic meatus. MIDDLE EAR: inflammation, otosclerosis. INNER EAR: Ménière's disease, syphilis, fevers, suppuration of the labyrinth, fracture at the base of the skull, acoustic nerve tumor, acoustic trauma. DRUGS: quinine, salicylates, aminoglycoside antibiotics.

The External Ear

The *pinna* or *auricula* is a flattened funnel with crinkled walls of yellow fibroelastic cartilage, beginning externally with a wide brim and narrowing internally to the external acoustic meatus. The prominent folds are readily identified, although there is considerable individual variation (Fig. 5-56A). The *helix* at its central end curves anteriorly as the *crus,* then winds upward, backward, and downward posteriorly, to form the funnel's brim. Above the midpoint of its posterior vertical portion, a fusiform swelling occasionally develops, the *darwinian tubercle.* An inner concentric fold, the *antihelix,* partially surrounding an ovoid cavity, the *concha,* divides into an upper and lower portion by the transverse helical crus. From the anterior brim of the funnel, below the crus, the *tragus* points backward toward the lower concha as a small eminence. From the lower portion of the antihelix, another eminence, the *antitragus,* points forward across the *intertragal notch* to the tragus.

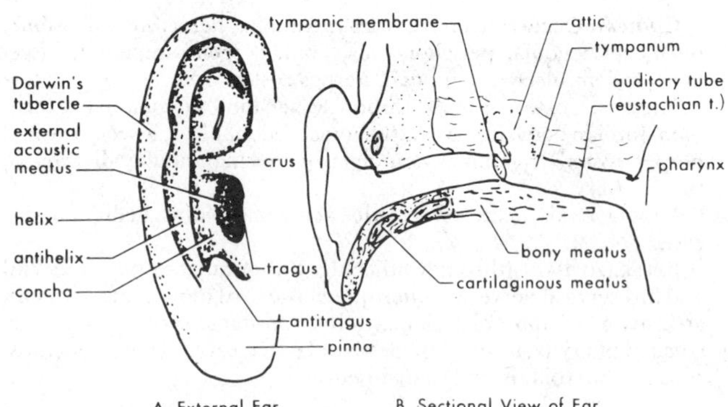

Fig. 5-56. Anatomy of pinna and middle ear. **A.** Surface of pinna. *The main features are depicted, but there are many individual variations. Darwin's tubercle is only occasionally present.* **B.** Middle ear. *Vertical section through the ear. Note the flexible cartilaginous portion of the external acoustic meatus and its bony segment. The upper edge of the tympanic membrane slants outward about 35° from vertical; the conical apex points inward and upward.*

The deep lower concha forms the mouth to the *external acoustic meatus.* At the junction of the inferior limbs of the helix and antihelix is a pendant *lobule* of adipose and areolar tissue, with no cartilage.

The external acoustic meatus is a canal about 2.5 cm (1 inch) long, extending from the bottom of the concha to the tympanic membrane (Fig. 5-56B). The superficial portion of about 8 mm is walled with cartilage; the deeper 16 mm runs through the temporal bone. From the concha, the canal forms a gentle S, in the general direction of inward, forward, and upward. About 20 mm in from the concha is a bony constriction in the canal, the *isthmus.* To view the tympanic membrane, the canal may be straightened by pulling *upward* on the superior border of the pinna so the flexible cartilaginous portion is raised to coincide with the axis of the bony canal.

The Middle Ear

Within the petrous portion of the temporal bone, the canal of the external acoustic meatus widens to form the tympanic cavity, surmounted by an *attic* providing room for movements of the ossicles. Separating the tympanic cavity and the external acoustic meatus, the *tympanic membrane* is an ovoid biconcave disk slanting across the canal in a plane 35° from the vertical, so its upper portion is more superficial than the deeper inferior attachment. Inside, the *manubrium of the malleus* is firmly attached to the tympanic membrane; viewed from outside, the attached portion appears as a smooth ridge forming a radius of the membrane, slanting upward and slightly anterior to the vertical. The tympanic membrane is a shallow cone whose apex points upward and inward into the tympanic cavity. When a beam of light shines into the canal, a brilliant wedge is cast upon the membrane; its apex is the center or *umbo* and its legs extend peripherally in the anterior inferior quadrant of the membrane, approximately at a right angle to the manubrium. This wedge is termed merely *the light reflex.*

EXAMINATION OF THE EAR. *Pinna:* **Inspect the pinna for size, shape, and color. Note serous, purulent, or sanguinous discharges from the meatus. Palpate the consistency of the cartilages and any swellings. Movements of the pinna and tragus are painful with external otitis, but not with otitis media.** ***Cleaning the External Acoustic Meatus:*** **Prepare the meatus for inspection by taking time to clean it properly. Remove liquid material with a cotton applicator. Remove solids through an ear speculum, with either a cotton applicator or a cerumen spoon *under direct vision.* *Using the Aural Speculum:* Use a speculum attached to a lighted otoscope, or a speculum and a head mirror. Select the largest speculum that will fit the cartilaginous canal. Insert the speculum while retracting the pinna *upward and backward* for adults; use *downward* traction for infants and young children (Fig. 5-57). Since the lining epithelium of the bony canal is very sensitive, use gentle manipulation. Before inspection is attempted, tip the patient's head toward his opposite shoulder to bring the canal horizontal. Examine the normal landmarks of the drumhead: the *manubrium* of the malleus that forms a smooth ridge from the umbo or center and runs radially upward and forward toward the circumference and ends in the *knob* of the short process; the two *malleolar folds,* diverging from the knob to the periphery; the *light reflex,* a bright wedge of light whose apex is the umbo and whose legs extend downward and forward at about five o'clock; the *shadow of the incus,* often showing through the membrane in the upper posterior quadrant; finally, look carefully around the entire *circumference of the annulus* for perforations just inside its border. Note the *color* and**

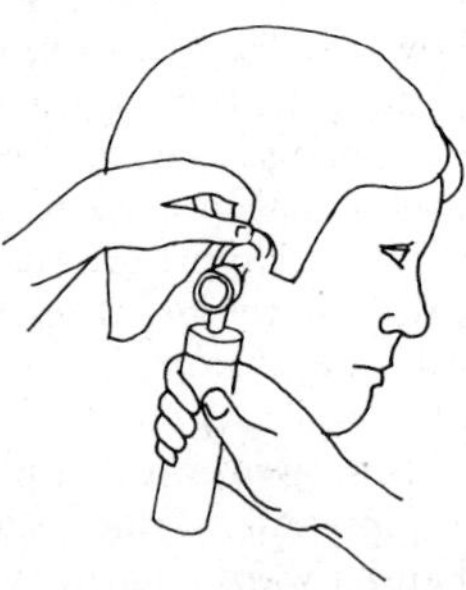

Fig. 5-57. Use of the electric otoscope. *Insert the ear speculum by pulling the upper edge of the pinna upward and backward to straighten the cartilaginous meatus so it coincides with the axis of the bony canal.*

***sheen* of the membrane, normally shiny and pearly gray. Serum in the middle ear colors it *amber* or *yellow;* pus shows as a *chalky white* membrane; blood appears as *blue.* Note changes in the *definition of the manubrium;* bulging makes the landmarks *indistinct* or completely *obscures* them. Inadequate function of the auditory (eustachian) tube produces *retraction* of the membrane that sharpens the outline of the manubrium and mallear folds; when fluid accumulates, the membrane looks *amber* and *air bubbles* may show through. The wedge of the light reflex may be *distorted* but interpretation is often difficult. When the incus is *visible* through the membrane, a normal middle ear is fairly certain.**

Malformations of the Pinna (Fig. 5-58). The pinna may develop smaller than normal, *microtia,* or unusually large, *macrotia.* Rarely, the pinna is absent, usually in association with *atresia* of the external acoustic meatus. The pinna may protrude at a right angle to the head, *lop ear* or *bat ear.* Failure of development of the lobule produces *Aztec ear* or *Cagot ear.* When an eminence occurs near the upper third of the posterior helix, the effect is termed *Darwin's ear.* A pointed pinna is a *satyr ear.* Curling of the pinna is called *scroll ear.* A small rudimentary *accessory pinna* may develop. Untreated hematomas heal as nodular and bulbous irregularities of the helix and antihelix, the *cauliflower ear.*

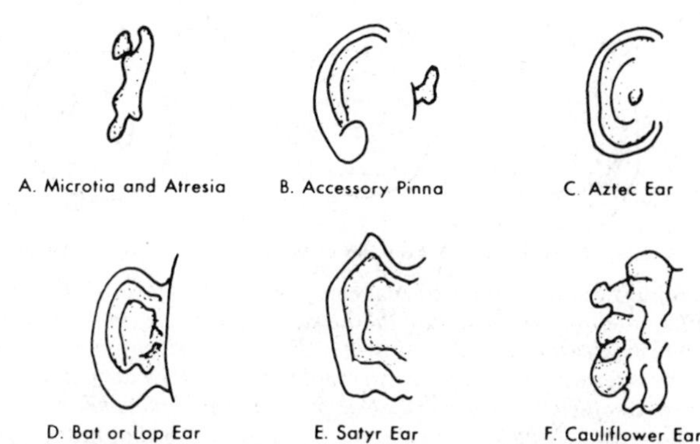

Fig. 5-58. Malformations of the pinna. **A.** *Microtia and atresia are associated congenital defects; only a ridge of skin and cartilage may represent the ear.* **B.** *An accessory pinna is usually small and rudimentary; it is commonly found anterior to the tragus of the well-formed ear.* **C.** *Aztec or Cagot ear is characterized by the absence of the lobe.* **D.** *The bat or lop ear stands out from the head at a right angle.* **E.** *A satyr ear has a point at the top of the helix.* **F.** *An acquired deformity, the cauliflower ear is misshapen by fibrosis from trauma.*

Pinnal Nodule: ***Darwin's Tubercle.*** A developmental eminence in the upper third of the posterior helix, this condition is harmless. It must be distinguished from acquired nodules, such as tophi.

Pinnal Nodule: ***Gouty Tophus.*** In long-standing gout, accumulations of sodium urate crystals may occur in the helix and antihelix; they also occur in the olecranon bursa, the tendon sheaths and aponeuroses of the extremities. The nodules are painless, hard, and irregular (Fig. 5-59A). They may burst to discharge their chalky contents.

Pinnal Nodule: ***Painless Nodules.*** In addition to gouty tophi, these may be basal-cell carcinomas, rheumatoid nodules, or leprosy.

Pinnal Nodule: ***Painful Nodule.*** A small indurated area of skin and cartilage may develop in the superior helix. The cause is unknown, but it usually follows trauma.

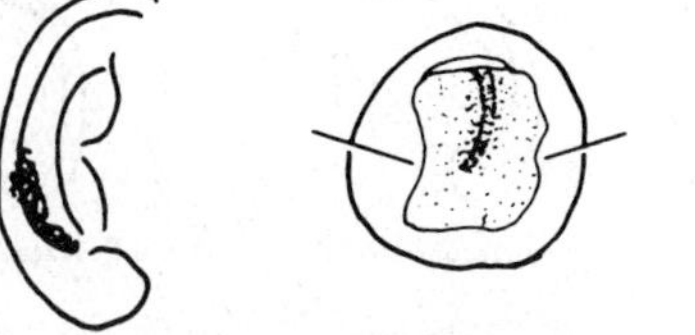
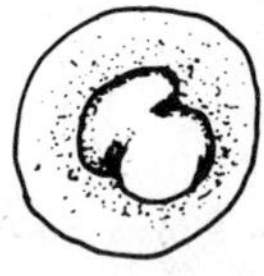
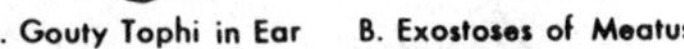

Fig. 5-59. Lesions of the external ear. **A.** *Tophi are hard, irregular, painless nodules usually near the helix. Occasionally, the skin breaks down to exude chalky crystals of urates.* **B.** *Bony swellings may protrude into the external acoustic meatus from the walls so the view of the eardrum is completely obscured.* **C.** *Polyps occasionally may be seen in the external meatus and ordinarily give no difficulty in diagnosis.*

Pinnal Nodule: ***Calcification of the Cartilage.*** This is a rare complication of Addison's disease. The nodule is not usually tender.

Pinnal Mass: ***Hematoma.*** Usually a result of trauma or a coagulation defect, blood accumulates between the cartilage and the perichondrium to form a tender, blue, doughy mass, usually without spontaneous pain. Early diagnosis is desirable for prompt incision and drainage of the blood to avoid suppuration or cauliflower ear.

Recurring Inflammation of Pinna: ***Relapsing Polychondritis.*** This is a rare disease with degeneration and inflammation of cartilage, especially the pinna; but there may be involvement of the nasal septum. Involvement of the laryngeal cartilages is indicated by *hoarseness.* The trachea, bronchi, and joint cartilages may be affected. *Blindness* may result from involvement of the sclerae; *tinnitus* and *deafness* from involvement of the middle ear. Rarely degeneration of the aortic ring has led to aortic regurgitation or aneurysm; similar involvement of the mitral ring has caused mitral valve leaflet prolapse. The involved ear is painful, swollen, and reddened, except over the lobule, which remains normal since there is no underlying cartilage. Although the exact etiology is unknown, symptoms remit after treatment with corticosteroids or Dapsone [J. Martin, et al.: Relapsing Polychondritis Treated with Dapsone, *Arch. Dermatol.,* **112:**1272, 1976.].

Postpinnal Mass: ***Dermoid Cyst.*** A favorite site is just behind the pinna. This lesion is soft and semifluctuant.

Pinnal Neoplasms. Squamous-cell carcinoma is common on the pinna, the basal-cell type is less frequent. Any small crusted, ulcerated, or indurated lesion that fails to heal promptly should be suspected and biopsied. In the advanced stages, the squamous-cell type produces fungating lesions while the basal-cell neoplasm tends to be flattened with elevated borders.

▼ *Key Sign:* ***Discharge from the Ear (Otorrhea).*** Discharge from the ear suggests a number of possibilities, depending upon the nature of the discharge:

Clinical Occurrence: YELLOW DISCHARGE: melting cerumen. SEROUS DISCHARGE: acute eczematous lesions in the meatal wall, early ruptured acute otitis media. BLOODY DISCHARGE: trauma of the external canal from without, or longitudinal temporal bone fracture causing tympanic membrane and external canal laceration. PURULENT DISCHARGE: chronic external otitis, chronic suppurative otitis media with or without cholesteatoma, tuberculous otitis media.

External Acoustic Meatus: ***Cerumen.*** Earwax normally forms in the cartilaginous portion of the meatal canal and protects the epithelium and captures foreign particles invading the canal. The wax migrates to the concha because of epithelial migration of ear canal skin in that direction. Either *excessive production* of wax or a *narrowed meatus* leads to *impacted cerumen,* causing partial or complete obstruction of the canal. When obstruction is complete, *partial deafness* results. *Tinnitus* or *dizziness* may accompany. A partial obstruction is often completed suddenly when water is forced into the meatus during bathing or swimming. The obstructing wax may be seen easily through the external meatus. As a result of external dermatitis, or spontaneously, the supply of wax may become *inadequate;* the accompanying dryness causes scaling and pruritus.

External Acoustic Meatus: ***Exostoses and Chondromas.*** Multiple exostoses form nodules in the osseous part of the meatus near the tympanic membrane (Fig. 5-59B). They rarely produce obstruction, although the view of the drumhead may be partially obscured. A single bony osteoma may also occur. Rarely, chondromas arise from the cartilaginous portion of the canal, usually without obstructing.

External Acoustic Meatus: ***Furuncle.*** When this lesion forms in the outer half of the canal, it produces *extreme pain.* It appears as a red tender eminence, with or without a pustule.

External Acoustic Meatus: ***Acute External Otitis.*** *Pain* may be mild or severe; it is accentuated by movement of the tragus or pinna. The epithelium appears either pale or red; it may swell to close the canal and impair hearing; the tragus may also swell. An aural discharge often results. Fever is not uncommon. Tender palpable lymph nodes may appear in front of the tragus, behind the pinna, or in the anterior cervical triangle. A variety of organisms can cause the inflammation, but the usual offender is *Pseudomonas aeruginosa* or less commonly streptococci, staphylococci or *Proteus vulgaris.* Often swimming in contaminated water initiates the disease.

External Acoustic Meatus: ***Chronic External Otitis.*** Instead of pain, *pruritus* is the chief symptom. Aural discharge may be present. The epithelium of the pinna and the meatus is thickened and red; it is abnormally *insensitive* to the pain of instrumentation. Bacteria and fungi are the chief causative agents, although the condition may accompany a chronic dermatitis, such as seborrhea or psoriasis.

External Acoustic Meatus: ***Foreign Body.*** Children often place objects in their ears, discovered later on routine examination. A purulent discharge from the canal or earache may be the first indication.

External Acoustic Meatus: ***Insect Invaders.*** Occasionally insects enter the canal where their movements cause great distress. To remove one, place a drop of oil or a pledget soaked with ether in the canal and extract the immobilized creature. By contrast, we have seen maggots in a thriving state in the ear of a patient with chronic external otitis with the usual insensitiveness.

External Acoustic Meatus: ***Polyps.*** A polyp may form a bulbous reddened pedunculated mass arising either from the meatal wall or from the middle ear (Fig. 5-59C). Gently moving the mass with the forceps frequently indicates its origin. In either site, the growth causes a *foul purulent discharge.*

External Acoustic Meatus: ***Glomus Tumor.*** Fibrovascular tumors arise from the glomus bodies in the jugular bulb or the middle ear mucosa. They present with pulsatile tinnitus in the involved ear or, sometimes the glomus jugulare type has paralysis of cranial nerves 9 through 11 (which pass through the jugular foramen). They appear as red masses behind the tympanic membrane. Identical tumors arise from the carotid artery bifurcation. Rarely, the tumors are multiple, malignant, or secrete vasoactive amines. If biopsied, they bleed profusely.

External Acoustic Meatus: ***Carcinoma.*** Either squamous-cell or basal-cell carcinoma can involve the meatal epithelium, producing aural *discharge* and *pain.* In advanced stages, deafness and facial paralysis may occur. The appearance of the neoplasm is similar to that in other regions.

Middle Ear: ***Eustachian Tube Block.*** Swelling of the orifice of the auditory (eustachian) tube during an upper respiratory infection prevents access of air to the tube. The patient experiences mild intermittent pain and a feeling of fullness in the ear. Hearing is temporarily impaired on swallowing, the patient may hear a popping sound. Inspection of the eardrum shows it to be *retracted* (Fig. 5-60B). Occasionally, bubbles may be seen behind the eardrum.

Middle Ear: ***Acute Suppurative Otitis Media.*** *Throbbing earache* is a prominent symptom; frequently there is fever. Hearing is impaired. Occasionally slight dizziness and nausea occur. The pain subsides when the pent-up pus is released by bursting of the eardrum. Before rupture, the tympanic membrane *bulges* to obliterate the normal landmarks (Fig. 5-60D); its surface is bright red and lusterless. After rupture, pus appears in the canal; a pulsatile stream of discharge may be seen emerging from the perforation in the drum. Usually, *light pressure* upon the mastoid process elicits *pain.* The disease usually accompanies a cold, influenza, scarlet fever, or measles. The fever and signs of constitutional disease are more prominent in children than in adults.

Middle Ear: ***Acute Serous Otitis Media.*** The symptoms may be simply fullness in the ear and impaired hearing. The tympanic membrane is normal or retracted. Through the membrane may be seen amber serous fluid (Fig. 5-60C). When the middle chamber is partially filled, the fluid meniscus appears as a *fine black line.* Sometimes air bubbles are visible (Fig. 5-60E). The condition usually accompanies upper respiratory infections, although it may occur alone. Reduction of barometric pressure, as in an airplane ride, may induce it.

Middle Ear: ***Acute Mastoiditis.*** Usually invasion of the mastoid

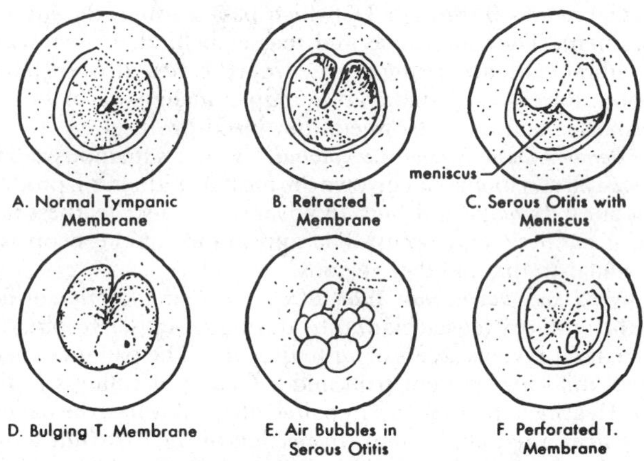

Fig. 5-60. Lesions of the tympanic membrane. **A.** *The normal tympanic membrane glistens; its disk contains a brilliant triangle, the light reflex, with its apex at the center or umbo and its base at the annulus; the tympanic membrane is slanted downward and forward. The handle of the malleus makes an impression on the disk from the umbo upward and forward.* **B.** *The retracted eardrum results from absorption of air from an obstructed auditory tube. The light reflex is bent, and the shadow of the malleus and its folds stand out in sharper relief than normally.* **C.** *Serous fluid in the tympanum shows through the membrane with an amber color; hairline menisci curve from the handle of the malleus to the annulus.* **D.** *The bulging drumhead shows the curves in the membrane that obscure normal landmarks of the malleus and distort the light reflex.* **E.** *When serous fluid is mixed with air, bubbles may be plainly seen through the drumhead.* **F.** *Perforations of the membrane look like oval holes through which a dark shadow may be seen.*

cells results from inadequate treatment of acute suppurative otitis media. The symptoms of otitis gradually increase. There is low-grade fever with a thick purulent discharge from the meatus. The eardrum is lusterless and edematous. *Deep bone pain* can be elicited by *firm pressure* upon the mastoid process. X-ray films confirm the diagnosis by showing clouding of the mastoid air cells, and bony destruction, which is only evident radiographically after two to three weeks of suppuration.

Complications: Extension outward can cause a subperiosteal abscess of the mastoid process. Less commonly, erosion of bone damages the facial (7th) nerve, with resulting facial paralysis. Extension through the inner table to cause meningitis, epidural abscess, abscess of the temporal lobe or cerebellum. Infection of the internal ear to produce labyrinthitis.

Middle Ear: ***Chronic Suppurative Otitis Media.*** By definition, the condition is associated with a *permanent perforation* of the eardrum (Fig. 5-60F). A marginal perforation of the annulus is more grave than a central defect. The chief symptom is *painless aural discharge.* Hearing is always impaired. The amount of discharge may wax and wane, but recurrence is invariable. Painless discharge accompanying an upper respiratory infection suggests previously existing perforation. Occurrence of pain or vertigo indicates development of a complication, such as subdural irritation, brain abscess, or labyrinthine involvement.

Middle Ear: ***Cholesteatoma.*** In chronic suppurative otitis media with a marginal perforation of the eardrum, the squamous epithelium of the meatus may grow into the attic of the tympanic cavity. Desquamation produces a caseous mass of cells, keratin, and debris, which slowly enlarges and extends into the mastoid antrum. The mass may ultimately erode bone. In the meatus, the mass appears shiny white and caseous. The x-ray picture is characteristic.

Hearing Losses. *Sensorineural losses* (nerve deafness) result from disorders of the cochlea or the acoustic (8th) nerve. Some of the causes are hereditary deafness, congenital deafness, trauma, infections, drug toxicity, and aging (presbycusis). *Conductive losses* occur from failure in transmission of sound vibrations to the sensory apparatus, as in obstruction of the external acoustic meatus, disorders of the eardrum and middle ear, overgrowth of bone with fixation of the stapes (otosclerosis).

ROUGH QUANTITATIVE TEST FOR HEARING LOSS. **Several methods are available. When the *whispered voice* is used, place your mouth at the side of the patient's head, about 2 feet (60 cm) from his ear; have him cover the near eye with one hand to prevent lip reading, while his other hand covers his far ear. After you exhale, strongly whisper test words and have the patient repeat them, or whisper questions that cannot be answered by "yes" and "no." Test consistently with loud, medium, and soft tones. Or, using the same intensity for all tests, find the maximal distance from the ear at which the whisper may be heard. Repeat the test with the *spoken voice* which**

is louder. Testing with the *ticking watch* involves only high-pitched sounds and depends on yes-or-no answers, unless the distance from the ear is varied. Hearing acuity may also be tested with the vibrations of a tuning fork; a fork with a frequency of from 512 to 1024 cycles per second is preferred; the usual 128-cycle fork for testing vibratory sense is too low-pitched.

TESTING DISTINCTION BETWEEN PERCEPTIVE AND CONDUCTIVE HEARING. **Use a tuning fork with frequencies from 512 to 1024 cycles per second. So the intensity of the test sound is *near the threshold,* set the fork in motion by pinching the ends and suddenly releasing, or by gently tapping the knuckle of the other hand. *Weber's Test* (Fig. 5-61A): Place the handle of the vibrating fork against the midline of the skull, and ask the patient whether the sound is louder in one ear than the other. With normal *perceptive* hearing and no *conductive* loss, the sounds are equal in the two ears. When hearing is equal bilaterally, the sound will lateralize to the side of *conductive* loss which shuts out the masking effect of room noises. *Perceptive* loss on one side makes the sound louder on the opposite. So lateralization of sound to the right ear means conductive loss on the right or perceptive loss on the left. *Rinne's Test* (Fig. 5-61B): Test one**

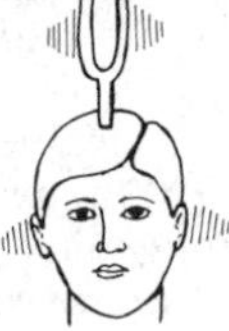

A. Weber's Test

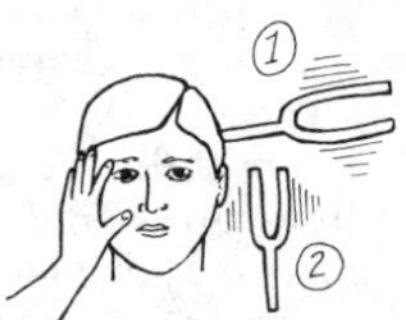

B. Rinne's Test

Fig. 5-61. Tests of hearing perception and conduction. **A.** *In Weber's test, place the handle of the vibrating tuning fork upon the midline of the skull and ask the patient to compare the intensity of the sound in the two ears. Lateralization of the sound to one ear indicates a conductive loss on the same side, or a perceptive loss on the other side.* **B.** *In Rinne's test, first place the handle of the vibrating tuning fork against the mastoid process while the patient covers his opposite ear with his hand. Have the patient signal when the sound ceases; then hold the still-vibrating tines near the external ear without touching the patient; have him indicate when the sound ceases. Normally, air conduction persists twice as long as bone conduction—called "Rinne-positive." When bone conduction persists as long or longer, the test is "Rinne-negative."*

ear by pressing the handle of a vibrating fork against the mastoid process and asking the patient to signal with his hand when the sound ceases. At the signal, remove the fork and hold the still-vibrant tines near his ear without touching him. At the signal for cessation of the sound by air conduction, hold the fork to your own ear to determine any residue of sound. Normally, air conduction persists longer than bone conduction (the sound undergoes progressive weakening as the fork dampens), in which case the result of the test is arbitrarily said to be *Rinne-positive*. The test is *Rinne-negative* when bone conduction persists the longer. With air conduction, the sound normally persists twice as long as with bone conduction, a ratio of 2:1. The test just described does not detect changes in the ratio between 2:1 and 1:1. A more selective test that demonstrates this range of defect is *timing* the persistence of sound with a separate trial of the fork for air and bone.

LABYRINTHINE TEST FOR POSITIONAL NYSTAGMUS. Have the patient seated on an examining table and inspect the eyes carefully for spontaneous nystagmus (p. 84). Then have him lie supine, wait 30 seconds, and look for nystagmus. Then assist him in turning his head and body to one side; after 30 seconds, look for nystagmus. Try the same test with turning to the other side. After a short rest, decline the head over the top of the table and look for nystagmus after 30 seconds. After another rest supine, have him sit up and inspect after 30 seconds. In each case, the *slow* component of the nystagmus is in the direction of the endolymph flow (contrarily, nystagmus is named for its *fast* component).

LABYRINTHINE TEST FOR PAST POINTING. Have the patient seated facing you, keeping his eyes closed during the test (Fig. 5-62). Have him point his forefingers toward you; place your forefingers lightly

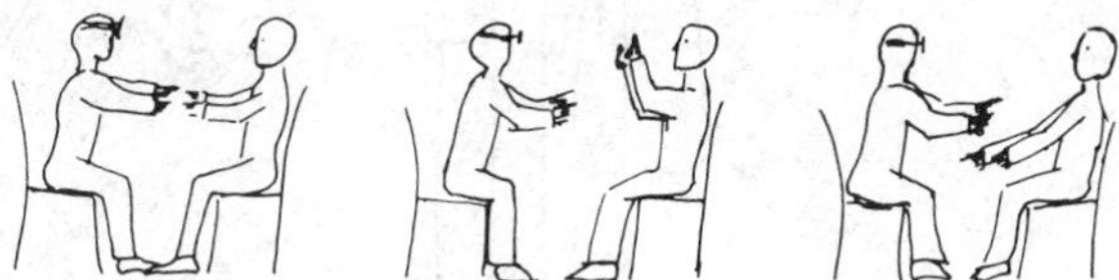

Fig. 5-62. Past pointing test for labyrinthine disorders. *Seat the patient opposite the physician (in the drawings, the creature with the head mirror); have him close his eyes and extend his index fingers toward you. Touch the fingers with yours and hold your position while the patient riases his hand above his head. Have him replace his fingers over yours without opening his eyes. Normally this maneuver can be performed accurately; past pointing indicates either loss of positional sense or labyrinthine stimulation.*

under his. Hold your fingers in constant position; ask him to raise his arms and hands, then have him return his fingers to yours. Normally, this maneuver is easily accomplished. Deviation to the right or left of the target fingers, *past pointing*, indicates either labyrinthine stimulation or loss of positional sense. The flow of endolymph is in the *same* direction as the past pointing.

LABYRINTHINE TEST FOR FALLING. **Have the patient stand with the inner aspects of his feet close together (heel and toe) (Fig. 5-63). Encircle his body with your arms but without touching him. Assure him that you will not let him fall, then have him close his eyes. With labyrinthine stimulation or loss of positional sense, he will tend to fall. With labyrinthine stimulation, he will fall in the *same* direction as the flow of endolymph. Falling during the test is *Romberg's sign*.**

OTHER LABYRINTHINE TESTS. ***Electronystagmography* and the *caloric stimulation test* are best reserved for the specialist.**

Dizziness: ***Unsystematized Dizziness.*** The patient has an alarming sense of disturbed relation to space. Frequently he cannot describe it further, other than that he is unsteady, weak,

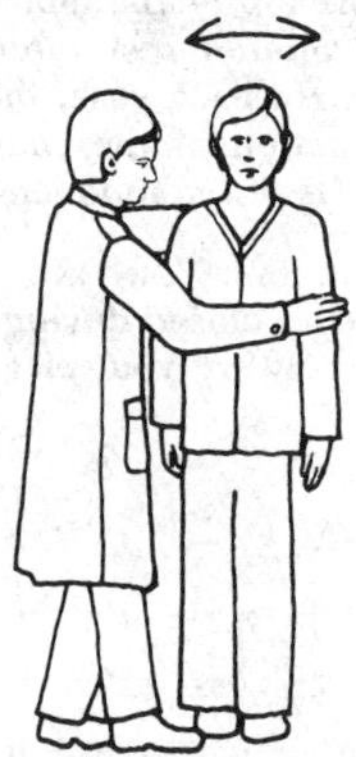

Fig. 5-63. Falling test for labyrinthine disorders (Romberg's sign). *Ask the patient to stand with his toes and heels together. Stand beside him with your arms surrounding, but not touching, him. After assuring him that that you will not let him fall, have him close his eyes. With labyrinthine stimulation, the patient tends to fall in the direction of the flow of endolymph. Falling may also indicate loss of positional sense as tabes dorsalis. Normally the patient will waver somewhat, but not fall.*

blank, or has a feeling of turning. There is no definite impression that his surroundings are whirling about him.

Clinical Occurence: EARS: vestibular neuronitis, utricular trauma from skull fracture, otosclerosis, leaks from tears in the oval or round windows, perilymph fistula. EYES: muscle imbalance, refractive errors, simple glaucoma. PROPRIOCEPTIVE System: pellagra, chronic alcoholism, pernicious anemia, tabes dorsalis. CENTRAL NERVOUS SYSTEM: mild cerebral anoxia (arteriosclerosis, hypertensive cardiovascular disease, chronic hypotension, anemia, paroxysmal atrial fibrillation, aortic stenosis with insufficiency, heart block, carotid sinus syndrome, simple syncope, postural hypotension), infections (meningitis, encephalitis, brain abscess, syphilis), trauma, tumors, migraine, absence seizures, endocrine conditions (hypothyroidism, menstrual-pregnancy-menopause pattern, hypoparathyroidism with tetany, paroxysmal hypertension with associated adrenal tumor, hypoglycemia), disorders of water metabolism, psychoneurosis.

▼ *Key Symptoms:* ***Vertigo.*** When his eyes are open, the patient's surroundings seem to be whirling about him. With the eyes closed, he feels in motion. Severe degrees of vertigo are accompanied by nausea and vomiting.

Clinical Occurrence: PERIPHERAL LABYRINTHINE SYSTEM: serous labyrinthitis, perilymph fistula, labyrinthine (otic capsule) fistula, viral labyrinthitis, otosclerosis, otitis media with effusion, benign paroxysmal positional vertigo, idiopathic endolymphatic hydrops (Meniere's disease), motion sickness, cholesteatoma, temporal bone fracture, postural vertigo.

CENTRAL LABYRINTHINE SYSTEM: migraine, vertebrobasilar insufficiency, brainstem or cerebellar hemorrhage or infarction, cerebellopontine angle tumors, intraaxial tumors (pons, cerebellum, medulla), craniovertebral abnormalities causing cervicomedullary junction compression, multiple sclerosis, intracranial abscess (temporal lobe, cerebellum, epidural, subdural).

EIGHTH NERVE: infections (acute meningitis, tuberculous meningitis, basilar syphilitic meningitis), trauma, tumors.

BRAINSTEM NUCLEI: infections (encephalitis, meningitis, brain abscess), trauma, hemorrhage, thrombosis of the posteroinferior cerebellar artery, tumors, multiple sclerosis.

— *Vertiginous Disorder:* ***Acute Toxic Labyrinthitis.*** In this most frequent cause of vertigo, the patient gradually develops a sense of whirling that reaches a climax in 24 to 48 hours. During the height of the symptoms, nausea and vomiting may occur. The patient seeks comfort in the horizontal position; raising the head may induce vertigo; thus, he is incapacitated for several days. The symptoms gradually subside, and they disappear in three to six weeks. There is *no accompanying tinnitus or hearing loss.*

Clinical Occurrence. Acute febrile illness, such as pneumonia, influenza, or acute cholecystitis. Other causes are certain drugs, alcohol, fatigue, allergy.

— *Vertiginous Disorder:* ***Vascular Disease.*** Transient vertigo may be caused by vascular spasm. More severe and prolonged symptoms occur from thrombosis or rupture of an artery or vein; there is sudden vertigo with nystagmus, *loud tinnitus,* and *sudden deafness.* Partial recovery is usual in three to four weeks.

— *Vertiginous Disorder:* ***Trauma.*** Skull fracture through the inner ear, concussion, or a loud noise may induce symptoms similar to a vascular accident. Tinnitus and hearing loss are present. Labyrinthine tests show delay and hypoactivity on the affected side.

— *Vertiginous Disorder:* ***Labyrinthine Hydrops*** (Ménière's Syndrome). This is characterized by *sudden attacks* of whirling vertigo, tinnitus, and perceptive hearing loss, with intervals of *complete freedom* from vertigo; but the hearing loss and the tinnitus persist. An attack lasts hours but not days. Hearing loss predominates on one side, is fluctuating but slowly progressive. Tinnitus also fluctuates, accentuating before an attack. The disease is self-limited. The cause of the hydrops is unknown. Labyrinthine tests are normal or hypoactive on the involved side.

— *Vertiginous Disorder:* ***Damage to the Eighth Nerve or Brainstem Nuclei.*** Lesions at either level produce vertigo and nystagmus. Disorders of the eighth nerve are accompanied by *hearing loss,* absent with lesions of the brainstem, except when other cranial nerves are also damaged.

The Scalp and Skull

The scalp has five strata: the skin, the subcutaneous tissue, the epicranius, a fascial cleft with connective tissue, and the pericranium (Fig. 5-64).* Surgically, the outer three strata are

* Mnemonic: S = skin, C = connective tissue, A = aponeurosis, L = loose connective tissue, P = periosteum.

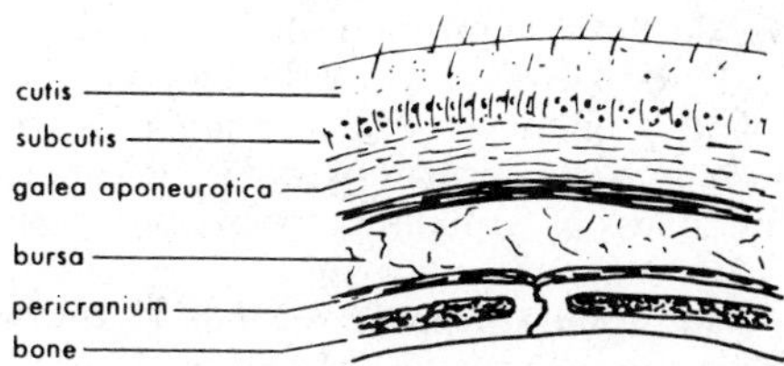

Fig. 5-64. Layers of the scalp. *For practical purposes, the cutis, subcutis, and galea aponeurotica constitute a single layer, thick and tough, with fibrous bands compartmenting the tissue and binding it to the galea, so the spread of infection is very limited. Between the galea and the pericranium is a bursa with little areolar tissue, so infections spread easily through the entire area covered by the galea and its attached muscles (in total, the epicranium). The pericranium is the periosteal layer covering the bones of the skull and dipping inward at the suture lines, so subperiosteal fluid is limited to the area over a single bone.*

a single layer, thick, tough, and vascular, whose strength is supplied by the epicranius. The *epicranius* is a sheet of tissue covering the vertex of the skull; it consists of the *frontalis muscle* attached to the supraorbital ridges, the *occipitalis muscle* fixed to the occiput, both connected by an intervening central aponeurosis, the *galea aponeurotica.* The skin and subcutaneous tissue are tightly bound to the galea by numerous fibrous bands that sharply limit the spread of blood and pus in the layer. The *pericranium* is the periosteal layer of the bones of the skull; it dips into the suture lines, limiting subperiosteal blood or pus to the surface of a single bone. Between the pericranium and the galea is a *fascial cleft* containing a little connective tissue. In this space, blood or pus spreads under the entire epicranius.

The scalp has three areas of *lymphatic drainage.* The region of the forehead and the anterior portion of the parietal bone drain to the *preauricular lymph node.* The midparietal region drains first to the *postauricular node* and thence to the nodes of the *posterior cervical triangle.* The occipital area drains first into the nodes at the origin of the Trapezius, thence to the *posterior cervical triangle.*

Wrinkling of the Forehead. Transverse wrinkles normally occur in the forehead with extreme upward gaze or in raising the eyebrows in facial expression. *Absence* of such furrowing is a sign of thyrotoxicosis. Deep wrinkling, with longitudinal furrowing, and prominence of intervening tissue constitute the *bulldog skin* in pachydermatosis and some congenital disorders. Unilateral loss of wrinkling results from facial nerve paralysis.

Bleeding from Scalp Wounds. Wounds in the scalp bleed profusely because the tissue is extremely vascular. The wounded scalp *does not gape* unless the galea aponeurotica has been severed. If gaping is noted, one should suspect a compound fracture of the skull, so the wound should not be explored without the strict asepsis of the operating room.

Fluctuant Scalp Masses: **Hematoma, Abscess, or Depressed Fracture.** When blood or pus accumulates in the skin or subcutaneous layer of the scalp, it is *sharply localized* and the mass readily slides over the skull. A boggy fluctuant mass in the entire adult scalp can be attributed to either blood or pus in the subepicranial fascial cleft; the same finding in a young child may also be evidence of fracture of the parietal bone. A fluctuant mass bounded by the suture lines of a skull bone indicates subperiosteal blood or pus, or a depressed fracture. A hematoma under the pericranium usually has a soft center that is plastic, but the edges are firm and closely resemble the feel of a depressed fracture.

Cellulitis of the Scalp. The scalp is tender, soft, and boggy. The infection extends rapidly, causing edema of the eyelids and pinnae; there are tender swollen regional lymph nodes.

Scalp Mass: **Sebaceous Cyst** (Wen). A common lesion, it is

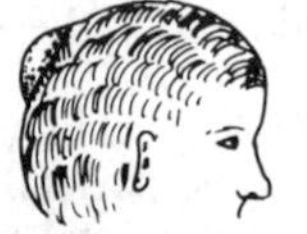
A. Sebaceous Cyst or Wen

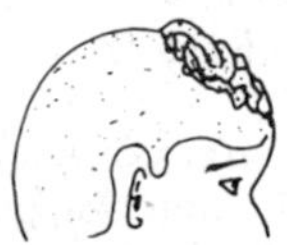
B. Cirsoid Aneurysm

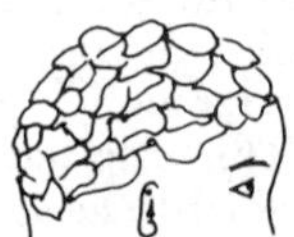
C. Turban Tumor

Fig. 5-65. Lesions of the scalp. **A.** *Sebaceous cysts are single or multiple smooth masses in the upper layer of the scalp; they slide easily over the underlying bursa.* **B.** *A cirsoid aneurysm is a rare lesion that presents as fluctuant sinuous vessels that may produce bruits.* **C.** *A turban tumor is also rare; it proliferates to form festoons over the scalp; it is red, lobulated, and does not support the growth of hair.*

either single or multiple. The mass is firm, nontender, nonulcerative, often hemispheric (Fig. 5-65A). It is a sebaceous cyst arising from obstruction of the sebaceous gland's orifice. Since it arises from the skin, it slides easily over the skull. When rare suppuration occurs, the tumor bleeds easily and may be mistaken for a squamous-cell carcinoma. Bailey describes *Cock's peculiar tumor,* a suppurating sebaceous adenoma that also must be distinguished.

Scalp Mass: ***Lipoma.*** A fatty tumor in the subcutaneous layer feels smooth; the finger slides around its edges. When it occurs beneath the pericranium, its movement is strictly limited, but the finger can detect a smooth rounded border.

Scalp Masses: ***Rare Tumors.*** Chronic cystic swellings of the scalp (Fig. 5-65B) include *cirsoid aneurysm,* which produces a bruit; *cavernous hemangioma* from a meningocele, which slowly refills after being denoted by pressure; *pneumatocele,* which is tympanitic with percussion. In the scalp, *neurofibromas* may occur as part of the generalized neurofibromatosis of von Recklinghausen. The lesions are discrete, sessile or pedunculated tumors that look solid but seem to collapse with pressure. Rarely, a proliferating scalp tumor forms a festoon hanging from the head; the effect is achieved by either a neurofibroma or a *turban tumor* of doubtful cause, growing slowly to produce a red lobulated, fissured cap, devoid of hair (Fig. 5-65C).

Skull Malformation: ***Oxycephaly*** (Steeple Skull, Craniosynostosis). Premature union of the cranial sutures leads to grotesque malformations, such as a skull with a pointed vertex (Fig. 5-66A). Surgical treatment in infancy can prevent deformity in adulthood.

Skull Malformation: ***Meningocele.*** An outpouching of the meninges may occur in the midline of the vertex or the occiput (Fig. 5-66D).

Skull Malformation: ***Parrot's Bosses*** (Hot-Cross-Bun Skull). An increased prominence of the frontal and parietal bosses produces intersecting grooves at the sagittal and transverse sutures (Fig. 5-66C). This deformity is usually a stigma of congenital syphilis.

Enlarged Infantile Skull: ***Hydrocephalus.*** The increased intracranial pressure from deficient spinal fluid circulation causes enlargement of the calvarium before the sutures are closed (Fig. 5-66B). In contrast, the bones of the face are normal in

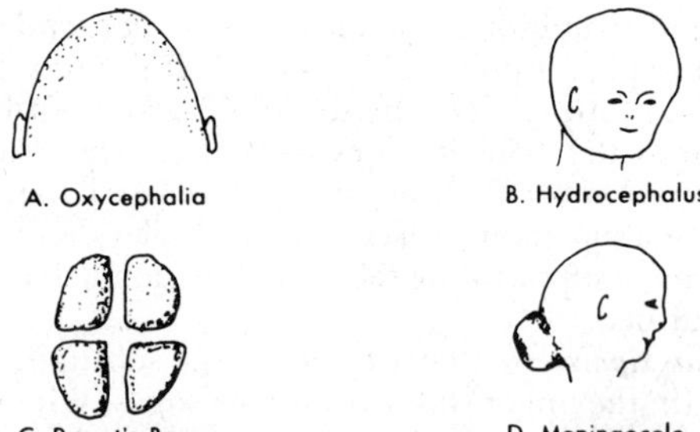

Fig. 5-66. Malformations of the skull. **A.** *Oxycephalia, oxycephaly, or steeple skull is pointed at the vertex as a result of premature fusion of the cranial sutures.* **B.** *Hydrocephalus shows enlargement of the calvarium as compared to the normal size of facial bones in the same subject. It results from increased intracranial pressure before the sutures have united.* **C.** *Parrot's bosses or hot-cross-bun skull is notable for the bulging prominence of four parietal and frontal bones, leaving contrasting deep fissures at the suture lines. It is usually the result of congenital syphilis.* **D.** *Meningocele is a fluctuating outpouching of the meninges in the vertex or occiput.*

size. With early detection, appropriate surgical treatment can prevent its occurrence and progression.

Enlarged Adult Skull: ***Osteitis Deformans*** (Paget's Disease of Bone). The bones of the skull thicken centrifugally by the replacement of normal osseous tissue with porous vascular osteoid. The calvarium is large compared to the facial bones (Fig. 5-67). A bruit is sometimes heard in the skull. The porous bone may form arteriovenous shunts affecting the general circulation. In addition to bone pains, the patient may complain that his hats have become too small. Other associated bone changes are acquired: kyphosis, bowed legs, shortening of the stature from flattened vertebrae.

Skull Masses: ***Osteomyelitis.*** Involvement of the frontal bone with osteomyelitis leads to a localized edematous swelling over the affected region. This condition is usually a sequel of acute or chronic suppurative sinusitis.

Skull Masses: ***Neoplasms.*** *Osteoma* frequently occurs in the outer table of the skull, producing a hard sessile eminence in the bone. A protuberance, soft or hard, in one of the bones of the vertex may be a *pericranial sarcoma,* diagnosed only by

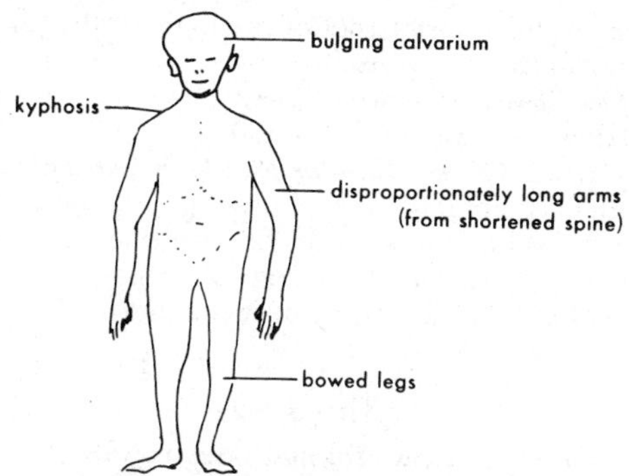

Fig. 5-67. Bony signs of osteitis deformans (Paget's disease of bone). *The chief osseous features of Paget's disease are the enlarged calvarium contrasting with the normal-sized face underneath, from thickening of the skull; kyphosis and shortening of the spine from flattening of the vertebral bodies; with shortening of the spine, the arms look proportionately longer than the trunk; and bowed legs.*

biopsy. Hard or soft masses in the cranial bones may be carcinomatous metastasis, lymphomas, leukemia, or multiple myeloma.

Skull Softening: ***Craniotabes.*** Firm digital pressure on the skull behind and above the pinna discloses yielding of the outer table of the skull. Softening of the outer table occurs in rickets, hydrocephalus, syphilis, and hypervitaminosis A.

The Cheeks

Swelling of the Cheek: ***Parotitis.*** This subject has been discussed with the examination of the mouth (p. 178).

Swelling of the Cheek: ***Preauricular Abscess.*** An abscess is formed by involvement of the preauricular lymph node in front of the tragus. The swelling is localized, tender, and sometimes warm. The chief diagnostic problem is to find the source in the region drained by the node. The area to be searched is the side of the face, the pinna, the anterior wall of the external acoustic meatus, the anterior third of the scalp, the eyebrows, and the eyelids. A *congenital preauricular sinus* may be the site of recurrent abscesses. This sinus opens through a tiny hole at the anterior root of the helix of the pinna, near the crus, or in the tragus itself.

Ulcer of the Cheek: ***Preauricular Ulcer.*** The ulcer results from the breakdown of a preauricular abscess.

Swelling of the Cheek: ***Masseter Muscle Hypertrophy.*** Either one or both masseter muscles may undergo spontaneous hypertrophy and produce swelling of the face that must be distinguished from parotid gland swelling. While palpating the mass, have the patient clench his teeth; if the entire mass hardens, the swelling is muscular.

The Jaws

Spasms of the Jaw Muscles: ***Trismus.*** See p. 148.

EXAMINATION OF THE TEMPOROMANDIBULAR JOINT. **Palpate over the joint while the patient opens and closes the mouth, feeling for clicking or crepitus (Fig. 5-68). The equivalent noises may be heard by placing the bell of the stethoscope over the joint during movement. To elicit joint *tenderness*, face the patient; place the tips of your forefingers behind the tragi in each external acoustic meatus; pull forward while the patient opens the mouth.**

Temporomandibular Joint: ***Rheumatoid Arthritis.*** This joint is a favorite site for the migratory polyarthritis of the rheumatoid type. *Tenderness* in this location is diagnostic and distinguishes the disease from rheumatic fever (Fig. 5-69A). Trismus may occur from muscle spasm.

Temporomandibular Joint: ***Osteoarthritis.*** The disease produces *crepitus* in the joint with movement. The patient may hear

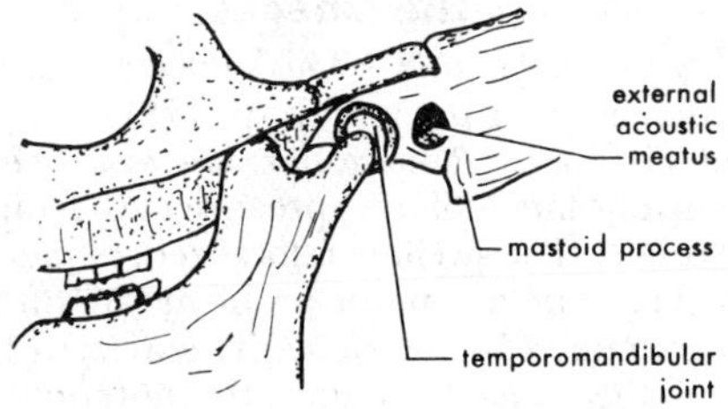

Fig. 5-68. Anatomy of the temporomandibular joint. *The drawing emphasizes the nearness of the joint to the external acoustic meatus, so the joint may be palpated by a finger in the meatus.*

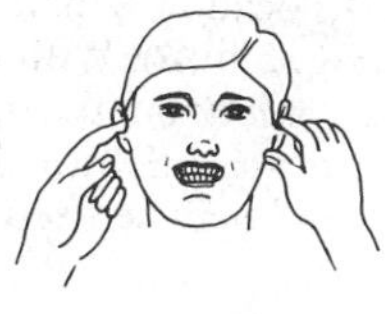

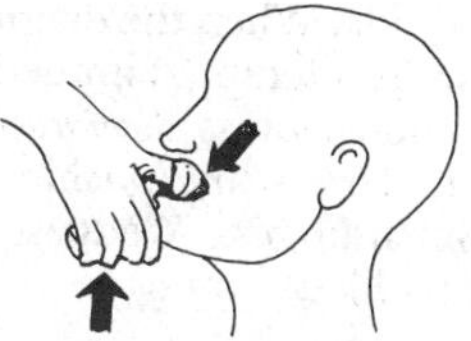

Fig. 5-69. Lesions of the temporomandibular joint. **A.** Testing for tenderness. *Place the tips of your index fingers in each external acoustic meatus and have the patient open his mouth. Rheumatoid arthritis of this joint will be tender with this maneuver, a helpful sign to distinguish from rheumatic fever.* **B.** Reduction of dislocated mandible. *Wrap your thumbs with padding, place them over the lower third molars, and press them downward while pulling the point of the chin upward with your fingers until the condyle of the mandible is felt to slide back into the joint socket.*

grating during chewing or talking. Other diseases that occasionally affect the temporomandibular joint are systemic lupus erythematosus, gout, Sjögren's syndrome, and Mediterranean fever. Osteoarthritis of the joint will produce crepitus when the patient chews which causes complaints.

Temporomandibular Joint: ***Displaced Cartilage.*** The patient may hear a snap in the ear. Thereafter, an annoying click occurs with each opening of the mouth. The clicking may be palpated as a sudden movement in the joint. Occasionally, the joint *locks* with sudden pain in the ear radiating to the pinna and the skin above; this is accompanied by salivation from stimulation of the auriculotemporal nerve. Pain persists until reduction of the cartilage.

Temporomandibular Joint: ***Dislocation.*** Usually after a wide yawn or an upward blow on the chin when the mouth is opened widely, the jaw is *fixed open.* The mandible protrudes so the lower teeth override the upper. Palpation discloses an abnormal *depression* or *pit* anterior to the tragus. The condition is more obvious when bilateral; in *unilateral dislocation* the pretragal depression occurs only on the affected side. Confirmation may be obtained by palpating through the external acoustic meati where no movement of the mandibular head is felt on the affected side. When the diagnosis of dislocation is made, reduction can be attempted immediately (Fig. 5-69B). With the padded thumbs, press *downward and backward* on the posterior lower molars, while pushing the chin *upward* with the third and fourth fingers. Wedges of soft wood may be used in place of the padded thumbs.

The Neck

▼ *Key Symptom: **Pain in the Neck.*** Pain in the neck is a common complaint whose cause is often readily diagnosed by a careful history, palpation of the neck, and examination of the oropharynx. Yet the more serious disorders are myriad and may be overlooked without careful consideration of more than 50 conditions in the following list. For example, carotid arteritis is rarely diagnosed, confirming the truth of Goethe's maxim "What one knows, one sees." In palpation of the neck each anatomic structure should be systematically examined. The enhancement of pain by certain bodily movements may be somewhat helpful in searching for the source of pain.

Clinical Occurrence: NECK PAIN ENHANCED BY SWALLOWING. *Pharynx:* pharyngitis, Ludwig's angina. *Tonsils:* tonsillitis, neoplasm. *Tongue:* ulcers, neoplasm. *Larynx:* laryngitis, neoplasm, ulcer, foreign body. *Esophagus:* inflamed diverticulum (demonstrated by esophagram), peptic esophagitis, radiation esophagitis. *Thyroid Gland* (*see* pp. 207–18): acute suppurative thyroiditis, subacute thyroiditis (pain often radiating to ear), hemorrhage into thyroid cystadenoma. *Carotid Artery:* carotid arteritis (p. 205), carotid body tumor (p. 225), inflamed thyroglossal duct or cyst (p. 218). *Salivary Glands:* mumps, suppurative parotitis.

NECK PAIN ENHANCED BY CHEWING. *Mandible:* fracture osteomyelitis, periodontitis. *Salivary Glands:* mumps, suppurative parotitis.

NECK PAIN ENHANCED BY MOVEMENTS OF THE HEAD. *Sternocleidomastoideus:* torticollis (p. 206), hematoma. *Nuchal Muscles:* viral myalgia, muscle tension, "crick" in neck. *Cervical Spine:* injury, herniated intervertebral disk, spinal arthritis, meningitis, meningismus craniovertebral junction abnormalities.

NECK PAIN ENHANCED BY SHOULDER MOVEMENT. *Superior Thoraic Aperture:* cervical rib (p. 431), scalenus anticus syndrome (p. 429), costoclavicular syndrome (p. 431).

NECK PAIN NOT ENHANCED BY MOVEMENT. *Skin and Subcutaneous Tissues:* furuncle, carbuncle, erysipelas. *Lymph Nodes:* acute adenitis (any cause). *Branchial Cleft Remnants:* inflamed pharyngeal cyst.

Salivary Glands: calculus in duct. *Subclavian Artery:* aneurysm. *Nervous System:* poliomyelitis, herpes zoster, epidural abscess, spinal cord neoplasm. *Spinal Vertebrae:* herniated intervertebral disk, metastatic carcinoma. *Referred Pain:* from Pancoast's syndrome (p. 726), angina pectoris, and other conditions in the six-dermatome band (pp. 227–51).

— ***Neck Pain Enhanced by Swallowing: Carotid Arteritis.*** Frequently, after the onset of a viral pharyngitis, the patient complains of *pain* in the side of the neck that is *intensified by swallowing*. The pain may extend to the mandible or the ear. It may be *constant* or *throbbing*. Fever may be an accompaniment. Some patients have no generalized symptoms; others exhibit *profound lassitude*. Several relapses may occur in a few months. ***Physical Signs.*** The bulb at the bifurcation of the carotid artery is exquisitely *tender,* and the trunk of the common carotid may be tender over its accessible course to the clavicle. In some patients the carotid bulb seems *dilated* and its pulsations *exaggerated.* Sudden digital compression of the carotid causes the pain to spread in the distal branches of the external carotid to jaw, ear, and temple (*Fay's sign*). One or both common carotid arteries may be involved. The pharynx and larynx may appear normal or slightly hyperemic and edematous. In a few cases *aphthous ulcers* have been present. ***Laboratory Findings.*** The leukocyte count and the erythrocyte sediment rate are normal. ***Pathophysiology.*** No biopsies of the carotid artery have been reported, but various writers tend to regard the condition as a variant of temporal arteries (giant-cell arteritis). This seems a premature conclusion since the complications of carotid arteries have been relatively benign. ***Distinction.*** The diagnosis is made by demonstration of the specific tenderness of the carotid artery; but unless this sign is sought, the neck tenderness is attributed to lymphadenitis or subacute thyroiditis. A "therapeutic test" with corticosteroids may promptly relieve pain and tenderness in either carotid arteritis or subacute thyroiditis, so relief is not diagnostic.

Carotid arteritis deserves wider recognition and study. Clinical descriptions differ remarkably, so one wonders whether there are several causes for the syndrome. All writers state that the disease is common but seldom diagnosed. Some associate it with migraine or psychoneurosis; others attribute it to a viral infection with a seasonal incidence. In some series of patients the disease has been predominantly unilateral, in others bilateral. Some clinicians report prompt relief with steroids; others have negative results. Most have accepted an analogy with temporal arteritis, but no histologic proof has been offered.

EXAMINATION OF CERVICAL MUSCLES AND BONES. **Take a careful history; it will usually exclude many in the long list of causes. Have the patient's neck and shoulders uncovered. Face the patient and note any swellings, especially in the Sternocleidomastoideus and the cervical spine. Note any asymmetry or fixed posture of the neck. Palpate the cervical vertebrae and the muscles for local tenderness and masses. Note the extent of movement and the pain elicited by cervical anteflexion, dorsiflexion, and rotation of the head. If the physical signs do not suffice, have x-ray examinations of the cervical spine with special attention to tender and painful sites. Special diagnostic maneuvers are discussed in the following.**

Stiff Neck. Pain in the neck and limitation of its motion are the usual signs directing attention to the muscles, bones, and joints of the cervical region. The disorders are so varied as to defy a routine approach to diagnosis.

Clinical Occurrence. CONGENITAL. Congenital torticollis. ACQUIRED. *Acute Infectious:* fibrositis (including common transient stiff neck), reflex spasm (adenitis from acute pharyngitis, meningitis, etc.), inflammatory bone lesions (including subluxation of the atlas, sudden onset of caries), calcific tendinitis of M. longus colli. *Acute Traumatic:* injuries of cervical vertebrae (fractures, dislocations, subluxations, strains), rupture of intervertebral disk, injuries to muscles and other soft parts. *Degenerative:* cervical spondylitis with fibrositis. *Chronic Infectious:* rheumatoid arthritis, infectious arthritis, tuberculous spondylitis, intramuscular gummas. *Chronic Posttraumatic:* untreated acute injuries, contractures from burns, nerve injuries. *Neoplastic.*

Lateral Deviation of the Head: ***Torticollis*** (Wryneck). One Sternocleidomastoideus may be more prominent than the other; the head may be tipped slightly to one side. If tipping is present, but the muscles are not prominent, ask the patient to straighten his head, whereat the sternal head of one muscle will tense more than the other (Fig. 5-70). If the torticollis is long-standing, the face and even the skull may be asymmetric. The *congenital type* is attributed to hematoma or partial rupture of the muscle at birth: this results in unilateral muscle shortening.

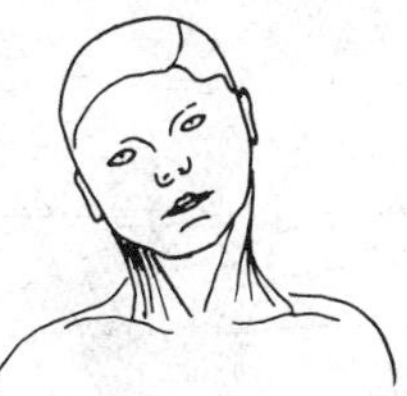

Fig. 5-70. Torticollis or wryneck. *The head is inclined to one side by the shortened sternocleidomastoid muscle, which is frequently more prominent than its mate. If the contrast between the two muscles is not evident, it may be accentuated by asking the patient to straighten his head.*

The tilt of the head from torticollis must be distinguished from the head posture assumed to correct for vertical squint (see p. 90), or an ocular muscle palsy, *ocular torticollis.* To demonstrate the latter, slowly but firmly straighten the neck with your hands while watching the eyes for the appearance of squint. In other patients the head is tilted to resolve diplopia from extraocular muscle imbalance. Another group of patients have asymmetric erosion of the occipital condyle from inflammatory (usually) rheumatoid arthritis or neoplastic disease with cranial settling in a tilted position.

Lateral Deviation of the Head: ***Tumor of the Sternocleidomastoideus.*** A mass can be felt in the belly of the muscle that is usually a hematoma.

Stiff Neck with Dorsiflexion: ***Meningitis.*** The neck is held stiffly in slight or extreme dorsiflexion from pain and muscle spasm. Forcefully anteflexing the neck results in involuntary flexing of the hips, knees, and ankles. This is *Brudzinski's sign,* an indication of meningeal irritation. It must be distinguished from cervical osteoarthritis.

The Thyroid Gland

The largest compact endocrine gland, the thyroid is a flattened structure in the neck. It consists of two *lateral lobes* whose upper halves lie on either side of the projecting prow of the thyroid cartilage; the lower halves are at the sides of the trachea (Fig. 5-71). A flat band of *isthmus* passes in front of the upper tracheal rings, joining the lateral lobes at their lower thirds.

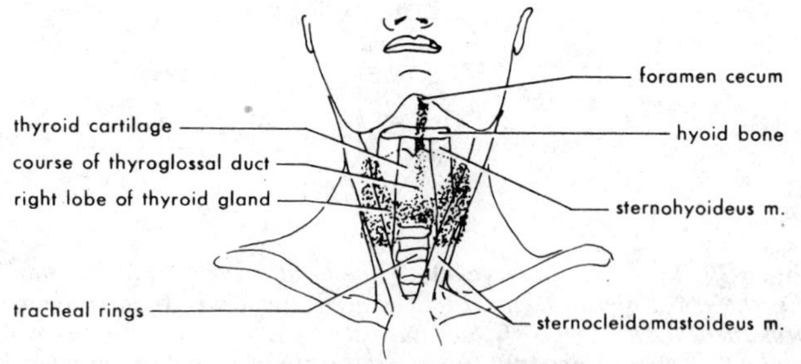

Fig. 5-71. Anatomic relations of the thyroid gland. *The drawing shows the anterior view. The stippled structures are the thyroid gland and the course of the obliterated thyroglossal duct that occasionally contains remnants that persist and become clinically important.*

The major outline of the gland is trapezoidal, with parallel top and bottom and the sides converging downward (the Greek *thyroid* means shield-shaped). The normal adult gland weighs about 25 to 30 gm; it is slightly larger in the female. Each lateral lobe is an irregular cone about 5 cm long; the greatest diameter is about 3 cm, the thickness about 2 cm. The right lobe is normally a fourth larger than the left. The lateral posterior borders touch the common carotid arteries. Usually, on the posterior lateral surfaces are the parathyroid glands. The recurrent laryngeal nerves lie close to the medial deep surface. Each lobe is covered anteriorly by the respective Sternocleidomastoideus, but the isthmus lies on the tracheal rings and is practically subcutaneous. Pairs of superior and inferior thyroid arteries supply an exceedingly vascular parenchyma. The gland is firmly fixed to the trachea and larynx, so that it ascends with them during swallowing; this movement distinguishes thyroid structures from other masses in the neck. The thyroid occupies the upper anterior mediastinum; downward enlargement by adenomatous growth extends behind the sternum, a *retrosternal goiter* (incorrectly termed *substernal*). The thymus gland also occupies the anterior mediastinum; some anatomists describe a suspensory ligament descending from thyroid to thymus. Thus a tumor of the anterior mediastinum may arise from either gland.

Usually the normal adult thyroid is not palpable. In a thin

neck, the normal isthmus may be felt as a band of tissue that just obliterates the surface outlines of the tracheal rings. A *goiter* is any enlarged thyroid gland. A few lymph nodes are regularly present in the thyrohyoid membrane; when enlarged, they are sometimes termed the *delphian nodes* because they lodge metastasis from thyroid carcinoma.

Knowledge of the embryonic development is necessary for the diagnosis of thyroid disorders. A median diverticulum, evaginating from the ventral pharyngeal wall, goes downward and backward as a tubular duct, bifurcating and further dividing into cords that later fuse to form the thyroid isthmus and lateral lobes. As the *thyroglossal duct,* the tube extends from the future foramen cecum in the tongue downward, passing in front of the trachea, to join the thyroid isthmus. Normally, the thyroglossal duct obliterates, but remnants may persist in the adult to form *thyroglossal sinuses* or *cysts.* At the duct's superior end, a *lingual thyroid gland* may form that functions normally. Inferiorly, ductal tissue frequently forms a *pyramidal lobe* of the thyroid gland. Arising from the isthmus or a lateral lobe, usually the left, the structure may ascend in front of the thyroid cartilage, as high as the hyoid bone. Occasionally, a normal glandular component, such as the isthmus or lateral lobe, may fail to develop. Rarely, the lingual growth may be the only active thyroid tissue in the body.

Anatomic alterations of the thyroid gland are frequently associated with disturbances of function. Excesses or deficits of thyroid hormone alter the physical structure of the body to produce physical signs. The examiner attempts (1) to determine the morbid anatomy of the thyroid gland, (2) to make an assessment of thyroid function. His examinations may be confirmed and elucidated by the proper use of laboratory tests.

Anatomic Disorders of the Thyroid Gland

PHYSICAL EXAMINATION FOR THYROID DISORDERS. **Have the patient seated in a good crosslight. Inspect particularly the lower half of the neck in the anterior triangles. Have him swallow to note any *ascending* mass in the midline or behind the Sternocleidomastoidei. If the patient is obese, or he has a short neck, tilt his neck back to be supported by his hands clasped at the occiput; ask him to swallow while in this posture. *Palpation from Behind:* Have the patient seated in a chair and stand behind him. Instruct him to lower the chin**

and rest the head against your body, to relax his neck muscles. Place your thumbs back of his neck, curl your fingers anteriorly so their tips rest over the thyroid gland (Fig. 5-72A). Whenever necessary, have the patient swallow to assist in defining a mass. It may be desirable to have him hold some water in his mouth and swallow on demand. Run the fingers up and down the tracheal rings, feeling for any tissue on their anterior surface; if found, it is likely to be hyperplastic thyroid isthmus. Palpate systematically the lower poles of both lateral lobes. Palpate the anterior surface of the lateral lobes through the Sternocleidomastoidei, the patient's head slightly inclined *toward* the side being examined to relax the muscles. Occasionally, the thyroid is more easily felt when the neck is dorsiflexed. If the findings need further elucidation, proceed to examine from in front. *Frontal Palpation:* Sit down to face the seated patient. Place the fingers of one hand at the back of the neck with your extended

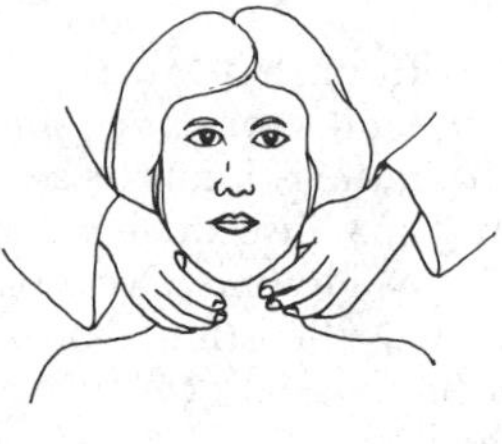

A. Palpation of Thyroid from Behind

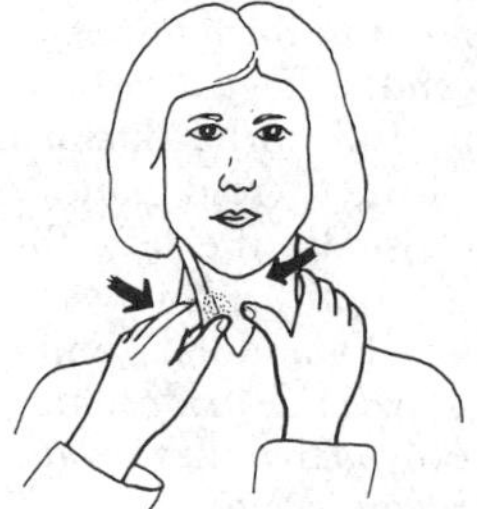

B. Palpation of Thyroid from in Front

Fig. 5-72. Palpation of the thyroid gland and adjacent structures. **A.** Palpation from behind. *Stand behind the sitting patient and have him rest his head against your body to relax the neck muscles. Place your thumbs behind his neck, curling your fingers anteriorly so your fingertips explore the trachea and the regions behind the sternocleidomastoid muscles. First feel for the thyroid isthmus applied to the anterior aspect of the tracheal rings; then palpate the lower poles of the lateral lobes; finally feel the upper poles of the lateral lobes. During the examination, shift the inclination of the patient's head to relax the neck muscles, and have the patient swallow to test the adherence to the trachea of palpated masses.* **B.** Frontal palpation of the thyroid gland. *Seat yourself facing the seated patient. With one thumb, push the trachea toward the opposite side while the other thumb and index finger are feeling deeply on either side of the sternocleidomastoid muscle in bidigital palpation of the lateral thyroid lobe that is behind the muscle. Have the patient swallow to test the adherence of the masses to the trachea.*

thumb forward at the base of the thyroid cartilage (Fig. 5-72B). With the pulp of this thumb, push the trachea gently away from the midline, while the fingers of your other hand are inserted behind the Sternocleidomastoideus of the opposite side, where they can feel the posterior aspect of the displaced lateral lobe; let the thumb feel medial to the muscle for the anterior surface of the mass. Having the patient swallow or depress the chin may further assist in the examination. Palpate the second lateral lobe in the same manner with the tasks of the two hands reversed. *Auscultation of a Goiter:* When the thyroid gland undergoes hyperplasia, the accelerated blood flow through the large tortuous thyroid arteries often produces vibrations, felt as a *thrill,* or heard with the bell of the stethoscope as a soft murmur, usually called a *thyroid bruit.* The bruit must be distinguished from a *carotid murmur* that may be heard proximal to the gland and an *aortic murmur* that originates at the base of the heart. The bruit is often confused with a *venous hum;* but the hum has a different pitch and is abolished by light compression of the jugular vein.

Small Diffuse Goiter. Less than twice normal size, both lobes and the thyroid isthmus are slightly enlarged, smooth, relatively soft. Usually the right lobe is larger than its mate, but all components share in the hyperplasia. Asymmetry may occur from congenital absence of a lobe or the isthmus. ***Physiologic Hyperplasia.*** (1)Before menstrual periods, (2) from puberty in the female until 20 years of age, (3) during pregnancy. ***With Hyperfunction.*** In most persons under 40 years of age with thyrotoxicosis the goiter is diffuse rather than nodular. The increased blood flow in the hyperplastic gland may produce a bruit. ***With Hypofunction.*** With iodine deficiency, or with excessive doses of thiouracil drugs, thiocyanates, para-aminosalicylic acid, phenylbutazone, lithium, cobalt salts; rarely, in certain patients taking iodides. In persons with inherited defects of thyroid enzymes. From chronic thyroiditis.

Large Diffuse Goiter. More than twice normal size, all parts of the gland are smooth, enlarged, and firm. The surface may be slightly irregular (bosselated); but small circumscribed nodules are absent. This type is frequently termed *colloid goiter,* or *endemic goiter,* although the terms are not always applicable, since sporadic cases occur in nongoitrous regions. This size of goiter may occur in any category listed for smaller diffuse glands, except that physiologic hyperplasia rarely becomes so large.

Multinodular Goiter. The gland may be small or large. The significant feature is the presence of *two or more distinct nodules* in the parenchyma. These are usually found in persons over 30 years of age. The nodules may vary in consistency in the same goiter; an occasional hard nodule is proved by x-ray films to be calcified. The nodules are thyroid adenomas. *With Euthyroidism.* A scintigram shows normal or sparse concentration of ^{131}I in the nodules. *With Thyrotoxicosis.* In addition to the symptoms and signs of thyrotoxicosis and the laboratory findings of hypermetabolism, the scintigram demonstrates excessive concentration of ^{131}I in the nodules, the so-called hot nodules. *Subacute Thyroiditis.* The gland is unusually firm, rather small (20 to 30 gm), but frequently contains one or more nodules, often *tender*. The patient may complain of *pain with swallowing*. The pain is frequently *referred to the ear*, so the physician may be consulted for earache. Within a few weeks a nodule may regress or another develop. *Chronic Thyroiditis.* Nodules may be present. The gland is hard, only slightly enlarged, nontender. The distribution of ^{131}I is usually patchy. *Carcinoma.* In a multinodular goiter of long-standing, one nodule or area may feel much harder than the rest, either from carcinoma or calcification. The diagnosis may be made only by biopsy. Sudden increase in the size of a nodule is frequently caused by *hemorrhage into a cyst*, usually an indication for surgical exploration. Ultrasonic examination will distinguish a cyst from a solid nodule.

Uninodular Goiter. About half the goiters, judged to contain solitary nodules by palpation, are found at operation to be multinodular and adenomatous. One goiter in 10 or 20, so explored, proves to be carcinomatous. A scintigram demonstration that the nodule concentrates ^{131}I poorly, weighs in favor of exploratory operation. Fine-needle aspiration of the nodule may be helpful in diagnosis. Frequently, the single nodule is found to be a *fetal adenoma*, regarded by some as precancerous.

Small, Hard, Smooth Goiters. These may occur in thyrotoxicosis, subacute or chronic thyroiditis, or carcinoma. The history, course, and laboratory function tests are fairly distinctive for thyrotoxicosis and subacute thyroiditis. Enlargement of the delphian nodes limits the choice to subacute thyroiditis and carcinoma, usually distinguished by laboratory tests. Almost always, surgical exploration must distinguish between carcinoma and chronic thyroiditis.

Masses Beneath a Thyroidectomy Scar. The masses of fibrosis in a previous operative scar often cannot be distinguished by palpation from thyroid tissue. An interpretation must be made on the history and the pathologist's report of the tissue removed at the operation. Rapid growth of a mass is often regeneration of thyroid tissue. A scintigram will show whether the tissue is functioning as normal gland. Enlargement of remote lymph nodes should weigh in favor of carcinoma. A fine-needle biopsy of the nodule will often suffice.

Tracheal Displacement from Goiter. Many patients with a small goiter complain of a sense of constriction of fullness in the neck, although the caliber or the position of the trachea is not altered; this must be ascribed to suggestion or the instinct to protect a vulnerable region. But a large or strategically located goiter may certainly cause either, or both, tracheal compression and displacement (Fig. 5-73A). *Trachael Compression.* Usually the trachea is narrowed in the transverse diameter.

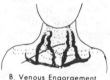

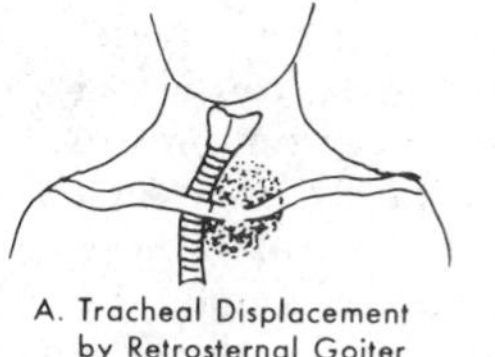

B. Venous Engorgement
from Retrosternal Goiter

Fig. 5-73. Two physical signs of retrosternal goiter. **A.** Tracheal displacement. *The diagram shows a typical situation in which retrosternal goiter on the patient's left compresses the trachea transversely and pushes it to the right. The tracheal deviation frequently can be demonstrated by palpation; compression of the trachea may be inferred from the history of dyspnea, or from Kocher's sign in which pressure on the lateral lobe produces stridor. In many cases tracheal compression must be proved by posteroanterior x-ray film of the chest.* **B.** Venous engorgement in the neck. *The compression of the external jugular vein by a retrosternal goiter produces engorgement of the superficial branches in the skin of the neck and clavicular regions, suggesting the possibility of obstruction of the superior vena cava. But the internal jugular vein is rarely impaired, so the cyanosis of the face and edema of the neck associated with superior vena caval obstruction are not present.*

Small degrees of compression cannot be diagnosed by history or physical examination. With a greater degree of embarrassment, *Kocher's test* is helpful, where slight pressure on the lateral lobes of the thyroid produces stridor. Posteroanterior and lateral x-ray views of the neck usually demonstrate the narrowing of caliber. ***Tracheal Displacement.*** Lateral deviation of the trachea can usually be shown by physical examination (see p. 286), except where the deviation begins at a level below the suprasternal notch, when x-ray examination must be made.

Retrosternal Goiter (Substernal, Intrathoracic, or Submerged Goiter). When the lower border of a goiter cannot be definitely palpated in the neck, consider the possibility of retrosternal extension, most frequently encountered when the neck is short and the goiter adenomatous. Usually, careful palpation of the gland during deglutition convinces the examiner of the extension. The shadow of goitrous extension is usually visible on the x-ray film of the region. Rarely, the goiter may be entirely retrosternal and rise only with increased intrathoracic pressure, such as with coughing; this is termed a *plunging goiter*. The patient's story may suggest the diagnosis. Increase in retromanubrial dullness seldom occurs. A goiter in the superior thoracic aperture may compress other structures, causing (1) cough; (2) dilated veins over the upper thorax from pressure on the internal jugular vein (Fig. 5-73B); rarely, also, edema of the face; (3) nocturnal dyspnea, from a posture of the neck assumed during sleep in which the goiter impinges upon the trachea; (4) dyspnea while awake, when the head is tilted to the side; (5) hoarseness, from pressure on the recurrent laryngeal nerve. The circulation may be tested by having the sitting patient *hold the arms* vertically, touching the face, for a few minutes. In this position, an obstructed thoracic inlet will cause congestion and cyanosis of the face, and dyspnea. Superior vena caval obstruction usually causes spontaneous edema of the face and arms. Rarely, a retrosternal goiter may be present without any accessible thyroid tissue in the neck. For reasons unknown, a high incidence of thyrotoxicosis is associated with retrosternal goiter.

Signs of Thyroid Function

Once the physician has assessed the gross pathologic changes in the thyroid, mostly by inspection and palpation, he turns to the evaluation of thyroid function by seeking symptoms and signs of two clinical entities, *myxedema* and *thyrotoxicosis*. The evidence is conclusive that myxedema is purely a deficit of thyroid hormone; hence *hypothyroidism* is an accurate equivalent expression. But thyrotoxicosis or Graves' disease is not necessarily synonymous with *hyperthyroidism* because some clinical features have never been reproduced in animals or man. Many ocular phenomena remain unexplained by the present knowledge of the thyropituitary axis. With this reservation, we prefer to tabulate the signs of the two diseases as opposite extremes of thyroid function, to assist the reader's memory. Rarely, metastatic carcinoma of the thyroid gland produces hyperthyroidism [J. M. Cerletty and W. J. Listwan: Hyperthyroidism Due to Functioning Metastatic Thyroid Carcinoma, *J.A.M.A.*, **242:**269–70, 1979].

Facies. In *thyrotoxicosis* the face is thin, the features sharp, the expression alert and vivacious; movements of the facial and neck muscles are frequent and fast. The responses to questions are quick; the emotions are labile. In contrast, the face of the *myxedematous* patient is rounded, relaxed, indefinably puffy without frank edema. The expression is placid and good-natured. His responses are slow.

Voice. The voice is normal in *thyrotoxicosis*. In *myxedema* its quality is frequently hoarse and coarse, from edema of the vocal cords. The singer can no longer sing; his friends are solicitous because of his "cold."

Neuromuscular System: Spontaneous Movement. In *thyrotoxicosis* the movements are excessive (hyperkinesia), and their speed faster than normal. Speech cadence is accelerated; the tongue and wrists can be flipped in alternating motion faster than normal. In *myxedema* there is paucity of unnecessary motion (hypokinesia), the motions are slow and deliberate. The speech is slow and distinct. The alternate motion rate of flipping tongue and wrists is retarded. *Muscle Strength.* In *thyrotoxicosis* there is some generalized muscle weakness but symmetric groups seem particularly involved. The Quadriceps femoris is most often affected, so the patient must push with arms on the chair or his thighs to arise from a sitting position. Both shoulder girdles may be weak; symmetric pairs of eye muscles may be paralyzed. In *myxedema,* there is some generalized weakness, but focal atrophy or disability is lacking. *Tendon Reflexes.* The reflexes in *thyrotoxicosis* are normal or hyperactive. In a patient with *myxedema,* when a knee jerk is elicited, one can see and feel the slow relaxing of muscles after the jerk. ***Tremor.*** Almost always in *thyrotoxicosis* the extended fingers and tongue exhibit a *fine* tremor. In addition, there may be a coarse tremor in a group of muscles in the calf or thigh as the result of weakness. The patient with *myxedema* has no opposite sign. ***Tongue.*** The tongue is normal in *thyrotoxicosis;* in some *myxedematous* patients the tongue seems large and awkward.

Integument. Changes in this tissue are more easily perceived in women than in men. ***The Skin.*** In *thyrotoxicosis* the skin feels softer than normal; it is thin, moist, and sweating. The skin over the shins may be the site of circumscribed elevated areas that are firm, nontender, and pink. Paradoxically, this is called *pretibial myxedema,* although it usually occurs in thyrotoxicosis in association with the exophthalmic syndrome. A counterpart of pretibial myxedema is thickening of the skin on the dorsa of the great toes. In *myxedema* the skin feels cold, dry, and thick; often there is scaling that is difficult to distinguish from ichthyosis. The palms and circumoral skin may be yellow from carotenemia. ***The Hair.*** In *thyrotoxicosis* the hair on the head is fine in texture, oily, and abundant. In *myxedema* the hairs on the head are dry and coarse, so they emit a crackling sound when lightly brushed. The texture is approached by that resulting from the so-called permanent wave. Looking at the profile of the forearm, one sees paucity or absence of lanugo hairs; or a few lonesome broken shafts may remain. The lateral thirds of the eyebrows are often thinned, but this occurs in many normal persons past middle age. ***The Nails.*** In *thyrotoxicosis* the fingernail may separate from its matrix (onycholysis); usually only one or two pairs of nails are involved. In *myxedema* the nails are dry and brittle; sometimes they are longitudinally ridged.

The Eyes. In about one fifth of the patients with *thyrotoxicosis,* various signs of the endocrine eye lesion may develop, usually after onset of hypermetabolism, but sometimes antedating it by some months; frequently the eye signs appear when hypermetabolism is subsiding after treatment with radioiodine or by thyroidectomy. Rarely, the eye lesions appear during full-blown myxedema. Occasionally, the emergence of the eye lesion is associated with the development of pretibial myxedema. The entire spectrum of eye lesions may not occur in a single individual. Often the signs are initially unilateral, the other eye being involved some months later. The signs are lid lag, lid spasm, lacrimation, chemosis, periorbital edema, periorbital solid infiltration with mucopolysaccharides, and exophthalmos (proptosis) (Fig. 5-6, p. 82). Often there is paresis of extraocular muscles, usually involving one or two symmetric pairs; isolated weakness of the two superior recti is common. In *myxedema* the only ocular sign is periorbital edema.

Cardiovascular System: Strength of Cardiac Contraction. In *thyrotoxicosis* the strength of myocardial contraction is augmented, as manifest by the accentuated precordial thrust and the sharpness of the heart sounds. In *myxedema* the precordial thrust is normal or feeble. ***Cardiac Rate.*** Tachycardia is almost the rule in *thyrotoxicosis;* the ventricular rate is normal or slow in *myxedema.* ***Cardiac Rhythm.*** *Thyrotoxicosis* is notorious for the high incidence of atrial fibrillation and atrial flutter. In *myxedema,* dysrhythmias are rare. ***Blood Pressure.*** In *thyrotoxicosis* the systolic pressure is slightly elevated, the diastolic diminished, so the pulse pressure is widened, thus a pistol-shot sound is often present in the femoral arteries. In *myxedema* the blood pressure is normal, or else there is moderate elevation of both systolic and diastolic values that may return to normal with treatment of the glandular defect.

Gastrointestinal System: Food Intake. The caloric intake is frequently increased in *thyrotoxicosis,* usually with contrasting weight loss; the weight depends upon whether the patient can take enough food to meet the increased caloric requirements. In *myxedema* food intake may be small with constant or gaining weight. ***Intestinal Motility.*** In *thyrotoxicosis* defecation may be more frequent; the onset of true diarrhea is a grave prognostic sign. Constipation is very common in *myxedema;* the resulting tympanites may suggest *ileus.*

Accumulation of Body Fluid. In *thyrotoxicosis* body fluid does not accumulate unless cardiac failure occurs. In *myxedema* pericardial effusion, ascites, and edema of the ankles all occur without cardiac failure.

Catemenia. In *thyrotoxicosis* the menses are usually normal; occasionally there is oligomenorrhea. In *myxedema,* menorrhagia is common.

The Blood. The erythrocytes are usually normal in *thyrotoxico-*

sis, but leukopenia sometimes occurs. In *myxedema* a normocytic or macrocytic anemia is frequent. The anemia is refractory to therapy with iron, vitamin B_{12}, or anything else but thyroid hormone.

The Psyche: Mentation. In *thyrotoxicosis* there is no disturbance. The patient with *myxedema* often complains of thinking more slowly; this can readily be confirmed by objective measurements. *Emotional Affect.* Patients with *thyrotoxicosis* are notoriously irritable and emotionally labile. Most patients with longstanding *myxedema* appear cheerful and placid; but those with recently acquired symptoms complain bitterly and are often dejected. *Psychoses.* Depressions are common in *thyrotoxicosis;* occasionally manic states develop. Patients with *myxedema* may develop depressions, though not so commonly as with thyrotoxicosis. *Myxedema coma* is a rare but grave occurrence.

Laboratory Tests of Thyroid Function. The most satisfactory tests now available for thyroid function are the radioactive-iodine uptake of the thyroid gland (RAI), the serum uptake of ^{131}I-labeled triiodothyronine (T_3 uptake), and the total serum thyroxin (total T_4), the free serum thyroxine (free T_4) and the serum thyroid stimulating hormone (TSH) concentration. *Thyrotoxicosis.* Elevated RAI, T_3 uptake, total T_4 and free T_4. The TSH is suppressed. *Myxedema.* Lowered RAI, T_3 uptake, total T_4 and free T_4. The TSH is elevated. *Subacute Thyroiditis.* An initial toxic phase with low RAI and high T_4 may be followed by a brief hypothyroid phase with low T_4 levels and high TSH. *Chronic Thyroiditis.* All tests normal until functional failure produces hypothyroidism.

Nongoitrous Cervical Masses and Fistulas

Once the thyroid gland has been excluded by inspection and palpation as the site of a cervical mass, the examiner can turn to consideration of other structures in the neck.

Midline Cervical Mass: ***Thyroglossal Cysts and Fistulas.*** A thyroglossal *cyst* may appear at any time in life, arising from remnants of the thyroglossal duct. Only a few of the cysts are translucent. A *fistula* results from bursting of an inflamed cyst or the incomplete excision of a thyroglossal remnant. Cysts at various levels present individual problems in diagnosis (Fig. 5-74). *Suprahyoid Level.* A thyroglossal cyst immediately above the hyoid bone must be distinguished from a sublingual der-

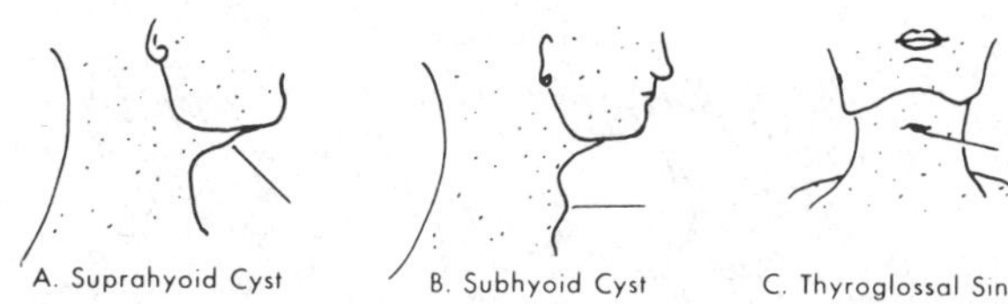

Fig. 5-74. Thyroglossal cysts and sinuses. *Normally the thyroglossal duct becomes completely obliterated before birth. But often segments of the duct persist and develop into cysts or even sinuses. Any of these derivatives will occur in the midline of the neck, a fact that is considered in diagnosis.* **A.** Suprahyoid cysts. *This is above the hyoid bone.* **B.** Subhyoid cyst. *A segment between the hyoid bone and the thyroid cartilage may give rise to a cyst.* **C.** Thyroglossal sinus. *This may develop anywhere from the foramen cecum at the base of the tongue to the thyroid gland; it drains through the skin and is always in the midline.*

moid cyst that may be visible under the tongue as a white opaque body shining through the mucosa. *Subhyoid Level.* The cyst is in the midline between the hyoid bone and the thyroid cartilage. Sometimes swallowing causes the mass to hide temporarily under the hyoid; to demonstrate, have the patient dorsiflex his neck and open his mouth, whereat the cyst reappears. *Thyroid Cartilage Level.* Only at this site does a thyroglossal cyst *deviate from the midline,* usually to the left; the forward pressure of the prowlike thyroid cartilage pushes it aside. To distinguish the mass from an enlarged lymph node have the patient protrude the tongue maximally. If the mass is connected with the thyroglossal duct structures, the maneuver gives it an *upward tug.* *Cricoid Cartilage Level.* A thyroglossal cyst in this region must be distinguished from an adenoma of the pyramidal lobe of the thyroid. The cyst tugs upward with protrusion of the tongue. Adenomas in other parts of the goiter lead to the presumption that the mass is pyramidal lobe. Biopsy may be necessary to decide.

Midline Cervical Mass: ***Pyramidal Lobe of Thyroid.*** See the preceding discussion on thyroglossal cyst at the cricoid level. The pyramidal lobe may extend from the isthmus of the thyroid to the hyoid bone (Fig. 5-75A), true to its name, its base on the isthmus is usually wider and can be felt as an isthmic projection.

Midline Cervical Mass: ***Delphian Nodes.*** These are lymph nodes

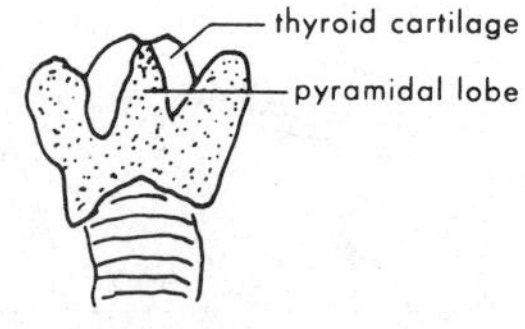

A. Pyramidal Lobe of Thyroid Gland

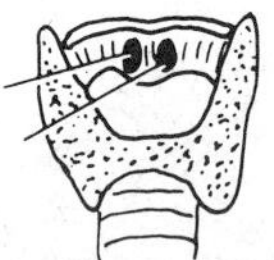

B. Delphian Nodes

Fig. 5-75. Associated thyroid masses. **A.** Pyramidal lobe of thyroid gland. *This is an upward projection of thyroid tissue, usually arising from the isthmus or left lobe. It may follow the course of the thyroglossal duct as far as the hyoid bone.* **B.** Delphian nodes. *These are enlarged lymph nodes in the thyrohyoid membranes. Usually they are involved only in thyroid carcinoma or in subacute thyroiditis.*

in the midline of the thyrohyoid membrane (Fig. 5-75B). They enlarge in subacute thyroiditis and in thyroid carcinoma. Examination of the main mass of the thyroid usually gives a hint of whether to suspect regional lymphadenopathy.

Mass in Suprasternal Notch: ***Dermoid Cyst.*** Frequently a nonpulsatile fluctuant mass in the suprasternal notch (Burns' space) proves to be a dermoid cyst. The mass is not adherent to the trachea nor does it move upward with protrusion of the tongue. The cyst may be confused with tuberculous abscess.

Fatty Tumor in Suprasternal Notch: ***Dewlap.*** In Cushing's syndrome from excess of adrenocorticosteroids, a soft, nontender fatty mass may form in the suprasternal notch. The term *dewlap* has been suggested because of its resemblance to a fold of skin in the cow.

Mass in the Suprasternal Notch: ***Tuberculous Abscess.*** This has the same physical characteristics as a dermoid cyst, except that it is slightly less fluctuant. It may arise from an abscess in the lung apex or by drainage from the deep cervical chain of lymph nodes.

Pulsatile Mass in the Suprasternal Notch: ***Aorta or Innominate Artery.*** Occasionally, elongation of the aortic arch or the innominate artery causes the vessel to bow upward into the suprasternal notch. This is not necessarily evidence of aneurysmal dilatation (see p. 445).

PALPATION OF THE CERVICAL LYMPH NODES. **Seat the patient in a chair and stand behind him to palpate the neck with your fingertips.**

Examine in sequence the sites of the various groups of lymph nodes (Fig. 5-76): (1) *Submental,* under the chin in the midline and on either side; (2) *submandibular,* under the jaw near its angle; (3) *jugular,* along the anterior border of the Sternocleidomastoideus; (4) *supraclavicular,* behind the midportion of the clavicle; (5) *poststernocleidomastoid,* behind the posterior border of the upper half of the Sternocleidomastoideus; (6) *suboccipital,* in the apex of the posterior cervical triangle; (7) *pretrapezius,* in front of the upper border of the Trapezius; (8) *postauricular,* behind the pinna on the mastoid process; (9) *preauricular,* slightly in front of the tragus of the pinna. When an enlarged lymph node is found, examine carefully the region drained by the gland for a primary lesion. For nodes in the anterior cervical triangle, include the anterior third of the scalp, as well as facial structures. For nodes in the posterior cervical triangle, examine the posterior two thirds of the scalp. Determine whether the lymphadenopathy is *localized* to the neck or *generalized,* by searching the regional lymph nodes in other parts of the body: axilla, epitrochlear region, inguinal and femoral regions. Characterize the enlarged nodes as to *size, consistency, tenderness;* whether they are *discrete* or *matted together;* whether *fixed* or *mobile*. **See also p. 467.**

Acute Cervical Lymphadenopathy: ***Localized Lymphadenitis.*** Commonly, infections of the scalp, face, mouth, teeth, pharynx, or ear cause localized lymphadenitis of the neck, in the particular group of nodes draining the involved region. Included in

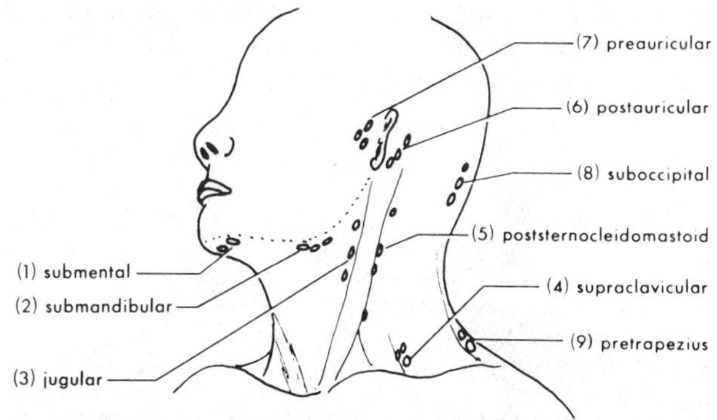

Fig. 5-76. Superficial lymph nodes of the neck. *Palpation of the neck for lymphadenopathy is accurate only when the region of each group of nodes is examined in systematic fashion. The drawing contains a numbered scheme for examining nine groups of nodes in sequence.*

localized lesions is chancre of the face with its regional lymphadenitis. Cervical adenopathy is also common in erythema nodosum, although the subcutaneous lesions are almost always limited to the legs.

Acute Cervical Lymphadenopathy: **In Generalized Lymphadenitis.** Frequently the discovery of cervical lymphadenitis leads to the search for enlarged nodes elsewhere in the body to establish a generalized distribution.

Clinical Occurrence. Secondary syphilis, rubella (German measles), infectious mononucleosis, generalized furunculosis, multiple bites from lice, serum sickness, drug allergy (serum sickness type) especially from penicillin, cat scratch disease, African trypanosomiasis (A. sleeping sickness), kala-azar, scrub typhus. The postauricular gland is seldom involved, except in secondary syphilis and rubella. Swelling of the posterior cervical nodes (*Winterbottom's sign*) is diagnostic in African trypanosomiasis.

Chronic Localized Cervical Lymphadenopathy: **Hodgkin's Disease.** The lymph nodes may enlarge rapidly over one to three weeks or slowly over a few months; the amount of swelling is much greater than in acute adenitis. The nodes are nontender and discrete; they do not suppurate. Although the disease may involve any lymph nodes in the body, frequently only a single group is affected for a long time, most often in the neck (Fig. 5-77A). Analysis of biopsy material establishes the histopathologic type, and subsequent clinical staging of the extent of disease permits selection of appropriate treatment.

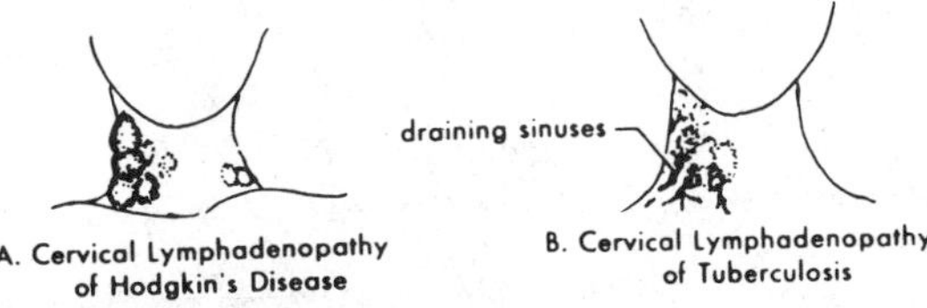

Fig. 5-77. Cervical lymphadenopathy. **A.** In Hodgkin's disease. *There is no specific pattern of involvement of the nodes. The neck is frequently affected first, often unilaterally, and such a case is represented here. The nodes are mostly on one side; they are large, firm, discrete, nontender, and nonsuppurative.* **B.** In tuberculosis. *One finds a matted mass of nontender lymph nodes; the nodes are firm, but some have suppurated and formed draining sinuses.*

***Chronic Localized Cervical Lymphadenopathy:* Tuberculosis** (Scrofula). Usually the disease is caused by the bovine strain of tubercle bacilli, although human strains have occasionally been implicated. The disease has a predilection for the cervical lymph nodes. The nodes are large, multiple, and nontender. Classically, the nodes should be matted together, but this is often difficult to determine by palpation (Fig. 5-77B). Frequently the nodes suppurate and form indolent sinus tracts. Extensive scarring of the neck often results. The diagnosis should be proved by biopsy and culture. The bacteriologic examination should establish whether the strain of tubercle bacilli is bovine or human.

***Chronic Localized Cervical Lymphadenopathy:* Gummas.** Tertiary syphilitic granulomas tend to involve a single group of nodes. The lymph nodes are large, nontender, discrete, nonsuppurating. Serologic tests for syphilis are usually positive, but this does not prove the syphilitic causation because the disease may be coincident with another cause for nodal involvement. Biopsy of a node is indicated. Classically, gummas regress rapidly or completely in a few weeks with the oral administration of iodides. There may be instances in which this therapeutic test is desirable.

***Chronic Localized Cervical Lymphadenopathy:* Actinomycosis.** The cervical lymph nodes may be involved by *Actinomyces bovis,* producing much enlargement. The nodes are prone to suppurate, forming sinuses with a bright red hue. The pus contains *sulfur granules,* 1 to 2 mm in diameter, which magnification shows to be of the fungi. Prolonged treatment with penicillin has been effective.

***Chronic Localized Cervical Lymphadenopathy:* Carcinomatous Metastasis.** The nodes are usually stony hard, nontender, nonsuppurative. Epidermoid carcinoma predominates. In *anterior jugular lymph node* involvement, primary malignancies are found in the upper aerodigestive tract including the maxillary sinus, oral cavity, tongue, tonsil, hypopharynx, and larynx. In the *submental region,* metastases occur from primary neoplasms in the lower lip, anterior tongue and floor of the mouth. In the *posterior triangle,* nasopharynx and scalp are common sites of origin. Careful examination of suspicious areas *and the remainder* of the upper aerodigestive is essential to assure biopsy of the primary tumor rather than the cervical metastasis [D. E. Schuller, et al.: The Prognostic Significance of Metastatic Cervical Lymph Nodes, *Laryngoscope* **90:**557, 1980.].

Chronic Localized Cervical Lymphadenopathy: ***Virchow's Node*** (Sentinel Node, Signal Node, Troisier's Node). This classic physical sign is an enlargement of a single lymph node, usually in the *left supraclavicular* group, frequently behind the clavicular head of the left Sternocleidomastoideus. Often it is so deep in the neck that it escapes casual examination. A purposeful search requires the patient's trunk to be erect and the examiner facing him; the fingers explore the region behind the muscle head. The node may rise to be palpated as the patient performs the Valsalva maneuver. The node is the site of carcinomatous metastasis from a primary lesion in the upper abdomen. When a primary carcinoma is found in the abdomen, demonstration of the sentinel node is proof of distant metastasis.

Lateral Cervical Cyst: ***Branchial Cyst.*** A tumor usually appears in adult life, not in childhood. Commonly there is a single cystic mass just anterior but deep to the upper third of the Sternocleidomastoideus (Fig. 5-78A). The mass feels resilient and slightly soft, except when intercurrent inflammation hardens it and makes it tender. Aspirated fluid appears to be pus, but spread on a watch glass, oil droplets may be seen floating on the surface. Microscopically, these droplets contain many cholesterol crystals, a diagnostic sign.

Lateral Cervical Fistula: ***Branchial Fistula.*** In the same location as branchial cyst, the fistula may either be congenital or developed later from an inflamed cyst. Probing the tract usually

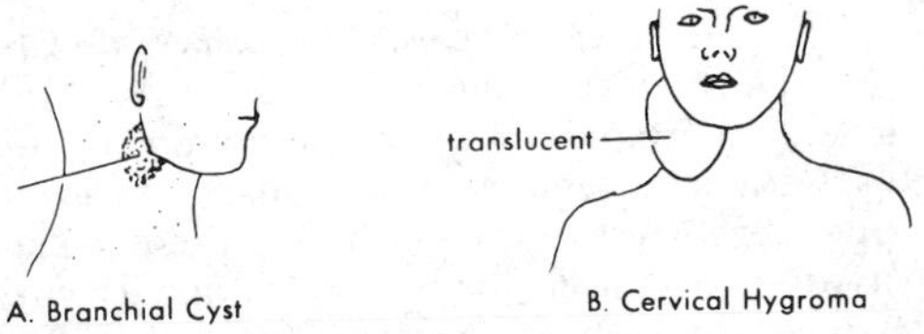

Fig. 5-78. Single tumors of the lateral neck. **A.** *The typical branchial cyst is anterior and deep to the upper third of the sternocleidomastoid muscle. The mass is resilient and fairly soft, except when hardened by infection. Sinuses may form and persist.* **B.** *A hygroma is a mass formed by occluded lymph channels. It is soft, irregular, and compressible. Brilliant translucence is the outstanding feature.*

discloses a blind end in the lateral pharyngeal wall. Fistulas become intermittently infected.

Lateral Cervical Cyst: ***Hygroma.*** Usually present from childhood, the mass is formed by many cysts of occluded lymphatic channels. The mass is soft, irregular, and partially compressible. Usually it occupies the upper third of the anterior cervical triangle, but it may extend downward and under the jaw (Fig. 5-78B). It is readily distinguished from all other cysts by its *brilliant translucence.* Its size may vary from time to time. It may become inflamed.

Lateral Cervical Cyst: ***Carotid Body Tumor.*** Arising from the chromaffin tissue of the carotid body, the mass can be palpated near the bifurcation of the common carotid artery (Fig. 5-79A). It is sometimes called a *potato tumor* because of its shape. Although growing in the carotid sheath, it does not always transmit arterial pulsations. It appears in middle life and grows very slowly. It may early feel cystic; later it becomes hard. The mass is mobile laterally, but movement vertically is restricted. Pressure on the tumor sometimes produces slowing of the heart rate and dizziness. Occasionally, the tumor produces vasoactive amines, and palpation can produce pupillary dilatation and hypertension, a diagnostic sign. In one fifth of

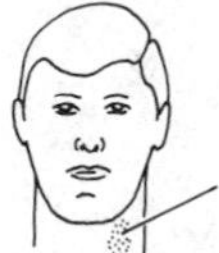

A. Tumor of Carotid Body

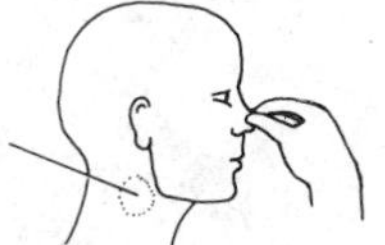

B. Intermittent Cervical Pouches

Fig. 5-79. Single tumors of the lateral neck (cont.). **A.** Tumor of the carotid body. *The mass usually arises near the bifurcation of the common carotid artery. Usually shaped like a potato, it is freely movable laterally, but it cannot be moved in the long axis of the artery.* **B.** Intermittent cervical pouches. *Some cystic masses will be found to be present at times and absent at others. This story suggests the presence of a diverticulum of the pharynx, if associated with eating, or if associated with forceful blowing of the nose; a diverticulum is likely to come from the larynx. To demonstrate in the former case, the patient should be asked to eat; in the latter, the patient should blow through the pursed lips with nose closed.*

the cases, regional metastasis eventually occurs upward along the sheath of the artery.

Lateral Cervical Cyst: ***Zenker's Diverticulum*** (Pharyngeal Pouch). The patient complains of gurgling in the neck, especially during swallowing. Regurgitation of food is common during eating or when lying on the side. An intermittent swelling in the side of the neck can be seen; usually the left side is involved (Fig. 5-79B). When not apparent, the swelling may be induced by swallowing water. Pressure on the filled pouch causes regurgitation of old food. The diagnosis is made from the esophagram.

Lateral Cervical Cyst: ***Laryngocele.*** Herniation of the laryngeal diverticulum through the lateral thyrohyoid membrane causes an intermittent swelling of the neck at that point. Blowing the nose will often induce an air-filled swelling that is resonant to percussion. Usually the condition occurs from chronic severe coughing or sustained blowing on musical instruments.

Lateral Cervical Cyst: ***Cavernous Hemangioma.*** As in other parts of the body, the swelling is soft; compression partially empties the cavity of blood and *refilling is slow.* A faint blue color under the skin may be discerned.

6

The Thorax and Cardiovascular System

Pain in the Chest

Thoracic pain is a presenting symptom with many different causes. Unless obviously the result of trauma, chest pain is likely to be exaggerated by fear of heart disease, so a precise diagnosis is necessary. If cardiac disease or other serious disorders are excluded, the physician should support his reassurances by demonstrating the factors that actually induce the patient's pain. Chest pain is often accompanied by few or no physical signs, so the examiner must secure diagnostic clues by searching questions about the *attributes of pain* (PQRST = provocative-palliative factors, quality, region, severity, and timing). The search must be made while reviewing a considerable list of possible causes, as arranged here for a diagnostic approach. The patient may recognize the pain as superficial rather than deep and may localize it rather sharply. Almost always this type of pain is accompanied by localized tenderness. The structures involved are the skin and subcutaneous tissues, the fat, or the breasts.

▼ *Chest Pain with Tenderness:* ***Skin and Subcutaneous Structures.*** Inflammation, trauma, and neoplasm in these tissues are similar to those of other regions and offer no special diagnostic problems, *provided* they are thought of and searched for. The presence of bruises, lacerations, ulcers, hematomas, masses, or tenderness is usually diagnostic.

— *Chest Pain with Tenderness:* ***Chest Wall Syndrome.*** This disorder has been further defined by subjecting the patient to four maneuvers: (1) *palpation of the chest wall for tenderness*, by applying firm steady pressure to the sternum, the costosternal junctions, the intercostal spaces, the ribs, and the pectoralis major muscles and their insertions, (2) *horizontal flexion of the arms* by lifting one arm after the other by the elbow and pulling it across the chest toward the ipsilateral side, with the head rotated toward the ipsilateral side, (3) *flexion of the neck*, by having the patient look toward the ceiling while his arms are pulled backward and slightly upward, (4) *vertical pressure upon the head.* If any of these tests reproduces the patient's pain, physiotherapy is given as a therapeutic test. Other tests of coronary function may be positive if there is concomitant disease [S. E. Epstein, L. H. Gerber, and J. S. Borer: Chest Wall Syndrome, *J.A.M.A.*, **241:**2793–95, 1978].

— *Chest Pain with Tenderness:* ***Thrombophlebitis of the Thoracoepigastric Vein*** (Mondor's Disease). The pain is felt along the anterolateral chest wall with radiation to the axilla or inguinal region. A tender cord 3 to 4 mm in diameter is usually palpable and often visible when the skin is stretched. The disease is self-limited and lasts two to four weeks [N. R. Thomford and W. J. Holaday: Mondor's Disease (Phlebitis of the Thoracoepigastric Vein), *Ann. Surg.*, **170:**1035–37, 1969].

— *Chronic Retrosternal Pain:* ***Xiphisternal Arthritis.*** The pain may be ascribed to myocardial ischema *unless* the xiphoid cartilage is palpated and the pain reproduced.

— *Chest Pain with Tenderness:* ***Fat.*** In a rare form of obesity, symmetric fat lobules on the trunk and limbs are painful and tender. The condition is known as *adiposis dolorosa* (Dercum's disease).

— *Chest Pain with Tenderness:* ***Breasts.*** Painful lesions are fissures of the nipples (p. 252), cystic mastitis (p. 261), fibroadenosis (p. 261), acute breast abscess (p. 264), and occasionally breast carcinoma (p. 263).

Chest Pain Intensified by Respiratory Motion

Thoracic movements displace ribs, muscles, nerves, and pleural surfaces. When these structures are inflamed or traumatized, the *pain is accentuated* by breathing, coughing, laughing, or sneezing. As with superficial pain, the regions may be *tender*, but the distinguishing feature of intensification by thoracic movement is designated here as *respiratory pain.* The structures to be considered are ribs, cartilages, muscles, nerves, and pleurae. A systematic inventory of causes of pain in each of these tissues should be considered in the examination.

▼ *Key Symptom:* ***Respiratory Pain.*** This is a complaint that introduces many conditions.

— *Respiratory Pain:* ***Chest Wall Twinge Syndrome*** (Precordial Catch, Rib S). This is the most common type of pain bringing the patient to the physician because of a fear of cardiac disease. The patient experiences brief episodes of sharp pains or "catches" in the anterior chest, usually on the left side, although they may occur elsewhere. No association with exertion has been noted, although some patients report the onset while assuming a bent-over posture. The pains last from one half to three minutes; they are aggravated by deep breathing, relieved by shallow respirations [A. J. Miller and T. A. Taxidor: The "Precordial Catch," a Neglected Syndrome of Precordial Pain, *J.A.M.A.*, **159:**1364, 1955]. The cause is unknown; speculation has considered intercostal muscle spasm and fleeting costochrondral pains. A series of 791 persons in the Omaha region indicated in questionnaires that 48% of the men and 70% of the women had experienced such pains; 9% had sought medical consultation [D. Stegman and B. Mead: The Chest Wall Twinge Syndrome, *Nebr. Med. J.*, pp. 528–33, Sept., 1970]. The condition is harmless, but the patient must be reassured that it is not due to heart disease.

— *Respiratory Pain:* ***Rib Fracture.*** The respiratory motions of broken fragments cause *well-localized, sharp, lancinating pain.* The patient may tell of a previous blow to the chest, but will seldom associate a history of coughing with a cough fracture (p. 288). The diagnostic signs of rib fracture are *point tenderness* at the fracture site, *bone crepitus* on palpation and induction of pain at the site by *remote pressure* on the rib (p. 288). When this lesion is not remembered and excluded, the history is likely to suggest pleurisy.

— *Respiratory Pain:* ***Periostitis of Rib.*** Although the bone marrow is relatively insensitive, inflammation of the periosteum is extremely painful. Trauma or acute osteomyelitis produces periostitis with *exquisite tenderness* and *severe sharp pain,* often affected by motion. It persists for hours; it is often worse at night. Acute osteomyelitis is usually accompanied by fever and leukocytosis, long before x-ray changes can be detected in the bone (p. 653).

— ***Respiratory Pain: Periosteal Hematoma of Rib.*** This likewise is very painful and tender. It usually follows direct trauma and its diagnosis is easy.

— ***Respiratory Pain: Costochondritis of Rib.*** This is a common cause of chest pain. The onset may be sudden or gradual. The pain is usually *dull;* it is intensified by respiratory motion and movements of the shoulder girdle. The sole physical sign is *tenderness* in the groove at the junction of rib and cartilage. There is no swelling, and there are no x-ray findings. A rare form is called *Tietze's syndrome,* in which a *tender fusiform swelling* appears in the cartilage, often that attached to the 2nd rib. The cause of the disease is unknown; it may subside in a few weeks or persist for months.

— ***Respiratory Pain: Slipping Cartilage.*** A costal cartilage, fractured from long-forgotten trauma, may slip over an adjacent rib causing *pain* with respiratory motion, or movement of the shoulder girdle. The slipping may be accompanied by an audible or palpable *click* (Fig. 6–17).

— ***Respiratory Pain: Stitch of the Intercostal Muscles.*** A *sharp pain* in the chest wall following severe exercise may be relieved by rest. The mechanism is unknown; it has been attributed to spasm of the diaphragm.

— ***Respiratory Pain: Intercostal Myositis.*** Severe *aching pain,* intensified by thoracic motion, results from inflammation of the intercostal muscles. The muscles are *tender; induration* and *palpable nodules* may ultimately appear.

— ***Respiratory Pain: Strain of the Pectoralis Minor.*** Irritation of this muscle from overuse, such as elevation of the arm, carrying a knapsack, or lifting a baby, causes *pain* in the chest. The involved muscle is *tender.*

— ***Respiratory Pain: Disorders of the Shoulder Girdle.*** Any of these may cause *pain* in the upper chest, augmented by thoracic motion. See p. 713.

— ***Respiratory Pain: Intercostal Neuralgia, Nonspecific.*** Irritation of an intercostal nerve produces *sharp, lancinating, stabbing pain* along the nerve's course. The pain is frequently intensified by respiratory motion or movements of the trunk; exposure to cold may accentuate it. *Tenderness along the nerve* is diagnostic. Usually the tenderness is maximal near the vertebral foramen, in the axilla, or at the parasternal line; these points correspond to the major cutaneous branches of the nerve.

Clinical Occurrence. Tabes dorsalis, mediastinal neoplasm, neurofibroma (where an intercostal mass may be felt), or in vertebral caries.

— ***Respiratory Pain:*** ***Herpes Zoster*** (Shingles). This is a specific type of intercostal neuralgia. There is sudden onset of the *neuralgic pain* described in the preceding paragraph. The physical findings are nondescript until *clusters of herpetic vesicles* appear in a few days along the course of nerve, imparting a *burning pain* and *erythema* to the involved skin. The vesicles burst and slowly heal. The distribution is always *unilateral,* and it does not cross the midline. The pain may subside in a week or so, or it may persist for months as *postherpetic neuralgia.* Before the appearance of the vesicles the clinician may be confused about the diagnosis.

— ***Respiratory Pain:*** ***Pleurisy*** (Pleuritis). Inflammation of the pleura produces *knifelike* or *shooting pains* in the skin of the adjacent thoracic wall. The pain is definitely intensified by *breathing, coughing, laughing.* Often a *friction rub* appears (p. 313) to be felt and heard, but this is not constantly present, so it may be missed for several examinations. Signs of *pleural effusion* (p. 316) may develop. ***Pathophysiology.*** The *visceral pleura* is *anesthetic,* but the parietal pleura contains many sensory fibers that join the trunks of adjacent intercostal nerves, giving off twigs to the overlying skin. Anesthetizing the skin will relieve pleural pain. Evidence suggests that pleural pain is caused either by stretching of the inflamed parietal pleura or by separation of fibrous adhesions between two pleural surfaces. It is difficult to credit the concept that pain is produced by the rubbing together of two pleural surfaces; pain often occurs without a friction rub, and a rub is often present without pain. *Distinction:* The diagnosis of pleurisy is made from the history of the typical pain and the presence of a friction rub. Other disorders such as rib fractures, myositis, and neuritis must be excluded by lack of appropriate tenderness, as they also respond to chest motion.

— ***Respiratory Pain:*** ***Diaphragmatic Pleurisy.*** Epitome: *sharp shooting pain, intensified by thoracic motions, in the epigastrium, lower retrosternal region, or in the shoulder.* The pain is sharp and lancinating, especially augmented by deep breathing, coughing, or laughing. It may be localized along the costal margins, the epigastrium, the lumbar region, or in the neck at the superior border of the Trapezius or the supraclavicular fossa. The painful areas are all on the same side. A pleural *friction rub* may be present. ***Pathophysiology.*** The peripheral portion of the diaphragmatic pleura is supplied by the 5th and 6th intercostal nerves, so involvement of their regions produces pain near the costal margins. The central area of the diaphragm is served by the phrenic nerve that also supplies the neck and the peritoneal surface of the diaphragm at its central area; thus pain in the neck may be caused from irritation of the diaphragmatic pleura by subphrenic abscess or splenic infarction or rupture (Fig. 6-1). ***Distinction.*** The diagnosis of pleurisy is probable when pain is accompanied by fever and friction rub; later, pleural effusion may appear. But judgment must be guarded because subphrenic abscess perforating the diaphragm can produce similar findings. Occasionally gastric herniation through the esophageal hiatus of the diaphragm may give similar pain. Pericarditis with pleuritic pain should be considered (p. 231). A previous history of dysphagia or intra-abdominal disease should suggest disorders of the esophagus, subphrenic abscess, peptic ulcer, or pancreatitis.

— *Respiratory Pain:* ***Epidemic Pleurodynia*** (Bornholm Disease, Devil's Grip). *Epitome: sudden severe pains in thorax or abdomen, with frequent shifting of loci and asymptomatic intervals; fever and*

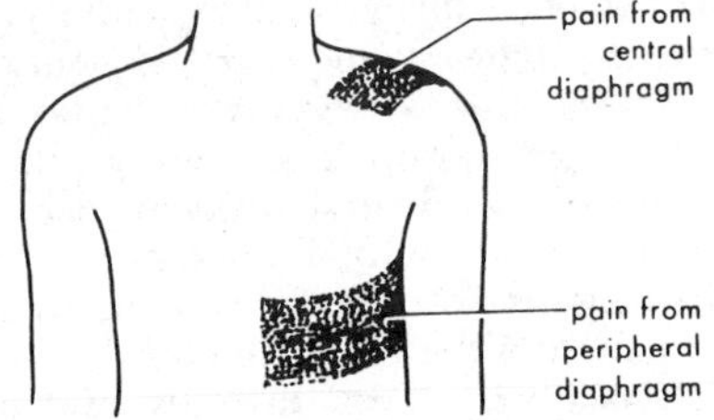

Fig. 6-1. Referral of diaphragmatic pain. *Irritation of the central portion of the diaphragm, either pleural or peritoneal surface, causes pain at the superior border of the trapezius muscle and the supraclavicular fossa. Stimulation of either surface of the peripheral portions of the diaphragm results in pain in the skin supplied by the T-6 dermatome.*

headache without leukocytosis; duration of a few days. After a nondescript prodrome of 1 to 10 days, the patient is suddenly seized with apparently *catastrophic sharp, knifelike pains* in the walls of the thorax or abdomen, intensified by breathing and other bodily motions; the thorax may be splinted and the thighs flexed upon the belly. Paroxysms of intense pain are separated by *intervals of complete comfort.* Severe *headache* is frequent. Cases may appear sporadically or in epidemic. Mild *pharyngitis* is often noted. The muscles of the neck, trunk, and limbs may be *tender.* In one quarter of the cases a *friction rub* is detected. *Orchitis* or *pericarditis* may complicate. X-ray films of the chest are usually negative. ***Pathophysiology.*** The usual cause is an infection with group B Coxsackie virus, although group A or an ECHO virus is occasionally implicated. ***Laboratory Findings.*** The leukocyte count is normal. The virus is frequent in the normal throat, so its presence is no proof of pathogenicity. Rising viral titers may help to confirm the diagnosis but are not helpful for early diagnosis. ***Distinction.*** The sudden retrosternal pain reminds the physician of myocardial infarction or dissecting aneurysm. The fever suggests pneumonia or acute appendicitis. Lacking an epidemic, the correct diagnosis may be suspected from the normal leukocyte counts. A period of several days of worried observation until symptoms subside is the usual method of making the diagnosis.

Deep Retrosternal or Precordial Pain—A Symptom of the Six-Dermatome Band

Deep visceral pain behind the sternum or in the precordial region is *not specific* for cardiac disorders; rather it should be regarded as *the prime symptom for the entire region supplied by dermatomes T-1 to T-6.* The neuroanatomy of the region furnishes the structural basis for this concept, and clinical experience confirms it.

Dermatomes T-1 to T-6 cover the thoracic surface from the neck to beneath the xiphoid process; they extend down the anteromedial aspects of the arms and forearms (Fig. 6-2). The upper four dermatomes are supplied by sensory afferent fibers to the posterior roots of T-1 to T-4; in the cord, the fibers communicate with one another superiorly and inferiorly. Practically all the thoracic viscera are served by sensory fibers in these pathways: myocardium, pericardium, aorta, pul-

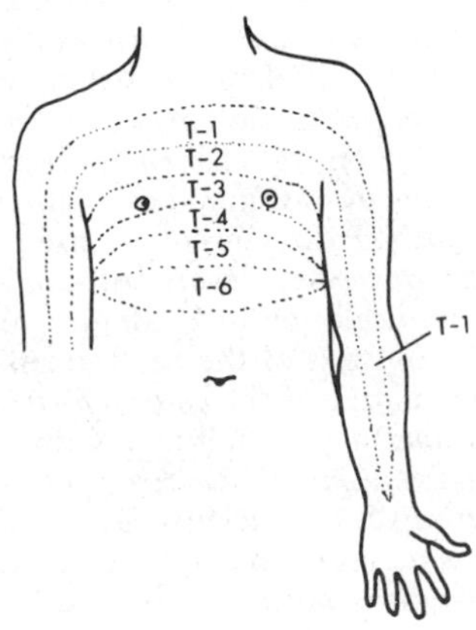

Fig. 6-2. The six-dermatome band. *Dermatomes T-1 to T-6 inclusive form a band that covers most of the thorax and extends down the anteromedial aspect of the arms and forearms. Sensory pathways from the viscera of this entire region are so interconnected axially that stimulation of any part can produce the same patterns of chest pain.*

monary artery, esophagus, and mediastinum. Lesions in any of these structures produce pain of the same quality, *deep, visceral, poorly localized.* Usually such pain is maximal in the retrosternal region or the precordium; it often extends with lesser intensity upward into the neck, to either the left or right hemithorax, downward on the anteromedial aspects of one or both arms and forearms.

The band made by dermatomes T-5 and T-6 comprises fibers from the lower thoracic wall, the diaphragmatic muscles and their peritoneal surfaces, the gallbladder, the pancreas, the duodenum, and the stomach. Inflammation in these structures causes *deep, visceral, poorly localized pain* precisely similar in quality to that from the upper band. Usually the maximal intensity is in the *xiphoid region* and in the *back, inferior to the right scapula.* But the pain may extend to the upper band of T-1 to T-4 through posterior connections in the sympathetics, so that the pattern may be indistinguishable from that arising above the diaphragm.

Diagnostic Modus Operandi. **To determine the cause of deep chest pain, (1) accept the *location* of the pain as indicating only**

that the source is *somewhere* in the six-dermatome band: the myocardium, pericardium, aorta, pulmonary artery, mediastinum, esophagus, gallbladder, pancreas, duodenum, stomach, or the subphrenic region; (2) shorten the list of possibilities by carefully searching for *provocative-palliative factors* and *timing;* (3) make appropriate tests to distinguish between the disorders on the shortened list.

▼ *Six-Dermatome Pain:* **Angina Pectoris** (Heberden's A., Effort A.). *Epitome: deep steady pain or discomfort for 1 to 10 minutes in the six-determatome region, initiated by exertion and relieved by rest and nitroglycerin.* The Pain. *Quality:* usually described as *burning, aching,* or a sense of *tightness* or *pressure.* To illustrate the sense of constriction, the patient frequently *clenches the fist,* a sign emphasized by Samuel A. Levine. *Severity:* the discomfort may be mild, moderate, or severe. It may be so slight as not to arouse concern of either the patient or his physician; or the patient may have a sense of impending death. *Timing:* the pain is *continuous,* not fleeting or lancinating. The duration of pain is usually *more than 1 minute but less than 10 minutes. Region:* the pain may occur *anywhere in the six-dermatome band.* Often it is most intense behind the sternum or in the precordium, radiating upward into the neck or throat or down the medial aspect of either arm, forearm, or hand. Ischemic pain arising from muscle in the distribution of the right coronary artery may radiate to the interscapular or high dorsal region of the back. Less frequently the pain occurs in the thoracic vertebrae, the right hemithorax and arm. Occasionally the patient denies having any chest pain, but complains of pain in the limbs or neck exclusively. *Provocative Factors:* (1) *Exertion,* such as walking, climbing, lawn mowing, and similar activities. But an important characteristic of exertional angina is the *lag period;* a certain amount of activity must be sustained *before* the pain occurs; and the pain subsides *only after* a period of rest has elapsed. Exertional pain without a lag period suggests a source in the musculoskeletal system. In a minority of cases, angina occurs with rest or sleep. (2) *Postprandial,* after eating a hearty meal. (3) *Intense emotion.* (4) *Tachycardia* of any origin. (5) *Cold environment,* with or without exertion, such as walking while breathing cold air or sleeping in cold bedclothes. (6) *Rest,* when blood pressure or heart rate changes occur during sleep. Vasospastic angina is also more likely to occur during rest than during activity. Hypertension caused by a pheochromocytoma. (7) *Hypoglycemia,* spontaneous or from insulin. (8) *Positive inotropic or chronotropic effects of drugs* (caffeine, catecholamines, etc.). (9) *Anemia* (reduced oxygen-carrying capacity when the hemoglobin is less than 10 grams per dL.). *Palliative Factors:* (1) rest, (2) warm environment, (3) the administration of nitroglycerin, or nifedipine sublingually, (4) the Valsalva maneuver. ***Physical Signs.*** Often no physical signs are found during an attack, but fourth heart sounds frequently occur during angina because of decreased compliance of the ischemic ventricle. The presence of an ectopic rhythm suggests a cause for the pain. In some cases a *precordial bulge* or thrust at the cardiac apex may be palpated. The phenomenon is attributed to temporary failure of the left ventricle from myocardial ischemia. Signs of aortic stenosis, syphilitic aortitis, or free aortic regurgitation suggest causes for the angina. ***Diagnostic Tests.*** The unequivocal relief of pain or other discomfort in the six-dermatome band by the administration of nitroglycerin (glyceryl trinitrate, USP) is strongly suggestive of angina pectoris, but not diagnostic.

Test with Nitroglycerin. The tablets of the drug should be fresh; age and exposure to light cause deterioration in potency. The dose should be proved *pharmacologically adequate* for the individual by causing *flushing* or *headache.* Instruct the patient to dissolve the tablet under the tongue at the onset of an attack of discomfort; he should take one tablet of 0.4 mg every three minutes for three trials. If flushing or headache, or the cessation of chest pain occurs within any three-minute interval, he is to discontinue the schedule. Relief of pain with a dose causing flushing or headache is strong evidence for angina pectoris. When headache or flushing occurs without relief of discomfort, simple angina is unlikely. If neither relief of discomfort nor pharmacologic headache or flushing is evoked, consider using larger doses. Sublingual nifedipine has also proved useful in relieving attacks of angina pectoris.

Electrocardiogram. Many patients have a normal ECG during rest, and some even during an attack of angina. An ECG during pain may show transient ischemic changes such as ST segment depression. A graded treadmill *exercise test* may be justified, provided the tracing is normal during rest. It is well to keep in mind that there are both false-positive and false-negative stress tests.

Distinction. The brevity of anginal attacks (less than 10 minutes) usually excludes consideration of myocardial infarction, dissecting aneurysm, pulmonary embolism, and neoplasm.

Esophageal pain may be related to swallowing. The supine position often initiates the pain of hiatal hernia: an esophagram, taken in the head-down position, usually demonstrates the hernia and/or gastroesophageal reflux. Like angina, pain from cholecystitis often occurs after meals; epigastric tenderness or a cholecystogram often indicates gallbladder disease. Walking induces pains in the shoulder girdle or spine, as well as angina; lack of a lag period favors muscle pains. Anginal pain is the only type promptly relieved by nitroglycerin. Chest pain often occurs in a patient with possible angina and with x-ray evidence of hiatal hernia, gallstones, or peptic ulcer. The complex problem is usually resolved by diagnostic procedures and therapeutic trials directed at each disorder in sequence. ***Pathophysiology.*** Anginal pain results from a *temporary* oxygen deficit in the myocardium. The underlying basis may be (1) narrowing of the coronary lumens by atherosclerosis, inflammation of the coronary ostia in syphilitic aortitis, embolus or thrombus in the lumen; (2) diminished coronary blood flow in aortic regurgitation, when low systemic diastolic pressure impairs diastolic filling of the coronary arteries; (3) in aortic stenosis, when a continual high demand for oxygen in the myocardium is caused by extra isometric work of the left ventricle. These structural defects are *permanent handicaps* that may permit adequate coronary circulation for a certain level of activity. When increased demands *temporarily* exceed the critical level, oxygen deficit is produced and angina ensues. Exertion, emotion, and digestion make such temporary demands. In addition, fast cardiac rates shorten the diastolic filling time and diminish blood flow, while simultaneously the ventricle requires more oxygen. So angina is encountered in tachycardia. Anemia still further diminishes the oxygen-carrying capacity, so lesser degrees of temporary demand trigger the anginal attack. Nitroglycerin causes dilatation of the coronary vessels and may redistribute myocardial blood flow, but the predominant effect of the drug is to reduce stroke volume, thus relieving anginal pain.

Clinical Occurrence. Coronary artery *narrowing* from atherosclerosis or vasospasm, syphilitic aortitis, embolism or thrombosis in the coronary artery; coronary *insufficiency* from aortic stenosis or free aortic regurgitation; *temporary* insufficiency during tachycardia or ectopic cardiac rhythms (paroxysmal tachycardia, flutter, and atrial fibrillation).

— *Six-Dermatome Pain:* ***Variant Angina Pectoris*** (Rest A., Prinzmetal's A.). The quality and location of the chest pain resemble the classic Heberden's angina, but the onset occurs *at rest* and with no obvious initiating factors. The pain recurs in cycles, waxing and waning, often at the same time each day. During a paroxysm the S-T segments of the ECG are elevated transiently, suggesting myocardial injury. The pain is promptly relieved by nitroglycerin or nifedipine sublingually. Recent reviewers agree that coronary artery spasm has been amply proved as the cause of the Prinzmetal variant angina. Some instigators of spasm have been isolated: direct irritation by a cardiac catheter, drugs (methacoline, ergonovine, a combination of propranolol and epinephrine), cold-pressor tests, quick withdrawal of a high concentration of nitroglycerin, irritation in the region of an atheromatous plaque [R. J. Luchi, R. A. Chahine, A. E. Raisner: Coronary Artery Spasm, *Ann. Intern. Med.*, **91**:441–49, 1979]. Definitive diagnosis can only be made by demonstrating the coronary spasm in angiography when spasm is demonstrated to be relieved by nitroglycerin or other vasodilator drugs. Or, a provocative test may be tried by the intravenous injection of ergonovine maleate, with standard coronary angiography before and after, showing the appearance and disappearance of spasm. There is an increased prevalence of migraine and Raynaud's phenomenon in patients with variant angina.

Relation of Angina to Myocardial Ischemia. The association of rest angina with coronary artery spasm in Prinzmetal's variant angina stimulated critical reexamination of the old hypothesis that angina was the result of coronary artery stenosis. Autopsies had proved that 10% of patients with myocardial infarction and sudden death did not have coronary stenosis. There was no correlation between the degree of coronary artery narrowing and the severity of angina, or the fatal prognosis. The degree of collateral coronary circulation could not be predicted by the presence or absence of symptoms. Animal experiments had shown that occlusion of 65% of the coronary artery lumen would still permit a fivefold increase of resting flow. With newer instruments and techniques A. Maseri and his Italian team in Pisa studied many patients by continuous ECG monitoring, stress testing, coronary arteriography, and regional myocardial scintigraphy [*Am. J. Cardiol.*, **42:**1018–35, 1978]. They proved that ECG changes definitely reflected coronary artery spasm; massive occlusion caused *elevation* of the S-T segments, while lesser amounts of spasm caused *depression* of S-T. Anginal pain occurred *after* the ECG changes, not simultaneously. Either type of ECG change could occur *with* or *without* angina; so the presence or absence of pain *is not a reliable indicator of myocardial ischemia.* They concluded that rest angina was caused by acute oxygen deficit from spasm or other mechanism.

— *Six-Dermatome Pain:* **Acute Myocardial Infarction.** *Epitome: steady deep pain or discomfort, usually lasting for more than 20 minutes, unrelieved by nitroglycerin, accompanied by electrocardiographic changes and laboratory findings of tissue necrosis.* *The Pain.* The thoracic discomfort is similar to angina pectoris in its quality, location, intensity, and its unremitting character, but it usually lasts from 20 minutes to many hours, even days. Simple angina is readily excluded by the lack of response to the administration of nitroglycerin. Often the pain is not induced by exertion, nor does it remit with rest. In moderately severe cases, the pain quickly accentuates to an intensity seldom experienced with angina. The patient often complains of a sense of constriction in the chest and nausea. The high intensity may be sustained for hours; thereafter the pain subsides to a dull ache that may last for days. Shortness of breath may reflect poor muscle compliance or a failing ventricle and high left-sided filling pressures. Nausea and vomiting may occur, particularly when the right coronary artery is involved. *Physical Signs.* The onset of pain is often followed by vomiting. *Sweating* and *pallor* accompany, so the skin is *cold* and *moist.* The heart rate *accelerates* and the blood pressure often *declines,* sometimes to shock levels. A *gallop rhythm* (p. 373) may be heard; the heart sounds often become *muted.* Fine and medium *rales* appear in the *lung* bases (p. 312). At any time, the condition may suddenly worsen with the onset of *ectopic cardiac rhythms* that require immediate therapy. A *pericardial friction rub* (p. 345) over the infarcted area appears in about 15% of cases. Occasionally myocardial infarction is symptomless; in mild cases, relatively few symptoms and signs appear. At the other extreme, rapid progression leads to shock, cardiac failure, and sudden death. *Complications.* Shock, pulmonary edema (p. 332), ectopic cardiac rhythms (pp. 355–64), myocardial rupture, ventricular aneurysm (p.

343), rupture of papillary muscles or the intraventricular septum (p. 392), thromboembolism. *Laboratory Findings.* Hours after onset the *temperature rises* slightly and necrosis causes *leukocytosis* and *acceleration* of the erythrocyte sedimentation rate (ESR). Confirmatory signs of necrosis are *elevation* of creatine phosphokinase (CPK), serum glutamic oxalacetic transaminase (SGOT), and lactic dehydrogenase (LDH); levels of these enzymes begin to rise in 6 hours, attain maximum in 48 hours, and decline in 4 to 7 days. An excessively high SGOT suggests hepatic necrosis. The serum bilirubin level remains normal. *Electrocardiogram.* When present, changes in the ECG are often diagnostic, but clinical findings are better indicators of the severity of myocardial damage. In four fifths of cases there are early elevation of the S-T segment, inversion of T waves, and the appearance of Q waves. In the remaining fifth, some changes usually occur within the first 10 days. *Distinction.* The diagnosis may not be conclusive until several days have elapsed during which intensive care is given and many examinations have been performed. The onset may be similar in *pulmonary infarction.* Enzyme changes may be helpful in differentiating. The serum bilirubin may be elevated in pulmonary infarction, contrasting with normal values in myocardial damage. X-ray films of the chest may show an area of increased density in the lungs with pulmonary infarction; lung scans (ventilation perfusion scans) may be helpful. The presence of thrombophlebitis in some remote region may suggest embolism. *Dissecting aneurysm* frequently begins with pain and prostration. The development of an aortic diastolic murmur transmitting down the right sternal border and/or asymmetric pulses may help to distinguish. In *acute pericarditis* the pain may be severe and resemble infarction, but soon the pain is intensified by bodily motions, breathing, swallowing; but pericarditis can be a sequel of myocardial infarction. *Acute pancreatitis* must be distinguished from myocardial infarction; the pain is similar, but a rise in the serum amylase and alkaline phosphatase suggests pancreatic disease. X-ray examinations of the esophagus, stomach, and gallbladder may disclose hiatal hernia, peptic ulcer, or gallstones that give pain similar to myocardial infarction. Sometimes the harried physician is confronted with the coincidence of two or three of these conditions, and the distinction of the cause of the pain must rest upon the results of appropriate tests.

Clinical Occurrence. Commonly, atherosclerotic narrowing of the coronary arteries with thrombotic occlusion. Less common are hemorrhage into a plaque, coronary artery embolism, or coronary arteritis.

— *Six-Dermatome Pain:* ***Preinfarctional Angina*** (Coronary Failure, Intractable Angina). These and other terms are practically synonymous; none is entirely descriptive. The condition may be considered an intermediate state between angina pectoris and myocardial infarction, frequently progressing to the latter. *Epitome: the pain of myocardial infarction without signs of necrosis, although there is a strong presumption that some degree of focal necrosis may be rather common.*
The Pain. Angina occurs with greater frequency, often with less effort and may occur at rest or during sleep. *Physical Signs.* Signs of infarction do not appear. *Laboratory Findings.* Fever and leukocytosis are absent; serum enzymes are normal. *Electrocardiogram.* The ECG changes are minor or absent. *Distinction.* In the early stages, it cannot be distinguished from myocardial infarction or the other conditions resembling it.

Clinical Occurrence. The condition may climax a long series of anginal attacks, with progressive shortening of asymptomatic intervals. Augmented fluid volume or cardiac failure may precipitate the symptoms in a patient with previous anginal attacks.

— *Six-Dermatome Pain:* ***Postmyocardial Infarction, Postcardiotomy Syndromes.*** Several weeks to a month or more after myocardial infarction, cardiac surgery, or penetrating and nonpenetrating injury to the heart, a hypersensitivity reaction to antigen derived from injured myocardium may produce a syndrome characterized by fever, pericarditis, pleuritis, pericardial or pleural effusions, and pneumonitis. Recurrences are common, usually with decreasing severity. These syndromes often respond dramatically to corticosteroids and other anti-inflammatory drugs. Recurrent myocardial infarction is a major consideration in differential diagnosis when the syndrome occurs in patients with ischemic heart disease. *Distinction:* The almost simultaneous appearance of a pericardial friction rub with the pain and the lack of new Q-waves on the ECG help distinguish the syndrome from recurrent infarction.

— *Six-Dermatome Chest Pain:* ***Gastroesophageal Hypercontracting Sphincter.*** Spasm of the sphincter may produce severe *retrosternal pain*, described as "pressure," "squeezing," or "burning," and suggesting angina pectoris. Or *dysphagia* may be the only symptom. A contraction may endure for 9 to 15 seconds. The condition is often associated with hiatal hernia of the stomach. But the contractions cannot be discerned by esophagram or esophagoscopy. Demonstration requires motility studies with an indwelling balloon [J. M. Garett and D. H. Godwin: Gastroesophageal Hypercontracting Sphincter, *J.A.M.A.*, **208:**992–98, 1969].

— *Six-Dermatome Pain:* ***Acute Pericarditis.*** *Epitome: deep constant or pleuritic pain, in the six-dermatome band or the phrenic distribution, often with pericardial friction rub or ECG signs.* *The Pain.* The pain or discomfort often closely resembles that of myocardial infarction in its location and quality. Or it may be *pleuritic* with accentuation by breathing, coughing, or changes in position. It may have the distinction of being *intensified by swallowing* from involvement of the esophagus. The pleuritic pain may be referred *to the shoulder* (Fig. 6-3). The chest discomfort may be prolonged for many hours; it is *not relieved* by

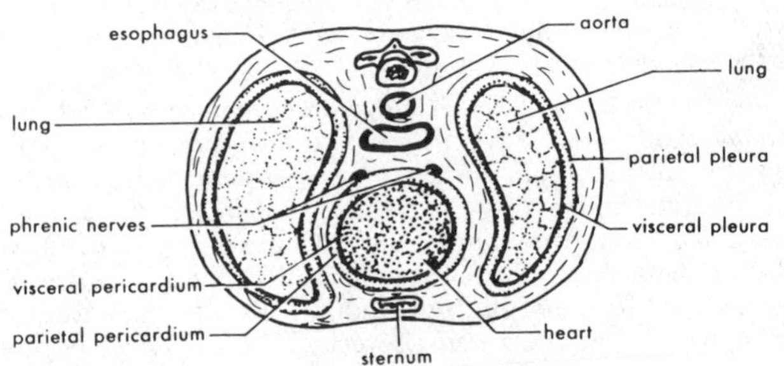

Fig. 6-3. Pleuropericardial relationships. *Diagram of a transverse section of the lower thorax with anesthetic serosal surfaces represented by heavy beaded lines and pain-sensitive surfaces by lighter beaded lines. Note the proximity of the phrenic nerves and esophagus to the parietal pericardium, so pericarditis can produce pain in the phrenic nerve distribution or pain on swallowing.*

nitroglycerin. Rarely, the pain is *throbbing* and synchronous with the heartbeat. The patient may be most comfortable sitting up and leaning forward. ***Physical Signs.*** The onset of pain is soon followed by *fever*. An inconstant *pericardial friction rub* (p. 345) is often heard and felt; usually this disappears with the formation of *pericardial effusion*. ***Laboratory Findings.*** Usually there are leukocytosis and elevation of ESR. There may be moderate elevation of the SGOT. ***Electrocardiogram.*** The ECG signs are fairly diagnostic: widespread elevation of the S-T segments followed by temporary or permanent inversion of T waves. The ECG signs of pericarditis must be differentiated from the injury currents of infarction and from early repolarization changes that represent a normal variant. ***Distinction.*** Until a pericardial friction rub appears or ECG signs develop, the steady pain suggests myocardial infarction, dissecting aneurysm, pulmonary infarction, cholecystitis, peptic ulcer. Pain on swallowing may suggest an esophageal lesion. The pleural pain must be distinguished from that of pleurisy, subphrenic abscess, and splenic infarction. The rare throbbing pain is distinctive. ***Pathophysiology.*** The visceral pericardium and the inner surface of the parietal pericardium are *anesthetic* (Fig. 6-3), but the outer surface of the lower parietal pericardium is *pain-sensitive*. Closely enveloping the anterior and lateral pericardium is the *sensitive* parietal pleura; this apposition explains the pleural involvement from pericarditis. Of clinical interest is the close proximity of the esophagus and the phrenic nerves, so that spreading inflammation can cause *dysphagia* and *phrenic pain*. All these sensitive regions supply nerve fibers to the six-dermatome band. Since afferent sensory fibers from the central area of the diaphragm run in the phrenic nerve, irritation of the lower pericardium may cause pain in the neck at the superior border of the Trapezius. The production of the constant crushing retrosternal pain has not been explained.

Clinical Occurrence. Painful pericarditis usually results from pyogenic or viral infections, rheumatic fever, collagen diseases, or trauma. *Painless* pericarditis occurs with uremia, tuberculosis, mycotic infection, myxedema, or chronic constrictive pericarditis.

— ***Six-Dermatome Pain:*** **Pulmonary Artery Embolism and Pulmonary Infarction.** *Epitome: sudden onset of dyspnea or pain in the six-dermatome band, sometimes with hemoptysis or "asthma," in a* *patient with thrombophlebitis, cardiac failure, or prolonged immobility.* **The Pain.** The pain is either *pleuritic* or a *deep crushing sensation* in the six-dermatome band. Sudden dyspnea is the key sign. There may be *dyspnea without pain.* **Physical Signs.** Systemic effects may predominate, with *weakness, prostration, sweating, nausea,* and *vomiting. Fever* and *tachycardia* are the rule. The *dyspnea* and *cyanosis* may be extreme. Sometimes *painless dyspnea* resembles asthma; this has been attributed to the release of serotonin from platelets in the blood clot. When present, *hemoptysis* and *bloody pleural effusion* are diagnostic. Massive infarction is often indicated by the onset of *shock, jaundice,* or *right-sided heart failure.* The onset of pulmonary hypertension is marked by the *increasing loudness* of the pulmonic 2nd heart sound and the appearance of a palpable *precordial thrust* of the right ventricle. Sudden death is not uncommon. Occasionally pulmonary embolism may be accompanied by *boardlike rigidity of the abdomen,* usually in the upper quadrant beneath the lung involved with the embolism. This is involuntary muscle spasm, so that the region is not tender. Its occurrence is confusing because it tends to focus attention upon intra-abdominal lesions. **Laboratory Findings.** Leukocytosis and a heightened ESR are usually present; the LDH and serum bilirubin rise, but the SGOT may be normal; this contrasts with the elevation of both enzymes in myocardial infarction and the normal bilirubin level. Arterial blood gases including a decreased P_aO_2 may be helpful in making the diagnosis. **Electrocardiogram.** The ECG findings include a shift in the electric axis to the right, an incomplete right bundle branch block, or inverted T waves in right precordial leads. **X-ray Examination.** An area of increased density may appear in the lung field; this is usually nonspecific in appearance, the typical wedge-shaped shadow is uncommon. The diagnosis is suggested by evidence of pleural effusion, atelectasis, dilatation of the pulmonary artery, elevation of the leaf of the diaphragm. Ventilation-perfusion scans may help to establish the diagnosis. **Distinction.** Sudden onset of pain in the chest or dyspnea or unexplained sinus tachycardia in a patient with a predisposing condition should raise the question of pulmonary embolism and infarction. Lacking an obvious source for an embolus, the symptoms and signs may suggest asthma, bronchopneumonia, pleurisy, pericarditis, spontaneous pneumothorax, myocardial infarction, acute pancreatitis, or perforated peptic ulcer. The laboratory findings assist in excluding myocardial infarction and several other conditions. Little precision has been added to the diagnosis of pulmonary embolism by the use of radiographic films of the chest. Danish workers concluded from double-blind tests that radiologists became prejudiced by the opinions of the clinicians [Herlev Hospital Study Group: Diagnostic Decision-Process in Suspected Pulmonary Embolism, *Lancet,* **1**:336–38, 1979]. In a persuasive article Robin argues that pulmonary embolism is greatly overdiagnosed because the pathologists have taught it is a very common malady on the basis of postmortem findings which, of course, only reflect the incidence in dead persons. He concluded that low P_aO_2 values are nonspecific; perfusion scans are most valuable to rule out pulmonary embolism, but the incidence of false-positive scans is high; pulmonary angiography is the most accurate diagnostic method now available. [E. D. Robin: Overdiagnosis and Overtreatment of Pulmonary Embolism: the Emperor May Have No Clothes, *Ann. Intern. Med.,* **87**:775–81, 1977.]

Clinical Occurrence. A *blood clot* may serve as an embolus in cardiac failure or atrial fibrillation; it may originate in an accessible or deep thrombophlebitis that has developed during the postoperative state or during prolonged bed rest, or from immobilization by a cast, or in normal persons sitting or standing in cramped positions for a long time. *Fat emboli* arise from the marrow of fractured bones (p. 652). *Air emboli* are expected from fractured ribs when they pierce the pleura (p. 288). *Amniotic fluid emboli* may occur during labor; when the fluid contains meconium, it is especially dangerous.

— *Six-Dermatome Pain:* ***Dissecting Aortic Aneurysm.*** *Epitome: sudden sharp crushing pain in the six-dermatome band, then progressive diminution of pulses in the aortic branches and loss of specific nerve functions.* *The Pain.* In four fifths of the cases the breakthrough in the intima is *sudden,* producing *sharp crushing* or *tearing pain* in the six-dermatome band, suggesting myocardial infarction. In the remainder, the onset is gradual, often without chest pain. *Physical Signs.* Usually the previous level of arterial blood pressure is *sustained,* in contrast to the hypotension in myocardial infarction. *Proximal Progression:* When the hematoma extends proximally from the tear in the aortic arch, it may (1) distort the aortic valve ring to separate the commissures and cause a *murmur* of aortic regurgitation (p. 386), often transmitting down the right sternal border, (2) occlude the coronary ostia and cause myocardial infarction (p. 239), (3) produce hemopericardium with a *pericardial friction rub* (p. 345) and *cardiac tamponade* with *dyspnea, cyanosis, low-volume pulses,* and *hypotension* (p. 402), (4) swell the base of the aorta causing a *pulsating sternoclavicular joint.* The latter sign distinguishes the condition from myocardial infarction; otherwise it occurs only with ruptured saccular aneurysm of the aorta, persistent right aortic arch, or fusiform aneurysms of the innominate, carotid, or subclavian artery [R. B. Logue and C. Sikes: *J.A.M.A.,* **148:**1209, 1952]. *Distal Progression:* When the hematoma extends away from the heart, its course may be indicated by the sequential appearance in the various aortic branches of *asymmetric diminution* or *loss* of arterial *pulses* and signs of deficient function in the nerves of the regions supplied; occlusion of the carotid artery may cause cerebral ischemia with localizing neurologic signs; loss of vertebral artery supply is indicated by spinal cord lesions, such as *paraplegias, anesthesias, cyanosis, pallor, pain;* occlusion of the renal artery may be marked by pain simulating *renal colic,* or *anuria* or *hematuria.* ***Pathophysiology.*** Cystic medial necrosis and intramural hemorrhage may lead to secondary intimal rupture, or intimal tears may be the primary event. Blood from the lumen penetrates the weakened media to produce a hematoma that splits the vessel wall into two layers. Rarely, compensation occurs by the development of a second intimal tear distally, usually at the aortic bifurcation. The distal rent provides egress from the channel in the media; so the aorta consists of two concentric tubes through which blood courses, a *double-barreled aorta.* ***X-ray Findings.*** Plain films of the chest are diagnostic when they show widening of the aorta, or when preformed calcific plaques in the intima are widely separated from the outer border of the aortic wall. Ultrasonic examination is diagnostic.

Clinical Occurrence. In men over 40 years, the most common causes are hypertension and/or cystic medial necrosis. In women, the hormonal state of pregnancy predisposes to rupture during labor. A rare cause in the young is Marfan's syndrome, in which there is an inherited defect in the media.

— *Six-Dermatome Chest Pain:* ***Spontaneous Esophageal Rupture*** (Boerhaave's Syndrome). During the course of vomiting, a *sudden pain* may occur in the chest or upper abdomen; this is accompanied by *extreme dyspnea.* The physical signs of mediastinal emphysema may appear, including a *crunching sound in the precordium* (Hamman's sign). X-ray films show air in the mediastinum. *Distinction:* the symptoms are common to myocardial infarction, perforated peptic ulcer, cholecystitis, pancreatitis, esophagitis, hepatitis, nonperforating ulcer, pneumonia. The x-ray demonstration of mediastinal emphysema should exclude all the foregoing in favor of ruptured esophagus.

— *Six-Dermatome Pain:* **Congenital Absence of Left Pericardium.** Although this is considered a rare condition the authors of a recent paper predict it will be found often when the diagnosis becomes familiar [J. R. Morgan, A. K. Rogers, and A. D. Forker: Congenital Absence of the Left Pericardium. Clinical Findings, *Ann. Intern. Med.*, **74**:370–76, 1971]. *Symptoms.* Nonspecific anterior *chest pain* often initiated by exertion or lying on the left side; the pain persists for a few seconds or minutes. *Physical Signs.* A *heaving apical impulse* displaced to the left axilla, often with a *sustained thrust. A systolic ejection murmur* at the second left intercostal space. *ECG Findings.* Vertical or right-axis deviation; leftward displacement of transition zone in the precordial leads. *X-ray Findings.* Posteroanterior films of the chest show prominent main pulmonary artery and displacement of the heart leftward while the trachea remains in midline. Interposition of a lung segment causing a translucent zone between inferior cardiac border and left hemidiaphragm.

— *Six-Dermatome Pain:* **Diaphragmatic Hernia** (Hiatal Hernia). *Epitome: dull steady or burning pain, without dysphagia, usually in the lower retrosternal or xiphoid region, sometimes initiated by recumbency.* *The Pain.* In most persons the hiatal hernia is symptomless. A minority complain of either *deep steady pain* in the retrosternal or xiphoid region, or occasionally *burning pain* in the same region, probably related to associated gastroesophageal reflux. The attacks of pain may closely resemble angina pectoris except that they are *not relieved* by nitroglycerin. In some patients the pain occurs after *lying horizontal* for an hour or so when the stomach slides upward into the thorax; but this is not a reliable symptom, as most patients with the complaint do not have hiatal hernia, and many with proved hernia do not notice any pain. Attacks of *burning pain* are usually caused by reflux of the gastric contents into the esophagus and indicate a local esophagitis. A third type of *extremely severe pain* in the same region may last for hours; it results from incarceration or strangulation of a herniated portion of the stomach in the hiatus. ***Physical Signs.*** Usually there are none. In congenital *eventration of the diaphragm,* where much of the stomach lies in the thorax, *peristaltic sounds* may be heard high in the left hemithorax. ***X-ray Findings.*** In the commonest type, the *sliding hernia,* the hiatal ring is enlarged and the gastric cardia slides through into the thorax, especially in the supine or head-down position (the latter posture should be employed for x-ray examination). In the less common *parahiatal hernia,* the gastric cardia protrudes into the thorax through a defect in the diaphragmatic muscle *beside* the esophagus, but not through the hiatus, so esophagus and cardia are separated by a fibrous band. With barium in the stomach, gastric reflux into the esophagus can be seen. ***Complications.*** Gastrointestinal hemorrhage, strangulation of the herniated stomach, severe esophagitis.

Esophageal Symptoms. Chest pain *with dysphagia* accurately points to a primary disorder of the esophagus, except in the case of acute pericarditis (p. 242). But when an esophageal lesion causes pain *without dysphagia,* attribution to the esophagus follows a more circuitous route that involves considering all structures in the six-dermatome band. Even when the patient experiences both pain and dysphagia, his attention is often so fixed upon the pain that the examiner is in doubt whether the difficulty in swallowing is emotional or organic. ***Esophageal Pain.*** The maximal intensity is usually retrosternal or in the xiphoid region, although it may occur anywhere in the six-dermatome band. The pain may be *sharp,* or it may be *steady* and *constrictive,* resembling angina pectoris. ***Dysphagia.*** Often the patient describes the "sticking" of food at a certain level in the chest, with or without pain. When the lesion is actually in the upper half of the esophagus, the patient's localization proves quite accurate, but lesions in the lower half are inaccurately located; so the occurrence of dysphagia merely calls attention to the esophagus as a whole. No physical signs are produced by lesions in the gullet so diagnosis depends upon symptoms, esophagram, and esophagoscopy. ***Other Symptoms.*** *Heartburn* is an intermittent burning constricting sensation that moves from the xiphoid region upward to the pharynx where an acid taste may be perceived; it is related to gastroesophageal reflux. *Belching* (gaseous eructation) is often the complaint of the air swallower; in *aerophagia* the patient gulps air immediately before belching, although he cannot be convinced of it. Aerophagia and belching are functional behaviorisms, but they often occur unconsciously when there is abdominal discomfort of a more serious nature. *Regurgitation of gastric juice* is the flow of gastric contents from stomach to mouth *without the effort of vomiting;* it may be functional, but it also occurs in cardiospasm.

— *Six-Dermatome Pain with Dysphagia:* ***Acute Esophagitis.*** There is *retrosternal pain* intensified by swallowing.

Clinical Occurrence. After prolonged vomiting, trauma from overlong contact with intragastric tubing, esophageal burns from corrosive substance, acute infections.

— *Six-Dermatome Pain with Dysphagia:* ***Chronic Esophagitis.*** Pain and dysphagia are similar in quality to those in the acute lesions, but the duration covers weeks or months. It may be complicated by *peptic ulceration* of the esophagus, especially with hiatal hernia. Esophageal stricture may occur secondary to the esophagitis.

Clinical Occurrence. Gastroesophageal reflux in hiatal hernia. During or long after x-ray radiation of the mediastinum for neoplasms.

— *Six-Dermatome Pain with Dysphagia:* ***Cardiospasm (Achalasia).*** A motor disturbance involves the lower two thirds of the esophagus, so the lower esophageal sphincter fails to relax normally and dilatation of the gullet results. *Dysphagia* is the prime symptom; this may be accompanied by *retrosternal pain,* but in some cases there is *no pain.* The dilatation of the esophagus permits *regurgitation* of food. The esophagram is diagnostic.

— *Six-Dermatome Pain with Dysphagia:* ***Cancer of the Esophagus.*** The early symptom is *dysphagia;* weeks or months later, pain *retrosternally* may be added. The pain sometimes radiates to the neck or back. The esophagram is diagnostic.

— *Six-Dermatome Pain with Dysphagia:* ***Foreign Body.*** Swallowed rigid objects may lodge at the level of the aortic arch, causing *pain* and *dysphagia.* Esophagoscopy is indicated.

— *Six-Dermatome Pain with Dysphagia:* **Diverticulum of the Esophagus.** Although pouches may form anywhere in the gullet, only *Zenker's diverticulum* regularly produces symptoms. This is an outpouching in the posterior hypopharynx protruding downward between spine and esophagus. It fills with food causing *dysphagia* and *regurgitation of putrefied food.* Occasionally there is retrosternal pain. The esophagram visualizes the pouch.

— *Six-Dermatome Pain with Dysphagia:* **Plummer-Vinson Syndrome.** This occurs in some women with severe iron deficiency. A weblike formation in the esophagus may be found to explain the *dysphagia* in some, although no anatomic basis can be discovered in many. The obstruction may be demonstrated in the esophagram.

— *Six-Dermatome Pain with Dysphagia:* **Dysphagia Lusoria** (Aberrant Right Subclavian Artery). Pain is rarely present, and *dysphagia* is the only symptom. This prompts the making of an esophagram that shows a transverse band of indentation in the esophagus produced by the anomalous right subclavian artery (p. 450).

— *Six-Dermatome Pain:* **Mediastinal Tumors.** Although mediastinal lesions rarely cause pain in the chest, they are considered here because of their location in the six-dermatome band. Most growths in the region attract attention by their physical signs from compression of normal structures, or they are found in the x-ray films of the chest. Physical signs that may indicate mediastinal tumors are *dyspnea* from retrosternal goiter (p. 214), *hoarseness* and *brassy cough* from compression of the recurrent laryngeal nerve (p. 170), *Horner's syndrome* (unilateral ptosis of the eyelid, *miosis* of the pupil, and *lack* of facial sweating from involvement of the superior cervical ganglion, (p. 800), *edema* of the arms and neck with cyanosis from obstruction of the superior vena cava (p. 451), *chylous pleural effusion* (p. 319). The tumors may be lymph nodes enlarged in Hodgkin's disease, carcinoma, or tuberculosis; retrosternal goiter; thymoma; or teratoma (dermoid cyst). When a dermoid forms an esophageal fistula, it may produce the elegant sign of spitting hair, *trichoptysis.* One of the few painful lesions of the mediastinum produces *Pancoast's syndrome* (superior sulcus tumor, p. 726), in which there is severe pain in the neck, shoulder, or down the arm, from neoplasm in the pulmonary apex, the upper mediastinum, or the superior thoracic aperture.

— *Six-Dermatome Pain:* **Spontaneous Pneumothorax.** Frequently there is *sudden severe pain* in the chest, often unilateral, rarely localized. It is immediately followed by progressive *dyspnea* and *cyanosis.* Shock may ensue. The first thought of the diagnostician is usually pulmonary embolism, but the physical signs are distinctive when a large amount of air enters the pleural cavity. The trachea is *deviated away* from the affected side; the breath sounds are *absent* and the percussion note *hyperresonant* on that side (p. 321). Pulmonary collapse may be such as to require urgent diagnosis and treatment to prevent suffocation. When the air leak is small (less than 50 cc), the only physical sign may be *decreased breath sounds;* then the condition must be distinguished from pulmonary embolism, myocardial infarction, and acute pericarditis. Sometimes the condition is *painless.* *X-ray Findings.* Films of the chest are diagnostic if there is enough air to separate the layers of pleura in an accessible location.

Clinical Occurrence. In "healthy" young persons with no discernible pulmonary lesion; rupture of a pleural bleb in pulmonary emphysema; occasionally, in nonsuppurative disease of the lungs, such as sarcoidosis, fibrosis, or silicosis. Puncture of the lung by a fractured rib is the most common traumatic cause.

— *Six-Dermatome Pain:* **Spontaneous Pyopneumothorax.** The onset is similar to that in spontaneous pneumothorax, but there is usually a known history of bronchiectasis, lung abscess, or tuberculosis with cavitation. The sudden spillage of pus into the pleural cavity produces severe *prostration, chills, fever,* or *shock.* The physical signs and x-ray examination show evidence of hydropneumothorax (p. 323), but *pus* can be aspirated from the pleural sac.

— *Six-Dermatome Pain:* **Subphrenic Diseases.** Although lesions below the diaphragm usually produce abdominal pain, the frequent exceptions make it imperative to consider subphrenic disorders also in the context of *pain in the six-dermatome band.* It is dangerous to the patient and embarrassing to the physician to overlook this possibility.

Clinical Occurrence. Subphrenic abscess (p. 518), acute cholecystitis (p. 546), peptic ulcer (p. 542), acute pancreatitis (p. 543), and splenic infarction (p. 550).

The Breasts

▼ *Key Symptom:* ***Pain in the Breast.*** The patient who consults the physician for pain in the breast often fears that cancer is the cause, when the actual disorder is usually something else. The physical examination often makes the diagnosis.

Clinical Occurrence. *Physiologic:* onset of puberty, menstruation, pregnancy. *Traumatic:* hematoma, pressure of clothes. *Nipples:* fissure, inflammation, epithelioma. *Breasts:* cysts, submamarry abscess, mastitis, galactocele, tuberculosis, mastodynia, late carcinoma of the breast.

The Female Breast

The importance of adequate breast examination, in women, is evidenced by the frequency of malignancy in that superficial organ, the high mortality rate in those with advanced disease, and the demonstrated improved survivorship among those diagnosed with small tumors.

Normally the mammary glands are rudimentary in children and men. In the woman, maximal development occurs in the early childbearing age, when the breasts become conical or hemispherical, extending from the second to the sixth or seventh ribs. Ductal growth, in the adolescent female, follows the production of estrogenic hormones by the ovary. With ovulation, the secretion and circulation of estrogen and progesterone result in alveolar development. Other hormones, including prolactin, adrenocorticotropic hormone (ACTH), corticosteroids, growth hormone, thyroxine, and androgens, appear to play facultative roles in completion of breast development and milk production. Any surgical intervention in the developing breast bud must be considered relative to possible gains and losses. Since malignancy is so uncommon in the prepubertal female and the consequences so great, i.e., to remove the entire breast "anlage" prior to maturation, biopsies of such girls/women must be done only with due consideration. The left mamma is usually slightly larger than the right. The breasts may engorge premenstrually, but almost certainly will during pregnancy. The cone or hemisphere contains from fifteen to twenty subdivided *lobes,* radially arranged, each with its own excretory *lactiferous tubule* discharging through a separate orifice in the nipple. Considerable fat surrounds the glands, so discrete lobes are not ordinarily palpable. Fibrous bands vertically infiltrate the breast tissue, forming *suspensory ligaments* (Cooper's ligaments) that attach the stroma to the skin. A *fascial cleft* separates the deep surface of the breast from the thoracic wall, permitting some mobility. Lying against the pectoral fascia, the breast tissue forms a circular area of contact; from this circle the *axillary tail* of gland tissue projects laterally and superiorly along the axillary and Serratus anterior fascia (Fig. 6-4). This extension must be understood to evaluate masses in the axilla.

The *nipple,* a conical or cylindrical structure, is slightly below and lateral to the center of the breast. The overlying skin is wrinkled and pigmented; it is roughened with papillae containing the orifices of the lactiferous tubules. The skin of the nipple extends for a radius of 1, 2 or more centimeters onto the surface of the breast to form the *areola.* Both nipple and areola vary from pink to brown, depending upon the person's complexion and parity. The color darkens progressively after the second month of pregnancy; coincidentally, the areola expands its circumference. Small elevations in the surface of the areola are produced by the sebaceous glands of Montgomery (*areolar glands*) that secrete a lipoid material to protect the nipples during nursing. Radial and circular muscle fibers are embedded in the subcutaneous tissue of the areola; light friction or mas-

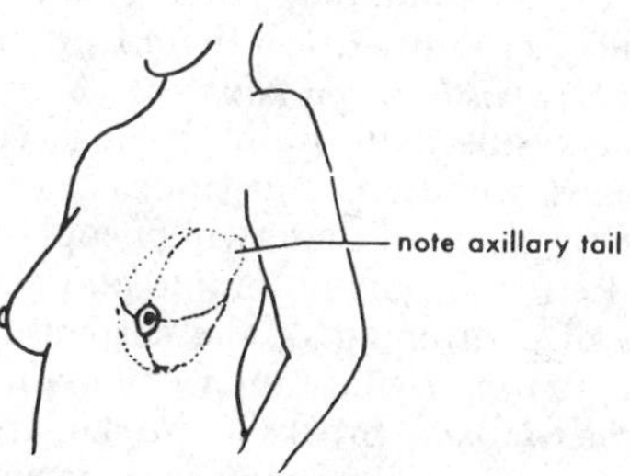

Fig. 6-4. Quadrants of the breast. *The hemisphere of the breast is divided into quadrants by imaginary vertical and horizontal lines intersecting at the nipple, named upper medial, upper lateral, lower medial, and lower lateral. Popularly, these quadrants are also respectively named upper inner, upper outer, lower inner, and lower outer. Note the protrusion of the upper lateral quadrant, called the "axillary tail," in which breast tissue extends to the axilla.*

sage stimulates them to contract, producing erection of the nipple.

In the routine physical examination, the breasts are usually inspected and palpated with the patient supine. Whenever the patient complains of a lump in the breast, or the routine methods hint at the possibility of a mass, special procedures should be utilized for more adequate search.

EXAMINATION OF THE NIPPLES. **No special posture of the patient is required. Inspect the skin of the anterior trunk for *supernumerary nipples*. Look for *retraction* of the nipple; ascertain whether the deformity is recent or old; recent ones suggest acquired disease. Look for *fissures* in the nipples. Search for *discharge* from the nipples by gently compressing the nipple and aerola between the thumb, and forefinger; note the *color* of the discharge. Look for *dry scaling* and *red excoriation* of the nipple. Palpate the periphery of the areola for tender nodules.**

Supernumerary Nipples and Breasts (Polythelia and Polymastia). Extra nipples occur frequently in both sexes as minor errors in development; rarely, they are associated with glandular tissue to form a complete breast. Commonly, supernumerary nipples are smaller than normal; often they are mistaken for pigmented moles, but close examination usually discloses a miniature nipple and areola. Most occur in the mammary or milk line on the thorax and abdomen; rarely, they are found in the axilla, on the shoulder, flank, groin, or thigh. Their only importance is to distinguish them from moles.

Retraction of Nipples: ***Inverted Nipples.*** A common developmental anomaly results in the nipple having a craterlike depression, a harmless variation. But appearance after maturity should arouse suspicion of underlying neoplastic or inflammatory disease. Retraction of the nipple and skin dimpling are consequences of shortening of the suspensory ligaments of the breast due to underlying tumor or inflammation.

Fissures in the Nipple. Breaks in the skin are usually caused by local infection; their presence may indicate a deep abscess otherwise unsuspected.

▼ *Key Sign:* ***Secretions of the Breast.*** The appearance of abnormal secretions of the breast leads to the consideration of a surprisingly large number of causes, as summarized from A. B. Barnes [Diagnosis and Treatment of Abnormal Breast Secretions, *N. Engl. J. Med.*, **275:**1184, 1966].

— ***Serous, Bloody, or Opalescent Breast Fluid.*** Such secretions may occur with benign or malignant lesions. The presence of bilaterality is very important. When pregnancy does not exist, the production of secretions are usually due to incompletely understood hormonal influences. It is when unilateral discharge is present that the examiner's index of suspicion of an underlying pathologic condition must be alerted. If the cause is not evident from the history or physical examination, cytologic examination of the fluid or biopsy of the breast tissue may be helpful, though invasive cancers of the breast do not ordinarily cause such discharges.

Clinical Occurrence. BENIGN LESIONS: fibrocystic disease, intraductal papilloma, sclerosing adenosis, chronic cystic mastitis, duct ectasia, galactocele (p. 263), papillary cystadenoma, breast abscess (p. 262), keratosis of nipple, fat necrosis (p. 262), acute mastitis (p. 264), tuberculosis (p. 263), toxoplasmosis, eczema of nipple.
MALIGNANT LESIONS: carcinoma of the breast (p. 263), adenofibrosarcoma, fibrosarcoma, neurosarcoma, Paget's disease of nipple (p. 255).

— ***Abnormal Lactation.*** Lactogenesis depends upon the action of lactogen of the anterior pituitary, progesterone and estrogen from the ovaries and placenta. Milk ejection is initiated by mechanical stimulation sending afferent impulses to the hypothalamus, causing release of oxytocin from the posterior pituitary. The role of prolactin and placental lactogens is not clear. Certain physiologic states and clinical disorders may be associated with the secretion of milk:

Clinical Occurrence. PHYSIOLOGIC STIMULATION: suckling, pregnancy, mechanical stimulation of nipples. BREAST TRAUMA AND INFLAMMATION: trauma to chest wall, thoracoplasty, pneumonectomy, mammoplasty, herpes zoster. PITUITARY DISORDERS: uterine atrophy with amenorrhea and lactation (Frommel's disease), irradiation of pituitary, section of pituitary stalk. MISCELLANEOUS: after encephalitis, costal metastasis from adrenal carcinoma, hypothyroidism in adolescent girls, hyperthyroidism in women, chorioepithelioma of testis. TRANQUILIZING DRUGS: phenothalazines, reserpine, methyldopa.

Scaling and Excoriation of the Nipple: Paget's Disease. This can be a manifestation of a slow-growing intraductal carcinoma. Early, a scaling eczematoid lesion involves the nipple. Later, the nipple becomes reddened and excoriated; complete destruction of the structure may result. The process extends along the skin as well as in the ducts. A deep-seated mass is present in half the cases representing an invasive malignancy, the cells of which have extended along the ductal system and the lactiferous tubules onto the surface of the nipple. As Paget described in his report of 1874, patients experience "tingling, itching, and burning."

Tender Nodule in the Areola: ***Abscess of the Areolar Gland.*** The sebaceous glands of Montgomery may become inflamed, forming tender palpable abscesses in the periphery of the areola. Usually single, these infections may become quite large and invade into the breast tissue proper unless incised and drained early in the course of events. As with all abscesses, when drained, a biopsy ought to be performed to rule out the presence of an underlying cancer, which has led to secondary infection.

EXAMINATION FOR BREAST MASSES. ***Inspection*** **of the breast includes observation of the surface and transillumination of masses.** ***Palpation*** **comprises compression of the tissue between thumb and forefinger, pressing the gland against the chest wall with the flat of the hand, testing the surface with the thermal sense, and moving the gland to test mobility. During examination, the patient should be required to assume several postures sequentially, the better to bring out certain signs. Especially to be noted are increased heat and redness of the overlying skin, tenderness, dilated superficial veins,** ***peau d'orange,*** **retraction (dimpling, asymmetry, decreased mobility), opaque and translucent masses.**

Patient Sitting with Arms Down **(Fig. 6-5A): Have the patient stripped to the waist and sitting on the table or in a chair facing you. Note** ***recent retraction*** **of the nipple. Look for** ***unilateral dilated superficial veins*** **as evidence of underlying disease. Observe whether the two nipples are** ***symmetricaly*** **placed; dislocation suggests retraction. Compare the** ***size*** **and** ***shape*** **of the breasts, remembering that the left may normally be slightly larger. Look for abnormal** ***bulging;*** **flattening of a lateral contour is also significant. Search for** ***dimpling,*** **a sign of retraction. Examine for** ***peau d'orange,*** **evidence of edema of the skin. If the patient has noted a lump, ask her to** ***point it out;*** **then palpate the opposite breast first. Palpate the tissue carefully in all four quadrants of both breasts between the thumb and forefinger for** ***increased heat, tenderness,*** **and** ***masses.*** **When a mass is found, ascertain its** ***location, size,*** **and** ***consistency.*** **Squeeze the breast between thumb and fingers to bring out** ***dimpling*** **(Fig. 6-6A). Gently pinch**

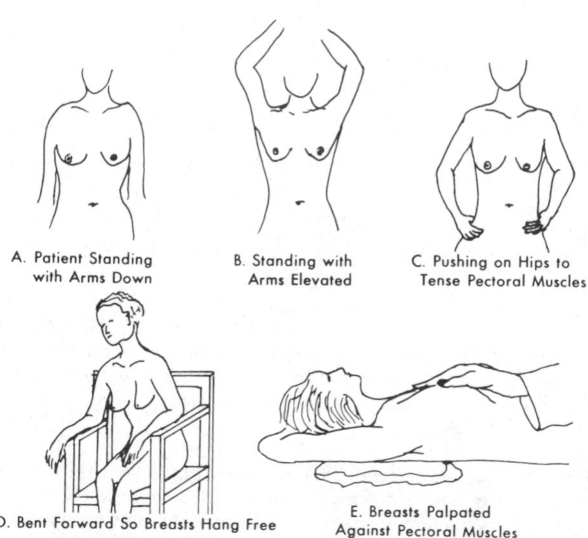

Fig. 6-5. Positions of the patient for examination of the breasts. *The patient is stripped to the waist and sits facing the examiner. In* **A** *The patient sits with arms at sides; the examiner looks for elevation of the level of a nipple, dimpling, bulging, and peau d'orange. When the patient raises her arms, as in* **B,** *dimpling and elevation of the nipple are accentuated when there is a mass fixed to the pectoral fascia. In* **C** *the patient pushes her hands down against her hips to flex and tense the pectoralis major muscles; the examiner moves the mass to determine fixation to the underlying fascia. When the breasts are large and pendulous, the patient is asked to lean forward, as in* **D,** *so the breasts hang free from the chest wall; retraction and masses become more evident. In the supine position,* **E,** *the examiner presses the breasts against the chest wall with the flat of his hand; the normal nodosity from the lobules is less prominent and significant masses are more distinctly felt.*

the overlying skin to determine *fixation* of the mass to the integument. *Transilluminate* the mass to find whether it is opaque or translucent (Fig. 6-6B).

Patient Sitting with Arms Raised* (Fig. 6-5B): Have the patient raise her arms over her head while you look for a *shift in relative position* of the two nipples and the disclosure of *dimpling, bulging,* or *peau d'orange.

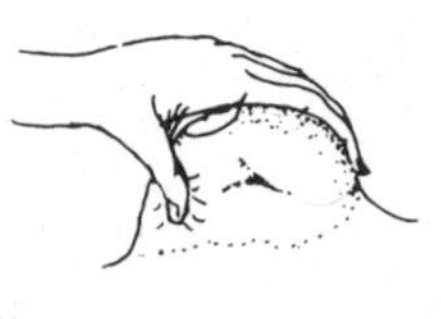

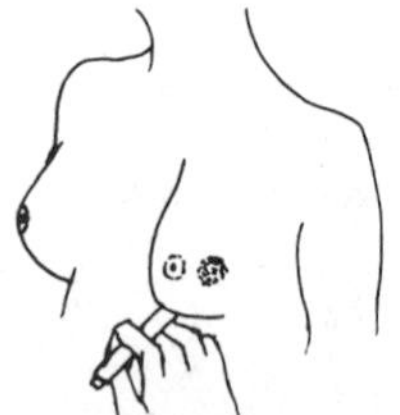

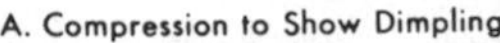

A. Compression to Show Dimpling B. Transillumination of Mass

Fig. 6-6. Further breast examination. **A.** Breast compression to accent dimpling. *Dimpling is a sign of shortening of the suspensory ligaments of the breast from neoplasm or inflammation.* **B.** Transillumination of the breast. *The density of a mass may, on occasion be ascertained by transillumination of the breast; transparency probably means a cyst full of fluid; other masses are opaque.*

Patient Sitting with Hands Pressing Hips **(Fig. 6-5C): Have the patient press her hands downward on her hips to tense the pectoral muscles. This maneuver brings out *dimpling* by putting tension on the breast ligaments, which arise from the Pectoralis major fascia. Grasp the mass between thumb and forefinger; move it back and forth transversely, then up and down, to test fixation to the underlying muscles. Perform this test *with* and *without* tensing the muscles. When the mass lies in the axillary tail, *tense* the Serratus anterior muscle by having the patient press her hand downward on your shoulder.**

Patient Sitting with Trunk Bent Forward **(Fig. 6-5D): When the breasts are large and pendulous, have the patient lean forward, supporting herself with her hands on chair arms or on her knees, so the mammae hang free from the chest wall. This posture sometimes facilitates inspection and palpation.**

Patient Supine **(Fig. 6-5E). When the breast is dependent it may feel nodular due to the constituent fat lobules. The nodosity is less apparent when the patient lies supine and the breast is pressed against the chest wall with the flat of the examining hand. Thus, significant masses become more distinct.**

Palpation of Regional Lymph Nodes: **When carcinoma of the breast is suspected, metastasis of the regional lymph nodes is sought. Expert clinicians advise examination with the patient sitting. Sit, facing the patient, and palpate the left axilla with your right hand (Fig. 6-7A). Place the hand in the axilla with the extended fingers approximated, and the palm toward the chest wall. Point your fingers**

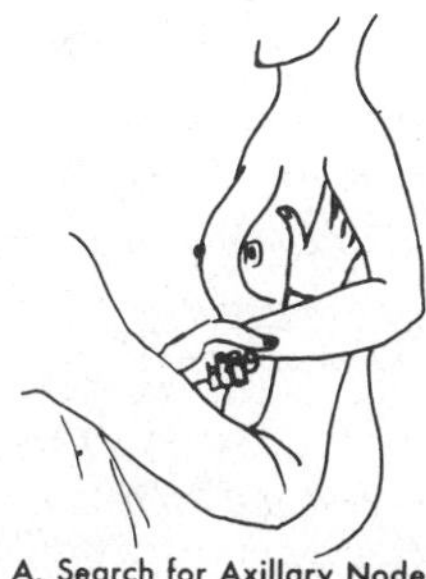

A. Search for Axillary Nodes

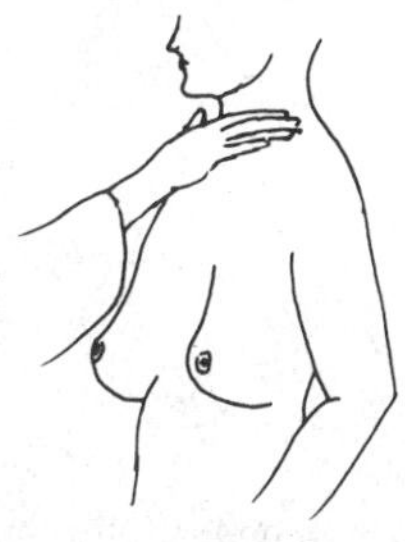

B. Search for Supraclavicular Nodes

Fig. 6-7. Palpation of lymph nodes in the breast region. **A.** *In palpation of the left axilla the examiner slides his right hand toward the axillary apex, with palm toward the chest wall and approximated fingers extended so the pulps feel the structures on the thoracic cage. With his left hand, he directs the patient's upper arm close to the chest to relax the axillary muscles. He asks her to rest her arm on his examining arm and he supports her shoulder with his left hand. The positions are reversed to examine the right side.* **B.** *The supraclavicular fossa is palpated for large nodes.*

obliquely toward the apex of the axilla. Have the patient relax her left arm while you grasp her left wrist with your left hand and direct her upper arm toward the chest wall to relax the axillary muscles. Then let her rest her left hand on your examining arm, while your released left hand is used to support her behind the shoulders. Slide the pulps of your examining fingers along the thoracic cage to feel enlarged lymph nodes. Note the size, location, consistency, and mobility of the nodes. The *central group* of nodes occurs near the middle of the thoracic wall of the axilla (Fig. 6-8). The *lateral axillary group* is located near the upper part of the humerus and is best demonstrated by having the patient's arm elevated so that you can feel along the axillary vein. With the arm still elevated, feel along beneath the lateral edge of the Pectoralis major muscle for the *pectoral group*. With the patient's arm raised, get behind her and palpate under the anterior edge of the Latissimus dorsi muscle for the *subscapular group*. Palpate under the clavicle for the *infraclavicular group*. Enlargement in the supraclavicular group is sought by feeling the clavicle (Fig. 6-7B). Thermography or mammography may assist in delineating abnormalities within the breast. [D. B. Kopans, J. E. Meyer and N. Sandowsky: Breast Imaging. *N. Engl. J. Med.*, 310:**960, 1984].**

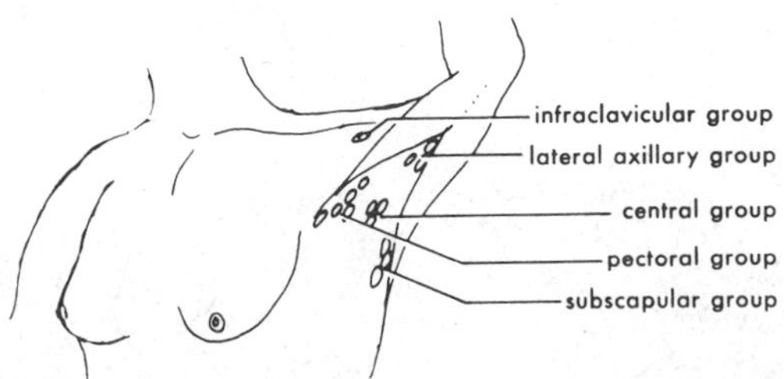

Fig. 6-8. Lymph node groups in the axilla. *Note that the lateral axillary group is on the inner aspect of the upper arm, near the axillary vein. The subscapular group lies deep to the anterior edge of the latissimus dorsi muscle. The pectoral group is behind the lateral edge of the pectoralis major muscle.*

Be certain to examine the crease under and between the breasts for neoplasms that may look like calluses [J. R. Watson and C. G. Watson: Carcinoma of the Mammary Crease, *J.A.M.A.*, 209:1718–19, 1969].

▼ *Key Sign:* ***Masses in the Breast.*** As the endometrium responds to the influence of the pituitary ovarian axis, so do the components of the breast parenchyma. While basically a highly complex and specialized sweat gland, the organ, in the adult, is in fact made up of four major components: stroma, ductal epithelium, glandular acini, and the myoepithelium. Each of these is influenced by a variety of hormonal signals. The signal may be abnormal, either too great or too small, or the receptor may be unable to respond to the "normal" signal. It may be overly responsive to a completely normal signal, in what has been called "hyperestrinism." Fibrocystic disease has, in both the professional and lay vernacular, been used to describe a broad spectrum of benign, nonmalignant, pathologic conditions of the female breast. A specific pathologic diagnosis is dependent upon the preponderance of one normal component over others.

Under the influence of estrogens, during the follicular phase of the menstrual cycle, minimal mitotic activity occurs within the breast. Progesterones provoke significantly greater cellular division. Periodic changes within the breast are then taking place at a continual if not predictable pace. Prior to the onset of menses, the breasts increase in size under the influence of the sex steroids. If conception takes place, under the influence of not only estrogens and progesterones, but prolactin as well, extensive alveolar and ductal proliferation occurs. With parturition, the epithelium becomes actively secretory, and milk is released [R. B. Greenblatt, J. S. Chaddha, A. Teran, and A. Lewis: Fibrocystic Breast Disease: Pathophysiology, Hormonology, Treatment. *Contemp. Surg.*, **24**:49, 1984].

Dependent upon the predominating abnormal cellular component and the individual pathologist interpreting the material, a variety of pathologic conditions may be identified. If the pathologic observation is confined to stromal proliferation, fibroadenoma, virginal hypertrophy of the breast, and intracanalicular fibroadenoma may be diagnosed. When the abnormality is predominantly located in the ductal system, micro- or macrocystic disease, cystic mastititis, sclerosing adenosis, intraductal papilloma, and ductal ectasia involving the sinus lactiferous are terms that can be used to indicate the nature of the changes. If the main source of change resides within the terminal ductules and glandular elements, lobular hyperplasia can be identified. Finally, changes within the myoepithelium, consisting of hyperplasia, lead to a diagnosis of myoepithelial hyperplasia of Reclus.

To the clinical diagnostician, the overriding issue to be kept in mind is that only the pathologist is capable of making the diagnosis, to the exclusion of all other possibilities. Neither the surgeon, radiologist, nor anyone else can speak with the certainty of the microscopist.

There is no particular virtue in making a diagnosis of a benign breast condition. Only by the removal of a discrete, dominant, even "biopsyable" lesion, however, can the abnormal process be identified as to its true character. It is unfortunately true that after palpating a lesion in the breast, individuals have been dissuaded from doing a biopsy on the basis of a normal radiographic finding. Any clinically identifiable discrete mass or process must be excised. False-negative imaging studies are too prevalent to be employed as a gold standard.

ASPIRATION OF BREAST CYSTS. **Under certain circumstances the decision may be made to aspirate clinically cystic lesions in the**

breast. Proponents of certain techniques have published descriptions of their approach to this common procedure [W. C. Barnes, Jr.: Management of Cystic Diagnosis of the Breast. Am. J. Surg., 129:324, 1975].

Many have found the use of the vacutainer blood tubes equally suitable. After cleansing the skin with an alcohol sponge, the needle is passed into the firmly held mass, and the tube then pushed onto the needle within the drawing container. This is certainly no more painful than first infiltrating the skin with a local anesthetic, which can be most unpleasant. If the fluid is nonbloody, the mass completely disappears, and does not recur in follow-up, no further treatment is required.

Solitary Translucent Breast Masses: ***Cyst of the Breast.*** Fluctuation can be demonstrated by holding the periphery of the mass tight to the chest wall with one hand and pressing the center of the mass with the fingers of the other; but lipoma and breast abscesses also fluctuate. The abscess is often quite tender and has other evidence of inflammation, while true lipomas are exceedingly rare, accounting for less than 1% of all breast lesions. Cysts, on the other hand, are very common. Transillumination may make the distinction by disclosing the translucent area.

Solitary Nontender Breast Mass: ***Fibroadenoma.*** This is usually found in a young woman with large breasts. The nodule is firm, elastic, or rubbery in consistency, ovoid or lobulated. It may be the size of a pinhead or quite large. The mass is nontender and freely movable, so palpation of moderate-sized nodules causes them to slip easily in the breast tissue. *Distinction.* The mass must be distinguished by biopsy from dysplasia, carcinoma, and cystosarcoma phylloides.

Solitary Nontender Breast Mass: ***Chronic Breast Abscess.*** Pus may become enclosed by a thick wall of fibrous tissue, presenting a nontender, irregular, firm mass requiring biopsy to distinguish from carcinoma.

Solitary Nontender Breast Mass: ***Fat Necrosis of the Breast.*** Trauma to the breast may produce a hematoma resulting in a scar that adheres to the surrounding tissue and causes retraction. The finding may suggest carcinoma. The history of trauma should not weigh too heavily in the diagnosis because the natural inclination of patients is to attribute neoplastic masses to some remote traumatic incident. While this lesion is inconsequential of and by itself, it must be removed and examined by the pathologist to determine its actual significance.

Solitary Nontender Breast Mass: **Tuberculosis of the Breast.** Early, the granulomatous mass may be localized, firm, irregular, and nontender, so that the findings suggest carcinoma. But the breast masses later become multiple and indurated, the skin becomes pigmented, and the infection may involve the axillary lymph nodes leading to break down and fistulous track formation.

Masses During Lactation: **Galactocele** (Caked Breasts). During or after lactation, one or more opaque cysts may form from blockage of ducts. Signs of inflammation are absent. When a single breast is involved, apply a breast pump to the other. If milk is obtained, then pump the affected breast and the mass will disappear.

Solitary Nontender Breast Mass: **Carcinoma of the Breast.** Usually there is a *dominant* nontender mass in the breast. Involvement of the suspensory ligaments results in *retraction*, revealed by dimpling, deviation of the nipples, and fixation to the pectoral muscles. *Flattening* of the nipple and a bloody or clear *discharge* indicates the presence of disease in the lactiferous tubules. Lymphatic obstruction produces edema of the tissues, manifested by *peau d'orange* (Fig. 6-9). Lymphatic spread is marked by regional lymphadenopathy and x-ray signs of metastasis to the lungs, spine, skull, and pelvis. A solitary breast mass mandates a diagnostic biopsy. Occasionally, the presenting signs are bloody discharge without a mass, enlarged lymph nodes in the axilla without a mass, or dermal inflammation without a mass.

Age of the patient with a palpable breast abnormality can

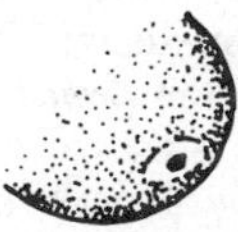

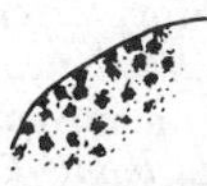

Fig. 6-9. Peau d'orange. *Edema of the breast is indicated when the skin is indented deeply with holes that are the accentuated orifices of the sweat glands. The holes are deepened by the surrounding edematous skin, which gives the appearance of an orange skin or a pig skin.*

assist in estimating the probable pathology. While the incidence of cancer in a woman less than 30 years of age is 1%, there is a steady rise with increasing age, and it is now estimated that one in eleven women will eventually develop breast cancer. The median age at which the various pathologic breast abnormalities appear in women is known, and upon that basis probabilities estimated. The following table is based on data from patients operated upon at New York Medical College-Flowers Fifth Avenue Hospitals during the period 1960–1975 [H. P. Leis, Jr.: The Diagnosis of Breast Cancer, Ca- A Cancer Journal for Clinicians, **27**:209–32, 1977.]:

Relationship of Breast Abnormalities and Age

Diagnosis	Age Range (Median)
Fibrocystic disease	20–49 (30)
Fibroadenoma	15–39 (20)
Intraductal papilloma and ductal ectasia	35–55 (40)
Carcinoma	40–71 (54)

Inflammatory Mass: ***Acute Mastitis.*** The breast is flushed, tender, hot, swollen, and indurated, frequently accompanied by chills, fever, and sweating. Usually *a single breast quadrant* is involved. Axillary lymphadenopathy is infrequent; when present it suggests the possibility of inflammatory carcinoma. Often the inflammation proceeds to abscess formation. In about two thirds of the cases, the disease occurs during lactation. *Distinction.* Inflammatory carcinoma must be distinguished.

Inflammatory Mass: ***Acute Abscess of the Breast.*** Usually this is the sequel of acute mastitis. There is a localized, hot, tender mass that is *fluctuant.* Frequently, the process produces chills and fever with leukocytosis.

Inflammatory Mass: ***Inflammatory Breast Carcinoma.*** Malignant neoplasm may present as an acute inflammatory disease, especially in the lactating breast. The signs are similar to those of acute mastitis, except that the entire breast is swollen and there is early involvement of the axillary lymph nodes. This is in distinction to acute mastitis in which the inflammation is usually limited to a single breast quadrant and lymphadenopathy is uncommon.

***Inflammatory Mass:* Juvenile Mastitis.** This disease occurs in young boys and in women between 20 and 30 years of age. Signs of inflammation are present in a firm mass beneath the nipple. Usually the involvement is unilateral. The course is only a few weeks.

The Male Breast

Because of its rudimentary structure, the male breast is more readily examined than the woman's. Unfortunately, examination is frequently neglected because the physician does not realize that the male breast may be the site of serious disease. The principles of examination are similar to those described for women. Residual anlage for breast development may remain in males, and can be responsive to hormonal influences at any time during life from adolescence to old age. Breast development may occur secondary to abnormal endocrine influences, including hyperthyroidism, prolactin-secreting adenomas, acromegaly, tumors of the testes and adrenals, and secondary to a variety of drugs including, of course, estrogens. It is not infrequently observed in alcoholic males as liver disease interferes with normal hormonal degradation processes.

Acute Mastitis in the Male Breast. This usually occurs from trauma. Bailey states that the most common cause is irritation from braces (suspenders). The signs are similar to the condition in women. More commonly, in this day and age, irritation and chafing of the nipple and breast occur in active sports, like jogging and similar activities.

Gynecomastia (Gynecomazia). This is defined as a transient or permanent noninflammatory enlargement of the male breast. The *idiopathic* type frequently appears at puberty and is usually unilateral. *Hormonal* stimulation causes bilateral enlargement in a variety of situations: the administration of estrogens in the treatment of prostatic cancer, with anorchism and after castration, in Cushing's syndrome, and in chorioepithelioma of the testis. Enlargement of the breasts may also occur in cirrhosis of the liver, probably from incomplete hepatic destruction of estrogen. *Refeeding* gynecomastia occurs when patients with severe malnutrition are given food. Gynecomastia is said to be frequent in leprosy; only the nipples are hypertrophied. Occasionally, it is encountered in leukemia, lymphoma, pulmonary carcinoma, familial lumbosacral syringomyelia, and thyrotoxicosis. Among the drugs occasionally causing gynecomastia are digitalis, isoniazid, spironolactone, phenothiazine, and diazepam. One author has described five cases of men whose breasts enlarged when their hips or shoulders were immobilized in spica casts for several months. The cause is unknown [H. H. Kaminsky: Gynecomastia in Patients Immobilized in Spica Casts, *J.A.M.A.*, **210**:2395–96, 1969].

Carcinoma of the Male Breast. About 1% or 2% of carcinomas of the breast occur in men. The mass is apparent early because of the paucity of breast tissue. The lesion begins as a painless induration and retraction of the nipple and fixation to the skin and deep tissues. The mass does not transilluminate.

The Thoracic Wall

The thoracic wall includes the bodies of the twelve thoracic vertebrae, the twelve pairs of ribs, and the sternum. The bones are arranged as a cage covered by skin subcutaneous tissue, fascia and muscles with accompanying blood vessels, nerves, and lymphatic channels. Certain anatomic facts are pertinent to the physical examination.

Bones of the Thorax

Each rib is a flattened, arched bone; its vertebral end has a *head, neck,* and *double tubercle;* the sternal end continues as a *costal cartilage.* In typical ribs, a bipartite arthrodial (gliding) joint binds the head to the bodies of the two adjacent vertebrae and their intervertebral disk. A second arthrodial joint connects the articular tubercle of the neck with the transverse process of the upper vertebra, so each rib has two adjacent connections with the vertebral column. The 1st, 10th, 11th, and 12th ribs are atypical; each articulates with a single vertebra.

The *sternum* is a flat bone in the anterior midline of the thorax (Fig. 6-10). Shaped like an ancient Greek sword pointing downward, it consists of the *manubrium* (handle), the *gladiolus* (blade), and the *xiphoid cartilage* (tip). The manubrium is joined to the gladiolus by a fibrocartilage that sometimes develops a

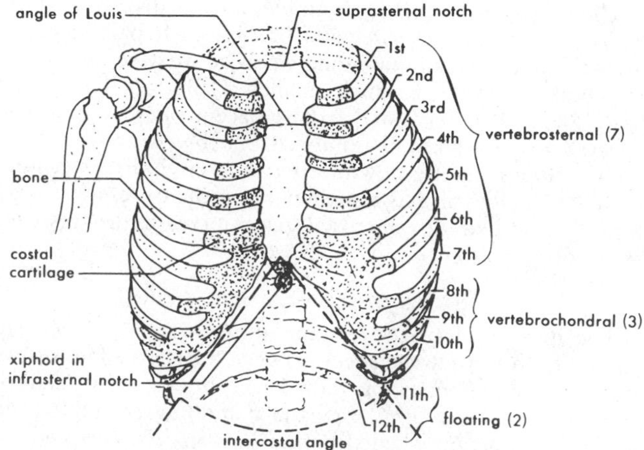

Fig. 6-10. The bony thorax. *The left clavicle is removed to expose the underlying first rib. The cartilages of the xiphoid and ribs are stippled. Note that the costicartilage of the 2nd rib articulates with the fibrocartilage between the manubrium and the gladiolus and with the edges of both bones. Note also the surface landmarks of the suprasternal notch, the angle of Louis, and the infrasternal notch. The two lower rib margins form the intercostal angle.*

synovial cavity; but mobility is slight. The 1st to 7th ribs, inclusive, are *vertebrosternal* (true ribs); their costal cartilages join the sternum. Of the others (false ribs), the 8th, 9th, and 10th ribs are *vertebrochondral,* each costal cartilage commonly joining the cartilage of the rib above, but many variations occur. The 11th and 12th ribs, free at their anterior ends, are termed *vertebral* (floating ribs). The costal cartilage of the 1st rib articulates with the manubrium by a synarthrodial (fixed) joint. The other six true ribs attach the sternum by arthrodial joints with synovial cavities. The 2nd rib is exceptional in having two synovial cavities by which it makes contact with interfaces on both the manubrium and gladiolus at their fibrocartilage. The *xiphoid cartilage* is fixed to the lower end of the gladiolus; usually it develops calcification during later life; commonly it is either lance-shaped or bifid; it may be mistaken for an abdominal mass when it angulates forward.

The shape of the thorax resembles a truncated cone whose varied circumferences are pairs of ribs, each pair having a greater diameter than that immediately above it, so the sterno-vertebral dimension is much smaller at the top than at the base. Each rib is separated from adjacent ones by *intercostal spaces;* the space takes its number from the rib above it. The 1st rib slopes slightly downward from vertebra to sternum; each succeeding rib has a greater slope than the one above; thus, the width of the intercostal spaces increases progressively from top to bottom.

Muscles of the Thoracic Wall

The intercostal spaces contain the *Intercostales externi* and *interni.* Each is a muscle sheet between adjacent edges of two ribs to draw the bones together. When the 1st rib is fixed by contraction of the *Scaleni,* the externi and interni pull the ribs upward; the action is aided by the *Levatores costorum* and the *Serratus posterior superior.* When the last rib is fixed by contraction of the *Quadratus lumborum,* the *Subcostales* and the *Transversus thoracis* draw the ribs downward.

Surface Anatomy of the Thorax

The anterior surface of the sternum is subcutaneous, so it presents landmarks for inspection and palpation. The separated heads of the clavicles form the sides of the *suprasternal notch* (jugular notch); its base is the superior edge of the manubrium (Figs. 6-10 and 6-11). The junction of the manubrium and gladiolus produces a slight angle protruding anteriorly,

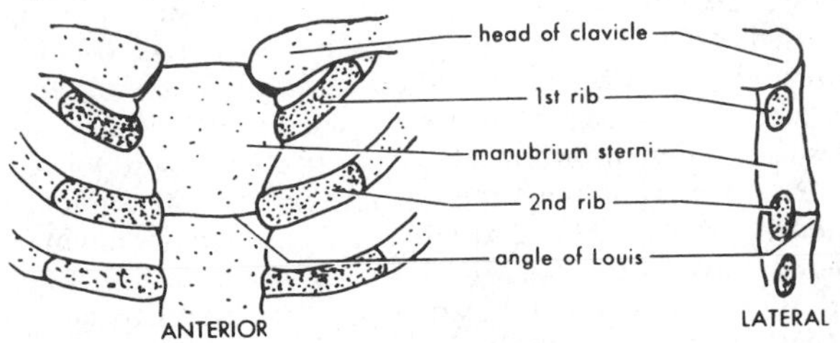

Fig. 6-11. Detail of the angle of Louis. *Note especially that the adjacent edges of the manubrium and gladiolus form the angle of Louis. In turn the angle serves as a landmark in counting ribs anteriorly because the 2nd rib abuts the junction that forms the angle.*

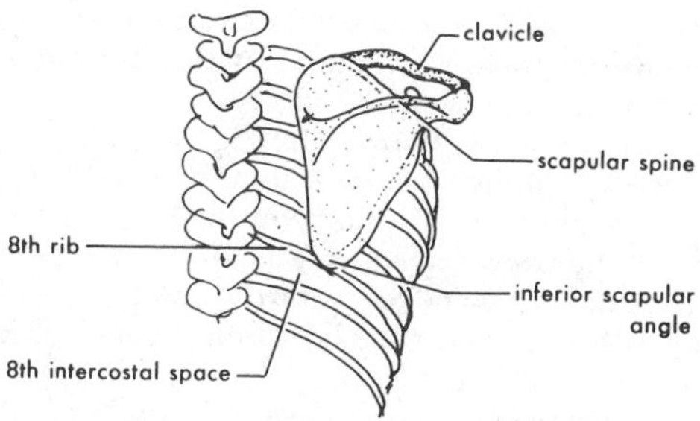

Fig. 6-12. Surface landmarks of the posterior thorax. *Note the relation of the scapulae to the ribs. The inferior angle of the scapula is usually at the 7th rib or interspace, or the 8th rib; this fact permits one to identify the 7th rib posteriorly when counting ribs in the back.*

the *angle of Louis* (angle of Ludwig, sternal angle). This marks the 2nd rib articulating with the manubrium-gladiolus. At the inferior end of the gladiolus is a slight depression, the *infrasternal notch,* formed by the junction of the costal cartilages of the two 7th ribs. Immediately beneath this, the *xiphoid cartilage* may be felt and, sometimes, seen.

Portions of most ribs can be seen or palpated, except the 1st rib, which is effectually overlaid by the clavicle. The Pectoralis major and the female breasts obscure palpation of parts of the ribs anteriorly; the Latissimus dorsi covers some ribs in the axillary line. Posteriorly, the scapulae cover parts of the 2nd to 7th ribs, inclusive. With the arms at the sides, the *inferior border of the scapula* is usually at the 7th or 8th intercostal space, serving as the usual landmark for counting ribs in the back (Fig. 6-12). The inferior margins of the 7th, 8th, and 9th costicartilages on the two sides meet in the midline to form the *infrasternal angle* (intercostal angle); the angle may be considerably more or less than 90°. The diagram (Fig. 6-10) shows that an oblique line drawn from the head of the clavicle to the anterior axillary line on the 9th rib locates approximately the costochondral junctions of the 2nd and 10th ribs, inclusive.

Respiratory Excursions of the Thorax

At the end of expiration, the volume of the thorax is minimal. Inspiration expands the thoracic volume by increasing the dimensions of the cavity anteroposteriorly, transversely, and vertically. Each integrated component of this movement will be considered separately.

Anterior Bulging of the Thorax. In Fig. 6-13A, consider the geometry of a cylindric pail with its wire handle bowed in a semicircle of slightly greater diameter than the cylinder. When the handle hangs down obliquely, the distance from its center to the cylindric axis coincides with the radius of the pail. As the handle is raised toward the horizontal, its periphery travels away from the sides of the pail. Now consider the model in Fig. 6-13B, where an arched piece of wood represents the thoracic spine, and a vertical stick is the sternum in the position of expiration (dotted). The two upright pieces are connected above by a hinged strut, representing the 1st rib. The dotted hoop represents a pair of ribs, acting together as a circle, whose plane slants downward from the axis of rotation through the spine (broken line). When the sternum and 1st rib are pulled upward, the costal ring rotates to push the sternum forward and upward. Anatomically, this movement is executed when the sternum and 1st rib are fixed by the scaleni, while contraction of the external and internal intercostal muscles narrows the interspaces. The ribs are pulled upward and the sternum thrust forward, increasing the anteroposterior dimension of the thoracic cavity.

Lateral Expansion of the Thorax. Consider a similar model in Fig. 6-13C, where the sternum and the 1st rib are fixed. Each rib of a pair is, this time, a separate semicircle rotating on an anteroposterior axis (broken line). During expiration the planes of the hoops slant downward on either side of the axis. When the hoops are pulled upward toward the horizontal, each hoop acts as a pail handle by moving farther from the center, increasing the transverse dimension. Anatomically, the narrowing of the interspaces by the intercostal muscles causes elevation of the rib curves to increase the transverse diameter of the thorax.

Thus fixation of the 1st rib and manubrium by the scaleni and the narrowing of the interspaces by the intercostal muscles cause rotation of each rib, except the 1st, on both an anteroposterior and a transverse axis, expanding the corresponding dimensions of the thoracic cavity. Since the lower ribs are longer and more oblique, and the interspaces are wider, the amplitude of movement is greater in the lower thorax.

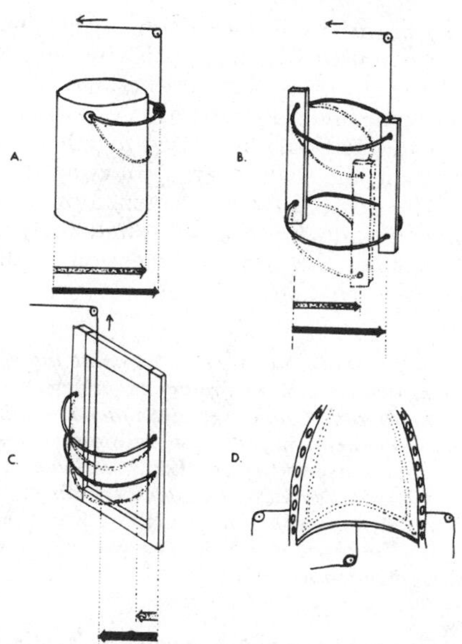

Fig. 6-13. Models illustrating the respiratory movements of the thorax. **A.** *This is a cylindric metal pail or bucket with its semicircular bail or handle. At rest, the handle hangs obliquely, so its center and the side of the pail are equidistant from the central axis of the cylinder. When the bail is raised to the horizontal, its bow diverges from the side of the pail by a distance represented by the two arrows.* **B.** *This is a model with two parallel hoops piercing two vertical sticks. The elevation of the front stick (representing the sternum) will increase the distance between it and the other stick (representing the spine). The differences in the points of the arrows show this change in the anteroposterior diameter. It should be noted that the hoops are rigid circles.* **C.** *This rack represents the sternum and the spine from which hang semicircular hoops, like ribs. When the hoops are elevated, the diameter from the midline of the frame increases, as shown by the arrows. Now the ribs actually have motions depicted in both* **B** *and* **C,** *so elevation of the sternum and the lateral bows of the ribs during inspiration increases both the transverse and the anteroposterior diameters of the thorax. In* **D** *is represented the way the volume of the thorax is still further augmented during inspiration by depression of the diaphragm.*

Vertical Elongation of the Thoracic Cavity. The diaphragm is an elliptic sheet of muscle whose center is a fibrous aponeurosis. The edges of the sheet are fixed to the lower ribs while the center forms a dome into the cavity. After expiration, the dome is high and the thoracic walls are closest together (Fig. 6-13D). During inspiration, the walls diverge, lowering the diaphragmatic dome. The dome is further flattened by contraction of the diaphragmatic muscle during inspiration. Lowering the diaphragm elongates the vertical dimension of the thoracic cavity to increase its volume.

INSPECTION OF THE THORACIC WALL. **Examine the skin over the thorax for *lesions* that restrict respiratory excursion. Note *structural deformities* of the thorax. Note cough and noisy breathing. Observe the respiratory movements in the chest, noting *rate, amplitude,* and *rhythm* of the entire respiratory act. Look for labored inspiration or expiration. Observe *retraction* of interspace during inspiration. Examine for localized disorders in the amplitude of thoracic excursions by applying the hands to the chest as markers. Note the amplitude of diaphragmatic movements.**

*Restrictive Soft Tissue: **Atrophy or myopathy.*** These disorders include the sequelae of poliomyelitis and the changes secondary to various myopathies that involve the chest wall.

*Restrictive Soft Tissue: **Cicatrix.*** Extensive scarring of the skin and soft tissue of the thorax from burns, operations, or lacerations may seriously restrict inspiration. The tidal volume is diminished, leading to alveolar hypoventilation.

*Restrictive Soft Tissue: **Scleroderma.*** The skin and soft tissues become stiff and tight, restricting inspiration. The skin elsewhere is similarly affected, especially over the fingers and face. Hyperpigmentation and vitiligo often coexist in the same region. Raynaud's syndrome is frequent.

*Thoracic Deformity: **Rachitic Rosary.*** A prominent structural feature of rickets is failure in hardening of the bones. The sternal ends of rachitic ribs bulge at their costochondral junctions. The bulging is mostly inward, but in severe cases there is enough outward bulging to be perceived as knobs at the costochondral junctions (Fig. 6-14A). The condition exists only during the activity of the rickets in the first two years of life; healing obliterates the knobs without a trace.

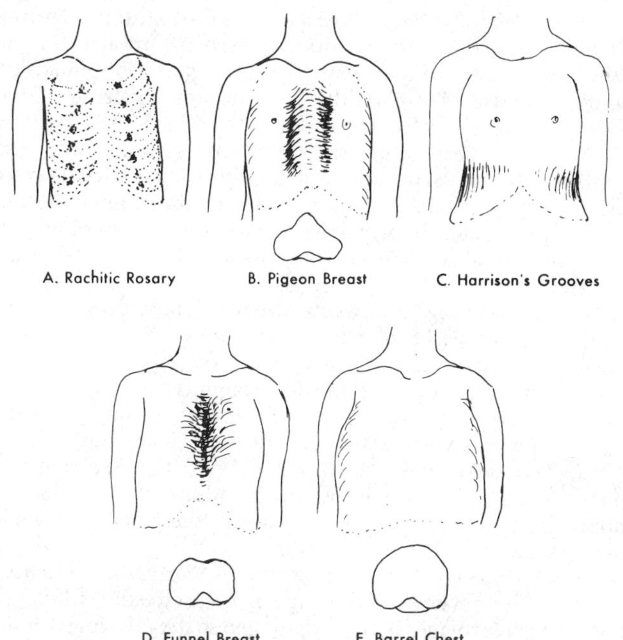

Fig. 6-14. Deformities of the thorax. **A.** Rachitic rosary. *The diagram illustrates the knobs occurring at the costochondral junctions during the activity of the disease of rickets. They disappear after healing.* **B.** Pigeon breast. *During active rickets the softening of the ribs permits the sternum and costicartilages to be pushed anteriorly in the shape of a ship's keel. The anteroposterior dimension of the thorax is increased, but the transverse diameter may be narrowed. Vertical grooves are formed in the line of the costochondral junctions, as depicted in the cross section. The deformity is permanent.* **C.** Harrison's grooves. *Transverse grooves in the lower thorax may occur during active rickets from the pull of the diaphragm at its thoracic attachments. The deformity is permanent.* **D.** Funnel breast. *In rickets and some congenital disorders, the softened ribs permit the lower part of the sternum to sink posteriorly, forming a pit or depression of varied size. The anteroposterior diameter is diminishing, as the cross section shows.* **E.** Barrel chest. *The augmented lung volume in emphysema causes the thorax to assume a permanent inspiratory position, with increase in both transverse and anteroposterior dimensions, as depicted in the cross section.*

Thoracic Deformity: ***Pigeon Breast*** (Pectus Carinatum). During active rickets, the softened upper ribs bend inward, forcing the sternum forward to increase the anteroposterior dimension at the expense of the width. The sternum protrudes from the narrowed thorax like the keel of a ship (Fig. 6-14B). Healing of the rickets perpetuates the deformity. Pigeon breast also occurs in Marfan's syndrome. Similar distortion occurs in severe primary kyphoscoliosis, but the sides of the thorax are not symmetric. Fusion abnormalities in the midline resembling pectus carinatus also occur in some forms of congenital heart disease.

Thoracic Deformity: ***Harrison's Groove*** (Harrison's Sulcus). During active rickets the protuberant rachitic abdomen pushes the plastic lower ribs outward on a fulcrum formed by the costal attachments of the diaphragm. The line of bending forms a *groove* or *sulcus* in the rib cage, extending from the xiphoid process transversely toward the axillae, and a *flaring* of the cage below the groove (Fig. 6-14C). The deformity remains when the rickets heals. In the adults, the condition is not serious, but patients worry about it; the examiner should not mistake it for a grave disorder.

Thoracic Deformity: ***Funnel Breast*** (Pectus Excavatum, Trichterbrust). The reverse of the pigeon breast results when the lower costal cartilages become deranged so the inferior sternum and xiphoid process are retracted toward the spine. In its rudimentary form, an oval pit occurs near the infrasternal notch. A more extensive distortion (Fig. 6-14D) is formed when the entire lower sternum sinks, to diminish seriously the anteroposterior dimension of the thoracic cavity, gravely compromising the heart and lungs. Rickets often produces this deformity, but many cases are unexplained, as in Marfan's syndrome. Funnel breast may be an occupational acquisition, as in *cobbler's chest,* where the workman habitually presses shoes against his sternum.

Thoracic Deformity: ***Barrel Chest.*** Either pulmonary emphysema or senile kyphosis may produce this. Both the anteroposterior and transverse dimensions of the thorax are enlarged, without bulges or depressions, so the arched ribs tend to form perfect circles in cross section (Fig. 6-14E). The permanently augmented volume of emphysematous lungs sustains the thorax continuously in the inspiratory position. The sternum is pushed forward, the ribs are horizontal, the diaphragmatic dome is depressed. The expiratory act is inhibited. Senile kyphosis of the thoracic spine produces a similar posture in the ribs, distinguished from emphysema only by lack of the auscultatory signs of lung disease.

Thoracic Deformity: ***Localized Bulges and Depressions.*** When acquired during early life, extreme cardiac enlargement may produce a bulge over the precordium. An example is bulging of the left anterior chest wall in patients with interatrial septal defects. Rachitic depressions in the thorax may occur without definite pattern. In the adult, a bulge may result from erosion of the thorax by aortic aneurysm. Neoplasm of the ribs may protrude, or burrowing abscesses may bulge through the wall. Localized depressions may result from retraction by underlying fibrosis.

INSPECTION OF THE THORACIC SPINE. **Have the patient stand or sit; inspect the profile of the spine from the side for *kyphosis, lordosis,* and *gibbus.* From the back, look for lateral deviation of the spinous processes, *scoliosis.* When the curvature is slight, or the patient is very fat, palpate each spinous process and mark its location with a skin pencil, whereat the deviation will be obvious. Consider the possibility of *kyphoscoliosis,* a combination of lateral and anteroposterior deviation. This is sufficient examination of the spine to evaluate the thorax; a more detailed functional approach is described on pp. 730–32.**

Spinal Deformity: ***Kyphotic Thorax.*** The normal posterior convexity of the thoracic spine may be accentuated in a *smooth curve* (Fig. 6-15A). Among the many causes are senile osteoporosis, ankylosing spondylitis (Marie-Strümpell disease), Paget's disease, and acromegaly. *Angular* kyphosis results from collapse of one or more vertebral bodies; the protruding angle is called a *gibbus* (Fig. 6-15A). Gibbus may result from compression fracture, tuberculosis of the bodies (Pott's disease), neoplasm of the bodies, or syphilis. In either curved or angular kyphosis, the spinal flexion may force the thorax to assume permanently the inspiratory position, with increased anteroposterior diameter and horizontal ribs. The thoracic distortion is identical with the barrel chest of pulmonary emphysema. In this case, the auscultatory signs of emphysema are absent.

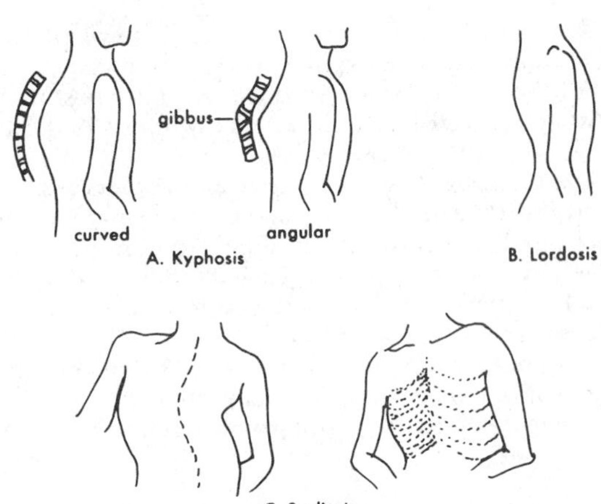

Fig. 6-15. Curvatures of the spine affecting the thorax. **A.** Kyphotic thorax. *The thoracic curve of the spine is accentuated either smoothly by disease of a number of vertebrae or in angular fashion by collapse of the body of a single vertebra from compression fracture, neoplasm, osteoporosis, or infection. The angle or gibbus is obvious in the physical examination. With the increased concavity of the spinal curve, the thorax is thrown into the inspiratory position with increased anteroposterior diameter.* **B.** Lordotic thorax. *Disease of the hips or lumbar spine results in increase of the backward concavity of the lumbar region. This deformity displaces the thoracic spine posteriorly; consequent pull on the lower thorax holds it in the expiratory position.* **C.** Scoliotic thorax. *Scoliosis is lateral deviation of the spine. An inclination of the thoracic spine to one side causes a compensating opposite displacement in the lumbar region, making an* S *curve. The curvature may be so slight as to be detected only by marking the tips of the spinous processes with a skin pencil and noting the deviation from the vertical. The displacement of the spinous processes underemphasizes the true condition because the bodies of the vertebrae are usually rotated considerably more than their spinous processes. The spinous processes always rotate toward the concave side, so the opposite side has widened intercostal spaces, anterior flattening of the thorax, and posterior bulging of the ribs; the shoulder on that side is elevated.*

Spinal Deformity: ***Lordotic Thorax.*** Usually the anterior convexity of the *lumbar spine* is accentuated from weakness of the back muscles, excessive weight of the abdomen, or ankylosis of the hips. Accentuation of the lumbar curve throws the thoracic spine backward and the thoracic cage becomes flattened from the pull of the abdomen, causing an expiratory position to be assumed (Fig. 6-15B).

Spinal Deformity: ***Scoliosis.*** Lateral curvature of the thoracic spine is usually accompanied by some rotation of the vertebral bodies, but only the lateral deviations of the spinous processes are visible (Fig. 6-15C). Minor functional scoliosis forms a *single* lateral curve, usually with convexity to the right. With structural changes, the lateral curve in the thorax produces an opposite compensatory curve inferiorly, so the line of spinous processes forms an S-shaped curve. The spinous processes always rotate toward the *concave side.* On the convex side, rotation of the vertebral bodies causes *flattening* of the ribs anteriorly and *bulging* of the chest posteriorly, raising of the shoulder, and lowering of the hip. Viewed from the patient's back, the posterior bulge is augmented with anteflexion of the spine. (See Fig. 9-31, p. 731.)

Spinal Deformity: ***Kyphoscoliosis.*** The thoracic deformity of scoliosis is accentuated and compounded when kyphosis is also present. The thoracic cavity may be so reduced as to compromise the heart and lungs.

▼ *Key Sign:* ***Cough.*** A cough is a sudden, forceful, noisy expulsion of air from the lungs. It may be single or paroxysmal. An *unproductive cough* is a short sharp noise of distinctive quality that experience teaches will not yield sputum. A cough in which sputum is raised is *productive,* recognized by everyone by its longer duration, its rattle, and the distinctive sound. A cough is said to be *brassy* when it is unproductive and has a strident quality, commonly heard in patients with laryngitis. It also occurs in any condition that narrows the trachea or glottal space, such as laryngeal paralysis, neoplasm of the vocal cord, aortic aneurysm. In pertussis, the *whooping cough* is characterized by the long strident inspiratory noise preceding the cough.

The three stages of coughing are preliminary inspiration, glottal closure and contraction of respiratory muscles, then sudden glottal opening to produce the outward blast of air. Coughing may be voluntary or involuntary. Stimuli to coughing are exudates in the pharynx or bronchial tree, the irritation of foreign bodies, or inflammation. The sensory nerve endings for the cough reflex are branches of the vagus in the larynx, trachea, and bronchi; but cough may also be induced by stimulation in the external acoustic meatus that is supplied by the auricular nerve (Arnold's nerve), a branch of the vagus. An anatomic classification of the causes of coughing follows:

Clinical Occurrences. LARYNX AND PHARYNX. Chronic pharyngitis, acute and chronic laryngitis, neoplasm, tuberculosis, syphilis. TRACHEA AND BRONCHI. Tobacco smoking, inhalation of noxious gases, dust, allergens, paranasal sinusitis, acute and chronic tracheobronchitis (especially measles and pertussis), typhoid fever, bronchiectasis, extrinsic pressure from osteophyte of cervical vertebra, carcinoma, asthma without asthmatic breathing. LUNGS. Pneumonia, pulmonary tuberculosis, lung abscess, pulmonary emphysema, carcinoma, chronic passive congestive, pulmonary infarction, pulmonary edema, hydatid disease. MEDIASTINUM. Aortic aneurysm, lymphadenopathy (tuberculous, carcinomatous, or lymphomatous), neoplasia (dermoid, teratoma, neurofibroma, retrosternal goiter, thymoma, foregut cysts). EXTRATHORACIC. Habit spasm, foreign body or wax in the ear, subphrenic abscess. Hair against the tympanic membrane [A. P. Wolff, M. May, and D. Nuelle: Tympanic Membrane. A Source of Cough Reflex, *J.A.M.A.*, **223:**1269, 1973].

▼ *Key Sign:* ***Hiccup (Singultus).*** *Hiccup* or *hiccough* is a sudden involuntary diaphragmatic contraction producing an inspiration interrupted by glottal closure to emit a characteristic sharp sound. These contractions occur about two or three each minute. The variety of clinical conditions with which hiccup is associated prompts the inference that the stimulus may be initiated centrally with mediation through the phrenic nerve, or by direct stimulation of the phrenic nerve, and perhaps by direct irritation of the diaphragm. The causes are listed for diagnostic purposes:

Clinical Occurrence. REFLEX STIMULATION WITHOUT ORGANIC DISEASE. Excessive laughter, tickling, aerophagia, excessive tobacco smoking, excessive intake of alcohol, hysteria (persisting for weeks, but ceasing during sleep.) DISEASES OF THE CENTRAL NERVOUS SYSTEM. Encephalitis, meningitis, vertebrobasilar ischemia, intracranial hemorrhage, intracranial tumor, uremia, senile changes in brain and medulla. MEDIASTINAL DISORDERS. Trauma to phrenic nerve, enlargement of lymph nodes (tuberculosis, malignant neoplasm, fibrosis), bronchial obstruction, adherent pericardium, excessive cardiac enlargement, myocardial infarction, esophageal obstruction. PLEURAL IRRITATION. Pneumonia with pleurisy. ABDOMINAL DISORDERS. Diaphragmatic hernia of stomach, subphrenic abscess, subphrenic peritonitis, involvement of liver (neoplasm, gumma, abscess), carcinoma of stomach, splenic infarction, acute intestinal obstruction, acute hemorrhagic pancreatitis, after operations in the upper abdomen. TABES DORSALIS. Mechanisms unknown. DIAPHRAGMATIC STIMULATION. Caused by an implanted cardiac pacemaker.

▼ *Key Sign:* ***Hemoptysis.*** Spitting or coughing of blood is hemoptysis. The bleeding lesions may be anywhere from the nose to the lungs. Expectorated blood comes from the upper respiratory tract; blood in the bronchial tree induces coughing. The patient may not be able to discriminate between the two actions, so the entire tract must be considered.

Clinical Occurrence. UPPER RESPIRATORY TRACT. Epistaxis in the nasopharynx, bleeding from the oropharynx, bleeding from the gums, laryngitis, laryngeal carcinoma, hereditary hemorrhagic telangiectasia. BRONCHIAL TREE. Acute and chronic bronchitis, trauma from coughing, bronchiectasis, bronchial carcinoma, broncholiths, erosion by aortic aneurysms. LUNGS: INFECTIONS. Pneubmonia (especially klebsiella), lung abscess, tuberculosis, fungal infections, amebiasis, hydatid cyst. TRAUMA. Foreign body. CARDIOVASCULAR. Pulmonary infarction, mitral stenosis, chronic passive congestion in cardiac failure, arteriovenous fistula, anomalous pulmonary artery, hypertension. HEMATOLOGIC. Thrombocytopenia, leukemia, hemophilia, uremia. OTHERS. Lipoid pneumonia, Wegener's granuloma, Goodpasture's syndrome, idiopathic pulmonary hemosiderosis.

Noisy Breathing: ***Stertorous Breathing.*** The term is derived from *stertor*, snoring. In its benign form, it is the noise produced by vibrations of the lax soft palate during sleep, known as snoring. It occurs during sleep apnea. A similar sound results from vibrations of secretions in the upper respiratory tract. When this occurs during severe illness, it is frequently a grave prognostic sign, the "death rattle."

Noisy Breathing: ***Stridulous Breathing.*** A high-pitched whistling or crowing sound is caused by passage of air through the partly closed glottis. It occurs in edema of the vocal cords, neoplasm, diphtheritic membrane, abscess of the pharynx, and foreign body in the larynx or trachea.

Respiratory Rate: ***Tachypnea*** (Fast Breathing). At rest, the normal respiratory rate in adults is between 14 and 18 cycles per minute; in the newborn, the rate is about 44; gradually the rate diminishes until maturity. Women have slightly higher rates than men. In waking patients, the respiratory rate should be counted *unobtrusively*, such as pretending to count the pulse, because many persons tend to breathe faster when their attention is directed to their respiratory functions. Tachypnea occurs with exertion, fever, cardiac insufficiency, pain, acute respiratory distress from infections, pleurisy, anemia, and thyrotoxicosis. Breathing is faster when restricted by pulmonary infiltration, abdominal distention, paralysis of the respiratory muscles, pulmonary emphysema, pneumothorax, or obesity.

Respiratory Rate: Bradypnea (Slow Breathing). When the rate is slow and the rhythm regular, breathing is usually deeper than normal. The rate is slowed in uremia, diabetic coma, from excessive alcohol or morphine, and in conditions with increased intracranial pressure.

Deep Breathing: Kussmaul Respiration (Air Hunger). The term *Kussmaul breathing* is applied to deep, *regular* sighing respirations, whether the rate be normal, slow, or fast. This type occurs in diabetic acidosis and uremia, as an exaggerated form of bradypnea. In addition, this pattern is a response to air hunger in generalized peritonitis, severe hemorrhage, and pneumonia.

Shallow Breathing. There is no special name for this. It occurs in circulatory failure, meningitis, and unconsciousness from many causes.

▼ *Key Sign:* ***Cheyne-Stokes Respiration.*** This is the commonest form of periodic breathing. Periods of apnea alternate regularly with series of respiratory cycles. In each series the rate and amplitude of successive cycles increase to a maximum; then there is progressive diminution until the series is terminated by another apneic period. Pallor may accompany the apnea, but the patient is frequently unaware of the irregular breathing. Patients are often somnolent during the apneic periods and then arouse and become restless during the hyperpneic phase. The disorder is a result of fluctuations in the P_aCO_2 of blood reaching the respiratory center and the loss of normal feedback controls to maintain a more constant P_aCO_2.

Clinical Occurrence. Normal. During the sleep of normal children and the aged. DISORDERS OF THE CEREBRAL CIRCULATION. *Cardiac failure:* left-sided failure from any cause. INCREASED CEREBRAL PRESSURE. Meningitis, hydrocephalus, brain tumor, subarachnoid hemorrhage, intracerebral hemorrhage. INJURY TO BRAIN TISSUE.

Cerebral thrombosis, cerebromedullary degeneration, atherosclerosis, syphilis, head injury. NARCOTICS. Morphine and its derivatives, barbiturates, alcohol. HIGH ALTITUDE. During sleep, before acclimatization.

Irregular Breathing: ***Biot's Breathing.*** An uncommon variant of Cheyne-Stokes respiration, periods of apnea alternate irregularly with series of breaths of equal depth that terminate abruptly. It is most often seen in meningitis.

Irregular Breathing. ***Painful Respiration.*** Otherwise normal respirations are interrupted by the pain of thoracic movement from pleurisy, traumatized or inflamed muscles, fractured ribs or cartilages, or subphrenic inflammation, such as acute cholecystitis or peritonitis.

Irregular Breathing: ***Sighing Respirations.*** The normal respiratory rhythm is occasionally interrupted by a long deep sigh. The patient complains of shortness of breath, without other visible signs of it. This is commonly encountered in psychoneurotic persons.

▼ *Key Sign:* ***Dyspnea.*** Literally the term *dyspnea* means difficult breathing; in this sense it is a symptom. The patient's complaint is likely to be "shortness of breath," "quickly out of breath," "can't take a deep breath," "smothering," or "tightness in the chest." But the term is also used as a physical sign, since dyspnea is often accompanied by tachypnea, increased respiratory excursions, tensing of the Scaleni and Sternocleidomastoidei, flaring of the ala nasi, and unequivocal facial expressions of distress. Sometimes the patient is not conscious of being dyspneic, and the first clue encountered by the examiner is that the patient pauses for breath in the middle of an average sentence. It is useful to distinguish several degrees, ranging from *exertional dyspnea* to *dyspnea at rest,* and *orthopnea.* ***Orthopnea.*** This is the most severe; the patient is prompted to assume a position at rest that elevates the head and thorax toward the vertical. Some clinicians refer to *two-pillow orthopnea* and *three-pillow orthopnea,* to describe the required elevation. Orthopnea is often overlooked when the patient does not mention it and he sits while being examined. The physician must specifically *ask* about it, or he must observe the patient supine. The mechanism of orthopnea is unknown, but the erect position lowers the domes of the diaphragm, permitting greater volume expansion. A diagnostic classification of the causes of dyspnea may be based upon anatomic and physical criteria.

Clinical Occurrence. I. OXYGEN INGRESS. *Oxygen Deficiency in the Air.* Breathing air at high altitudes. *Obstruction in the Airways. Larynx and trachea:* infectious (laryngeal diphtheria, acute laryngitis, Ludwig's angina), allergic (angioneurotic edema), trauma (hematoma or laryngeal edema), neuropathic (abductor paralysis of vocal cords), foreign body, tumors of the neck (goiter, carcinoma, Hodgkin's disease, aortic aneurysm), ankylosis of the cricoarytenoid joints. *Bronchi and bronchioles:* acute bronchitis, asthma, asthmatic bronchitis, retrosternal goiter, multiple foreign bodies (e.g., aspirated food particles), extensive bronchiectasis, bronchial stenosis. *Pulmonary alveoli:* pulmonary edema from left heart failure or noxious gases, pulmonary emphysema, pulmonary fibrosis, cystic disease of the lungs, pulmonary infiltrations (pneumonia, carcinoma, granuloma), excessive resection of the lungs, pulmonary alveolar proteinosis. *Compression of the Alveoli.* Massive atelectasis, pneumothorax, hydrothorax, abdominal distention. *Malfunction of the Thorax.* Paralysis of the respiratory muscles (especially the intercostals and the diaphragm), thoracic deformities (kyphoscoliosis, thoracoplasty), scleroderma of the thoracic wall.

II. DEFICIT IN OXYGEN UPTAKE: *Circulation of the Lungs.* Passive congestion (cardiac failure), pulmonary artery stenosis, arteriovenous shunts in heart or lungs, pulmonary infarction, emboli (blood clots, fat globules, air bubbles), arteriolar stenosis (pulmonary hypertension, Ayerza's disease, x-radiation of lungs). *Hemoglobin Deficiency.* Anemia, carbon monoxide poisoning (carboxyhemoglobinemia), methemoglobinema and sulfhemoglobinemia, cyanide and cobalt poisoning.

III. ABNORMAL NERVOUS STIMULI. Pain from respiratory movements, exaggerated consciousness of respiration (effort syndrome), hyperventilation syndrome, respiratory arrhythmia (increased intracranial pressure, acidosis).

INSPECTION OF THE RESPIRATORY EXCURSIONS. **Abnormalities in the amplitude of respiratory movements in various regions of the thorax direct attention to lesions in the chest wall, or underlying pleura and lungs. The method of inspection is described at this juncture because it is employed in this sequence of the examination. Later, the findings from inspection are interpreted when they are supplemented by signs obtained with palpation, percussion, and auscultation.**

Movement of the Chest in One Piece. During respiratory movements, the entire thorax appears to move as a unit. This may result from increased lung volume in pulmonary emphysema or ankylosis of the joints of the thoracic cage.

Inspiratory Retraction of Interspaces. The inward movement is usually more evident in the lower thorax. The finding suggests fibrosis of the underlying lung, or pulmonary emphysema. *Sudden, violent* retractions occur in tracheal obstruction and severe paroxysms of asthma.

TESTING EXCURSION OF THE UPPER THORAX. **Place a hand on each side of the patient's neck with palms against the upper anterior thoracic wall. Curl the fingers firmly over the superior edges of the Trapezii. Move the palms downward against the skin, to provide slack, until the palms lie in the infraclavicular fossae. Then extend your thumbs so their tips meet in the midline (Fig. 6-16A). Have the patient inspire deeply; permit your palms to move freely with the chest while your fingers are anchored firmly above on the Trapezii. The upper four ribs move forward with inspiration, so your thumbs *diverge* from the midline. Normally, the thumbs move laterally for equal distances. Asymmetric excursions suggest a lesion on the lagging side in the chest wall, the pleura, or the upper lobe of the lung.**

TESTING EXCURSION OF THE ANTERIOR MIDDLE THORAX. **With your fingers high in each axilla and your thumbs abducted, place the palms on the anterior chest. Move the hands medially, dragging skin to provide slack, until the thumb tips meet in the midline at the level of the 6th ribs (Fig. 6-16B). Have the patient inspire deeply; let your hands follow the chest movements; the thumbs diverge and serve as markers. A unilateral lag indicates a nearby lesion in the wall, pleura, middle lobe of the right lung, or lingula of the left lung.**

TESTING EXCURSION OF THE POSTERIOR LOWER CHEST. **Have the patient sit or stand with his back toward you. Place your fingers in each axilla, with the palms applied firmly to his chest, so your forefingers are one or two ribs below the inferior angles of the scapulae. To provide slack, press the soft tissues and pull your hands medially until your extended thumbs meet over the vertebral spines (Fig. 6-16C). Have the patient inspire deeply; follow the lateral movements of the chest with your hands so your diverging thumbs serve as markers. A unilateral lag indicates a lesion in the nearby wall, pleura, or lower lobes of the lung.**

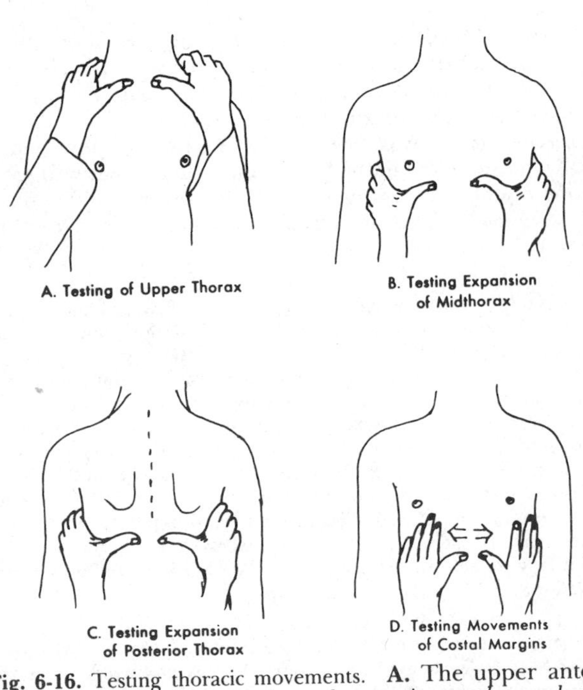

Fig. 6-16. Testing thoracic movements. **A.** The upper anterior thorax. *The fingers are hooked over the trapezius muscles, one hand on each shoulder. The thumbs are extended and their tips approximated. When the patient inspires deeply, the hands are permitted to travel passively with the anterior chest wall, while divergence of the thumbs from the midline is noted for distance and timing.* **B.** Expansion of the anterior midthorax. *A hand is placed in each axilla with the palmar surface against the chest wall. The abducted thumbs are pointed medially along the 6th ribs until their tips approximate. When the patient inspires deeply, the hands follow the chest wall passively and the thumbs are watched for divergence from the midline in distance and timing.* **C.** Expansion of the posterior thorax. *A hand is placed in each axilla with palmar surface against the chest wall. The abducted thumbs are approximated. During deep inspiration the divergence of their tips from the midline is noted for distance and timing.* **D.** Movement of costal margins. *A thumb is placed along each costal margin so the tips approximate. During deep inspiration the thumbs passively follow the margins, and the divergence of their tips from the midline is watched for distance and timing.*

Diminished Local Excursion of the Thorax. This points to a lesion in the underlying wall, pleura, or lung. The restricted movement may be caused by pain, fibrosis, or consolidation.

Localized Bulging of the Thorax During Expiration: Flail Chest. The fracture of several nearby ribs or the separation of several contiguous costal cartilages results in an abnormal movement of that region of the wall, with local bulging during expiration and retraction during inspiration. Since rigidity of the wall is destroyed, the increased negative intrathoracic pressure during inspiration pulls the injured segment inward; the rise in intrathoracic pressure during expiration causes it to bulge.

TESTING EXCURSION OF THE COSTAL MARGINS. **With the patient supine, place your hands so the extended thumbs lie along the inferior edges of the costal margins, with their tips nearly touching (Fig. 6-16D). Have the patient inspire deeply; let your thumbs follow the costal margins. Normally, the thumbs diverge from the upward pull on the ribs by the diaphragm. Diminished divergence indicates depression of the dome of the diaphragm; convergence results when the dome is considerably flattened.**

Inspiratory Convergence, or Lessened Divergence of Costal Margins. When the dome of the diaphragm is flattened, the direction of its pull on the costal margins is changed from upward to medially. The degree of outward flare of the margins is lessened or, in extreme cases, the margins are pulled inward. Lowering of the diaphragm may be caused by pulmonary emphysema or by accumulations of fluid or air in the pleural space.

Exaggerated Costal Margin Flare During Inspiration. Elevation of the dome of the diaphragm increases the pull upward. The most common causes are hepatomegaly and subphrenic abscess.

PALPATION OF THE TRACHEA. **Assess the position of the trachea by palpating its relations to the tissues in the suprasternal notch. Direct the forefinger through the suprasternal notch and feel the size of the space between the head of the right clavicle and the right aspect of the trachea; compare this space with that on the other side. *Alternate Method:* Direct the pronated finger exactly posteriorly through the middle of the suprasternal notch until the fingertip touches the tracheal rings. The curvature of the rings touches the finger on the center of its tip, the trachea is in the midline.**

Lateral Deviations of the Trachea. At the level of the clavicle, lateral tracheal deviation may be caused by a mass higher in the neck, such as cervical goiter or a group of enlarged lymph nodes. Below the suprasternal notch, a retrosternal goiter, eccentrically located, may push the trachea to one side. The trachea and mediastinum deviate to the opposite side with pleural effusion and spontaneous pneumothorax. Displacement of the trachea to the ipsilateral side occurs in pulmonary atelectasis or fibrosis of the lung or pleura. Carcinoma of the lung rarely causes displacement except by producing atelectasis.

Axial Fixation of the Trachea. While the patient's head is held in the customary position, one grasps the cricoid cartilage or tracheal rings with the thumb and index finger and lifts the structure cephalad. Normally, there is considerable axial mobility. Fixation of the trachea occurs normally when the neck is dorsiflexed, and abnormally in pulmonary emphysema, adhesive mediastinitis, aortic aneurysm, mediastinal neoplasm.

PALPATION OF THE THORACIC WALL. **This procedure is frequently neglected, resulting in many errors in diagnosis. Palpation is certainly indicated by (1) any pain in the chest, (2) masses seen in the chest wall, (3) masses apparently in the breast, (4) draining sinuses in the thorax. *Examination of Soft Tissue:* Press or pinch the large muscles of the thorax to elicit *tenderness;* if tender, try to determine the movements that elicit *pain.* Feel for *soft-tissue crepitus.* Palpate the interspaces for *tenderness* and *masses. Examination of Costal Cartilages:* Palpate the costochondral junctions. Test them for *tenderness, swelling,* and *mobility. Ribs:* Palpate for point *tenderness, swelling, bone crepitus,* and remote pain on compression. *Xiphisternal Joint:* Palpate for tenderness.**

Tender Muscle in the Thorax. Frequently a tender muscle is mistaken by the patient and the physician for intrathoracic disease. A competent woman physician told one of us that she was certain that the pain in her left chest was angina pectoris until she found that her left pectoralis muscle was tender and she realized that she was lifting her heavy child too frequently.

Soft-Tissue Crepitus: ***Subcutaneous and Mediastinal Emphysema.*** Trauma to the chest may produce subcutaneous emphysema of the thoracic wall. Air may invade the chest wall from the neck or directly from the lung. In the first case, rupture of pulmonary alveoli permits air to travel beneath the visceral pleura to the hilum of the lung, thence along the trachea to the neck, where dangerous swelling may occur; the thoracic wall is involved secondarily by migration from the neck. Massive swelling of the neck and face is accompanied by cyanosis, directing attention to the condition. When a fractured rib punctures the pleura, ingress of air through the visceral pleura to the thoracic wall causes emphysema. In this case, *soft-tissue crepitus* may be the first clue. This is a sensation imparted to the pressing finger by small globules of air moving in the tissues (see p. 501). The air may invade the mediastinum where it produces a distinctive *systolic crunching* in the precordium known as *Hamman's sign.* Vomiting seems to produce this condition without esophageal rupture [P. M. Beigelman, L. V. Miller, and H. E. Martin: Mediastinal and Subcutaneous Emphysema in Diabetic Coma with Vomiting, *J.A.M.A.,* **208:**2315–18, 1969].

Mass in the Interspace: ***Hodgkin's Lymphadenopathy.*** Involvement of a lymph node along the internal mammary artery in Hodgkin's disease produces swelling in an upper parasternal interspace. Bailey states that this is pathognomonic of the disease.

Mass in the Interspace: ***Fluctuant Masses.*** These are usually abscesses. A *cold abscess* is tuberculous, so named because it lacks surrounding inflammation. It usually arises from a nearby rib. Actinomycosis frequently produces abscesses in the lung that burrow through the chest wall. An abscess may result when an untreated pleural empyema points through the interspaces, termed *empyema necessitans.*

Sinuses in the Thoracic Wall. Chronic sinuses discharging through the intercostal spaces may result from a variety of conditions, including empyema, tuberculosis, actinomycosis, and necrosis of ribs. The sinus tract should be probed from the exterior to ascertain the extent and direction. Actinomycosis produces a sinus with a peculiar dusky color around its mouth; the organism may be found by microscopic examination of the pus. X-ray examination is necessary for more detailed information of all sinuses.

Tender Costal Cartilage: ***Costal Chondritis*** (Tietze's Syndrome). Pain and fusiform swelling of one or more costicartilages may occur gradually or suddenly. The overlying skin is reddened. Pain may radiate to the shoulder, neck, or arm. There is no lymphadenopathy. The swelling may persist for months after the pain and tenderness subside. X-ray findings are lacking. The cause is unknown. The condition must be distinguished from osteitis, periostitis, rheumatic chondritis, and neoplasm of the ribs. Injection of the lesion with procaine relieves the pain.

Pain in the Chest: ***Fractured Rib.*** The patient complains of pain in the chest with respiratory movement. Inspiration is limited by pain. Palpation discloses *point tenderness* on a rib. The edges of the fracture may be *felt,* but bone crepitus is usually absent because the fragments are well apposed. With one hand supporting the back, compression of the sternum with the other elicits pain at the untouched fracture site (Fig. 6-17A). The physical signs are diagnostic, although x-ray examination may not reveal a fresh fracture. The diagnosis is made readily when the patient gives a history of trauma to the thorax that prompts appropriate examination. But many fractures are missed because physicians have not yet learned of *cough fracture,* described by Robert Graves sometime before 1833. There is no history of a blow; but rather, the patient has been coughing for some time with an upper respiratory infection. Pain begins to occur with respiratory movements. The typical signs of fracture of a rib are present, *provided* the physician

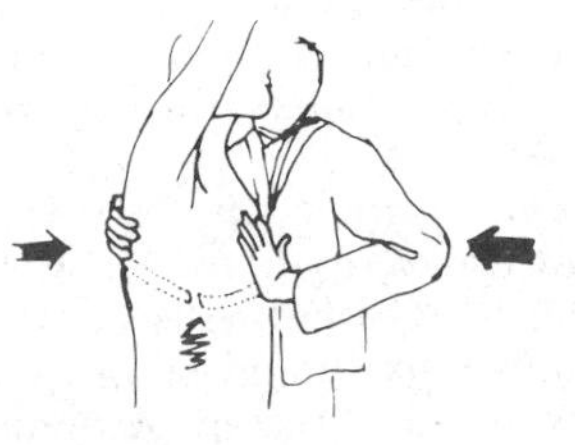

A. Compression Test for Rib Fracture

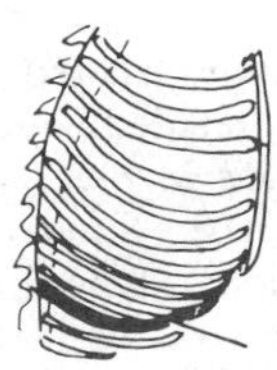

B. Slipping 10th Rib

Fig. 6-17. Examining for rib pains. **A.** Compression test for rib fracture. *When the site of suspected rib fracture is located by point tenderness, the sternum is pushed toward the spine with one hand while the other supports the patient's back. The maneuver will elicit pain at the untouched fracture site.* **B.** Slipping 10th rib. *When the 10th rib lacks an anterior attachment, it can slip forward upon the 9th rib during respiratory movements and cause pain.*

palpates the ribs. Any ribs from the 5th to the 10th are likely to break, usually anterior to the attachments of the Serratus anterior that pulls the rib upward, and posterior of the fixations of the Obliquus externus abdominis that pulls the rib downward; thus a shearing force is exerted on the rib. A single cough is not enough to produce fracture; breaking is attributed to the fatigue from repeated stressful movements. When palpation of the ribs is not performed, the condition is usually diagnosed as pleurisy. Fractures of several contiguous ribs are usually caused by external violence; the chest wall may be so weakened as to produce the flail chest described on p. 285.

Pain in the Chest: ***Slipping Rib.*** The 10th rib is usually affected. The interchondral ligament between the 9th and 10th costicartilages becomes weakened and elongated, permitting the 10th rib to override the 9th (Fig. 6-17B). The slipping rib may cause pain, falsely attributed to intra-abdominal disease. The increased mobility can be palpated.

Pain in the Chest: ***Palpable Pleural Friction Rub.*** The inflamed pleural surfaces lose their lubricating fluid ("dry pleurisy") and rub together during movements of the lungs. Sometimes the vibrations from the two rubbing surfaces can be felt, similar to that of two pieces of dry leather rubbing together. The rub is also heard with the stethoscope or the unaided ear as a creaking sound.

Mass in a Rib. Some causes of masses on ribs are callus around an old fracture or fibrous dysplasia; neoplasm of ribs, such as chondrosarcoma, metastasis of carcinoma, angioma, and eosinophilic granuloma; bone cysts, including osteitis fibrosa cystica. A neurofibroma arising from an intercostal nerve causes a swelling near the neck of the rib. X-ray examination usually distinguishes the various lesions.

Tender Sternum: ***Normal.*** Many normal persons have *slight tenderness* in the lower third of the sternum, elicited when the finger is drawn over it.

Tender Sternum: ***Chronic Myelocytic Leukemia.*** Firm pressure, systematically applied with the finger to various parts of the sternum may disclose a small or large area of tenderness, more intense than normal, in some patients with chronic myelocytic leukemia, according to Bailey. The tender site is usually in the lower third of the bone.

Tender Sternum: ***Fractured Sternum.*** The profile of the sternum usually bears some abnormal angulation, the site of which is tender. Pain prompts the patient to bend the head and thorax forward with the shoulders rotated inward.

Tender Xiphoid: ***Xiphisternal Arthritis.*** This causes chest pain sometimes mistaken for angina pectoris, but *tenderness* is distinctive.

The Lungs and Pleura

The airways of the respiratory system include the nasal passages and nasopharynx, the mouth and oropharynx, the larynx, the trachea, and the branches of the bronchial tree supplying the pulmonary alveoli.

The Bronchial Tree

The trachea bifurcates asymmetrically into the *right* and *left bronchus.* Viewed through the bronchoscope, the dividing septum is the *carina.* The right bronchus deviates but slightly from the axis of the trachea, but the left bronchus diverges at a greater angle, making it less accessible to the bronchoscope and explaining why foreign bodies are more likely to lodge in the right main stem bronchus. The right bronchus sends a *lobar bronchus* to each of three pulmonary lobes; the left bronchus forms two lobar bronchi. Each first branch of a lobar bronchus supplies a *bronchopulmonary segment* of lung. Surmounting the trachea, the larynx is a frequent site of obstruction, either from intrinsic swelling or by paralysis of its vocal cords. The heart lies in front of the tracheal bifurcation and the aorta arches over the left bronchus from front to back. Interposed between the aorta and bronchus is the *left recurrent laryngeal nerve,* which descends in front of the aortic arch, loops under it, and ascends beside the trachea to the neck. The dilated aorta may produce a tracheal tug by pulsating against the left bronchus, or it may compress the left recurrent laryngeal nerve against the left bronchus with resulting paralysis of the left vocal cord.

The Lungs

The lungs may be regarded as clusters of pulmonary alveoli around the subdivisions of the bronchial tree. The right lung has three major masses: the *right upper lobe,* the *right middle lobe,* and the *right lower lobe,* each about its lobar bronchus.

The left lung has but two lobes: the *left upper lobe* and the *left lower lobe,* each with its lobar bronchus. Each lobe is separated from others in the same lung by a *lobar fissure,* an infolding of visceral pleura. Molded by the contour of the thoracic cavity, the shape of both lungs is similar, but the medial edge of the left lung has an inferior indentation, the *cardiac notch.*

For convenience of the bronchoscopist, the thoracic surgeon, and the radiologist, each lung lobe is further divided into *bronchopulmonary segments,* each consisting of the cluster of alveoli supplied by a single *first branch* of the lobar bronchus (Figs. 6-18 and 6-19). Anatomically, these divisions are not grossly demarcated by fissures; their limits are demonstrable only by special dissections with injected preparations. When present, extra fissures do follow these boundaries.

In the practice of thoracic surgery, the *lingula* tends to be regarded as a separate lobe, homologous to the right middle lobe.

The Bronchopulmonary Segments

Right Upper Lobe
- Apical
- Posterior
- Anterior

Right Middle Lobe
- Lateral
- Medial

Right Lower Lobe
- Superior
- Medial basal
- Anterior basal
- Lateral basal
- Posterior basal

Left Upper Lobe
- Superior Division
  - Apical-posterior
  - Anterior
- Inferior Division or Lingula
  - Superior
  - Inferior

Left Lower Lobe
- Superior
- Anterior-medial-basal
- Lateral basal
- Posterior basal

The topography of the five lung lobes has some clinical applications. In Fig. 6-20 note that the anterior aspect of the right lung is formed almost entirely of the right *upper* and *middle* lobes; the posterior aspect contains only the *upper* and *lower* lobes. The wedges of the upper and middle lobes have their apices pointed posteriorly, while the apex of the lower lobe points anteriorly. In the left lung, the *upper* and *lower*

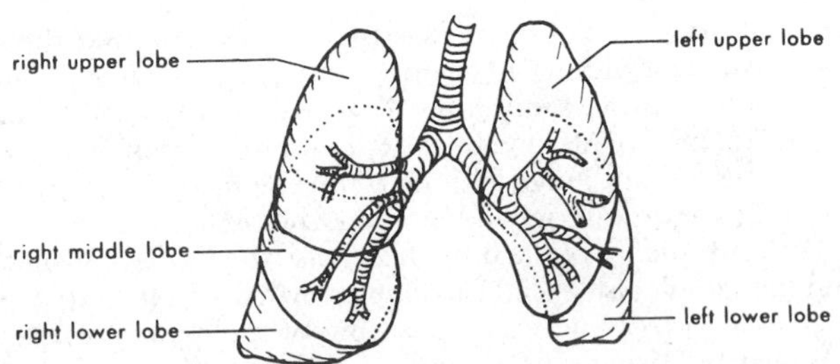

Fig. 6-18. The lobes of the lungs. *The transparent diagram shows the anterior aspects of the pulmonary lobes, together with their main bronchi. Note the three divisions of the right main bronchus, and the more direct line with the trachea on the right side.*

lobes present both back and front. The apex of the upper lobe faces posteriorly; the lower lobe apex is anterior.

The Pleura

The relations of a single lung to its pleura can be visualized by imagining a sphere of thin plastic material from which

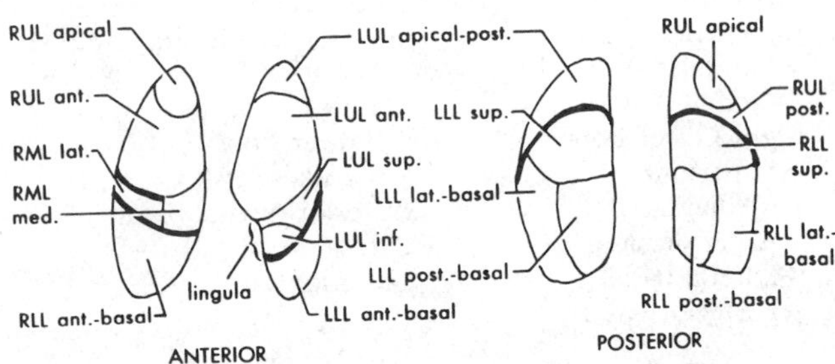

Fig. 6-19. Segmental divisions of the lungs. *The thick lines are the gross pulmonary fissures, readily identified on inspection of the lung and sometimes in the x-ray films. The thinner lines are established only by careful dissections of injected preparations. In the abbreviations the first capital letter designates "right" or "left"; the second, "upper," "middle," and "lower"; the third L is for "lobe." Note that the lingula, composed of the superior and inferior segments of the left upper lobe, is near the heart and corresponds in many respects to the right middle lobe.*

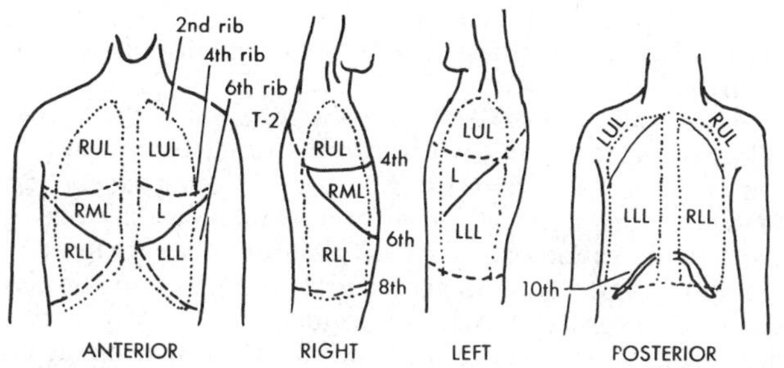

Fig. 6-20. Topographic location of the five lobes of the lungs. *The heavy solid lines are actual pulmonary fissures; the broken lines are projections, except for the boundary of the lingula (L.), which is hypothetic.*

the air is being evacuated (Fig. 6-21). As the sphere collapses, one part invaginates to form a hollow hemisphere with convex and concave layers in apposition. Imagine the convex layer cemented to the inside of the thoracic cavity, to represent the *parietal pleura.* Place the lung in the concavity of the hemisphere and cement its surface to the concave layer of plastic, to represent the *visceral pleura.* Arrange the invagination of

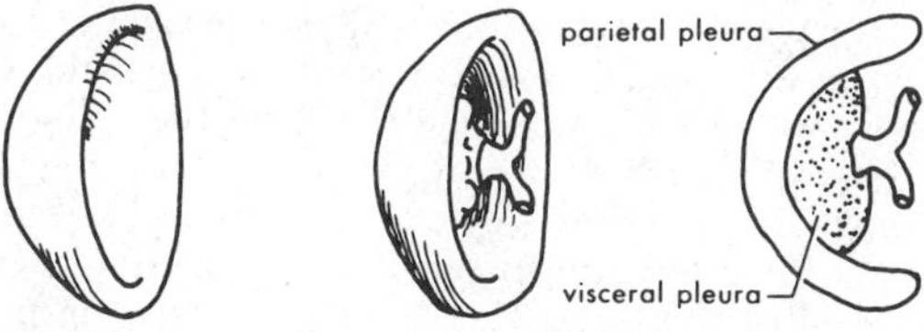

Fig. 6-21. Models illustrating relations of pleura to lung. *Deflate a rubber or plastic sphere so it assumes a hemisphere with a concave and convex surface. Place the model lung in the concavity and cement the lung surface to the inner surface of the hemisphere. In cross section, the parietal pleura will be represented by the convex surface of the hemisphere; the cemented layers represent the visceral pleura. The analogy is continued by exhausting the hemisphere of air and replacing with a little fluid to lubricate the inner surfaces. This geometry should be visualized in the examination of the chest and in looking at x-ray films, remembering that the pleural surfaces are anterior as well as lateral.*

the sphere so the parietal pleura has a greater area than the visceral pleura, permitting the lung some mobility in the thoracic cavity.

Anatomically, the parietal pleura is adherent to the thoracic wall; the visceral pleura is fixed to the lung surface and also lines the interlobar fissures. The two apposing layers form the *pleural cavity,* devoid of air and containing only enough fluid for lubrication. The parietal pleura has the greater area, extending inferiorly on the ribs and diaphragm some distance below the lower tip of the lung to form the *costophrenic sinus.* The lung descends partway into this sinus during deep inspiration.

Mechanics of the Lung and Pleura

When the otherwise normal lung is removed from the thoracic cavity, it partially collapses from the *elastic recoil* of its tissue. Even so, the lung contains enough trapped air to make it float on water. The organ feels tough, elastic, spongy, light in weight, and crepitant—i.e., it crackles from the movement of air bubbles under the pressing fingers. The volume of the collapsed lung is much smaller than the hemithorax from whence it came. When the lung is in the closed thorax, its volume is much greater because its surface is held against the thoracic wall by the apposition of the parietal and visceral pleurae. Contact between the two pleural layers is maintained because the pleural sac is devoid of air, so the layers are pressed together by the weight of the atmosphere upon the thoracic wall and parietal pleura on one side, and the column of air under atmospheric pressure in the airway pressing through the alveoli on the other side. So the atmospheric pressure resists any force tending to separate the pleural layers. The elastic recoil of the lungs exerts such a separating pull. If a needle attached to a water manometer is inserted into the empty pleural space, the pressure during expiration registers about −5 cm of water, roughly a measure of the elastic recoil of the lung and thorax during rest. During inspiration, the negative pressure increases to about −15 cm of water because additional elastic recoil is produced by stretching the lung as its volume increases.

The parietal pleura contains sensory nerve endings, but the visceral pleural is anesthetic. This fact is significant in performing thoracentesis. The pain of pleurisy has been attributed to two dry surfaces of pleura rubbing together, but clinical observation discloses patients with painless pleural friction rubs and pleural pain without rubs; pleural pain is ascribed to stretching of the inflamed parietal pleura during respiratory excursions.

Physical Assessment of Lungs and Pleura

Some clinicians argue that physical examination of the lungs and pleura is no longer necessary, since x-ray examination is readily available and discloses many lesions without physical signs. The advantages of x-ray examination are acknowledged; the procedure should be employed, but its deficits still make physical examination necessary. Early pneumonia can be diagnosed by the clinician before x-ray signs appear. A fractured rib may be obvious to palpation weeks before callus is evident in the x-ray film. The radiologist cannot diagnose asthma. The friction rub of pleurisy can appear and subside without x-ray signs. Pulmonary emphysema may be evident clinically long before the radiologist can recognize it. Obstruction of the airway by a radiolucent object may not give early signs in the x-ray film to assist the bronchoscopist.

The physical examination of the pleura seeks to detect evidence of pleural inflammation, pleural adhesions, increases in pleural thickness, and the presence of air or excessive fluid in the pleural cavity. The lungs are examined to judge their volume, extensibility, density, deviations in the caliber of the bronchial tree, and abnormal secretions in the airways. As already indicated, inspection and tactile palpation give some information. Examination is extended by observing the vibratory qualities of the thorax and its contents. Some vibrations may be perceived by vibratory palpation, using the deep sensibility in the joints and muscles of the examiner's hands. Other vibrations are perceived as sound by the examiner's unaided ears in sonorous and definitive percussion, or through the stethoscope in auscultation. Vibrations are produced by the patient's spoken voice and by the examiner tapping the patient's chest. The caliber of the airways and their contained secretions modify the breath sounds or produce extraneous noises heard through the stethoscope.

Vibratory Palpation of the Lungs and Pleura

Since palpation perceives many different types of sensation with the examiner's hands, we have chosen to introduce a more selective term, *vibratory palpation*, to designate specifically the use of the examiner's vibratory sense. This seems justified because a different technique is required. Set a tuning fork in vibration and apply the handle first to the fingertip and then to the palmar base of the finger over the metacarpophalangeal joint; this readily demonstrates the superior sensitivity of the basal part of the finger to vibrations.

During speech, the patient's vocal cords set up vibrations in the bronchial air column that are conducted to the chest wall where they may be perceived by vibratory palpation, as *vocal fremitus* (or tactile fremitus). Diminished vocal fremitus can be caused by blockage of the airways or sound screens of fluid or air in the pleural cavity, or by fibrosis of the pleura itself. Increased transmission of vocal fremitus occurs with consolidation of the lungs about the bronchial tree. The density of the tissues is determined by percussion. Since the intensity of vocal fremitus is compared in various regions of the chest, equal pitch and loudness must be employed in each spoken test word. Vocal fremitus is normally more intense in the parasternal region in the right second interspace where it is closest to the bronchial bifurcation. The interscapular region is also near the bronchi and registers increased fremitus. High-pitched voices produce unsatisfactory vibrations for vocal fremitus, so some women must be instructed to lower the pitch of the spoken test words.

PROCEDURE IN VIBRATORY PALPATION. **If able, have the patient seated or standing. Test for *vocal fremitus* by applying the palmar bases of the fingers of one hand to the interspaces (Fig. 6-22). Ask the patient to repeat the test word "ninety-nine" or "one-two-three," using the same pitch and intensity of voice each time. If vibrations are not well felt, have the patient lower the pitch of the voice. Compare symmetric parts of the chest sequentially with the *same hand*, such as left infraclavicular fossa, then right; left 4th interspace, then right. It is easier to compare two sensations sequentially from the same hand than to compare simultaneous sensations from two hands. When the lower thorax is reached, use the ulnar surface of the hand in the interspaces to ascertain the point at which fremitus is lost. In the absence of a pleural lesion, this maneuver should indicate the**

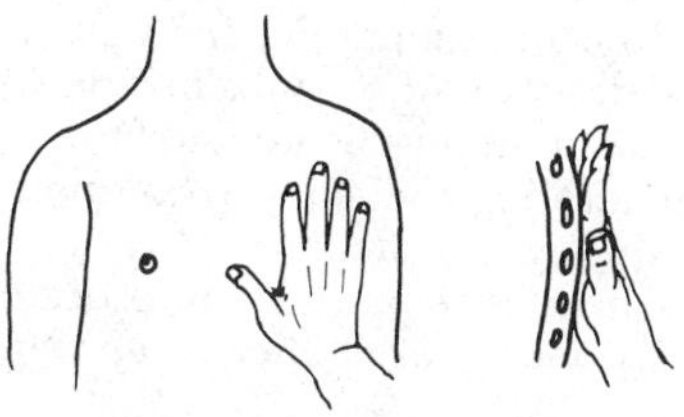

Fig. 6-22. Detection of vocal fremitus by vibratory palpation. *Symmetric points on the chest are palpated sequentially with the same hand and the strength of vocal fremitus is compared in different regions. The palpating hand is applied firmly to the chest wall with palm in contact with the wall and vibrations are sensed with the bases of the fingers, the most acutely sensitive.*

position of the *lung bases;* the site should be compared with that obtained by resonance by percussion, and the transmission of breath sounds by auscultation. With the same method, feel for pleural *friction rubs* (*friction fremitus*) over the thorax.

Vocal Fremitus Diminished or Absent. Since the palpable vibrations of the chest wall register movements of the bronchotracheal air column, failure of the vocal cords or blockage of the airways results in absent vocal fremitus. The interposition of filters of variable quality such as thickened pleura, pleural effusion, or pneumothorax, obstructs transmission of vibration through the chest wall, with diminished or absent vocal fremitus.

Vocal Fremitus Increased. Consolidated tissue in pneumonia or inflammation around a lung abcess, when in contact with a bronchus or cavity in the lung, transmits bronchotracheal air vibrations with greater efficiency than do the air-filled pulmonary alveoli; hence vocal fremitus is increased.

Percussion of the Lungs and Pleura

Percussion may be defined as the act of striking the surface of the body either to elicit a sound by which the density of the underlying tissue may be judged, or to determine the extent of an organ of constant density. *Sonorous percussion* is employed to detect changes from the normal density of an organ. For example, striking an air-filled lung produces one quality of sound; quite another sound is emitted from a lung filled with exudate; the contrasting sounds depend upon different densities. When the density of an organ is invariable and contrasts with that of the surrounding tissue, the borders of the organ are disclosed by locating the site of transition of one sound quality to the other; this is *definitive percussion.* For example, percussion of the heart is employed only to locate its boundaries with the lung; the density of neither tissue is in question.

Sonorous Percussion

When the body surface is struck in the practice of sonorous percussion, the underlying tissues vibrate to produce so-called *percussion notes* having mixed frequencies, so they are actually noises. These sounds vary with the density of the organ and the overlying tissue. Language is utterly inadequate for recognizable descriptions of sound, and attempts to describe these notes as high-pitched or low-pitched are futile and confusing. Nor do visual records of sound vibrations convey information that assists the reader to recognize sound quality. We prefer to present the subject, unadorned with acoustic verbiage, by merely stating that certain tissues emit sounds with arbitrary names; their recognition must be gained by listening.

The percussion note from the air-filled lung is termed *resonance.* Percussing the gastric air bubble yields a sound of quite different pitch and timbre, called *tympany;* the word is derived from the Greek for "drum," and the sound vaguely resembles a drumbeat. *Dullness* is a distinctive noise elicited by percussion over the heart when not covered by inflated lung. Percussion of the thigh muscles yields *flatness.* Absent in the normal body, *hyperresonance* is emitted by the emphysematous lung; it is intermediate between resonance from the lung, filled with small air sacs and septa, and tympany from the large undivided bubble in the stomach.

In a nontechnical sense, the percussion sounds may be regarded as constituting the notes of a scale, which progresses from tissues of great density to tissues of slight density in the following sequence: *flatness* from the thigh muscles, *dullness* from the blood-filled heart and overlying chest wall, *resonance* from the normal lung of small air pockets and septa, *hyperresonance* from the emphysematous lung with larger air pockets, and *tympany* from a single large bubble of air in the stomach. The *duration* of emitted sound correlates well with the density producing it; flatness can be perceived as a very *short* sound; each succeeding note in the scale is longer than its predecessor, as the density lessens. The pitch and timbre of the sounds must be learned by listening.

Modified tympanitic notes have limited value in special situations. In suspected pneumothorax, the *coin test* may be used. An assistant percusses the front of the affected hemithorax by holding a coin flat to the chest wall and striking it with the edge of a second coin (Fig. 6-23). The examiner listens with his stethoscope over the back on the same side for a clear ringing note, termed *bell tympany*. Although not always present, bell tympany is diagnostic of pneumothorax. Percussion over a pneumothorax, or a large pulmonary cavity, sometimes yields a hollow low-pitched sound, termed *amphoric*. Occasionally, a superficial pulmonary cavity has a small bronchial exit through which percussed air is forcefully expelled to produce *crackedpot resonance*. The name is descriptive, as the sound is dull, clinking, and closely approximates the effect obtained by percussing the cheek when the mouth is slightly opened. The zone of lung above a level of pleural fluid may be *tympanitic;* the sound is termed *skodaic tympany*. It arises from dilated air sacs in the lung just above the part compressed by the pleural fluid.

An abnormal *distribution* of sounds of normal quality can be pathologic. The lung is normally resonant; while being consolidated with exudate, its density increases to yield, successively, impaired resonance, dullness, and flatness. Ordinarily,

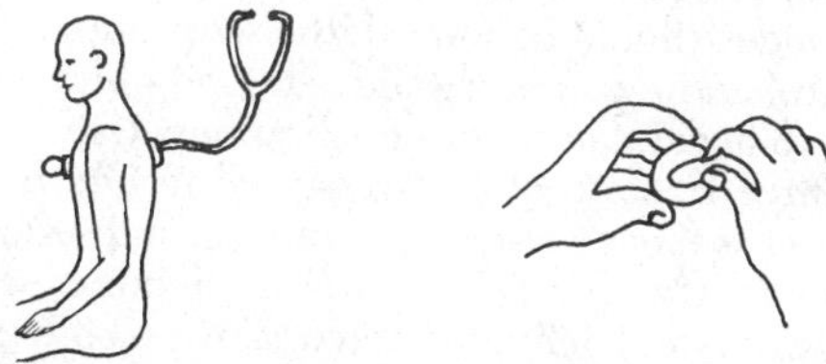

Fig. 6-23. Coin test for pneumothorax. *An assistant places a coin flat on the anterior chest wall and strikes it with the edge of a second coin. The examiner applies the chestpiece of his stethoscope to the back of the same hemithorax. In pneumothorax, the note is transmitted as a clear ringing sound, called bell tympany.*

the pleura contributes little to the percussion note, but fluid in the pleural cavity produces a dense layer that gives dullness to flatness in a characteristic distribution.

Definitive Percussion

In the examination of the thorax, definitive percussion is employed to outline the borders between lung resonance and dullness of the heart, the spleen, the upper border of the liver, the lumbar muscles below the lung bases. The boundary between resonant lung and tympanitic gastric bubble outlines Traube's semilunar space. Krönig's isthmus over the lung apices is defined by percussing the area of resonance in the supraclavicular fossae.

Two Methods of Thoracic Percussion

When the examiner elicits sound by striking the chest directly with his fingers or hand, the procedure is called *direct or immediate percussion*. Striking the percussion blow on an inanimate object or the examiner's finger is *indirect* or *mediate percussion*.

Indirect or Mediate Percussion. Physicians in the United States commonly employ this method. The palmar surface of the left long finger is firmly pressed into an intercostal space, as a *pleximeter;* only the distal phalanx should touch the wall. As a *plexor,* the tip of the right long finger strikes a sharp blow on the distal interphalangeal joint of the pleximeter finger (Fig. 6-24A). The examiner holds the plexor finger partly flexed and rigid; he delivers the blow by bending *only* the wrist, so the weight of the hand lends momentum to the stroke to ensure repetitive blows of precisely equal force. Neither the elbow nor the shoulder should be moved, the wrist must be relaxed. After the stroke, the plexor should rebound quickly from the pleximeter, to avoid damping the vibrations. Usually, a series of two or three staccato blows are struck in one place; then the pleximeter is moved elsewhere for a second series to compare the sounds. Most physicians employ this bimanual method for both sonorous and definitive percussion, on both the thorax and the abdomen. Sonorous percussion requires a strong blow, estimated to vibrate tissue in the chest for a radius of 6 cm, 3 cm in the thoracic wall, and 3 cm in the lung parenchyma. A lighter blow should be struck by this method for definitive percussion.

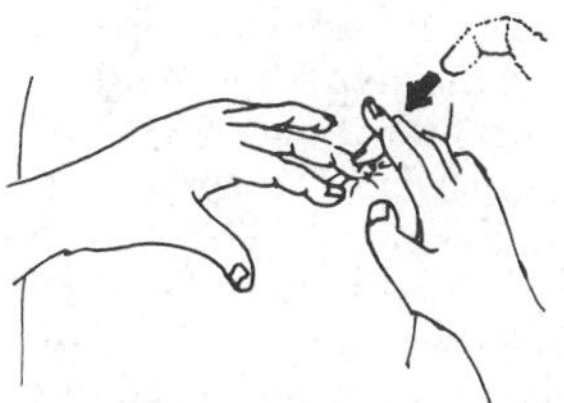

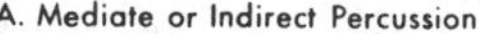

A. Mediate or Indirect Percussion

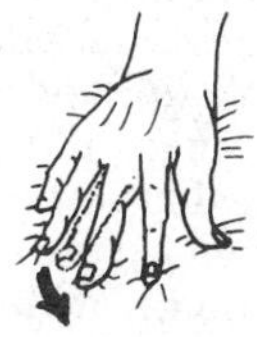

B. Direct or Damped Percussion

Fig. 6-24. Two methods of percussion. **A.** Indirect (bimanual) percussion. *The terminal digit of the left long finger is firmly applied to the interspace as a pleximeter. The distal interphalangeal joint of that finger is struck a sharp blow with the tip of the flexed right long finger. The fingers of the right hand are held partly flexed and the wrist is loose so that the striking hand pivots exclusively at the relaxed wrist to furnish blows of equal intensity. After striking the blow, the plexor hand is withdrawn rapidly from the pleximeter so as not to dampen the vibrations. The method is best suited for deep sonorous percussion of thorax and abdomen. It is somewhat inferior for definitive percussion.* **B.** Direct percussion (Hoover's damped percussion). *The percussing hand, either right or left, touches the body wall with the hypothenar eminence, the tip of the abducted thumb, and the abducted little finger. The long finger serves as the plexor; no pleximeter is used. Holding its interphalangeal joints in rigid extension, the long finger is flexed only at its metacarpophalangeal joint. The percussing finger strikes the interspace sharply and remains in contact with the surface to dampen the vibration. The method is superior for definitive percussion; it is satisfactory for sonorous percussion of the chest. It is not for the abdomen.*

Hoover's Direct Damped Percussion. Direct or immediate percussion is not widely employed in this country. Many writers condemn it without qualification, construing it to mean the forceful striking of the thorax with the full hand, swinging from the elbow or shoulder. The textbooks have completely ignored a method of direct damped percussion developed by Charles F. Hoover and successfully practiced by his students at Western Reserve University [C. F. Hoover: Definitive Percussion and Inspection in Estimating the Size and Contour of the Heart, *J.A.M.A.*, **75:**1626–30, 1920]. The practice has spread by word of mouth, and undoubtedly many physicians use it. There are many variations in detail, so the senior author has described the procedure as learned in Cleveland over 50 years ago.

The fingers and thumb of the right hand are moderately

abducted and rigidly extended (Fig. 6-24B). The hand rests on the chest wall at three points: the hypothenar eminence, the thumb tip, and the tip of the little finger. As a plexor, the long finger in rigid extension strikes the chest wall with its tip, flexing at the metacarpophalangeal joint. The finger retains contact with the chest wall for a short time *to damp* the vibration. One must learn to ignore the slap from striking the skin, and listen for the deeper note from the underlying tissue. The author states that the differences in resistance of the tissues can also be sensed, but I have never consciously learned to do this. The left hand may stretch the tissues at the percussion site or lift a pendulous breast out of the way. For definitive percussion of cardiac and lung borders, Hoover's method is much more accurate than the indirect methods. The procedure is faster and less fatiguing than the bimanual method. Since only one hand is engaged, the other may support a weak patient or hold a struggling child. When facing the patient to percuss his chest, the left hand may percuss the left chest and, alternately, the right hand may be used for the right side. Although not as vigorous as indirect percussion, the ease of Hoover's method also recommends it for light sonorous percussion of the chest; the damped stroke is somewhat inferior for deep sonorous percussion. I have not found the procedure satisfactory for percussion of the abdomen.

PROCEDURE IN THORACIC PERCUSSION. **Ideally, the patient should lie supine on an examining table, with the physician at his right side. After percussion on the front of the chest, the table should be broken so that the patient may sit up, when the borders of the heart are outlined, and both sonorous and definitive percussion are applied to the back. The entire examination can be conducted from the patient's right side, a convenience to the physician. When the patient sits on a stool, the examiner usually sits directly facing him. This position is optimal for examining the back; it is inconvenient for percussing the front with Hoover's damped percussion, and it is decidedly awkward for bimanual percussion. With the patient ill in bed, the examiner usually works from the patient's right side on both the anterior and posterior chest.* If the patient is too ill to**

* Some consider it undignified, discourteous, or unmannerly, for the physician to sit on the patient's bed in making an examination. This etiquette originated in the good old days when the height of hospital beds was designed for the convenience of the physician and

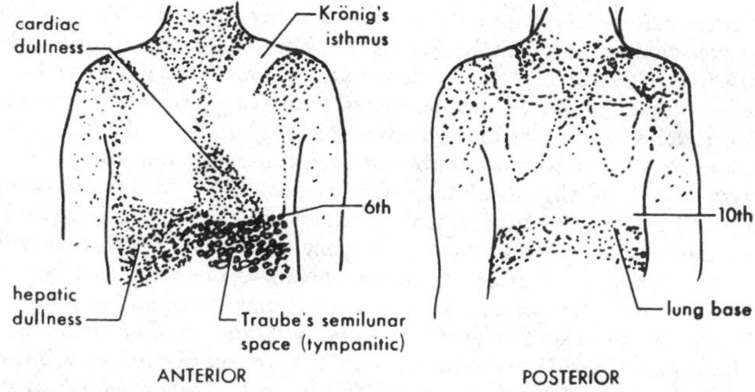

Fig. 6-25. Percussion map of the thorax. *The entire lung surface is normally resonant. At the apices, a band of resonance runs over the shoulders like shoulder straps and is known as Krönig's isthmus. Definite hepatic dullness ranges downward from the level of the right 6th rib to merge into hepatic flatness. Traube's semilunar space of tympany extends downward from the left 6th rib; it is variable in extent, depending upon the amount of gas in the stomach. Posteriorly, the dullness below the lung bases begins at about the 10th rib.*

sit up, he must be examined in the right or left *lateral decubitus*. This position introduces special pitfalls in the interpretation of percussion sounds. Changing the position of the ill patient may prove painful to him and laborious to the attendant, so the examiner may choose to inspect, palpate, percuss, and auscultate the front, then repeat the sequence on the next aspect that is presented on moving.

A routine sequence for thoracic percussion will be described; many other plans are equally good. A physician interrupts his routine whenever a finding is disclosed that needs further search or introduces new problems (Fig. 6-25).

***Percussion of Cardiac Dullness:* Usually, we prefer to do this after inspection and palpation of the precordium, and before examination of the lungs and pleura; many use different sequences. The procedure entails definitive percussion, for which we recommend Hoover's damped stroke. For details of the examination of cardiac borders see p. 346.**

---

the other numerous bedside attendants rather than for the safety of the patient. We challenge the physician with an unstable spine to lean over a low bed, or sit by a modern stainless-steel hospital structure with built-in dependent side rails to block his legs, and make an adequate examination of the chest. Sitting on the bed is a modern necessity.

Percussion of the Anterior Lungs: This procedure calls for sonorous percussion, either with *heavy* indirect bimanual percussion or with the *lighter* stroke of Hoover's direct damped method. When the latter is employed, it may be supplemented with heavy indirect percussion for detailed examination of a suspected region. To make the lateral aspects of the thorax accessible in the supine position, the patient's arms should be slightly abducted; when standing or sitting, his hands should rest on his hips. Starting under the clavicles, compare the percussion sound from each interspace sequentially with that from the contralateral region. Work downward to the region of hepatic dullness on the right and Traube's semilunar space on the left (Fig. 6-25). Percuss also the lateral aspects of the thorax. The entire anterior region should be resonant, except for the area of cardiac dullness.

Percussion of Hepatic Dullness: The domed superior aspect of the liver normally produces a transverse zone of *dullness* from the 4th to the 6th interspaces in the right midclavicular line. Since a wedge of lung, edge downward, intervenes between the upper border of the liver and the chest wall, the transition in the 6th interspace from lung resonance to hepatic dullness is subtle and gradual. The lower border of the dull zone merges into *hepatic flatness* when percussion is carried below the edge of the lung.

Percussion of Gastric Tympany: Normally, the stomach contains an air bubble of variable size that yields tympany in an area known as *Traube's semilunar space*. The upper tympanitic border is somewhat lower than the upper border of the liver on the opposite side, because the left diaphragm is lower. The anterior horn of the halfmoon ends in the lower border of cardiac dullness. The variable volume of air in the stomach vitiates the diagnostic value of this area.

Percussion of Splenic Dullness: The spleen, normal in size and location, is an oval between the 9th and 11th ribs in the left midaxillary line. Frequently, it can be delineated accurately as an area of splenic dullness by its size and shape. But gastric or colonic tympany often obscures it completely. Or, the area of dullness in the region may be greatly enlarged by fluid or solids in the stomach or colon or by pleural effusion. The splenic area is worthy of percussion, however, because an enlarged spleen is seldom obscured by gas, and an increased area of splenic dullness prompts more searching palpation for the organ.

Percussion of the Lung Apices: At this juncture, the patient must be sitting or standing. The apices of the lungs normally extend slightly above the clavicles, producing a band of resonance over each shoulder, widening at its scapular and clavicular ends. The narrowest part, termed *Krönig's isthmus,* lies on the shoulder top, where its normal width is between 4 and 6 cm. Fibrosis or infiltration of the lung narrows or obliterates the isthmus of resonance. We have not been able to percuss the borders with satisfactory accuracy and have given up; many others have also. We merely sound each supraclavicular fossa by modified indirect percussion. For the pleximeter in the left fossa, the examiner's left arm is put around the patient's back, and the *left long finger* is curled anteriorly over the trapezius muscle into the fossa, where it is struck by the plexor finger of the right hand (Fig. 6-26B). For the pleximeter on the right, the examiner's *left thumb* is pressed into the fossa from above (Fig. 6-26A).

Percussion of the Posterior Lungs: This is an exercise in sonorous percussion. The patient is sitting or standing. His arms are folded in front and he is requested to pull his shoulders forward ("hump the shoulders"), with the spine slightly anteflexed. Percussion of each hemithorax is begun at the top, working downward to compare symmetric regions sequentially. The scapular muscles and bones impair resonance in proportion to their mass, so interpretation of percussion notes is difficult. The zone of resonance ends inferiorly at about the 9th rib, the left being lower than the right (Fig. 6-25).

Percussion of the Posterior Lung Bases: During quiet respiration, the inferior lung edges are relatively high in the costophrenic sulci, usually at about the 9th rib on the left and the 8th interspace on

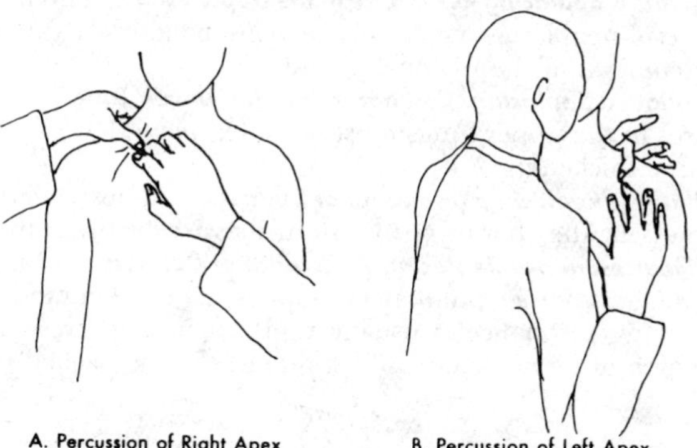

Fig. 6-26. Percussion of the lung apices. *Bimanual indirect percussion is applied in the usual fashion except for the use of the pleximeter. As the examiner faces the patient he uses the left long finger as the pleximeter for the left apex, but he puts his arm around the patient's back and hooks the pleximeter finger over the left supraclavicular fossa from behind. In percussing the right apex, the left thumb is used as a pleximeter. It is applied to the right supraclavicular fossa by sliding it down from the edge of the trapezius muscle.*

the right. The transition between lung resonance and muscle dullness or flatness is gradual over the wedge-shaped lung borders. Light percussion is required; Hoover's direct damped stroke is the better. After the lung bases have been located during quiet respiration, mark the level, have the patient inspire deeply and hold the breath, while you percuss the level after descent. Normally, the bases should move downward 5 or 6 cm.

Dullness in the Lateral Decubitus. When the patient cannot sit up in bed, the best compromise is frequently to percuss the back while the patient lies on one side or the other. Decidedly, the position is not optimal because it is difficult to interpret the percussion sounds. The damping effect of the mattress causes a band of dullness in the part of the thorax nearest the bed (Fig. 6-27). Directly above this band is an irregular area of dullness caused by compression of the downward lung by the body weight. The lengthwise sag of the mattress from the body weight flexes the spine laterally to compress the thoracic wall and underlying lung on the upward hemithorax, yielding another area of dullness.

Dullness Replacing Resonance in the Upper Lung. This finding suggests neoplasm, atelectasis, or consolidation of the lung, or neoplasm of the regional pleura.

Dullness Replacing Resonance in the Lower Lung. To the causes in the upper lungs must be added pleural effusion and pleural thickening.

Flatness Replacing Resonance or Dullness. Almost invariably, flatness in the thorax results from massive pleural effusion.

Hyperresonance Replacing Resonance or Dullness. This finding suggests either pulmonary emphysema or pneumothorax. The lung resonance is usually replaced by hyperresonance; the area of hepatic and cardiac dullness is encroached upon.

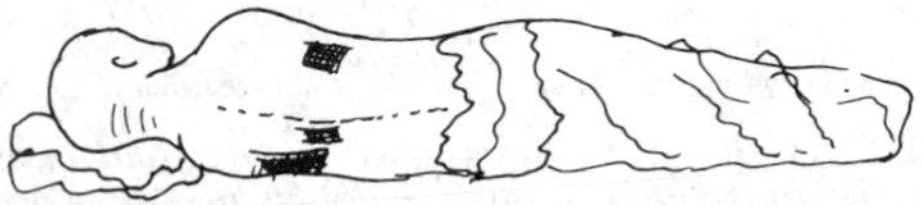

Fig. 6-27. Areas of dullness created by the lateral decubitus position. *The lowest cross-hatched area is dull from compression of the thorax against the mattress. Immediately above, dullness is produced by compression of the lung from the body weight. In the opposite lung, dullness results by lateral deviation of the spine as it follows the sag in the mattress and compresses the lung.*

Tympany Replacing Resonance. This occurs practically only with a large pneumothorax.

Use of the Stethoscope

The stethoscope is an instrument that conveys a vibrating column of air from the body wall to the ears. Binaural models are commonly used in the United States; reception of sound in two ears results in greater transmission of intensity than when a single ear perceives. The usual stethoscope does not amplify sound; it merely assists in excluding extraneous noises, but the instrument invariably modifies the sound to a greater or lesser degree. Sounds from the lungs and heart have a frequency range between 60 and 3000 cycles per second. [For detailed information on the physics of the instrument, the reader should consult M. B. Rapport and H. B. Sprague: Physiologic and Physical Laaws That Govern Auscultation and Their Clinical Application, *Am. Heart J.*, **21**:257, 1941.]

The binaural instrument consists of a chestpiece, rubber or plastic tubes, and two earpieces held in the ears by a connecting spring. Two types of chestpiece are indispensable, each receiving a different range of sound pitch. The *bellpiece* (Ford model) is a hollow cone with a rim of hard rubber or plastic as a base. At the conical apex are hollow metal connecting tubes for either one or two segments of tubing. The bellpiece transmits *all* sounds from the chest, but the *low-pitched* sounds come through particularly well. The low-pitched murmur of mitral stenosis and the fetal heart sounds may be audible only with this pickup. The diameter of the bell's meatus has acoustic qualities—the wider the opening, the lower the pitch of sounds permitted transmission. The *Bowles chestpiece* is a flat cup covered with a semirigid diaphragm of Bakelite that serves as a filter to exclude low-pitched sounds, so the isolated *high-pitched* sounds seem amplified. The Bowles piece should be considered a special-purpose device for high-pitched sounds from the heart, such as regurgitant aortic murmurs; breath sounds are also well heard. The material of the diaphragm is acoustically important; x-ray film or other improvised substitutes are not as satisfactory as Bakelite or other special plastics now furnished. Cracks in the diaphragm impair its properties. The Sprague chestpiece (Fig. 6-28) is now a popular and convenient

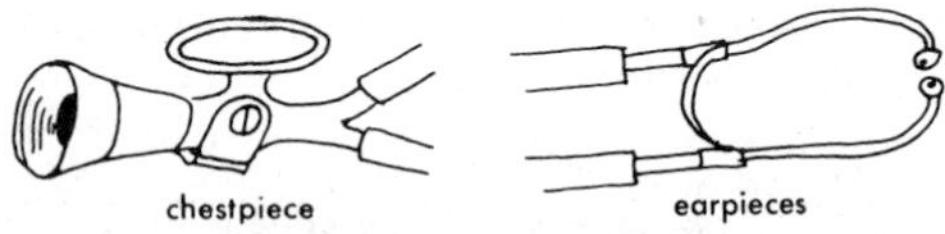

Fig. 6-28. The Sprague stethoscope. *The chestpiece combines the bell and diaphragm receiver, with a valve to direct the air through either. The earpieces are connected by a spring that holds them in place.*

combination of the bell and diaphragm types with a valve that can shunt the air column from one to the other.

The soft *rubber tubing* should be thick-walled; its inside diameter should not be smaller than the caliber of the connecting tubes. For optimal acoustics, the length of the rubber tubing should not exceed 30 cm, but many physicians compromise for a greater and more convenient length.

Of prime importance, the stethoscope should *fit the user's ears.* The plastic or rubber earpieces should impinge upon the external auditory meati without discomfort or pain, yet they should fit tightly to permit no air leakage.

More art than meets the eye is required to use the stethoscope. The diaphragm should be pressed *tightly* against the chest wall in contrast, the rim of the bell should touch the chest wall *lightly,* but completely. Heavy pressure with the bell stretches the underlying skin over the bell's circumference so the skin becomes a diaphragm excluding low-pitched sounds. The entire rim of the bell must touch the skin, otherwise a *roaring sound* from extraneous noise warns the examiner of a leak. At first use, the listener is distracted by extraneous noises coming through the walls of the tubing; he soon learns to ignore these completely. The breath of the examiner on the tubing produces noise; try this, so the sound may be recognized and eliminated. Rubbing of the skin or hair with the chestpiece produces sounds like rales. Wet the hair, or place a soft rubber rim on the bell. Movements of muscles, joints, or tendons sound like friction rubs; be certain that you can recognize them so they can be eliminated. If you do not hear the expected sounds with the first attempt, do not discredit your instrument; your ears are probably normal and the stethoscope satisfactory, but you need *practice.* Use the bell for narrow spaces like the supraclavicular fossae. Thin-walled chests present difficulties in fitting the chestpiece into the interspaces without leakage; remove the broad rim of the bellpiece and use the exposed narrower part of the cone to fit. Examine the instrument occasionally to ensure that it has no leaks or plugs of cerumen or other debris [read Oliver Wendell Holmes' "Song of the Stethoscope"].

Auscultation of the Lungs and Pleura

The movements of the bronchotracheal air column produce vibrations that may be perceived as sounds. Vibrations may occur from air eddies in quiet breathing through normal airways, from air moving in dilated or constricted tubes, from the behavior of fluid moved by the air, from the interruptions of the air column from movement of the vocal cords. The absence of the sounds normally produced by the bronchotracheal air column indicates blockage in the airways or an abnormal screening of sound in the pleural cavity.

Breath Sounds

Several types of breath sounds produce distinctive qualities. All are characterized by rising pitch during inspiration, falling

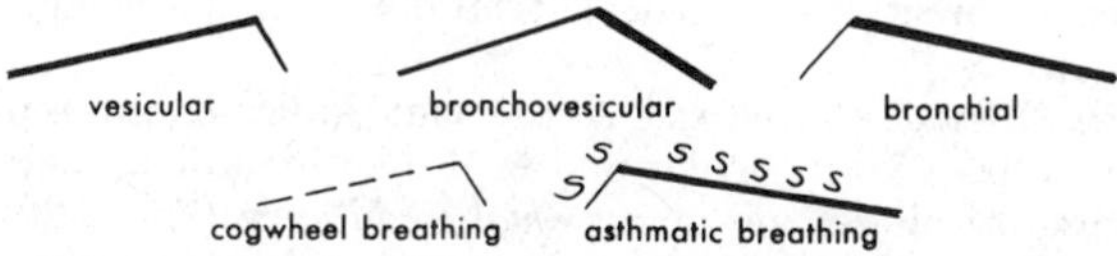

Fig. 6-29. Distinguishing features of breath sounds. *In the diagrams, the vertical component indicates rising and falling pitch. The thickness of the lines indicates loudness. The horizontal distance represents duration. Inspiration is longer in vesicular breathing; expiration in bronchial breathing. Bronchovesicular breathing is a mixture of the two. Normally vesicular breathing is heard over most of the lungs, except that bronchovesicular breathing occurs over the thoracic portion of the trachea, anteriorly and posteriorly. Bronchial breathing does not occur in the normal lung. In cogwheel breathing the inspiratory sound is interrupted with multiple breaks. Asthmatic breathing is characterized by a much prolonged and higher-pitched expiratory sound than is found in bronchial breathing. Asthmatic breathing is usually, but not always, accompanied by sibilant and sonorous rales.*

pitch during expiration. *Duration* of the two phases of respiration is the distinguishing feature of the various breath sounds. The longer the phase, the louder the sound in that phase.

Vesicular Breathing. The shallow breathing during quiet respiration produces a whishing noise that can be heard over the surface of the lungs. Vesicular breath sounds are characterized by having a *long inspiratory phase* and a *short expiratory phase* (Fig. 6-29). They are heard normally over the entire lung surface, except beneath the manubrium sterni and in the upper interscapular region, where they are replaced by bronchovesicular breathing. The breath sounds are faintest over the thinner portions of the lungs.

Bronchial Breathing (Tubular Breathing). In direct contrast to vesicular breathing, bronchial breath sounds have a *short inspiratory phase* and a *long expiratory phase* (Fig. 6-29). They are usually louder, but not always; intensity should not be relied upon to distinguish. Bronchial breathing does not occur in the normal lung; it results from consolidation or compression of pulmonary tissue that facilitates transmission of sound from the bronchial tree. The closest normal counterpart is *tracheal breathing,* heard in the suprasternal notch and over the 6th and 7th cervical spines; but it is harsher and more hollow than true bronchial breathing. Tracheal breathing has no pathologic significance.

Bronchovesicular Breathing. As the name indicates, this is intermediate between vesicular and bronchial breathing. The two respiratory phases are about *equal in duration* (Fig. 6-29), although expiration is frequently a bit longer. Normally, it is heard at the manubrium sterni and in the upper interscapular region. In other parts of the lung, bronchovesicular breathing is *pathologic* and indicates a small degree of pulmonary consolidation or compression that transmits sounds from the bronchial tree with increased facility. As the degree of compression or consolidation increases, bronchovesicular breathing is converted to bronchial breathing.

Asthmatic Breathing. Like bronchial breathing, *inspiration is short, expiration prolonged,* but despite this description, there is no confusing the two (Fig. 6-29). In asthma the expiratory phase is several times longer than in bronchial breathing, and the pitch is much higher. The listener is impressed with the great effort of expelling the air. Frequently, but not always, asthmatic breathing is accompanied by musical rales.

Amphoric Breathing. The Latin word for jug is *amphora.* Amphoric breath sounds have the quality generated by blowing air over the mouth of a bottle. In the lungs, this sound is produced by a large empty superficial cavity that communicates with a bronchus or an open pneumothorax. When the pitch is relatively low and the sound hollow, it is called *cavernous breathing* with the same pathologic significance.

Cogwheel Breathing. This is identical with vesicular breathing, except that the inspiratory phase is *broken by short pauses,* giving the impression of jerkiness (Fig. 6-29). The pauses are attributed to irregular inflation of the alveoli; it has no pathologic significance.

Metamorphosing Breathing. The breath sounds suddenly change in intensity in different parts of the cycle. This is usually caused by movement of a loose bronchial plug.

Voice Sounds

Because of their pitch and loudness, whispered and spoken voice sounds are somewhat more valuable than breath sounds in detecting pulmonary consolidation, infarction, and atelectasis. In the normal lungs, whispered test words are faint and their syllables are not distinct, except over the main bronchi. Increases in loudness and distinctness have pathologic significance. Spoken voice sounds are not quite so satisfactory as whispered sounds because they are too loud for careful distinction.

Whispered Pectoriloquy. Pulmonary consolidation transmits whispered syllables distinctly, even when the pathologic process is too small to produce bronchial breathing. Particularly valuable is the sign in detecting early pneumonia, infarction, and pulmonary atelectasis.

Bronchophony. Normally, the spoken syllables are indistinctly heard in the lungs. In the presence of pulmonary consolidation, syllables are heard distinctly and sound very close to the ear.

Egophony. This is a form of bronchophony in which the spoken syllables have a peculiar nasal or bleating quality. Often the tone quality is imparted by compressed lung below a pleural effusion, although it occasionally is heard in pulmonary consolidation.

Adventitious Sounds

Sounds in the lungs that are not modifications of breath or voice are termed adventitious sounds. Their origins are various, as will be described.

Rales. This word, pronounced "rahls," refers to sounds in the lungs from the movement of fluid or exudate in the airways or from the passage of air through constricted tubes. Rales may disappear on breathing deeply or coughing. When they are induced by coughing, they are *posttussive rales;* the patient is requested to expire and cough at the end of expiration. The qualitative names for rales are myriad and their classifications chaotic, scarcely worth the effort. We prefer the relatively simple designations of Cabot and Adams. There are two chief categories: *moist rales* from relatively thin secretions in the airways, and *dry rales* (a misnomer) produced by thick secretions or the vibrations of membranes. **Moist Rales.** *Coarse rales* or *rhonchi* or *gurgling rales* occur in the larger bronchi. They gurgle and usually occur in the moribund patient, too weak to clear fluid from the larger airways. Moist *medium* or *crepitant rales* arise from relatively thin fluid moving in the bronchi or bronchioles; they sound like clicks or small bubbles and occur in bronchitis, pneumonic consolidation, infarction, the cavities of lung abscesses and bronchiectasis, and tuberculosis. Moist *fine, crackling,* or *subcrepitant* rales are supposed to arise from fluid in the alveoli; their sound is imitated by rubbing several hairs between the thumb and forefinger; their significance is the same as for crepitant rales. Since rubbing the stethoscope on the chest hair produces the same sound, the hair must be wetted or the chestpiece rimmed with soft rubber. **Dry Rales.** These are produced by the movements of thick exudate or the vibration of inflamed or edematous membranes; if high-pitched, they are *musical rales;* if low-pitched, they are termed *sonorous rales.* Commonly, they are heard in asthma or pulmonary edema; their quality is distinctive. A dry coarse rale is called a *rhonchus.*

Inspiratory Crackles (Rales, Crepitations, Moist Sounds.) Views based upon research have been stated in an editorial [Inspiratory Crackles, *Lancet,* **1**:969–70, 1974]. The term *rales* is discarded in favor of the more descriptive *inspiratory crackles.* Workers are now agreed that the crackles are "miniature explosions which occur when previously closed airways open suddenly, allowing pressure upstream and downstream to equalise." The former concept that the sounds arose from fluid in the airways is rejected. Nath and Capel demonstrate that a clinically important fact is whether the crackles appear *early* or *late* in inspiration. *Early Inspiratory Crackles.* These sounds are conducted to the mouth; they are not altered by coughing. They are caused by delayed elastic recoil that allows the airways to shut during expiration. They are encountered in conditions where the airways are seriously obstructed: chronic bronchitis, emphysema, asthma. *Late Inspiratory Crackles.* These noises are not conducted to the mouth; they are dependent on gravity, so they are found at the bases of the lungs. They are heard when lung compliance is reduced and elastic recoil is augmented, as in fibrosing alveolitis, pulmonary sarcoid, scleroderma, congestive cardiac failure.

Audible Pleural Friction Rub. Inflammation of the pleura may result in loss of lubricating fluid so the apposing pleural surfaces rub together producing a sound similar to that from rubbing two dry pieces of leather together. The sound may also be imitated by firmly rubbing the thumb against the forefinger near the ear. A friction rub is frequently mistaken for rales until the characteristic quality is recognized. The rub may be constant, lasting for only a few respiratory movements, then disappearing for a while.

Special Sounds in Hydropneumothorax. Movement of fluid is noiseless in a cavity devoid of air. When the cavity contains *both* air and fluid, body movements cause a *succussion splash,* audible to the patient and the examiner. Such a splash is normally present in the stomach or bowel; pathologically, it occurs in hydropneumothorax where its presence is diagnostic. To elicit, the physician grasps the patient's shoulders and shakes the thorax while listening with or without a stethoscope. A fluid-filled stomach protruding into the thorax through a diaphragmatic hernia may also produce the splash. Hippocrates described the sign, but the physician should hesitate to shake a very ill patient in doing homage to the Father of Medicine. Occasionally, one hears a *falling-drop sound* resembling a drop of water hitting the surface of fluid; this has been attributed to the obvious, but it is occasionally encountered in the collapsed lung. A *metallic tinkle* may be heard when air bubbles emerge through a small bronchopleural fistula below the fluid level;

when the fistula is larger, the air may gurgle to cause a *lung-fistula sound.*

Bone Crepitus. The movements of fractured ends of a rib may produce a grating sound, leading to a correct diagnosis.

Systolic Popping, Clicking, or Crunching Sounds. Such sounds may be heard near the heart in *mediastinal emphysema.* Often the sign first suggests the diagnosis. The air bubbles may invade the tissues of the neck and produce subcutaneous crepitus.

Bruit in the Lungs. A rare finding is a *continuous bruit* from an arteriovenous fistula of pulmonary vessels. The intensity of the murmur is *increased with inspiration,* diminished with expiration. Usually the condition is associated with hereditary hemorrhagic telangiectasia. An abnormal but undiagnostic shadow may be seen in the x-ray films of the chest; arteriography is diagnostic.

PROCEDURE IN AUSCULTATION OF THE LUNGS AND PLEURA. **Seek a quiet place. The room should be warm to eliminate shivering as a cause of muscle sounds. Have the patient sitting or supine. When recumbent, the back should be examined by turning from side to side. The Bowles chestpiece is convenient to slip between the bed and the chest wall. Demonstrate to the patient how you wish him to *breathe through the mouth,* deeper and more forcefully than usual. Some normal persons cannot cooperate; when their attention is called to their respiration, they heave and puff irregularly, making noises with their mouths. Some actually induce hyperventilation tetany. Make certain that the patient is actually breathing deeply, rather than making prodigious movements of the chest without exchanging much air. Start listening with the stethoscope anteriorly at the apices and work downward, comparing symmetric points sequentially. Then listen to the back, starting at the apices and working downward. Inferiorly, note where the breath sounds disappear; compare these sites with those determined by vocal fremitus and percussion, to decide where the lung bases lie.**

At all points on the chest, *identify the breath sounds,* whether vesicular, bronchovesicular, bronchial, asthmatic, cavernous, or absent, by their duration of inspiration and expiration, their quality and pitch (Fig. 6-30). If spontaneous rales are heard, note whether they persist or disappear after a few deep breaths. If rales are *not* heard, test for *posttussive rales* by listening while the patient coughs at the end of expiration. Then, go over the front and back again, while the patient whispers test words, such as "one-two-three" or "ninety-nine," to determine the absence or the presence of *whispered pectoriloquy.* Test similarly with the *spoken voice for bronchophony.* Listen

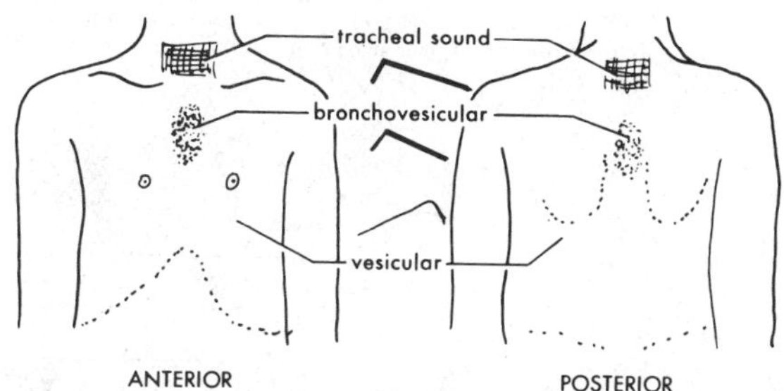

Fig. 6-30. Map of breath sounds in the normal chest. *The areas of the lungs that are unlabeled yield normal vesicular breathing.*

for friction rubs, bone crepitus, and other special sounds. Either before or after examination of the lungs, auscultate the heart (see pp. 349, 375, 377).

Interpretation of Pulmonary and Pleural Findings

The findings disclosed by inspection, palpation, percussion, and auscultation of the lungs and pleura may now be synthesized to attain a certain level of diagnosis. Frequently, the signs of altered density serve as a starting point for the differential diagnosis, so the subject will be presented in terms of altered density and the transmission of vibrations to the periphery.

Dullness and Diminished Vibrations: ***Small Pleural Effusion*** (Fig. 6-31). Unless the fluid is loculated, dullness always occurs in the lowermost part of the thorax. The dull region is a transverse band, broadest posteriorly and laterally because the costophrenic sulcus is higher in front. The superior border of the dullness may be difficult to percuss accurately because the fluid layer is an upward-pointing wedge. Shifting dullness is not usually demonstrable. Since air is absent, there is no succussion splash. With a small amount of fluid, the respiratory excursions of the thorax are normal. In pleurisy, an antecedent friction rub disappears when fluid forms. Pleural fluid baffles vibrations from the bronchotracheal column of air, so vocal fremitus, breath sounds, whispered and spoken voice are transmitted poorly to the stethoscope. The mediastinum is not shifted with small pleural effusions. *Distinction.* Unless the fluid has recently appeared, the signs cannot be distinguished from thickened pleura, except by diagnostic thoracentesis. X-ray

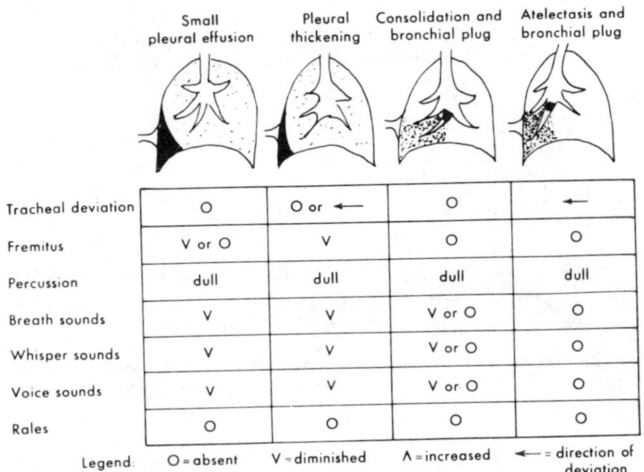

	Small pleural effusion	Pleural thickening	Consolidation and bronchial plug	Atelectasis and bronchial plug
Tracheal deviation	O	O or ←	O	←
Fremitus	V or O	V	O	O
Percussion	dull	dull	dull	dull
Breath sounds	V	V	V or O	O
Whisper sounds	V	V	V or O	O
Voice sounds	V	V	V or O	O
Rales	O	O	O	O

Legend: O = absent V = diminished Λ = increased ← = direction of deviation

Fig. 6-31. Thoracic disorders with dullness and diminished vibration.

films frequently disclose small amounts of pleural fluid undetected by physical examination. The radiologist cannot always distinguish between effusion and thickening, but the fluid can usually be seen to shift with changes of position. ***Definition.*** During the physical examination, any liquid in the pleural cavity is referred to as "fluid." Later, diagnostic thoracentesis reveals the liquid to be pus (pyothorax or empyema thoracis), blood (hemothorax), chyle (chylothorax), or a yellow fluid (the same word, but a different sense) that further testing discloses to be a transudate or an exudate.

▼ *Key Sign:* ***Pleural Fluid (Hydrothorax)*** (Fig. 6-32). The pleural fluid produces a dull or flat note to percussion; the lung immediately over the fluid may be hyperresonant (skodaic resonance) from distention of the alveoli above a compressed region. The distribution of dullness is typical of fluid. The trachea may be pushed to the unaffected side. Vocal fremitus is absent. Occasionally, loud bronchial breathing is heard through the fluid from the compressed lung; the unwary mistake it for consolidation. Even when breath sounds are inaudible through the stethoscope, direct auscultation, with the unaided ear laid directly to the chest wall, will reveal faint

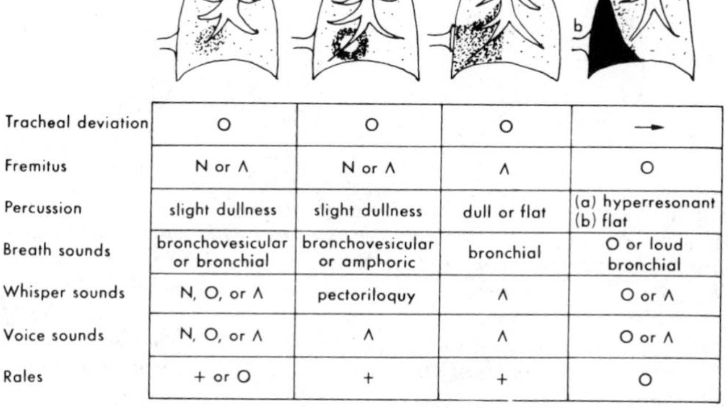

	Small consolidation	Thick-walled cavity	Massive consolidation	Large pleural effusion
Tracheal deviation	O	O	O	→
Fremitus	N or Λ	N or Λ	Λ	O
Percussion	slight dullness	slight dullness	dull or flat	(a) hyperresonant (b) flat
Breath sounds	bronchovesicular or bronchial	bronchovesicular or amphoric	bronchial	O or loud bronchial
Whisper sounds	N, O, or Λ	pectoriloquy	Λ	O or Λ
Voice sounds	N, O, or Λ	Λ	Λ	O or Λ
Rales	+ or O	+	+	O

Legend: O = absent N = normal + = present Λ = increased ← = direction of

Fig. 6-32. Thoracic disorders with dullness and accentuated vibration.

bronchial breathing. ***Distinction.*** Fluid is distinguished from consolidation by displacement of the trachea and, if necessary, by diagnostic thoracentesis. ***Diagnostic Hydropneumothorax.*** Massive pleural effusion obscures the lung fields in the x-ray films, so that no appraisal of the parenchyma is possible. A satisfactory film may be obtained by aspirating some of the fluid and injecting 5 to 100 cc of air into the pleural cavity, producing a hydropneumothorax. When the patient stands, the fluid level falls below much of the lung, permitting its visualization (Fig. 6-33).

During the physical examination any liquid in the pleural cavity is called "fluid." But subsequent thoracentesis reveals the liquid to be clear (*transudate* or *exudate*), purulent (*pyothorax* or *empyema thoracis*), bloody (*hemothorax*), or chylous (*chylothorax*). After gross inspection, the aspirated fluid should be examined by obtaining total and differential leukocyte counts, specific gravity, content of protein and glucose, and bacteriologic cultures. When neoplasm is suspected, a cytologic examination is indicated, although the results are frequently difficult to interpret. A pleural biopsy may be made with a Cope or a Vim-Silverman needle. The biopsy of scalene lymph nodes

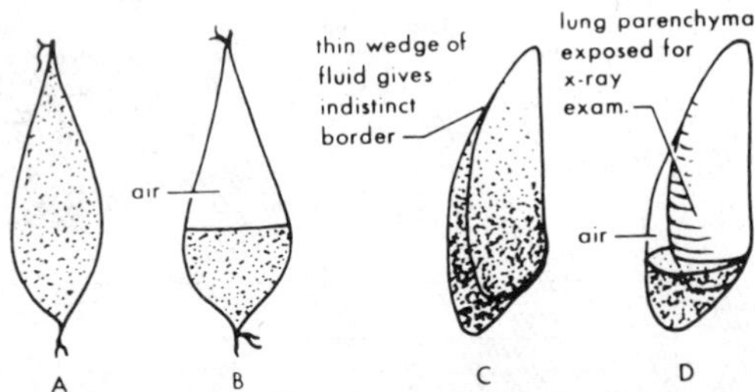

Fig. 6-33. Models illustrating pleural effusion and diagnostic pneumothorax. *In* **A** *is suspended a plastic bag filled with water; note its contour. When air is introduced in* **B,** *a fluid level forms, the contour changes, and a succussion splash occurs with shaking. An uncomplicated pleural effusion is represented in* **C;** *note the upper wedge of water. When air is let in, in* **D,** *the fluid level forms, removing much of the layer overlying the lung, so x-ray examination of the parenchyma is facilitated.*

may provide the necessary evidence. Pleural effusion can often be detected with the M-mode ultrasonogram in the absence of physical findings or roentgenogram indications [F. V. Adams and V. Galati: M-mode Localization of Pleural Effusion. *J.A.M.A.*, **239:**1761–64, 1978].

Clinical Occurrence. TRANSUDATES (clear yellow fluid, specific gravity less than 1.015, protein less than 2.5 gm per 100 mL). Congestive cardiac failure, nephrotic syndrome, portal vein obstruction, benign ovarian fibroma (Meigs' syndrome). When hydrothorax is associated with ascites, leakage of ascitic fluid through diaphragmatic holes lined with endothelium may be the mechanism. Such defects were observed in microscopic sections; the gradient of labeled albumin declined from pleural fluid to thoracic duct lymph; and bubbles of air were observed through the thoracoscope coming from the diaphragm in the presence of pneumoperitoneum [F. L. Lieberman, R. Hidemura, R. L. Peters, and T. B. Reynolds: Pathogenesis and Treatment of Hydrothorax Complicating Cirrhosis with Ascites. *Ann. Intern. Med.*, **64:**341, 1966]. CLEAR EXUDATES (clear yellow fluid, specific gravity more than 1.015, protein more than 2.5 gm per 100 mL). *Predominance of Granulocytes:* bacterial pneumonia, pulmonary infarction, rheumatic fever, rheumatoid arthritis (glucose less than 20 mg per 100 mL), infection with Coxsackie A virus, pulmonary abscess, subphrenic abscess, carcinoma, systemic lupus erythematosus, sclerodema. *Predominance of Lymphocytes:* tuberculosis, fungal infections, myxedema, carcinoma. *Predominance of Eosinophils:* contusions, pulmonary infarction, induced pneumothorax, Hodgkin's disease, echinococcal (hydatid) infection, rheumatoid arthritis, Loeffler's syndrome. CLOUDY EXUDATES (fluids with higher leukocyte counts than clear exudates). Same causes as for clear exudates. BLOOD-TINGED EXUDATES. Carcinoma, benign or malignant mesothelioma of pleura, pulmonary infarction, contusion, hemopneumothorax, tuberculosis, infection with Coxsackie A virus, hemorrhagic pancreatitis, strangulated omentum in diaphragmatic hernia. BROWN EXUDATES (from degenerating erythrocytes). Amebic abscess of liver, old cholesterol effusions. RED BLOOD. Trauma, contusion, hemopneumothorax. MILKY FLUID. *Chylous* (with fat droplets): disruption or obstruction of the thoracic duct. *Pseudochylous* (without fat droplets): empyema (cloudy from leukocytes, cholesterol effusion from tuberculosis or idiopathic) (crystals may be present). RECURRENT BILATERAL EFFUSION: asbestosis. DRUG SENSITIVITY: acute nitrofurantoin reaction; systemic lupus erythematosus, chemotherapeutic drugs, methylsergide [E. C. Rosenow, III: Drug-Induced Lung Disease: Causes and Diagnosis. *Pract. Cardiol.*, **5**:41–51, 1979].

Dullness and Diminished Vibration: ***Thickened Pleura*** (Fig. 6-31). Since pleural fibrosis results from the organization of pleural effusion, the distribution of dullness is the same. The pleura may attain a thickness of 5 or 6 cm. The thicker it is, the more it obstructs air transmission and the more the percussion note indicates denseness. Extensive fibrosis may pull the trachea to the affected side. *Distinction.* Diagnostic thoracentesis is frequently needed to distinguish from pleural effusion, or ultrasonic examination may be conclusive.

Clinical Occurrence. Any long-standing pleural effusion may organize. Neoplastic involvement may stimulate thickening.

Dullness and Diminished Vibration: ***Pulmonary Consolidation with Bronchial Plug*** (Fig. 6-31). The consolidated lung produces dullness. A bronchial plug prevents vibrations of the air column, so there is absence of vocal fremitus, breath sounds, whispered and spoken voice. The trachea is not displaced. *Distinction.* Usually, plugging of a bronchus is a transitory occurrence in lobar pneumonia, so its nature is recognized by the sudden loss of air transmission. X-ray films can usually distinguish between pleural effusion and pulmonary consolidation. If the dullness is in the upper lobe, effusion is excluded on physical examination.

Dullness with Diminished Vibration: ***Atelectasis with Bronchial Plug***

(Fig. 6-31). The volume of the atelectatic lung is diminished; the dense mass is pulled toward the chest wall by the negative intrathoracic pressure, so the trachea shifts to the affected side. The collapsed lung is dull because its density is increased. The bronchial plug prevents air vibration, so vocal fremitus, breath and voice sounds are absent. *Distinction.* The tracheal deviation distinguishes from consolidation with bronchial plug and from pleural effusion. Usually, atelectasis is accompanied by fever that distinguishes it from thickened pleura with fibrotic traction on the mediastinum.

Dullness with Accentuated Vibration: ***Small Consolidation*** (Fig. 6-32). A small deeply placed region of consolidation may produce impaired resonance or dullness, depending on its size and depth from the chest wall. The dense lung transmits the air column with increased facility, so vocal fremitus is increased, bronchovesicular or bronchial breathing is heard. Whispered pectoriloquy and bronchophony are produced by the consolidation. *Distinction.* Small consolidation must be distinguished from a small cavity lying near a bronchus by the amount of purulent sputum produced and the absence of other signs of cavity. X-ray films are usually diagnostic.

> **Clinical Occurrence.** Pneumonia, granulomatous infiltrates of the lung, neoplasm about a bronchus, rheumatoid arthritis, sarcoidosis.

Dullness with Accentuated Vibration: ***Thick-Walled Cavity*** (Fig. 6-32). The signs of pulmonary consolidation are present—dullness, increased vocal fremitus, bronchovesicular breathing, pectoriloquy. Usually distinctive, but most infrequent, is amphoric breathing or cracked-pot resonance. Even these signs may be present in consolidation without cavity. X-ray films usually are diagnostic.

Dullness with Accentuated Vibration: ***Massive Consolidation*** (Fig. 6-32). The dense lung yields dullness or flatness on percussion. The solid mass in contact with a bronchus transmits vibrations with increased facility, so vocal fremitus is pronounced, there is bronchial breathing, whispered and spoken voice produce pectoriloquy and bronchophony. Crepitant and subcrepitant rales are frequently present. The lung volume is unchanged, so the trachea remains in the midline. *Distinction.* Occasionally consolidation may be confused with a thick-walled cavity, and the distinction must be made by x-ray films. Massive pleural effusion gives dullness and may transmit loud bronchial breath sounds, but the trachea is usually displaced to the unaffected side.

Clinical Occurrence. Classically, in lobar pneumonia; occasionally in neoplasma of the lung.

Resonance and Hyperresonance: ***Pulmonary Emphysema*** (Fig. 6-34). Loss of interstitial elasticity and interalveolar septa leads to air trapping, so the volume of the lungs is increased. The augmented volume holds the thoracic walls continuously in the inspiratory position, producing the increased anteroposterior diameter of the barrel chest. The diaphragm is pushed downward so the costal margins move out sluggishly or actually converge during inspiration. The lungs are hyperresonant throughout because of their density. Air pockets are poor transmitters of vibrations, thus vocal fremitus, breath sounds, whispered and spoken voice are impaired or absent. When the breath sounds are audible, they are faint and harsh, lacking the rustling quality of vesicular breathing. This absence of the vesicular quality is distinctive; it may antedate recognizable x-ray evidence of emphysema. Rales are not necessarily present.

THE MATCH TEST OF RESPIRATORY FUNCTION. **In emphysema, the vital capacity is usually, but not always, impaired. A more reliable bedside indicator is the *match test* [T. H. Snider, J. P. Stevens, F. M. Wilner, and B. M. Lewis: Simple Bedside Test of Respiratory Function, *J.A.M.A.,* 170:1631, 1959]. From a standard paper matchbook, detach a match and light it; when it burns steadily, hold it 6 inches (15 cm) from the patient's open mouth.**

Have the patient breathe deeply and then blow through the wide-open mouth to extinguish the match. Caution him not to purse the lips. Of the patients with a maximum breathing capacity of less than 60 liters per minute, 80% failed to extinguish the match. Of those with one-second vital capacity less than 1.6 liters, 85% could not perform the test.

Resonance or Hyperresonance: ***Closed Pneumothorax*** (Fig. 6-34). When the leak between lung and pleura becomes sealed or when air is instilled into the pleural cavity for diagnosis or therapy, a *closed pneumothorax* is formed. If the volume of enclosed air is small, the lung remains partially inflated and the mediasatinum is not displaced. Or in an open pneumothorax, a similar situation may be created by pleural adhesions which

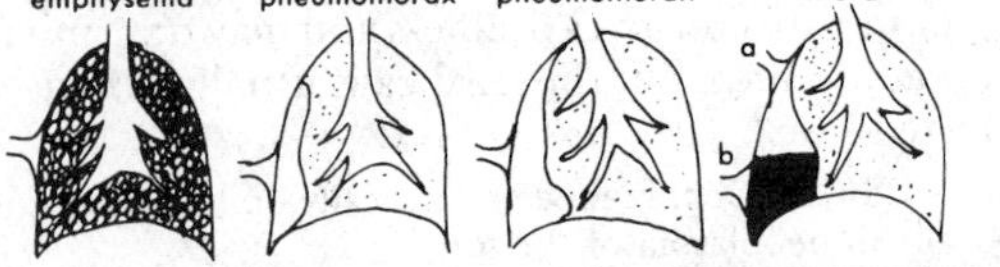

	Pulmonary emphysema	Closed pneumothorax	Open pneumothorax	Hydropneumothorax
Tracheal deviation	O	O	→	→
Fremitus	V	O	O	O
Percussion	hyperresonant	resonant or hyper	hyperresonant	(a) hyperresonant (b) flat
Breath sounds	V or O	V or O	V or O	O
Whisper sounds	V or O	V or O	V or O	O
Voice sounds	V or O	V or O	V or O	O
Rales	+ or O	O	O	O
		coin sound	coin sound	coin sound
				succussion splash
				shifting dullness

Legend: O = absent V = diminished + = present ← = direction of deviation

Fig. 6-34. Thoracic disorders with resonance and impaired vibration.

prevent collapse of the lung and displacement of the trachea. Vocal fremitus, breath sounds, whispered and spoken voice are usually inaudible or impaired. The chest wall is resonant or hyperresonant. *Distinction.* Frequently this cannot be distinguished from a normal or emphysematous chest by percussion. The disparity between the breath sounds on the two sides is the clue that leads to an x-ray film to make the diagnosis. There may be a pendular deviation of the trachea *toward* the affected side during inspiration. A tear in the pleura may be *spontaneous* or the result of *trauma* to the thorax. Very rarely a right-sided pneumothorax recurs with menstrual periods [G. A. Lillington, S. P. Mitchell, and G. A. Wood: Catamenial Pneumothorax, *J.A.M.A.,* **219:**1328–32, 1972].

Resonance or Hyperresonance: ***Open and Tension Pneumothorax*** (Fig. 6-34). With continual communication between lung and pleural cavity, the air in the *open pneumothorax* is under atmospheric pressure. The collapse of the affected lung is complete, and the mediastinum is drawn to the unaffected side by the contraction of the normal lung. Overlying the pneumothorax, the chest wall is hyperresonant or tympanitic. Fremitus, breath and voice sounds are absent. Usually, the patient is severely dyspneic and cyanotic. The physical signs of *tension pneumothorax* resemble those of the open pneumothorax, although the condition is actually a modified closed type. A wound of ingress serves as a valve permitting air to be sucked in during inspiration, preventing loss during expiration. Thus the pressure in the cavity builds up in excess of the atmosphere, causing extreme tracheal deviation and compression of the normal lung. This situation is accompanied by deep cyanosis, severe dyspnea, and shock that demands aspiration of air from the cavity as a lifesaving measure.

Resonance and Hyperresonance: ***Hydropneumothorax*** (Fig. 6-34). Hyperresonance or tympany in the upper part of the thorax, with dullness inferiorly, suggests either hydropneumothorax or a massive pleural effusion. In either case, the trachea is displaced to the unaffected side. In hydropneumothorax, the hyperresonant region does not transmit fremitus, breath or voice sounds, whereas the lung over hydrothorax transmits well. When air is present, the fluid level can be sharply demarcated by percussion, the level is vague in simple effusion. Shifting dullness is readily demonstrated by percussion in the presence of air; this is not the case in hydrothorax. The air-filled cavity carries bell tympany, and a succussion splash may be demonstrated.

Resonance and Dyspnea: ***Asthma.*** Between attacks, the patient is perfectly well and his chest contains no abnormal findings. A paroxysm of asthma frequently begins with an unproductive cough and rapidly progressing dyspnea. The patient rises to a sitting position, frequently leaning over a table or chair back. The facial muscles express anxiety. The respiratory rate does not increase, but expiration becomes prolonged and laborious; wheezing may be heard at a distance. Often sweating is profuse. The previously resonant chest becomes hyperresonant and the lung bases descend. The thorax is held in the inspiratory position; the costal margins diverge but slightly, or they may actually converge during inspiration. In severe paroxysms, the sternocleidomastoid and platysma muscles tense and the alae nasi flare with each expiratory effort. Asthmatic breathing is readily heard: the inspiratory phase is short, the expiration is prolonged greatly. Breathing is accompanied by coarse and musical rales. Localized disappearance of breath sounds can occur temporarily from bronchial plugging. As the attack subsides, clear tenacious sputum is raised, and the breathing gradually becomes less labored. Asthma *can occur* without the distinctive breath sounds. The only sign that consistently identified severe impairment of pulmonary function was *retraction of the sternocleidomastoideus muscle* [E. R. McFallen, Jr., R. Kiser, and W. J. de Groot: Acute Bronchial Asthma. Relation Between Clinical and Physiologic Manifestations, *N. Engl. J. Med.*, **288:**221–25, 1973]. *Distinction.* Although most writers describe this clinical picture as "distinctive," it can be confused with other conditions. The musical rales occur in acute bronchitis without the labored respiration. When "asthmatic" breathing is limited to a single region, bronchial obstruction from foreign body or neoplasm should be suspected. The sudden occurrence of left-sided cardiac failure may closely simulate asthma. In this case, there are musical rales; labored breathing may prevent auscultation of the heart. The symptoms and signs of asthma are often relieved in a few minutes by epinephrine or other bronchodilators. If *circulatory overload* is suspected, immediate distinction *at the bedside* is imperative to save life. Tourniquets have been applied to all four extremities in the past, just tight enough to obstruct venous flow but not eliminate arterial pulses. About 15% of the blood volume can be pooled in the extremities in this manner. This procedure can result in prompt subsidence of the symptoms and signs of circulatory overload, but is seldom used in present day treatment.

Resonance and Dyspnea: **Pulmonary Edema.** Edema of the lungs may be caused by left-sided cardiac failure, pulmonary disease, or injury to pulmonary epithelium by noxious gases. In cardiac failure, the condition is usually chronic and the diagnosis fairly obvious. Occasionally, paroxysmal nocturnal dyspnea in cardiac patients may closely resemble asthma. The onset is sudden with coughing and wheezing. Breathing is labored, with cyanosis and frothy sputum, occasionally bloody. The chest is resonant, but the bronchi are filled with bubbling rales and sometimes musical sounds. *Distinction.* The prolonged expiratory phase may resemble asthma, and the distinction may be made by the response to the injection of epinephrine (see discussion under Asthma).

Clinical Occurrence. CARDIOVASCULAR: mitral stenosis, left-sided cardiac failure, pulmonary embolism, circulatory overload with electrolyte solutions intravenously or blood transfusions. NEUROLOGIC: postictal, head trauma, subarachnoid hemorrhage. INTRAVENOUS NARCOTICS. NOXIOUS GASES. OBSTRUCTION: hanging, suffocation. MISCELLANEOUS: uremia, at high altitudes, systemic lupus erythematosus, snakebite, heroin intoxication.

Resonance and Dyspnea: ***Pulmonary Fibrosis.*** In chronic dyspnea with normal thoracic resonance, the possibility of fibrosis of the lungs must be considered. The breath sounds are faint, the volume and density of the lungs appear normal to physical examination. Rales may be present. X-ray films will disclose evidence of fibrosis.

Clinical Occurrence [this is a collection of ill-defined disorders producing interstitial pneumonitis/fibrosis; many are undoubtedly hypersensitivity reactions to unusual antigens]: cystic fibrosis, allergic alveolitis (farmer's lung or silo-filler's disease), rheumatoid arthritis, Sjögren's syndrome, Hamman-Rich disease, occupational diseases (miner's, bagassois—sugar cane, suberosis—cork dust, sequoiosis—redwood dust, wheat weevil disease—from wheat flour, mushroom workers, malt workers, cheese workers, furrier's disease, coffee workers), ornithosis, diffuse pulmonary carcinoma, disseminated lupus erythematosus, polyarteritis nodosa, sarcoidosis, tuberculosis, fungus infections, drugs (chemotherapeutic agents, corticosteroids, gold, azulfide [drugs cited by E. C. Rosenow, III: Drug-Induced Lung Disease; Causes and Diagnosis, *Pract. Cardiol.*, **5**:44–51, 1979]).

Resonance and Dyspnea: ***Acute Tracheal or Bronchial Obstruction.*** Complete obstruction of the trachea is incompatible with life. Partial obstruction by a foreign body, neoplasm, diphtheritic membrane, or other plug produces violent prolonged inspiratory movements with extreme retraction of the intercostal spaces, suprasternal notch, supraclavicular fossae, and epigastrium. A low-pitched rhonchus, the *asthmatoid wheeze,* may be heard over the chest and at the opened mouth during inspiration and expiration. In a *ball-valve* obstruction, the rhonchus occurs only during inspiration. Another indication of partial bronchial obstruction is the *bagpipe sign:* when the patient is required to cut short a forced expiration while the stethoscope is on the chest, the sound of expelling air is heard *to continue* after his effort has ceased. If the inspiratory rhonchus is audible on both sides of the chest, the affected side is the one with the *palpable rhonchus.* In obstruction of a large bronchus or a large pneumothorax, there is a *pendular movement* of the trachea, moving *toward* the affected side during *inspiration*, away from it with expiration. Movements of a foreign body may cause an *audible slap* with coughing or breathing. Slow development of bronchial obstruction may be symptomless; sudden closure causes severe dyspnea. Higher-pitched rhonchi arise from smaller bronchi.

Resonance and Rales: **Bronchitis.** Secretions in the bronchi and trachea produce rales, usually coarse, occasionally musical. Secretions high in the trachea produce rales that are heard throughout the entire thorax. The cough may be unproductive; tenacious or mucoid sputum may be raised. Usually, there is no impairment of the airways, so breath sounds are normal. Occasionally, asthmatic breathing occurs, disappearing after epinephrine is given. X-ray films show no distinctive findings in bronchitis.

Resonance and Rales: **Bronchiectasis.** In a resonant chest, with rales at the lung bases, bronchiectasis should be considered. The display of copious purulent sputum by coughing or by diagnostic postural drainage practically clinches the diagnosis. Frequently the x-ray film lends little confirmation unless bronchograms are made. The lower left lobe, behind the heart, is particularly inaccessible to x-ray examination, so physical signs are essential. *Diagnostic postural drainage* can be done on the examining table (Fig. 6-35). Have the patient lie prone across the table with the shoulders lowered and resting on the seats of two chairs, so the thorax is sloping downward from the abdomen. Place a pan on the floor in front of the patient's head, and urge the patient to cough several times. Frequently, in bronchiectasis, the pus will roll out and the diagnosis is achieved.

BEDSIDE INSPECTION OF THE SPUTUM. **Inspection of the sputum discloses many valuable diagnostic clues in pulmonary disease. The modern habit of expectorating into pieces of disposable paper tissue seriously interferes with proper examination. Have a paper sputum cup on the bedside stand and order 24-hour collections of sputum, free from chewing gum, matchsticks, chewing tobacco, ashes, cigar and cigarette stubs. Estimate the daily *volume*. Note the *color, turbidity*, and *viscosity*. Ascertain whether it is *bloody, frothy*, or *odoriferous*. Place a sample in a Petri dish to look for caseous masses, Dittrich's plugs, Curschmann's spirals, bronchial casts, and concretions. When-**

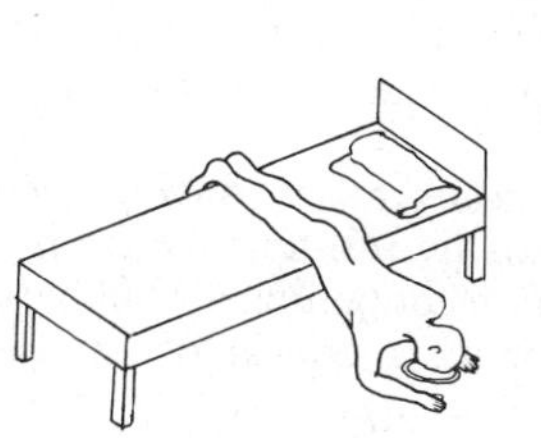

On a bed 24 inches (60 cm) high

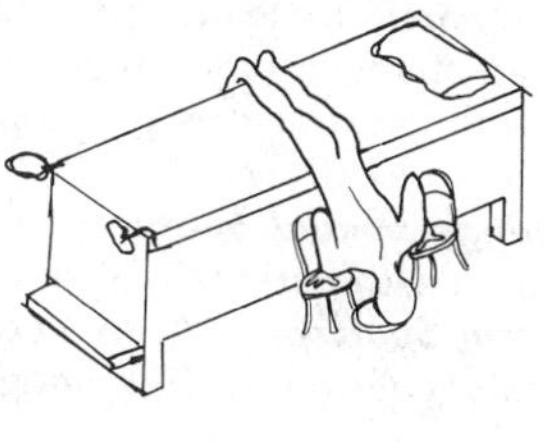

On an examination table 40 inches (100 cm) high

Fig. 6-35. Postural drainage. *The figures indicate two arrangements for postural drainage of a lung abscess or bronchiectasis. The procedure imposes hard work on a patient, so he may need assistance to keep from falling. The entire trunk should be declining cephalad, with the hips flexed so the thighs rest on the horizontal plane of the table. The position should be assumed for 5 to 15 minutes while the patient is urged to cough and expectorate into a basin or upon a newspaper spread upon the floor.*

ever indicated, send specimens to the bacteriologist for culture and other examinations.

Bloody Sputum. Blood in the sputum usually impresses the patient enough to bring him to the physician, and the first problem is to decide the anatomic site of the hemorrhage. *Blood-Streaked Sputum.* This is usually caused by inflammation in the nose, nasopharynx, gums, or larynx. Sometimes it occurs only after severe paroxysms of coughing and may be attributed to trauma. *Pink Sputum.* Usually a result of blood mixing with secretions in the alveoli or smaller bronchioles, it most frequently occurs in pneumonia or pulmonary edema. *Massive Bleeding.* Among the causes are pulmonary tuberculosis, lung abscess, bronchiectasis, pulmonary infarction, pulmonary embolism, bronchogenic carcinoma, and erosion from a broncholith. Not infrequently, frank bleeding from the lungs occurs early in mitral stenosis. Abscesses in pulmonary actinomycosis and blastomycosis may bleed.

Bloody Gelatinous Sputum (Currant-Jelly Sputum). Copious quantities of tenacious bloody sputum are almost pathognomonic for pneumonia caused by *Klebsiella pneumoniae* (Friedländer's bacillus) or type III pneumococcus.

Rusty Sputum (Prune-Juice Sputum). Purulent sputum containing changed blood pigment is typical of the pneumococcal pneumonias, but it is frequently antedated by small amounts of frank blood.

Stringy Mucoid Sputum. Typically raised during recovery from an asthmatic paroxysm, this sputum may be frothy.

Frothy Sputum. A thin secretion containing air bubbles, frequently colored with hemoglobin, is typical of pulmonary edema.

Purulent Sputum. The exudate may be yellow, green, or dirty-gray. *Small Amounts.* This is typical of pneumonia during resolution. It may arise in small tuberculous cavities or from lung abscess. *Large Amounts.* Copious purulent sputum suggests lung abscess, bronchiectasis, bronchopleural fistula. If antibiotics have not been given, the sputum is often fetid. Many lung abscesses do not yield much sputum because their bronchial communications are inadequate for complete drainage. In bronchiectasis, the daily volume is often from 200 to 500 ml. On standing, bronchiectatic sputum typically separates into three layers with mucus on top, separated by clear fluid from pus on the bottom. Copious sputum from a patient with signs of pleural effusion means *bronchopleural fistula.*

Broncholiths. Occasionally, calcified particles are found in the sputum, by either the patient or his physician. These are usually broncholiths, derived from calcified lymph nodes eroding the bronchi or from calcareous granulomas in silicosis or histoplasmosis. Their discovery may explain the source of pulmonary hemorrhage. Some hemorrhages have been fatal [C. S. Lin and W. H. Becker: Broncholith as a Cause of Fatal Hemoptysis, *J.A.M.A.*, **239:**2153, 1978].

Pulmonary Infiltrations: ***Lymphomatoid Granulomatosis.*** This is a disease belonging to the group of necrotizing vasculitides (for classification see p. 466). *Pathophysiology:* a variegated array of lymph cells, atypical lymphocytoid, plasmacytoid, and reticuloendothelial cells invade various tissues and vessels. *Lungs: always involved,* in contrast to Wegener's granulomatosis. Nodules of various sizes occur in the lungs, skin, kidneys, and central nervous system; but *usually spared* are the spleen, lymph nodes, and bone marrow. In contrast with Wegener's granuloma, the upper respiratory tract is seldom involved. *Prognosis and Therapeutic Response:* rapidly progressive to death; but long-time remissions obtained with corticosteroids plus cyclophosphamide.

The Heart

Functionally, the circulation includes the heart, the blood and its conducting vessels, the lymph and its ducts, and the cell walls; a system that pervades the entire body. But practical clinical diagnosis necessitates separate categories based upon convenience; for example, the facts of the cardiovascular system are mostly elicited by physical examination, but the examination of the blood is performed in the laboratory. In the procedures of physical examination, convenience dictates an assessment of the body by anatomic regions, so the heart and blood vessels are tested sequentially. Vascular phenomena are further divided into those dependent upon cardiac action and those caused by local disorders of blood vessels. The examination of the cardiovascular system is presented here in much the same sequence as the physician finds convenient in the search for a diagnosis.

A complete cardiac examination includes history taking, physical examination, and supplementary procedures that seem indicated, such as electrocardiography, fluoroscopy, phonocardiography, cardiac catheterization, and aortography. Although special emphasis is directed to the precordium in the physical examination, the entire body must be carefully examined for the remote effects of cardiac dysfunction.

Fourfold Diagnosis Required for Heart Disease

A proper assessment of the patient with heart disease necessitates a diagnosis that includes four categories: the etiology, the anatomic abnormalities, the physiologic disorders, and the functional cardiac capacity. The formal statement of such a diagnosis should follow this example: "rheumatic heart disease, inactive (= etiologic); mitral stenosis, right ventricular hypertrophy, dilatation, pulmonary congestion (= anatomic); atrial fibrillation (= physiologic); functional class II, dyspnea with moderate exertion (= functional capacity)." The categoric descriptions conform to the standards commonly accepted in the U.S. [Criteria Committee of the New York Heart Association: *Diseases of the Heart and Blood Vessels—Nomenclature and Criteria for Diagnosis*, 6th ed. Little, Brown & Co., Boston, 1964].

1. Etiologic Cardiac Diagnosis. Congenital defects. Infections. Rheumatic fever. *Vascular:* essential hypertension, atherosclerosis, systemic lupus erythematosus. *Renal:* hypertension from renal ischemia, uremia. *Hematologic:* anemia. *Endocrine:* acromegaly, hyperthyroidism, hypothyroidism. *Neoplastic:* carcinoid, tumors of the heart. *Metal poisoning:* iron, cobalt. Fibroelastosis.

Making the Etiologic Diagnosis. In some cases the cause may be diagnosed from the history of antecedent disease (rheumatic fever) or the duration of symptoms (congenital). More frequently, the anatomic disorder points to the etiology (syphilitic aortic regurgitation, rheumatic mitral stenosis, congenital patency of the ductus arteriosus). The manifestations of concomitant disease often explain the cardiac disorder (anemia, endocrine disorders, hypertension). Thus the anatomic diagnosis frequently leads directly to an inference of causation.

2. Anatomic Cardiac Diagnosis: Acquired Disease. *Aorta and pulmonary arteries:* aneurysm, aortitis, arteriosclerosis, dissecting aneurysm, embolism, thrombosis, injury, rupture of aorta. *Coronary arteries:* arteritis, atherosclerosis, embolism, thrombosis. *Endocardium and valves:* endocardial fibroelastosis, bacterial or indeterminant endocarditis, mural endocarditis, mural thrombosis, endocardial neoplasm (myxoma), rupture of valves or chordae tendineae, valvular deformities (stenosis, prolapse, or regurgitation), valvular sclerosis, active valvulitis. *Myocardium:* aneurysm, cardiac dilatation and hypertrophy, fibrosis, infarction, myocarditis, neoplasm, rupture, thrombus in cardiac chamber, trauma, infarction. *Pericardium:* calcification, hemopericardium, hydropericardium, pneumopericardium, neoplasm, pericarditis. ***Congenital Disease.*** *Noncyanotic group:* Examples include uncomplicated left to right shunt lesions, such as atrial and ventricular septal defects and patent ductus arteriosus; congenital aortic and pulmonary valvular stenosis, coarctation of the aorta, vascular rings, corrected transposition of the great vessels, anomalous coronary artery. *Cyanotic group:* Tetralogy of Fallot, tricuspid atresia, transposition of the great vessels, total anomalous pulmonary venous return, truncus arteriosus, single atrium, single ventricle. *Potentially cyanotic groups:* examples include intracardiac communications associated with occlusive hypertensive pulmonary vascular disease, Ebstein's anomaly (downward displacement of the tricuspid valve).

Making the Anatomic Diagnosis. The assessment of anatomic abnormalities rests heavily upon the physical examination. The signs usually yield sufficient information to diagnose acquired abnormalities of single valves, patent ductus arteriosus, and some septal defects; fluoroscopic examination may be partially confirmatory; the ECG assists but little. Cardiac dilatation and hypertrophy may be diagnosed by the physical examination in many cases; cardiac enlargement is evident in the x-ray films, and hypertrophy occasionally is revealed by the ECG findings. But many congenital anomalies of valves and vessels are too complicated to be distinguished by physical examination alone; they require cardiac catheterization or specialized imaging procedures, such as echocardiography. Pain is frequently the key symptom in the diagnosis of myocardial ischemia and infarction, pericarditis, and myocarditis; the symptoms are supplemented by serial changes in the ECG.

3. Physiologic Cardiac Diagnosis: *Disturbances in Cardiac Rhythm and Conduction.* Premature beats, atrial fibrillation or flutter, paroxysmal atrial tachycardia, junctional (AV nodal) rhythms, intraventricular conduction delays, ventricular tachycardia, atrioventricular (AV) block, ventricular fibrillation, Wolff-Parkinson-White syndrome. *Disturbances in Myocardial Contractility.* Cardiac insufficiency (cardiac failure), valve annulus incompetency, gallop rhythm, pulsus alternans, pulmonary hypertension. *Clinical Syndrome.* Anginal syndrome, carotid-sinus syndrome, Wolff-Parkinson-White syndrome, cyanotic crisis, cardiac tamponade, intracardiac ball-valve obstruction.

Making the Physiologic Diagnosis. Many disturbances of cardiac rhythm can be diagnosed by their physical signs and confirmed by the ECG; but some conduction defects require the ECG. Most disorders of myocardial contractility have distinguishing physical signs. Of the clinical syndromes, all can be detected by the history or physical examination, except the Wolff-Parkinson-White syndrome, which requires ECG confirmation.

4. Functional Cardiac Diagnosis: *Class I (no incapacity).* Although the patient has heart disease, the functional capacity is not sufficiently impaired to produce symptoms. *Class II (slight limitation).* The patient is comfortable at rest and with mild exertion. Symptoms occur only with more strenuous activity. *Class III (incapacity with slight exertion).* The patient is comfortable at rest but dyspnea, fatigue, palpitation, or angina appears with slight exertion. *Class IV (incapacity with rest).* The slightest exertion invariably produces symptoms, and symptoms frequently occur at rest.

Making the Functional Cardiac Diagnosis. The requisite information can be obtained from the history, or from actual observation of the patient.

Therapeutic Classification. To a statement of the functional class, a letter may be appended to indicate the physician's prescription for limitation of activity. CLASS A. No restriction of activity. CLASS B. Restriction of severe activity. CLASS C. Restriction of moderate activity. CLASS D. Sharp restriction of ordinary activity. CLASS E. Restriction to complete rest in a chair or bed.

Diagnosis of Cardiac Failure

Acute Pulmonary Edema (Acute Left-Ventricular Failure). *Paroxysmal Dyspnea (Cardiac Asthma).* This is characterized by sudden seizures of breathlessness. When sleep is interrupted, it is termed *paroxysmal nocturnal dyspnea.* These mild attacks are attended by *orthopnea* and *coughing, rales* in the *lung bases.* The rales are coarse rhonchi or wheezes and gurgles. The patient often finds that walking a few minutes relieves the dyspnea, permitting him to resume sleep. Such an episode can be distinguished from true asthma by finding that the lungs do not clear when he inhales a bronchodilator. *Generalized Acute Pulmonary Edema.* This is a more severe and dangerous degree in which *intense dyspnea* and *cyanosis* are accompanied by rhonchi and gurgles *throughout* the lungs. The discomfort intensifies, and he coughs copious *frothy blood-tinged sputum.* Sudden death may ensue. *Pathophysiology.* When produced by circulatory disorders, the condition is termed *left-ventricular failure.* It may occur from a sudden *decrease in myocardial function* accompanied by rising left ventricular filling pressures resulting from infarction, ectopic tachycardia, hypertension, or myocarditis. More commonly, the cause is *increased filling load* from augmentation of the blood volume in assuming the horizontal position, or hypervolemia from the intravenous administration of crystalloid or colloidal solution or blood transfusion. Whether by increased load or decreased myocardial contractility, the left ventricle cannot maintain a normal left ventricular end-diastolic pressure. The pulmonary capillaries become engorged, so plasma or water passes from their lumens into the alveoli to impair the ingress of oxygen.

Clinical Occurrence. Paroxysmal dyspnea is more likely to occur in hypertension, aortic valvular disorders, or coronary artery disease. Generalized pulmonary edema may occur from myocardial infarction, ectopic tachycardia, or circulatory overload with parenteral fluid administration. The noncardiac conditions producing pulmonary edema are nephritis, the inhalation of noxious gases, and the hypoxia of high altitudes.

Chronic Congestive Cardiac Failure. Usually this starts as left-ventricular failure that produces pulmonary congestion with *dyspnea, orthopnea,* and *cough. Nocturia* is often an early symptom. Medium or coarse *rales* are heard in the lung bases. The congestion extends backward to cause right-ventricular failure with elevated venous pressure, indicated by *engorged jugular veins.* Even before the increase in venous pressure, a *hepatojugular reflux* can be demonstrated. Frequently a *protodiastolic gallop* (S_3) *rhythm* develops. Later, the liver becomes *large, tender,* and *painful.* After hepatomegaly from congestion has been present for some time, the liver capsule becomes thickened and tenderness disappears. Edema fluid accumulates as right-sided or bilateral *hydrothorax, ascites,* and pitting *edema of the ankles.* The level of dependent edema gradually ascends from ankles to thighs; the vulva or scrotum and penis may become grossly swollen. Edematous skin may extend to the heart level, seldom above it. The lips, ears, and nailbeds may be *cyanotic.* Impaired cerebral circulation may result in *mental aberrations* and *periodic breathing.* ***Laboratory Findings.*** The circulation time from arm to tongue is prolonged, but this is seldom tested now. The ventricular ejection fraction is low. Often some proteinuria is present. Erythrocytosis may develop. ***X-ray Findings.*** Films of the chest may show cardiac enlargement (dilatation), pleural effusions, and the exaggerated parenchymal markings of pulmonary congestion. But hydrothorax may obscure one or both borders of the heart. ***Distinction.*** The clinical picture just described is frequently considered pathognomonic when, as a matter of fact, it is not. A patient with portal vein obstruction may present a similar syndrome, except that the cirrhotic patient may lie flat comfortably. But this clue is not entirely reliable; occasionally a patient with cardiac failure is unaccountably comfortable in the reclining position, and one with cirrhosis may be dyspneic from hydrothorax. Metastasis from carcinoma may produce fluid in the abdominal and thoracic cavities with a distribution similar to that in cardiac failure.

▼ *Key Symptom:* ***Palpitation.*** In medicine *palpitation* is applied to the symptom in which the patient is conscious of his heart action, whether it be fast or slow, regular or irregular. Although often caused by trivial disorders, it nevertheless frightens the patient, as does any symptom referable to the heart. So the cause must be found and carefully explained. The sensation is usually described as "pounding," "fluttering," "flopping," "skipping a beat," "missing a beat," "stopping," "jumping," or "turning over." The frequency, regularity, rate, and intensity depend upon the underlying cause. To anyone who examines patients it is obvious that many dysrhythmias do not reach consciousness. Heartbeats that are felt usually have an abnormally loud 1st heart sound. This occurs when the diastolic filling time of the ventricle is shortened and the next contraction begins while the AV valves are far apart; so the valve leaflets must travel a greater distance to close and are pushed by a rapidly augmenting intraventricular pressure.

Clinical Occurrence: BEATS AT IRREGULAR INTERVALS (ABOLISHED BY EXERTION). Premature beats with or without a twinge of "pain" or discomfort in the chest. REGULAR BEATS IN PAROXYSMS (WITHOUT EXERTION OR INDUCED BY IT). *Exertion:* strenuous exercise in normal persons, slight exercise with anemia, effort syndrome. *High cardiac output at rest:* anxiety, hypertension, thyrotoxicosis, fever, arteriovenous shunts (congenital, traumatic, infectious, or in Paget's disease of bone), cor pulmonale, beriberi. *Pressure on the heart:* mediastinal tumor, tympanites, aerophagia. *Drugs:* tobacco, tea, coffee, alcohol, morphine, cocaine, atropine, amyl nitrate, insulin, epinephrine, ephedrine, aminophylline, carbon monoxide poisoning, thyroid hormones, digitalis.

— *Palpitation:* ***Hyperkinetic Heart Syndrome*** (Effort S., Neurocirculatory Asthenia). This condition is found in young persons with increased ejection rate from the left ventricle and bounding arterial pulse. It is attributed to excessive stimulation of beta-adrenergic receptor sites because it responds to the administration of propranolol. *Symptoms:* disturbing palpitation, tachycardia, inappropriate exertional dyspnea. *Physical Signs:* tachycardia at rest, systolic hypertension, chest pains. *Distinction:* exclude thyrotoxicosis, idiopathic hypertrophic subaortic stenosis, pheochromocytoma, porphyria. The condition responds to the administration of propranolol while small doses of isoproterenol precipitate frank hysteria [E. D. Frohlich, R. C. Tarazi, and H. P. Dustan: Hyperdynamic Beta-Adrenergic Circulatory State, *Arch. Intern. Med.*, **123:**1–7, 1969].

GENERAL INSPECTION. **Many signs outside the precordium and blood vessels give valuable information about cardiac function; these are seen when surveying the entire patient.**

Dyspnea and Hyperpnea (Shortness of Breath). See p. 281.

▼ *Key Sign:* ***Pallor.*** Pallor is the lack of the normal red color imparted to the skin and mucous membranes by the blood in the lumina of the superficial vessels. The skin color is modified by the thickness of the avascular epidermis and the amount of melanin and other pigments in the dermis. So inspection of the skin for an assessment of generalized pallor is always supplemented by observing the color of the conjunctivae and the oral mucosa. In persons deeply pigmented because of race or other factors, the color of the mucosa may be the only reliable physical sign. Pallor can be produced by edema or myxedematous tissue surrounding the superficial blood vessels, by vasoconstriction, by dilution of erythrocytes in the blood, or by subnormal concentrations of hemoglobin in the red cells, or any combination of these.

Clinical Occurrence: LOCALIZED PALLOR. Exposure to cold, vasoconstriction (e.g., Raynaud's phenomenon), arterial insufficiency (narrowed lumina, thrombosis, embolism), edema. GENERALIZED PALLOR: *Peripheral Vasoconstriction. Acute:* exposure to cold, severe pain, vomiting, hemorrhage and shock, hypoglycemic reactions, low cardiac output syndrome with decreased tissue perfusion. *Paroxysmal:* apneic periods in periodic breathing, hypertensive periods from pheochromocytoma, vertiginous periods in Ménière's disease, migraine. *Chronic:* normal in some persons, glomerulonephritis (anemia may contribute). *Obscuration of Skin Vessels.* Edema, myxedema (anemia may contribute), scleroderma. *Cardiac.* Asystole (Adams-Stokes attacks, syncope), myocardial infarction, aortic stenosis (severe). *Erythrocytopenia.* Deficient numbers of red cells.

▼ *Key Sign:* ***Cyanosis.*** Cyanosis is the blue color seen through the skin and mucous membranes when concentrations in 100 mL of blood exceed 5.0 gm of reduced hemoglobin, 1.5 gm of methemoglobin, or 0.5 gm of sulfhemoglobin. The amount of oxyhemoglobin does not affect the color. *Local cyano-*

sis occurs when blood is deoxygenated in the vessels in venous stasis or in the tissues from extravasation. Many normal persons have localized venous stasis in some parts of the body. *Generalized cyanosis* is seen in the lips, nailbeds, ears, and malar regions; its presence indicates an abnormality of the systemic circulation. Since the blue color is within the venules, capillaries, and arterioles of the subpapillary plexis, it fades with superficial pressure, distinguishing it from *argyria,* in which silver sulfide has been deposited in the skin by the action of light on ingested silver compounds.

Clinical Occurrence: LOCAL CYANOSIS. Localized venous stasis, extravasations of blood in superficial tissues. GENERALIZED CYANOSIS FROM INSUFFICIENT OXYGENATION. *Tracheobronchial obstruction:* foreign body, compression. *Alveolar barrier:* asthma, atelectasis, pulmonary edema, pneumonia from *Pneumocystis carinii. Defective alveoli:* pulmonary emphysema, pulmonary fibrosis, pulmonary consolidation (lobar pneumonia). *Ineffective circulation:* pulmonary artery stenosis, arteriovenous shunts in heart or lungs, cardiac failure. *Nonoxygenated hemoglobin compounds:* methemoglobinemia, sulfhemoglobinemia, hemoglobinopathies with failure to bind oxygen. GENERALIZED CYANOSIS FROM INCREASED DEOXYGENATION. Stasis from exposure to cold.

▼ ***Key Sign: Edema.*** Excessive accumulation of interstitial fluid is termed *edema,* either *localized* or *generalized.* When the amount of generalized edema is great, the condition is termed *anasarca* or *dropsy.* In the adult, fluid accumulates to the amount of about 10 pounds (4.5 kg) before it is detectable by the examiner as *pitting edema.* To demonstrate the presence of edema the physician's thumb is pressed into the skin of the patient against a bony surface, such as the subcutaneous aspect of tibia, fibula, or sacrum. When the thumb is withdrawn, an indentation persists for a short time. The *depth* of the pit *should be estimated and recorded in millimeters,* shunning such meaningless expressions as "three-plus."

The *distribution* of edema should be noted, since the amount of fluid is roughly proportional to its extent as well as its thickness. In response to gravity, dependent edema first appears in the feet and ankles of the walking patient. When the patient is bedfast, the examiner should search for early edema by turning him over and indenting the posterior surface of the calves and the skin overlying the sacrum. As the amount of fluid increases, a faint *water level* may be detected under the skin; seldom does dependent edema rise higher than the heart. Anasarca can be recognized at a glance by the obliteration of superficial landmarks under the skin. When edema of the legs has been present for a long time in walking patients, the subcutaneous tissues and the skin become fibrotic, so they no longer pit on pressure; this is sometimes called *brawny edema* (i.e., musclelike).

Normally the distribution of water between blood and interstitial tissues is maintained by an equilibrium among several components. Fluid flows from vessels to the interstices in response to the intravascular hydrostatic pressure and the colloid osmotic pressure of the interstitial fluid. In the opposite direction, fluid enters the blood because of the interstitial tissue tension and the oncotic pressure of the plasma proteins. Interstitial fluid is also returned to the blood as lymph. Alteration of any of these components upsets the equilibrium. An increase in the systemic venous pressure in congestive heart failure produces generalized edema; occlusion of a vein may result in localized edema. Obstruction of lymphatic channels produces *lymphedema* with physical signs indistinguishable from those produced by edema from other mechanisms. Reduction in the plasma albumin (the plasma protein with the highest osmotic pressure) results in lowering the oncotic pressure of the plasma, permitting edema to form. Increased capillary permeability in acute nephritis may cause edema that is not dependent. Tissue inflammation by bacterial, chemical, thermal, or mechanical means increases capillary permeability to make localized edema.

Clinical Occurrence: LOCALIZED EDEMA: *Inflammatory. Infectious:* boils, carbuncles, cellulitis, abscesses, erysipelas, osteomyelitis, gas gangrene. *Metabolic: gout. Venous Obstruction. Intraluminal:* thrombophlebitis, thrombosis, metastatic neoplasm growing in veins. *Mural:* varicosities, mural tumors, arteriovenous fistulas. *External pressure:* lymph nodes, aneurysms, tumors, garters, garter belts.

Lymphatic Obstruction. Intraluminal: filaria, metastatic carcinoma. *Mural:* cellulitis. *External pressure. Surgical excision. Traumatic:* bruises, sprains, fractures. *Chemical or Physical Injuries. Excessive heat or cold:* frostbite, sunburn, scalds, burns. *Stings:* insects, snakes, plants. *Irritants or corrosives. Angioneurotic Edema. Congenital:* amniotic bands, arteriovenous fistulas. *Hereditary.* Milroy's disease. BILATERAL EDEMA ABOVE THE DIAPHRAGM: *Inflammatory. Infec-*

tious: erysipelas, cellulitis, anthrax, Ludwig's angina, trichinosis. *irritants:* contact dermatitis. *Superior Vena Caval Obstruction.* Thoracic aneurysm, mediastinal neoplasm, thrombosis from infection of hand or arm, intraluminal metastasis from hypernephroma. *Increased Capillary Permeability.* Acute nephritis, angioneurotic edema. Scleroderma. BILATERAL EDEMA BELOW THE DIAPHRAGM: *Cardiovascular.* Congestive cardiac failure, constrictive pericarditis, portal vein obstruction, obstruction of the inferior vena cava, venous obstruction from intraluminal metastatic carcinoma, thrombophlebitis. *Loss of venous tone:* convalescence, lack of exercise. *Hypoalbuminemia.* Nephrosis, anemia, cachexia, beriberi. *Ascites.* Any cause. *Compression of Veins.* Garter belts, etc.

Exercise Edema. Development of facial and ankle edema has been studied in healthy men undergoing severe exercise and its mechanism discussed [Editorial: *Lancet,* **1:**261–62, 1979].

Idiopathic Edema. Recurrent and chronic edema is frequently observed in middle-aged women in which the mechanism has so far defied explanation; it cannot be placed under the foregoing categories. This has been discussed in several letters in the *Lancet,* **1:**1979 on pp. 826, 1188, and in *Lancet,* **2:** 1979, p. 355.

High-Altitude Edema. Many women and fewer men experience facial and lower-limb edema when hiking at altitudes exceeding 2400 m. A high-salt intake will augment this effect. With return to lower levels diuresis occurs and the edema disappears [H. N. Hultgren: High-Altitude Edema, *J.A.M.A.,* **239:**2239, 1978].

Tropical Edema. Pitting edema of the ankles often occurs abruptly in normal adults within 48 hours after they have traveled from a temperate climate to the heat of the tropics. It spontaneously resolves in a few days of acclimatization [R. F. Buchan: Ankle Edema of Tropical Climes, *J.A.M.A.,* **218:**99, 1971; F. X. Schloeder: Ankle Edema in Tropical Climes. *Ibid.,* **218:**1705, 1971].

Periodic Edema (Cyclic E., Idiopathic E.). Many women experience periods of edema and abdominal distention for years. There is no evidence of cardiac, renal, or electrolyte disorder. *Symptoms.* Absent or minor, such as headache, irritableness, depression. *Diagnosis.* (1) Demonstration of intermittent fluid retention and sudden weight gain, (2) exclusion of organic disease, (3) evidence of substantial psychologic or emotional disorder [G. W. Thorn: Approach to the Patient with "Idiopathic Edema" or "Periodic Edema," *J.A.M.A.*, **206:**333–38, 1968].

The Precordium

The anterior surface of the chest closest to the heart and aorta is conveniently termed the *precordium*. Normally, this area extends vertically from the 2nd to the 5th intercostal space, transversely from the right border of the sternum to the left midclavicular line in the 5th and 6th interspaces. The upper epigastrium is occasionally included. When the heart is enlarged or displaced, the boundaries of the precordium shift accordingly. In dextrocardia, all signs described herein are located in the opposite hemithorax.

Anatomic Relations of the Heart and Precordium

The projections of the normal heart upon the precordium are depicted in Fig. 6-36A. Behind the manubrium sterni are the arch of the aorta and other mediastinal structures. The right border of the heart corresponds roughly to the right edge of the sternum from the 3rd to 5th interspaces. The right atrium forms the right border, but the right ventricle is very close to it. The left ventricle forms the cardiac apex and a slender area of the left border. Thus the greatest area between these two boundaries represents the projection of the right ventricle.

Movements of the Heart

The fibrous sac of the pericardium suspends the heart from the great vessels and anchors it below to the central tendon of the diaphragm (Fig. 6-36B). In descending, the diaphragm elongates the vertical cardiac axis while narrowing its transverse diameter. During quiet breathing, this effect is unimportant, but deep inspiration delays the filling of the right cardiac chambers perceptibly. This mode of suspension permits lateral displacement of the heart with changes in posture, so the patient should be erect to delineate the cardiac borders accurately. When the diaphragm is pushed upward by abdominal distention or the sitting posture, the heart becomes more horizontal and the apex moves leftward.

The myocardial fibers form a complete spiral, so contraction

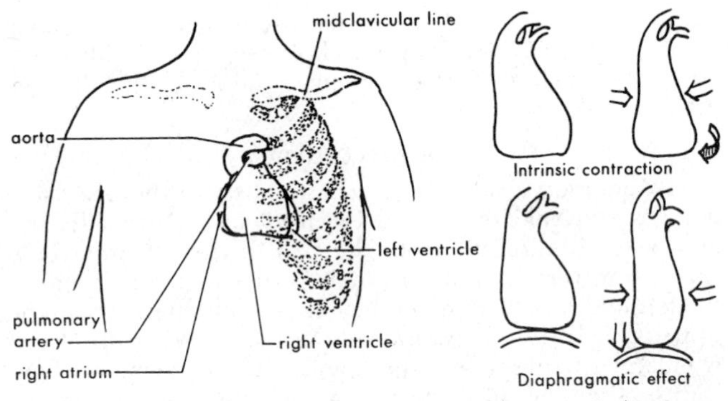

Fig. 6-36. Location of the heart and its contours. **A.** Precordial projections of the anterior surface of the heart. *Note that the entire central area of the precordium is the projection of the right ventricle. The left border and apex are formed by the left ventricle; the right atrium constitutes the right border.* **B.** Normal changes in the cardiac contour. *The intrinsic contraction of the cardiac chambers diminishes all diameters. During inspiration, the descending diaphragm stretches the heart from its superior anchorage in the fascia surrounding the aorta and pulmonary artery; the vertical cardiac axis is elongated; the transverse dimension is narrowed, delaying the filling of the right ventricle.*

produces a decrease in all diameters during systole (Fig. 6-36B). The apex rotates forward and to the right, approaching the chest wall and frequently causing a visible and palpable thrust, the *apical impulse.* Occurring early in systole, this thrust serves the examiner as a marker for the onset of cardiac contraction.

Cardiac Dilatation and Hypertrophy

Enlargement of the heart occurs either from dilatation of its chambers or from hypertrophy of its muscle walls; frequently both causes operate. Some clinicians refuse to distinguish between the two possibilities, preferring the noncommittal diagnosis of "cardiac enlargement." But closer attention to the precordium enables distinction between the two conditions in many cases. Increase in the overall size of the heart from myocardial hypertrophy is usually *imperceptible.* For example, if concentric hypertrophy should double the thickness of the ventricular walls, leaving the chamber volumes normal, the left border would be moved leftward by 10 mm and the right border would shift rightward by only 4 mm (Fig. 6-37). Since the percussing finger is at least 15 mm wide, this difference could not be detected by percussion, nor by the roentgenogram. Frequently ventricular hypertrophy is not diagnosed by the electrocardiogram. Enlargement of the heart, perceptible by percussion or roentgenogram, must be attributed to *dilatation of the chambers,* although an element of hypertrophy may be present.

The elongated fibers of the dilated heart cause only weak impulses in the anterior chest wall, although left ventricular dilatation can cause an increase in the area of the apical impulse. But hypertrophied cardiac muscle produces a thrust more powerful than normal that the skilled examiner can distinguish by palpation. An accentuated apical thrust may mean hypertrophy of the left ventricle; a palpable thrust in the projection of the right ventricle upon the precordium may be produced by right ventricular hypertrophy. These are reliable criteria of diagnosing ventricular hypertrophy.

Precordial Inspection. **The examiner should stand or sit at the patient's right side. Good illumination comes from a single source, shining transversely toward the examiner across the anterior chest surface. Alternate arrangements are to have the single light source**

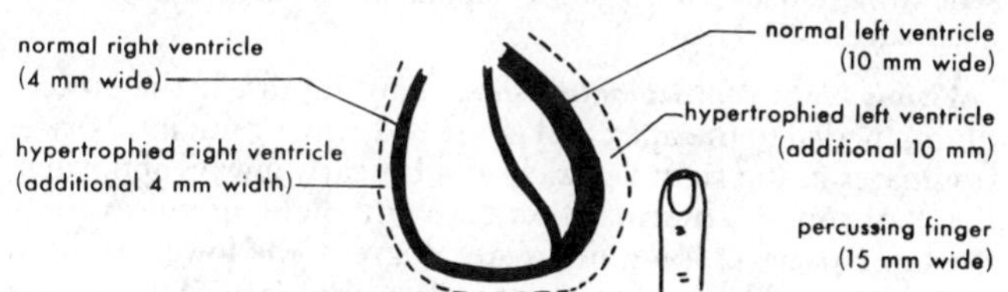

Fig. 6-37. Contribution of myocardial hypertrophy to the area of cardiac dullness. *Without dilatation of the chambers, concentric hypertrophy of the cardiac muscle to twice its normal thickness and weight cannot cause enough increase in an area of cardiac dullness to exceed the width of the percussing finger. Therefore, increase in the area of dullness must be attributed to dilatation when pericardial effusion is excluded.*

shining from head to foot of the patient, or from foot to head, with the observer on the right side. When possible, the patient should be examined both supine and erect. First, look for an apical impulse, then shift your head so your line of sight is across the sternum to detect heaving of the precordium. Finally, inspect the manubrial area.

The physical signs from inspection, palpation, and percussion of the precordium depend for their interpretation upon relatively normal anatomic relations between the heart and the chest wall. In gross distortions of the thoracic cage, such as kyphoscoliosis, funnel breast, or thoracoplasty, conclusions must be formed cautiously.

Visible Apical Impulse. In about one fifth of normal persons one sees an impulse, synchronous with the beginning of ventricular systole, in the left 5th interspace 7 to 9 cm from the midsternal line (or about 1 to 2 cm medial from the mid-clavicular line). *Pathophysiology.* The impulse is caused by the forward and rightward rotation of the heart at the onset of ventricular systole, bringing the apex against the chest wall.

Clinical Occurrence. The normal finding has been described. Increased amplitude may be caused by left ventricular hypertrophy (arterial hypertension, aortic stenosis, aortic regurgitation, mitral regurgitation); an increased impulse is associated with heightened myocardial tone (exertion, emotion, thyrotoxicosis, digitalization). The location may be shifted to the left (cardiac dilatation, right pneumothorax, right hydrothorax, left pleural adhesions). The impulse may be shifted to the right (left pneumothorax, right pleural adhesions). Severe pulmonary emphysema may force the heart downward to give an epigastric impulse just inferior to the xiphoid cartilage.

Visible Right Ventricular Impulse. Any impulse in the precordium, medial to the apex and in the 3rd, 4th, or 5th interspace, originates in the right ventricle and is nearly always abnormal, if felt through a normal thorax. With slight impulses, only the interspaces pulsate; in greater degrees, the lower sternum may heave with the heartbeat. *Pathophysiology.* The muscle of the normal right ventricle is not strong enough to produce a visible impulse on the normal chest wall, but a dilated and hypertrophied right ventricle frequently does.

Clinical Occurrence. Right ventricular hypertrophy (mitral stenosis, pulmonic stenosis, pulmonic regurgitation, tricuspid regurgitation, right-to-left shunts); right ventricular dilatation from pulmonary hypertension; forward displacement of the heart (tumors behind the heart); protuberance of the right ventricle (aneurysm of the right ventricular wall); transient impulse (during an attack of angina pectoris).

Precordial Bulge. In both children and adults, a protrusion of the bony thorax over the right ventricle may occur from great cardiac enlargement of congenital heart disease. In the adult, a bulge near the upper sternum may be produced by erosion from a syphilitic aneurysm of the aorta.

Retraction of the 5th Interspace. In some normal persons, a systolic retraction of the 5th interspace near the apex can be noted. This is not a reliable sign of disease.

Clinical Occurrence. It is often present with considerable right ventricular hypertrophy.

Epigastric Pulsation. This occurs in many normal persons, especially after exertion. Occasionally, displacement of the heart in pulmonary emphysema causes it. Most frequently it is produced by pulsation of a normal abdominal aorta.

PRECORDIAL PALPATION. **Pulsation and other sensations can be perceived in the precordium by the examiner's sense of touch and vibration. The palmar bases of the fingers are most sensitive to vibrations. Demonstrate this by holding the handle of a vibrating tuning fork alternately to the fingertips and palmar aspects of the metacarpophalangeal joints (Fig. 6-38). Accordingly, palpate the precordium with the palm of the hand. First, examine the areas where pulsations are visible; later feel each part of the precordium systematically. Determine the presence and strength of right and left ventricular**

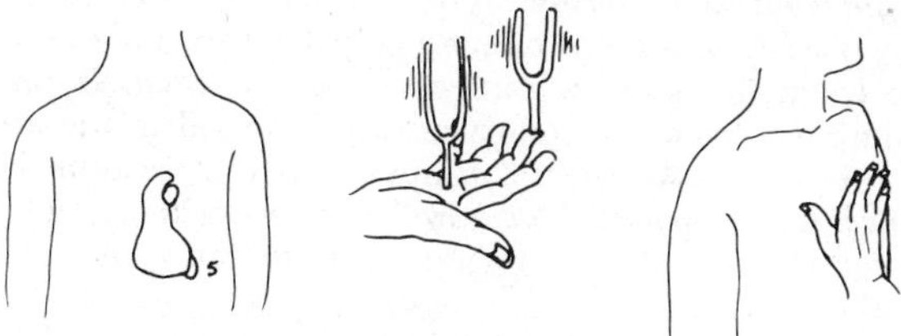

Fig. 6-38. Vibratory acuity in various parts of the hand. *Place the handle of a vibrating tuning fork sequentially on the fingertip and on the palmar aspects of the metacarpophalangeal joint to demonstrate that the palmar base is the more sensitive. This part of the hand should be applied to the precordium to detect thrills and ventricular thrusts.*

thrusts. Pulsations over the base of the heart should be carefully felt. Thrills should be identified and times as systolic or diastolic by their relation to the apical impulse. Recognize and time pleural and pericardial friction rubs.

Apical Thrust (Point of Maximum Impulse [PMI].). This is the impulse at the apex of the heart that is caused by the forward rotation at the beginning of ventricular systole. Normally, it is maximum from 7 to 9 cm to the left of the midsternal line in the 5th interspace (1 to 2 cm medial to the left midclavicular line). The strength of the normal impulse must be learned by examining many hearts. *Pathophysiology.* A hypertrophied left ventricle strikes the precordium with more-than-normal force. A weak myocardium produces an apical impulse of lesser intensity, although dilatation of the heart may cause it to be perceived over a wider area than normal. Increased myocardial tone from any cause accentuates the impulse.

Clinical Occurrence. Normally, an apical impulse may be felt in about one fifth of adults and a higher proportion of children, when the chest wall is not too thick, nor the breast too large. Frequently the impulse may be felt when it is not visible. Accentuated thrust occurs in heightened myocardial tone (exertion, emotion, thyrotoxicosis, digitalization); left ventricular hypertrophy (arterial hypertension, aortic stenosis, aortic regurgitation, mitral regurgitation, patent ductus arteriosus, coarctation of the aorta). The location may be shifted to the left (cardiac dilatation, right pneumothorax, left pleural adhesions); it may be displaced to the right (left pneumothorax, right pleural adhesions).

Right Ventricular Thrust. The normal right ventricle, normally placed, does not produce a palpable thrust in the resting state when the thoracic dimensions are normal. If present, the impulse from the right ventricle is found in the area of the precordium between the apex and the sternum in the 4th or 5th interspaces. *Pathophysiology.* Overactivity, right ventricular hypertrophy, or forward protuberance may give an impulse.

Clinical Occurrence. Hyperdynamic circulation (exertion, emotion, thyrotoxicosis); right ventricular hypertrophy (mitral stenosis, pulmonic stenosis, pulmonic regurgitation, tricuspid stenosis or regurgitation, right-to-left shunts); pulmonary hypertension from any cause; forward displacement of the heart (tumor behind the heart);

transient thrust (during an attack of angina pectoris); anterior displacement from enlarged left atrium [G. H. Manchester, P. Block, and R. Gorlin: Misleading Signs in Mitral Insufficiency, *J.A.M.A.*, **191:**87, 1965].

Pulsations at the Base. In pulmonary hypertension an impulse may be felt over the pulmonary conus in the 2nd or 3rd interspace just to the left of the sternum.

Clinical Occurrence. In severe mitral stenosis; rarely in aneurysm of the aorta. Pulsations in the right 2nd interspace may occur from an aneurysm at the base of the aorta or in conditions leading to pulmonary hypertension.

Thrills. These are vibrations felt over the precordium that have been likened to the sensation elicited by placing the hand on the chest of a purring cat. In the human body, the closest normal analogy is the sensation when the thorax is palpated while the person is speaking. Thrills have the same significance as murmurs and are usually associated with them. They should be located accurately and timed with respect to their sequence in the cardiac cycle, employing the apical impulse for reference. *Pathophysiology.* Eddies from blood coursing through an abnormal heart or arteries produce vibrations that are transmitted to peripheral structures, audible as murmurs, palpable as thrills. Since the ear is more sensitive to vibrations of this frequency, most murmurs are unaccompanied by thrills.

Clinical Occurrence. In mitral stenosis diastolic and presystolic thrills may be felt at the apex. Severe aortic stenosis causes a systolic thrill in the 2nd right interspace and in the carotid arteries. Less frequently, thrills accompany other organic murmurs, as a patent ductus arteriosus, where it is continuous throughout the cardiac cycle. Thrills may be produced by a ruptured chorda tendinea or valve leaflet.

Palpable Friction Rubs (Friction Fremitus). A friction rub occasionally may be felt, although more reliance is placed upon its detection by auscultation. The tactile sensation can be likened to the feel of two pieces of leather being rubbed together. A rub over the precordium that is synchronous with the heartbeat is presumed to be of pericardial origin; pleural rubs usually correspond with respiratory movements. Pericardial rubs are inconstant; they may be revived by shifting the posture of the patient. Both types are accompanied by distinctive sounds heard with the stethoscope. ***Pathophysiology.*** Inflammation of the pericardium or the pleura may cause loss of the normal lubricant so the two pericardial layers rub together.

Clinical Occurrence. Pericarditis may be caused by infection or may occur over an area of myocardial infarction. Pleurisy may occur as a result of pulmonary infarction or from inflammation secondary to infection or neoplasm.

PRECORDIAL PERCUSSION. **The precordium is percussed to define the cardiac borders. Since this is a problem in definitive percussion, we prefer Hoover's method of direct damped percussion, described on p. 301, which we believe to be more accurate than the methods employed for sonorous percussion. To avoid interference with the examination, the left arm of the supine patient is placed in elevation of about 90°; the erect patient is asked to put his left hand on his hip. The sitting woman is requested to hold up her left breast with the homolateral hand, when the examiner is using two-handed indirect percussion; with direct percussion, one of the examiner's hands is free to lift the breast and stretch the skin taunt over the area being percussed.**

With either method of percussion, delineate the *left border of cardiac dullness* (LBCD) by percussing in the 5th, 4th, and 3rd left interspaces sequentially, starting over resonant lung near the axilla and moving medially along an interspace until relative cardiac dullness is encountered (Fig. 6-39). The beginner should mark with a skin pencil where the note changes. The distance from the midsternal line to the LBCD in the 5th interspace should be measured and recorded. Measurement should be made along a straight line parallel to the transverse diameter of the thorax, not following the curvature of the chest wall; thus the measurement can be directly compared with posteroanterior film of the chest. The *right border of cardiac*

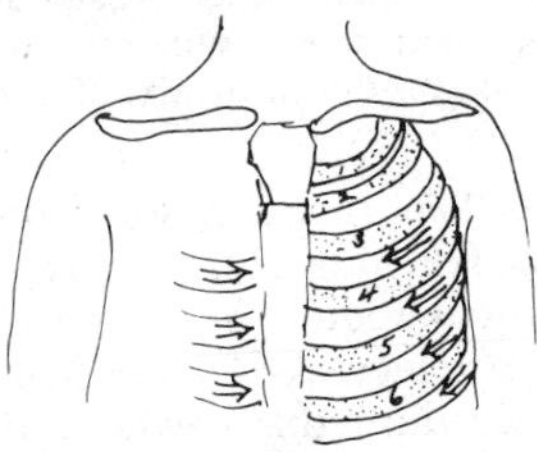

Fig. 6-39. Pattern of precordial percussion. *The 5th, 4th, and 3rd intercostal spaces on the left are percussed sequentially, as indicated by the arrows, starting near the axilla and moving medially until cardiac dullness is encountered.*

dullness (RBCD) is sought near the right edge of the sternum; hence the change from resonant lung to cardiac dullness cannot be clearly discerned in the normally placed right border. When the right border is displaced rightward, the change in percussion note in the right hemithorax is definite and accurate. If the right border is behind the sternum, the examiner cannot be certain of its position; it may be displaced leftward. A good maneuver is to compare the sternal percussion notes at the level of the 5th rib and at the 3rd costal level. Normally, the note at the lower level is duller; if it is more resonant, the right border may be shifted to the left edge of the sternum. No conclusion about the size of the heart should be made by percussing *only the left border;* the position of the right border must also be established. In the presence of hydrothorax or thickened pleura, percussion of one border of the heart may be impossible.

In the examination of the precordium, the width of the *retromanubrial dullness* is conveniently measured. Normally, its width should not exceed 6 cm in the adult; an excessive width suggests a mass in the mediastinum.

To interpret the findings from cardiac percussion, the *position of the trachea* should be determined. The examining finger is held straight and inserted into the suprasternal notch, exactly anteroposteriorly, until the fingertip encounters the curved surface of the tracheal rings. If the curvature of the trachea does not meet the center of the fingertip, the trachea is displaced. Merely a local segment of the trachea may be deviated, or its position may indicate displacement of the entire mediastinum and heart. X-ray examination may be necessary to distinguish (Fig. 6-40).

Left Border Shifted to Left. The LBCD is normally 7 to 9 cm to the left of the midsternal line (MSL).

Clinical Occurrence. Dilatation of the left ventricle (RBCD normally placed or shifted to right); pericardial effusion (RBCD shifted to right, muffled heart sounds, paradoxical pulse); displacement of normal-sized heart to left by right pneumothorax, right hydrothorax, left pleural adhesions, atelectasis of left lung with mediastinal shift to left.

Left Border Shifted to Right. Consider pulmonary emphysema with small heart in midline, or cardiac lingula of lung that prevents accurate percussion of LBCD; displacement to right by atelectasis of right lung, left pneumothorax, left hydrothorax; dextrocardia.

Right Border Shifted to Right. Distinguish between cardiac dilatation and pericardial effusion (cf. Left Border Shifted to

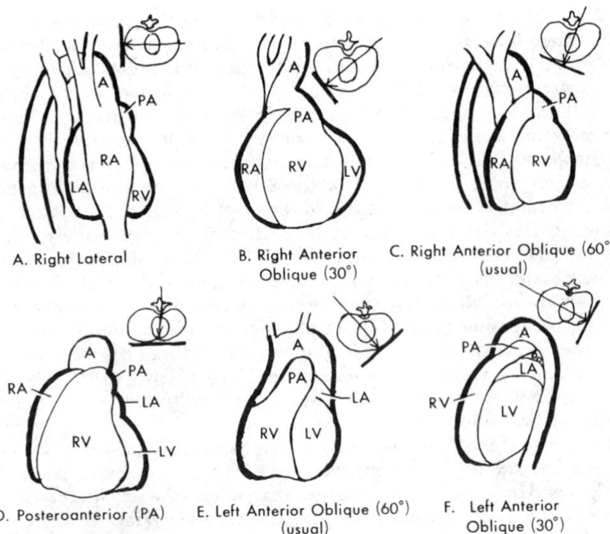

Fig. 6-40. X-ray silhouettes of the heart. *The positions are named for the aspect of the patient's thorax that faces the cassette (except in the PA view). Angles are measured between the direction of the x-ray beam and the plane of the patient's back. Heavy lines on the silhouettes indicate distinctive segments used in diagnosis.*

Left); left pneumothorax, left hydrothorax, right lung atelectasis, right pleural adhesions; dextrocardia.

Right Border Shifted to Left. Distinguish between left atelectasis, left pleural adhesions, right pneumothorax, right hydrothorax.

Widened Retromanubrial Dullness. The width in excess of 6 cm suggests aortic aneurysm, retrosternal goiter, thymic tumor, lymphoma, or metastatic carcinoma. There may be blood or pus in the mediastinum.

Widened Area of Cardiac Dullness. The area of cardiac dullness is judged to be expanded when its transverse diameter has been increased by (1) lateral displacement of the right or left border with the opposite border normally situated, or (2) lateral displacement of both borders in opposite directions.

An expansion of the area is caused by either cardiac dilatation or pericardial effusion.

Variations in Ventricular Rate and Rhythm

The emphasis is deliberately placed upon ventricular phenomena; the atria usually function silently, contributing no important diagnostic signs to auscultation of the precordium except for their role in generation of the 4th heart sound, the variations in loudness of the first heart sound that accompany AV dissociation and the atrial sounds sometimes heard in AV heart block. The diagrams explaining both atrial and ventricular phenomena somehow impart information that seems difficult to organize for diagnostic purposes. Electrocardiographic classifications, although logical and fundamental, are not suitable aids because they do not describe the physical findings. Initially, many experience difficulty in diagnosing cardiac dysrhythmias because they fail to realize that the physical signs of the heart's action are practically all ventricular. We believe that most clinicians examine the heart by diagnosing the dysrhythmia before they identify and describe the heart sounds; however illogical, this order will be followed.

The *sinoatrial* (*SA*) *node* lies in the right *atrial* wall near the entrance of the superior vena cava (Fig. 6-41). As the normal pacemaker of the heart, it originates rhythmic waves of excitation that spread quickly through the wall of both atria until they reach the *atrioventricular* (*AV*) *node* near the posterior margin of the interatrial septum. Here there is slight delay, while atrial systole is completed. The excitation then passes down a specialized conducting tissue, the *bundle of His,* that divides into right and left branches, each passing down the corresponding side of the interventricular septum to excite the muscle of the right and left ventricles more or less simultaneously. Deviations in timing and in the pathways taken by these waves cause changes in rate and rhythm that can be analyzed with considerable accuracy in the electrocardiogram. Most abnormalities can be diagnosed, or at least suspected, by close attention to the auscultatory signs from the ventricles.

Auscultation for Cardiac Rate and Rhythm. **When one listens at the precordium, pairs of sounds can be heard in seemingly endless repetition. Each member of a pair usually differs from its mate in intensity and pitch. Without further analysis at this time, one can**

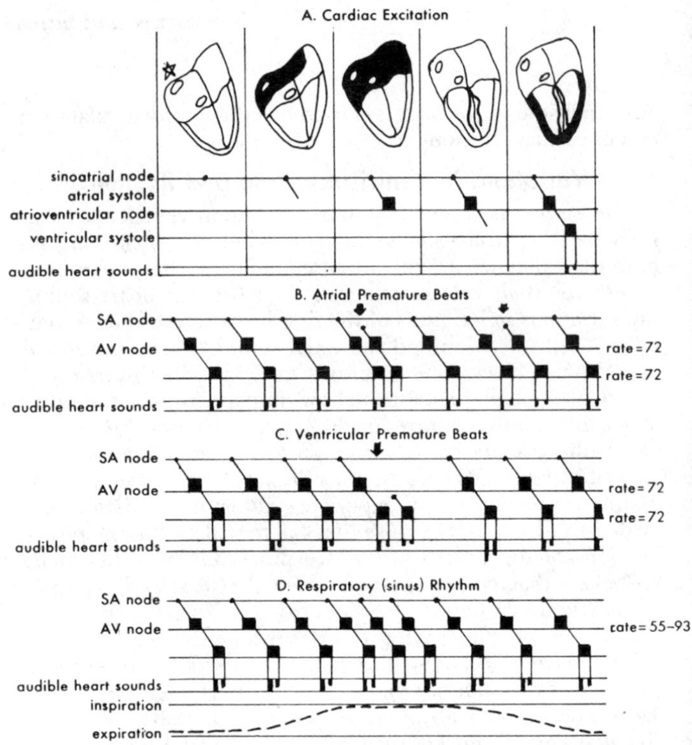

Fig. 6-41. Disturbances of cardiac rate and rhythm I. **A.** *Diagram illustrating the spread of excitation over the heart. The stimulus starts in the sinoatrial node and spreads throughout the walls of the atria, finally reaching the atrioventricular node where there is a short delay. The stimulus then proceeds down the His bundle by its two branches along the right and left wall of the interventricular septum to the apex, spreading thence to the muscle of the right and left ventricles. The atria contract before the impulse has left the AV node; ventricular systole occurs when the impulse has spread over the walls of the lower chambers. Note that the heart sounds that result from ventricular systole are the only perceptible physical signs of this process.* **B.** *Atrial premature beat is represented as originating outside the SA node, an ectopic beat. This is followed by a short compensatory pause that cannot ordinarily be detected by the ear.* **C.** *An ectopic ventricular beat with an audible compensatory pause, a physical sign of its origin.* **D.** *Respiratory or sinus arrhythmia or dysrhythmia is represented. There is acceleration of the heart rate near the height of inspiration; this acceleration originates in the SA node. In any dysrhythmia the heart sounds of a*

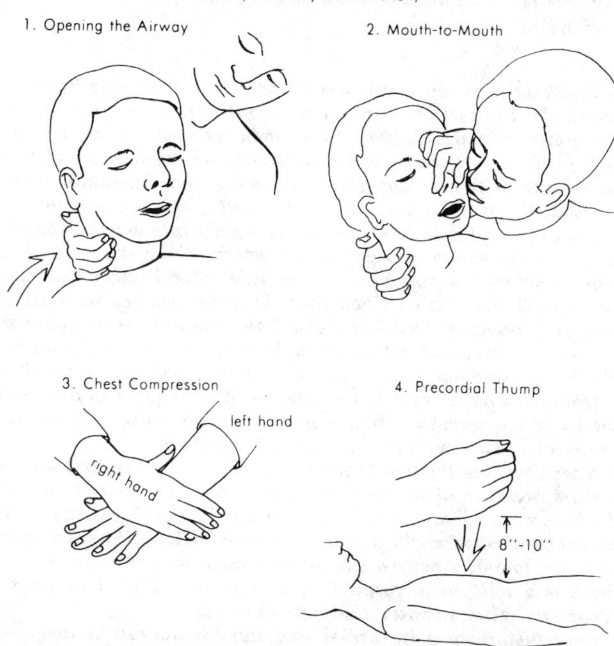

beat following a shortened interval are often fainter than normal; beats following an abnormally long pause are louder than normal. **E.** Cardiopulmonary resuscitation (CPR). *With the subject supine and horizontal, stand at his left side.* **1. Opening the airway.** *Lift his neck with your left hand with his head tilting backward and clear the mouth of foreign material.* **2. Mouth-to-mouth breathing.** *Hold the subject's head with your right palm while your index finger and thumb pinch the nostrils closed. Take a deep inspiration and place your lips over the subject's; blow forcefully into the subject's lungs. Then disengage and watch him exhale passively as his chest sinks. Repeat the blowing every five seconds, counting as "one thousand-one, etc."* **3. External cardiac compression.** *If the heart beat is imperceptible in the carotid pulse, or elsewhere, put the heel of your left palm over the subject's lower sternum, avoiding the fragile xiphoid process, and top with your other hand. Holding your elbows extended and stiff, press vertically on the sternum by depressing your shoulders to move it downward one or two inches. Relax the pressure immediately and repeat 80–100 times a minute.* **4. Precordial thumping.** *When cardiac arrest is obvious, raise your fist 20 or 25 cm (8 or 10 in.) above the precordium and deliver to it a single quick blow. If there is no immediate response, resort to chest compression.*

assume that each represents a heart sound, and the pair indicate a ventricular contraction. The *ventricular rate* is measured by counting the number of pairs in 10 or 15 seconds and multiplying the value by 6 or 4, as the case may be, to determine the number of beats per minute. With very slow rates, a longer period of counting should be used. Guessing at the heart rate is fallacious and fraught with error. In the same fashion, the *arterial pulse rate* may be counted, palpating the waves in a peripheral artery. If the counting of the ventricular rate is possible, we see little value in also measuring the arterial pulse rate. When there is a discrepancy between the two, it is termed a *pulse deficit*. Pulse deficit has been overemphasized as a sign of atrial fibrillation when, in fact, it occurs whenever ventricular contraction occurs before enough blood has accumulated to produce a pulse wave in the arteries; it is frequent in premature beats and bigeminal rhythm. Nurses should be instructed to count ventricular rates in all cardiac patients routinely.

After counting the heart rate, listen carefully for several minutes for the presence of an *irregularity of rhythm*. The slower the rate, the longer and more intently should one listen; dysrhythmias are harder to detect when the diastolic intervals are long. When irregularities are found, a *pattern* should be sought to determine whether there is a relation to respiratory movements or whether there is recurrence after a constant number of beats.

Most disturbances in cardiac rate and rhythm can be diagnosed or suspected during physical examination. The following conditions have distinctive physical signs; others have been omitted because they can be detected only with the aid of the electrocardiogram. The order selected for presentation is designed for diagnostic use and is a classification of physical signs rather than one of conductive mechanisms.

Orderly Rhythm (Rate, 60–120): ***Sinus Rhythm.*** This is the beat of the normal heart. Ventricular systoles are equally separated in the series. With heart rates less than 100 beats a minute, diastole is longer than systole; the two intervals become equal at about 100 beats per minute; above 100, systole is the longer. Exertion causes acceleration to rates of 150 to 160. Vagus stimulation by holding the breath, pressure on the eyeballs, or massage of the carotid sinus produces slowing of the rate in a steplike manner. ***Pathophysiology.*** In sinus rhythm, the impulse originates in the SA node, spreads throughout the walls of the atria, causing their contraction; then it reaches the AV node. The impulse then follows the two branches of the His bundle to spread into the two ventricles, causing them to contract. *Distinction.* Regular rhythm with similar rate also occurs in atrial flutter with 3:1 or 4:1 block. Rather than sinus rhythm, flutter should be suspected when digitalis has been given to a patient with flutter and 2:1 block; digitalis is more likely to increase the degree of block than to convert the rhythm to normal. In sinus rhythm, exertion produces smooth acceleration of the heart rate, but it causes sudden increases in flutter; the ventricular rate may jump from 120 to 180 as the block is diminished from 3:1 to 2:1.

Clinical Occurrence. Normal.

Emergency: Cardiac or Respiratory Arrest

The recognition of this condition demands from the nearest informed bystander immediate treatment for survival until professional staff arrives. Public education seeks to inform all adults and children in this first aid. Early Symptoms of a Heart Attack: prolonged severe *pain behind the sternum* often radiating to the neck, jaw, shoulder, or arm; *sweating; nausea and vomiting; shortness of breath. Clinical Occurrence:* ventricular fibrillation, cardiac standstill, myocardial infarction, automobile accidents, and other trauma, drowning, electrocution, suffocation, drug intoxication.

CARDIOPULMONARY RESUSCITATION (CPR) **(To be given by any informed adult or child available).**

WHEN VICTIM IS UNCONSCIOUS: ***Lay the patient flat* on a bare hard surface with his *back downward* (in accidents from automobiles or diving, suspect the possibility of a *fractured neck* before much manipulation; in such cases avoid moving the head in any direction). Otherwise,**

OPEN THE AIRWAY: ***Lift up the neck* with the head *tilting backward. Clear the mouth* of foreign material. Listen and watch for *breathing;* if none,**

GIVE MOUTH-TO-MOUTH BREATHING: **Kneel beside the patient's head while holding it *tilted backward* with your palm while *pinching his nose. Take a deep breath, place your lips tight* against those of the patient, and *blow your breath* into the patient's mouth and watch the patient *exhale passively* as his chest falls. *Repeat every 5 seconds* (count a second as the time taken to say "one-thousand-one" or "one-thousand-two", etc.). Continue as long as assistance is needed, indicated by your feeling of resistance and compliance in the airway as you breathe into it; by feeling his chest rise and fall; and by** hearing air escaping from his mouth. When the patient's lips cannot be opened, use the following:

MOUTH-TO-NOSE BREATHING. Kneel beside the patient's head while holding it *tilted back with your hand,* use the other hand to *lift his jaw. Seal his lips* by this position of his jaw, but it may be necessary to open his lips to permit exhaling. *Take a deep breath* and place your mouth over his nose and *blow into the nostrils; withdraw your mouth promptly* after each blow. *Repeat the cycle every 5 seconds.*

MOUTH-TO-STOMA BREATHING. When the patient has a tracheostomy, blow through the stoma as with mouth-to-nose breathing.

EXTERNAL CARDIAC COMPRESSION: Ascertain whether the heart is beating by *palpation of the peripheral pulses,* especially *that of the carotid artery,* located in the groove between the trachea and the slanting medial border of the sternocleidomastoideus muscle (or more precisely, the pulsation is felt in the *carotid triangle* with the sternocleidomastoideus posteriorly, the omohyoid muscle anteriorly, and the posterior belly of the digastricus superiorly). In addition to the artificial breathing; with the patient lying in the same position, *kneel close by the side* of the patient, *place the heel* of your hand on the lower half of the patient's sternum with the transverse axis of your wrist parallel to the long axis of the sternum, *avoiding any pressure on the xiphoid process* which is easily fractured. Put your *other hand on top of* the first one. With your *elbows held stiffly, press your arms from the shoulders down* vertically on the sternum to *depress it* at a minimum of 1½ to 2 inches. Follow compression *by immediate relaxation, keeping your hands in place.* The *compression rate* should be 80–100 cycles per minute when there is one rescuer. If there are two rescuers, five chest compressions should be given to one breath (5:1 ratio). With only a single rescuer, he should give *2 quick breaths* after *each 15 chest compressions,* given at the rate of 80–100/*min.* (When properly performed this procedure can produce a systolic blood pressure of 100 mm Hg but a diastolic pressure of 0—a blood flow of ¼ to ⅓ normal.)

PRECORDIAL THUMP. (This is recommended in witnessed cases of cardiac arrest, monitored patients, and in known atrioventricular block. A single blow may restore the beat in ventricular dysrhythmias and in some cases of heart block; the fist may serve as pacemaker until mechanical means are provided.) With the fleshy part of your fist, *strike a sharp quick blow* over the *middle* of the sternum, swinging *from a distance* of 8 to 12 inches. This should be given *within the first minute* of cardiac standstill. If there is no immediate response,

begin external cardiac compression at once. [For more detailed discussions read Standards and Guidelines for Cardiopulmonary Resuscitation (CPR) and Emergency Cardiac Care (ECC), *J.A.M.A.*, 255:2905–84, 1986.].

Orderly Dysrhythmia (Rate, 60–120): ***Atrial Flutter with 3:1 Block.*** The rate of the ventricle may be between 90 and 120, depending on whether there is 3:1 or 4:1 block. The ventricular contractions are perfectly spaced, with no differences in the intensity of heart sounds from beat to beat. Digitalis increases the degree of block in flutter, a possibility to consider in taking the history. Vagus stimulation may produce sudden drops in ventricular rate as the degree of block is increased from 2:1 to 3:1, while the atrial rate remains constant. *Pathophysiology.* Regular impulses are generated in the atria at extremely high rates, causing atrial contractions from 255 to 360 times per minute (Fig. 6-42D). The ventricles rarely respond to such rapid stimuli, so 2:1 block develops. An atrial rate of 360 results in a ventricle beating 180 times a minute.

Clinical Occurrence. Digitalis intoxication, rheumatic heart disease; diphtheria, coronary artery disease, thyrotoxicosis, and other forms of heart disease.

Orderly Rhythm (Rate Less Than 60): ***Sinus Bradycardia.*** This is the natural rate for a few persons. Rates usually range from 50 to 60, rarely as low as 40. The rhythm is normal. The rate accelerates smoothly with exertion. *Pathophysiology.* The excitation follows the normal pathways from the SA node. The slowness of the rate is attributed to vagus influence on the node. *Distinction.* Bradycardia suggests the possibility of AV heart block, either 3:1, 4:1, or complete. Sinus bradycardia, in contrast to these, has normal acceleration to exercise and slowing to vagus stimulation.

Clinical Occurrence. Some normal persons, especially long-distance runners. Occasionally in severe infections. Jaundice.

Orderly Dysrhythmia (Rate Less Than 60): ***Second-Degree AV Block*** (Mobitz II). Ventricular systoles occur at regular intervals with rates of 35 to 60 per minute. Each beat has the same intensity. The only distinctive physical sign may be faintly audible atrial contractions in the cycles not resulting in ventricular beats (Fig. 6-42A). Sometimes two *a-waves* for each ventricular

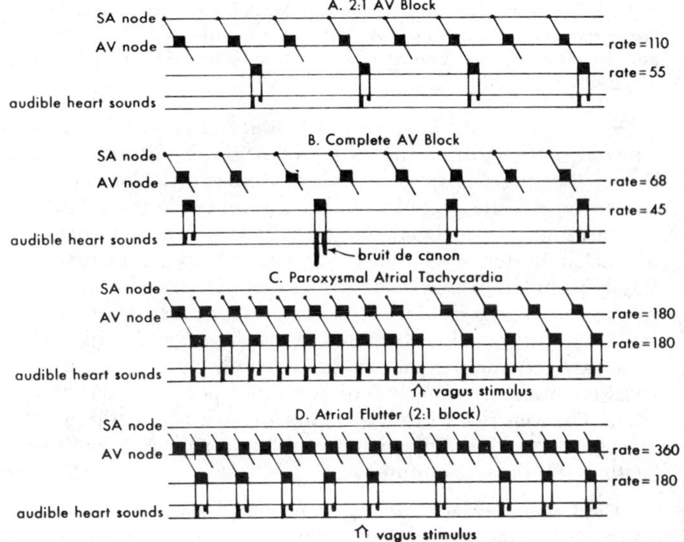

Fig. 6-42. Disturbances of cardiac rate and rhythm II. *In all diagrams the audible heart sounds are the only physical signs to indicate the presence and operation of the mechanisms.* **A.** *Second-degree AV block is depicted with 2:1 ratio. Alternate stimuli from the atria are blocked in the AV node so the ventricles beat only half as fast as the atria. The only physical sign is a slow regular heartbeat with first sounds of equal intensity.* **B.** *Complete AV block is depicted in which the ventricles beat independently of the atria and usually assume a slow rate, below 50 per minute, that accelerates little with exertion. A louder-than-common first sound occurs when ventricular filling is augmented by an atrial contraction occurring by chance at the optimal time; this is called by the French the "bruit de canon."* **C** *and* **D.** *When ventricular beats are regular with rates between 160 and 220 per minute, two conditions must be distinguished. In* **C** *is represented paroxysmal atrial tachycardia and* **D** *shows atrial flutter. Vagal stimulation may convert paroxysmal atrial tachycardia to normal rhythm, but there is no temporary slowing. In contrast, the only response of flutter to vagus stimulus is slowing for a few beats.*

contraction may be seen in the jugular vein. An electrocardiogram is often needed for diagnosis. *Pathophysiology.* In 2:1 AV block, alternate impulses from normally functioning atria are blocked, so the atrial rate is twice that of the ventricles. A 3:1 block occurs when every third beat from the atrium is transmitted through the AV node. *Distinction.* In both sinus bradycardia and second-degree heart block, the rate is accelerated with exertion, but complete heart block exhibits little response.

Clinical Occurrence. Acute infections, especially rheumatic fever and diphtheria; valvular heart disease; digitalis intoxication; coronary artery disease.

Orderly Dysrhythmia (Rate Less Than 60): ***Third-Degree AV Block.*** The ventricular contractions are evenly timed, but the intensity of the heart sounds is augmented when an atrial systole happens to precede ventricular contraction (Fig. 6-42B). With especially coincidental timing, there is a loud booming sound, *bruit de canon;* it may come infrequently, so auscultation should be prolonged for 60 seconds or more. More frequently, there are less spectacular variations in intensity of the first sounds. *Distinction.* This is the only bradycardia in which exertion does not accelerate the ventricular rate. The variation in intensity of the first sounds is distinctive. *Pathophysiology.* The atria beat regularly and at normal rates in response to stimuli from the SA node, but no excitation is transmitted through the AV node to the ventricles. The ventricles set up an autonomous rhythm with rates of 25 to 60 per minute.

Clinical Occurrence. Same as in second-degree heart block.

Orderly Dysrhythmia (Rate Less Than 60): ***Atrial Fibrillation with Digitalis Intoxication.*** Actually, this is a dysrhythmia, but fibrillation with slow ventricular rate is often mistaken for regular rhythm because the examiner does not listen long enough to detect the occasional irregularity that reveals the diagnosis. When the rate is slow, one should listen for several minutes before concluding that the rhythm is normal.

Orderly Rhythm (Rate More Than 120): ***Sinus Tachycardia.*** The rate is between 120 and 160 beats per minute with a perfectly regular rhythm. Vagus stimulation produces smooth deceleration. *Pathophysiology.* The impulses originate in the SA node and are transmitted normally throughout the conducting system. *Distinction.* Especially with rates of more than 140, sinus tachycardia must be distinguished from atrial flutter with 2:1 block. In flutter, vagus stimulation slows the rate in jerky fashion; paroxysmal atrial tachycardia does not slow, but may convert to normal rhythm and rate.

Clinical Occurrence. Exercise, emotional states, thyrotoxicosis, anemia, fever, hyperkinetic heart syndrome, and many debilitated states.

Orderly Dysrhythmia (Rate More Than 120): ***Paroxysmal Atrial Tachycardia.*** The attack begins and ends suddenly, lasting for a few minutes to many days. The ventricular rate is usually between 150 and 225 beats per minute. All ventricular beats have the same intensity and are equally spaced. Vagus stimulation by massage of the carotid sinus or a Valsalva maneuver *does not* produce temporary slowing; either there is no response, or the attack is terminated abruptly and normal rhythm resumes within a single cycle (Fig. 6-42C). Pressure on the eyeball is not an acceptable method of vagal stimulation because of potential damage to the eye. *Pathophysiology.* The arrhythmia is most often a reentrant or reciprocating form of tachycardia involving the AV node. True ectopic atrial tachycardia does occur. *Distinction.* The condition must be distinguished from sinus tachycardia that exhibits vagus slowing smoothly and from atrial flutter in which vagus slowing is often associated with varying AV block.

Clinical Occurrence. In apparently normal hearts; frequently in the Wolff-Parkinson-White syndrome, in various types of heart disease.

Orderly Dysrhythmia (Rate More Than 120): ***Paroxysmal Ventricular Tachycardia.*** Bedside diagnosis is *urgently needed* because this condition may induce ventricular fibrillation and death. There is complete atrioventricular dissociation with the ventricles beating faster than the atria. The onset and ending are abrupt. The ventricular rate usually is between 150 and 250 per minute. The rhythm is regular; but it is *not* influenced by vagal stimulation. So the condition must be distinguished from atrial flutter and paroxysmal atrial tachycardia. The variable relationship of atrial to ventricular systole furnishes the most distinctive sign: *variation in the intensity of the first sounds*. Some sounds are especially loud *cannon sounds* resulting from near superimposition of atrial and ventricular systole. Only the first heart sound may be audible, so mistakes in counting result in half the actual value. The cannon sounds are absent when the atria are fibrillating. Occasionally the ventricular rate is slower than 150.

Clinical Occurrence. Acute myocardial infarction, coronary artery disease, overdoses of drugs (digitalis, quinidine, procaine amide). Trauma to the heart from surgery or catheterization.

Emergency Treatment. See p. 354 for Precordial Thumping.

Orderly Dysrhythmia (Rate More Than 120): ***Atrial Flutter.*** The ventricular rhythm is perfectly regular with constant rates between 150 and 180, usually more than 120 with 2:1 block. Vagus stimulation should be attempted by having the patient hold his breath, perform a Valsalva maneuver, or by compression on the carotid sinus. Slowing for a few beats may result, to be followed by a transition of several irregular beats, and finally resumption of the previous rate and rhythm. Spontaneous shifts in ventricular rate may occur in large increments or decrements, e.g., from 120 to 180, or vice versa. This suggests a changing ratio of heart block between 2:1 and 3:1. *Pathophysiology.* Rapid regular stimuli are fired from an ectopic focus in the atrial wall, causing atrial contractions at rates between 250 and 360 per minute (Fig. 6-42D). The ventricles usually do not respond with such rapidity, so every alternate stimulus is stopped in the AV node, a 2:1 block. Vagus stimulation may cause a temporary increase in the degree of block. *Distinction.* In sinus tachycardia vagus stimulation causes smooth slowing. Paroxysmal atrial tachycardia cannot be slowed by the vagus, but vagus impulses may convert the rhythm to normal.

Clinical Occurrence. Usually in organic heart disease; sometimes in thyrotoxicosis.

Random Dysrhythmia: ***Premature Beats.*** Isolated or infrequent premature beats are quickly recognized by auscultation. Among a series of normal beats, a premature contraction from an *atrial* impulse is heard as a beat coming through before its expected time (Fig. 6-41B). It may be followed by a compensatory pause shorter than that usually associated with ventricular premature beats, but differentiation is difficult if not impossible at the bedside. If the premature beat occurs soon after a normal emptying of the chamber, little blood has accumulated to be ejected during the premature systole; the resulting heart sounds are less intense, and the stroke volume may be insufficient to produce an arterial pulse wave that can be felt. When premature beats are very frequent, they present the effect of a chaotic rhythm constituting a diagnostic problem (Fig. 6-43A). As the heart rate accelerates, "benign" ventricular premature beats tend to decrease, and the irregularity is temporarily abolished. So the response to exercise may distinguish between fibrillation and premature contractions. Careful listening reveals that a long pause is *always* preceded by a very short pause. ***Pathophysiology.*** An excitation arises from an ectopic focus in the atrium or ventricle; it is transmitted to the ventricles where the premature contractions are evident. ***Distinction.*** Exercise increases the irregularity of fibrillation but may abolish the premature contractions. In atrial flutter with varying degrees of block making a chaotic rhythm, exertion may result in a sudden excessive increase in ventricular rate resulting from a change in the ratio of the block. Premature beats occur in normal hearts, frequently in patients with organic heart disease; in response to adrenergic stimulation and digitalis; in electrolyte disturbances (hypokalemia).

Random Dysrhythmia: ***Atrial Fibrillation.*** Every student can glibly recite that fibrillation is an "irregular irregularity," but experience in teaching demonstrates this statement to be misleading. The inexperienced student has great difficulty in recognizing fibrillation; he is impressed by the fast runs of apparently normal spacing. He has not learned to listen for the breaks in these runs, followed by a few irregular beats, which actually indicate the condition to the experienced. The fast runs are also irregularly spaced, but this cannot be recognized by the examiner's sense of rhythm; it can only be indicated in the electrocardiogram where it can be measured accurately. Since ventricular contractions occur at all stages of chamber filling, the heart sounds from ventricular contractions vary in intensity. The ventricular rate is accelerated by exertion; the rhythm becomes more chaotic. With ventricular rates of less than 70, irregularities in rhythm are more difficult to detect.

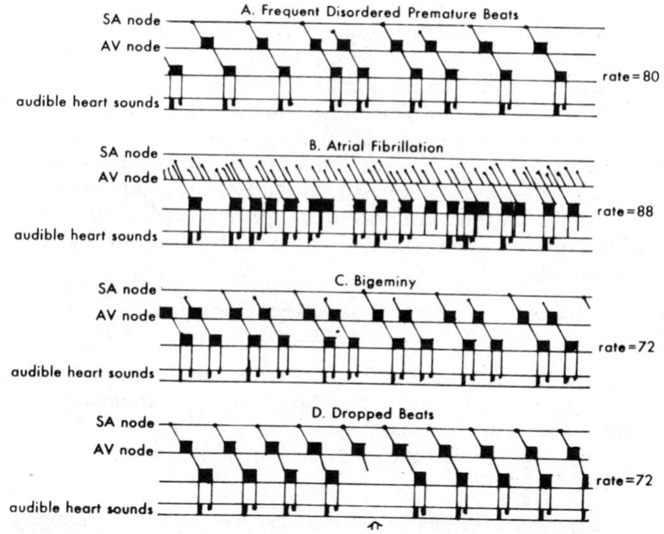

Fig. 6-43. Disturbance of cardiac rate and rhythm III. *As in previous diagrams, only the audible heart sounds are the physical signs of these disorders.* **A.** *Normal rhythm is interspersed with two random premature beats. If such beats are very frequent, the ear may not be able to distinguish them from atrial fibrillation unless some maneuvers are employed. The rhythm becomes regular as the rate accelerates to about 120 beats per minute.* **B.** *Atrial fibrillation is represented. The ventricular rhythm is grossly irregular and continues so when the rate is accelerated by exercise to more than 120 per minute.* **C.** *An example of bigeminy is shown with a normal beat followed by a premature beat and this pattern repeated many times. The premature beats tend to fall out when exercise accelerates the rate to over 120 per minute.* **D.** *Dropped beats in second-degree AV block are shown. Each successive impulse going through the AV node produces a longer interval until one fails to induce ventricular contraction. In contrast to premature beats, exercise tends to increase the number of dropped beats.*

Careful listening reveals a series of beats that seem to be evenly spaced until finally one occurs too soon or too late, and one realizes that the supposed regularity was an illusion. An occasional long pause is *not* preceded by a short pause. With rates less than 60, fibrillation is very difficult to detect; one should listen longer. ***Pathophysiology.*** The atria do not contract as units; different muscle segments contract separately, so the cardiac surface resembles the turbulence of the surface of boiling water. Stimuli from all parts arrive in complete disorder at the AV node, and a variable minority are transmitted to the ventricles at irregular intervals (Fig. 6-43B). Accordingly, ventricular rhythm presents no pattern. ***Distinction.*** Multiple premature beats without pattern tend to drop out when the ventricular rate is accelerated to 120 by exertion. In flutter with variable AV block, exercise increases the rate by large increments.

Clinical Occurrence. Organic heart disease; acute infections including rheumatic fever; thyrotoxicosis; digitalis intoxication.

Random Dysrhythmia: ***Ventricular Fibrillation.*** The ventricular beats are grossly irregular, but the sounds from them are inaudible. The patient usually dies before an electrocardiogram can record them; but they may be anticipated by cardiac monitor.

Emergency Treatment. See p. 354 for Precordial Thumping.

Orderly Dysrhythmia: ***Respiratory (Sinus) Dysrhythmia.*** The ventricular rate accelerates as inspiration approaches its maximum (remember: *a-i*) and decelerates during expiration (*d-e*) (Fig. 6-41D). The relation to phases of respiration is diagnostic; when the overall ventricular rate is slow, the association may not be as evident as expected. At rates less than 60, the rhythm may at first appear to be a series of premature beats, until the examiner remembers to check the respirations. ***Pathophysiology.*** The excitations originate in the SA node and are conducted normally through the heart. ***Distinction.*** The relation to respirations is diagnostic.

Clinical Occurrence. Normal in children, persists throughout life in some; occurs in many disorders but is not diagnostic of any.

Orderly Dysrhythmia: ***Bigeminy*** (Coupled Rhythm). The ventricular beats are grouped in pairs, the first a normal beat, the second premature; the compensatory pause after the premature beat separates the pair from its successor. If auscultation of the heart is performed, this dysrhythmia cannot be missed; but if only the arterial pulse is palpated, the premature beat of the couple may not be palpable, and a regular rhythm with half the ventricular rate may be diagnosed. This occurs whenever the premature beats follow the regular beats by an interval so short as not to permit adequate ventricular filling. As with other premature beats, exercise may cause the rhythm to resume a normal pattern. *Pathophysiology.* Each normal beat is followed by a premature beat arising from an ectopic focus in the atrium or ventricle. *Distinction.* A similar pattern is formed by second-degree AV block with a ratio of 3:2. This is not converted to normal by acceleration of the heart beat.

Clinical Occurrence. In normal hearts. In organic disease of the heart. In digitalis intoxication.

Orderly Dysrhythmia: ***Trigeminy.*** The rhythm sounds as if there were three normally spaced beats followed by a pause. Acceleration of the heart usually converts to normal rhythm. *Pathophysiology.* Systematic recurrence of either ventricular or atrial premature beats produces this dysrhythmia (Fig. 6-43C). Two normal beats are followed by a premature beat whose compensatory pause separates the triplet from its successor; or a single normal beat is followed by two premature beats with compensatory pauses. *Distinction.* AV block with a ratio of 4:3 presents a similar pattern; but the rhythm is not converted to normal with exercise.

Clinical Occurrence. In normal hearts, organic heart disease, and digitalis intoxication.

Orderly Dysrhythmia: ***Dropped Beats.*** A series of two, three, four, or more beats is followed by a pause. The pattern may recur regularly. The rhythm is not materially changed by acceleration of the heart rate. *Pathophysiology.* (1) Sinus pauses or sino-atrial block. (2) During the series of equally spaced ventricular beats, each impulse from the atrium takes progressively longer to pass through the AV node until one fails completely, causing a dropped ventricular beat (Fig. 6-43D). This type of second-degree AV block is termed the *Wenckebach phenomenon.* The ratio of block is usually 3:2, 4:3, 5:4, or 6:5. The denominator of the fraction is never 1 or the ventricular rhythm would appear entirely normal. *Distinction.* Bigeminy and trigeminy convert to normal rhythm when the heart accelerates.

Clinical Occurrence. Infectious diseases including rheumatic fever; digitalis intoxication; organic heart disease.

Daytime Somnolence and Fatigue: ***Sleep Apnea Syndromes*** (Pickwickian S.). This title probably includes more than one clinical entity. Early accounts (1965) described the pickwickian syndrome, named after the fat boy in Charles Dickens' writings, as a grossly *obese male* with *daytime somnolence, polycythemia, alveolar hypoventilation,* and sometimes *right ventricular failure.* With more clinical experience, physicians realized that the daytime somnolence was the result of nocturnal interruptions of sleep by many intervals of apnea interspersed with loud snoring. Still later, observations revealed that the periods of apnea were accompanied by, if not caused by, attacks of cardiac dysrhythmias (bradycardia, tachycardia, especially ventricular) that sometimes caused sudden death. Some writers described two types of dyspnea: commonly, *obstructive dyspnea* when expiratory movements persist during apnea, and, rarely, *central apnea* when respiratory movements cease with the lack of air flow through the bronchial tree. More symptoms have been added: *depression or hostility,* transitory *pulmonary and systemic hypertension.* A familial type has been reported [Editorial: Sleep Apnea Syndrome, *Lancet,* **1:**25–26, 1979]. More perspective has been achieved from a study of 30 asymptomatic men and 19 women also without symptoms. Each was monitored during a night's sleep. Twenty men had 264 episodes of nocturnal oxygen desaturation or abnormal breathing; but no women had desaturation and only three had nine periods of apnea. There was no statement about cardiac dysrhythmia [A. J. Block, *et al.:* Sleep Apnea and Oxygen Desaturation in Normal Subjects, *N. Engl. J. Med.,* **300:**513–17, 1979].

Cardiac Sounds: A Synopsis

In writing this section the authors have depended heavily upon several papers to which the reader is referred for more details [J. J. Leonard and F. W. Kroetz: *Examination of the Heart, Part IV: Auscultation,* 1966, New York, American Heart Association; J. Abrams: Current Concepts of the Genesis of Heart Sounds, *J.A.M.A.,* **239:**1287–92, 1978].

Intracardiac Sounds

Normal Heart Sounds

Most experts seem to have accepted the view of Robert F. Rushmer that all four heart sounds result from vibration of the left ventricular muscle, the cardiac skeleton, the valves, the great vessels, and from momentum and velocity of the blood mass as it flows through the elastic system. This supersedes the hypothesis that vibrations from the closing valves evoke sounds.

At the onset of systole the contraction of the ventricles suddenly increases the intraventricular pressure, closing the mitral and tricuspid valves and opening the aortic and pulmonic leaflets (Fig. 6-44). Closure of the cuspids causes the blood to rebound in the ventricles, transmitting vibrations to the chest wall that are heard as the *first heart sound* (S_1). After brief reverberation, the blood courses silently into the aorta and the pulmonary artery until the ventricles are nearly empty. Then the ventricles relax in diastole, the intraventricular pressure falls, the resulting jet tail approximates the leaflets, and the arterial back pressure completes the closure. The sudden arrest of the backflow sets up another series of vibrations, audible as the *second heart sound* (S_2). The names of the heart sounds are often qualified by the valve areas where they are heard (Fig. 6-45), as *mitral first sound* (M_1), *pulmonic second sound* (P_2). The heart sounds are usually loudest in the part of the precordium nearest the point of origin; the first sound from the cuspid valves, at the apex; the second sound from the semilunar valves, at the base. Invariably the second sound is louder than the first *at the base;* but *at the apex* M_2 may be as loud or louder than M_1. The intensity of the heart sounds deviates from the normal when more or less stress is put upon the valve leaflets by anatomic or physiologic abnormalities.

Onset of Systole: First Heart Sound (S_1). *Pathophysiology.* The sound is produced by vibrations in the left ventricular muscle, the mitral valve apparatus, and the left ventricular outflow tract, and from acceleration and deceleration of the blood mass during early ventricular systole. S_1 has three components: (1) the early rise in left ventricular pressure, (2) the opening of the aortic valve, and (3) the rapidly rising intra-aortic pressure.

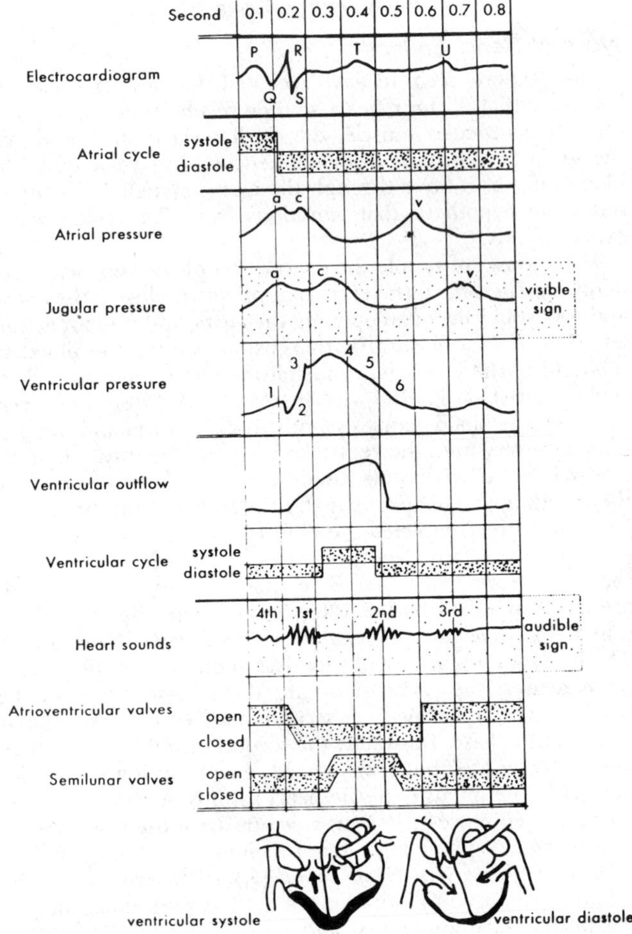

Fig. 6-44. Relation of the heart sounds to other events in the cardiac cycle. *Of all these phenomena, only one visible and one audible sign are produced.*

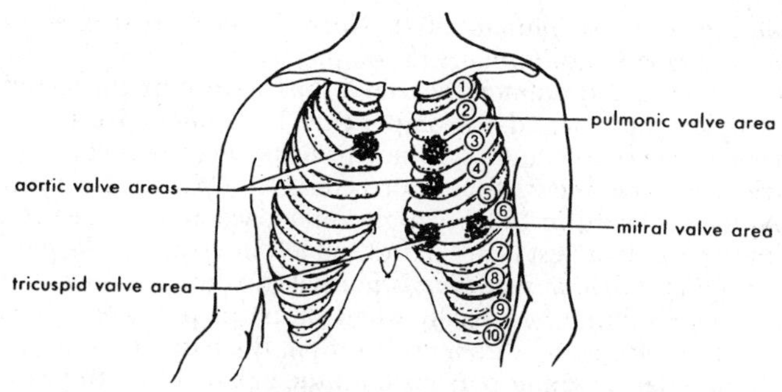

Fig. 6-45. Locations of all cardiac valve areas for auscultation of the precordium. *Situated where the sounds originating from the valves are best heard, the areas are not necessarily closest to the anatomic location of the valves. Usually, but not always, the locations are at the point of maximum intensity from the valves for which they are named.*

It seems doubtful that there are separate mitral and tricuspid components of S_1. *Optimum Audibility.* Normally heard over the entire precordium, S_1 is usually louder than S_2 at the cardiac apex (left 5th interspace near the midclavicular line); at the base of the heart, it is fainter than S_2. *Timing.* It marks the beginning of ventricular systole. Prolongation of S_1 is called *splitting,* although most workers deny it is true splitting. *Distinction.* S_1 is synchronous with the visible apical impulse and the palpable precordial thrust.

Clinical Occurrence: *Accentuated* S_1. Normally S_1 is louder than S_2 at the apex but accentuation is pathologic when it occurs in mitral stenosis, tachycardia from fever, hyperthyroidism, exercise, emotion, and hypertension. *Diminished* S_1 occurs in thick chest wall of the obese person, pulmonary emphysema, pericardial effusion, pleural effusion, first-degree AV block, acute rheumatic fever, atherosclerotic heart disease, weak ventricular contraction from myocardial infarction, cardiac failure, shock. *Varied Intensity of Heart Sounds:* atrial fibrillation, atrial flutter with varying degrees of block, complete AV block, ventricular tachycardia. *Widening or Splitting of* S_1: in normal persons, in right-bundle-branch block.

***Onset of Diastole:* Second Heart Sound (S_2).** *Pathophysiology:* Most workers now believe that S_2 is caused by vibrations in the great vessels, the closed valves, and the ventricular outflow tract, and by rapid deceleration of the blood mass from the closing of the semilunar valves. Normal *inspiratory splitting* of S_2 is ascribed to differences in compliance or distensibility between aorta and pulmonary artery, thus separating the sound complex into A_2 and P_2 components. The interval between ventricular systole and A_2 is much shorter than between ventricular systole and P_2; thus A_2 precedes P_2. *Optimum Audibility:* A_2 is best heard in the 2nd right interspace and the 3rd left interspace; P_2 is best heard in the 2nd left interspace. *Respiratory Effect: Inspiratory splitting* is normal in young persons, but *expiratory* splitting, especially when sitting, is pathologic (Fig. 6-46). *Intensity:* S_2 is greater than S_1 at the base of the heart; P_2 is louder in young persons until the age of 15 or 16 years, when A_2 gradually becomes louder.

Clinical Occurrence: *Accentuated A_2*: arterial hypertension, aortic regurgitation, aneurysm of the ascending aorta; rarely aortic stenosis. *Accentuated P_2:* pulmonary hypertension, mitral stenosis, left ventricular failure, atrial septal defect, truncus arteriosus. *Di-*

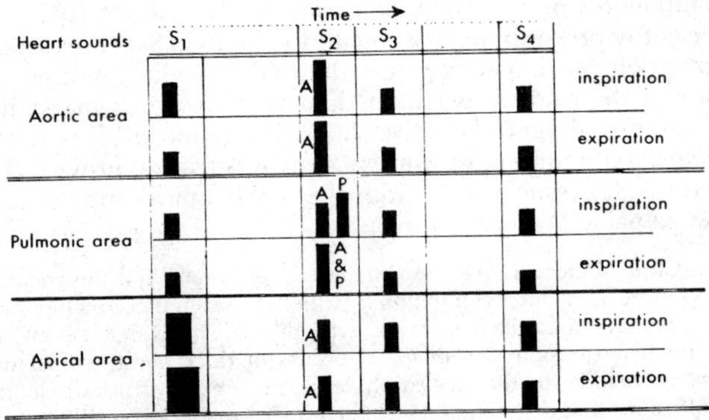

Fig. 6-46. Normal physiologic variations in the heart sounds. *Duration is represented on the horizontal axis, and intensity of the heart sounds is indicated on the vertical axis. The 1st sound (S_1) is prolonged during inspiration. The aortic component of the 2nd sound (S_2) is audible over the entire precordium, but the weaker pulmonic component is heard only in the left 2nd intercostal space. During expiration, the aortic and pulmonic components of S_2 are fused. But with inspiration the right ventricle becomes more distended and contracts later, thus delaying the pulmonic component and splitting S_2. Splitting of S_2 is normal only in this pulmonic area; it is pathologic elsewhere.*

minished S_2: pulmonic stenosis (congenital or acquired), atrial septal defect, A_2 sometimes absent in aortic stenosis. *Widened Inspiratory Splitting of P_2:* delayed closure of pulmonic valve, right-bundle-branch block, atrial septal defect; pulmonic stenosis, early closure of aortic valve, mitral regurgitation. *Expiratory Splitting of P_2:* Left-bundle-branch block, aortic stenosis, pulmonary hypertension, atrial septal defect. *Reversed or Paradoxic Splitting of A_2:* delay of A_2 will cause this in idiopathic hypertrophic subaortic stenosis, valvular aortic stenosis, left bundle branch block (Fig. 6-47).

Abnormal Systolic Sounds

When systole and diastole have been identified by employing S_1 and S_2 as markers, the examiner listens for sounds in the systolic interval with the knowledge that any abnormal sound must be either *a murmur* or *a systolic click.*

Basal Systolic Murmur: ***Valvular Aortic Stenosis*** (cf. p. 378).

Basal Systolic Murmur: ***Hypertrophic Subaortic Stenosis*** (cf. p. 381).

Basal Systolic Murmur: ***Supravalvular Aortic Stenosis*** (cf. p. 382).

Basal Systolic Murmur: ***Hypertension or Atherosclerosis*** (cf. p. 382).

Basal Systolic Murmur: ***Valvular Pulmonic Stenosis*** (cf. p. 382).

Basal Systolic Murmur: ***Infundibular Pulmonic Stenosis*** (cf. p. 383).

Basal Systolic Murmur: ***Atrial Septal Defect at Ostium Secundum*** (cf. p. 383).

Basal Systolic Murmur: ***Coarctation of Aorta*** (cf. p. 385).

Basal Systolic Murmur: ***Cardiopulmonary M.*** (cf. p. 385).

Basal Systolic Murmur: ***Benign Murmurs*** (cf. p. 385).

Midprecordial Systolic Murmur: ***Ventricular Septal Defect*** (cf. p. 389).

Midprecordial Systolic Murmur: ***Tricuspid Regurgitation*** (cf. p. 389).

Apical Systolic Murmur: ***Mitral Regurgitation*** (cf. p. 390).

Apical Systolic Murmur with Midsystolic Click: ***Mitral Leaflet Prolapse*** (cf. p. 391).

Apical Systolic Murmur: ***Papillary Muscle Dysfunction*** (cf. p. 392).

Apical Systolic Murmur: ***Benign M.*** (cf. p. 385).

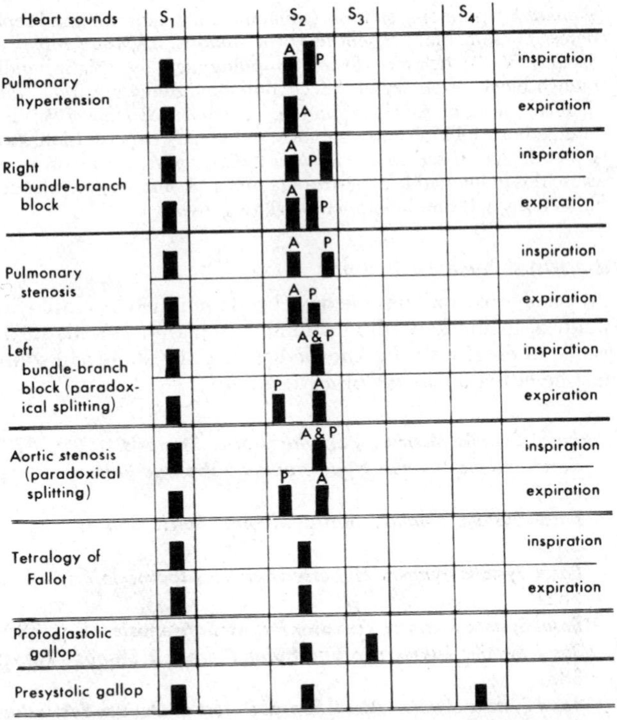

Heart sounds	S_1	S_2	S_3	S_4	
Pulmonary hypertension		A P			inspiration
		A			expiration
Right bundle-branch block		A P			inspiration
		A P			expiration
Pulmonary stenosis		A P			inspiration
		A P			expiration
Left bundle-branch block (paradox-ical splitting)		A & P			inspiration
		P A			expiration
Aortic stenosis (paradoxical splitting)		A & P			inspiration
		P A			expiration
Tetralogy of Fallot					inspiration
					expiration
Protodiastolic gallop					
Presystolic gallop					

Fig. 6-47. Pathologic variations in the heart sounds. *Pathologic splitting of the 2nd sound (S_2) is diagnostically important, because it occurs when undue stress is placed upon the pulmonic valve leaflets; so splitting occurs during expiration, and increases during inspiration. In pathologic splitting of S_2, the aortic component is so delayed that it becomes the second element of the couplet instead of the first. This explains the greater splitting during expiration. The two types of gallop rhythm are produced by augmentation to audibility of either the 3rd or 4th heart sounds (S_3 or S_4). The appearance of the protodiastolic gallop signals a grave prognosis; the presystolic gallop may also reflect abnormal physiologic change.*

Systolic Click: ***Aortic Ejection Click.*** *Pathophysiology.* A click is sometimes heard at the onset of ejection from the left ventricle. This is attributed to sudden tensing of the roots of the aorta and pulmonary artery, at the onset of ejection. In other cases the opening of the semilunar valves may cause it. *Optimal Audibility:* at the base and apex; usually louder at the apex. *Timing:* early in systole. *Respiratory Effects;* no change.

Clinical Occurrence. Dilatation of the aortic root in aneurysm of the ascending aorta; coarctation of aorta; hypertension with aortic dilatation; valvular aortic stenosis; aortic regurgitation.

Systolic Click: **Pulmonic Ejection Click.** *Pathophysiology.* This is a click at the onset of pulmonary ejection occurring when the pulmonary artery is dilated. *Optimal Audibility:* at the base of the heart in the left 2nd interspace. *Timing:* variably in systole. *Respiratory Effects:* decreases or disappears with inspiration; augmented with expiration.

Clinical Occurrence. Dilated pulmonary artery from any cause. In some cases with a loud click, the latter is fused with S_1 and the sound is interpreted as loud S_1.

Apical Late Systolic Murmur and Midsystolic Click: **Mitral Valve Prolapse** (cf. p. 391).

Clinical Occurrence: Marfan's syndrome, myxomatous changes of the mitral valve and other forms of mitral valve prolapse.

Mid- or Late Systolic Clicks: **Papillary Muscle Dysfunction.** This occurs with variable degrees of mitral regurgitation when there is transient or permanent stretching and attenuation of a papillary muscle due to myocardial ischemia or infarction and fibrosis. *Optimal Audibility:* at apex. *Timing:* mid- or late systole, sometimes at the beginning of a systolic murmur. *Respiratory Effects:* none.

Clinical Occurrence. During angina or an acute ischemic episode; following myocardial infarction.

Abnormal Diastolic Sounds

After the systolic interval has been examined, the observer should attend to the diastolic interval between S_2 and S_1, with the knowledge that sounds in this segment can be *murmurs, opening snaps, third heart sounds* (S_3), *audible* S_4, or *pericardial knocks.*

Basal Diastolic Murmur: **Aortic Regurgitation** (cf. p. 386).
Basal Diastolic Murmur: **Pulmonic Regurgitation** (cf. p. 387).

Midprecordial Diastolic Murmur: ***Coronary-Artery Stenosis*** (cf. p. 387).
Midprecordial Diastolic Murmur: ***Tricuspid Stenosis*** (cf. p. 390).
Apical Diastolic Murmur: ***Mitral Stenosis*** (cf. p. 394).
Apical Diastolic Murmur: ***Secondary Mitral Stenosis*** (cf. p. 395).

Diastolic Snap: ***Mitral Opening Snap.*** *Pathophysiology.* In mitral stenosis, when the left intraventricular pressure drops to equality with the atrial pressure, the AV valve ring starts descending, but the descent is suddenly stopped, producing the snap. The diastolic rumble begins a few hundredths of a second later. *Optimal Audibility:* best at apex, but radiates to base.

Diastolic Snap: ***Tricuspid Opening Snap.*** *Pathophysiology.* Usually this is difficult to identify because it is associated with other valve involvements of rheumatic fever.

Clinical Occurrence. Rheumatic heart disease; atrial septal defect.

Diastolic Sound: ***Pericardial Knock.*** *Pathophysiology.* In constrictive pericarditis the ventricular filling stops abruptly early in diastole, producing vibrations and a sound. *Optimal Audibility:* heard widely over the precordium. *Pitch and Intensity:* high-pitched with less constriction; low-pitched with more constriction; may exceed S_1 or S_2 in loudness. *Timing:* earlier in diastole than S_3. *Respiratory Effect:* marked.

EXAMINATION FOR GALLOPS OR TRIPLE RHYTHMS. **Listen for triplets of heart sounds, resembling a horse's gallop, consisting of couplets alternating with single sounds. The couplet may be either a normal S_2 followed closely by an audible S_3, or an audible S_4 preceding a normal S_1. This calls for an accurate identification of S_1 and S_2. If the ventricular rate is less than 90/min, listening at the base will furnish a loud S_2 that should be unmistakable. At the apex, the louder sound is likely to be S_1. If the heart rate exceeds 90/min, Levine and Harvey advise vagus stimulation by momentary carotid pressure. Analysis is possible during the brief ensuing bradycardia.**

Early Diastole: ***Audible Third Heart Sound (S_3)*** (Ventricular or Protodiastolic Gallop). An audible S_3 closely follows S_2 in early diastole at the transition from the rapid phase of ventricular filling to the slow filling phase as the left ventricular septum and posterior free wall reach the limits of diastolic excursion. The resulting reverberations of ventricular muscle and blood mass cause the sound. *Optimal Audibility:* Best heard at the apex with the patient lying on his left side, in a quiet room. *Respiratory Effect:* Expiration augments. Accentuated by exercise, abdominal pressure, or flexing the knees upon the abdomen.

Clinical Occurrence. Normal in children and young adults. Serious in older persons where it indicates myocardial dysfunction, with increased LV filling pressure and elevated pressure in the left atrium. Less serious, when caused by diastolic overload in anemia, thyrotoxicosis, and atrioventricular shunts.

Late Diastole: ***Audible Fourth Heart Sound (S_4)*** (Atrial Sound; Presystolic or Atrial Gallop). *Pathophysiology:* An audible S_4 may be caused by vibrations of the left ventricular muscle, the mitral valve apparatus, and the LV flow tract. *Timing:* Occurs after atrial contraction but before S_1. Audibility is said to be frequent. It reflects a decrease in ventricular compliance.

Clinical Occurrence. Often heard in normal persons; also in aortic stenosis, subaortic stenosis, hypertension, coronary artery disease as in acute ischemia or infarction, myocardiopathy, anemia, hyperthyroidism, AV fistula.

Diastolic: ***Audible S_3 and S_4*** (Summation Gallop, Mesodiastolic Gallop). The sounds are so close together that they may give the impression of a single sound or a rumbling murmur. Vagus stimulation by carotid pressure may slow the rate enough to distinguish four sounds per cycle.

Pancyclic Sounds

Basal Continuous Murmur: ***Patent Ductus Arteriosus*** (cf. p. 388).

Midprecordial Continuous Murmur: ***Coronary Arteriovenous Fistula***, or ***Ruptured Aortic Sinus Aneurysm*** (cf. p. 393).

Extracardiac Sounds

Because they are relatively uncommon and are heard in the precordial region, the extracardiac sounds are very often mistaken for murmurs unless their quality differs so widely from the usual murmur that no similarity exists. Once the possibility is considered, the distinctions can usually be found.

The conclusive difference is that extracardiac sounds *are not strictly synchronous* with a specific part of the cardiac cycle.

Systolic and Diastolic: **Pericardial Friction Rub.** *Pathophysiology.* The sound arises from rubbing together of two dry pericardial surfaces that have lost their lubrication from an inflammatory process. This definition does not preclude the existence of rubs with a pericardial effusion; the effusion often does not cover the entire pericardial sac. *Optimum Audibility:* Have the patient prone and listen at the precordium during deep expiration. When the sound is not immediately heard, have the patient move to another position. *Pitch and Intensity:* usually the sound is high-pitched, like two pieces of leather rubbing together. Often the sound is scratchy, grating, rasping, or squeaky. *Timing:* The sound may be present during the entire cardiac cycle; usually it is not restricted to systole or diastole; often it is inconstant. Through the stethoscope the sounds seem closer to the ear than murmurs.

Clinical Occurrence. Infectious pericarditis; the tissue adjacent to a myocardial infarction; after cardiac surgery; in uremia; rarely in pulmonary infarction.

Systolic and Diastolic: **Mediastinal Crunch** (Hamman's sign). *Pathophysiology.* Pneumothorax may give rise to a sound in the mediastinum from air bubbles in the tissues. *Optimal Audibility:* near the precordium and over the mediastinum. *Pitch and Intensity:* a crunchy sound, usually rather loud. *Timing:* at random, or synchronized with the heart beat. *Distinction:* the quality of the sound is unique. It is best heard when the patient is in the left lateral recumbent position. There may be palpation crepitus in the supraclavicular fossae.

Clinical Occurrence. Pneumothorax from trauma or cardiac surgery.

Systolic and Diastolic: **Venous Hum** (Humming Top Murmur; *bruit de diable*). *Pathophysiology.* High velocity flow in the internal jugular veins, especially the right, produces vibrations in the tissues that are heard as sound. *Optimal Audibility:* usually in both supraclavicular fossae, often in the 2nd and 3rd interspaces near the sternum. *Pitch and Intensity:* low-pitched hum throughout the cardiac cycle with frequent augmentation during diastole. It is intensified by having the patient sit or stand. *Respiratory Effect:* none. *Distinction:* the hum is readily abolished by light pressure on the jugular veins beside the trachea. The hum is frequently mistaken for an intracardiac murmur.

Clinical Occurrence. Some normal children and adults; thyrotoxicosis; anemia (a combination of venous hum and intracranial bruit suggests the presence of intracranial malformations).

AUSCULTATION OF THE HEART SOUNDS. **When the stethoscope is applied to the precordium, one hears pairs of sounds that follow in endless series. As previously indicated, the first task is to diagnose the rhythm. Then attention is directed toward the individual sounds. *Positive identification* of the first and second sounds must first be made, because they serve as audible markers of the beginning and ending of cardiac systole. When an apical impulse is visible or palpable, the sound synchronous with it is the first sound; this is the best association to make. In the absence of an apical impulse, the carotid pulse wave may be palpated, realizing that there is a perceptible interval between cardiac systole and the arrival of the resulting wave in the neck. If the ventricular rate is less than 100, the diastolic interval is longer than the systolic, so the first sound can be accepted as the first of the pair. When identification of the heart sounds or timing of murmurs is difficult because the tones are muffled or the rate is fast, *slow the heart* for a few beats by having the patient take a deep breath, or *massage* either carotid sinus. The initial sound after a long pause must be the first sound followed by a systolic interval (S. A. Levine and V. S. Mathur). Finally, at the base of the heart the second sound is almost invariably louder than the first. The radial pulse should never be used in timing because it is too far removed from the heart in distance and time, so it is misleading. When the two heart sounds have been identified at the base, the stethoscope should be moved short distances toward the apex, called *inching*, tracing each sound through changes in intensity and quality, identifying them in each of the classic valve areas.**

During another journey of the stethoscope over the precordium from base to apex, attention should be directed toward the *intensity* of the two sounds, whether they are accentuated or diminished as compared to norms established by experience in examining normal hearts.

In a third precordial journey, one should note the *duration* of the first sound and the *splitting* of the second sound during *inspiration* and *expiration*. In examining for duration and splitting, one should think of the typical heart sound as being the shortest sound that can be perceived; any sound that exceeds this must be either pro-

longed, split, or a murmur. Prolonged sounds can be differentiated from murmurs by their abrupt beginning and ending, where murmurs have gradual onset and end. A sound that begins abruptly but ends gradually is probably a heart sound followed by a murmur.

Cardiac Murmurs

Normal blood flows silently at normal velocity through normal vessels. Audible murmurs result from vibrations set up by vortices developing near the mural interfaces of the bloodstream after it passes an obstruction or dilatation (vortex-shedding theory). For a model, attach two feet (60 cm) of pliable rubber tubing to a laboratory water faucet. Palpate the tubing with the thumb and finger on one hand and turn on the water with the other. A velocity can be attained that will not vibrate the walls of the tubing, because the flow is laminar and smooth. With this velocity, constricting the tubing slightly with the fingers will cause vibrations in the distal part. Or, with no constriction, increase the velocity until the tubing vibrates. One can also demonstrate that a less viscous fluid, such as alcohol, will set up vibrations at less velocity than water. In a normal heart, murmurs may be induced when the velocity of normal blood is *increased* by exercise or thyrotoxicosis, a *flow murmur.* In anemia, blood with *lessened viscosity* may produce murmurs at normal velocity. Normal blood flowing over *abnormal obstruction* or through *unusual openings* in the circulation sets up turbulence and collision currents that result in murmurs. Trained observation of these murmurs for their location, pitch, and relations to the cardiac cycle can lead to remarkably accurate diagnoses of the anatomic derangements within the heart and vessels.

Systolic murmurs are described chronologically according to the part of the systolic interval in which they occur, as *early systolic* (or *protosystolic*), *midsystolic,* and *late systolic.* When the murmur occupies the entire systole it is termed *pansystolic* (or *holosystolic*). Leatham has taught us a more interpretive classification of systolic murmurs by associating the configuration of the murmurs with the pressure relations that produce them. When vibrations are set up by forcing blood from regions of high pressure to those initially low but rising, *ejection murmurs* are produced. An example is aortic stenosis where the murmur starts soon after the first sound, intensifies to a maximum at midsystole, and tapers off to disappear before the second sound when the intraventricular pressure equals that in the aorta before diastole begins. In contrast, *regurgitant murmurs* occur when blood leaks continuously from a high-pressure region to one of low pressure during systole, producing a pansystolic murmur of almost uniform intensity. This is typified in mitral regurgitation. With these criteria it is possible to distinguish many of the systolic murmurs of organic disease from those occurring only in early systole, midsystole, or late systole that are of little significance and are called *benign* (or functional, innocent, accidental, physiologic, nonpathologic).

Diastolic murmurs are practically always pathologic. Chronologically, they are classified as *early diastolic* (protodiastolic), *middiastolic,* and *presystolic* (late diastolic). Nearly all diastolic regurgitant murmurs are prolonged because the pressure in the great vessels remains higher than that in the ventricles during their entire relaxation. The ejection diastolic murmur of mitral stenosis does not start with the onset of diastole because pressure in the ventricle must fall before becoming less than that in the atrium.

The quality of murmurs is of some diagnostic value. Ventricular filling murmurs are relatively *low-pitched* because they are produced by blood flowing under relatively little pressure, while blood flowing through narrow orifices under higher pressure causes *high-pitched* murmurs.

AUSCULTATION OF CARDIAC MURMURS. **Search for cardiac murmurs only after the heart sounds have been positively identified, so they may be employed as audible markers for the onset and ending of systole. Decide whether a sound of abnormal length is a split heart sound or a heart sound and murmur. Now turn your attention to the systolic interval between the first sound and the second. Decide whether there is any audible sound in this interval, using the assumption that a heart sound is the shortest perceptible sound; anything appreciably longer may be heart sound and murmur. In such a combination, remember that a heart sound *begins and ends abruptly.* A prolonged sound starting abruptly and dwindling is probably a heart sound followed by murmur; one developing gradually and ending abruptly is likely murmur and heart sound. Carefully examine each valve area on the precordium with *both bell and diaphragm* chestpieces of the stethoscope. Cover the intervening space on the precordium by *inching.* Once the presence of a murmur is established, ascertain the following characteristics:**

***Timing:* Determine in what part of the cardiac cycle the murmur**

occurs and whether it is early, middle, or late in the interval, by reference to the first and second heart sounds.

Location: **Ascertain at what point on the precordium the murmur exhibits maximum intensity. Several scales are in use; we recommend Levin's with six gradations: *Grade 1,* barely audible with greatest difficulty; *Grade 6,* so loud is can be heard with the stethoscope off the chest; *Grade 2,* just easily audible; *Grade 5,* loudest requiring a stethoscope; *Grades 3* and *4,* intermediate. The recording of Grade 3, for example, should be *Grade 3/6* to show the scale of 6 is being used.**

Pattern or Configuration: **Decide whether the murmur is uniform in intensity throughout, whether the pitch increases, *crescendo,* or diminishes, *decrescendo* or *diminuendo.* The term *diamond-shaped* murmur is taken from the graphic representation on the screen of the phonocardiograph; the maximum intensity is midsystolic with crescendo preceding and diminuendo following the apex (Fig. 6-48).**

Pitch: **Determine whether the murmur is high-pitched or low-pitched. To the inexperienced and nonmusical, the simplest method is to find whether the murmur is heard better with the bell chestpiece (low-pitched) or the diaphragm (high-pitched). Last but important, ask the question of whether the pitch seems more like a murmur or a pericardial friction rub. The latter, being rare, is frequently misdiagnosed as a murmur; the only distinction is by the quality of the sound. In using the bell chestpiece, press it very *lightly* on the skin; heavy pressure stretches the skin taut to form a diaphragm that filters out low-pitched sounds, leaving only those of higher pitch. The diaphragm should be pressed *firmly* against the skin.**

Posture and Exercise: **When possible, the heart should be auscultated in both the supine and erect positions. In addition, the left lateral position of the patient should be employed, with the precordium downward, to demonstrate certain murmurs, especially the presystolic murmur of mitral stenosis. Exercise sometimes brings out otherwise inaudible murmurs.**

After the systolic interval has been thoroughly explored, turn the attention to the diastolic interval; carry out the same procedures and ask the same questions.

Basal Systolic Murmur: ***Valvular Aortic Stenosis*** (Fig. 6-49C). The lesion may be symptomless until constriction of the orifice is severe; then exercise induces *dyspnea, anginal pain,* or *syncope.* *Murmur.* Classically the murmur is heard in the 2nd *right* interspace, but almost as often it is audible along the *left* sternal border in the 3rd and 4th interspaces. In about

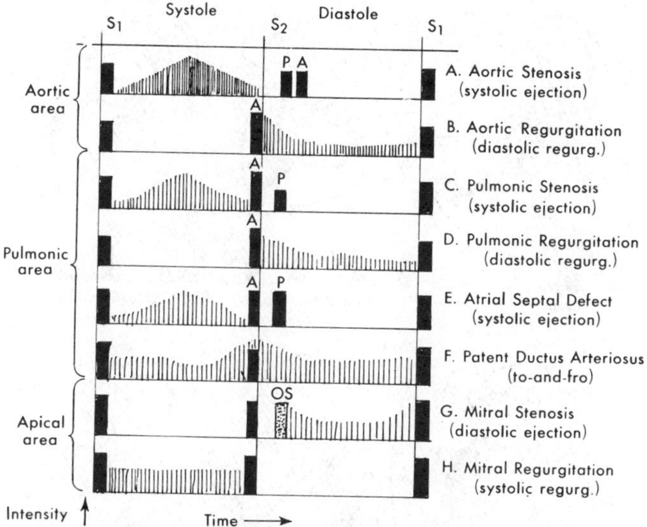

Fig. 6-48. Common pathologic heart murmurs. *The diagrams are drawn to represent intensity of the heart sounds and murmurs on the vertical axis and duration on the horizontal axis. The exceptionally low-pitched murmur is depicted by widely spaced shading. "A" and "P" refer to the aortic and pulmonic components of the 2nd sound (S_2); "OS" indicates the opening snap of the mitral valve in mitral stenosis. Note that the systolic ejection murmurs are inaudible at either end of systole and attain maximum intensity at midsystole (in this diagram they form the upper halves of "diamond-shaped" figures of the phonocardiogram). The systolic regurgitant murmurs are pansystolic. The configuration of the diastolic ejection murmur of mitral stenosis terminates in a crescendo caused by superimposition of atrial contraction. Although the diastolic regurgitant murmurs are pandiastolic, in aortic and pulmonic regurgitation the late diastolic part is seldom heard.*

15% of cases, it is loudest at the apex. Regardless of the point of maximal intensity, it is transmitted *to the carotid arteries*. Loud murmurs are often accompanied by *systolic thrills* over the base and in the carotids. It is a typical *ejection murmur* with onset a short interval after the 1st sound, during the rise of the intraventricular pressure; it ceases *before* the 2nd sound, when the intraventricular pressure falls below aortic pressure. Its con-

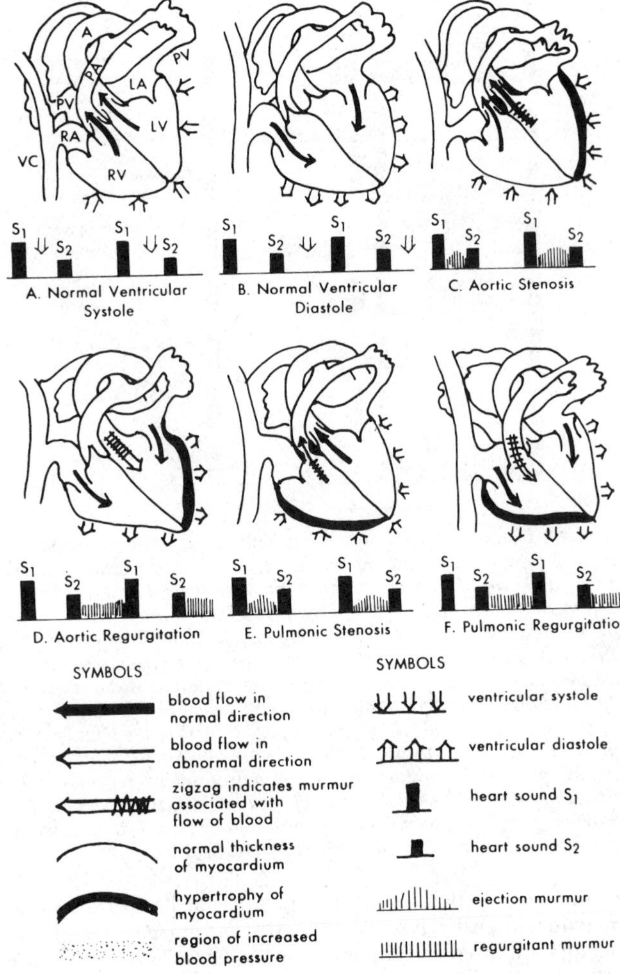

Fig. 6-49. Anatomic bases for cardiac murmurs I.

figuration in the phonocardiogram furnishes the murmur with its description of *diamond-shaped;* the first half *rises* in pitch, *crescendo,* the remainder falls in pitch, *diminuendo* or *decrescendo* (Fig. 6-48). The murmur is usually *medium-pitched,* so it is audible with either the bell or the diaphragm chestpiece. Although usually *harsh,* occasionally it has a peculiar quality that prompts the term *seagull murmur,* like the call of a gull or the cooing of a dove. *Heart Sounds.* In moderate or severe stenosis, A_2 *is diminished* or *absent.* During expiration, P_2 may be split, called *paradoxical splitting,* from delayed closure of the aortic valve that furnishes a component of the 2nd sound (p. 368). Often the murmur is preceded by an *ejection click* made by the opening snap of the aortic valve; this disappears when the valve becomes calcified. The 4th heart sound is frequently audible, producing a *presystolic gallop.* *Precordial Thrust.* Hypertrophy of the left ventricle produces an *accentuated precordial apical thrust.* In the left lateral recumbent position a *double (bifid) apical thrust* is sometimes felt; the first impact comes from atrial contraction, the second from left ventricular systole. *Arterial Pulse.* Occlusion of more than 75% of the orifice produces a *plateau pulse* (p. 406) and diminished pulse pressure. A decrease in the rate of rise as well as a decrease in amplitude is often perceptible. In tight aortic stenosis *pulsus bisferiens* may be present. *X-ray Findings.* Calcification of the aortic valve may be seen on the films. *Distinction.* The systolic murmurs of hypertension or atherosclerosis are accompanied by normal heart sounds at the base; the murmurs are not transmitted to the carotids. The *apical* systolic murmur of aortic stenosis is *diamond-shaped;* but the murmur of mitral regurgitation is *pansystolic* or *holosystolic* and the basal heart sounds are normal. The apical systolic murmur from calcific aortic stenosis is *intensified* and *prolonged* during inhalation of amyl nitrite; this distinguishes it from the murmur of mitral regurgitation. An apical systolic diamond-shaped murmur may occur in valvular aortic stenosis or hypertrophic subaortic stenosis (see latter).

Clinical Occurrence. Rheumatic valvulitis, calcific disease of the aortic valve, congenital anomalies.

Basal Systolic Murmur: ***Hypertrophic Subaortic Stenosis.*** The lesion results from hypertrophy of the left ventricle and the interventricular septum: this obstructs the outflow tract *intermit-*

tently. Males are more often affected; sometimes a familial incidence is suggested by many unexplained sudden deaths in the kindred. The condition should be suspected when the signs of aortic stenosis are atypical. A *systolic ejection murmur* is heard along the left sternal border and the apex, rather than in the *right* 2nd interspace and the carotids. In contrast to the plateau pulse of valvular stenosis, the arterial pulse wave has a *sharp upstroke*. Pulsus bisferiens is often present. As in valvular stenosis, a *presystolic gallop* is frequent. *Absence* of a systolic ejection click is distinctive in subaortic stenosis. Unlike fixed valvular stenosis, the symptoms and signs *vary* because of the differing effects of changes in peripheral resistance and the influence of inotropic agents. The outflow obstruction and consequent signs are *intensified* by exercise, the Valsalva maneuver, or the administration of nitroglycerin, digitalis, or isoproterenol. The diagnosis is confirmed by cardiac catheterization or echocardiography.

Basal Systolic Murmur: ***Supravalvular Aortic Stenosis.*** A rare congenital anomaly, this is the result of narrowing of the ascending aorta, or a small-holed diaphragm distal to the valve. It produces most of the signs of valvular stenosis, but A_2 *is accentuated* and the *carotid murmurs* are *unusually loud*. The diagnosis is confirmed by cardiac catheterization.

Basal Systolic Murmur: ***Hypertension or Atherosclerosis.*** A murmur of medium pitch and moderate intensity is frequently heard in the aortic region of persons with hypertension or arteriosclerosis. It may be transmitted to the apex. It is never as loud as some murmurs of aortic stenosis. The basal heart sounds are not diminished. The murmur may be faintly heard in the carotids. *Pathophysiology.* The murmur may be caused by tortuosity or dilatation of the aorta or by arteriosclerotic plaques. *Distinction.* Loud murmurs of aortic stenosis are easily excluded, because the arteriosclerotic type is seldom loud. Normal heart sounds at the base are incompatible with stenosis.

Clinical Occurrence. Arteriosclerosis.

Basal Systolic Murmur: ***Valvular Pulmonic Stenosis*** (Fig. 6-49E). Maximal in the 2nd left interspace, this murmur is otherwise similar to that of aortic stenosis in intensity, configuration, and pitch. Transmission may be into the carotids, the left side more than the right. The P_2 is widely split (Fig. 6-48C) but difficult to bear. Commonly there is an *ejection click;* its presence distinguishes the lesion as valvular rather than infundibular pulmonic stenosis. Right ventricular hypertrophy is indicated by an accentuated precordial thrust in the area of projection of the right ventricle, but is not often detectable if there is concentric hypertrophy without dilatation. *Pathophysiology.* This is a systolic ejection murmur with diamond-shaped contour. The delayed ejection through the pulmonic orifice delays or abolishes the pulmonic component of the second heart sound. *Distinction.* The murmur is usually higher pitched than that of an atrial septal defect.

Clinical Occurrence. Congenital, singly or in the tetralogy of Fallot; acquired carcinoid tumor.

Basal Systolic Murmur: ***Infundibular Pulmonic Stenosis.*** The funnel-shaped portion of the right ventricular chamber that leads to the pulmonary artery is the *infundibulum.* Congenital narrowing of the funnel produces a form of pulmonic stenosis. In contrast to valvular stenosis, the ejection murmur and the systolic thrill are usually *in the 3rd left interspace* and there is *no ejection click.* Although this lesion may be isolated, it is usually accompanied by a ventricular septal defect, as in the tetralogy of Fallot.

Basal Systolic Murmur: ***Atrial Septal Defect at the Ostium Secundum*** (Fig. 6-50A). A medium-pitched murmur is nearly always heard in the 2nd or 3rd left interspace. The configuration frequently resembles that of pulmonic stenosis with maximum intensity a little before midsystole (Fig. 6-48E). P_2 is widely split. *Pathophysiology.* The systolic murmur is produced when the blood courses with high velocity through the pulmonary artery from an overfilled right ventricle. The pulmonary outflow tract murmur is sometimes accompanied by a low-pitched diastolic flow murmur heard along the lower left sternal border, resulting from increased flow through the tricuspid valve. *Distinction.* Sometimes the murmur is indistinguishable from that of pulmonic stenosis, but the murmur usually attains maximum earlier in systole and is lower pitched, leaving a longer pause before the second sound. The murmur rarely becomes very loud, in contrast to that in pulmonic stenosis. The degree of splitting of P_2 is the same during inspiration and expiration; the split is wide and fixed.

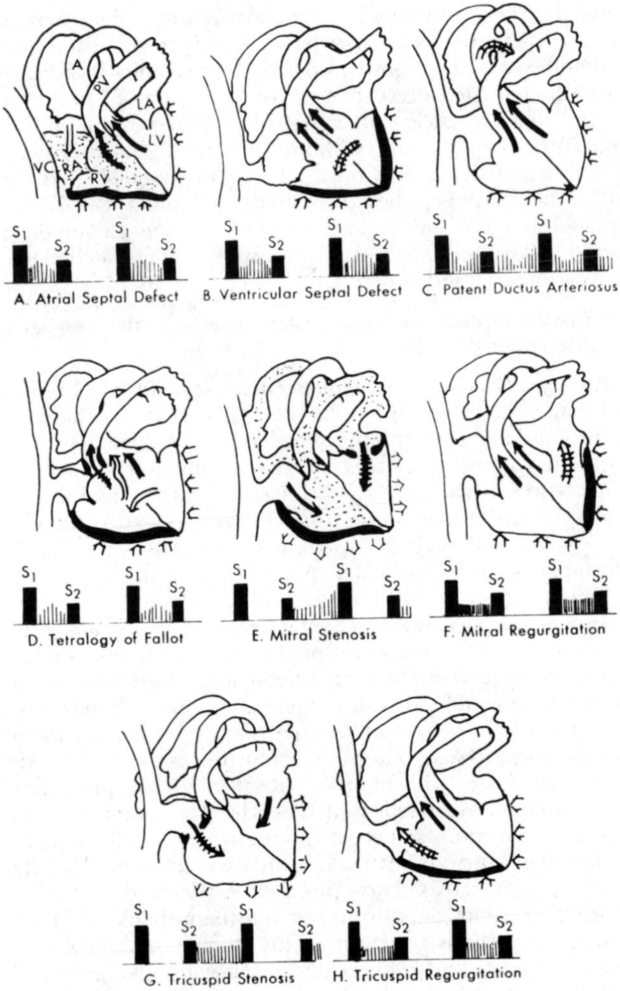

A. Atrial Septal Defect

B. Ventricular Septal Defect

C. Patent Ductus Arteriosus

D. Tetralogy of Fallot

E. Mitral Stenosis

F. Mitral Regurgitation

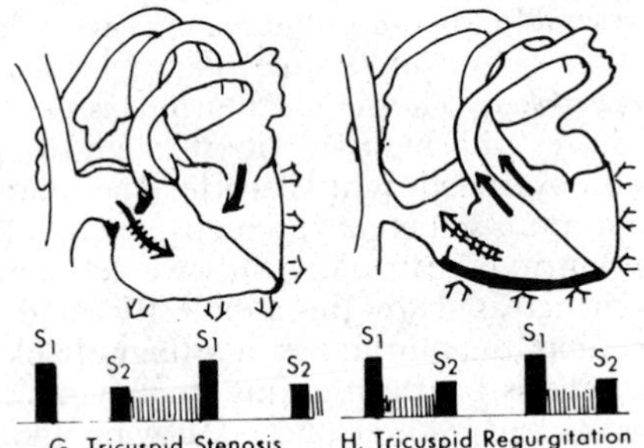

G. Tricuspid Stenosis

H. Tricuspid Regurgitation

Fig. 6-50. Anatomic basis for cardiac murmurs II. (*Same symbols as in Fig. 6-49.*)

Clinical Occurrence. Congenital.

Basal Systolic Murmur: ***Coarctation of Aorta.*** When audible anteriorly, this murmur is faint and maximal in either the left or right 2nd interspace. Usually, it is heard much better over the thoracic spine. A continuous bruit can sometimes be heard over the sternum from the dilated internal mammary arteries. When the back is not routinely auscultated for murmurs, the condition is first suggested by finding *diminished* or *absent femoral pulses*. Palpable pulsations of the intercostal arteries in the posterior thorax confirm the diagnosis. *Pathophysiology.* The most common site of coarctation is just distal to the origin of the left subclavian artery, so the circulation to the head and arms is not affected. The pulse waves in the distal aorta and its branches are impaired; this is most easily discovered by routinely palpating the femoral arteries when examining the abdomen. The collateral circulation develops through the internal mammary and the intercostal arteries (Fig. 6-69, p. 448). The latter become dilated enough to be palpated in the intercostal spaces in the back of the thorax and produce notching in the inferior rib margins posteriorly, visible in x-ray films. The site of constriction is remote from the precordium, so the murmur is faintly heard, if at all, on the anterior chest.

Clinical Occurrence. Congenital.

Basal Systolic Murmur: ***Cardiopulmonary.*** Occasionally a faint systolic sound resembling a murmur may be heard along the heart borders during inspiration. It disappears during expiration or when the breath is held. *Pathophysiology.* This is ascribed to the air being forcefully expelled from the margins of the inflated lung by pulsations of the heart.

Clinical Occurrence. Not significant except that it must be distinguished from a true murmur.

Basal Systolic Murmur: ***Benign Murmurs*** (Innocent, Physiologic, Functional, Nonpathologic). Many names are employed. Most common in the second left interspace, they are characterized as medium-pitched and generally grade 1 or 2, although occasionally louder. Usually they are short, occurring early, in the middle, or late in systole. When maximal in the 2nd interspace, they are infrequently transmitted to the neck. The

P_2 is always normal. They are best heard in the supine position and tend to disappear sitting or standing. Have the patient sit upright with the shoulders back. The murmur may persist if the patient sits in a "slouched" position. *Pathophysiology.* Some authors believe that most are produced by increases in velocity or decreases in viscosity of the blood. *Distinction.* Their short duration without accompanying changes in the heart sounds assists to distinguish these murmurs from those of organic disease.

Clinical Occurrence. In anemia, fever, emotional disturbances, exercise, thyrotoxicosis, pregnancy. In about 50% of normal children.

Basal Systolic Murmur: ***Benign Thoracic Outlet Bruit.*** Most common in well-developed, muscular young men, this systolic bruit is maximal in the supraclavicular fossa. It is usually heard in the first right intercostal space as well, but attenuates as the so-called aortic area is approached. It may also radiate to the right carotid. Manipulation of the shoulder during auscultation may modify the bruit. It has no clinical significance but has been confused with aortic stenosis.

Basal Diastolic Murmur: ***Aortic Regurgitation*** (Fig. 6-49D). This is a high-pitched blowing murmur, heard best with the diaphragm of the stethoscope held firmly against the chest wall. The point of maximum intensity is in either the 2nd right interspace or the 3rd left. Transmission down the right rather than the left sternal border should suggest aneurysmal dilatation of the aortic root. The first heart sound is usually normal; A_2 is often accentuated. The murmur immediately follows the second sound and exhibits a rapid diminuendo during the first third or so of diastole; it recedes to inaudibility or is pandiastolic at very low intensity (Fig. 6-48B). When faint, the murmur is best heard with the patient leaning forward. Usually, there is an accompanying aortic systolic murmur. Accentuation of the precordial apical thrust indicates the accompanying left ventricular hypertrophy and dilatation. Usually there are signs of vasodilatation, high pulse pressure, and pistol-shot sounds. *Pathophysiology.* The murmur is typically diastolic regurgitant. The diminuendo from the beginning is caused by the high initial pressure in the aorta at the initiation of ventricular diastole; this also causes the accentuated A_2. The high pitch is caused by blood being forced through a relatively small orifice at high pressure. ***Distinction.*** The quality and location of the murmur in the 2nd right interspace cannot distinguish it from the murmur of pulmonic regurgitation, but the maximal intensity in the aortic area, an accentuated precordial apical thrust, increased pulse pressure with a Corrigan pulse, pulsus bisferiens, and Duroziez's sign, all favor the diagnosis of aortic regurgitation.

Clinical Occurrence. Rheumatic valvulitis, syphilis of the aorta, ruptured valve leaflet from bacterial endocarditis. Marfan's syndrome, dissecting aorta, aneurysm of the sinus of Valsalva, annular ectasia of the aorta (diastolic murmur often most prominent in *right* parasternal region).

Basal Diastolic Murmur: ***Pulmonic Regurgitation*** (Fig. 6-49F). This is frequently termed the *Graham Steell murmur*. It is indistinguishable in quality and timing from the murmur of aortic regurgitation (Fig. 6-48D). It is usually less loud and is transmitted less widely than the aortic murmur. The point of maximum intensity is usually in the 2nd or 3rd left interspace. The P_2 may be accentuated. A precordial thrust of the right ventricle may be palpated. ***Pathophysiology.*** This is practically always caused by dilation of the ring of the pulmonic valve by hypertension in the pulmonary circuit. ***Distinction.*** Usually the diagnosis is made by the absence of peripheral signs of aortic regurgitation.

Clinical Occurrence. Pulmonary hypertension from mitral stenosis, left-sided heart failure, pulmonary emphysema, idiopathic pulmonary hypertension, congenital heart lesions.

Midprecordial Diastolic Murmur: ***Coronary-Artery Stenosis.*** Phonocardiography and coronary arteriography have proved that a stenotic coronary artery can produce an audible diastolic murmur of diagnostic significance. The physical findings in two patients may prove typical [T. O. Cheng: Diastolic Murmur Caused by Coronary Artery Stenosis, *Ann. Intern. Med.*, **72:**543–46, 1970]. Both men had *exertional angina pectoris*. In both the examiner heard a high-pitched, *middiastolic murmur, crescendo-diminuendo,* at the left 4th intercostal space, sharply localized to the sternal border; S_1 was accentuated. S_4 was audible in both (atrial gallop rhythm). In both, the diastolic murmur *decreased in intensity* after the inhalation of amyl nitrite. Coronary arteriography showed stenosis in the anterior descending branch of both left coronary arteries. In both, the murmurs disappeared with the onset of myocardial infarction. *Distinction.* Middiastolic murmurs with accentuated S_1 occur in both mitral stenosis and coronary artery stenosis; but the coronary murmur is high-pitched while the mitral murmur is low-pitched. The valvular murmur is diminuendo-crescendo, the reverse sequence of the coronary murmur. An audible S_4 was heard in both cases of coronary stenosis; such a finding is incompatible with mitral stenosis. The inhalation of amyl nitrite augments the intensity of the mitral murmur, but diminishes the loudness of the coronary murmur.

Basal Continuous Murmur: ***Patent Ductus Arteriosus*** (Fig. 6-50C). A murmur heard continuously throughout systole and diastole in the 2nd or 3rd left interspace is typically caused by a patent ductus. Usually there is a crescendo late in systole and a diminuendo after the second sound, producing a *machinery murmur* (Fig. 6-48F). Sometimes the noise runs from first sound to first sound, with a second sound buried in the crescendo. Frequently there is a short pause between the first sound and the onset of the murmur. Occasionally the murmur is transmitted down the left sternal border; sometimes it can be heard at the apex. Most frequently, transmission is to the interscapular region. The murmur is medium-pitched and rumbling, heard with either bell or diaphragm. Louder murmurs are harsh. Shunts of considerable degree produce accompanying diastolic murmurs at the apex from high flow through the mitral valve, Corrigan pulse with wide pulse pressure, and pansystolic murmurs in the tricuspid area. The precordial thrust of both the right and left ventricles may be accentuated. *Pathophysiology.* A patent ductus is a variety of arteriovenous fistula, except that the leak is between an arterial circuit of high pressure and an arterial system of lesser pressure. If the leak is large, the peripheral pulse wave may be the collapsing variety encountered in aortic regurgitation. The continuous murmur results from blood flowing into the lesser pressure region of the pulmonary circuit during the entire cycle, with greater pressure during ventricular systole and a consequent higher pitch to the murmur. Tricuspid regurgitation may develop from the pulmonary hypertension. The increased volume of left-sided flow through the mitral orifice may produce a diastolic rumble simulating mitral stenosis. The pressures may be modified by the presence of other congenital anomalies. *Distinction.* When the diastolic component of the murmur is absent because of pulmonary hypertension or other reasons, the condition can be distinguished from pulmonic stenosis only by cardiac catheterization. The continuous murmur should be distinguished from a venous hum in the internal jugular vein; the sound in the vein is abolished by digital compression of the vein.

Clinical Occurrence. Congenital.

Midprecordial Systolic Murmur: ***Ventricular Septal Defect*** (Fig. 6-50B). The uncomplicated type of this lesion is called *Roger's disease.* The high membranous defects are more common than the ones in the muscular septum. Typically the murmur is pansystolic with peak intensity in midsystole. The pitch is high, heard with the diaphragm firmly pressed. Usually maximum intensity is found in the 3rd or 4th left interspace. Loud murmurs are accompanied by thrills. When the defect is large, P_2 may be accentuated. The murmur may be transmitted over the entire precordium and to the interscapular region. With the development of pulmonary hypertension, the intensity and harshness of the murmur diminish. *Pathophysiology.* The murmur has the diamond-shaped configuration of a typical ejection systolic murmur because the blood flows at high pressure through a relatively small opening into a region of much lower pressure. The midsystolic accentuation is lost when right ventricular pressure is augmented in pulmonary hypertension. *Distinction.* In the presence of pulmonary hypertension, ventricular septal defect may require cardiac catherization or imaging techniques to be distinguished from patent ductus arteriosus in which the diastolic murmur has been lost because of high pulmonic pressure. Faint murmurs must be distinguished from benign systolic murmurs.

Clinical Occurrence. Singly and in the syndromes of Eisenmenger and Fallot.

Midprecordial Systolic Murmur: ***Tricuspid Regurgitation*** (Fig. 6-50H). The point of maximum intensity is nearly always near the left sternal border at its inferior end. It may be sharply localized or transmitted to the apex. Faint murmurs are *early systolic;* loud ones are heard throughout systole. The pitch is high, the quality harsh, heard best with the diaphragm firmly pressed. *Inspiration makes the murmur audible or accentuates it.* There are no characteristic changes in the heart sounds. Right ventricular hypertrophy may be present as shown by a palpable right ventricular precordial thrust. In severe grades of tricuspid insufficiency, striking engorgement of the neck veins and a pulsating liver may occur. *Pathophysiology.* This is a systolic regurgitant murmur in which the blood flows out of the ventricle during the entire systolic interval. Flow is accentuated during inspiration. *Distinction.* The location of maximum intensity and the effect of inspiration are characteristic and diagnostic.

Clinical Occurrence: ACQUIRED: rheumatic valvulitis, right-sided cardiac failure from any cause, pulmonary infarction. CONGENITAL. Ebstein's deformity of the tricuspid valve.

Midprecordial Diastolic Murmur: ***Tricuspid Stenosis*** (Fig. 6-50G). The murmur is low-pitched, rumbling, diastolic with a presystolic crescendo when atrial fibrillation is absent. It is best heard with the bell chestpiece lightly placed. The point of maximum intensity is quite sharply localized at the lower left sternal border in the 4th or 5th interspace. The first heart sound is accentuated in that region. Sometimes an opening snap of the tricuspid valve can be identified. In lesser degrees, the murmur is late diastolic; with greater degrees it also occupies middiastole and even early diastole. A diagnostic characteristic is its *accentuation with inspiration.* *Pathophysiology.* The presystolic accentuation is the result of atrial contraction. Since right ventricular filling is augmented during inspiration, the murmur becomes louder accordingly. *Distinction.* The murmur can usually be distinguished from that of mitral stenosis by its location and its accentuation during inspiration.

Clinical Occurrence. Rheumatic valvulitis, congenital heart disease, carcinoid tumor.

Apical Systolic Murmur: ***Mitral Regurgitation*** (Fig. 6-50F). A loud, high-pitched, pansystolic murmur with maximum intensity at the apex is typical (Fig. 6-48H). Fainter murmurs may occur only in early systole. The murmur begins with the first sound, which it may mask, and continues at approximately the same intensity throughout. Occasionally, an apical murmur occurs late in systole. Fainter murmurs are well localized; louder murmurs of central mitral insufficiency are transmitted to the axilla. There is little variation with the phases of respiration. No diagnostic changes occur in the heart sounds in moderate insufficiency; in extreme cases there may be splitting of S_2 with inspiration. Left ventricular hypertrophy and dilatation may be present as indicated by accentuation of the apical thrust. An increased thrust or lift at the left parasternal line may sometimes result from systolic expansion of the left atrium rather than from right ventricular dilatation and hypertrophy. A *ventricular knock* is sometimes found in severe cases, as a loud noise coming at the time of the third heart sound; it is felt as a diastolic thrust at the apex. ***Pathophysiology.*** This is the prototype of the systolic regurgitant murmur. Blood is forced backward through the mitral orifice with almost constant velocity during the entire systolic interval. In extreme degrees, the left ventricle empties prematurely, so the aortic component of the second sound is early, causing a widened splitting of the second sound. ***Distinction.*** The murmur must be distinguished from that of aortic stenosis, which is often loud at the apex, as well as at the base. The duration and quality of the murmur and comparison of murmurs at the apex and base will make differentiation possible. Benign murmurs at the apex are usually short and limited to a segment of the systolic interval; they are usually medium-pitched.

Clinical Occurrence: IMPROPER FUNCTIONING OF THE MITRAL VALVE: rheumatic valvulitis. DILATATION OF THE MITRAL VALVE RING: any condition producing left ventricular dilatation.

Apical Late Systolic Murmur after Midsystolic Click; ***Mitral Valve Leaf Prolapse.*** (Of 16 synonyms in the literature, we have selected these six for their descriptive qualities: Myxomatous Degeneration of Mitral Valve; Billowing Posterior Mitral Leaflet Syndrome; Syndrome of Balloon Deformity of Mitral Valve; Aneurysmal Protrusion of Mitral Leaflet; Ballooning Mitral Valve with Precordial Honk or Whoop; Floppy Valve Prolapse.) *Pathophysiology:* The valve undergoes myxomatous degeneration producing redundant valve tissue (especially the posterior valve) with consequent enlargement of the valve annulus and elongation of the chordae tendineae. This is believed a very common condition (6–20%), much more frequent in women. It can be inherited, probably as an autosomal dominant with reduced male expressivity. Since the leaflets and annulus become too large for the ventricle, systole causes one or more scallops of the valve leaflets to be propelled backward into the atrium and billow out. The chronic stretching weakens the leaflets and chordae to produce mitral regurgitation. *Symptoms:* Most persons are without symptoms. The minority develop *easy fatigue, shortness of breath, nonanginoid chest pain, palpitation,* or *syncope.* *Signs:* HABITUS. Usually normal. Some patients show stigmata of *Marfan's syndrome* with arachnodactylism, hyperextensible joints, ectomorph build. HEART SOUNDS. Wide splitting of S_2, and sometimes audible S_3. MURMURS. Heard best at the apex, the systolic murmur classically occurs late in systole. It is usually short and relatively high-pitched, giving the impression of a crescendo sound. It may be transmitted to the back to the left of the spine. Its quality is described as "cooing," "honking," or "whooping." It may be inaudible or so loud it can be heard away from the chest without a stethoscope. It is *louder* with the patient standing, *softer* and *shorter* with him squatting. Auscultation in the erect position after exercise may elicit a murmur that could not be heard at rest with the patient supine. CLICK OR GALLOP. A snapping or clicking sound is heard and sometimes palpated during midsystole; at the same time, a retraction of the apical region may be observed. *Diagnosis:* diagnostic signs may occur in the ECG, the echocardiogram, and the cineangiogram. *Associated Dysrhythmias:* Ventricular premature beats, paroxysmal atrial tachycardia, atrial fibrillation, sinus bradycardia, periods of sinus arrest, positional atrial flutter. *Complications:* strokes, myocardial infarction, rupture of chordae tendineae, congestive cardiac failure, endocarditis, sudden death.

Apical Systolic Murmur: ***Papillary Muscle Dysfunction.*** *After Acute Myocardial Infarction.* Injury to a papillary muscle may cause a pansystolic apical murmur of grade I-II/VI. *After Rupture of Papillary Muscle.* Suddenly a *pansystolic murmur of grade* II-IV/VI may appear; it is roughened and often accompanied by a *precordial thrill,* but massive mitral insufficiency may be associated with a surprisingly soft murmur. An *audible* S_4 is common to both situations. The ECG findings are variable and nonspecific. X-ray films of the chest may show pulmonary edema. Cardiac catheterization is usually diagnostic [R. F. DeBusk and D. C. Harrison: The Clinical Spectrum of Papillary Muscle Disease, *N. Engl. J. Med.,* **281:**1458–67, 1969]. Ultrasonic examination distinguishes such lesions.

Abrupt Loud Systolic Murmur: ***Rupture of Interventricular Septum or Papillary Muscle.*** When during the course of a myocardial infarction a sudden loud systolic murmur appears, it suggests either rupture of the interventricular septum or of a papillary muscle. In the latter prompt *massive pulmonary edema* follows. This is not like a ruptured septum in which signs of right-sided failure as well as low cardiac output with poor peripheral perfusion occur. The situation is a grave emergency and prompt diagnosis is needed. Bedside catheterization of the right heart has been done to distinguish between the two conditions [S. G. Meister and R. H. Helfant: Rapid Bedside Differentiation of Ruptured Interventricular Septum from Acute Mitral Insufficency, *N. Engl. J. Med.,* **287:**1024–25, 1972].

Midprecordial Continuous Murmur: ***Coronary Arteriovenous Fistula or Ruptured Aortic Sinus Aneurysm.*** Similar physical signs in these two conditions require a precise diagnosis by aortography. A *continuous murmur* with *late systolic accentuation* (machinery or to-and-fro) is audible at the lower portion of the sternum, on either or both sides. It is often accompanied by a *systolic* or *continuous thrill.* *Distinction.* Although the to-and-fro murmur has the same quality as that in ductus arteriosus, the location is sufficiently different to be distinctive. A midprecordial to-and-fro murmur can occur in the combination of interventricular septal defect and aortic regurgitation, but this murmur lacks the late systolic accentuation. Although a *venous hum* may be audible behind the upper sternum, its accentuation is diastolic and it is abolished by pressure on the internal jugular vein. [For further rare causes to be considered see J. C. Holmes, N. O. Fowler, and J. A. Helmsworth: Coronary Arteriovenous Fistula and Aortic Sinus Aneurysm Rupture, *Arch. Intern. Med.,* **118:**43, 1966.]

Apical Systolic Murmurs: ***Benign Murmurs.*** Although heard at the apex, these murmurs are usually louder near the sternal border in the 3rd and 4th left interspaces. They are low-pitched, heard best with the bell held lightly. Generally they are shorter than organic murmurs; they are never pansystolic but may occur during any third of the systolic interval. Often they are better heard when the patient is supine. *Pathophysiology.* Unknown. See also p. 376.

Clinical Occurrence. Very frequent in normal children; common in normal adults. Some late apical systolic murmurs are produced by mitral regurgitation.

Apical Diastolic Murmur: ***Mitral Stenosis*** (Fig. 6-60F). This murmur is heard best in the supine position; it should not be excluded until proved absent when the patient is in the left lateral position. It is usually sharply localized to an area near the apex; the diameter of the area may be critical, so that the bell must be placed directly on it to hear the murmur; only by carefully inching the bell over the entire apex can a loud murmur sometimes be discovered. The murmur is *low-pitched* and *rumbling*, sometimes only heard with the bell held lightly. The sound may resemble the roll of a drum. In early stenosis, the murmur occurs in middiastole; as the orifice narrows, the murmur starts earlier and ends later, until it almost covers the diastolic interval, but there is always a *pause* after the second sound before the onset of the murmur. In the absence of fibrillation, the long murmur has a *presystolic crescendo* that disappears when fibrillation intervenes (Fig. 6-48G). But clinicians know it occasionally persists [J. M. Criley and A. J. Hermes: The Crescendo Presystolic Murmur of Mitral Stenosis with Fibrillation, *N. Engl. J. Med.*, **285:**1284–87, 1971]. The murmur is often accompanied by a thrill at the apex when the patient is in the left decubitus. The first sound at the apex is usually *accentuated.* If there is pulmonary hypertension, the *P_2 is accentuated.* When the murmur is loud, there is usually an *opening snap* of the mitral valve shortly after the second sound, heard best at the left sternal border between the 2nd and 4th interspaces; this is commonly mistaken for a split second sound. The P_2 has only the normal splitting. The opening snap disappears when the mitral cusps become rigid. Often there is a palpable *right ventricular thrust* to indicate right ventricular hypertropy. *Pathophysiology.* In early mitral stenosis, ventricular filling is slightly delayed and the period of rapid filling is shortened so a mid-diastolic murmur is produced. Since there is adequate ventricular filling, the pressure is little increased by atrial contraction, and no presystolic murmur is produced. With a narrower orifice, ventricular filling is prolonged, so that atrial systole contributes an augmentation of pressure in the ventricle and a presystolic crescendo; this added boost is absent in fibrillation. The accentuated M_1 is caused by the prolonged filling time that places the valves low in the ventricle when they are snapped shut by systole. Pulmonary hypertension produces the accentuated P_2. The audible opening snap of the mitral valve is attributed to the heightened pressure in the atrium. *Distinction.* Tricuspid stenosis produces a similar murmur, but it is localized nearer the sternum. The murmurs of aortic and pulmonic regurgitation also occur at the apex. Ultrasonic examination resolves diagnostic questions and furnishes further details about degree of involvement.

Clinical Occurrence. Nearly always from rheumatic heart disease; rarely congenital.

Apical Diastolic Murmur: ***Shuddering of the Anterior Leaflet of the Mitral Valve*** (Austin Flint Murmur). Some patients with severe grades of aortic regurgitation and normal mitral valves have murmurs at the cardiac apex, similar in pitch and timing to those produced by organic disease of the mitral valve. When the examiner is confronted with this combination of aortic and mitral murmurs he attempts to decide whether the mitral valve is normal. Authors vary on the criteria for diagnosis; the indications of Levine and Harvey are cited here. When the aortic lesion is undoubtedly syphilitic, the murmur is the Flint type (Figs. 6-49D and 6-50E). The presence of atrial fibrillation favors an organic lesion of the mitral valve, as the dysrhythmia is rarely associated with an aortic lesion. M_1 is not accentuated with the Flint murmur. Accentuation of P_2 favors organic mitral stenosis. The opening snap of the mitral valve is absent in the Flint murmur. Notching of the P waves in the electrocardiogram favors an organic lesion of the mitral valve. *Amyl Nitrite Test.* When tachycardia and diminished systolic blood pressure have been produced by the inhalation of amyl nitrite, the apical diastolic rumbling of the Flint murmur becomes *fainter,* but the murmur of organic mitral stenosis becomes *louder* [W. Nasser, M. E. Travel, H. Feigenbaum, and C. Fisch: Austin-Flint Murmur Versus the Murmur of Organic Mitral Stenosis, *N. Engl. J. Med.,* **275:**1007, 1966]. *Pathophysiology.* The murmur is thought to be due to shuddering of the anterior leaflet of the mitral valve as the aortic regurgitant jet flows past it. This can be demonstrated by echocardiography.

Clinical Occurrence. With aortic regurgitation from rheumatic valvulitis or syphilis.

Congenital Complex: ***Eisenmenger's Syndrome.*** This consists of interventricular septal defect, pulmonary hypertension, right ventricular hypertrophy. This may be suspected when the pertinent valvular signs are coupled with cyanosis, right-to-left shunt, clubbing of the fingers. X-ray examination and cardiac catheterization are required to make an exact diagnosis.

Congenital Complex: ***Tetralogy of Fallot.*** The addition of pulmonic stenosis to the three components of Eisenmenger's complex constitutes the tetralogy (Fig. 6-50D). The condition should be considered when multiple lesions are associated with cyanosis, polycythemia, and clubbing of the fingers. X-ray and catheterization studies must make the diagnosis.

Congenital Complex: ***Lutembacher's Complex.*** This is a combination of acquired mitral stenosis and congenital interatrial septal defect. It should be suspected when the pertinent physical signs are encountered in a patient with a childhood history of heart disease.

Congenital Complex: ***Ebstein's Anomaly of the Tricuspid Valve.*** A congenital deformity of the tricuspid valve occurs in which the cusp is extremely thin and inadequate. There is downward displacement of a portion of the valve below the level of the AV ring, producing so-called "ventricularization" of the right atrium. Tricuspid regurgitation is not a prominent feature.

The Blood Vessels

In making the physical examination the physician must have precise knowledge of the location of the accessible arteries and veins, their relations to other parts of the vascular system, and their responses to cardiac action. The usually palpable arteries are temporal, external carotid, brachial, radial, ulnar, arch of aorta and innominate (in the suprasternal notch under certain conditions), abdominal aorta, common iliac, femoral, popliteal, dorsalis pedis, and posterior tibial (Fig. 6-51). The veins frequently visible in the normal person are the external jugular, cephalic, basilic, median basilic, great saphenous, and the veins on the dorsa of the hands and feet. Other veins become visible during increases in general venous pressure or in the formation of collateral circulations.

Vascular Signs of Cardiac Activity

Cardiac action maintains blood pressure in both veins and arteries. Left ventricular activity produces pulses in all accessible arteries. Movements of the right ventricle originate venous pulses only in the upper part of the body. Since arterial pressure is normally about 16 times as high as pressure in the large veins, visible arterial pulsations are *palpable;* venous pulsations are usually *not palpable.* This fact is useful in determining the origin of visible pulsations in the upper part of the body.

Arterial Signs of Cardiac Action

The overall function of the ventricles as pumps is reflected in the arterial blood pressure, modified by the caliber of the vessels forming the peripheral resistance. The contour of the arterial pulse waves is affected partially by the action of the left ventricle and the condition of the aortic valve orifice. Note that abnormalities of the other heart valves do not have this effect. Disturbances of the cardiac rate and rhythm are transmitted to the arterial pulses in somewhat modified form.

MEASUREMENT OF ARTERIAL BLOOD PRESSURE. **The intra-arterial blood pressure can be measured directly by inserting a needle into the lumen of the artery, but this method is impractical and is rarely employed in bedside examination except in intensive care units. Clinically, the indirect method is used in which external measured pressure is applied to the overlying tissues and the compression necessary to occlude the artery is assumed equal to the intra-arterial tension. For this procedure the sphygmomanometer is employed, consisting of a flat rubber bag enclosed in a cuff of indistensible fabric or plastic. A rubber pump inflates the bag with air; tubing connects the pump to the bag and also to a manometer, either mercury or anaeroid, to measure the applied air pressure in millimeters of mercury. The arm cuff should be at least 10 cm wide; for the thigh, a width of 18 cm is preferable. The tension to compress the overlying tissues is usually regarded as negligible; but a thick arm will yield readings 10 to 15 mm higher than the actual pressure unless a wide cuff is used.**

For routine measurements, the patient may be either sitting or lying in the supine position. In special cases, the pressure may be quite different with changes in posture. The patient should have been resting for some time. Bare the arm and affix on it the collapsed

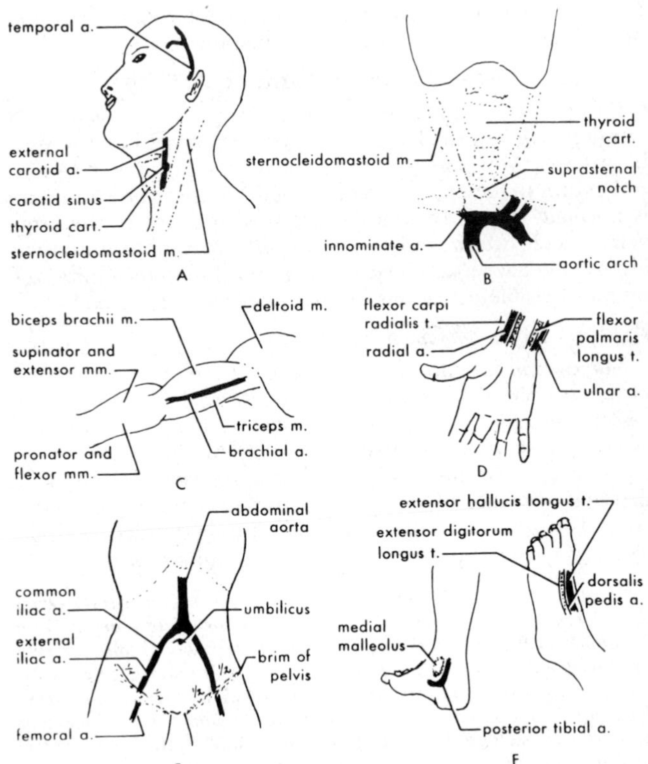

Fig. 6-51. Sites of palpable arteries. **A.** *The temporal artery is anterior to the ear and overlies the temporal bone, one of the few normally tortuous arteries. The common carotid is deep in the neck near the anterior border of the sternocleidomastoid muscle. The bifurcation of this artery is opposite the superior border of the thyroid cartilage. The carotid sinus is at the bifurcation.* **B.** *Slight elongation of the aorta or its dilatation makes this vessel accessible to palpation in the suprasternal notch. With slight shifting to the right or left, the innominate or left carotid arteries may also be felt in the notch.* **C.** *Near the elbow, the brachial artery lies deep in the biceps-triceps furrow on the medial side of the arm. It courses toward the midline of the antecubital fossa where it is usually just medial to the biceps tendon.* **D.** *The radial artery is just medial to the outer border of the radius and lateral to the tendon of the*

cuff snugly and smoothly, so the distal margin of the cuff is at least 3 cm proximal to the antecubital fossa. *Then rest the supinated arm on the table or bed with the antecubital fossa approximately at the level of the heart.* Palpate for the exact location of the brachial arterial pulse; it is usually medial, but occasionally lateral, to the insertion of the Biceps brachii tendon. Inflate the cuff to a pressure about 30 cm of mercury above the point where the palpable pulse disappears. Open the valve slightly so the pressure drops gradually. From this point, observations may be made by either auscultation or palpation.

The preferable choice is usually the *auscultatory method* in which vibrations from the artery under pressure, called *Korotkoff sounds,* are utilized as indicators. Press the bell of the stethoscope lightly over the brachial artery and note the pressure reading at which sounds first become audible; this reading is taken as the *systolic pressure.* As deflation proceeds, the sounds become louder and maintain a maximum for a considerable range; then they become muffled; take a reading at the point of muffling. Take another reading at the point where the sounds disappear; but continue listening to zero pressure to detect the presence of an occasional blank range known as an *auscultatory gap.* If the gap is not detected, the diastolic reading may be erroneously high. Record the three readings thus: 130/80/75, where the first value is the point of appearance of sounds, the second point is where muffling occurs, and the third reading is when the sounds disappear (disregarding the auscultatory gap). The highest value is the systolic pressure; but disagreement is prevalent as to whether the second or third value represents the closest approximation to the intra-arterial *diastolic pressure.* By recording all three values, any reader can draw his own conclusions, and he is not forced to guess at the criterion employed by the examiner for the diastolic pressure. The American Heart Association now recommends the point of disappearance for the diastolic pressure in most instances. Occasionally, the sounds persist to zero pressure,

---

flexor carpi radialis, where the finger can press it against the bone. The ulnar artery is in a similar position to the ulna but it is buried deeper, so often it cannot be felt. **E.** *The abdominal aorta and parts of the iliac arteries can usually be felt as generalized pulsations through the abdominal wall. The femoral artery is palpable at the inguinal ligament midway between the anterior superior iliac spine and the pubic tubercle.* **F.** *The posterior tibial artery is palpable as it curves forward below and around the medial malleolus of the fibula. The dorsalis pedis artery is felt usually in the groove between the first two tendons on the medial side of the dorsum of the foot.*

as in thyrotoxicosis and aortic regurgitation. In such cases, accept the second value because a diastolic pressure of zero is impossible.

Palpation is an alternate method, employed to check the results by auscultation; and when Korotkoff sounds are imperceptible, it is the only method available. Palpate the radial artery distal to the cuff, and take the systolic pressure as the point in which pulse waves first appear. Recently, an old observation to determine diastolic pressure by palpation has been validated [C. D. Enselberg: *N. Engl. J. Med.*, 265:272–74, 1961]. During deflation of the cuff as the level of diastolic pressure is approached, a peculiar single vibration is felt in each pulse wave that the author calls a *whip*. The pressure at which the whip disappears has been shown to be close to the true *diastolic pressure*. This method may be used by patients in taking their own pressure readings.

When the blood pressure has been measured with the manometer cuff overlying a very fat arm, it is advisable to check the value by measuring the pressure at the wrist. The cuff is wrapped around the forearm and the stethoscope bell is placed over the radial artery.

In taking the arterial pressure in the femoral artery, have the patient lie *prone* on a table or bed. Wrap a wide cuff (18 cm or more) around the thigh so the lower margin of the cuff is several centimeters proximal to the popliteal fossa. Inflate the cuff and auscultate the popliteal artery in its fossa. Considerable difficulty may be encountered in holding the cuff on the conical thigh to get even compression.

Blood pressure measurements may be obtained more conveniently *at the ankles* than at the popliteal fossae. A. G. Hocken advises the auscultatory method with a standard-sized manometer cuff [*Lancet*, 1:466, 1967]. Have the patient lie *supine* and apply the cuff just above the malleolus. Place the chestpiece of the stethoscope distal to the cuff and behind the medial malleolus (posterior tibial artery), or on the dorsal extensor retinaculum of the ankle (dorsalis pedis artery). Pressure values by this method were found comparable to those from the brachial artery. The Korotkoff sounds were audible in 27 of 30 consecutive patients. The obvious advantages of this method merit its extensive trial.

In hypotensive states with coincident intense peripheral vasoconstriction, the sphygmomanometric method may seriously underestimate the true intra-arterial pressure. This situation often occurs in shock. J. N. Cohn caused disappearance of Korotkoff sounds when the blood flow in the arm of a normal subject was diminished by an intravenous infusion of levarterenol, although the intra-arterial pressure remained normal [*J.A.M.A.*, 199:972, 1967]. With smaller degrees of vasoconstriction the Korotkoff sounds underestimate the systolic pressure and overestimate diastolic values.

Normal Arterial Tension. The precise bounds of the normal blood pressure are difficult to define. The experienced clinician usually has certain criteria that may be altered by special circumstances. Most regard a systolic pressure over 140 mm Hg as slightly high. A systolic pressure of less than 100 mm Hg may be encountered in an otherwise normal person, but the value must be evaluated from the presence or absence of other signs of disease. Many place 90 mm Hg as the upper limit of normal diastolic pressure and 60 mm as the lower limit of normal range. The diastolic pressures between 90 mm and 100 mm are often regarded as borderline, but not definitely elevated. Statistical data show an increase in the average systolic pressure with increases in age, but this is of little value to the physician concerned with an individual patient. As in other biologic variations, his patient shows no evidence of whether he is near the mean, or still normal at two standard deviations from the mean in the distribution curve. Normal adults exhibit a *circadian variation* in the blood pressure; it is highest in midmorning, falling progressively during the day, and reaching lowest about 3 A.M. [M. W. Millar-Craig, C. N. Bishop, and E. B. Raftery: Circadian Variation of Blood-Pressure, *Lancet,* **1**:795–97, 1978].

Systolic Hypertension. In this condition the systolic pressure is in excess of 150 mm Hg, but the diastolic pressure is normal. ***Pathophysiology.*** The increased systolic pressure is the result of either increased stroke volume of the ventricles or increased rigidity of the aorta and other large arteries.

Clinical Occurrence. INCREASED CARDIAC OUTPUT: thyrotoxicosis, anemia, arteriovenous fistulas, aortic regurgitation, emotional states. RIGID AORTA: atherosclerosis.

Diastolic Hypertension. Both the systolic and diastolic pressures are elevated, but the heightened diastolic pressure is the more important because it represents the minimal continuous load to which the vascular tree is subjected. ***Pathophysiology.*** The diastolic pressure is the result of increased peripheral resistance by narrowing of the lumina of the blood vessels, either by vasoconstriction or by thickening of their intima.

Clinical Occurrence. Renal disease. ENDOCRINE DISORDERS: pheochromocytoma, adrenocortical hyperfunction, acromegaly, carcinoid, aldosteronism. NEUROGENIC CONDITIONS: brain tumor, cerebrovascular accidents, poliomyelitis, lesions of the diencephalon, emotional disorders. CONDITIONS OF UNKNOWN CAUSE: essential hypertension, possibly coarctation of the aorta, eclampsia.

Prognostic Significance of Systolic and Diastolic Pressures. Formerly the systolic pressure was considered relatively unimportant in the evaluation of atherosclerotic disease. This opinion is gradually changing. Workers at the University of Manitoba in a study of 3983 men found that systolic pressure showed stronger association than diastolic with the development of cerebrovascular disease, especially between the ages of 40 and 50 years [S. W. Rabkin, S. A. L. Mathewson, and R. B. Tate: Predicting Risk of Ischemic Heart Disease and Cerebrovascular Disease from Systolic and Diastolic Blood Pressures, *Ann. Intern. Med.*, **88**:342–45, 1978; R. C. Tarazi: Clinical Import of Systolic Hypertension, *Ann. Intern. Med.*, **88**:426–27, 1978].

Paroxysmal Hypertension. The patient's blood pressure is normal except for episodes of diastolic hypertension associated with pallor, anxiety, sweating, palpitation, nausea and vomiting. *Pathophysiology.* In one third of the patients with pheochromocytoma, the tumor secretes epinephrine or norepinephrine intermittently, producing the characteristic symptoms and signs. *Distinction.* The condition must be distinguished from temporary emotional disorders.

Hypotension. Both the systolic and diastolic pressures are diminished below the *accustomed* level for the patient. This may mean that values within the normal range are hypotensive for the patient who has previously had essential hypertension.

Clinical Occurrence. Myocardial infarction, hemorrhagic or neurogenic shock, hypovolemia, atrial thrombus, vena caval obstruction, cardiac tamponade, adrenal hypofunction, vasovagal disturbances, panhypopituitarism.

Orthostatic or Postural Hypotension. The blood pressure is normal in the recumbent position, but when the patient arises both the systolic and diastolic pressures fall to levels producing faintness or syncope. *Pathophysiology.* Either the normal sympathetic discharges to the heart and blood vessels are diminished, or the blood is pooled in the lower extremities by varices or hemangiomas, so that venous return to the heart is deficient.

Clinical Occurrence. After long illnesses in bed; after the postural reflexes are abolished by sympathectomy; in tabes dorsalis and diabetic neuropathy; with large varices or hemangiomas of the legs; with the use of ganglionic blocking agents in the treatment of arterial hypertension.

Widened Pulse Pressure. The pulse pressure is the difference between the systolic and diastolic values in millimeters of mercury. The normal pulse pressure is between 30 and 40 mm Hg. Values in excess of this may occur within the upper limits of normal systolic pressure and the lower limits of the diastolic pressure. In addition, widened pulse pressure is regular in both systolic and diastolic hypertension, but is accepted with these and usually not spoken of as being abnormal.

Clinical Occurrence. Besides hypertension, widened pulse pressure may occur in aortic regurgitation, thyrotoxicosis, patent ductus arteriosus, arteriovenous fistulas, beriberi heart, coarctation of the aorta, emotional states.

Narrowed Pulse Pressure. Pressures less than 30 mm Hg may occur in tachycardia, severe aortic stenosis, constrictive pericarditis, pericardial effusion, or ascites.

Inequality of Blood Pressure in Arms. This is frequently encountered and sometimes cannot be explained. Causes to be considered are atherosclerotic occlusion of subclavian artery, scalenus anticus syndrome, cervical rib, superior thoracic aperture syndrome, malposition of patient when supine on table, after open-heart surgery [W. P. Zmyslowski: Disparity in Blood Pressure Between Arms, *J.A.M.A.*, **238:**2495, 1977].

Manometric Detection of Pulse Wave Disturbances. During measurement of the blood pressure, changes in the volume of individual waves may be detected that are too subtle to be palpated. These include atrial fibrillation, pulsus paradoxus, pulsus alternans. They are described under the appropriate items.

Diastolic Pressure Sign in Aortic Regurgitation (Mayne's Sign). Moderate or mild degrees of aortic regurgitation may be detected by demonstrating a diminution of more than 15 mm Hg in the diastolic pressure in the arm when it is elevated over the head, as compared with values taken when the arm is at heart level. This is attributed to increased hydrostatic pressure at the aortic orifice. [B. Mayne: On Aortic Regurgitation. A New Physical Sign, *Irish J. Med. Sci.*, **6:**80–81, 1953].

PALPATION OF THE ARTERIAL PULSE. **The pulse may be palpated in any of the accessible arteries (Fig. 6-51). To the anesthesiologist in the operating room, the temporal arteries or the arteries in the**

foot may be most convenient. To the physician at the bedside the brachial or radial pulse is usually accessible. The radial artery is pressed lightly against the radius with the examining finger; or the wrist may be encircled by the fingers and hand. The examiner ascertains the *contour* of the pulse wave and its *volume, rate,* and *rhythm;* the latter two are discussed under heart action (p. 349). He also looks for *patterns* of variability in the pulse volume.

Contour: ***Normal Arterial Pulse.*** The *primary wave* starts with a swift upstroke to the peak of systolic pressure, followed by a more gradual decline. Approximately at the end of ventricular systole, a secondary and normally smaller upstroke occurs, the *dicrotic wave,* set up by a rebound against the closing aortic valve (Fig. 6-52A). Normally the dicrotic wave is impalpable; it is demonstrated only by the sphygmograph. One feels merely a sharp upstroke and a more gradual downstroke. The systolic pressure measures the peaks of the waves, and the diastolic pressure the troughs. One can also feel the difference between a full and slight wave volume.

Contour: ***Pulsus Bisferiens*** (Dicrotic Pulse). This is an arterial pulse wave with a dicrotic element approaching the height of the primary element, thus effecting a double wave (*bis,* twice + *ferire,* to beat) (Fig. 6-52B). In many cases this wave pattern may be perceived by simple *light palpation,* preferably over the carotid artery. Lesser impalpable degrees can be shown by *auscultation of the compressed brachial artery.* With the patient supine or sitting, his extended arm is placed horizontally on a flat surface with forearm supinated. A large stethoscope bell is applied over the artery in the antecubital fossa. With the proximal arc of the bell, pressure is gradually increased over the artery. Under low pressure a *knock* appears, followed by a short *systolic crescendo-diminuendo bruit.* Further pressure abolishes first the bruit, then the knock. In the presence of a palpable or impalpable pulsus bisferiens, this maneuver produces a *double systolic bruit,* with a very short silent interval between elements of the couplet and a much longer silence during diastole. The same maneuver is employed to elicit Duroziez's sign, a *systolic-diastolic bruit* (p. 409), but in the latter the two bruits are widely separated, one in systole, the other in diastole. Occasionally the distinction between the two signs cannot be made by auscultation, but the phonocardiograph is diagnostic.

In free aortic regurgitation, a *triple bruit* may be heard when this maneuver is applied. The triplet is thought to be a combination of the double-systolic bruit of pulsus bisferiens and the systolic-diastolic bruit of Duroziez [R. N. MacAlpin and A. A. Kattus: Brachial-Artery Bruits in Aortic-Valve Disease and Hypertrophic Subaortic Stenosis, *N. Engl. J. Med.,* **273:**1012, 1965].

Clinical Occurrence. Aortic stenosis with moderate aortic regurgitation, tight aortic stenosis, free aortic regurgitation, hypertrophic subaortic stenosis, hyperthyroidism, anxiety states.

Contour: ***Bounding or Collapsing Pulse*** (Corrigan Pulse, Water-Hammer Pulse). With high pulse pressure the upstroke of the waves may be very sharp and the downstroke falls precipitously (Fig. 6-52C). This type of pulse wave is encountered in essential hypertension, thyrotoxicosis, emotional states, aortic regurgitation, patent ductus arteriosus, and arteriovenous fistula. The same conditions give rise to the pistol-shot sound (p. 409).

Contour: ***Plateau Pulse*** (Pulsus Tardus). The upstroke of the wave is gradual and the downstroke is prolonged; the peak is blunted and forms a plateau (Fig. 6-52D). This is encountered in severe degrees of aortic stenosis, where ejection through the narrowed orifice is seriously impaired.

Volume Changes: ***Pulsus Alternans.*** With normal rhythm and normal interval between beats, the pulse waves *alternate* between those of greater and lesser volume. This is a sign of myocardial weakness (Fig. 6-52E). In lesser degrees, the difference may not be palpable, but it is readily detected in measuring the blood pressure by the auscultatory nethod. As the cuff is deflated from high pressure, the sounds from alternate beats are first audible; as the pressure declines, the number of sounds is suddenly doubled. This phenomenon must be distinguished from bigeminal rhythm, in which the intervals between members of a couplet are shorter than between pairs.

Volume Changes: ***Pulsus Bigeminus*** (Coupled Rhythm). The intervals between members of the couplet are shorter than the time between the pairs, in contrast to the normal rhythm of pulsus alternans (Fig. 6-52F). The second or premature beat of the pair may have less volume than the preceding normal beat, because contraction occurs before complete ven-

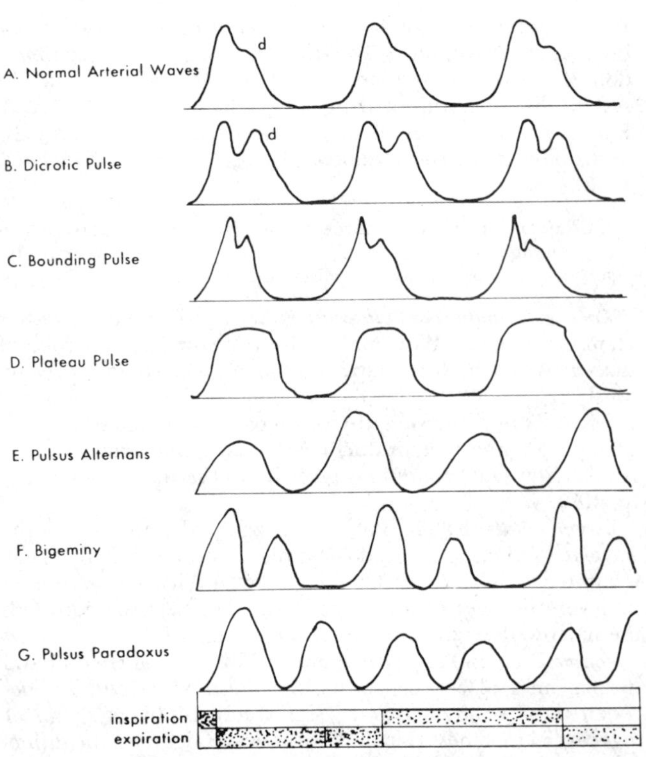

Fig. 6-52. Arterial pulse waves. **A.** *Normal arterial waves showing primary elements, followed by a small dicrotic element that is too weak to be palpable; it is caused by rebound against the closing aortic valve leaflets.* **B.** *The dicrotic pulse is formed by a palpable accentuation of the dicrotic wave in febrile or toxic conditions.* **C.** *The bounding or collapsing pulse is caused by a fast upstroke and downstroke, typically encountered in aortic regurgitation, thyrotoxicosis, and essential hypertension.* **D.** *The plateau pulse occurs in severe aortic stenosis from the slow ejection of blood through a narrowed orifice.* **E.** *Pulsus alternans is characterized by a normal rhythm; the pulse waves alternate between high and low volumes, an indication of serious myocardial weakness.* **F.** *Pulsus bigeminus also may have alternating waves of high and low volume, but the intervals between elements of a couplet are shorter than those separating the couplets. The waves with low amplitude are formed*

tricular filling. Occasionally, the premature beats follow regular beats so closely that they do not produce waves in the peripheral arteries, so the radial pulse rate is half the ventricular rate. Errors in diagnosis may be avoided if the rhythm is first evaluated over the precordium by auscultation.

Volume Changes: **Pulsus Paradoxus.** Under normal conditions of rest there is an *inspiratory fall* of less than 10 mm Hg in the arterial systolic pressure and an accompanying *inspiratory fall* in venous pressure. These changes are scarcely perceptible in the physical examination. A *paradoxical pulse* differs from normal in two respects: (1) the inspiratory diminution in arterial pressure *exceeds* 10 mm Hg, and (2) the inspiratory venous pressure *remains steady* or *increases* (Kussmaul's sign). The exaggerated waxing and waning in the pulse volume can usually be palpated (Fig. 6-52G); it can also be more precisely demonstrated with the sphygmomanometer. To be significant, the sign must occur *during normal cardiac rhythm,* and with respirations of normal *rhythm* and *depth.* *Pathophysiology.* Normally, inspiration diminishes the intrathoracic pressure, so more blood flows into the thorax, and the inflow to the right ventricle is increased. Although right ventricular output is thus augmented, the inspiratory expansion of the pulmonary bed accommodates a volume exceeding the output of the right ventricle. The net result is a diminution of blood delivered to the left ventricle and a reduction in arterial and venous pressure during inspiration. When a pericardial effusion is interposed, the inspiratory descent of the diaphragm exerts traction on the taut pericardium to further impede the left ventricular outflow during inspiration. But traction on the right heart also restricts its filling, so that normal diminution in venous pressure does not occur, and it may actually increase [W. Dock: Inspiratory Traction on the Pericardium, *Arch. Intern. Med.,* **108:**837, 1961]. Incompletely evaluated is the lack of distensibility of the left atrium that may interfere with left ventricular

---

by premature ventricular contractions when the chambers are incompletely filled. **G.** *Pulsus paradoxus, or inspiratory weakening of the pulse, is a sign of pericardial effusion, constrictive pericarditis, or cardiac tamponade. It is attributed to traction of the diaphragm on a distended pericardium, although the mechanism has been disputed for a long time.*

filling [W. H. Resnik and T. R. Harrison, in *Principles of Internal Medicine,* 5th ed., McGraw-Hill Book Co., New York, 1966, p. 848].

Clinical Occurrence. Pericardial effusion, adhesive pericarditis, cardiac tamponade, pulmonary emphysema, severe asthma, paramediastinal effusion, endocardial fibrosis, fibroelastosis, myocardial amyloidosis, scleroderma. More recent additions to the list are mitral stenosis with right-sided cardiac failure, tricuspid stenosis, hypovolemia, massive pulmonary embolism [editorial by Samuel Vaisrub: Pulsus Paradoxus Pulmonale, *J.A.M.A.,* **228:**1030–31, 1974]. Contrary to previous clinical belief, the presence of pulsus paradoxus was reported in mild as well as severe cases of airway obstruction in asthma [C. Shim and M. H. Williams, Jr.: Pulsus Paradoxus in Asthma, *Lancet,* **1:**530–31, 1978].

Volume Changes: ***Inequality of Contralateral Pulses.*** Disparity between the volumes of the two radial pulses, for example, may be perceived by palpating both simultaneously. A diminution in one suggests an aneurysm or partial obstruction.

Disordered Changes in Pulse Volume or Rhythm. Many dysrhythmias produce arterial beats of greater or lesser volume and disordered timing. It is preferable to diagnose the disturbance from the precordial findings, rather than attempting a judgment from the peripheral pulse alone. One should realize that any ventricular contraction occurring before the ventricle has had time to fill will produce a peripheral pulse wave of diminished volume, or none at all.

Arterial Sound: ***Arterial Murmur or Bruit.*** Normally, arteries are silent when auscultated with the bell chestpiece placed *lightly* over them. Interference with the normal laminar blood flow through the vessel may cause eddies that set the arterial wall in vibration, heard as a *systolic murmur* and palpated as a *thrill.* Although *murmur* and *bruit* are literally synonymous, there is a tendency among Americans to reserve *bruit* for certain specific arterial sounds, or especially soft murmurs.

Clinical Occurrence. Arteries become tortuous from arteriosclerosis or other circumstances; arteries constricted congenitally, by intimal proliferation, or by an arteriosclerotic plaque; arterial aneurysm; dilatation of the thyroid arteries and increased blood flow in thyrotoxicosis (here, the word *bruit* is often used); blood flow through an arteriovenous fistula or large arterial collaterals as in aortic coarctation. A *continuous murmur* is produced by either an arteriovenous fistula (p. 434) or a partially obstructed artery when the diastolic pressure is *lowered,* so that the collateral circulation is deficient distal to the obstruction [J. D. Myers, H. V. Murdough, H. D. McIntosh, and R. K. Blaisdell: Observations on Continuous Murmurs over Partially Obstructed Arteries, *Arch. Intern. Med.,* **97**:726, 1956].

Arterial Sound: Pistol-Shot Sound. When the stethoscope bell is placed *lightly* over an artery, particularly the femoral, a sharp sound like a gunshot may be heard. This is produced by the front of an arterial pulse wave, of higher-than-normal pulse pressure, striking the arterial wall in the region of auscultation.

Clinical Occurrence. Although commonly associated with aortic regurgitation, it also occurs in conditions with high pulse pressure, such as essential hypertension, thyrotoxicosis, and anemia.

Arterial Sound: Duroziez's Sign. When the femoral artery is somewhat compressed by *pressure* on the overlying stethoscope bell, eddies are created by the stenosis to produce a *systolic murmur* in normal persons. Whenever such compression produces a *second murmur* closely following the first and giving the impression of a to-and-fro murmur, it is *Duroziez's sign.*

Although usually attributed to retrograde flow of blood in the vessel, the second murmur occurs only when a dicrotic pulse wave is present, suggesting that the second phase is caused by onward acceleration of blood flow. Most commonly encountered in aortic regurgitation of severe grades, it may also occur in other conditions with high pulse pressure. *Method of Listening.* Listen through the stethoscope while pressure on the bell is *gradually* increased. First the normal systolic murmur appears; with further pressure a critical point is reached when the second murmur becomes audible.

Venous Signs of Cardiac Action

Cardiac action produces physical signs in the venous system by (1) alteration of the venous pressure in the periphery, (2) production of venous congestion in the viscera, (3) alteration of the venous pulse waves.

Venous Pressure. A feature of right-sided heart failure is an increase in the venous pressure of the greater circulation that is demonstrable by physical examination. Peripheral venous pressure is usually measured from the *level of the right atrium.* In normal persons, direct measurements seldom show venous pressures in excess of 10 cm of water. Any peripheral veins below this level are *normally filled with blood;* those above are *collapsed.* In the erect position, the level of the right atrium is at the 4th intercostal space. Vertically from this point, a direct venous channel extends through the superior vena cava, the two subclavian veins, thence to the two external jugulars that emerge from the thorax at the superior borders of the clavicles to become subcutaneous and visible in the neck. With normal venous pressure in the erect position, a column of blood distends the superior vena cava to a height of about 10 cm above the right atrium. But in most adults, the upper border of the clavicles is from 13 to 18 cm above the right atrium, so the visible segment of this channel in the neck is collapsed when erect (Fig. 6-53C). The visible veins in the dependent arms and forearms are distended with blood up to the same level as in the vena cava. When the thorax reclines at 45°, the column of blood rises higher in the venous channel, so the head of the column may be visible in the jugulars. In the horizontal position, all peripheral veins are filled. If the arm is raised slowly, the distal portions of the veins collapse as they attain the height of 10 cm above the level of the right atrium.

ESTIMATING VENOUS PRESSURE. **Since the superior border of the clavicle in the adult is usually from 13 to 18 cm above the 4th interspace, distention of the external jugular vein in the neck when the body is *vertical* is valid evidence of increased venous pressure, *provided* there is not compression of the venous channel distal to the atrium. Factors that must be excluded are increased intrathoracic pressure from dyspnea, coughing, laughing, crying, and other movements involving the Valsalva phenomenon. A large cervical goiter may obstruct; a retrosternal goiter must be excluded by palpation and perhaps x-ray examination. The presence of venous waves in the jugular excludes obstruction centrally; but tense distention of the jugulars may prevent venous waves from being apparent. A few persons do not develop peripheral veins that are large enough to inspect. From the dimensions of the thorax, it is evident that the jugulars can be collapsed in the erect position and the thorax will conceal an abnormally high column of blood (Fig. 6-53C). Methods of measurement are desirable.**

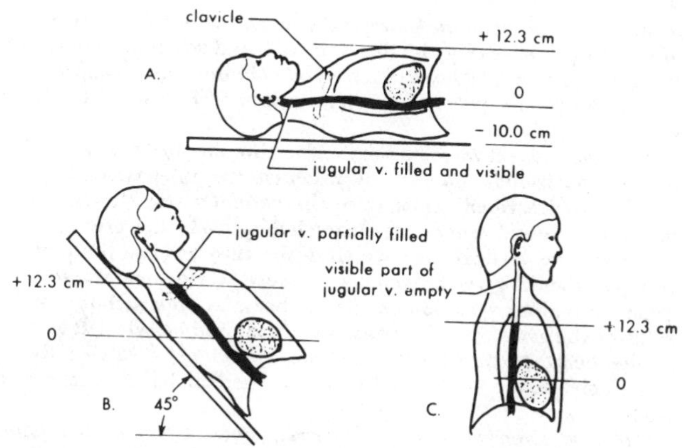

Fig. 6-53. Behavior of the jugular blood column with changes in posture. *The sagittal section is drawn to scale from a lateral x-ray film of a normal adult male thorax. The anteroposterior diameter of the thorax at the level of the 4th interspace is 20 cm; from this point, the vertical distance to the superior border of the clavicle is 15 cm in the erect position. The right atrium is located at the midpoint of an anteroposterior line from the 4th interspace to the back. In any posture, a horizontal plane through this point is the "phlebostatic" or "zero level." In this figure, a slightly elevated venous pressure of 12.3 cm is assumed.* **A.** *With the patient supine, the horizontal plane, 12.3 cm above the zero level, is above the neck so the jugular vein is filled; normal venous pressure also should fill the vein in this position.* **B.** *With the thorax at 45°, the blood column extends midway up the jugular, so the head of the column is visible.* **C.** *In the erect position, the head of the column is concealed within the thorax, 2.7 cm below the upper border of the clavicle, although the venous pressure exceeds the normal.*

Indirect Measurement of Venous Pressure. **When the head of a column of blood is visible in the vertical position and obstruction or temporary increases in pressure are excluded, the vertical distance in centimeters from the head of the column to the 4th interspace is an approximate measure of venous pressure. When the jugulars are collapsed in the vertical position, put the patient on an examining table or hospital bed with a movable back rest. Starting from the sitting position, slowly lower the thorax until the head of the blood column appears in the jugular vein. Establish the location of the right atrium in this position by running an imaginary anteroposterior line from the 4th interspace halfway to the back; a horizontal plane**

through this point is the *phlebostatic* or *zero level* for measurement of venous pressure (Fig. 6-53B). The vertical distance in centimeters from this plane to the head of the blood column gives an approximation of the venous pressure [T. Winsor and G. E. Burch: *Am. Heart J.*, 31:387; 1946].

Alternate Indirect Measurement. **The thorax can be at any angle between horizontal and vertical. Establish the phlebostatic level, as previously described. Then raise the patient's arm slowly until a position is found where the distended veins in the arm or hand collapse. The vertical distance from the zero level to the point of collapse should give the venous pressure. Unfortunately, there is great individual variation in the caliber and superficiality of the veins of the arms. For observation veins should be selected as close to the heart as possible to exclude blockage by valves; this is less likely in the cephalic, basilic, or median basilic veins (Fig. 6-54B).**

Direct Measurement of Venous Pressure. **If any doubt exists, venous pressure can be measured directly. This requires simple sterilized apparatus: a hypodermic needle of 23 or 25 gauge, a 20-mL Luer syringe, a three-way stopcock, and a small-bore glass tube graduated in centimeters that fits the outlet of the stopcock (Fig. 6-54D). Place the patient on a bed or table in the supine position with his arm supinated and resting upon a support that places the antecubital vein well below the reference point at half the anteroposterior diameter of the chest. Using sterile heparinized isotonic saline, fill the syringe with the solution, adjust the stopcock appropriately, and expel the solution into the manometer tube to the height of about 20 cm. Then turn the stopcock to make a channel from syringe to needle, and insert the needle aseptically into the vein, permitting a little blood to return to the syringe. Adjusting the cock for a channel from vein to manometer. Blood will run out or solution run in until the height of the column is equal to the venous pressure. Read off the height of the column in centimeters of water or blood above the reference level.**

Heightened Venous Pressure. When the venous pressure exceeds 10 or 12 cm of water under resting conditions, it should be considered elevated. *Pathophysiology.* In cardiac failure the venous pressure rises as the result of peripheral venous constriction and increased blood volume. In congestive failure when venous pressure exceeds 22 cm, the liver is always enlarged; above 25 cm, there are always ascites, edema, and orthopnea. The venous pressure is always high during increasing failure, but it falls before other signs of failure diminish. *Dis-*

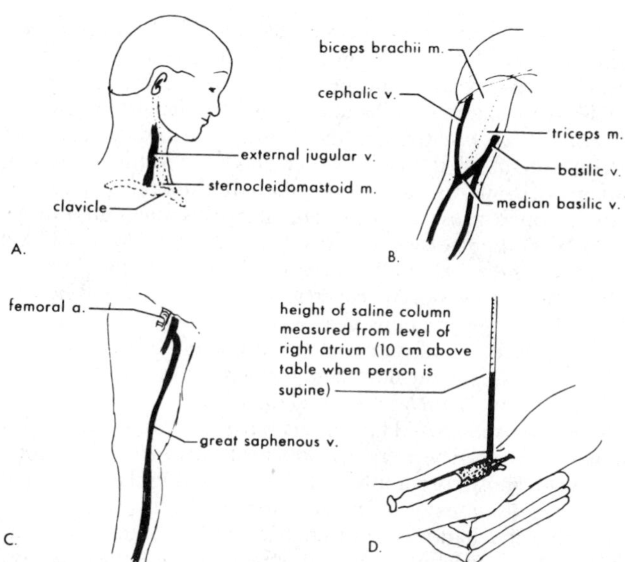

Fig. 6-54. Visible veins and venous pressure measurements. **A.** *Veins of the neck.* **B.** *Veins of the arm.* **C.** *Veins of the thigh and leg.* **D.** *Direct measurement of venous pressure in a peripheral vein.*

tinction. A generalized increase in venous pressure must be distinguished from venous obstruction of the channels to the right atrium. Obstruction may be caused by a large cervical or retrosternal goiter, thrombosis or neoplasm in the subclavian veins or the vena cava, or extrinsic pressure on the veins from granuloma or neoplasm.

Diminished Venous Pressure. The peripheral veins are collapsed when the patient is supine. *Pathophysiology.* This occurs in peripheral circulatory failure that is part of the shock syndrome, usually associated with hypovolemia, diminished venous tonus, or peripheral pooling.

Clinical Occurrence. Extreme cardiac failure, myocardial infarction, hemorrhagic shock.

Hepatojugular Reflux. This is an early sign of venous constriction that may be present before increased venous pressure is demonstrable by other means employed in the physical examination. Place the patient on a bed with movable back rest; lower the thorax until the head of the blood column is just visible in the jugular veins above the clavicle. Admonish the patient to keep breathing at the normal rate and depth. Then place the hand in the right upper quadrant of the abdomen, and press firmly upward under the costal margin. If venous constriction is present, displacement of this small amount of blood from the liver will cause a rise in the head of the blood column in the neck. ***Pathophysiology.*** This phenomenon probably is caused by venous constriction; it can be abolished by drugs that relieve venous spasm. It occurs not only in early cardiac failure, but also in cardiac tamponade from pericardial effusion, hemopericardium, and concretio cordis [G. E. Burch and C. T. Ray: *Am. Heart J.*, **48:**373, 1954].

Venous Pulsations. The venous pulse wave is a *normal* phenomenon that can be demonstrated near the heart in any superficial vein, most commonly in the external jugulars. In a few persons, pulsations occur in the superficial veins of the arms, forearms, and hands; the mechanism of this extension is unknown. The pulsation of a vein is readily distinguished from an arterial pulse by being *impalpable,* because the normal venous pressure is only about one sixteenth that in the arteries. Venous pulses are best seen at the head of a blood column, but visibility depends upon the amount of overlying tissue. Under ideal conditions, one can see three components of the wave (Fig. 6-55). The *a-wave* results from rebound of atrial systole; the *c-wave* is caused by bulging backward of the AV cusps at the beginning of ventricular systole; the *v-wave* is produced by filling of the atria while the AV valves are still closed, together with the upward (hence backward) movement of the AV valve ring at the end of ventricular systole. Since the a-wave arises from atrial activity it is the only direct physical sign of such action. Occasionally, a disproportion in the number of a-waves and ventricular systoles gives direct indication of a dysrhythmia. But the waves are difficult to see consistently and proper examination of the precordium usually leads to a diagnosis. In the *erect* position, the presence of a venous pulse is abnormal because it means that the blood column is higher than it should be, if temporary increased intrathoracic pressure can be excluded. When the geometry of posture has been so arranged

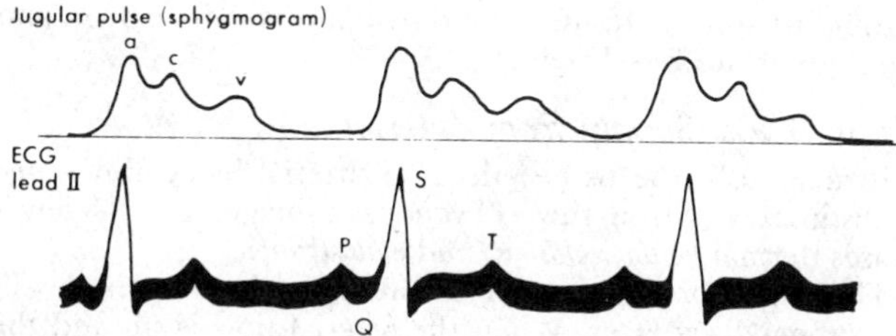

Fig. 6-55. Waves in the jugular vein. *The heart action is reflected in the jugular vein. The waves should be compared with the electrocardiogram, remembering that a perceptible time elapses between cardiac events and their signs in the neck. The "a" wave is the rebound from atrial systole; the bulging of the AV valve cusps after closure produces the "c" deflection; the "v" wave is the resultant of atrial filling while the cuspid valves are closed, together with an upward movement of the AV valve ring at the end of ventricular systole.*

as to expect a normal pulse wave, the *absence of venous pulse* is a sign of obstruction of the channel to the right atrium.

Capillary Pulsation. This has been widely advertised as a sign of aortic regurgitation, despite the repeated demonstrations of Thomas Lewis and others that it is a normal phenomenon, seen in most normal persons. To elicit, press down on the tip of the fingernail until the distal third of the pink nailbed has paled: with each heartbeat the border of pink extends and recedes. Forget it, except for answering examination questions.

Circulation of the Limbs

In the routine physical examination, most physicians test the circulation of the extremities by (1) palpation of the walls of the brachial or radial arteries and inspection of the retinal vessels for signs of arteriolar sclerosis or spasm; (2) palpation of the pulse volume in the pairs of brachial, radial, femoral, dorsalis pedis, and posterior tibial arteries; (3) inspection for varicose veins, edema, and ulceration of the arms and legs. Complaints of pain, coolness, or numbness in an extremity, or signs of enlarged veins, masses, swellings, localized pallor, rubor, or cyanosis, initiate special examinations of the peripheral circulation. When circulatory deficit is found, the cause is sought from the history, the distribution of the deficit, and the state of the vessel walls.

Tissue Blood Supply from Arteries

In diagnosis, the tissue effects of arterial blood flow must be distinguished from those of venous drainage. Arterial deficit causes dermal *pallor, coldness,* and *malnutrition.*

The *skin color* is imparted by the blood in the venules of the subpapillary layer. When the arterial flow is nil and the veins empty, the skin is chalky white. Partial but inadequate arterial supply may produce red or cyanotic skin, depending on the effect of external temperature and other factors upon the pooled blood in the venules. Since the degree of deoxygenation varies directly with the temperature, the same pooled blood may be *red* in the cold and *blue* at higher temperatures.

The *skin temperature* is a reliable indicator of the *blood flow rate* in the dermal vessels. Normally, flow is governed principally by the constriction or dilatation of the arterioles. The internal body temperature is maintained within narrow limits, partly by the regulated dissipation of heat from the dermal vessels. In clothed persons, the skin of the head, neck, and trunk is warmer than that of the extremities; the digits, in turn, are colder than their respective hands and feet. Peculiarly, the normal digits adjust to only two levels of temperature. The fingers are usually nearer blood temperature (90°F, or 32° C) when the air temperature exceeds 68° F, or 20° C. If the room temperature is below 60° F, or 16° C, the fingers adjust to a level of about 72° F, or 22° C; there are no intermediate levels of adjustment. Thus, the physician must distinguish between physiologic responses to external temperatures and the results of disease. Most reliable are the discrepancies between symmetric parts when they have been sufficiently exposed to the same external temperature.

When the affected part is below heart level, the pooled venous blood masks the effect of arterial flow to the part. Venous pressure rarely sustains a column higher than 30 cm above the right cardiac atrium, whereas the systolic arterial pressure produces a blood column more than 150 cm above the same reference point. Thus, when the hand or foot is lifted above the right atrium to a height exceeding the venous pressure, the masking venous blood pool is drained, permitting evaluation of the tissue color produced by the arterial blood. When the arterial deficit is unilateral, the color of the impaired extremity may be directly compared with its normal homologue. If the pair are affected equally, the examiner must judge the change in color from his experience with other patients.

Chronic arterial deficit also affects the nutrition of the integument and the underlying tissues, so that localized malnutrition furnishes signs of peripheral vascular disease.

In the physical examination, inspection and palpation impose a sharp distinction in the size of blood vessels. In this context, we shall consider *large arteries* as those normally carrying visible or palpable pulses and those with anatomic names whose occlusion can be recognized by the region of ischemia produced. Since *minute arteries* and the *arterioles* are observable only in the superficial layers of the skin, or in the retina, methods of their examination are quite different. Small vessel disturbances are recognizable as patterns in the skin and are detected by the methods of dermatologic description. Since most diseases of tissues involve the circulation incidentally, it is only practical to consider the diseases of the larger vessels as diagnostic entities.

DERMAL EXAMINATION FOR ARTERIAL DEFICIT. **In a draftless room at about 72° F, or 22° C, place the patient on an examining table or bed and expose the extremities for ten minutes. If the room temperature much exceeds 78.8° F, or 26° C, coldness in the skin is not demonstrable. Have the patient sit, hanging the legs from the table or bed; compare both feet for pallor, deep redness, pale blueness, deep blueness, or a violaceous color (Fig. 6-56). With the back or your hand or fingers, feel the *skin temperature* from the feet up the legs. Compare similar sites on each leg in sequence; in moving proximally, note whether the increase in temperature is gradual or sharply demarcated. Then have the patient lie supine. Grasp both his ankles and elevate the feet more than 12 inches, or 30 cm, above the estimated level of the right cardiac atrium. Note any change in the color of the feet. If the color does not change, have the patient dorsiflex the feet five or six times, wait several minutes, then observe the feet for *latent color changes* induced by exercise. Allow the feet to hang down again and note the *time of color return* to the skin. Note the time of return of color to an area blanched by finger pressure. Inspect the feet carefully for evidence of *malnutrition:* atrophy of the skin, loss of lanugo hair on the dorsa of the toes, thickening or transverse ridging of the nails, ulceration, patches of gangrene. Apply**

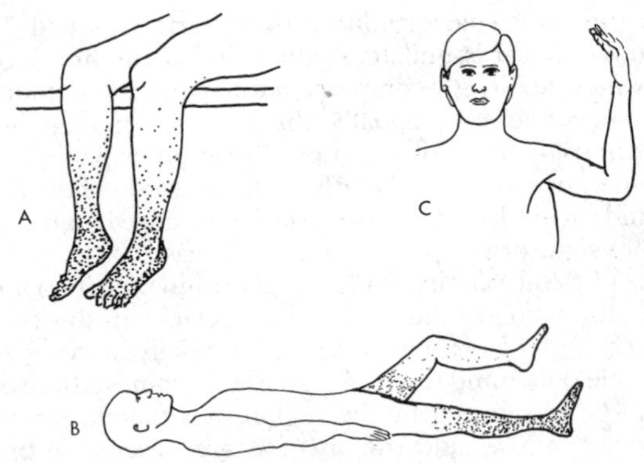

Fig. 6-56. Circulation of the skin in the extremities. **A.** *The legs are dependent to observe the color of the skin. Arterial deficit produces a violaceous color from pooling of the blood in the venules because of loss of venomotor tone associated with hypoxia.* **B.** *While the patient is supine, the foot is elevated above the level of venous pressure (15 cm above the right heart or 25 cm above the table when the patient is supine). Elevation drains the feet of venous blood so the skin color reflects only the presence of arterial blood. The observed is compared with opposite extremity, or with a concept gained from experience.* **C.** *The hand is raised above the heart level so the skin color is produced exclusively by arterial blood.*

the same principles in examining the upper extremities. Expose the hands for ten minutes, then observe the *color* in dependency and when elevated well above heart level. Have the hands opened and closed to disclose *latent color changes*. Note the *time of return of color* in dependency. Seek evidence of dermal malnutrition.

Feet Dependent: ***Warm Skin.*** The normal skin temperature indicates adequate arterial flow. The normal color is *red* or *pink*. If warm feet are blue, the warmth has been externally applied to feet with inadequate arterial flow.

Feet Dependent: ***Cold Skin.*** The arterial flow is inadequate. Uncomplicated, the situation produces pallor. When the skin is *blue* or *purple*, the inadequate arterial flow has been unable to displace the venous blood that contains reduced hemoglobin.

Feet Elevated: ***Cold Skin.*** The blue venous blood drains away to unmask tissues made *pallid* by insufficient arterial flow. When the elevated foot is lowered, the pink color normally returns in 20 seconds. Return of color in 45 to 60 seconds confirms the fact of arterial deficit.

Skin Atrophy. The skin is thinner than normal, as demonstrated by its shiny appearance and the fine texture of the wrinkles produced when it is pinched. The normal fine furrows in the dermis are absent. The lanugo hair on the backs of the hands and feet and the dorsa of the fingers and toes fails to grow.

Malnourished Nails. The nails grow slowly or not at all. They are dry, brittle, and contain transverse ridges. Later, they become thickened (Fig. 6-57B).

Skin Scars. On an extremity with arterial deficiency, the skin may contain round scars, covered with atrophied skin that may be pigmented (Fig. 6-57A). These develop without trauma as the result of obstruction of small arteries.

Skin Ulcers. Ischemic ulcers occur over the tips of the toes, the malleoli, the heels, the metatarsal heads, and the dorsal arches. They are termed *cold ulcers* because they lack the warm erythematous areola characteristic of *warm ulcers,* caused by infection. Frequently the borders of cold ulcers appear punched out.

Skin Gangrene. In the earliest stage, the lesions are round, less than 1 mm in diameter, with pitted centers of black skin (Fig. 6-57C). The areas may spread to involve the entire foot. When the skin is black, wrinkled and dry, the condition is

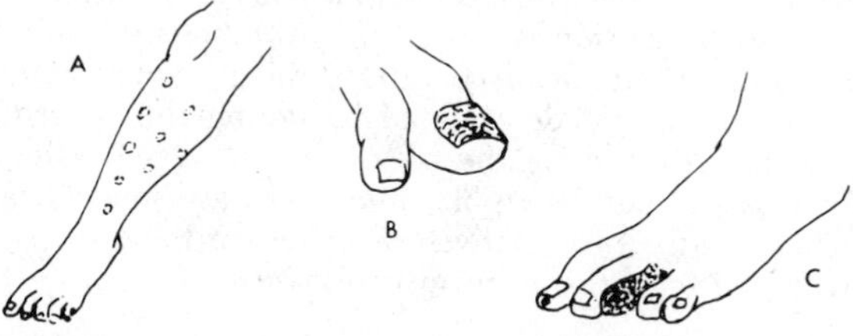

Fig. 6-57. Dermal lesions from arterial deficit. **A.** *The skin over the legs contains round areas of dermal atrophy, with or without pigmentation. These result from small superficial infarctions.* **B.** *The toenails grow more slowly than normal and the nail plates become thickened and laminated; the layers form transverse ridges.* **C.** *Gangrene of the distal parts may develop from arterial deficit. The sketch shows a round spot of gangrene on the tip of the great toe, and the middle toe blackened from dry gangrene.*

termed *dry gangrene.* If secondary infection occurs, the dead area becomes swollen with fluid oozing onto the surface; this is *wet gangrene.*

Disorders of Large Limb Arteries

Arterial disorders are either *occlusive* or *nonocclusive.* The occlusion may be partial or complete. When arterial deficit in tissues has been demonstrated, two etiologic factors are involved: (1) the *mechanism of arterial occlusion,* whether by compression of the vessel, vasospasm, narrowing of the lumen by intimal thickening, or plugging of the lumen by thrombus or embolus; (2) the *intrinsic disease of the artery* that promotes occlusion. Frequently, *compression* of an artery is related to a certain position of the extremity and is temporary. The condition may be demonstrated by maneuvers based on knowledge of the anatomy of the adjacent bones and muscles. Also transient is *vasospasm,* frequently recognized by the sharp border produced between ischemic and normal tissue. Usually *proliferation of the arterial intima* is inferred when the blood flow is diminished but still present. When the occlusion is complete, the cause is usually embolism or thrombosis. The onset of thrombosis is usually gradual and painless, whereas embolism occurs suddenly, with severe localized pain. The underlying intrinsic disease of the artery is usually inferred from the total clinical picture, the demonstration of characteristic findings in accessible arterial walls, the distribution of lesions in the arterial tree, and whether occlusion is caused by thrombosis or embolism.

In examining an involved artery, the proximal extent of the occlusion is first determined by noting the presence or absence of pulses along the course of the vessel. When the entire vessel is not accessible, inferences are made from its branches and the proximal vessels. Afterward, the vessel walls are palpated for signs of intrinsic disease.

EXAMINATION OF LARGE ARM AND LEG ARTERIES. **Through the ophthalmoscope, inspect the retinal arteries for widening of the stripes, spasm of the walls, arteriovenous nicking (Fig. 5-28, p. 120). Palpate the *walls* of accessible arteries, such as the brachial and radial, for increased thickness, tortuosity, and beading. A spastic artery feels like a small cord. Systematically compare the pulse volumes at similar levels of symmetric arteries.**

Upper Extremities. **Palpate the *subclavian artery* in the supracla-**

vicular fossa; feel for a thrill; listen for a bruit. With the forearm in about 90° flexion, palpate the *brachial artery* on the medial aspect of the arm, in the groove between the biceps and triceps muscles (Fig. 6-58A). Feel the *radial artery* on the flexor surface of the wrist, just medial to the distal end of the radius. Palpate the *ulnar artery* on the flexor surface of the wrist, just lateral to the lower end of the ulna; it lies deeper than the radial artery and frequently it is impalpable in the normal subject. Examine the *patency* of the radial and ulnar arteries with *Allen's test* (Fig. 6-58B): Have the patient sit with his hands supinated on his knees; stand at the patient's side with your fingers around each of his wrists and your thumbs on the flexor surfaces of his wrists; compress the tissue over both radial arteries with your thumbs while the patient opens and closes his hands several times; with the radial arteries still compressed, have him open the hands for inspection of his palms; look for the normal pink contributed by blood from the ulnar artery via the volar arch; an occluded ulnar artery will produce a pallid palm until the radial artery is released. Repeat the procedure, but compress the ulnar arteries instead.

Lower Extremities. With the *dorsal aspects* of your fingers, palpate the skin of the thighs and legs for abnormal distribution of skin

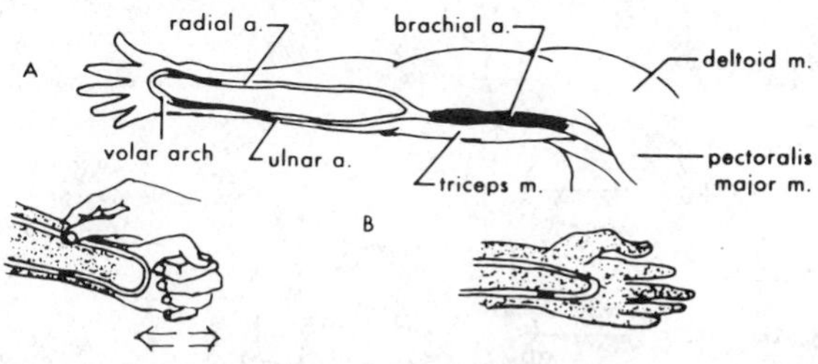

Fig. 6-58. Testing for patency of the arteries of the arm. **A.** *The arteries of the arm and forearm are palpable only in a segment of the brachial artery in the upper arm and segments of the radial and ulnar arteries in the wrist (segments in solid black). Frequently the ulnar pulse is not accessible to palpation in normal persons.* **B.** *The arteries in the volar arch and its contributing radial and ulnar arteries can be evaluated by Allen's test. The patient rests his supine hand on his knee and the examiner compresses the radial artery with one thumb and the ulnar artery with the other thumb. The patient is required to clench and open the fist three times; when finally held open, the radial artery is released to see how fast color will return to the palm from the arterial supply of the radial. The test is repeated releasing the ulnar artery first. The contributions of each artery can thus be assessed.*

temperature, comparing symmetric areas. When the feet are abnormally cold, find a sharp line of demarcation with a proximal region of normal temperature. Especially feel for a warm area over the knees or the anteromedial aspect of the thighs that indicates collateral circulation via the geniculate artery. Palpate the *abdominal aorta* deeply between the xiphoid and the umbilicus, where the aorta bifurcates. Feel the *common iliac arteries* from the bifurcation to the midpoint of the inguinal ligaments. Palpate the *common femoral arteries* just below the inguinal ligaments, equidistant between the anterior superior iliac spines and the pubic tubercles (Fig. 6-59). Feel for the pulse of the *popliteal arteries* with the patient supine and the legs extended. Place one of your hands on each side of the patient's knee with your thumbs anteriorly near the patella and the fingers

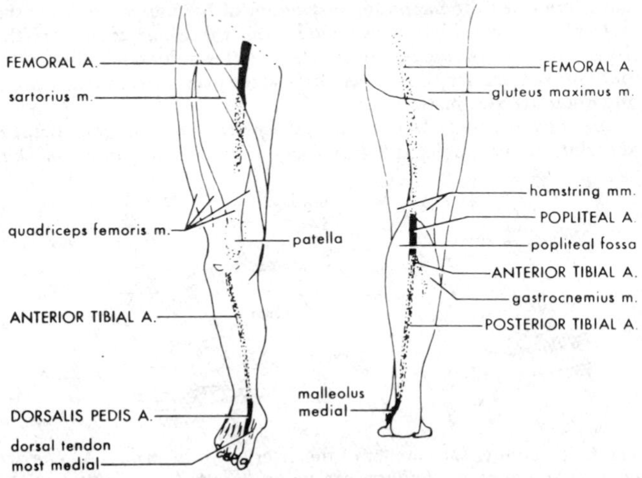

Fig. 6-59. Palpable arteries of the lower limb. *The palpable segments of the arteries are in solid black; the other parts are stippled. The femoral artery is palpable only a short distance below the inguinal ligament; it courses beneath the ligament at the midpoint between the anterior superior iliac spine and the pubic tubercle. The popliteal artery lies vertically in the popliteal fossa, near the end of the femur; it can be felt only by compressing from behind the contents of the fossa against the bone. The posterior tibial artery can be felt as it curls forward and under the medial malleolus. The palpable segment of the dorsalis pedis artery lies just lateral to the most medial of the dorsal tendons of the foot (the flexor of the great toe); the accessible portion is over the arch of the foot.*

curling around each side of the knee so the tips rest in the popliteal fossa. Press the fingers of both hands forward hard to compress the tissues and the artery against the lower end of the femur or the upper part of the tibia; feel for pulsation of the artery. Frequently the pulse of a normal popliteal artery is impalpable. For the pulse of the *posterior tibial artery*, feel in the groove between the medial malleolus and the Achilles tendon. It may be more accessible with passive dorsiflexion of the foot. Locate the *dorsalis pedis artery* on the dorsum of the foot, just lateral to and parallel with the tendon of the Extensor hallucis longus (the most medial of the dorsal pedal tendons and the one that runs to the great toe). In apparently normal persons over 45 years old, frequently either the dorsalis pedis or the posterior tibial pulses will be impalpable, but not both on the same foot. In feeling for the patient's pulse, carefully guard against mistaking the pulse in your own fingertips for that of the patient. Test the patency of the dorsalis pedis and posterior tibial arteries with *Allen's maneuver*, using the same principles as described for the pulses of the wrist, except compress the pedal artery while the foot is elevated, than let the foot hang down to observe the color.

Ultrasonic Examination Employing the Doppler Shift Technique. Small portable instruments for use at the bedside make it possible to evaluate the arterial circulation more precisely, especially when the pulses are not readily palpable.

Arteriography. When surgical treatment of a chronic occlusion seems possible, arteriography is usually required. Radiopaque medium is injected into the artery above the obstruction; the resulting x-ray films visualize not only the site of occlusion but also the collateral circulation.

Palpability of Pedal Pulses [G. E. Garrison: Pedal Pulses in Diagnosis of Arterial Disease, *J.A.M.A.*, **210**:908, 1969]. Congenital absence of a palpable dorsalis pedis pulse is a common and clinically insignificant finding. Barnhorst and Barnes found 12% of 1000 children without other vascular disease having absence of one or both dorsalis pedis arteries; Silverman encountered similar findings in 17% of 1014 soldiers. Congenital absence of the posterior tibial pulse is uncommon in the white race, but it occurred in 9% of 106 Black soldiers. If either arterial pulse is present, the circulation to the limb may be normal. But the author reports that both ipsilateral pulses may be normal *at rest* and disappear after exercising the limb when there is some stenosis of the ipsilateral common iliac or femoral artery. Thus the absence of one pedal pulse on a side is of doubtful clinical significance *unless it has been known to be previously present.*

Acute Arterial Plugging: ***Embolism and Arterial Thrombosis.*** Usually, the patient experiences sudden excruciating *pain* in the extremity, followed by *numbness* and *weakness* in the part. Occasionally, anesthesia and myasthenia precede the pain that appears more gradually. The distal portion of the extremity becomes *pallid* and *pulseless.* One or two hours later, the distal skin becomes *blue,* while *mottling* occurs proximally. Cyanosis lessens when the limb is elevated. The skin of the affected part soon becomes *colder.* The pulseless artery may be felt as a tender cord that must be distinguished from a similar finding caused by reflex vasospasm in adjacent arteries. Tenderness in the calf muscles or the anterior leg indicates involvement, respectively, of the posterior tibial or the dorsalis pedis artery. Occasionally, the pain may be quite mild. Early the muscles are flaccid; later the foot assumes plantar flexion. *Distinction Between Thrombosis and Embolism.* Thrombosis is inferred when there are signs elsewhere of diffuse vascular disease, or the history discloses symptoms of arterial insufficiency, such as claudication. Embolism is suspected when atrial fibrillation is present, since dislodgment of a thrombus from the left atrium is the most common cause. When atherosclerosis and fibrillation coexist, the distinction may be impossible. Ultrasonic examination assists in the diagnosis and localization.

Clinical Occurrence of Thrombosis. Atherosclerosis, thromboangiitis obliterans, and other arteritides; blood sludging from polycythemia, hemoconcentration, and hyperglobulinemia; infection; trauma.

Clinical Occurrence of Embolism. Atrial fibrillation, mitral stenosis, myxomas of the left atrium, a mural thrombus following infarction, dislodgment of a thrombus from a traumatized artery.

Chronic Arterial Plugging: ***Occlusive Vascular Disease.*** Usually this term applies to the lower extremities. The patient complains of *continuous pain, night pain, intermittent claudication* (p. 744), or *coldness of the feet.* *Skin.* Arterial insufficiency may cause skin pigmentation, pallor, purplish discoloration that fades with elevation, coldness, warm areas of collateral circulation, local hair loss, malnutrition of toenails, ulceration, or gangrene. *Arterial Pulses.* Absence of pulsations in the femoral, popliteal, dorsalis pedis, or posterior tibial arteries. *Muscles.*

Atrophy may be present. With occlusion of the popliteal artery, collateral circulation may develop in the branches of the geniculate artery, producing the combination of *cold feet and warm knees.* The unusually warm skin from these collaterals may be *on the knee* or in an area on the *anteromedial aspect of the lower thigh,* with pulseless popliteal, posterior tibial, and dorsalis pedis arteries. Ultrasonic examination assists in the localization.

Arterial Plugging: ***Atherosclerosis.*** The term *arteriosclerosis* includes three entities: (1) atherosclerosis, (2) medial calcification of Mönckeberg, and (3) arteriolar sclerosis. Of the three, atherosclerosis is the only process that causes plugging of medium-sized arteries. It is characterized by medial degeneration and fibrosis, together with occlusive proliferation of the intima. Occlusion may also be caused by the formation of intimal plaques composed of lipoid material and calcium salts. The walls become less compressible; the unyielding tactile sensation is interpreted as *thickening.* The arterial segments lengthen. When the ends of a segment are anchored by surrounding tissue, the elongated vessel buckles in the middle, producing visible and palpable *tortuosity.* But the disease may be spotty throughout the body; frequently it is much more advanced in the vessels of the lower extremities. Involvement of the vessels of the upper extremities does not necessarily prove the cause of ischemia in the lowers; frequently it is the best evidence available. To explain occlusive vascular disease of the lower extremities, atherosclerosis is usually diagnosed by exclusion of other diseases, when the patient is over 45 years old. In diabetes mellitus, atherosclerosis frequently occurs at a much earlier age. *Atheromatous plaques* may be felt in the walls of accessible arteries, and the calcium can be seen in x-ray films; but plaques are not common in the vessels of the upper extremities. *Distinction.* Atherosclerosis must be distinguished from Mönckeberg's medial calcification, which is characterized by annular calcified plaques in the media of larger vessels. The plaques are readily palpated in the brachial and radial arteries as *beads* or *rings.* But this disease does not cause occlusion and seldom involves smaller vessels. It frequently coexists with atherosclerosis, but not invariably. Its plaques are readily seen in x-ray films. Arteriolar sclerosis is a disorder of small vessels, associated with arterial hypertension, but it does not cause occlusive vascular disease.

Arterial Evaluation with Doppler and Treadmill Tests. The accuracy in evaluation of the circulation of the lower limbs has been greatly enhanced by the addition of three testing methods to the physical examination: (1) the measurement of the blood pressure with the Doppler probe, (2) treadmill exercise, and (3) Doppler velocimetry. In a careful study of many patients with diabetes mellitus at the University of Washington, about one third having no history of claudication exhibited signs of arterial insufficiency with the noninvasive tests; one fifth considered normal by physical examination had positive tests [M. R. Marinelli *et al.*: Noninvasive Testing vs. Clinical Evaluation of Arterial Disease, *J.A.M.A.*, **241**:2031–34, 1979].

Arterial Plugging: ***Thrombosis of Aortic Bifurcation*** (Leriche's Syndrome). This is an atherosclerotic occlusion of the aortic bifurcation, causing loss of femoral and all distal pulses (Fig. 6-60A). It achieves the rank of a syndrome because the anatomic location permits surgical implantation of an aortic graft, if the distal vessels are proved patent by arteriography. The syn-

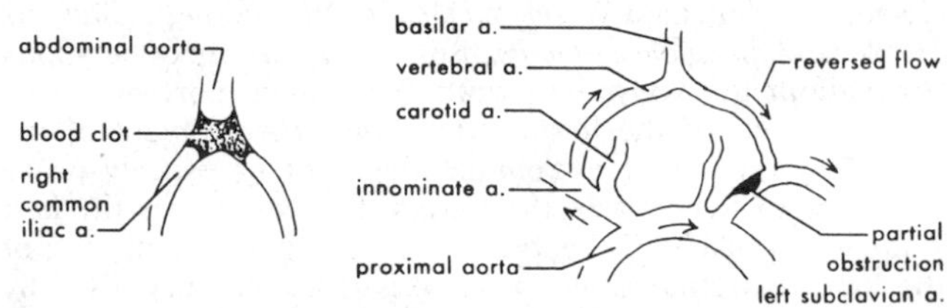

Fig. 6-60. Two syndromes of large-artery obstruction. **A.** Plugging at the aortic bifurcation (Leriche's syndrome). *A short thrombus closes the lower part of the abdominal aorta and extends a variable distance down the common iliac arteries. The accessible segments of the femoral, popliteal, dorsalis pedis, and posterior tibial arteries are rendered pulseless. Pain in the legs and intermittent claudication are the common symptoms.* **B.** Subclavian steal syndrome. *In this diagram is shown the most common site of narrowing, the left subclavian artery, although other sites have also been reported. The lowered pressure in the distal subclavian, together with anomalies of the vertebral and basilar arteries, produces a reversal of flow in the vertebral artery that results in ischemia of the brain stem. Surgical relief of the obstruction causes disappearance of symptoms. Since the closure of the artery is incomplete, the symptoms may be induced only with exertion of the left arm.*

drome is also caused by the chronic use of methysergide or ergot. Ultrasonic examination assists in localization of lesion.

Arterial Plugging: ***Thromboangiitis Obliterans*** (Buerger's Disease). The process begins as an acute panarteritis, involving all three layers of some medium-sized arteries. Granulation tissue in the intima ultimately causes gradual arterial plugging, producing arterial deficiency in the tissues. Commonly, only segments of an artery or arteries are affected. *Distinction.* There are no physical signs, as such, that distinguish the process from atherosclerosis. The *distribution* of affected vessels may differ from that in atherosclerosis; in addition to the vessels of the lower extremities, thromboangiitis has some predilection for the radial, ulnar, or the digital arteries of one or more fingers, as demonstrated by the Allen test. The *age incidence* in thromboangiitis is usually between 20 and 40 years, younger than in atherosclerosis. The disease occurs predominantly in *males*. Thromboangiitis is often associated with venous involvement, manifest as *superficial migrating thrombophlebitis*.

Nodular Vessels Without Asthma or Eosinophilia: ***Polyarteritis Nodosa—Classic*** (Periarteritis N.). This is the prototype for a large group of segmented necrotizing vasculitides [see p. 465 for classification and pathophysiology]. *Age and Sex:* all ages, both sexes, but peak incidence in the 5th to 6th decades, with slight female predominance. *Antigen:* usually unknown. *Involved Vessels:* small and *intermediate muscular arteries;* segmented distribution; sites especially at arterial bifurcations and branchings; sometimes processes extend to arterioles and adjacent veins. All layers of mural infiltration furnish sites for fibrinoid necrosis, thrombi, ischemia, and infarction; all stages are present simultaneously. *Asthma:* none. *Aneurysms:* present, up to 1 cm in diameter, in intermediate vessels demonstrated by angiograms of kidneys, liver, and viscera [these also occur in the overlap syndrome, systemic lupus erythematosus, and fibromuscular dysplasia]. *Allergic History:* uncommon. *Involved Organs:* LUNGS AND SPLEEN: not involved. GASTROINTESTINAL: visceral infarction. CORONARY ARTERIES: thrombosis in children. LIVER: acute to chronic hepatitis. PERIPHERAL NERVES: mononeuritis multiplex. SKIN: subcutaneous nodules on superficial vessels, palpable purpura, livido reticularis. JOINTS AND MUSCLES: myalgias, arthralgias, but not arthritis. *Laboratory:* no eosinophilia. *Symptoms and Signs* [none distinctive]: *fever, tachycardia,* *pain in viscera* and *muscles; glomerulitis, hypertension, myocardial infarction. Response to Therapy and Prognosis:* large doses of corticosteroids can sometimes suppress and perhaps prolong life; but treatment is unsatisfactory. There is progressive destruction of organs and often death from thrombosis.

Nodular Vessels with Asthma and Eosinophilia: ***Allergic Granulomatosis (G. of Churg and Strauss)*** (for classification and pathophysiology see p. 466). This disorder resembles closely the classic polyarteritis nodosa *except* that it has *associated asthma* and *eosinophilia* with an *allergic diasthesis* revealed by the family history. The lungs are involved with pneumonitis or exceptionally refractory asthma.

Atypical: ***Systemic Necrotizing Vasculitis (Overlap Syndrome).*** This category is necessitated by the seeming imperfections of the present classification (see p. 465 for classification and pathophysiology). It includes some of the characteristics of each the classic polyarteritis nodosa and the allergic granulomatosis. *Involved Blood Vessels: small* and *intermediate* muscular arteries, arterioles, capillaries, and veins. *Aneurysms:* angiograms may show aneurysms in small vessels. *Allergic History:* may be present. *Lungs:* may contain granulomata or infiltrates. *Eosinophilia:* may be present.

Plugging of Vessels of the Aortic Arch: ***Pulseless Disease*** (Takayasu's Disease). This is an arteritis of unknown cause that produces progressive thrombosis of the aortic arch and the innominate, carotids, and subclavians. A characteristic triad of signs is (1) absent pulse in a vessel of the upper extremity or the neck, (2) carotid sinus sensitivity wherein movements of the head induce syncope, (3) ocular disorders, such as cataract and retinal defects. Other occlusive disorders of the aortic arch must be distinguished.

Subclavian Stenosis: ***Subclavian Steal Syndrome.*** With increasing frequency patients are found with atherosclerotic stenosis of either subclavian artery, proximal to the origin of the vertebral artery. In addition to the expected low volume flow in the affected arm, retrograde flow from the ipsilateral vertebral artery induced cerebral ischemia in the brain stem and consequent neurologic signs (Fig. 6-60B). On the occluded side a *bruit* was always heard in the supraclavicular fossa, occasionally a *thrill* was felt in the same place. The arterial *pulse volume* and *blood pressure* were diminished in the affected arm. Manifestations of *cerebral ischemia* were intermittent or continuous; in various cases, they ranged from vertigo and vague dizziness to slurring of speech and hemiparesis. The cerebral signs and symptoms could be induced by *exercising* the affected arm. After precise localization with arteriography, endarterectomy was successful in relieving the condition. [See M. Reivich, H. E. Holling, B. Roberts, and J. F. Toole: Reversal of Blood Flow Through the Vertebral Artery and Its Effect on the Cerebral Circulation, *N. Engl. J. Med.,* **265:**878–85, 1961. Editorial: A New Vascular Syndrome—"The Subclavian Steal," *N. Engl. J. Med.* **265:**912–13, 1961. J. A. Mannick, C. G. Suter, and D. M. Hume: The "Subclavian Steal" Syndrome: A Further Documentation, *J.A.M.A.,* **182:**254–58, 1962.] Ultrasonic examination localizes site of obstruction and direction of flow.

Subclavian Compression Syndromes. Although compression of the subclavian artery is primarily a circulatory disturbance, the concomitant pressure on the brachial plexus produces symptoms and signs that bring the patient to the physician. Hence, the true nature of the disorder is usually diagnosed by considering the causes of peripheral neuritis in the upper extremities and making appropriate maneuvers that demonstrate brachial compression.

Subclavian Compression: ***Scalenus Anticus Syndrome.*** This condition is suggested by intermittent or constant pain in the ulnar aspect of the arm and hand, numbness or tingling in the same distribution, wasting or weakness of the arm or hand muscles. *Anatomy.* The anterior side of a cervical triangle is formed by the belly of the scalenus anticus muscle stretching from the 3rd, 4th, 5th, and 6th cervical vertebrae anteriorly and downward to the 1st rib (Fig. 6-61A). This posterior side is formed by the scalenus medius muscle; the base is the 1st rib. Between the two Scaleni emerge the subclavian artery and the brachial plexus. *Adson's Test.* Have the patient sit with pronated forearms on the knees, chin raised high and pointed toward the side being examined, holding his breath during inspiration; determine whether the radial pulse is abolished or diminished by this posture; check with the breath held in similar fashion, but the head held pointed straight forward. The latter posture should not cause compression.

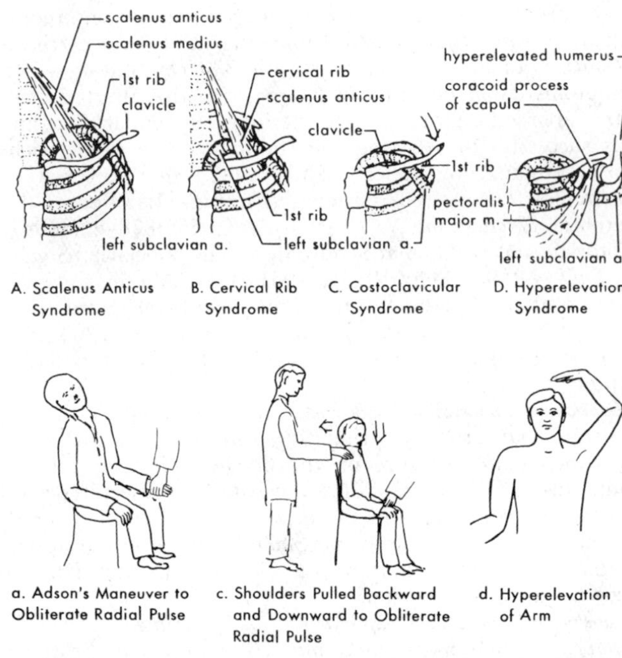

Fig. 6-61. Compression syndromes of the superior thoracic aperture. **A.** Scalenus anticus syndrome. *The scalenus anticus muscle has attachments to the transverse processes of the cervical vertebrae above and below to the first rib. Posteriorly and behind the subclavian artery, the scalenus medius attaches to the same bones. Hypertrophy of the bellies of the two muscles causes compression of the artery between them, with motions such as turning the head to the ipsilateral side. This is tested by Adson's maneuver* (a) *where the patient sits with chin raised, head rotated to the left, and chest held in the inspiratory position. A positive test is marked by diminution or disappearance of the left radial pulse. The other side is tested similarly.* **B.** Cervical rib syndrome. *The diagram shows a cervical rib compressing the right scalenus anticus muscle and indirectly the subclavian artery. This may produce diminution in the radial pulse or a peripheral neuritis of parts of the brachial plexus.* **C.** Costoclavicular syndrome. *The geometry of the aperture may be such that rotation of the clavicles downward and backward compresses the subclavian arteries against the first rib. This is tested* (c) *by having the patient seated in a chair*

Clinical Occurrence. Hypertrophy or edema of the muscle may occur after unusually vigorous use in normally sedentary persons, or in those with unusual occupations, such as weight lifters. Spasm of the muscle may result from poor posture, anomalous 1st rib, or cervical rib.

Subclavian Compression: ***Cervical Rib.*** In addition to producing spasm of the scalenus anticus muscle (see the preceding), cervical rib may directly compress the subclavian artery to produce diminution in the radial pulse in any position (Fig. 6-61B). Occasionally, the extra rib may be palpated directly in the supraclavicular fossa, but usually the examiner is uncertain, so that he relies upon the x-ray film for the diagnosis. The rib may also compress the brachial plexus to produce pain or paresthesias in the hand.

Subclavian Compression: ***Costoclavicular Syndrome.*** The symptoms are similar to those produced by compression of the scalenus anticus muscle. *Costoclavicular Maneuver.* This tests for compression of the subclavian artery by the 1st rib. Have the patient sit with his radial pulses palpated by an assistant; stand behind the patient and force his shoulders downward and backward, so that the thoracic outlet is narrowed (Fig. 6-61C). If there is sufficient disproportion to cause symptoms, the pulse volumes will be diminished. Recent studies have shown that the maneuver just described does not disclose the costoclavicular syndrome with many patients. Another test is recommended in which the patient stands with elbows flexed at 90°. In the coronal plane of the body (arms in 90° of abduction), the arms are placed successively in three positions, at 45°, 90°, and 135° of elevation (the latter position by placing the hands on the head). At each position, the radial pulse is palpated and the point beneath the midportion of the clavicle is auscultated. In a series of normal subjects, 5% had obliteration

---

and the examiner standing behind him. The physician pushes the shoulders downward and backward while an assistant feels for diminution of the radial pulses. **D.** Hyperelevation of the arm. *The geometry of the thorax in some persons is such that hyperelevation of the arm causes the coracoid process of the scapula to impinge and compress the subclavian artery. This is tested by* (d) *demonstrating that the radial pulse is lost with hyperelevation.*

of the radial pulse at 90° elevation and 15% at 135°. Patients with costoclavicular syndrome had pulse obliteration in at least one of the three positions; but in positions where the pulse was palpable, partial obstruction was shown by the presence of a *subclavicular systolic murmur* [T. Winsor and R. Brow: Costoclavicular Syndrome, *J.A.M.A.*, **196**:967, 1966].

Clinical Occurrence. Situations in which the shoulders are forced downward and backward, such as a long march with a heavy pack on the shoulders.

Subclavian Compression: ***Ischemia from Hyperelevation of the Arm.*** The patient usually complains of *numbness* and *tingling* in one or both hands or arms, either intermittent or constant. Questioning discloses that he sleeps supine with arms elevated so the hands are behind or over the head; or he has engaged in some occupation requiring elevation of the arms, such as painting ceilings. *Anatomy.* In some persons, elevation of the arm causes impingement on the subclavian artery by the coracoid process of the scapula, so the vessel is compressed (Fig. 6-61D). *Hyperabduction Test.* Lift the patient's hand over his head in approximately the position assumed in sleeping; have him open and close his hand several times; note whether the radial pulse volume is diminished or abolished.

White and Blue Fingers: ***Raynaud's Disease and Phenomenon.*** Paroxysmal constriction of the *digital* arteries and minute der-

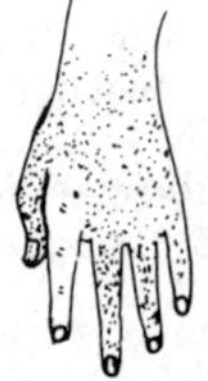

A. Blanching of Finger

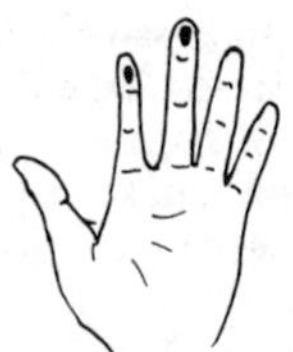

B. Gangrene on Fingertips

Fig. 6-62. Signs of Raynaud's disease. **A.** *Blanching of the finger induced by exposure to cold may produce the classic sequence of color changes where a sharply demarcated area at the end of a finger becomes chalky-white, then blue, and finally red, before it returns to normal. It may not be very painful.* **B.** *In long-standing cases, gangrenous spots at the fingertips occur; the area around the fingernail may ulcerate.*

mal vessels usually occurs bilaterally; commonly affecting the fingers, additionally involving the toes in half the cases. About four fifths of the patients are young women. The attacks are induced by exposure to cold or when experiencing emotional stress. Eventually, the digits of the hands and feet are symmetrically affected. Early attacks may involve only the tips of the digits; later, the process may extend proximally. From one to four fingers of each hand may be included, rarely the thumbs. In the classic picture, lasting from 15 to 60 minutes, the terminal digits become *chalky white* and numb (Fig. 6-62A). The pallid skin is covered with sweat. Soon the pallor is succeeded by *intense cyanosis* and pain. Sometimes either pallor or cyanosis is absent, never both. During recovery, either spontaneously or after immersion in warm water, projections of hyperemia from the unaffected skin invade the cyanotic regions until all blueness has been replaced by *brilliant red.* Hyperemia is accompanied by tingling, throbbing, and some swelling of tissues. After many attacks, trophic changes may appear in the nails and adjacent skin. Small areas of gangrene develop on the tips of the fingers and toes (Fig. 6-62B). *Pathophysiology.* The pallor is produced by tight constriction of the digital and smaller arteries of the part. Soon the capillaries dilate greatly to hold stagnant blood that becomes deoxygenated, producing the blue skin. *Distinction.* The sequence of pallor, cyanosis, and rubor is diagnostic when induced by exposure to cold. Currently, the term *Raynaud's disease* is reserved for cases in which the classic color changes are symmetric and there is no other associated disease. The same signs are attributed to *Raynaud's phenomenon* when they are associated with thromboangiitis obliterans, atherosclerosis, trauma to nerves of the arms from crutches or air hammers or cervical ribs, disseminated lupus erythematosus, polyarteritis, and various types of peripheral neuritis. Raynaud's phenomenon occurs more frequently in patients with migraine (26%) than in persons without that affliction (6%) and may represent the expression of a generalized vasospastic disorder. [I. Zahavi, A. Chagnac, R. Hering, S. Davidovich, and A. Kuritzky: Prevalence of Raynaud's Phenomenon in Patients with Migraine, *Arch. Intern. Med.,* **144:**742–44, 1984].

Blue Hands and Feet: ***Acrocyanosis.*** This is a benign affection in which the skin of the hands and feet is persistently cyanotic, cold, and sweating. The condition is most common in young women; it is seldom encountered in middle age in either sex. The skin is uniformly blue; the color is intensified by exposure to cold. The cyanosis is abolished when the part is elevated or when the patient sleeps. There is no discomfort; the patient consults the physician because of the cosmetic effect. *Pathophysiology.* The excessive arteriolar constriction is ascribed to increased tone of the sympathetic nervous system, although humoral agents may contribute.

Gangrene of Fingertips. Often gangrene of the fingertips is the end result of chronic Raynaud's disease or phenomenon, so this occurs in a variety of conditions.

Clinical Occurrence. Scleroderma, pneumatic-hammer disease, obstruction of the superior thoracic aperture (scalenus anticus syndrome, cervical rib, mediastinal tumor or abscess), atherosclerosis, thromboangiitis obliterans, cold agglutination causing blood sludging, ergotism, methylsergide medication, chronic renal failure and hemodialysis, possibly hyperphosphatemia, thrombocythemia.

Symmetric Gangrene of the Digits: ***Ergotism.*** An intense constriction of the peripheral blood vessels is caused by the ingestion of large amounts of ergot by normal persons or of small amounts by those who are sensitive. Ergot may be taken as a drug or eaten in grain that has been contaminated with the fungus. The first symptom is often burning pain in the extremities *(St. Anthony's fire),* with loss of arterial pulses in the hands or feet. Mottled cyanosis of the extremities and coldness of the skin follow. Finally, symmetric gangrene of the fingers and toes occurs, which may extend proximally. Symptoms of headache, weakness, nausea, vomiting, visual disturbances, and angina pectoris may accompany the signs.

Arteriovenous Fistula, Acquired. A communication between an artery and an adjacent vein may be caused by a stab or gunshot wound or by erosion from neoplasm or infectious arteritis. The hemorrhage after trauma is profuse but easily controlled. A thrill and bruit may develop some hours later. After wound healing has occurred, the signs of chronic circulatory disturbance develop. Although fistulas may occur in many parts of the body, the greatest variety of signs are evident when an extremity is involved (Fig. 6-63). *Venous deficit* is manifested by the development of varicose veins in the extremity,

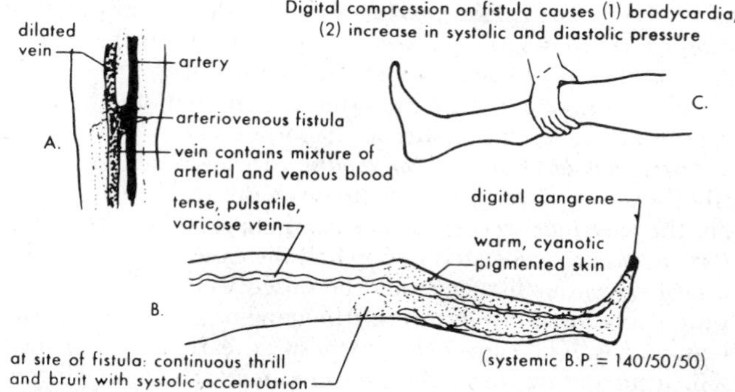

Fig. 6-63. Signs of arteriovenous fistula. *As an example, a fistula between the popliteal artery and vein is represented.* **A.** *Shows the communication between artery and vein behind the knee joint.* **B.** *The lesion is in the left leg; the superficial veins are greatly dilated from blood under arterial pressure, so they are tense to the touch and sometimes pulsatile. Distal to the fistula, the skin is warm from the arterial blood in the veins, cyanotic and pigmented from hemostasis. Distal gangrene may occur. At the site of the leak a thrill and bruit may be found; these are continuous throughout the cardiac cycle, with systolic accentuation. The arterial pulse pressure is greater than normal if the orifice of the fistula is large enough.* **C.** *Closure of the fistula by digital compression produces slowing of the heart rate (Branham's bradycardiac reflex) and augmentation of both systolic and diastolic arterial pressures in the general circulation.*

peripheral edema, stasis pigmentation of the skin, stasis ulceration in the foot, indurative cellulitis. The pedal ulcers are usually in the distal parts, in contradistinction to simple varicose ulcers that are over pressure points. *Arterial disorders* produce gangrene of the distal parts and hypertrophy of the extremity when the injury occurs before the epiphyses have closed; throughout the cardiac cycle a *thrill* and *bruit* occur locally with systolic accentuation; the skin temperature is increased distal to the fistula. When the shunt is large, the dilated superficial veins may be less compressible than normal, and the venous pressure may approach the magnitude of arterial pressure; the velocity of venous blood is increased; the right heart becomes dilated and cardiac failure may result. The *diastolic arterial pressure may be lowered* by an extensive shunt. Compression, so as to close the fistula, produces a sharp slowing of the pulse rate, called *Branham's bradycardiac sign,* and both the systolic and diastolic pressure may increase. Shunts deep in the abdomen or thorax yield only the bruit and the remote effects on venous and arterial pressure as diagnostic signs.

Arteriovenous Fistula, Congenital. Developmental shunts from arteries to veins may occur in many parts of the body, but they are most accessible to examination in the extremities. *Birth marks* are associated in one half the cases, so the question of arteriovenous fistula should be raised when one sees port-wine spots, blue-red cavernous hemangiomas, or diffuse hemangiomas. The signs are evident at an early age, and there is no history of trauma to the part. Frequently congenital fistulas are quite small, so the signs associated with the acquired type are not evident; thrills and bruits may be absent; the bradycardiac sign of Branham is less pronounced. The affected limb may be hypertrophied, and it may exhibit increased sweating and hypertrichosis.

Disorders of Large Limb Veins

Adequate drainage of blood from the extremities requires (1) *patency* of the venous lumina, (2) *voluntary muscle contractions* to furnish the pumping action by compressing the adjacent veins (Fig. 6-64), (3) *competent valves* in the veins so venous compression moves the blood proximally. A deficit in any of

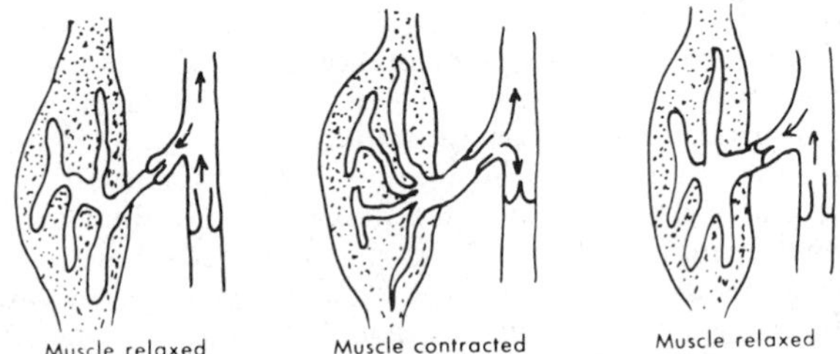

Fig. 6-64. Venous flow caused by muscular contraction. *When the muscle is relaxed, it is filled with blood, but no blood emerges into the collecting veins. Muscle contraction expels blood into the collecting veins and closes the valves so the blood is propelled toward the heart. Thus venous return from muscles depends upon patent vessels, competent valves, and muscular contractions.*

these three may result in *venous stasis,* indicated by *edema* of the extremities from increased filtration pressure in the capillaries, *stasis pigmentation* of the skin from capillary dilatation and damage, *ulceration* of the skin from bacterial invasion of poorly nourished tissues.

Venous occlusion results either from external compression of the walls or from plugging of the lumina by fibrosis, thrombi, or neoplasms growing in the vessel cavities. The pumping action of voluntary muscles may be dangerously inhibited by complete bed rest or by immobilizing an extremity with a cast. Excessive caliber of vessels may produce stasis as well as when the lumina are narrowed; varicose veins dilate to such a degree that their valves become incompetent.

EXAMINATION OF LARGE ARM AND LEG VEINS. **With the patient supine, look for signs of venous stasis: pitting *edema* of the extremity, stasis *pigmentation* of the skin, and *ulceration*. Have the patient stand, and look for *dilated veins* in the arms and legs. Demonstrate *venous occlusion* by elevating the extremity to determine whether the veins collapse promptly. If occlusion is present, palpate the venous walls for *hard plugs* of thrombus or *hard cords* of fibrosis. If patent varicose veins are present, use the special tests for *incompetency* of valves.**

Varicose Veins. This term is usually applied to dilated veins from all causes except angiomas. *Primary* varicosities are venous dilatations that develop spontaneously; *secondary* varicosities are dilatations resulting from proximal obstruction in pregnancy, trauma, thrombophlebitis, compressing tumors, congestive heart failure, portal obstruction, or arteriovenous fistulas. Whenever varicose veins occur in only one extremity the possibility of local compression or an arteriovenous fistula should be considered. In the latter condition, pulsations are frequently present in the dilated veins. When varicose veins are massive, assumption of the erect position may pool enough blood to cause orthostatic hypotension and faintness. ***Anatomy.*** Since varicosities are most common in leg veins, their anatomic relations are important to examination (Fig. 6-65). The *great saphenous vein* begins at the mediodorsal side of the foot and courses upward along the medial edge of the subcutaneous aspect of the tibia, going medial to the patella and posterior to the median epicondyle of the femur; in the thigh, its course is slightly lateralward and upward to the femoral canal, where

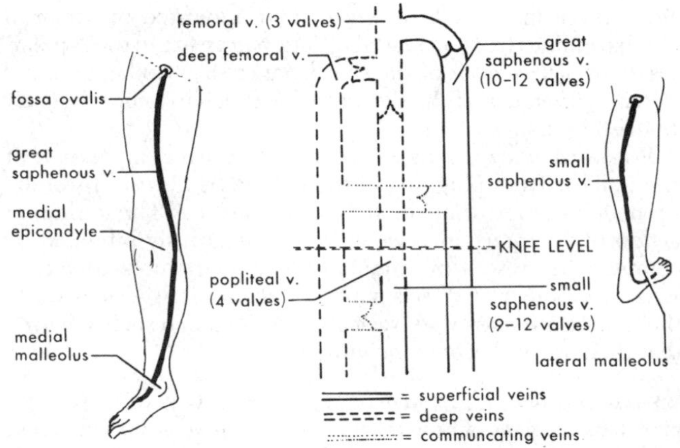

Fig. 6-65. Large superficial veins of the lower limb. *The great saphenous vein begins on the medial aspect of the foot, courses backward under the medial malleolus, up the medial aspect of the calf, behind the medial epicondyle, then obliquely across the anterior thigh to the femoral vein as it enters the femoral canal beneath the inguinal ligament. The small saphenous vein begins on the lateral side of the foot, curves backward beneath the lateral malleolus, then upward on the posterior surface of the calf to enter the popliteal fossa and joins with the popliteal vein. The middle figure diagrams the communications between the superficial veins (in heavy solid lines) and the deep veins (in broken lines) and the communicating vessels (in dotted lines).*

it empties into the *femoral vein.* The *small saphenous vein* begins at the lateral side of the foot, curving under and back of the lateral malleolus, going upward to assume a position in the midline of the belly of the gastrocnemius muscle; finally abandoning its superficial location, it dives deeply into the popliteal fossa to empty into the *popliteal vein.* Several *communicating veins* run between the great saphenous and the femoral vein. To summarize: the great saphenous vein emerges from the femoral canal and runs down the anteromedial aspect of the lower extremity to the medial side of the foot; the small saphenous vein emerges from the popliteal fossa and runs down the posterior aspect of the calf to curl under the lateral malleolus.

TEST FOR COMPETENCE IN GREAT SAPHENOUS VEIN (PERCUSSION TEST). **With the patient standing and the varicose veins filled with**

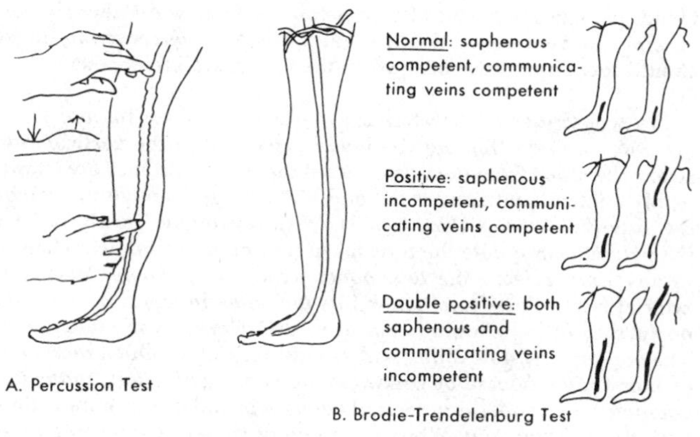

C. Perthes' Test

1. Vein size diminished: normal
2. Vein size unchanged: both saphenous and communicating veins incompetent
3. Vein size increased with pain: deep veins obstructed, communicating veins incompetent

Fig. 6-66. Tests of varicose veins. **A.** Percussion test. *This tests valvular competence. With the patient standing and the vein full of blood, the vessel is struck sharply above the knee with the left hand (1) while the right hand palpates a segment (2) to perceive an impulse indicating incompetence of the intervening valve.* **B.** Brodie-Trendelenburg test for competence. *This tests both the great saphenous vein and the branches communicating with the deep femoral vein. The lower limb is elevated vertically until drained of venous blood; then a tourniquet is applied at midthigh and the patient stands upright. The tourniquet is removed in 60 seconds. Normally arterial flow from below fills the vein in about 35 seconds. When the tourniquet is applied, faster filling indicates incompetence of the communicating veins. Normally, when the tourniquet is released, no further increment of blood is added from above; additional flow indicates saphenous valve incompetence.* **C.** Perthes' test for competence of the deep femoral vein. *A tourniquet is applied at midthigh when standing with the veins filled with blood. The patient walks for 5 minutes with tourniquet in place. Normally the size of the veins will reduce, indicating competent valves and patent lumens.*

blood, palpate a segment of vein below the knee while sharply percussing the vein above the knee (Fig. 6-66A). The receiving finger should feel an impulse only when the valves are incompetent.

TEST FOR COMPETENCE IN SAPHENOFEMORAL COMPLEX (BRODIE-TRENDELENBURG TEST). **Elevate the lower extremity to the vertical, and stroke the blood from the veins toward the heart until they are empty. Apply a tourniquet around the midthigh, snugly enough to occlude the superficial veins (Fig. 6-66B). With tourniquet in place, have the patient stand; note the time taken for venous filling from below; in any case, release the tourniquet within 60 seconds. Normally, arterial blood flow from below fills the veins in about 35 seconds; no further filling should occur after the release of the tourniquet. The sequence of slow filling with occlusion, and no added increment of blood after release of compression, is a *negative* test, indicating competence in both the great saphenous vein and its communications with the femoral vein. When occlusion of the great saphenous vein results in slow filling, but release of compression is followed by quick filling from above (1 to 10 seconds), the test is *positive* from incompetence of the great saphenous vein. A *double positive* test is marked by rapid filling during compression, together with an added increment of blood from above when pressure is released, indicating incompetence in both the saphenous vein and its femoral communications.**

TEST FOR OBSTRUCTION OF DEEP VEINS (PERTHES' TEST). **Have the patient walk about; then inspect the varicosities. Apply the tourniquet to the midthigh when the patient is standing and the veins are filled with blood; have him walk for five minutes (Fig. 6-66C). If the veins *collapse* below the tourniquet, the deep veins are patent and the communicating veins are competent. If the venous caliber remains *unchanged*, incompetence is present in both saphenous and communicating veins; competent veins would direct blood flow into the deep veins during muscular contractions. If the veins *increase in prominence* and *pain occurs*, the deep veins are occluded. The level at which incompetence is present in the communicating veins may be located by the *Ochsner-Mahorner modification* of Perthes' test. After the previous maneuvers, the tourniquet is applied at the knee and at the midcalf, sequentially, to determine the level of occlusion at which the veins will collapse with walking.**

ULTRASONIC EXAMINATION. **The competence of veins, deep as well as superficial, is accurately assessed with the Doppler-shift technique.**

Cavernous Hemangioma of the Leg. This congenital tumor may occur anywhere in the body. When a massive angioma involves the leg, it may be confused with varicose veins. The affected leg is usually enlarged circumferentially. The dilated ill-defined blood sinuses raise the surface of the normal skin, under which are seen purplish masses that are readily compressible. They are distinguished from varicosities by their distribution, which does not correspond to that of the large leg veins. In the erect position enough blood may be pooled to cause orthostatic hypotension.

Thrombophlebitis. As the name implies, thrombosis and inflammation of the venous walls are associated; inflammation may either precede or follow clot formation. The lesion may occur without previous cause, or it may result from mechanical or chemical trauma, suppurative disease, ischemia, anemia, polycythemia, or leukemia. When *acute,* the veins are painful and tender; the overlying skin is red and hot. Cramps are incited in adjacent muscles. Fever and leukocytosis are common. Involved superficial veins feel like firm cords. When thrombophlebitis involves an extremity, edema and dependent cyanosis result from venous occlusion. In a *chronic* process, pain and tenderness are slight and there are less reddening and heat in the overlying skin. *Special Varieties.* Sudden thrombophlebitis of the femoral vein presents a clinical picture termed *phlegmasia alba dolens,* because of the excruciating pain, the massive edema of the extremity, and the pallor from arterial spasm. These signs suggest arterial embolism, but the pallor is less intense; there is more cyanosis; the femoral vein is tender; no anesthesia is produced; when the arterial pulses are impalpable, they can usually be demonstrated by Doppler examination. A rare variant is *phlegmasia caerulea dolens,* caused by the involvement of the entire venous return of an extremity. It is characterized by extreme pain, massive edema, and deep cyanosis of the entire limb. Circulatory collapse may abolish the arterial pulses, but the deep blue of the skin distinguishes the condition from arterial embolism. Ultrasonic examination assists in diagnosis.

Deep-Vein Thrombophlebitis (Silent T., Phlebothrombosis). This term is usually applied to thrombosis of the deep veins of the legs. The sparse associated inflammation facilitates dislodgment of clots that provide the commonest missiles for the pulmonary embolism that so frequently kills bedridden patients. The symptoms and signs are often obscure or absent, but early diagnosis is sometimes lifesaving. For example, one investigator reported that one third of all patients over 40 years old undergoing surgery developed deep-vein thrombosis, as detected by radioactive fibrinogen; one half of these were not detected clinically. This inaccuracy in diagnosis could presumably be improved if physicians increased the number of clinical tests they customarily employ. [The authors acknowledge a debt for much of the following information to N. Shafer: Thrombophlebitis: Early Physical Signs, *Med. Counterpoint,* Feb., 1972, pp. 57–59.] ***Symptoms.*** *Pain* or a *sense of fullness* in the leg, aggravated by standing or walking. ***Systemic Signs.*** Restlessness, fever, tachycardia. "When there is a concomitant rise in temperature, pulse, and respiration in an otherwise normal course of events, we can be reasonably sure that thrombosis is present" [A. W. Alen and G. A. Donaldson: Venous Thrombosis, *Bull. N.Y. Acad. Med.,* **24:**619, 1948]. ***Cyanosis.*** Deep-vein thrombosis is often accompanied by cyanosis of the skin on the lower third of the leg or on the foot, especially when the leg is dependent. ***Elevated Skin Temperature.*** Expose the lower limbs to the room air for 10 minutes and then test the skin temperature of both legs with the back or your hand, comparing the two limbs. In half the cases of thrombophlebitis there is elevated skin temperature around ankle or calf. ***Edema.*** Pitting edema of the foot, ankle, or leg, persisting after a good diuresis or two weeks after the removal of a plaster cast, suggests deep-vein thrombophlebitis. ***Venous Engorgement of the Feet.*** Veins on the dorsa of the feet that remain distended when the legs are elevated to 45° suggest deep-vein thrombosis. *Pratt's sign* is the presence of three dilated veins over the tibia, called *sentinel veins.* The venous distention should persist when the legs are elevated to 45°. Small dilated veins just below the knee or above the ankle are usually communicating veins between the long and short saphenous systems, distended by blockage of intramuscular veins. ***Cough or Sneeze Pain in the Calf.*** Pain in the leg along the course of the thrombosed vein can be induced by sneezing or coughing *(Louvel's sign).* The pain disappears with digital compression of the vein proximal to the obstruction. ***Local Tenderness.*** Palpation of the leg to detect segments of thrombosis should be made for tenderness at several points, prompted by knowledge of anatomy. The deep veins of the plantar surface drain mainly into the posterior tibial vein, deep to tendo Achillis. The anterior tibial vein lies in a groove between tibia and fibula; it penetrates the interosseous membrane to join the popliteal vein. The majority of deep veins of the calf are in the soleus muscle [I. J. T. Davies: Clinical Signs of Deep-Vein Thrombosis, *Lancet,* **2:**321, 1972]. So the following regions should be palpated for tenderness: the soles; the region deep to tendo Achillis; in the groove between tibia and fibula (anterior tibial vein); bimanual palpation of the soleus muscle below the largest swelling of the calf made by the gastrocnemius; in the popliteal fossa; over the adductor muscles of the medial thigh; over the femoral veins above and below the inguinal ligaments; by digital examination of the rectum test for tenderness of the iliac veins. ***Calf Tenderness with Digital Compression*** *(Bancroft's Sign,* and *Moses' Sign).* Consists of compressing the calf forward against the tibia and comparing the resulting pain with that elicited by transverse compression while the gastrocnemius is lifted from the tibia by grasping both sides of the muscle. Thrombophlebitis causes more pain with forward compression. ***Calf Tenderness with Cuff Compression*** *(Lowenberg's Sign)* requires a sphygmomanometer cuff to be wrapped around each calf and simultaneous inflation of the two. The more sensitive calf is the site of thrombosis. Most normal persons tolerate pressures of 180 mm Hg. ***Calf Pain with Passive Congestion*** *(Ramirez's Sign)* requires the patient to be supine with knees slightly flexed. A sphygmomanometer cuff is placed above the knee and inflated to 40 mm Hg. The resulting venous pressure provokes pain at the site of the thrombophlebitis. If the pressure is sustained for 5 minutes, the intensity of the pain is increased, but it disappears promptly when the pressure is released. ***Weight and Consistency of Calf.*** With the patient's knee flexed to 90° and his foot on the bed, use the flat of your supine hand and lift the calf gently up and down to test *increased weight* and *hardness* for inflammatory edema of the limb. ***Bone Tenderness.*** Percuss the subcutaneous surface of the tibia, medial to the crest, using the tip of a flexed finger and a force similar to that employed to percuss a chest. Bone tenderness (Lisker's sign) is present in about 65% of persons with deep-vein thrombosis. Since the sign does not occur with herniated intervertebral disk or other lumbosacral affections, bone pain serves to distinguish thrombosis, because both conditions give a positive Homan's sign. ***Calf***

Spasm (*Homan's Sign*). The patient's knee is put in flexion and the examiner forcefully and abruptly dorsiflexes the ankle. This produces pain in the calf or popliteal region in about 35% of the patients with deep-vein thrombosis. But the sign is also positive with herniated low intervertebral disk and other lumbosacral affection. The absence of bone tenderness excludes the skeletal causes of Homan's sign. *Peabody's Technique.* This tests for spasm of the calf muscles by the presence of exaggerated plantar flexion. With the patient supine in bed, the examiner places his thumbs on the patient's soles at the ends of the second metatarsals. Enough pressure is applied to lift the feet about 20 inches (50 cm) off the bed. When the two medial malleoli are elevated and apposed, the two bunions should be opposite; calf spasm will lower the ipsilateral bunion. *Superficial Thrombophlebitis.* The presence of this may mask the coincidental occurrence of deep-vein disease. When available, ultrasonic examination greatly simplifies diagnostication of this condition.

Diagnosis of Chronic Painless Enlargement of the Legs. Several causes must be distinguished: *Adiposity* commonly occurs in women. Although some evidence of obesity is present elsewhere in the body, the fat about the ankles may be disproportionately great. The tissue has the consistency of fat, and pitting edema is absent. *Deep venous obstruction* usually is preceded by a history suggesting thrombophlebitis. The venous deficit may produce pain in the legs. Some pitting edema is usually present, although it may be obscured by thickening of the skin from the long duration. The skin is usually pigmented and cyanotic. Superficial veins may be dilated. *Varicose* veins are readily recognized when they are the cause of edema. *Lymphedema* causes a firm nonpitting swelling with no venous engorgement or cyanosis. In a large series of cases the authors concluded that the diagnosis of deep vein thrombosis necessitated venography only in patients with chronic venous insufficiency who had a normal Doppler ultrasonogram and an abnormal impedence plethysmogram, and in patients with abnormal hemodynamics [D. P. Flanigan *et al.:* Vascular-Laboratory Diagnosis of Clinically Suspected Acute Deep-Vein Thrombosis, *Lancet,* **2**:331–34, 1978]. Richards *et al.* concluded that when the Doppler ultrasonogram and impedence plethysmogram were both positive the diagnosis was certain [Richards *et al.:* Noninvasive Diagnosis of Deep Vein Thrombosis, *Arch. Intern. Med.*, **136:**1091–95, 1976].

Thrombosis of the Axillary Vein. The entire arm swells and aches, usually following trauma or intensive use of the arm in hyperabduction. The tissues are firm and there is no pitting edema. The superficial veins at the superior thoracic aperture may be dilated. Poor collateral circulation produces cyanosis of the skin. ***Distinction.*** In chronic cases, it must be distinguished from lymphedema. Both conditions produce solid, nonpitting swelling, but venous obstruction causes some cyanosis of the skin; the skin is pallid in lymphedema. Lymphedema of the arm is most common after radical mastectomy.

Circulation of the Head, Neck, and Trunk

The large arteries and veins in the head, neck, and trunk are less accessible to precise examination than are those in the extremities, so vascular disorders in these regions frequently must be inferred from evidence less direct than inspection and palpation of the vessels (Figs. 6-67 and 6-68A). In many instances, complexes of physical signs serve to indicate vascular lesions.

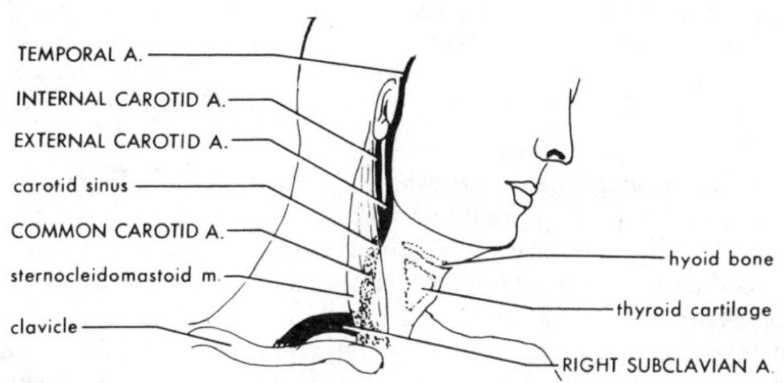

Fig. 6-67. Large superficial arteries of the head and neck. *The accessible arterial segments are diagrammed in solid black; inaccessible parts are stippled. The temporal artery courses anterior to the ear and upward to the temporal bone. The carotid arteries are deep to the anterior margin of the sternocleidomastoid muscle. The carotid sinus, at the bifurcation of the common carotid, is located by being level with the upper margin of the thyroid cartilage. A short segment of the subclavian artery is often palpable in the supraclavicular fossa.*

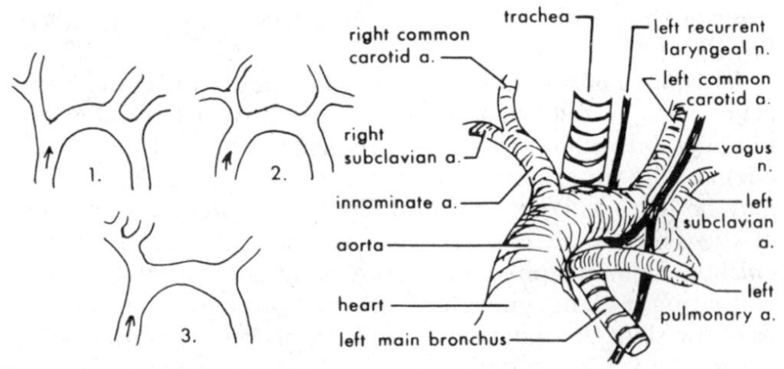

Fig. 6-68. Varieties and relations of the aortic arch. **A.** Varieties of the aortic arch. *The "normal" pattern (1) is only slightly more common than the other two; it has a right innominate artery, branching into the subclavian and common carotid. There is no left innominate artery; the left subclavian and common carotid originate from the aorta itself. In variation, there may be both a right and left innominate (2) or the right innominate may give off the left common carotid (3), in addition to the right carotid and subclavian.* **B.** Anatomic relations of a dilated aortic arch. *Aneurysm of the aortic arch or dilatation of the left atrium may compress the left recurrent laryngeal nerve against the cervical vertebrae or the left main bronchus, to produce paralysis of the left vocal cord, resulting in hoarseness or a brassy cough. Expansion of the arch downward impinges upon the left main bronchus so the trachea is depressed with each pulse wave, giving a physical sign called the tracheal tug.*

Arterial Aneurysms. Permanent abnormal dilatations of arteries occur as congenital anomalies or from weakening of the vessel walls. The forms of aneurysms are *fusiform, saccular,* and *dissecting*. Essentially similar physical signs are produced by fusiform and saccular dilatations, but the dissection of an artery presents an entirely different clinical picture. 2D echography, computerized tomography (CT) and magnetic resonance imaging (MRI) can be employed to examine the large arteries.

Thoracic Aneurysms. Whether saccular or fusiform, aneurysms of the thoracic aorta are caused by either syphilis or atherosclerosis. In either disease, the arch is commonly involved. Syphilis usually produces a lesion in the ascending aortic limb; rarely, it involves the descending limb.

Aneurysms of the Aortic Arch. Retrosternal *pain* is frequent, radiating to the left scapula, the left shoulder, or the left neck. Dilatation of the arch may compress the left recurrent laryngeal nerve against the trachea or the left main bronchus to cause *hoarseness* and a *brassy cough* (Fig. 6-68B). When the arch is dilated near the origin of the left subclavian artery, it may cause delay of the pulse wave to the left arm and reduction of more than 20 mm in the arterial pressure in that limb, so that there is *palpable diminution in pulse volume* in the left radial artery. The dilated aortic arch may push down the left main bronchus with each pulsation to produce a *tracheal tug,* perceived by lightly grasping the cricoid cartilage with the thumb and forefinger and feeling the trachea dip with each pulse (Fig. 6-68B). X-ray films of the chest usually confirm the diagnosis.

Aneurysms of the Ascending Aortic Limb. Cystic medial necrosis and Marfan's disease often involve the ascending aorta. The earliest sign is a *tympanitic aortic second heart sound* in the absence of arterial hypertension, from syphilitic aortitis. Later, the aortic valve becomes incompetent, so signs of *aortic regurgitation* appear. The murmur characteristically transmits down the right sternal border rather than the left. A palpable *thrust* may develop in the right second or third intercostal spaces. The *width of retromanubrial dullness is increased.* Erosion of ribs and protrusion of a *pulsatile mass* may occur in the region. X-ray films of the chest and aortography assist in the diagnosis.

Aneurysms of the Descending Aortic Limb. Frequently, these are silent and are discovered only by x-ray examination of the chest. They may erode the bodies of the vertebrae, when they cause pain in the back radiating around the chest through the intercostal nerves.

Aneurysms of the Abdominal Aorta. Atherosclerosis predominates as the cause. Frequently there is persistent or intermittent *pain* in the middle or lower belly, often radiating to the lower back. A *mass* with expansile pulsation can be felt in the region of the abdominal aorta; its expansile nature is demonstrated by showing lateral, as well as anteroposterior, movement to distinguish it from a solid tumor in front of the aorta that transmits the pulsation. The mass cannot be moved cephalad or caudad. A tortuous aorta must be distinguished by carefully palpating its course. In one tenth of the cases, a *bruit* may be heard over the aneurysm. A plain x-ray film of the abdomen may assist in the distinction, if sufficient calcium is present in the vessel walls to outline its course. Otherwise, aortography is indicated. Echography and computerized tomography are precise methods of diagnosis of this lesion—noninvasive methods that record the diameter of the aorta.

Aneurysms of the Upper Limbs. The subclavian, axillary, and brachial arteries are most commonly affected; the carotids are rarely involved. Trauma to the vessel wall is the most common cause; rarely, the vessels are involved by mycotic, necrotizing, or atherosclerotic aneurysms. The dilatations may be readily palpated in this region.

Aneurysms of the Lower Limbs. The most common sites are the femoral artery in Scarpa's triangle and the popliteal artery in its fossa. Atherosclerosis is the most common cause. The lesions are readily palpable.

Dissecting Aneurysm of the Aorta. Most commonly caused by atherosclerosis but also a consequence of cystic medial necrosis, a rupture of the intima occurs commonly in the ascending aorta; the blood extravasates into the media to separate the mural layers as the process extends distally. During progression, the mouths of the aortic branches may be occluded sequentially, with ischemia in the parts supplied. The onset is usually sudden, with *excruciating pain* that frequently begins in the infrascapular region and shifts successively to the lower back, the abdomen, the hips, and the thighs. *Shock* often results, with hypotension and collapse. Ischemia in various parts of the nervous system may produce syncope, convulsions, coma, hemiplegia, or paralyses of the lower limbs. Occasionally, arterial *murmurs* are heard. X-ray films of the thorax and abdomen may demonstrate separation of the aortic layers, if calcium is present as a marker. Usually the conditions is rapidly fatal. Rarely, healing occurs. One of us had a patient who died of another disease, having lived for years with an aorta composed of two concentric blood-filled tubes with communications at the proximal and distal ends. The diagnosis of dissection should be suspected in a sudden catastrophe in which there is sequential involvement of various bodily regions with loss of arterial pulses, when the distribution is compatible with extension distally along the aorta.

Mycotic Aneurysms. This term is applied to saccular aneurysms caused by weakening of the arterial walls from infectious processes other than syphilis. Mural involvement may develop as an extension of localized suppuration, actinomycosis, or tuberculosis. More frequently, an embolic arteritis occurs in the course of subacute bacterial endocarditis or septicemia. In one of our patients, an aneurysm of the femoral artery appeared as a complication of subacute bacterial endocarditis from brucellosis. Mycotic aneurysms usually involve vessels subject to much bending and lightly protected by overlying muscles, such as the axillary, brachial, femoral, and popliteal arteries.

Coarctation of the Aorta. Congenital strictures of the aortic arch may occur either proximal or distal to the point where the ductus arteriosus joins the aorta (*preductal* or *postductal*). Usually the constriction is distal to the mouth of the left subcla-

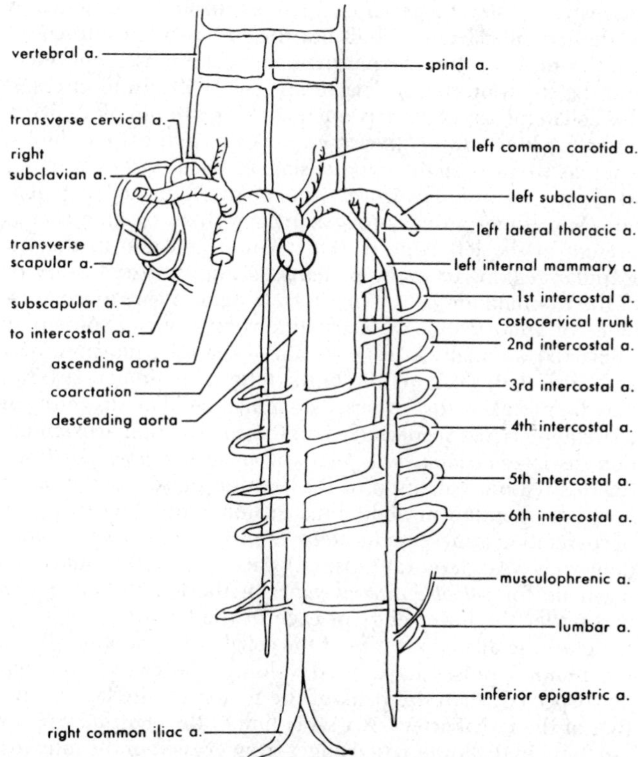

Fig. 6-69. Collateral circulation in coarctation of the aorta. *The diagram shows the collateral channels that cause dilatation of the intercostal arteries from the costocervical trunk and the internal mammary artery. The circulation around the scapula is augmented by blood through the transverse cervical artery. The pulse volume in the arms is normal; in the femoral arteries it is diminished or absent. The dilated scapular and intercostal arteries may be palpated in the back.*

vian artery, so the left arm is well supplied. When associated with an open ductus, there are usually additional congenital defects that cause early death; so almost invariably, the *adult* type has a closed ductus. Coarctations with closed ductus form extensive collateral arterial circulations through the branches of the left subclavian and all but the first two left intercostal arteries to meet the internal mammary, the musculophrenic, and the superior epigastric arteries (Fig. 6-69). In most cases, the collateral circulation is adequate for symptomless living into adult life. *Arterial hypertension* develops in the upper limbs, whereas there is slight hypotension in the lower extremities where the *diminished pulse waves* can be distinguished by palpation. Sometimes a midsystolic *murmur* with an ejection click is present at the left edge of the sternum and also in the left scapular region. In many patients, nothing in the history or in the examination of the heart itself yields a clue to the existence of abnormality. A bicuspid aortic valve is a commonly associated anomaly so that an aortic diastolic murmur may be heard. Bruits originating in the internal mammary arteries may be mistaken for intracardiac murmurs. The diagnosis of coarctation is first suspected when routine abdominal examination discloses *diminution in pulse volume in both femoral arteries;* for this reason, palpation of the femoral pulses should be an invariable routine in abdominal examination. The suspicion of coarctation is increased when *hypertension in the arms* is coincident with weak femoral pulses. A careful search should then be made for *palpable arterial pulses* in the left *scapular region* and under the lower edge of each of the left ribs posteriorly to detect the dilated arteries of the collateral circulation. When the femoral pulses have good volume, the coarctation may be suspected when the peak of the femoral pulse lags behind that of the radial artery. An x-ray film of the chest may reveal notching of the lower costal edges from erosion of the intercostal arteries. A young man or woman with hypertension should suggest the possibility of aortic coarctation. Finding coarctation of the aorta in an apparent female should suggest the possibility that "she" has the *gonadal dysgenesis syndrome of Turner,* in which this anomaly is common.

Aberrant Right Subclavian Artery (Dysphagia Lusoria). Anomalous development of the aortic arch may result in the *right* subclavian artery arising from the *descending* limb of the aorta, *distal* to the origin of the *left* subclavian (Fig. 6-70). To attain a position in the right axilla, the anomalous artery crosses the midline, obliquely and upward, either posterior to the esophagus, between the esophagus and the trachea, or rarely

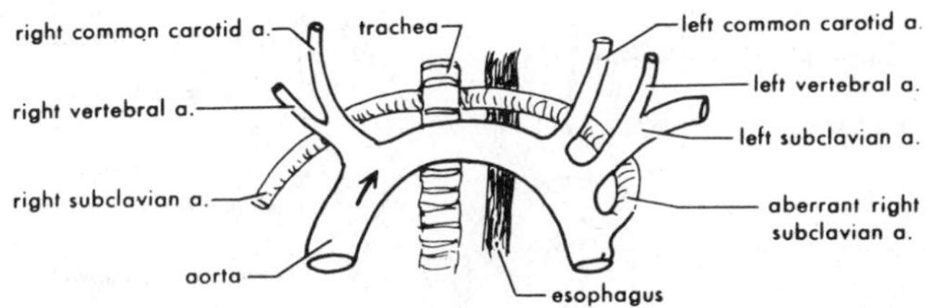

Fig. 6-70. Aberrant right subclavian artery. *The right subclavian artery arises in the descending aorta, distal to the origin of the left subclavian. It crosses the midline either behind the esophagus, between the esophagus and the trachea, or anterior to the trachea. In either of the first two patterns the artery may compress the esophagus, producing difficulty in swallowing, "dysphagia lusoria." A transverse compression band in the esophagram discloses the diagnosis.*

anterior to the trachea. If the artery is in contact with the esophagus as the patient attains adulthood, the aberrant vessel may produce intermittent pressure on the esophagus, resulting in *difficulty in swallowing* of solid food, the only symptom or sign leading to the diagnosis. The condition is termed *dysphagia lusoria* from the Latin *lusus naturae,* "a natural anomally." The diagnosis is made when dysphagia prompts an esophagram showing a pressure notch in the esophagus.

Temporal Arteritis. See p. 69.

Carotid Arteritis. See p. 205.

Superficial Migrating Thrombophlebitis. Successive episodes of thrombophlebitis involve different veins in widely separated parts of the body. In a single episode, a segment of vein becomes tender, reddened, and indurated; involution begins in a few days; the adjacent tissues become blue and yellow; some pigmentation of the skin may finally remain. Veins of the extremities are most commonly involved, but the subcutaneous veins of the abdomen and thorax may be affected. Although the lesions do not cause serious discomfort, this complex should prompt a search for other underlying associated disease: thromboangiitis obliterans; carcinoma of the pancreas or other abdominal organs; hematologic disorders, especially paroxysmal nocturnal hemoglobinuria.

Superior Vena Caval Obstruction (Fig. 6-71). The principal signs are intense *cyanosis* of the head, neck, and both arms;

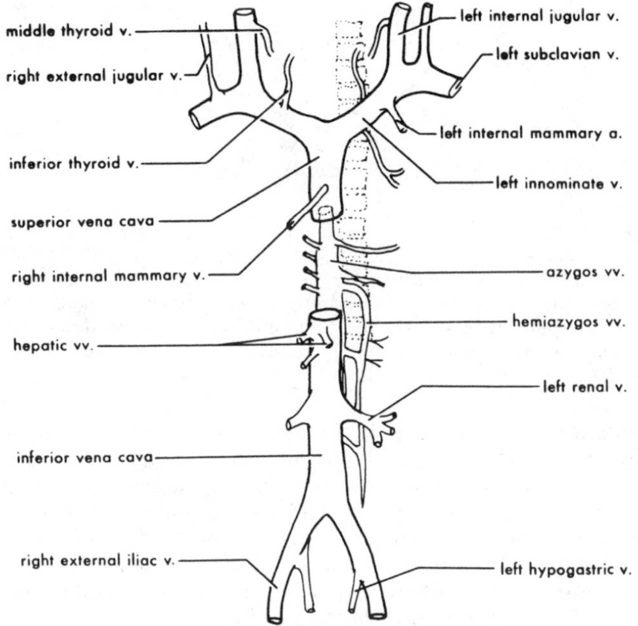

Fig. 6-71. Superior and inferior venae cavae.

engorgement of the veins in the cyanotic region with lack of the venous pulsations that normally originate in the right atrium of the heart; *edema* of the face, both arms, and the upper third of the thoracic wall. The circumference of the neck is enlarged by nonpitting edema *(Stokes' collar)*.

Clinical Occurrence. Neoplasms of the mediastinum; aortic aneurysms in the thorax; chronic mediastinitis from tuberculosis, syphilis, or pyogenic organisms; thrombophlebitis; constrictive pericarditis.

Inferior Vena Caval Obstruction (Fig. 6-71). The single physical sign most likely to lead to a diagnosis of *chronic* vena caval obstruction is the presence on the abdomen of *dilated superficial collateral veins* with *cephalad flow.* The visibility of the superficial veins may be facilitated by viewing them through red goggles;

still better is photography, using film sensitive to infrared light. Visible evidence of collaterals may appear within a week after complete obstruction and the veins may attain maximal size in three months. To localize the *site* of obstruction, the vena cava is considered in three segments. ***Lower Segment*** (below the renal veins). *Venous collaterals:* distributed over thighs, groins, lower abdomen, and flanks. *Edema of lower limbs:* originally pitting, this ultimately results in brawny indurations of the skin with dermatitis, varicosities, and ulcers. The *plasma protein* levels may rise to augment the oncotic pressure and offset the production of edema. *Pelvic congestion:* with obstruction at a higher level in the segment, pelvic congestion may produce *low back pain* and *edematous genitalia.* ***Middle Segment*** (above the renal veins and below the hepatic veins). *Venous collaterals:* large central abdominal veins with absence of lateral abdominal collaterals. *Occlusion of renal veins:* this produces the *nephrotic syndrome* with *generalized edema* and *massive proteinuria:* there is chemical evidence of hypoproteinemia and hypercholesterolemia. *Gastrointestinal manifestations:* nausea, vomiting, diarrhea, abdominal pain. The *malabsorption syndrome* may develop. ***Upper Segment*** (above the hepatic veins). *Venous collaterals:* prominent periumbilical plexus and large veins over the xiphoid region. ***Budd-Chiari Syndrome:*** hepatosplenomegaly, ascites, jaundice, chemical evidence of hepatic insufficiency. ***Special Examinations.*** Venography is indicated at all levels of obstruction. With proteinuria or hematuria, intravenous pyelography should be performed, but the interpretations should be made with the knowledge that obstruction of the vena cava is suspected.

Clinical Occurrence. *Intraluminal:* thrombosis, embolism, neoplastic metastases. *Intramural:* rare benign or malignant neoplasms of the venous wall. *External pressure:* enlargement of the liver, paravertebral lymphadenopathy, aortic aneurysm, surgical ligation. [For further details see M. E. Missal, J. A. Robinson, and R. W. Tatum: Inferior Vena Cava Obstruction, *Ann. Intern. Med.,* **62:**133, 1965].

Chronic Obstruction of the Portal System. Any obstruction to the outflow of portal blood in the hepatic vein, the liver, or the portal vein produces *portal hypertension,* indicated by only two physical signs: *splenomegaly* and *collateral venous circulations* of the portal system (Fig. 6-72). Collaterals are accessible to examination in the anus, the abdominal wall, and the esophagus. *Hemorrhoids* may be portal collaterals, but their occurrence from local causes is so common that their presence is rarely diagnostic. Dilatation of the paraumbilical vein produces a venous rosette around the navel, a *caput medusae,* but the occurrence is rare. Commonly, the demonstrable collaterals are *dilated superficial veins* in the abdominal wall between the umbilicus and the lower thorax; they contain blood flowing upward in the normal direction. When the veins are greatly dilated, one may hear a *venous hum* with systolic accentuation below the xiphoid process, over the epigastric surface of the liver, or around the navel. Formerly, this hum was attributed to a patent umbilical vein in the *Cruveilhier-Baumgarten syndrome;* now it is recognized as coming from varices in the falciform ligament. Dilated veins in the lower esophagus and gastric cardia produce *esophageal varices,* frequently visible in the esophagram. When the diagnosis of portal hypertension has been established, the following causes should be considered: thrombosis of the hepatic veins, portal cirrhosis of the liver, intrahepatic tumors and cysts, granulomatous diseases of the liver, thrombosis of the portal vein. *Hepatic Cirrhosis.* Although cirrhosis is by far the most common cause of portal hypertension, the signs of hepatic disease are necessary to distinguish it from other possibilities. Ascites is the most familiar sign of hepatocellular failure. The fluid in the abdomen, the pleural cavity, and the legs is caused by the combination of metabolic defects producing hypoproteinemia, sodium and water retention, increase in aldosterone secretion, *plus* increased capillary pressure from portal hypertension. Other signs of hepatic cellular disorders are jaundice, clubbed fingers, palmar erythema, vascular spiders, gynecomastia, testicular atrophy, loss of axillary and pubic hair, hemorrhages from defects in coagulation. Early in the development of cirrhosis, the *liver may be moderately enlarged;* as fibrosis occurs, the viscus shrinks somewhat and becomes *nodular* and *hard;* in late stages, it may be *impalpable.* Lacking the signs of hepatic insufficiency, the rarer causes of portal obstruction should be sought. *Chronic Hepatic Vein Occlusion.* This is one phase of the *Budd-Chiari syndrome.* The findings resemble very closely those of hepatic cirrhosis, so the condition is rarely diagnosed correctly during life. The signs of portal hypertension are present, together with ascites, hepatomegaly, and evi-

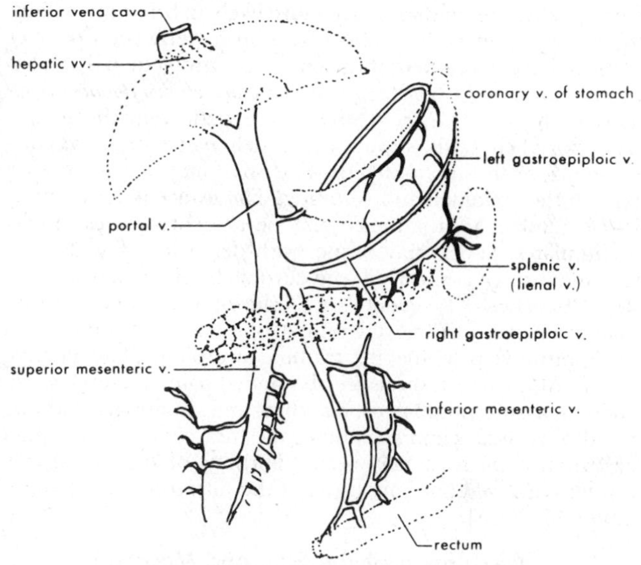

Fig. 6-72. The portal venous system.

dence of secondary hepatocellular failure. Only a sudden onset, or the lack of alcoholic intake or hepatitis, may give a clue to the correct diagnosis. ***Chronic Portal Vein Obstruction.*** Gradual thrombosis of the portal vein, producing portal hypertension, also may closely resemble the findings in hepatic cirrhosis. The occlusion may occur in polycythemia or from neoplastic invasion of the vein lumen. Knowledge of the underlying disease should suggest the disorder in the portal vein. ***Distinction Between Portal Obstruction and Cardiac Failure.*** Portal obstruction with ascites and edema of the ankles is frequently mistaken for the more common cardiac failure. Both conditions may present pleural effusion to obscure the size of the heart, hepatomegaly, ascites, edema of the ankles. Often, the first clue that one is not dealing with cardiac failure comes on finding that the patient is *not orthopneic.* This prompts an intensive search for overlooked signs of parenchymal disease of the liver.

Acute Obstruction of the Portal System. When occlusion occurs rapidly, the symptoms are more likely to bring the patient to the physician before signs of portal hypertension or liver damage have developed; thus, a different problem in diagnosis is presented (Fig. 6-72). *Acute Occlusion of the Hepatic Veins.* This is the *Budd-Chiari syndrome* of hepatic vein thrombosis from portal cirrhosis, suppuration, malignancy, trauma, polycythemia, or thrombophlebitis. The onset may be abrupt, with pain in the abdomen and vomiting. The liver enlarges rapidly and is tender. Mild jaundice may be present. Ascites rapidly accumulates. Shock may ensue, with death in a few days. If the initial stage is survived, the chronic findings may appear. *Acute Thrombosis of the Portal Vein.* Occlusion usually occurs after manipulation of the portal vein at operation, or is the result of suppurative pylephlebitis, trauma, or prolonged debilitating illness. At the onset, there are abdominal pain and tenderness, abdominal distention, ileus, diarrhea, and vomiting. Following rapidly are ascites and splenomegaly. Infarctions of the upper gastrointestinal tract may occur. Portions of the portal vein can be visualized and measured in the ultrasonogram [*Lancet,* **1**:656–57, 1978].

Circulation of the Skin and Mucosa

Most lesions of the skin and mucous membranes involve the vascular system to some extent, so a comprehensive discourse on the superficial circulation would encompass the entire field of dermatology, a subject for a much larger book. Some disorders of dermal vessels furnish signs of generalized disease; these will be considered together with local abnormalities from which they must be distinguished. The selected lesions contain enough blood so their red or blue color readily identifies them as vascular disorders.

Intradermal Hemorrhage. Extravasation of blood in the skin produces an area that is first red, then blue; in a few days, the degeneration of hemoglobin changes the color to green or yellow and fades. Since the blood in the area is extravascular, the color *does not blanch* with pressure. A *petechia* (pl., petechiae) is a round, discrete hemorrhagic area less than 2 mm in diameter; a larger spot is an *ecchymosis* (pl., ecchymoses). When hemorrhages of either size occur in groups, the condition frequently is termed *purpura.* Purpuric lesions may become confluent; they do not elevate the skin or mucosa. Spontaneous purpura from defects in platelets or other coagulating agents usually occurs on the lower extremities, although slight trauma to the skin may induce it elsewhere. When the capillaries are involved by infectious disease, the resulting purpura may predominate on the thorax and abdomen. In polyarteritis nodosa there may be *palpable* purpura from the hemorrhagic nodules. *Isolated petechiae* from bacterial emboli occur anywhere in subacute bacterial endocarditis. In the skin, they may be distinguished from small angiomas by not blanching under pressure; doubtful spots can be circled with ink so that their disappearance in a few days can be noted. Bacterial emboli frequently appear in the mucosa of the palate, buccal surfaces, and conjunctiva, where changes in color during resolution are not evident; in the conjunctiva, the petechiae sometimes have gray centers. A *hematoma* is an area in which underlying hemorrhage causes elevation of the skin or mucosa; extravasated blood frequently colors the surface.

Clinical Occurrence. Vascular abnormalities, as eroded or traumatized large vessels, hereditary hemorrhagic telangiectasia, allergic purpuras, infections, scurvy, Schamberg's disease. Extravascular abnormalities, as atrophy of subcutaneous tissues, increased dermal fragility in Cushing's syndrome. Intravascular abnormalities, as quantitative or qualitative deficits in platelets, and other coagulation defects. [For an extensive classification of the purpuras and the causes of hemorrhage, consult M. Winthrobe *et al.*, *Clinical Hematology,* 8th ed. Lea & Febiger, Philadelphia, 1981, pp. 1052–58.]

TOURNIQUET TEST FOR CAPILLARY FRAGILITY. **Moderate stasis produces a few petechial hemorrhages in the skin of normal persons; the same degree of trauma causes many more hemorrhages when the capillaries are fragile, the *Rumpel-Leede phenomenon.* Stasis may be produced with a tourniquet or, better, with an inflatable cuff. Place the cuff of a sphygmomanometer around the arm in the usual manner and inflate to a pressure halfway between systolic and diastolic levels. Maintain compression for five minutes, then release the pressure and wait two minutes or more before observation. Describe a circle 2.5 cm in diameter (the size of an American quarter-dollar) on the volar surface of the forearm, 4 cm distal from the antecubital fossa. Count the petechiae within the circle. Normally, the number of hemorrhages does not exceed five in men or ten in women and children. Capillary fragility is commonly increased in (1) platelet disorders, as thrombocytopenic purpura and thrombocytasthenia, (2) vascular disorders, as scurvy and senile purpura.**

Purpura and Arthralgia: ***Schönlein-Henoch Purpura*** (Anaphylactoid P.). This vasculitis is most commonly encountered in children, often coincident with streptococcal infections (see p. 466 for classification and pathophysiology). A *purpuric rash* occurs in company with *urticaria, arthralgias, abdominal pain, nausea and vomiting*, and *glomerulitis*. The platelet count remains normal. *Response to Therapy and Prognosis:* The disease is self-limited in children; corticosteroids are believed helpful in severe cases.

Dermal Hemorrhage: ***Scurvy.*** Punctate hemorrhages may occur in the skin; they are distinguishable from the usual petechiae by being *perifollicular*. Close inspection discloses that each petechia surrounds a hair follicle. The lesions are most common in the lower extremities.

Dermal Hemorrhage: ***Rocky Mountain Spotted Fever.*** On about the fourth day of fever, an eruption appears, composed of *erythematous macules,* 2 to 6 mm in diameter; they *blanch* on pressure. In two or three days, the lesions become *maculopapular,* assume a deep red color, and finally become *petechial hemorrhages* that resolve with the usual color changes. The rash begins on the wrists, ankles, palms, and soles; it spreads *centripetally* to the trunk, face, axillae, and buttocks. In contradistinction, the eruption of typhus fever, with similar individual lesions, begins on the trunk and extends *centrifugally,* rarely involving the face, palms, or soles.

Dermal Hemorrhage: ***Meningococcal Meningitis.*** Occurring in three quarters of the cases, the eruption involves the trunk and extremities with *petechial hemorrhages,* together with bright pink, tender *maculopapules,* 2 to 10 mm in diameter. Some maculopapules develop hemorrhagic centers. Large ecchymoses and hemorrhagic vesicles may form.

Dermal Hemorrhages: ***Disseminated Intravascular Coagulation.*** (DIC, Defibrination, Consumption Coagulopathy). The diagnosis of this disorder is often an emergency. The onset may be sudden or gradual. It is characterized by *shock,* the appearance of *ecchymoses, purpura,* or *petechiae,* often *fever,* and unusual bleeding from multiple sites. LABORATORY FINDINGS: the combination of thrombocytopenia, prolonged prothrombin and partial thromboplastin time and a low level of fibrinogen make the diagnosis a strong possibility.

Clinical Occurrence. Complications of pregnancy (dead fetus, placenta previa, abruptio placenta, attempted abortion), peritonitis, immunosuppressive drugs, radiotherapy and chemotherapy for cancer, snake bite, hepatic failure.

Pink Papules: ***Rose Spots of Typhoid Fever.*** These are erythematous *papules,* 2 to 4 mm in diameter, that *blanch* with pressure. They appear in the second week of the fever, usually in crops, few in number. Commonly on the upper abdomen and lower thorax, each lesion persists for two or three days, then disappears, leaving a faint brown stain.

Red Macule or Papule: ***Cherry Angioma.*** (Ruby Spot, de Morgan Spot, Senile Angioma, Papillary Angioma, Capillary Angiectasis, Papillary Telangiectasis). Usually less than 3 mm in diameter, often no larger than a pinhead, the cherry angioma is *bright red,* discrete, irregularly round. Larger lesions may be slightly elevated; occasionally they are pedunculated. The growth is surrounded by a narrow *halo* of pallid skin. Pressure induces only *partial blanching.* Small lesions may be distinguished from petechiae only by their permanence, when observed for several days. The angiomas occur in greatest profusion on the skin of the thorax and arms, next on the face and abdomen; they are less frequent on the forearms and on the lower extremities. In elderly persons, some lesions become atrophic and faded.

Clinical Occurrence. Everyone has a few; the number increases after the age of 30 years. They are associated only with the aging process. Bean states, "The cherry angioma is not the latter day imprint of witches and not the hallmark of cancer which naive and too hopeful physicians have desired."

Blue Papule: ***Venous Lakes.*** Thin-walled papules are filled with venous blood. Gentle pressure forces them to empty, leaving lax indentations beneath the level of the skin. They rarely occur before the age of 35; their numbers increase with age. They are ten times more common in men. Most frequent on the ears and face, next in frequency on the lips and neck, they are uncommon elsewhere. Aging is the only condition with which they are associated.

Sublingual Varices: ***Caviar Lesions.*** The superficial sublingual veins may develop varicosities with aging. Frequently they resemble a mass of purple caviar under the tongue (Fig. 6-73A). They are of no clinical significance.

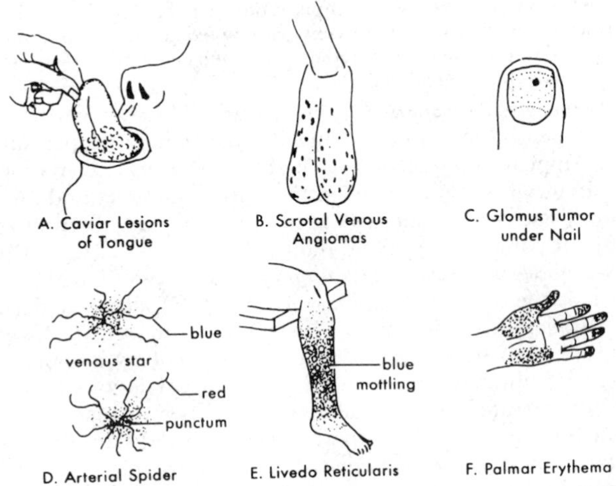

Fig. 6-73. Superficial vascular lesions with specific names. **A.** Caviar lesions of the tongue. *Varicose veins under the tongue form bluish masses that appear as bunches of caviar.* **B.** Scrotal venous angioma. *When the scrotum is spread out multiple papules may be demonstrated, 3 to 4 mm in diameter, dark red or blue.* **C.** Glomus tumor under the nail. *An elevated nodule, 2 to 10 mm in diameter, may occur any place in the skin, frequently under the nail plate. It is extremely painful.* **D.** Venous stars and arterial spiders. *One form of venous star is depicted; the lesions may also appear as cascades, flares, rockets, comets, or tangles. A typical form of arterial spider, with punctum and radicles, is presented. While venous stars are bluish, spiders are fiery red. Both lesions fade with pressure. Pressing the center with a pencil tip will not blanch the branches of a star; the radicles of the spiders will fade with pressure on the punctum. The star always overlies a large vein; the spider is not associated with a visible large vessel. As seen through a pressing glass slide, the venous star does not pulsate; the arterial spider fills from the center with pulsatile spurts.* **E.** Livedo reticularis. *Seen most often on the legs, the skin is mottled with deeply cyanosed areas interspersed with round pale spots. In one type, the discoloration disappears with warming; in others, it does not.* **F.** Palmar erythema. *An intense diffuse erythema occurs, deepest over the hypothenar eminence, less pronounced on the thenar eminence and the distal segments of the fingers. The erythema is not mottled.*

Blue Papules: ***Scrotal Venous Angioma*** (Fordyce Lesion). Not infrequently venous angiomas develop in the superficial veins of the scrotum in men over 50 years of age. The papules are usually multiple, 3 to 4 mm in diameter, and filled with venous blood that colors them dark red, blue, or almost black (Fig. 6-73B). Bean could find no relation to trauma.

Punctate Macules: ***Hereditary Hemorrhagic Telangiectasia*** (Osler's Disease). The first glance at the patient often discloses a pale face, spotted with dull red lesions. The pallor is caused by the anemia of almost continual hemorrhage from the lesions. The average lesion is punctate, about 1 to 2 mm in diameter. Usually, it is *not elevated;* some appear slightly depressed. The overlying skin may be covered with a fine silvery scale. Pressure causes *fading,* although blanching is incomplete in some. Through a compressing glass slide, the spots may be seen to pulsate. Occasionally, one or two fine superficial vessels may radiate from the punctum, but the radicles in arterial spiders are more numerous and the centers smaller. The mucosa is practically always involved; lesions are almost invariably found in Kiesselbach's area on the anterior portion of the nasal septum, giving rise to frequent *epistaxis,* for which the disease is famous. The tip and dorsum of the tongue are favorite sites. Most frequently affected in the skin are the palmar surfaces of the hands and fingers, the skin under the nail plates, the lips, ears, face, arms, and toes. The trunk is least involved. Since any structure may be the site of these lesions, bleeding may cause epistaxis, hemoptysis, hematemesis, melena, hematuria. There is a high incidence of *pulmonary arteriovenous fistulas* accompanied by polycythemia and clubbing of the fingers. The disease is hereditary, transmitted as a mendelian dominant character. It is believed that most lesions develop after childhood. The development and regression of some individual lesions have been observed, although most lesions are probably permanent. It is not uncommon for an affected child to have repeated epistaxis before other lesions appear in the skin and mucosa to establish the diagnosis.

Blue Nodule: ***Rubber-Bleb Nevi of Skin and Gastrointestinal Tract.*** Nevi of the skin may be accompanied by similar lesions in the gastrointestinal tract that are sites of serious *hemorrhage.* The dermal lesions may be few, or they may be scattered throughout the body. The condition is not hereditary. Bean describes three types of lesions: a large disfiguring angioma, a fluctuant thin-skinned bleb containing blood that leaves a rumpled sac when compression empties it into venous channels, an irregular blue area that gradually merges with the surrounding skin fading only partially with pressure.

Painful, Red or Blue Nodule: ***Glomus Tumor.*** This a benign neoplasm, thought to arise from the pericyte in the vessel walls of the glomus body. The lesions are more common in the hands and fingers, especially beneath the nail (Fig. 6-73C). The red or blue tumor is an elevated nodule, from 2 to 10 mm in diameter. It is *exquisitely painful,* completely disproportionate to its size. The pain may occur in paroxysms. The physician should learn to suspect a small spot that is very painful, because relief must be obtained by surgical excision.

Irregular Spongy Tumor: ***Cavernous Hemangioma.*** The tumor occurs in any tissue and varies in size from the microscopic to the huge where an entire extremity may be involved. Usually present at birth, it tends to enlarge with age. The tumor may involve skin, subcutaneous tissue, muscle, and even bone. The surface presents an irregular nodular mass, frequently bluish, and fluctuant. Raising the involved extremity above the heart level may result in partial emptying. A patient of ours pooled enough blood in a tumor of the lower extremity to cause dyspnea and tachycardia in the erect position; this was relieved by a compression bandage on the tumor.

Pulsating Tumor: ***Metastasis from Hypernephroma.*** Rarely, a metastatic lesion from hypernephroma involves the subcutaneous surface of bone in such a manner as to produce a functional arteriovenous fistula in the medulla. When the subcutaneous tissue is also involved, the pulsation is transmitted to the surface.

Pulsating Tumor: ***Cirsoid Aneurysm.*** A cavernous angioma eroding bone may form a congenital arteriovenous fistula. The overlying subcutaneous tissue is swollen into a visible pulsatile tumor that writhes like a nest of snakes.

Stellate Figure: ***Venous Star.*** The lesion occurs as part of the aging process or as a result of venous obstruction. Branches of small superficial veins radiate from a central point (Fig. 6-73D). Bean describes the patterns he has seen as stars, angular Vs, cascades, flares, rockets, and tangles. The entire figure may vary from a few millimeters to several centimeters in diameter. The vessels are *bluish,* whereas arterial spiders are bright red. When pressed upon, the color *fades;* the figure refills from the center when pressure is released, as do arterial spiders. In contrast to arterial spiders, pressure on the central point with a pencil *does not blanch* the radicles. The figure always overlies a larger vein, whereas the spider is not associated with a larger vessel. Venous stars are more common in women. The predominant sites are the dorsum of the foot, the leg, the medial aspect of the thigh above the knee, the back of the neck. They also occur in the skin swollen from obstruction of the superior vena cava. Their clinical importance is to be distinguised from arterial spiders.

Stellate Figure: ***Arterial Spider*** (Vascular Spider, Nevus Araneus, Nevus Arachnoideus, Nevus Arachnoides, Spider Angioma, Spider Telangiectasis). Typically, the *fiery red* vascular figure in the skin consists of a central *body* or punctum, varying from a pinpoint to a papule, 55 mm in diameter (Fig. 6-73D). Radiating from the body are superficial branching vessels forming the *legs* or *radicles.* The vessels may dip into the tissue to reappear further on, forming short visible segments, likened by Bean to the silk threads in American paper money. An *area of erythema* surrounds the body and extends several millimeters beyond the radicular tips. The lesion feels *warmer* than the surrounding skin. Rarely, the body is *visibly pulsatile;* occasionally the pulsation may be felt. Invariably, pressure over the body with a glass slide discloses the blood emerging from the punctum in pulses. When the body is pressed with a pencil tip, the radicles *fade;* they fill centrifugally when pressure is released. Spiders occur commonly on the face and neck and, in diminishing order of frequency, on the shoulders, anterior chest, back, arms, forearms, dorsa of the hands and fingers; rarely are they found below the umbilicus. **Pathophysiology.** The cause of arterial spiders is unknown. Anatomic studies demonstrate that a coiled vessel arises perpendicularly from a deep artery, its distal end forming the central body from which the legs radiate in the plane of the skin, branching and rebranching.

Clinical Occurrence. Spiders occasionally occur in apparently normal persons. They are seen sporadically in a variety of diseases. In greatest profusion and frequency, they are seen in patients with hepatic disease and during pregnancy. Those associated with pregnancy usually disappear after delivery. In both conditions, spiders are frequently accompanied by palmar erythema.

Reticular Pattern: ***Costal Fringe.*** Particularly in older men, the superficial veins near the anterior rib margins and the xiphoid process form networks, sometimes in the pattern of bands with rough correspondence to the attachments of the diaphragm. The condition has been attributed to pulmonary emphysema, but Bean finds no accurate relationship to the structures of the underlying thoracic cage. The lesion is merely another evidence of aging.

Reticular Pattern: ***Facial Telangiectasis.*** The vessels of the nose and face may be dilated in older persons. They are prominent in patients with hepatic disease. Frequently, but not always, they are associated with exposure to the wind and cold, as in farmers and sailors. They have no firm diagnostic significance.

Reticular Pattern: ***Radiation Telangiectasis.*** Large therapeutic doses of x-rays produce changes in the skin that occur months after exposure. The chief signs of x-ray dermatitis are *pigmentation, skin atrophy,* and *telangiectasis;* the last is the most conspicuous. Fine red or blue vessels appear in the skin, forming a disordered network. The border is sharply marked in the shape of the port from which the x-rays issued; this points to the artificial nature of the lesion and establishes the diagnosis.

Reticular Pattern: ***Livedo Reticularis.*** The skin of the arms and legs is mottled with round patches of normal skin set in a background of cyanotic hue (Fig. 6-73E). Three types are described. In *cutis marmorata* the mottling appears on exposure to cold; it *disappears with warming.* The other types *persist when warmed.* They are *livedo reticularis idiopathica,* which is not associated with other disease but occurs in persons with unstable nervous systems; and *livedo reticularis symptomatica,* a frequent accompaniment of periarteritis nodosa and other allied conditions. Ulceration is sometimes a complication of the two types that persist with warming.

Diffuse: ***Palmar Erythema.*** A fixed diffuse erythema involves the hypothenar eminence and, with less intensity, the thenar prominence (Fig. 6-73F). In severe cases, the palmar surfaces of the terminal digits and the thumb are similarly reddened. Rarely, the normal motting of the palms becomes accentuated and fixed. Palmar erythema is most common in hepatic disease and during pregnancy; the overall incidence in both conditions closely parallels the occurrence of arterial spiders, although both lesions may not be present in the same patient. The erythema tends to disappear after delivery.

Paroxysmal Flushing, Blanching, and Cyanosis: ***Metastatic Carcinoid.*** Usually a benign tumor of the ileum, carcinoid may metastasize to the liver where it produces excessive amounts of serotonin (5-hydroxytryptamine). Circulating serotonin causes paroxysms of *erythema* in the skin, intermixed with areas of *pallor* and *cyanosis*. A given area of skin may exhibit all three colors in rapid succession, a bewildering display reminding the observer of the aurora borealis. The eruption is most pronounced on the face and neck, although it may extend to the chest and abdomen. The excessive serotonin also causes hypotension, cramps in the abdomen, diarrhea, and bronchospasm. Late fibrosis in the right heart may result in pulmonary stenosis, tricuspid stenosis and insufficiency. The diagnosis is confirmed by demonstrating with a simple chemical test (*Udenfriend's test*) an increased excretion in the urine of 5-hydroxyindolacetic acid. The flush has been reproduced by the administration of pentagastrin and inhibited by somatostatin, but the authors consider these reactions too dangerous for diagnostic use [J. C. Fröhlich *et al.:* The Carcinoid Flush, *N. Engl. J. Med.*, **299:**1055–56, 1978].

Red Burning Extremities: ***Erythromelalgia*** (Erythermalgia). The patient complains of painful red skin of the hands or feet when exposed to heat. Temperatures above 31° C usually initiate the attacks. During a paroxysm the limbs are *red, warm, swollen*, and *painful*. The arterial pulses are present and normal. *Pathophysiology.* The manifestation occurs from excessive dilatation of arteries and arterioles.

Clinical Occurrence: PRIMARY TYPE: no known cause. SECONDARY TYPE: atherosclerosis, hypertension, frostbite, immersion foot, trench foot, peripheral neuritis, disseminated sclerosis, hemiplegia, chronic heavy metal poisoning, gout. The syndrome may antedate by many years the onset of myeloproliferative disorders, such as polycythemia vera [D. Alarcon-Segovia, R. R. Babb, J. B. Fairnairn II, and A. B. Hagedorn: Erythermalgia, *Arch. Intern. Med.*, **117:**511, 1966].

Segmental Necrotizing Vasculitides. In 1866 Kussmaul and Maier described the first case of periarteritis nodosa (now called classic polyarteritis nodosa) that became the prototype for a large group of vasculitides. Lacking the knowledge for an etiologic classification, the present categorization depends upon anatomic detail such as size and location of involved vessels and their correlation with clinical manifestations. This has not been entirely satisfactory when one finds categories overlap in an inexplicable manner. Despite its faults, the present classification has proven helpful in selecting appropriate treatment for many patients. *Pathophysiology.* Evidence has steadily accumulated in support of the concept that most of the necrotizing vasculitides are the result of immune reactions. The present theory holds that soluble antigen-antibody complexes, with excess antigen not cleared by the reticuloendothelial system, are deposited in the vessel walls, making the latter more permeable. The process is furthered by vasoactive amines from platelets and basophils triggered by IgE proteins. The immune complex activates components of complement that serve as chemotactic agents for polymorphonuclear leukocytes, which then infiltrate the vessel walls. These aggregates release collagenase and elastase that cause mural damage and necrosis, coincident with occlusion, thrombosis, hemorrhages, and ischemic tissues. The sites of the vascular lesions are, to a great extent, determined by blood flow turbulence, hydrostatic pressure in the lower limbs, the position of branching vessels, and the survival time of the immune complex. The involvement of blood vessels is segmental. Cell reactivity may also damage vessel walls. *Physical Signs:* The occurrence of these varies somewhat in each of the categories; none are pathognomonic. SKIN: Thrombosis in cutaneous vessels, especially the venules, produces areas of extravasation with centers of small thrombi, perceived as *palpable purpura.* DEEPER VESSELS: involvement of the larger arteries causes *spontaneous pain, tenderness,* and *pulselessness.* Venous thrombi may be palpable. *Acrogangrene* results in the tips of the digits from arteriospasm. *Asthma* is a frequent feature in some vasculitides.

Working Classification [after A. S. Fauci, B. E. Haynes, and P. Katz: The Spectrum of Vasculitides, *Ann. Intern. Med.*, **89:**660–76, 1978]. POLYARTERITIS NODOSA GROUP: classic polyarteritis nodosa; allergic granulomatosis; systemic necrotizing "overlap syndrome." HYPERSENSITIVITY VASCULITIS: serum sickness; Henoch-Schönlein purpura, essential mixed cryoglobulinemia with vasculitis, vasculitis associated with malignancy, vasculitis associated with other primary disorders. WEGENER'S GRANULOMATOSIS: LYMPHOMATOID GRANULOMATOSIS; GIANT-CELL ARTERITIS: temporal and carotid arteritis, Takayasu's arteritis; THROMBOANGITIS OBLITERANS (Buerger's disease); MUCOCUTANEOUS LYMPH NODE SYNDROME; MISCELLANEOUS VASCULITIDES.

The Lymphatic System

The lymph channels and their nodes make up a discontinuous auxiliary circulation for the blood vessels. Disorders of the lymphatics furnish but three physical signs: *palpable lymph nodes, red streaks in the skin* from superficial lymphangitis, and *lymphedema.* Palpable lymph nodes are the signs of *lymphadenopathy.* The procedures for palpating lymph nodes are described elsewhere in our book: p. 220 for *cervical nodes;* p. 259 for *axillary nodes;* p. 521 for *abdominal nodes;* p. 469 for *epitrochlear nodes.*

▼ *Key Sign:* ***Lymphadenopathy.*** Enlargement of the lymph nodes may be the presenting sign in many diseases. The nodes may be *tender* or *painless, discrete* or *matted together;* in some disorders the nodes *suppurate* (as indicated by *fluctuation*) and form *sinuses.*

Clinical Occurrence: GENERAL LYMPHADENOPATHY (three or more anatomic node groups involved). *Bacterial or viral:* scarlet fever, brucellosis, rubella (German measles), rubeola (measles), infectious mononucleosis (glandular fever), secondary syphilis, tularemia, bubonic plague, cat-scratch fever. *Protozoal:* African sleeping sickness, Chagas' disease, kala-azar, toxoplasmosis. *Fungal:* sporotrichosis. *Insect invasion:* scabies. *Metabolic:* Niemann-Pick disease, Gaucher's disease. *Neoplastic:* Hodgkin's disease, lymphosarcoma, lymphocytic leukemia, myelocytic leukemia, histiocytic medullary reticulosis. *Collagen disorders:* rheumatoid arthritis, Still's disease, dermatomyositis, systemic lupus erythematosus. *Drugs:* diphenylhydantoin. *Miscellaneous:* sarcoidosis, amyloidosis, serum sickness.

REGIONAL LYMPHADENOPATHY (one or two node groups involved). Any condition in which a local infection or neoplasm involves the regional lymph nodes.

LYMPH NODE SYNDROMES. *Inoculation sore with satellite node and generalized disease:* streptococcal infections, syphilitic chancre, inoculation tuberculosis, sporotrichosis, anthrax, erysipeloid, tularemia (ulceroglandular type), bubonic plague, rickettsial diseases (scrub typhus, boutonneuse fever, South African tick fever, Kenya typhus, rickettsialpox), filariasis, rat-bite fever, cat-scratch fever, primary neoplasm.

Pharyngitis with satellite nodes and generalized disease: streptococcal infections, diphtheria, scarlet fever, infectious mononucleosis (glandular fever), oral syphilitic chancre, oral histoplasmosis. *Genital lesion with satellite nodes and generalized disease:* syphilis, gonorrhea, chancroid, lymphogranuloma venereum, tuberculosis, cancer of penis.

SUPPURATIVE LYMPHADENOPATHY. The following diseases commonly cause suppuration of lymph nodes: streptococcal infections, staphylococcal infections, tuberculosis (bovine type), lymphogranuloma venereum, coccidioidomycosis, anthrax, cat-scratch fever, sporotrichosis, plague, tularemia.

The Regional Lymph Nodes

Suboccipital Nodes: *Location.* Midway between the external occipital protuberance and the mastoid process (Fig. 5-76), near the great occipital nerve. *Drainage.* *Afferents from* back of scalp and head; *efferents to* deep cervical nodes. *Symptoms.* Impingement of the enlarged nodes upon the great occipital nerve may produce *headache.* *Examination.* By palpation.

Clinical Occurrence. Any lesions within regional drainage, especially ringworm of scalp, bites in pediculosis capitis, seborrheic dermatitis of scalp, secondary syphilis, cancer.

Postauricular Nodes: *Location.* On mastoid process and at insertion of Sternocleidomastoideus, behind pinna (Fig. 5-76). *Drainage.* *Afferents from* external acoustic meatus, back of pinna, temporal scalp; *efferents to* superior cervical nodes. *Symptoms.* Mastoid tenderness simulating mastoiditis. *Examination.* By palpation.

Clinical Occurrence. Any lesion within regional drainage, infections of the acoustic meatus, herpes of the meatus. Often involved in rubella but not in rubeola.

Preauricular Nodes: *Location.* In front of the tragus of the external ear (Fig. 5-76). *Drainage.* *Afferents from* lateral portions of eyelids and their palpebral conjunctivae, skin of temporal region, external acoustic meatus, anterior surface of pinna. *Examination.* By palpation.

Clinical Occurrence. Lesions within regional drainage, especially rodent ulcer, epithelioma, chancre of face, erysipelas, ophthalmic herpes zoster, rubella, trachoma. *Ocular-glandular syndromes:* gonorrheal ophthalmia, tuberculosis, syphilis, sporotrichosis, glanders, chancroid, epidemic keratoconjunctivitis, adenoidal-pharyngeal-conjunctivitis virus (APC), leptothrix infection, lymphogranuloma venereum, tularemia, cat-scratch fever, Chagas' disease.

***Jugular Nodes:** Location.* Along anterior border of Sternocleidomastoideus, from angle of mandible to clavicle (Fig. 5-76). *Drainage. Afferents from* tongue except apex, tonsil, pinna, parotid gland; *efferents to* deep jugular nodes. *Examination.* By palpation.

Clinical Occurrence. Infection or neoplasm of tonsil, and other affections within regional drainage.

***Mandibular Nodes:** Location.* Under the mandible (Fig. 5-76). *Drainage. Afferents from* tongue, submaxillary gland, submental nodes, medial conjunctivae, mucosa of lips and mouth; *efferents to* superficial and deep jugular nodes. *Examination.* By palpation.

Clinical Occurrence. Infection and neoplasm within regional drainage.

***Submental Nodes:** Location.* In midline under apex of mandibular junction (Fig. 5-76). *Drainage. Afferents from* central lower lip, floor of mouth, tip of tongue, skin of cheek; *efferents to* mandibular nodes, deep jugular nodes. *Examination.* By palpation.

Clinical Occurrence. Infections or neoplasms within drainage region.

***Poststernocleidomastoid Nodes:** Location.* Along the posterior border of the Sternocleidomastoideus are the posterior cervical and inferior deep cervical nodes, not readily separated clinically (Fig. 5-76). *Drainage. Afferents from* the scalp and neck, upper cervical nodes, axillary nodes, skin of arms and pectoral region, surface of the thorax. *Examination.* By palpation.

Clinical Occurrence. Infections and neoplasms within regional drainage. Bilateral enlargement in trypanosomiasis is *Winterbottom's sign.*

***Scalene Nodes:** Location.* These are part of the inferior deep cervical nodes that lie deep in the supraclavicular fossa behind the Sternocleidomastoideus. *Drainage. Afferents from* the thorax. *Examination.* Not palpable; biopsy of the supraclavicular fat pads necessary.

Clinical Occurrence. Intrathoracic granulomas and neoplasms.

Supraclavicular Nodes: *Location.* Part of the inferior deep cervical chain, behind the origin of the Sternocleidomastoideus (Fig. 5-76). *Drainage. Afferents from* head, arm, chest wall, breast. *Examination.* By palpation.

Clinical Occurrence. On the *right side* granuloma or neoplasm from lung or esophagus; on the *left side* neoplasm from the abdominal cavity (see *Virchow's node,* p. 224).

Axillary Nodes: *Location.* Five groups lie on the medial aspect of the humerus, the axillary border of the scapula, the lateral border of the Pectoralis major (Fig. 6-8). *Drainage. Afferents from* the upper limb, the thoracic wall, and the breast. *Examination.* By palpation. In women, enlarged axillary nodes on the thoracic wall must be distinguished from axillary tail of the mammary gland (p. 256).

Clinical Occurrence. Many normal persons have slight permanent enlargement of the axillary nodes from previous infections. Infections or neoplasms within the regional drainage may produce them.

Epitrochlear Nodes: *Location.* About 3 cm proximal to the medial humeral epicondyle, in the groove between Biceps and Triceps brachii. *Drainage. Afferents from* ulnar aspect of forearm and hand, and entire little and ring fingers, the ulnar half of the long finger.

Clinical Occurrence. Acute local infections within the regional drainage, inoculation of generalized infections within the drainage area.

Mediastinal Nodes: *Location.* These include several groups, but those near the trachea and bronchi are not accessible clinically. *Examination.* Not palpable. X-ray films of the chest show widening of the mediastinum and masses in the hilar regions. Lymphangiography may assist, but azygograms are better.

Clinical Occurrence. Tuberculosis, coccidioidomycosis, histoplasmosis, sarcoidosis, silicosis, beryllium poisoning, erythema nodosum, Hodgkin's disease, lymphocytic leukemia.

Abdominal Nodes: *Location.* Distinction between intra-abdominal and retroperitoneal nodes cannot be made clinically. *Examination.* Occasionally large nodes may be palpated as vague masses in the abdomen (p. 521). Calcified nodes may be seen in the x-ray films.

Clinical Occurrence. Infections or neoplasms within the regional drainage, especially in Hodgkin's disease.

Inguinal Nodes: *Location.* A *horizontal* group lies along the inguinal ligament and a *vertical* group is beside the great saphenous vein in its upper segment. ***Drainage.*** *Afferents* of the horizontal group come from the skin of the lower anterior abdominal wall, retroperitoneal region, penis, scrotum, vulva, vagina, perineum, gluteal region, and lower anal canal; *afferents* of the vertical group come from the lower limb, along the great saphenous vein, penis, scrotum, and gluteal region. *Examination.* By palpation.

Clinical Occurrence. Regional infections and neoplasms. *Exception:* tumors of the testis metastasize directly to the para-aortic nodes and do not involve the inguinal nodes. Many persons have moderately enlarged nodes from chronic inactive infections.

Lymph Nodes of Hodgkin's Disease. In this disease the nodes are resilient or rubbery; they soften after x-ray or chemotherapy. Increasing size and firmness of the nodes signal recurring activity of the disease and further therapy. The ingestion of alcohol may produce severe pain in the nodes; frequently the pain is so severe and predictable that patients voluntarily abstain from alcohol.

Hodgkin's disease spreads from node to node, rather than arising multicentrically; so the disease may be arrested by irradiating the involved nodes. A thorough and detailed examination of all accessible groups of nodes by physical examination is required. Deeply situated nodes may be evaluated by lymphangiography, CT scanning or a magnetic resonance imaging. To histologically stage a patient properly, that is to identify the extent of involvement, a surgical exploration of the abdomen and retroperitoneal nodes may be required. Splenectomy, nodal biopsies, liver biopsy, and bone marrow biopsy, if not done previously, will be necessary.

STAGE I: disease confined to one node or one group of nodes in a single anatomic region, on one side of the diaphragm. STAGE II: disease confined to two or more lymph node regions on one side of the diaphragm. STAGE III: disease confined to lymphatic tissue, including lymph nodes, Waldeyer's ring, and spleen, on both sides of the diaphragm. STAGE IV: disease present in extralymphatic tissue, e.g., liver, bone marrow, stomach, eye. Subscripts affixed to the stage number are *A* for absence of symptoms of fever, pruritus, night sweats, malaise; *B* for the presence of some of the symptoms, as II_B.

7

The Abdomen and Rectosigmoid

The Abdomen

Skillful examination of the abdomen is a learned skill with productive consequences. In comparison with the chest, the abdomen encloses more organs that can become sites of disease. Examination of the belly must follow a less rigid pattern than that employed in some other regions; signs are often encountered that call for special maneuvers deviating from the routine. Evaluation of some findings demands alternation among the four basic methods of inspection: palpation, percussion, and auscultation. Although auscultation is the most useful method applied to the chest, the significance of inspection and palpation predominates in the abdomen. Physical signs in the chest can be interpreted with an elementary knowledge of physiology and pathology, but correct assessment of abdominal findings requires thorough competence in gross pathology. Surgeons are likely to excel in abdominal examination as their findings often play a major role in the decision to operate. Their manipulations are often more gentle because they deal with painful conditions. Abdominal diagnosis relies heavily upon skillful extraction of a meaningful history describing the nature and site of pain, the occurrence of nausea and vomiting, diarrhea, and constipation.

In the supine position, the abdominal cavity resembles an oval basin with a rigid bottom of vertebral column and back muscles. The brim is formed by the intercostal angle at one end, the pubes and ilia at the other. Heavy muscles constitute the long sides. The cover is formed by the flat muscles and fascia of the anterior wall, reinforced and thickened by two parallel bands of rectus muscles suspended from the ends of the basin.

In palpation of the abdominal cavity, the anterior wall resists the examining fingers by various degrees of muscle strength and tone. The examiner must minimize this resistance by gentleness and reassurance to secure relaxation. Usually the muscle tone is enough to give the examiner an illusion of a cavity of great depth, when actually it is very shallow.

When a mass is encountered in the abdominal cavity, the first problem is to determine what anatomic structure is involved, since practically no mass generates *de novo,* but arises from previously normal tissues. Most intra-abdominal viscera are attached by mesenteries or ligaments, permitting them to move with the diaphragm. Movement with respiration suggests association with a mobile organ in the cavity rather than a location behind it or attached to the wall.

In evaluation of masses in the abdomen, it is useful to consider the viscera as solid or hollow, because each has distinctive physical signs. The *solid viscera* are liver, spleen, kidneys, adrenals, pancreas, ovaries, and uterus. Most are composed of glandular parenchyma with characteristic shapes that tend to be retained during enlargement. Many are clustered under the protecting eaves of the lower thorax. The *hollow viscera* are the stomach, small intestines, colon, gallbladder, and urinary bladder. They are normally impalpable; but their lesions can often be felt; they may be distended by gas or fluid.

Two systems of topographic regions have been employed to describe locations in the abdomen (Fig. 7-1). Most physicians prefer the simpler division into quadrants by an axial and a transverse line through the umbilicus; we have employed it in this book.

Examination of the Abdomen

In general, employ the methods of physical examination in the following sequence: first, inspection; second, auscultation; third, palpation and percussion. Ensure a warm room or adequate covering, so the patient does not shiver and tense the abdominal wall. For most purposes have the patient lie

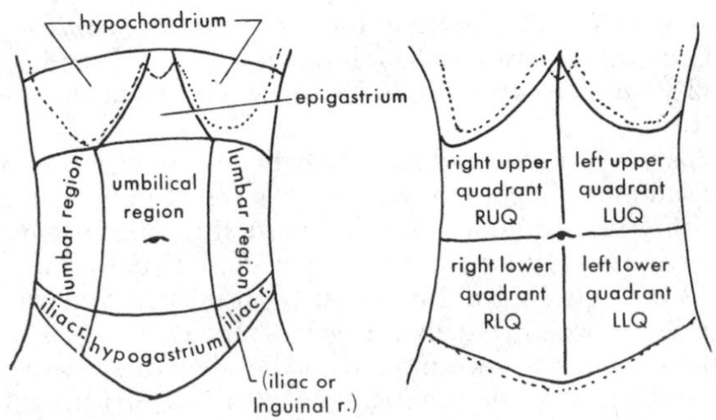

Fig. 7-1. Topographic divisions of the abdomen. *On the left are the regions of the abdomen as defined in the BNA terminology. Most of the nine regions are too small so that enlarged viscera and other structures occupy more than one. On the right is a simpler plan with four regions; it is preferred by most clinicians and is employed in this book. Many occasions arise when the quadrant plans need supplementing by reference to the epigastrium, the flanks, or the suprapubic region.*

supine, resting comfortably on an examination table or bed. Place one pillow under the head; patients with kyphosis require more elevation of head and shoulders. Another pillow under the knees may lend additional comfort and relaxation. When orthopnea is present, raise and support the trunk by a back rest to relax abdominal muscles. Drape the abdomen with a sheet or blanket, covering the lower limbs up to the pubes (Fig. 7-2). In addition, cover a woman's breasts with a folded towel. For most purposes, stand at the right side of the patient. Directions will be given only for right-handed examiners.

ABDOMINAL INSPECTION. **This rewarding procedure is frequently slighted because all physicians experience an obsessive desire to place their hands on the abdomen and start palpating. Conscious effort and self-discipline are required to force oneself to inspect properly, thoroughly, and unhurriedly (Fig. 7-3). If possible, arrange a single source of light to shine across the abdomen toward you, or alternatively have the light shine lengthwise over the patient. Inspect the abdomen sequentially for contour, scars, engorged veins, visible peristalsis, abnormal contour, and visible masses.**

Scars: ***Striae.*** Multiple scars, 1 to 6 cm long, run axially under the epidermis. When recent, they are pink or blue;

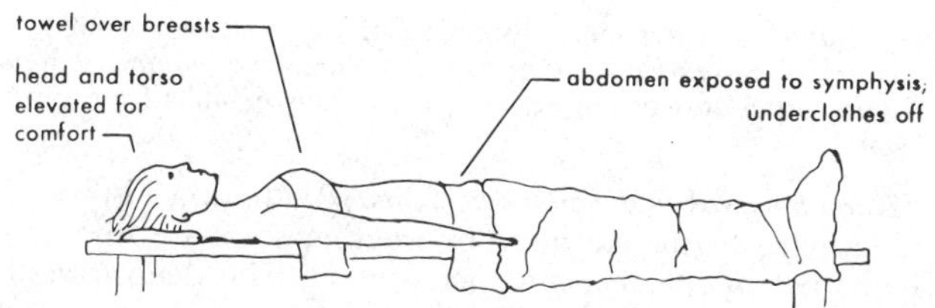

Fig. 7-2. Draping for abdominal examination. *The nude patient lies supine on the examining table with a sheet or blanket covering the lower extremities up to the pubes. For women, the breasts are covered with a folded towel or pillowcase. A small pillow supports the head. To secure further relaxation of the abdominal muscles, a pillow can be placed to support the knees in slight flexion.*

older scars are silvery. They occur in skin regions undergoing chronic stretching. Although striae are most common in the abdomen, deposition of adipose tissue or edema produces them also on the shoulders, thighs, and breasts. *Pathophysiology.* In normal skin, stretching causes rupture of the elastic fibers in the reticular layer of the cutis. In adrenal hypercorticism, the skin itself becomes fragile and easily breaks from normal stretching.

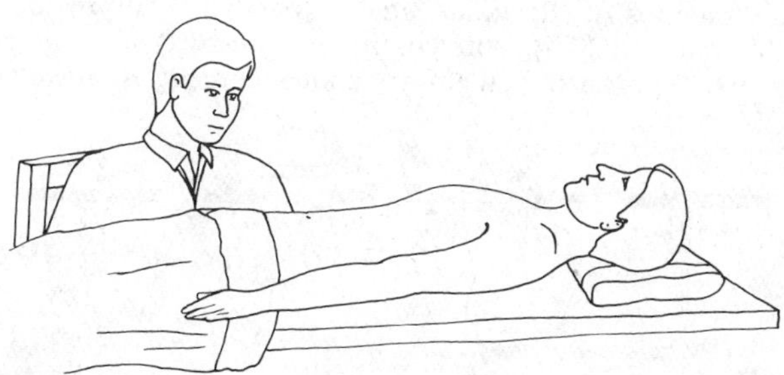

Fig. 7-3. Inspection of the abdomen. *The patient should be placed in a supine position with a single source of light shining across from feet to head, or across the abdomen toward the examiner. The examiner should take his ease by sitting in a chair at the right of the patient with his head only slightly higher than the abdomen. In this manner, the physician can concentrate his attention on the abdomen for several minutes in searching for signs of visible peristalsis or masses.*

Clinical Occurrence. Distention of the abdomen from pregnancy, obesity, ascites, tumors, or subcutaneous edema. Adrenal hypercorticism (Cushing's syndrome) usually exhibits fresh purple scars.

Scars: ***Surgical and Traumatic Scars.*** Without a history, the cause may only be surmised by whether scars are smooth or jagged, when suture marks are present. The deep irregular scars of burns are easily recognized. All scars are initially red, then pink; they fade to skin color in about six months. Finally they become pallid, as the vascularity of the fibrous tissue diminishes. Wounds healing by *first intention* produce thin scars because there is a minimum of fibrosis, lacking infection; a wide area of fibrosis separates the normal skin edges when the wound has healed by *second intention,* from irritation by drains or infection. In certain persons, scars may tend to heal with ridges of hyperplastic fibrous tissue; when the growth becomes exuberant and dense, it may attain a stage called *keloid.*

Engorged Veins. Ordinarily the veins in the abdominal wall are scarcely visible. But normal veins may be prominent when the panniculus adiposus is thin. Engorged veins are frequently visible through the normal abdominal wall. Above the umbilicus, the blood flow in the veins is normally *upward;* below the navel, it is *downward.* To demonstrate direction of flow, place the tips of the index fingers together, compressing a visible vein (Fig. 7-4). With continuous pressure, slide the fingers apart, producing an empty venous segment. Remove one

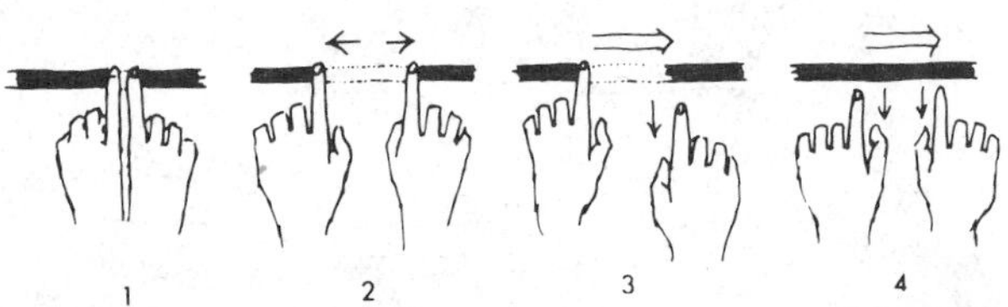

Fig. 7-4. Testing direction of blood flow in superficial veins. *The examiner presses the blood from the veins with his index fingers in apposition* (**1**). *The index fingers are slid apart, milking the blood from the intervening segment of vein* (**2**). *The pressure upon one end of the segment is then released* (**3**) *to observe the time of refilling from that direction. The procedure is repeated and the other end released first* (**4**). *The flow of blood is in the direction of the faster flow.*

finger to observe the time of filling from that direction; repeat the maneuver from the other end. ***Pathophysiology.*** Obstruction of the inferior vena cava causes a flow *upward* from the lower abdomen. In the upper abdomen, portal obstruction causes a normal upward flow; but obstruction of the superior vena cava causes a *downward flow* (reversal). Very rarely, engorged veins form a pattern around the umbilicus called *caput medusae;* knowledge of this establishes you as a scholar of Latin and mythology, but the finding has no more significance than the more common pattern of engorgement.

Clinical Occurrence. Emaciation, obstruction of the superior or inferior vena cava, portal vein obstruction, superficial venous thrombosis.

Visible Peristalsis. When the abdominal wall is thin, normal contractions of the stomach and intestines may be visible as slow undulations under the skin (Fig. 7-5A). When observed through a wall of normal thickness, the peristaltic waves are usually increased in amplitude and strength. The waves are slow; to see them, watch the abdomen for several minutes. Sit beside the bed with your eyes near the level of the abdominal profile. Tapping the wall with the fingers may initiate contractions. Borborygmus, intestinal rumblings heard without a stethoscope, in conjunction with visible peristalsis and evidence of the patient experiencing pain, are most suggestive of intestinal obstruction, either partial or complete. When the contractions are strong enough to cause the gut to feel hard, obstruction should be considered.

Clinical Occurrence. Pyloric obstruction, obstruction of small or large bowel. Normal in some thin persons.

Visible Pulsations. Normally the abdominal aorta causes a slight pulsation in the epigastrium. The amplitude is increased with widened pulse pressure, tortuous aorta, or aneurysm. The pulse may be transmitted to the surface with increased facility by a solid mass overlying the aorta. Often the caliber of the aorta may be established by palpation; tortuosity may be distinguished from dilatation. Feeling a pulsatile mass raises the question of aneurysm or a solid structure adjacent to the aorta. An aneurysm is expansile *laterally,* as well as anteroposteriorly. A murmur near the mass suggests aneurysm. Ultrasonic examination with the B-mode is often diagnostic.

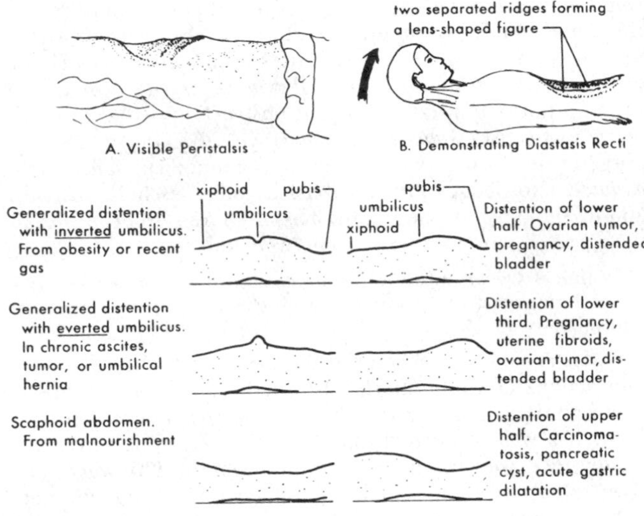
two separated ridges forming a lens-shaped figure
A. Visible Peristalsis
B. Demonstrating Diastasis Recti
xiphoid
pubis
umbilicus
Generalized distention with inverted umbilicus. From obesity or recent gas
Distention of lower half. Ovarian tumor, pregnancy, distended bladder
Generalized distention with everted umbilicus. In chronic ascites, tumor, or umbilical hernia
Distention of lower third. Pregnancy, uterine fibroids, ovarian tumor, distended bladder
Scaphoid abdomen. From malnourishment
Distention of upper half. Carcinomatosis, pancreatic cyst, acute gastric dilatation
C. Abdominal Profiles

Fig. 7-5. Visible abdominal signs. **A.** Visible peristalsis. *Peristaltic waves in the stomach or small bowel sometimes can be seen in the upper abdomen. They usually appear as oblique ridges in the wall that begin near the left upper quadrant and gradually move downward and rightward. Occasionally parallel ridges form a "ladder" pattern. Visibility may be caused by normal waves showing through a thin abdominal wall or by abnormally powerful waves beneath a normal wall. The latter indicates obstruction of a tubular viscus.* **B.** Diastasis recti. *This is abnormal separation of the abdominal rectus muscles. It is frequently not detected when the patient is supine unless the patient's head is raised from the pillow so the abdominal muscles are tensed.* **C.** Abdominal profiles. *Careful inspection from the side may give the first clue to abnormality, directing attention to a specific region and prompting search for more signs.*

Clinical Occurrence. Widened pulse pressure in arterial hypertension, aortic regurgitation, or thyrotoxicosis. Tortuous aorta. Aortic aneurysm. Solid mass overlying the aorta.

Diastasis Recti. The two abdominal rectus muscles may be separated from their normal juxtaposition. With the supine abdomen relaxed, no abnormality may be noted; or the examiner may suspect distention. Request the patient to raise his head from the pillow; this causes the abdominal recti to tense and reveal the separation of the pair (Fig. 7-5B).

Clinical Occurrence. Congenital. Acquired in pregnancy and other conditions producing abdominal distention or loss of muscular tone.

Everted Umbilicus. Without a hernia, this is a sign of increased intra-abdominal pressure from fluid or masses in the cavity.

Umbilical Fistula. This may discharge (1) urine through a patent urachus, or (2) pus from a urachal cyst or tract or an abscess in the abdominal cavity, or (3) feces from a connection with the colon.

Umbilical Calculus. This is not a true stone. In persons with poor hygiene, a hard mass of dirt and desquamated epithelium may accumulate in the umbilical cavity and cause inflammation.

Nodular Umbilicus (Sister Mary Joseph's Nodule). Abdominal carcinoma, especially gastric, may metastasize to the navel.

Bluish Umbilicus (Cullen's Sign). A faintly blue coloration may occur as the result of hemoperitoneum from any cause.

Ecchymoses on Abdomen and Flanks (Grey Turner's Sign). Discoloration caused by massive nontraumatic ecchymoses may occur in the skin of the lower abdomen and flanks. The color may be blue-red, blue-purple, or green-brown, apparently depending upon the degree of degradation of hemoglobin in the tissues. The mechanism is in doubt, but clinical evidence supports the view that it results from infiltration of the extraperitoneal tissues with blood. The blood coagulation mechanism is usually normal.

Clinical Occurrence. First associated with hemorrhagic pancreatitis, it also occurs with strangulated bowel, extravasation of hemorrhages from abscesses, and probable infarction of muscle in myxedema.

▼ ***Key Sign: Jaundice.*** Both *jaundice* and *icterus* designate a syndrome in which body tissues and fluids are stained by excesses in the blood of the bile pigments, *conjugated* and *unconjugated bilirubin.* Although the synonyms merely mean "yellow," medical use reserves them for this syndrome. But yellow skin is also caused by carotene, quinacrine (Atabrine, a malarial-suppressant dye), dinitrophenol and tetryl (both used in the manufacture of explosives); these conditions must be distinguished from jaundice. The bile pigments stain all tissues, but jaundice is most intense in the face, trunk, and sclerae. The presence of melanosis (tanning) in the skin from exposure to sunlight accentuates the yellow of jaundice. Slight degrees of jaundice can first be seen in the white frenulum of the tongue. The yellow in jaundice is frequently invisible in artificial light, whereas daylight plainly reveals its presence. Jaundice is usually visible when the concentration of conjugated bilirubin is 2 to 4 mg per 100 mL of serum. But repeated inspection of the skin in daytime may be misleading in estimating changes in intensity of the yellow, since the illumination of sunlight varies daily and hourly. When the jaundice is long-standing, the deep yellow may acquire a *green* hue. *Scleral Color.* Bilirubin is distributed uniformly throughout the sclera, in contrast to the yellow subscleral fat that collects in the periphery, farthest from the limbus; the color of quinacrine is said to be most intense near the limbus. Carotene *does not stain* the sclerae, but it accumulates in the skin of the forehead, around the alae nasi, and in the palms and soles (p. 678). *Pruritus.* Itching often accompanies obstructive jaundice; it may become an excruciating symptom that dominates the patient's consciousness. It is caused by injury of the sensory nerves in the skin from accumulation of bile pigments. The intensity of the itching is usually proportional and bears some relation to the concentration of bile pigments and their duration in the skin. *Bradycardia.* Obstructive jaundice is sometimes accompanied by sinus rhythm with ventricular rates between 40 and 50 beats per minute. *Dark-Colored Urine.* High concentrations of conjugated bilirubin in the urine as a consequence of failure of bilirubin excretion impart a dark yellow to brown color. Shaking a specimen in a test tube produces *yellow foam.* *Acholic Feces.* In complete biliary obstruction or severe hepatocellular degeneration, the stools are malodorous and lack the normal brown color; instead they appear *white* or *gray.* This appearance is often called clay-colored, but the term is a poor one; clay can be red, yellow, or black as well.

Normal Bile Pigment Cycle. When erythrocytes are destroyed in the circulation during the normal aging process, the freed hemoglobin is bound by the haptoglobin of the plasma as *haptoglobin-hemoglobin.* This is transported to the reticuloendothelial system where it is broken up to yield unconjugated bilirubin, iron, globin, and haptoglobin. The *unconjugated (free) bilirubin* circulates in the blood plasma in concentrations of 0.5–1.2 mg/100 mL; it is *insoluble* in water and bound to plasma albumin. The liver takes up the unconjugated bilirubin and combines it with glucuronic acid to form *water-soluble* bilirubin monoglucuronate and diglucuronate, together called *conjugated bilirubin.* The conjugate is excreted into the gut with the bile where bacterial enzymes convert it to the complex *urobilinogen.* Most urobilinogen is lost in the feces (100–200 mg/day), but small portions are reabsorbed by the intestine and reexcreted, some in the bile, and 0.5–1.4 mg/day in the urine. When pathologic processes cause conjugated bilirubin to enter the bloodstream, it is excreted in the urine; but excesses of unconjugated bilirubin in the blood cannot be filtered through the kidneys because the substance in insoluble in water. Excesses of urobilinogen in the blood appear in the urine.

NONINVASIVE TESTS FOR OBSTRUCTIVE AND INTRAHEPATIC JAUNDICE. **Much accuracy has been gained by the use of the newer ultrasonography and computerized tomography (CT). The former should be attempted initially because it is less expensive than the latter and nearly as accurate. One criterion for the diagnosis of obstructive jaundice by these methods is the presence of dilated bile ducts [Editorial: Non-invasive Methods for Diagnosis of Jaundice, *Lancet,* 2: 18–20, 1979].**

— *Jaundice:* ***Unconjugated Hyperbilirubinemia (Hemolytic Jaundice).*** An excess of unconjugated bilirubin in the serum causes an increase in urobilinogen in the urine. The urine contains no bilirubin. Confirmatory tests of intrinsic liver disorders are negative. The transaminase and alkaline phosphatase values are not elevated. The syndrome is usually caused by the production of an increased amount of unconjugated bilirubin overwhelming the hepatic capacity to conjugate; rarely is it due to diminished uptake by the liver or a defect in hepatic conjugation. The stools are normal in color.

Clinical Occurrence. *Increased production:* transfusion hemolysis, erythroblastosis, hemolysis from chemicals or infections, secondary hemolysis in pregnancy, congenital hemolytic icterus, sickle-cell anemia, thalassemia major, pulmonary infarction, absorption of hematoma, hyperbilirubinemia from portal-caval shunt. *Deficient hepatic uptake:* Gilbert's disease. *Deficient hepatic conjugation:* physiologic jaundice of the newborn, Crigler-Najjar syndrome inhibition of glucuronyl transferase, competitive inhibition by drugs detoxified as glucuronides.

— *Jaundice:* **Conjugated Hyperbilirubinemia (Obstructive Jaundice).** The feces are often *acholic*. The urine lacks urobilinogen, but it contains bilirubin. The serum alkaline phosphatase is definitely elevated, but the serum transaminases are usually normal or slightly increased. The obstruction may be in the biliary tree or in the canaliculi *(cholestasis)*. With ultrasonography dilatation of the bile ducts can be detected in most cases of obstructive jaundice, thereby clinching the diagnosis.

Clinical Occurrence. *Excretory obstruction:* gallstones, stricture of the duct, carcinoma at the head of the pancreas, cholestasis from drugs. *Liver-cell deficiency:* excretory defects, Dubin-Johnson syndrome, Rotor syndrome.

— *Jaundice:* **Extravasation Hyperbilirubinemia.** This syndrome has been reported after operations for massive hemorrhages into the tissues, followed by shock and the transfusion of large quantities of blood. In four cases, jaundice appeared from the 2nd to the 8th postoperative day. High concentrations of *conjugated* bilirubin and alkaline phosphatase were found in the serum. Although the findings suggested obstructive jaundice, autopsies showed no signs of obstruction and minimal liver damage. The mechanism has not been identified [P. A. Kantrowitz, W. A. Jones, N. J. Greenberger, and K. J. Isselbacher: Severe Postoperative Hyperbilirubinemia Simulating Obstructive Jaundice, *N. Engl. J. Med.*, **276:**591–98, 1967].

— *Jaundice:* **Mixed Hyperbilirubinemia.** The cause may be difficult to ascertain by laboratory tests; heavy reliance must be placed upon clinical evidence and liver biopsy. The plasma may contain both conjugated and unconjugated bilirubin; the elevation of the serum transaminases may depend upon the degree of liver damage incurred from both obstruction and infection. The stools may be acholic.

Clinical Occurrence. Acute hepatitis, prolonged biliary tract obstruction, hemolysis with secondary liver damage, familial and immaturity defects.

Distended Abdomen

EXAMINATION OF DISTENDED ABDOMEN. **The experienced observer easily recognizes that the abdomen is distended. The next task is to select from the following list the condition that best fits the physical signs: obesity, tympanites, ascites, pregnancy, feces, and neoplasms. As a mnemonic device, these are approximated as the *six f's:* fat, fluid, flatus, fetus, feces, and fatal growths. The abdominal distention may be contributed to by several simultaneous conditions, so the examiner must seek the entire gamut of signs and make a judgment. Distinction begins with inspection, but soon palpation and percussion are interspersed freely to bring out the attributes of each condition (Fig. 7-5C).**

Abdominal Distention: ***Obesity.*** The abdomen is uniformly rounded with an increase in girth. The umbilicus is buried deeply in the wall because it is adherent to the peritoneum; the layer of fat is superficial to it. Concurrently, fat accumulates in other parts of the body. Estimate the thickness of the panniculus adiposus by grasping a double layer between thumb and index finger; measure in centimeters half the thickness of the resulting fold at the base. In addition to the thickened panniculus, contributions to the girth of the belly in fat persons are made by the fat in the mesentery, omentum, and perirenal pads. Since generalized obesity is obvious, usually the problem is to determine whether any other causes of abdominal distention are also present.

▼ *Key Signs:* ***Tympanites*** (Meteorism). Tympanites or meteorism is the presence of excessive air or gas *within* the lumen of the stomach and intestines, or *free* in the peritoneal cavity. In either place, the physical signs are *abdominal distention* and a *large area of tympany.* The profile describes a single curve (Fig. 7-5C). Voluntary or involuntary *muscle spasm* of the abdominal wall may accompany, especially if free air is present.

Intestinal obstruction and ileus are synonyms for the condition in which the flow of intestinal contents is diminished, reversed, or arrested, with resulting *constipation* or *obstipation;* but normal fecal passage persists in local obstruction until the distal gut is emptied. The causes of obstruction are (*1*) *mechanical* (*local*), which may be either *high* or *low,* depending upon its distance from the duodenum, and (*2*) *nonmechanical* (*diffuse*), either *dynamic* or *adynamic.* Tympanites is the common sign of all types except in high intestinal obstruction where the proximal gut is too short to contain much air. Since the proximal gut is normal in a local obstruction, it reacts to produce *vomiting, colicky pain,* and *hyperperistalsis.* These signs are lacking in diffuse obstruction because the entire gut is affected. Frequently in the course of abdominal disease both types of obstruction occur sequentially.

— *Noisy Tympanites with Colic and Vomiting:* **Mechanical (Local) Ileus.** *Tympanites* is present when the locus is remote enough from the duodenum. Hyperperistalsis above the locus is indicated by *frequent loud peristaltic sounds* (*borborygmi*) accompanied by *colicky pain.* The characteristic *vomiting* comes sooner and is more intense the higher the locus of obstruction. Bile-stained vomitus indicates an obstruction distal to the second portion of the duodenum. Low obstruction may ultimately result in *fecal vomiting* and is classically indicative of colonic obstruction in a person with an incompetent ileocecal valve. Dehydration and exhaustion from pain and vomiting produce the picture of a *gravely sick* patient.

Clinical Occurrence: INTRALUMINAL: foreign bodies, neoplasm, gallstones eroding into the gut, meconium, bezoars, enteroliths, worms. VISCERAL COMPRESSION: adhesions, stenosis, hernias (p. 489), volvulus (p. 559), intussusception (p. 557), tumor, atresia.

— *Silent Tympanites Without Colic and Vomiting:* **Nonmechanical (Diffuse) Ileus.** A constant sign is *tympanites.* The peristaltic sounds are *diminished* or *absent.* When present, *abdominal pain* is slight and not colicky; *vomiting* is uncommon. Consequently, the patient often lacks the *appearance of sickness* characteristic of mechanical (local) obstruction. Although the signs are the same for both, nonmechanical (diffuse) ileus may be either *dynamic* or *adynamic,* depending upon whether fecal movement is impeded by spasm or atony of musculature:

Clinical Occurrence: ADYNAMIC (PARALYTIC) ILEUS: *Manipulation or Trauma:* surgical operations in the abdomen, retropyelography, trauma to the abdomen or axial skeleton, aerophagia. *Chemical:* HCI and gastric contents from perforated stomach or duodenum, enzymes released by acute pancreatitis, bile peritonitis, belladonna poisoning. *Metabolic:* hypokalemia, defective acetylcholine synthesis, myxedema, ganglionic blocking agents, diabetic acidosis. *Reflex Vascular:* thrombosis, embolism, ischemia, cardiac infarction, pulmonary embolism. *Mechanical:* adhesions, tumors, volvulus, intussusception, toxic megacolon, ascariasis. DYNAMIC (SPASTIC) ILEUS: uremia, heavy metal poisoning, infarctions, porphyria, ruptured abdominal viscera, typhoid fever, staphylococcal enterocolitis.

— *Tympanites Without Ileus:* ***Pneumoperitoneum.*** A small amount of air in the peritoneal cavity cannot be demonstrated by physical signs. With a larger quantity, *the area of tympany is extended. Pain* may be absent depending upon the presence of contaminants. The activity of the gut is normal if peritonitis is absent. Pneumoperitoneum may be distinguished from other states with tympanites only by the presence of free air under the diaphragm in the x-ray film of the abdomen taken in the erect or decubitus position.

Clinical Occurrence: Traumatic rupture of the gut. Perforation of the gut by ulcer, diverticulitis, foreign body, or neoplasm. Therapeutic pneumoperitoneum. Pneumatosis cystoides intestinalis. Infection with *Escherichia coli* or other gas-forming organisms.

— *Tympanites Without Ileus:* ***Aerophagia.*** This offers little diagnostic difficulty. The patient can be observed to *swallow* and *belch* air, although he is generally not conscious of it. A grave clinical error is to assume that the basis is always "neurotic"; air swallowing may be a response to abdominal discomfort from organic disease.

▼ *Key Sign:* ***Ascites:*** (Abdominal Dropsy). Unless distorted by surgical scars, diastasis recti, or hernia, the profile of the fluid-filled abdomen describes a single curve from xiphoid process to pubes (Fig. 7-5C). The umbilicus is frequently *everted.* The following signs are characteristic of free fluid (Fig. 7-6): *Bulging flanks* are produced in the supine position from the weight of the fluid pressing on the side walls; this may also occur in relaxation of the walls. An area of *tympany at the top* of the abdominal curve is caused by gas-filled mobile intestines floating to the surface of the fluid. A *fluid wave* can be demonstrated by tapping a flank sharply with the right hand while the left hand receives an impulse when placed against the opposite flank. There is a perceptible time lag between the tap and reception of the impulse. Fat in the mesentery produces a similar wave, so the fat must be blocked by having the patient or an assistant press the ulnar surface of the hand along the midline of the abdomen. A wave passing this block is usually

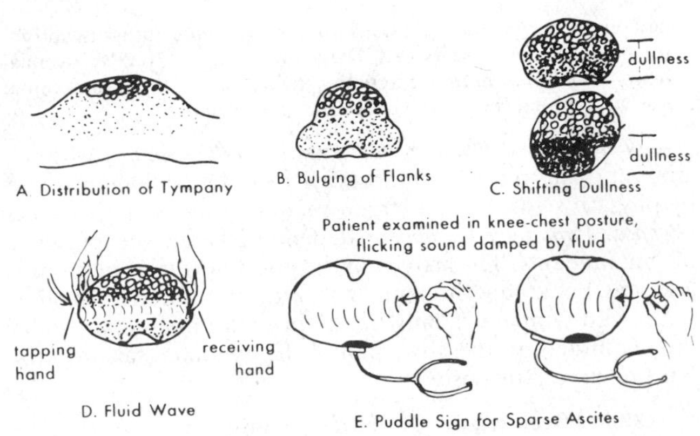

Fig. 7-6. Signs of ascites. **A.** Distribution of tympany. *In the supine position, free fluid causes the gas-filled gut to float, so an area of tympany forms at the top of the bulging wall.* **B.** Bulging flanks. *The weight of free fluid pushes the flanks outward so they bulge toward the table or the bed; fat in the mesentery also will cause this when the abdominal muscles are weak.* **C.** Shifting dullness. *The dependent fluid causes an area of dullness in the lowest part; this shifts to remain lowest with changes in position of the body.* **D.** Fluid wave. *A wave in the fluid, elicited by tapping one side of the abdomen, in transmitted to the receiving hand laid on the opposite side; the wave takes perceptible time to cross the abdomen. Fat in the mesentery may cause a similar wave, but it can be blocked by having an assistant press the wall downward; this does not block the fluid wave.* **E.** Puddle sign. *The previously mentioned signs are present with relatively large amounts of fluid; the puddle sign is present when there is as little as 120 mL of fluid. With the patient on his hands and knees for several minutes, the fluid accumulates in the most dependent part of the abdomen. The diaphragm of the stethoscope is placed on the skin at this point, and the examiner listens to the sound made by flicking the side of the abdomen with the finger. The flicking is repeated while the chestpiece is moved farther away; when the edge of the puddle is passed, the sound becomes accentuated, even though the distance be greater.*

caused by free fluid. Free fluid produces *shifting dullness.* With the patient supine, percuss the level of dullness in the flanks and mark it on the skin. Then turn the patient on one side for a minute, and percuss the new level of dullness; considerable shift indicates the probability of fluid, but fat in the mesentery may also shift in this manner, and feces in the bowel may give similar signs. These signs of fluid will not detect much less than 500 mL of free fluid in the abdominal cavity; in obese persons paracentesis abdomini may be necessary for diagnosis.

A *puddle sign* has been described, said to detect as little as 120 mL of free fluid in the abdominal cavity. The patient lies *prone* for five minutes, then rises on the elbows and knees. The diaphragm of the stethoscope is applied to the most dependent part of the abdomen, and the examiner repeatedly flicks the near flank with his finger, using constant intensity. Flicking at the same spot, the chestpiece is moved across the abdomen *away* from the examiner. When the farther edge of the puddle is reached, the intensity of the sound becomes louder. When the patient sits up, the difference in sound transmission disappears. The sign is not impaired by adipose tissue.

Clinical Occurrence: *Congestive cardiac failure:* from any cause. *Obstruction of portal vein:* portal cirrhosis of the liver, hepatic amyloidosis, hilar lymphadenopathy of the liver from infection or neoplasm. *Obstruction of hepatic veins or inferior vena cava above them* (physical signs indistinguishable from portal obstruction): endothrombophlebitis of hepatic veins (Budd-Chiari syndrome), thrombosis of inferior vena cava from infection or neoplasm. *Peritoneal irritation:* acute or chronic peritonitis, neoplastic implants, tuberculosis, hydatid disease. *Hypoproteinemia:* nephrosis, some anemias. *Obstruction of thoracic duct or receptaculum chyli* (chylous ascites): injuries to thorax or abdomen, tuberculosis, filariasis. *Others:* myxedema, primary amyloidosis, benign ovarian adenoma with ascites and hydrothorax (Meigs' syndrome), hunger edema and wet beriberi (thiamine deficiency and hypoproteinemia are only contributing factors).

— *Milky Ascitic Fluid:* ***Chylous Ascites*** (Chyloperitoneum). This is a rare condition with milky-looking fluid. The appearance results from the presence of fat as triglycerides and small amounts of cholesterol and phospholipids. *Pathophysiology.* The thoracic duct drains all body lymph channels except those served by the right lymphatic duct, which drains the right side of the head and neck, the right arm, and the right hemithorax. But obstruction of a single large lymph vessel rarely causes chyloperitoneum because of the many collateral lymph-lymph and lymph-vein communications. So obstruction depends upon the number of branches involved and the person's supply of collaterals. *Diagnosis.* The fluid usually has a *lipid content* in excess of that in the plasma; its *protein content* is more than half that of plasma; fat droplets are large enough to be visible in the light microscope. The quantities of lipid and protein vary with the diet, and the visibility of the fat globules depends on the physical state of the lipid. *Lymphangiography* may assist in demonstrating lymph node lesions leading to a biopsy, or it may show severance of ducts from trauma. Determination of the urinary output of 5-hydroxyindole acetic acid for carcinoid should be made; and the fluid should be analyzed for hyaluronic acid from a possible mesothelioma. Appropriate examinations should be made for other conditions in the following list:

Clinical Occurrence: Malignant lymphoma, other malignancies, liver diseases, nephritis, vascular thromboses, adhesive bands in the peritoneal cavity, tuberculosis, amyloidosis, benign neoplasm. It may occur iatrogenically following aortic surgery, staging laparotomies with lymph node biopsies, and following sympathectomies.

Abdominal Distention: ***Ovarian Cyst.*** Large ovarian cysts fill much of the abdominal cavity and *must be distinguished from ascites.* Since they are thin-walled and filled with fluid, they evert the umbilicus, produce fluid wave and shifting dullness. A trochar piercing the abdominal wall yields fluid that resembles ascites. The pelvic examination is not diagnostic. Three signs distinguish the cysts (Fig. 7-7): In the supine position the tympanitic intestines are pushed superiorly, so the top of the abdomen may be *dull.* Careful inspection of the abdominal profile reveals *two curves,* instead of one. A cyst *transmits the aortic pulsation anteriorly,* ascites does not. To demonstrate, press a ruler transversely on the abdomen below the umbilicus; the ruler moves visibly with each pulse wave. Ultrasonic B-mode examination distinguishes a cyst from ascites.

Abdominal Distention: ***Pregnancy.*** In advanced pregnancy the uterus has many mechanical attributes of an ovarian cyst, from which it must be distinguished. The diagnostic features of advanced pregnancy include: the breasts are engorged, fetal movements may be felt, the cervix uteri is softened, the small parts, head, or back of the fetus are palpable, the fetal heart may be audible.

Abdominal Distention: ***Feces.*** An accumulation of large amounts of feces, as in megacolon, may cause distention. The

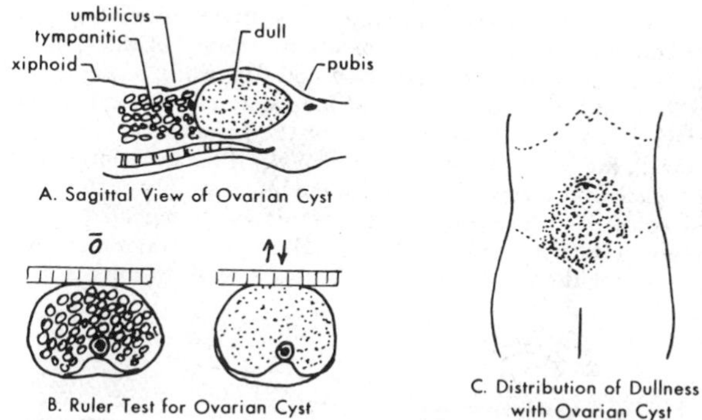

Fig. 7-7. Signs of ovarian cyst. **A.** *The profile of the abdomen shows a curve more pronounced in the lower half. The gas-filled intestines, producing tympany, fill the superior half of the cavity, instead of floating to the top.* **B.** The ruler test. *When the ruler is pressed transversely across the abdomen with free fluid, the pulsations of the abdominal aorta are not transmitted; but if the fluid be enclosed in a tight cyst, the aortic pulsation will move the ruler.* **C.** Distribution of dullness with ovarian cyst.

plastic nature of the masses can often be palpated through the abdominal wall.

Abdominal Distention: ***Visceral Enlargement.*** A large liver or spleen may fill much of the abdominal cavity. Masses of neoplasm may distend. The nature of the situation must be evaluated by palpation.

Depressed Abdomen: ***Scaphoid Abdomen.*** In extreme malnutrition, the abdominal wall sinks inward toward the vertebral column, forming a depression, pointed superiorly by the costal angle and inferiorly by the wings of the ilia. This has the shape of an ancient boat for which the Greek word is *skaphē.* The abdominal contents are more visible and more readily felt than normal, so the examiner is warned against attaching undue significance to the feel of structures that are unfamiliar because normally impalpable.

Abdominal Hernias

Examination for Abdominal Hernias. **The protrusion of a structure through a weak point in the abdominal wall is a *hernia.* In**

most cases, a hernia has a peritoneal sac that is often empty, but it may contain bowel, stomach, omentum, urinary bladder, colon, or even liver. Omentum feels soft and nodular, while bowel is smooth and fluctuant. Gas in a herniated loop may cause creptitation and peristaltic sounds. If the contents of the hernial sac can be easily replaced, the hernia is said to be *reducible;* if they cannot, the hernia is *irreducible or incarcerated.* When the blood supply of the incarcerated contents is interrupted, the hernia is *strangulated;* gangrene may quickly ensue (Fig. 7-8A). Pinching and strangulation of only a portion of the circumference of the gut wall produce a *Richter's*

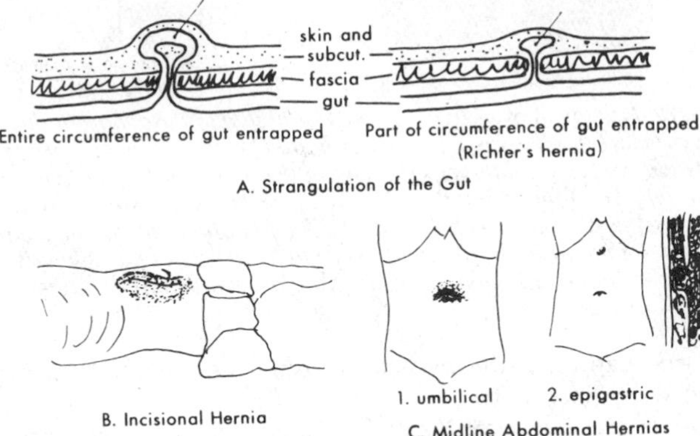

Fig. 7-8. Some hernias and their complications. **A.** Strangulation of the gut. *A loop of gut protruding through a fascial opening so the edges of the opening impinge upon the blood supply of the entire circumference of the lumen is the usual mechanism of strangulation of a hernia. If only a part of the circumference of the gut is pinched in the opening, the condition is called a Richter's hernia.* **B.** Incisional hernia. *A bulge near an operative scar usually indicates an incisional hernia. The lack of fascial support can be readily palpated. In the abdomen, the bulge may not be apparent when the muscles are relaxed and the patient is in the supine position. But it is readily seen when the patient is asked to raise the head or put some other type of tension on the abdominal muscles.* **C.** Midline abdominal hernias. *The adult type of umbilical hernia is depicted in which the fascial ring is incomplete so the bulge is superior to the umbilicus. An epigastric hernia is a small bulge of fat protruding from the deep layers through an opening in the linea alba. This hernia usually does not have a sac. It may not be detected unless the patient is examined in the standing position and the examining finger is run down the linea alba.*

hernia. Strangulated bowel feels firm, but it is usually not tender. The examiner *should not use force* to reduce a hernia because the result may be rupture of strangulated gut or *reduction en masse*, so that the sac accompanies the loop and the strangulation is not relieved.

Inspection is the first procedure in examination for hernia. If the condition is previously suspected, have the patient stand so the abdominal contents bulge through the hernial ring. Many hernias are encountered unexpectedly during routine examination of the supine patient. A bulge may be seen during relaxation, or it may appear during maneuvers that increase intra-abdominal pressure. Palpate the ring and its contents; insert the finger in the ring and feel an impulse when the patient coughs or blows against the lips closed by apposition to the back of his hand with the nose occluded.

Incisional Hernia. When an operative scar is present in the abdomen, test it by having the patient perform the Valsalva maneuver, or raise the head from the pillow when supine. Protrusion occurs adjacent to the scar (Fig. 7-8B).

Epigastric Hernia (Fatty Hernia of the Linea Alba). A small protuberance may be seen, but more often is felt, in the midline of the epigastrium. Attention may be called to the region by pain resembling that of chronic peptic ulcer. The hernia consists of a bit of properitoneal fat protruding outward between the fibers of the linea alba (Fig. 7-8C, 2). If the bulge cannot be seen, Bailey advises having the patient stand while the examiner runs a finger down the midline to discover a small nodule that is occasionally reducible. Usually this hernia does not have a peritoneal sac.

Umbilical Hernia. The navel may protrude, either during relaxation or when intra-abdominal pressure is increased by standing or the Valsalva maneuver. The *congenital type* is distinguished by protrusion through the umbilical scar; palpation of the ring reveals a complete fibrous collar continuous with the linea alba. In the *adult type* of hernia, the collar is lacking; the upper part of the hernia is covered only by skin (Fig. 7-8C, 1). It is properly termed a *paraumbilical hernia.* These are soft, except when chronic inflammation has caused thickening.

Clinical Occurrence. These defects are very common in infants and tend to resolve spontaneously by about 4 years of age. Frequently the adult type develops during pregnancy, in long-standing ascites, or when intrathoracic pressure is repeatedly increased as in asthma, chronic bronchitis, and bronchiectasis.

Indirect Inguinal Hernia (Fig. 7-9). The lateral end of the inguinal canal is the internal inguinal ring, lying just above the *midpoint* of the inguinal ligament. Through this ring the spermatic cord of the male emerges from the abdominal cavity into the canal. The cord courses medialward through the canal, emerging through the subcutaneous (external) ring, just lateral to the pubis. Thence the cord droops over the brim of the bony pelvis into the scrotum. In the male, a hernia follows the course of the cord. From the abdominal cavity, it may enter the canal for only a slight distance, or it may descend to the bottom of the scrotal sac. In the female, the hernia follows a similar course in the canal that contains the round ligament, corresponding to the spermatic cord. In either sex, a small indirect inguinal hernia may produce a bulge over the *midpoint* of the inguinal ligament, at the abdominal (internal) inguinal ring. To palpate the length of the canal in the male, place the fingertip at the most dependent part of the scrotum and invaginate the slack scrotal wall to insert the finger gently into the subcutaneous (external) inguinal ring (Fig. 7-10A). If the ring is sufficiently relaxed, guide the finger laterally and cephalad through the canal and have the patient cough or strain. A small hernia causes an impulse felt on the end of the fingertip. A larger hernia may feel like a mass in the canal. In the female, palpation of the inguinal canal is usually unsatisfactory, lacking the slack tissue of the male.

Direct Inguinal Hernia. A hernia through the posterior *wall* of the inguinal canal is termed *direct.* The site of the weakness is Hesselbach's triangle, bounded laterally by the inferior epigastric artery and medially by the lateral border of the rectus muscle, and the inguinal ligament; thus it lies nearly directly behind the subcutaneous (external) inguinal ring. A bulge is produced *close* to the pubic tubercle, just above the inguinal ligament; this is medial to the site of the bulge for an indirect hernia. With the finger in the inguinal canal, coughing or straining causes an impulse to be felt not at the tip or end of the finger, but rather on the pad of the distal phalanx. A direct hernia seldom causes pain. It is always acquired and usually occurs in the male.

Scrotal Hernia. An indirect hernia may enter the scrotum; there is doubt whether a direct hernia may do so. The two are said to be distinguished by palpating the lumen of the inguinal canal and following the hernial sac to the point of its emergence from the abdominal cavity, either close to the pubis in the direct, or at the midpoint of the inguinal ligament in the indirect.

Femoral Hernia. Just inferior to the midpoint of the inguinal ligament lies the femoral artery. In a few persons, its pulsation is visible; in most, palpation is required to detect it. Adjacent and medial to the artery lies the femoral vein, not demonstrable by physical examination. Immediately medial to the vein, is the femoral canal, a continuation of the femoral sheath, through which a small hernia may bulge when intra-abdominal pressure is increased. Larger femoral hernias become irreducible and may push *upward* in front of the inguinal ligament, so they must be distinguished from inguinal hernias. When the neck of the hernial sac can be palpated just lateral to and *below* the pubic tubercle, a femoral hernia is demonstrated; the neck of an inguinal hernia's sac is found *above* the inguinal ligament. A bulge just below the femoral canal may be caused by a *varix of the saphenous vein;* this fills upon standing and empties in the supine position; palpation of the filled varix yields a distinctive *thrill.* Inflammation and swelling secondary to hyperplasia of a lymph node or nodes can cause a mass in the area of the femoral vessels below the inguinal ligament, the so-called *bubo.* It occurs commonly in chancroid, syphilis, and lymphogranuloma venereum.

Mass in Femoral Triangle: ***Obturator Hernia.*** Rarely, and almost always in an emaciated woman over 60 years old, a peritoneal sac protrudes through the obturator foramen of the pelvis, causing a *fullness* or *mass* in the femoral triangle. The fullness is not sharply defined because the sac is covered by the pectineus muscle. The swelling can sometimes be palpated through the vagina. When only a portion of the circumference of the bowel is strangulated (Richter's type), the resulting pain may provide such a late warning that death results before diagnosis can lead to proper treatment. In almost half the cases of strangulation the genicular branch of the obturator nerve is compressed, producing *pain down the medial aspect of the thigh to the knee* (Romberg-Howship's sign). On the affected side the *thigh is usually held in semiflexion;* all hip motion is *painful.* *Distinction.* The condition must be distinguished from the far more common femoral hernia. When a mass from the obturator hernia

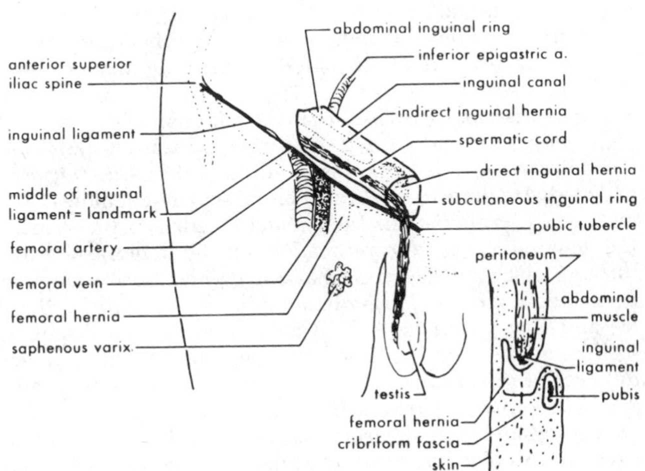

Fig. 7-9. Hernias in the inguinal region. **A.** Inguinal hernias. *The inguinal ligament stretches from the anterior superior spine of the ilium to the pubic tubercle. Just above and parallel to it the inguinal canal lies as a flattened tube between the superficial and deep layers of abdominal muscles. It is 1.5 inches (3.5 cm) long. The lateral end of the canal opens posteriorly into the abdominal cavity through the abdominal inguinal ring (internal ring). The ring is not palpable, but it is accurately located just above the midpoint of the inguinal ligament. The medial end of the canal opens anteriorly into the subcutaneous tissue through the subcutaneous inguinal ring (external ring), located in the male where the spermatic cord emerges from the abdominal muscles. A hernia is "indirect" when it enters the canal from the abdominal cavity through the abdominal inguinal ring; a hernia entering medial to this ring is "direct." In small hernias the relation of the bulge to the midpoint of the inguinal ligament is diagnostic of direct or indirect. If the hernia is large, palpation of the inguinal canal through the scrotum may determine its site of entrance into the canal. The direct hernia is represented as an anterior bulging of the posterior wall of the inguinal canal.* **B.** Femoral hernia. *Beneath the midpoint of the inguinal ligament the femoral artery and vein emerge from the abdomen where the artery's pulsation is palpable. Immediately medial to it is the impalpable and invisible femoral vein. The femoral canal lies medial to the vein, so the canal is about 2 cm medial to the pulsating artery. A bulge in the region of the femoral canal is produced by a femoral hernia, especially on coughing or*

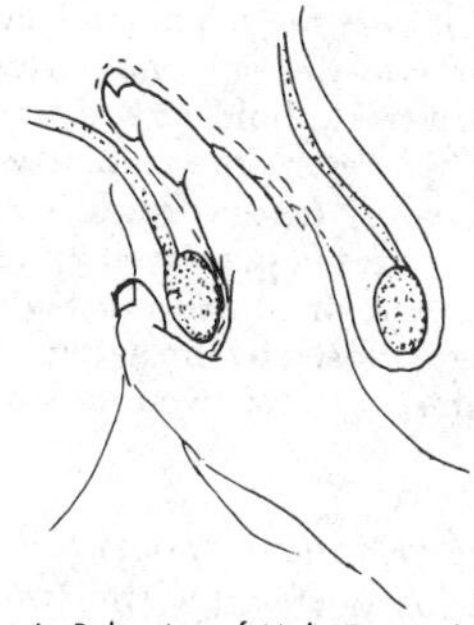
A. Palpation of Male External Inguinal Ring

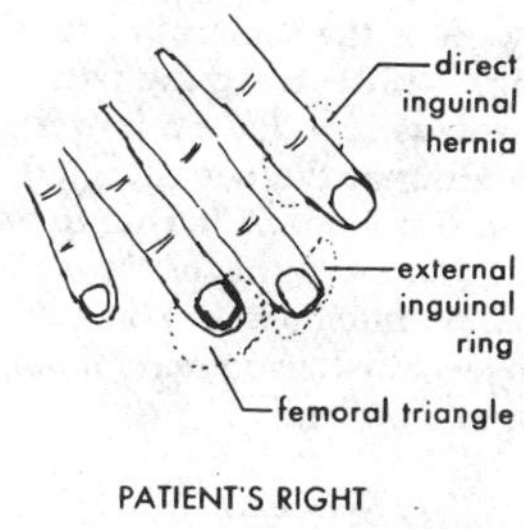

B. Zieman's Tridigital Examination for Hernia

Fig. 7-10. Examination of the inguinal regions for hernia. **A.** Palpation of the inguinal ring in the male. *The tip of the index finger is placed at the most dependent part of the scrotum and directed into the subcutaneous inguinal ring by invaginating the slack scrotum with it. The patient coughs or strains so an impulse from the hernial sac may be felt on the fingertip.* **B.** Zieman's tridigital examination for hernia. *The examiner stands by the patient's right side with his right hand placed near the right inguinal ligament so the tip of the long finger is in the external inguinal ring, the overlying index finger is in the vicinity of the internal inguinal ring, and the ring finger is in the femoral triangle. When the patient coughs, the fingers can detect a hernia in any of the three locations. The left side of the patient is examined from his left and with the examiner's left hand.*

is present, no pain is elicited when the fingers press just above the mass against the pubic ramus.

ZIEMAN'S INGUINAL EXAMINATION FOR HERNIA. **This procedure reveals direct and indirect inguinal hernias, and hernias of the femoral triangle. With the patient standing, stand at his right side and place the palm of your right hand in apposition to his right lower abdomen. Spread your fingers slightly so your *long finger* lies along the inguinal ligament with its pulp in the external inguinal ring, your *index finger***

---

straining. A varix of the saphenous vein may produce a bulge just below that fills on standing and empties when the patient reclines; palpation during coughing produces a distinctive thrill. The inset shows the protrusion of a femoral hernia upward in front of the inguinal ligament, so it may be confused with an inguinal hernia. Palpation in such cases demonstrates the inguinal canal to be empty.

is over the internal inguinal ring, and your *ring finger* palpates the region of the femoral canal and the opening of the saphenous vein (Fig. 7-10B). Have the patient take a deep breath, hold it, and bear down, as if to have a bowel movement. Then repeat the maneuver, standing at the patient's left side and palpating his left groin with your left hand. A hernia in any of the three sites is perceived either as a *gliding motion of the walls* of the empty sac or as a *protrusion of a viscus* into the sac. When the internal ring is closed by the palpating finger, any hernia mass must be other than secondary to an indirect inguinal hernia.

Mass Above the Inguinal Ligament: ***Spigelian Hernia.*** A peritoneal sac with considerable extraperitoneal fat perforates the linea semilunaris to lie within the abdominal wall; it is covered only by skin, subcutaneous fat, and the aponeurosis of the external abdominal oblique muscle. It is usually symptomless until it strangulates, when it produces a *tender mass* within the abdominal wall about 3 to 5 cm above the inguinal ligament. This should be inspected and palpated while the patient stands.

Abdominal Sounds

ABDOMINAL AUSCULTATION. **Frequently auscultation of the abdomen is omitted, but evidence accumulates that valuable signs can be elicited by including the procedure in the routine examination. Many physicians prefer to auscultate the abdomen before palpation disturbs the viscera to abnormal activity, thus obscuring vascular murmurs.**

Abdominal Murmurs. The presence of a murmur in an abdominal vessel indicates turbulent blood flow in a dilated, constricted, or tortuous artery. A murmur is often present in an aortic aneurysm. Primary hepatic carcinoma frequently produces an arterial bruit. In one report the murmurs were harsh, unlike a venous hum, and either purely systolic, or continuous with systolic accentuation. They could not be distinguished from those of alcoholic hepatitis [D. Clain, K. Wartnaby, and S. Sherlock: Abdominal Arterial Murmurs in Liver Disease, *Lancet,* **2**:516–19, 1966]. Rarely a venous hum may be audible over a hemangioma in the liver or in the dilated periumbilical circulation in Cruveilhier-Baumgarten's syndrome. A continuous systolic-diastolic bruit may occur from an arteriovenous fistula in renal vessels. The findings of murmurs should be

in this region. Bimanual palpation is necessary to detect moderate enlargement of these viscera. Palpation is employed as in the left upper quadrant, except that the left or lifting hand must be *supinated*, instead of pronated, to curl the fingers around the lower thorax near the examiner (Fig. 7-20). Also, the right or pushing hand must be directed so the tips of the index and long fingers are parallel to the right costal margin and the expected liver edge.

RUQ Mass: ***Rotated Liver.*** Pathologists report that many clinical diagnoses of hepatomegaly are not confirmed at autopsy because clinicians do not appreciate the ability of the normal-sized liver to rotate. The liver may be visualized as a body with a convex and concave surface, preempting the entire anterior portion of the right upper quadrant behind the ribs, and extending its left lobe to the left midclavicular line. The plane of the concave surface is tipped backward and downward. Although the anterior margin of the liver extends across the intercostal angle, the left third of the edge is rarely felt because of the taut suspension of fascia and muscle across the angle. The liver is heavy but its suspension is relatively meager. The coronal ligaments, attaching it to the diaphragm, arise posterior

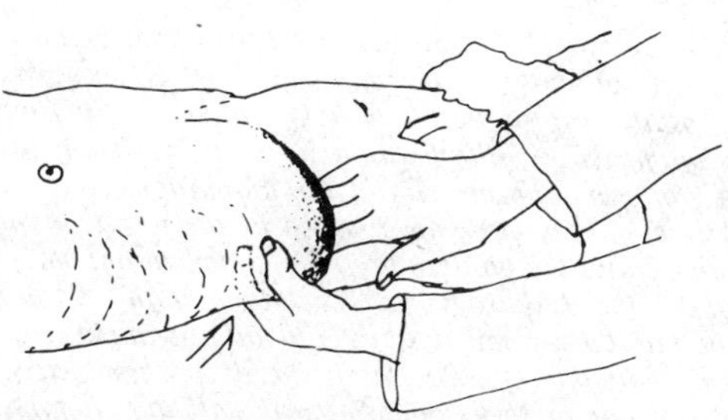

Fig. 7-20. Bimanual palpation of the right upper quadrant. *The right hand with fingers adducted is inserted under the right rib margin with the volar surface of the hand touching the abdominal surface; the tactile sensations are received with the fingertips of this hand. The supinated left hand is placed under the right lower thorax. When the patient inspires deeply, the right hand is moved farther upward and inward as the height of inspiration is approached. Simultaneously the right thorax is lifted by the left hand in the direction of the arrow. The maneuver is employed especially in feeling for the liver or right kidney.*

to the dome of the viscus (Fig. 7-21). The diaphragm is not strong enough to support the weight; it is aided by the negative pressure in the thorax resisting downward pull, by the vessels at the liver hilum to the left of the center of mass, and by the pressure of the abdominal muscles on the viscera and fat in the cavity. Two axes of rotation may be envisioned: a *transverse axis* through the liver near the attachment of the coronary ligaments, and an *anteroposterior axis* near the hilum, to the left of the center of mass. Downward rotation through the transverse axis causes a normal-sized liver to present more of its anterior surface below the costal margin. Downward rotation about the anteroposterior axis results in a tongue of liver

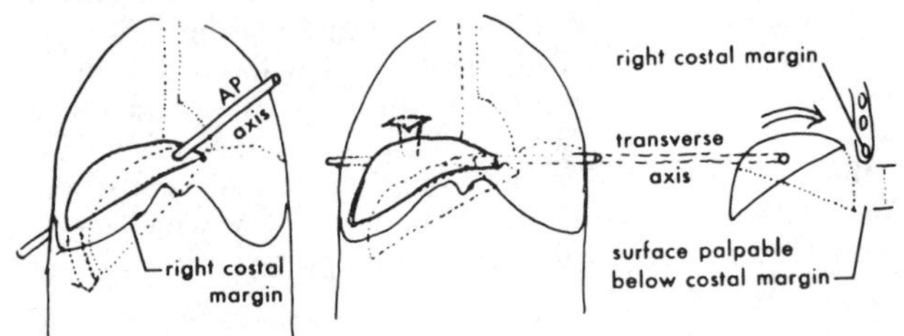

Fig. 7-21. Rotations of the normal-sized liver that make it palpable beneath the costal margin. *Normally the liver is maintained behind the right costal margin, inaccessible to palpation, suspended by its coronary ligaments and the fixation to the prevertebral fascia by its hilar blood vessels. The muscles of the diaphragm could not hold a 1500-gm liver if they were not assisted by the negative intrapleural pressure above and the positive pressure of abdominal contents below. Depression of the diaphragm or relaxation of the intra-abdominal pressure permits the normal-sized liver to fall beneath the costal margin and become palpable (ptosis). With the diaphragm fixed, the liver may rotate on one or two axes to become palpable; depression of the diaphragm increases the amount of palpable surface permitted by rotation.* **A.** *The liver may rotate on an anteroposterior axis near its left side. With this counterclockwise rotation the lower border appears below the costal margin with its edge presenting and forming an angle with the costal margin.* **B.** *When the normal-sized liver rotates on a transverse axis, the edge presenting below the costal margin is approximately parallel to it. This can only be distinguished from enlargement of the liver by the fact that the anterior surface curves inward.*

appearing in the right flank (Fig. 7-21A). Rotation may be expected in any condition that lowers the dome of the diaphragm, depletes the normal amount of fat in the abdominal cavity, or impairs the tone of the abdominal muscles. To establish the diagnosis of hepatomegaly the upper border of *hepatic flatness* must be percussed in the 6th right intercostal space or higher. The lower border of the liver should be palpable well below the costal margin; the liver of some normal persons is readily palpable just below the costal margin. The palpable margin should be roughly parallel to the costal margin, rather than descend almost vertically in the flank (Fig. 7-21A). If the lower border cannot be definitely felt, only a tentative diagnosis of hepatomegaly is justified; a conclusion based solely on the extent of liver dullness is hazardous. The palpable surface should be examined for consistency and nodularity. Tenderness can be elicited by direct palpation or by *fist percussion* (Fig. 7-22). The latter procedure is accomplished by placing the palm of the left hand on the thorax in the region of normal liver dullness; a *light* blow is struck on the dorsum of the hand by the right fist. *Percussion tenderness* occurs in acute cholecystitis. The size and shape of the liver and defects from abscesses and neoplasms may be shown by radioisotope scintigram, ultrasonography, and CT scanning.

Palpate the surface of the liver for *friction rubs* and auscultate it for *bruits*. The coincidence of these two signs indicates a

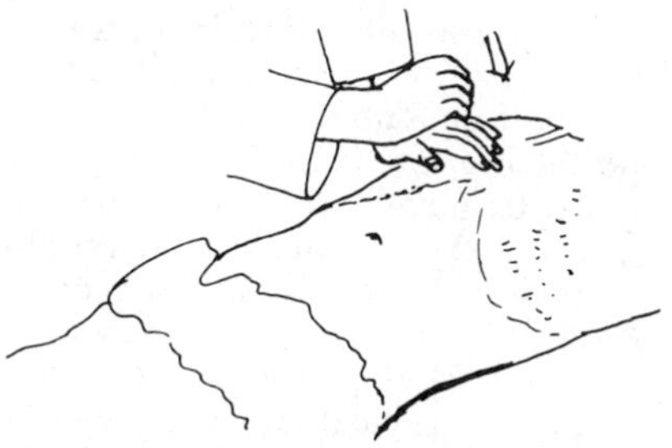

Fig. 7-22. Fist percussion over the liver. *The palm of the left hand is applied anteriorly to the lower ribs of the right hemithorax. The back of the applied hand is struck lightly with the fist of the right hand. This impact is painful in acute hepatitis and acute cholecystitis.*

high probability of hepatic carcinoma as the cause [H. I. Sherman and J. E. Hardison: The Importance of Coexistent Hepatic Rub and Bruit, *J.A.M.A.*, **241:**1495–96, 1979].

Clinical Occurrence: SMOOTH AND NONTENDER: fatty infiltration of the liver, late passive congestion of the liver, portal cirrhosis, lymphoma, portal obstruction, hepatic vein thrombosis, lymphocytic leukemia, rickets, amyloidosis, schistosomiasis, kala-azar. SMOOTH AND TENDER: early congestive cardiac failure, acute hepatitis, amebic hepatitis, amebic abscess of the liver, multiple hepatic abscesses. NODULAR: late portal cirrhosis of the liver tertiary syphilis, hydatid cysts of the liver, metastatic carcinoma. VERY LARGE: metastatic carcinoma, chronic myelocytic leukemia. VERY HARD: carcinomatosis.

RUQ Mass: ***Pulsatile Liver.*** An enlarged liver may move with each arterial pulsation. The movement can be *transmitted* by direct contact of the solid organ with the abdominal aorta, or it can be the object of the true pulsation from an intrinsic expansion and contraction of the liver parenchyma receiving excessive amounts of blood. *Expansile pulsation,* proving true pulsation, is demonstrated by placing the hands on opposite sides of the liver and showing that the opposite surfaces alternately diverge and converge.

Clinical Occurrence. Extreme tricuspid regurgitation.

RUQ Mass: ***Enlarged Tender Gallbladder.*** The gallbladder lies on the inferior surface of the liver, lateral to the right midclavicular line; normally, it is not palpable. In acute cholecystitis the gallbladder is usually exquisitely tender to fist percussion; in the early stages it may not be palpable. When distended, it is felt behind the liver border as a smooth, firm sausagelike mass. Palpation is frequently difficult because of the intense involuntary spasm of the abdominal muscles. Fist percussion over the liver is painful, but this is also a sign of acute hepatitis (Fig. 7-22). A valuable sign of acute cholecystitis is *inspiratory arrest* (Murphy's sign). The patient is asked to inspire while the examining fingers are held under the liver border where the gallbladder may descend upon them. Inspiration is arrested in midcycle by painful contact with the fingers. Carcinoma of the gallbladder produces a hard irregular mass that is moderately tender.

Clinical Occurrence. Acute cholecystitis, empyema, carcinoma.

RUQ Mass: ***Enlarged Nontender Gallbladder.*** A gallbladder filled with stones may occasionally be felt without pain to the patient. It resembles a smooth mass, shaped like a sausage. The same finding occurs in *hydrops* of the gallbladder in which mucous cells continue to secrete in the face of obstruction of the cystic duct. Painless distention of the gallbladder also occurs in many cases of carcinoma at the head of the pancreas. *Courvoisier's law* states that dilatation of the gallbladder does not occur in obstructive jaundice due to stone in the common duct because previous scarring of the wall has taken place; in obstruction from carcinoma at the head of the pancreas, there is no previous restrictive scarring, so dilatation of the gallbladder occurs. There are many exceptions, so the *law* should be changed to *sign*.

Clinical Occurrence. Cholelithiasis, hydrops of the gallbladder, distention due to carcinoma of the Ampulla of Vater or at the head of the pancreas.

RUQ Mass: ***Enlarged Right Kidney.*** Normally this organ lies 1 or 2 cm lower than its left counterpart because of the superimposed liver (cf. Fig. 7-19 and enlarged left kidney, p. 511). In many normal persons, the lower pole of the right kidney is palpable while the left is not. Since the shapes of the kidney and liver are so dissimilar, there is usually no difficulty in distinguishing them with bimanual palpation. Rarely a protruding renal mass may be confused with hydrops of the gallbladder or pancreatic pseudocyst. Kidney tumors may be smooth or irregular; when they become large they extend anteriorly and downward.

Clinical Occurrence. Hydronephrosis, neoplasm, cysts.

RUQ Mass: ***Ptotic Right Kidney.*** Bimanual palpation readily identifies the characteristic shape and size of the kidney, whether it be under the liver or in the pelvis.

Epigastric Smooth Masses. Occasionally acute gastric dilatation produces a slight visible enlargement of the epigastrium; the patient usually appears to be very ill. A smooth mass in the epigastrium of a person not acutely ill suggests a pancreatic cyst or a pseudopancreatic cyst. The profile of the epigastrium is quite typical (Fig. 7-5C). The tumor is not mobile or tender.

Epigastric Irregular Masses. Either infections or neoplasms in this region cause masses by involvement of the omentum, stomach, pancreas, left lobe of liver, and transverse colon. A polycystic or horseshoe kidney sometimes presents as a midline epigastric mass. Gastric or pyloric edema may be palpable. Usually the separate components of the mass cannot be distinguished by physical examination or x-ray diagnosis.

Upper Abdomen: ***Subphrenic Abscess.*** In the spaces under each diaphragm pus may accumulate from suppurative lesions elsewhere in the abdomen, such as perforated peptic ulcer or appendix. Usually there are no symptoms to direct attention to the subphrenic region. The patient has an unexplained fever or anorexia, after an acute inflammation localized elsewhere in the abdominal cavity. From his knowledge of the migration of pus in the abdomen, the examiner must learn to *suspect* abscesses under the diaphragm and *search* for the local signs. *Elevation* of either leaf of the diaphragm may be demonstrated by percussion; more certainly x-ray examination will disclose it. Inspection of the phrenic movements by fluoroscopy is especially helpful. *Pleural effusion* may occur on the affected side, as demonstrated by percussion dullness, impaired breath sounds, and x-ray films. *Air under the right diaphragm* may be suspected when percussion over the normal area of hepatic dullness in the right axilla yields tympany. Further localization in the involved subphrenic spaces may be obtained by palpation for *tenderness* and *edema* in specific locations as follows (Fig. 7-23). *Right Anterior Superior Space.* Under the right costal margin *in front of* the liver, between the 6th and 10th right intercostal spaces anteriorly. *Right Anterior Inferior Space.* Below the right anterior costal margin *behind* the liver. *Left Anterior Superior Space.* Under the left costal margin anteriorly, between the 6th and 10th left interspaces in the midclavicular line. *Left Anterior Inferior Space.* Under the left costal margin in the midaxillary line. *Left Posterior Inferior Space.* Over the left 12th rib. Computed tomography and, to a lesser extent, ultrasonography provide detailed anatomic localization of intra-abdominal abscesses that permit precise percutaneous placement of catheters large enough to effect drainage [W. C. Johnson, S. G. Gerzof, A. H. Robbins, and D. C. Nabseth: Treatment of Abdominal Abscesses. *Ann. Surg.* **194:**510–20,

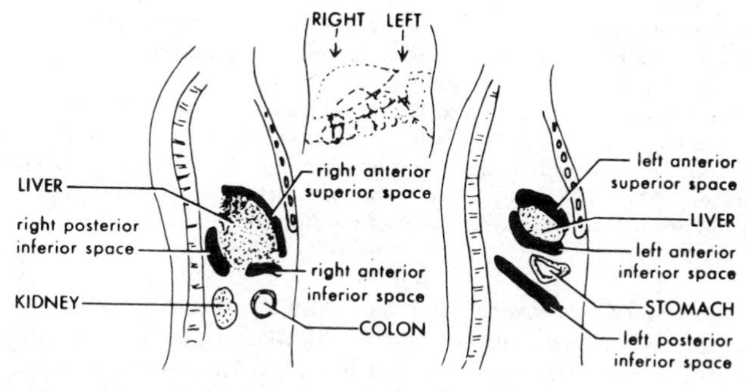

Fig. 7-23. Possible locations of subphrenic abscesses. *Reference to the diagrams will show the locations where tenderness and masses may be palpated from subphrenic abscesses. The various loci are in the right midclavicular line, behind the costal margin, and the left upper quadrant of the abdomen. Posteriorly, the region of the right kidney should be examined.*

1981]. The authors feel such an approach is as effective as operative drainage.

Lower Paramedial Mass: ***Hematoma of Rectus Abdominis Muscle*** (A Psychological Trap). This condition is considered with the intra-abdominal masses because it is often mistaken for one. Experienced clinicians have felt a mass in the sheath of the Rectus abdominis and projected its location *into* the abdominal cavity. If one thinks of it, the diagnosis is easy; the mass remains palpable *when the abdominal wall is tensed* by having the patient raise his head from the pillow, a maneuver that obscures intra-abdominal masses. The tumor is *below the umbilicus* and *beside* the midline. The mass may be *tender* and *painful.* [For beautiful colored lithographs by the master, Max Brodel, see T. S. Cullen and M. Brodel: Lesions of the Rectus Abdominis Muscle Simulating an Acute Intra-Abdominal Condition: I. Anatamony of the Rectus Abdominis Muscle, *Johns Hopkins Med. J.*, **61:**295, 1937]. The diagnosis is readily proved by ultrasonography [G. M. Wyatt and H. B. Spitz: Ultrasound in the Diagnosis of Rectus Sheath Hematoma, *J.A.M.A.*, **241:**1499–1500, 1979].

Clinical Occurrence: TRAUMA: severe coughing or sneezing, direct blows to the abdomen, abdominal paracentesis, operative injury, pregnancy, labor, ascites, abdominal masses. PREDISPOSING FACTORS: debilitating diseases, administration of anticoagulants. Vigorous palpation of the abdomen in a patient taking anticoagulants was the cause in one case [K. H. Borkovich and E. S. Stafford: Acute Anema and Abdominal Tumor Due to Hemorrhage in Rectus Abdominis Sheath Following Anticoagulant Therapy. *Arch. Intern. Med.,* **117**:103, 1966]. It has also occurred postoperatively when retention sutures have inadvertently injured the inferior epigastric artery.

Masses in Cecal Region. Occasionally the normal cecum can be felt as an indistinct soft mass, slightly tender, usually fluctuant. A firmer mass may be felt from involvement by tuberculous granuloma, pericecal or appendiceal abscess, Crohn's disease involving the distal ileum, or carcinoma.

Masses in Sigmoid Region. A *spastic sigmoid colon* feels like a cord about the diameter of the little finger, lying vertically about 5 cm medial to the left superior anterior iliac spine; the cord can be rolled under the fingers and is slightly or moderately tender. Ordinarily spastic sigmoid is not confused with *neoplasm* that produces a globular mass having dilated colon above it. Irregular plastic *masses of feces* may be a palpated in the sigmoid; they are occasionally mistake for neoplasm until movement or disappearance is demonstrated in one or two days.

Suprapubic Mass: ***Distended Urinary Bladder.*** Amazingly, the bladder may extend up to the level of the umbilicus, usually in the midline. The profile of the abdomen bulges in that region. The swelling is fluctuant and disappears with catheterization. It is sometimes mistaken for other tumors because of the extreme size or because a lateral diverticulum destroys its symmetry. It must be distinguished from ovarian cyst in the female.

Suprapubic Mass: ***Ovarian Cyst.*** The largest cysts simulate ascites, and their distinction is discussed elsewhere (p. 488). Those that extend just above the pelvic brim are always in the midline and resemble distended bladder. Often the cyst cannot be palpated vaginally because it is too high. Persistence of the fluctuant mass after catheterization suggest ovarian cyst or gravid uterus. Ultrasonograms are diagnostic.

Suprapubic Mass: ***Uterine Fibroid.*** When large enough, a uterus with leiomyomas may be felt above the symphysis pubis as a hard multinodular mass. Vaginal examination readily demonstrates the masses to move with cervix uteri and hence are attached to the fundus.

Shallow Abdominal Cavity. With deep palpation, the impression is gained of a cavity shallower than normal, but without definite masses. This finding results from enlargement of the preaortic and mesenteric lymph nodes, termed *retroperitoneal lymphadenopathy*. The hyperplastic nodes are covered with fascia and abdominal viscera, so the floor of the abdominal cavity seems more accessible than normal; discrete nodes cannot be felt (Fig. 7-24). The retroperitoneal nodes may be involved by lymphomas or granulomas visualized on CT scans.

Masses in the Groin. Among the structures to be considered when an indefinite mass is found in the groin are lymph nodes, hernia, varix, lipoma, ectopic testis, ectopic spleen, inguinal endometriosis (Solnitzke and Jehgers).

Nondescript Abdominal Masses. The masses previously described involve tissues more or less localized to a certain abdominal region. But the abdominal cavity is filled with coils of the gastrointestinal tract that may have a localized lesion anywhere in its length that may form a palpable mass. *Volvulus* is a twisting of the bowel that produces intestinal obstruction. The site is usually in the sigmoid colon (90%) or the cecum (10%). Vascular compromise secondary to circulatory impairment by twisting of the mesenteric root, distention of the involved segment, and formation of a closed loop make early diagnosis and treatment imperative. A vague tender mass may be felt, but frequently the only findings are distended bowel that produces

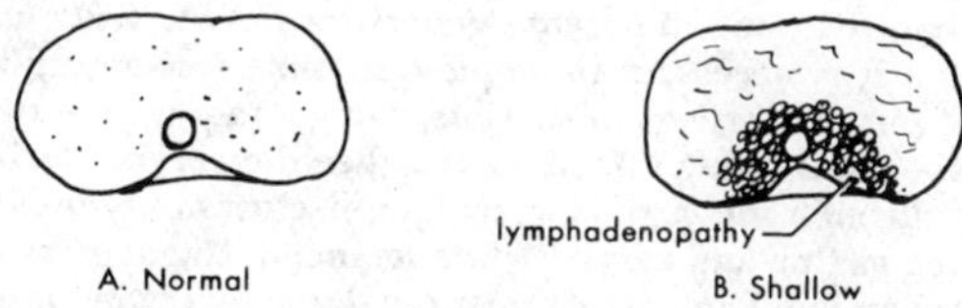

Fig. 7-24. Shallowness of the abdominal cavity. *Massive enlargement of prevertebral and preaortic lymph nodes cannot be distinguished as discrete masses by palpation through intervening tissues and viscera. The condition merely gives the examiner an impression that the abdomen is shallower than normal. The nodes are usually enlarged by lymphoma or carcinoma.*

tympany, pain, violent peristalsis, and vomiting. *Intussusception* occurs primarily in the pediatric population, especially in infants. It is the invagination of one portion of the gut into another, producing obstruction. The most frequent type occurs as prolapse of the distal small bowel into the cecum—the ileocolic type. Most frequently intussusception is preceded by a viral syndrome. Intermittent colicky pain is common; the site is painful and tender. The pathognomonic sign is an oblong mass in the right or upper midabdomen and absence of bowel in the right lower quadrant (Dance's sign). Bloody fluid may be expelled from the rectum late in the course. *Abscesses* may be present as palpable masses in many parts of the peritoneal cavity. They have no distinctive form, but they are suspected when a mass is palpated in a region normally devoid of solid organs. With the exception of intussusception, none of these conditions has characteristic physical findings; the diagnosis is made by the history of symptoms, the state of the patient, the signs of peritonitis and intestinal obstruction (Fig. 7-31).

Lower Abdomen

ABDOMINAL EXAMINATION PER RECTUM AND VAGINAM. **Digital examination of the rectum and vagina serves three purposes: (1) to detect intrinsic disease of the rectum and vagina, (2) to gain information about adjacent structures of the male and female genitourinary tract, (3) to examine the lower part of the peritoneal cavity. Although complete examinations of the rectum and vagina accomplish all three purposes, errors in diagnosis of abdominal conditions are notoriously common because these routes of palpation have not been employed. Through delicacy or haste, the pelvic examination in the female is especially often omitted because generations of students have been taught that it is necessary to employ the time-consuming inconvenience of putting the legs in stirrups, using a vaginal speculum, and having special lighting effects to visualize the cervix uteri. But inspection through the vaginal speculum discloses only intrinsic disease of the vagina and cervix, while its inconvenience has deterred the busy examiner from palpation through the vagina in the examination of the abdomen. We would urge routine vaginal palpation,** ***without the use of the vaginal speculum,*** **as part of every abdominal examination, reserving inspection through the speculum for special occasions, in the hope that more frequent palpation of the lower part of the peritoneal cavity would result.**

Since the peritoneal cavity extends into the pelvis, masses in the

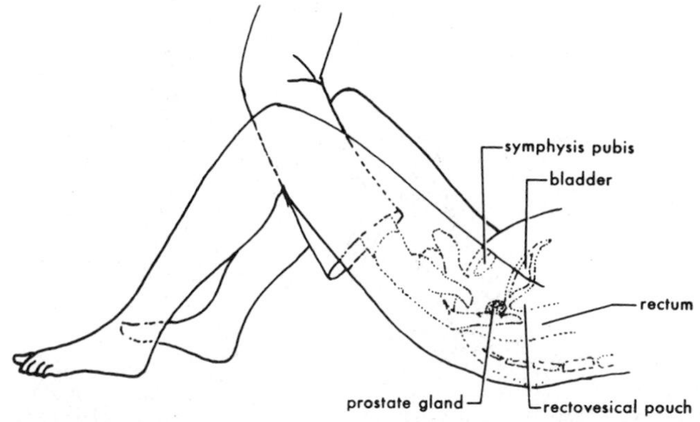

Fig. 7-25. Palpation of the male abdomen per rectum. *The lubricated index finger of the gloved right hand is inserted into the rectum of the male in the lithotomy position. The examining hand is supinated. Anteriorly the finger pad feels the prostate gland and seminal vesicles. Superiorly on the anterior rectal surface the fingertip reaches the location of the rectovesical pouch of the peritoneum. Normally, this pouch is not palpable; but the presence of pus or a tender mass may be perceived. Carcinoma cells may migrate to this pouch from the abdominal cavity, producing a hard, nontender, transverse ridge, called a rectal shelf, or Blumer's shelf.*

lower abdomen must always be palpated from below the pelvic brim as well as from above (Figs. 7-25 and 7-26). For this purpose, the *lithotomy position* is preferred for both vagina and rectum because masses in the cavity tend to fall upon the examining finger to become accessible more often than in other positions. With the patient lying supine, have the thighs and knees flexed so the feet rest upon the bed or in stirrups. Draw a rubber glove on the exploring* hand and lubricate the fingers well with surgical jelly, the index finger for a rectal examination, the index and long fingers for the vagina. In a woman, palpate the vagina first, then the rectum, so the same lubrication serves both orifices. Some clinicians insist on separate gloves for each orifice. Spread the labia minora apart with the index and long fingers; if the hymen does not prevent, insert both fingers into the vagina. Palpate the cervix uteri, the fundus, the adnexa.

* Surgeons and others using instruments advise training the nondominant hand for palpation in orifices to leave the dominant hand free to manipulate instruments.

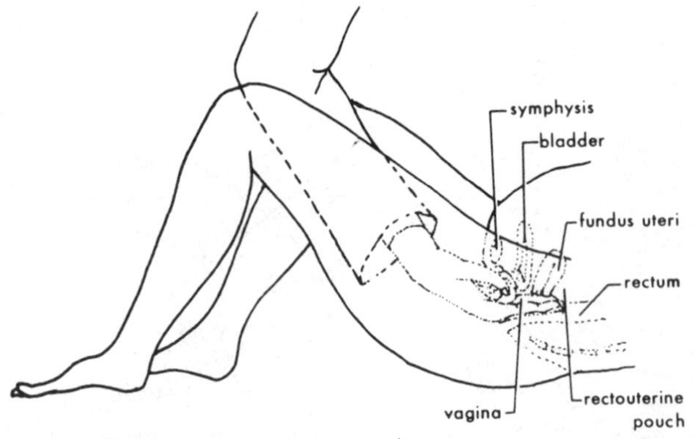

Fig. 7-26. Palpation of the female abdomen per rectum. *With the woman in the lithotomy position, the lubricated finger of the gloved right hand is inserted into the rectum with the hand supinated. The finger pad feels the cervix uteri and the fundus uteri through the anterior rectal wall. Passing the finger inward, superior to the cervix, the fingertip reaches the location of the rectouterine pouch (Douglas' pouch). Normally, this is not palpable, but a tender mass is evidence of pus in that structure. Carcinoma cells from the abdominal cavity may migrate to this region, forming a transverse ridge of hard, nontender tissues, called the rectal shelf or Blumer's shelf. Inflammatory tissue or pus in the adnexa may be felt through the rectum, but it is more distinctive when felt per vaginam.*

Especially, palpate the lateral fornices and the rectouterine pouch (Douglas' pouch) for masses and tenderness. In the rectal examination of both sexes, place the palm of the supinated examining hand toward the perineum and lay the *pulp* or *pad* of the index finger gently *upon* the anus, gently pressing so the anal spincter spreads to admit *first* the finger pad, *then* the tip of the finger. To avoid anal spasm, gently and slowly push the finger into the anal canal as far as possible. Press the fingers of the left hand upon the suprapubic region of the abdominal wall to accomplish bimanual palpation. Have the necessary materials ready to perform tests for occult fecal blood and be courteous enough to either clean the anus or provide papers or sponges for the patient to do so.

Pelvic Mass: ***Pelvic Abscess.*** In the male, a tender rounded mass, felt through the anterior rectal wall, superior to the prostate gland, is likely to be a pelvic abscess in the rectovesical pouch. Similarly in the female, a mass felt through the anterior rectal wall, superior to the cervix uteri, is probably an abscess in the rectouterine pouch. Commonly these abscesses result from perforation of the appendix or a colonic diverticulum, salpingitis, prostatitis.

Pelvic Mass: ***Colonic Neoplasm.*** In a person with a long mesocolon, a carcinoma of the colon may prolapse into the rectovesical or rectouterine pouch and be palpated as a firm mass.

Pelvic Mass: ***Redundant Bowel.*** Occasionally a loop of normal colon can be felt in the pelvic pouches. The mass is quite soft and freely movable; once felt the sensation is distinctive and will not be confused with cancer.

Pelvic Mass: ***Rectal Shelf*** (Blumer's Shelf). Carcinomatous metastasis from a primary site high up in the peritoneal cavity, e.g., the stomach, may accumulate in the pelvis. This accumulation is felt through the anterior rectal wall as a hard shelf in the rectovesical or rectouterine pouch. Although usually caused by neoplasm, Bailey states that it can also occur in pelvis inflammation in the female and prostatic abscess in the male.

Pelvic Mass: ***Mistaken Normal Structures.*** If a vaginal examination has not preceded, the unwary examiner may interpret as neoplasm a mass that feels hard through the anterior rectal wall, only to find (or worse, have someone else find) that it was the normal cervix uteri, much less distinctive when palpated through the rectal wall. When the uterus is retroverted, the normal fundus has been mistaken for cancer. A vaginal tampon or pessary may mislead when felt through the rectal wall.

▼ *Key Symptoms:* ***Anorexia and Polyphagia.*** A lack of appetite for food is *anorexia; polyphagia* or *bulimia* means an excessive or insatiable appetite. Although disorders of the appetite have limited diagnostic significance, they rate as key symptoms because the degree of anorexia provides a useful index of the severity of many diseases. When the metabolic rate is normal, anorexia results in a loss of body weight; the weight increases with polyphagia. With the true bulimic, weight loss may occur if engorgement is followed by forced vomiting to empty the stomach prior to any caloric utilization.

Clinical Occurrence: POLYPHAGIA. *Thyrotoxicosis:* often the patients present the paradox of increased food intake with loss of weight; occasionally a patient actually gains weight by excessive food intake. *Diabetes Mellitus:* occasionally hunger is excessive, but glycosuria prevents weight gain. *Fat Starvation:* a diet abnormally deficient in fat and protein does not assuage the hunger. *Emotional Disturbances:* some persons exhibit abnormal hunger when experiencing anxiety. *Migraine:* bulimia or polyphagia sometimes precedes a paroxysm of migraine by a day.

ANOREXIA. *Infectious Hepatitis:* anorexia is a presenting symptom; its disappearance is often the first indication of improvement. *Gastric Carcinoma:* anorexia is frequently an early symptom. *Anorexia Nervosa:* this is a psychotic state in which the patient refuses food and extreme cachexia results. *Miscellaneous:* anorexia is common to a myriad of febrile and debilitating diseases so that its presence has little diagnostic value.

PERVERTED APPETITE (PICA). *Pregnancy:* the gravid woman often develops cravings for certain foods. *Children:* some develop cravings to eat dirt, paint, or other materials; pica often accompanies hookworm infestation. When lead paint is ingested, the person may develop lead poisoning.

▼ *Key Sign:* ***Vomiting.*** The violence and discomfort of *vomiting* or *emesis* often make it a presenting complaint, impelling one to search for the cause although the possibilities are numerous and diverse. Vomiting is usually preceded by *nausea,* an unpleasant sensation referred to the stomach and suggesting that vomiting is imminent. ***Pathophysiology.*** Vomiting is an involuntary act of integrated movements: closure of the glottis, contraction and fixation of the diaphragm is inspiration, closure of the pylorus together with relaxation of the gastric wall and cardiac orifice, violent contractions of the abdominal muscles that forcefully expel gastric contents up through the relaxed esophagus. ***Variants of Vomiting.*** *Projectile Vomiting:* a particularly forceful type, unique in lacking antecedent nausea; it is associated with increased intracranial pressure. *Retching:* the involuntary act that involves all movements of vomiting, except that the cardiac orifice remains closed, so gastric contents are not expelled. *Water Brash or Pyrosis:* the expulsion of clear, burning fluid from the stomach by reverse gastric peristalsis, without accompanying contractions of abdominal muscles. *Regurgitation of Food:* the nonviolent backward flow of ingested food from the obstructed esophagus, an esophageal diverticulum, or an overfilled stomach, without accompanying contraction of abdominal muscles.

Clinical Occurrence: DIGESTIVE: numerous irritative disorders of the alimentary canal, biliary system, and pancreas. PERITONEAL: irritating disorders. GENITOURINARY: especially acute nephritis and acute pyelonephritis. AURAL: irritation of the external acoustic meatus, Ménière's disease. OCULAR: glaucoma. CRANIAL: cerebral and intracranial lesions. GENERALIZED: radiation sickness, uremia, trauma, diabetic acidosis, pregnancy, severe pain. Acute infectious diseases. DRUGS: digitalis, morphine, apomorphine, most chemotherapeutic agents. Poisons. PSYCHIC: offensive tastes, odors, and sights.

▼ *Key Sign:* ***Hematemesis.*** When blood is vomited soon after hemorrhage, it is *bright red.* But if the blood has been retained long in the stomach, digestive processes change the hemoglobin to a brown pigment that gives rise to *coffee-ground vomitus.* The sudden appearance of blood in the vomitus is emotionally upsetting and a small amount spreads over a large area, so the patient frequently overestimates the volume of loss. Occasionally the patient has difficulty in distinguishing between hematemesis and hemoptysis, especially when a coughing paroxysm induces vomiting. Bleeding in hematemesis may occur in the upper respiratory tract or in the alimentary canal as far down as the duodenum. Sites in the alimentary tract are usually found by x-ray examination of esophagus, stomach, and duodenum, or by esophagoscopy or gastroscopy. A history of hematemesis following prolonged and violent retching or vomiting, not infrequently associated with alcoholism, is characteristic of the Mallory-Weiss syndrome. Linear tears of the mucosa of the esophagogastric junction occur, esophagoscopy and gastroscopy confirm the diagnosis, and surgery may be lifesaving.

Clinical Occurrence: SWALLOWED BLOOD. From epistaxis, hemoptysis, or bleeding from mouth or gums.

ESOPHAGUS. Ulcerations, neoplasm of the wall, esophageal varices from portal obstruction (in hepatic cirrhosis, congestive splenomegaly, or pressure on the portal vein), aortic aneurysm eroding into esophagus, rupture of esophagus from vomiting, foreign body.

STOMACH. Peptic ulcer, gastric carcinoma, hiatal hernia of stomach, gastritis (from alcohol, arsenic, lead, antimony, cortisone), hereditary hemorrhagic telangiectasis, erosion of gastric ulcer or neoplasm into pancreaticoduodenal or splenic artery.

DUODENUM. Peptic ulcer, carcinoma, diverticulum, erosion of gallstone into the duodenum.

SYSTEMIC DISEASE. *Infections:* malignant variola or scarlet fever, syphilis, malaria, yellow fever, dengue, cholera, endocarditis. *Hematologic:* thrombocytopenia from any cause, hemophilia, vitamin K deficit in obstructive jaundice or hepatic disease. *Traumatic:* severe retching, abdominal injury, operations. Scurvy. Chronic nephritis.

▼ *Key Sign:* ***Acute Diarrhea.*** Defecation of *watery* or *loose* stools is called diarrhea. The definition emphasizes the consistency of the stools, not the frequency; the passage of many formed stools is not diarrhea. *Symptoms. Tenesmus:* cramping pains with straining and ineffectual or incomplete evacuation. *Cramping pain:* this may occur along the course of the colon where localization is accurate; but cramping from the small bowel is usually referred to the umbilical region. *Passage of flatus:* an explosive expulsion of gas often accompanies the watery stool. *Signs. Borborygmus* (plural, borborygmi): a rumbling noise made by the passage of gas in the intestine can often be heard by the patient and bystanders. *Hyperperistalsis:* the peristaltic sounds are increased in frequency and intensity. *Abdominal Distention:* the accumulation of gas in the gut lumen produces slight abdominal distention and an increased area of tympany. *Diarrheal Stools.* Examination of the stools frequently detects the cause of diarrhea. Inspection reveals the proportion of water to solids, the presence of fecal fragments, blood, pus, fat globules, and mucus. Microscopic examination is employed to identify pathogenic protozoa and undigested food particles. Stool cultures are obtained to discover the bacteria causing dysentery. *Sigmoidoscopic Examination.* Reveals evidence of inflammation, sometimes distinctive (pp. 580–87). *X-ray Examination.* The barium enema discloses distinctive appearances in some chronic diarrheas.

— *Acute Nonbloody Diarrhea:* ***Viral Gastroenteritis.*** This is a common epidemic disease caused by various viral agents that are generally not identified. The onset is often heralded by sudden nausea and vomiting, and explosive diarrhea, with or without abdominal cramps. Myalgia, malaise, and anorexia, usually without fever, often accompany. The diarrhea and vomiting subside within 48 hours; lassitude may persist for several days. *Laboratory Findings.* The leukocyte count is generally normal. The stools consist of water and fecal remnants; blood, pus, and mucus are absent. *Diagnosis.* The pattern of symptoms is readily recognized during an epidemic. But the isolated interpreted cautiously in the present lack of knowledge on the subject. ***Renal Artery Stenosis:*** Selective aortography has recently directed attention to the systolic murmurs in the renal arteries; about two thirds of them have been found to indicate renal artery stenosis. The murmurs are soft, medium- or low-pitched, most commonly heard just above and slightly to the left of the umbilicus (Fig. 7-11). A few patients with renal artery stenosis also have murmurs over the renal regions posteriorly. For examination, the patient should be supine with the abdominal muscles relaxed. The bell of the stethoscope should be employed; the room should be quiet.

Peristaltic Sounds. Place the stethoscope bell just below and to the right of the umbilicus and listen for gurgles; occasional weak tinkles are not evidence of good peristaltic waves. If they are not immediately audible, sit down and listen for at least five minutes measured by your watch. Stimulation by flicking the abdominal wall with the finger or dropping a volatile liquid on the skin should be tried.

Clinical Occurrence. *Absence of Sounds:* ileus from peritonitis, mesenteric thrombosis, pneumonia, myxedema, electrolyte abnormality, uremia, spinal cord injury, or advanced intestinal obstruction. Although peristalsis may be present, the sounds are diminished or inaudible in pneumoperitoneum. *Increased Peristalsis:* brisk diarrhea, early pyloric obstruction, early intestinal obstruction.

Succussion Splash. The combination of air and fluid in the normal stomach frequently produces audible splashes when

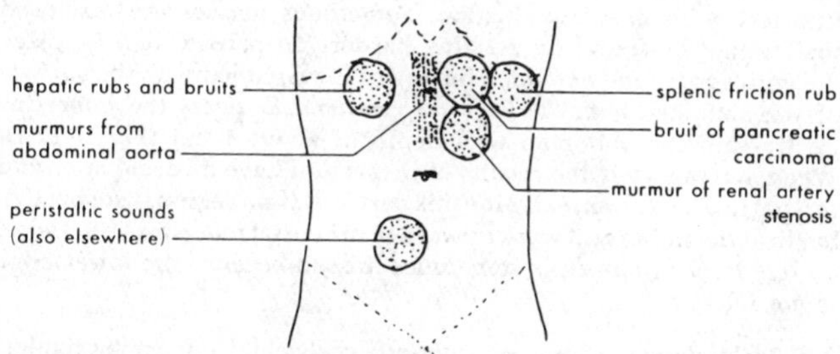

Fig. 7-11. Sounds heard in the abdomen. *Stippling indicates the optimum areas for the auscultation of the various identifiable sounds in the abdomen.*

the patient moves or the viscera are disturbed by palpation. But a very loud splash indicates much fluid and suggests obstruction in the stomach or gut or gastric dilatation.

Peritoneal Friction Rub. Like its pleural counterpart, this sound resembles that of two pieces of leather rubbing together. Frequently the rub is also palpable. Its presence indicates peritoneal inflammation.

Clinical Occurrence: splenic infarction, carcinoma of the liver (when accompanied by a bruit), liver abscess, syphilitic hepatitis, gonococcal perihepatitis, after liver biopsy.

Light Abdominal Palpation

METHOD OF LIGHT ABDOMINAL PALPATION. **Prior to palpation of the abdomen, the patient may be encouraged to locate the area of maximum tenderness. With the abdomen uncovered, the patient is encouraged first to *suck* his abdomen in as a Marine at attention. The patient should direct the examiner's attention to any area of discomfort. The examiner's hand is then positioned over the abdomen some 6 to 8 inches and the patient asked to *blow* his stomach out so as to touch the examiner's hand. Again the patient is directed to demonstrate the locality of discomfort. Finally, the patient is asked to cough. All these maneuvers are designed to cause movement of peritoneal surfaces, without direct contact of patient or examiner. Before attempting deeper palpation, palpate the entire abdomen *lightly*. This scouting expedition will discover regions of tenderness and increased resistance, to be examined later in detail. Forewarned by this gentle preliminary, the examiner can avoid producing some pain that would otherwise result in voluntary rigidity of muscle to interfere with deeper palpation. Sometimes masses are disclosed that cannot be found by pushing harder. To palpate lightly, place the entire palm and extended fingers of the right hand on the surface of the abdomen *with the fingers approximated;* press the fingertips gently into the abdomen to a depth of about 1 cm (Fig. 7-12A). When symptoms or the results of inspection have directed attention to a particular region, examine this part *last*. If no region is suspected, begin at the pubes and work upward to the costal margins. Otherwise, a huge liver or spleen is sometimes missed because the lower edge is not felt.**

Ticklishness. Some persons, especially children, exhibit tenderness or ticklishness from the lightest abdominal palpation; they flinch, grimace or tense the muscles so the examiner cannot evaluate underlying tenderness or masses. But such patients tolerate an equal amount of pressure from the bell of the stethoscope to elicit tenderness [S. M. Mellinkoff: Stethoscope Sign, *N. Engl. J. Med.*, **271:**630, 1964]. Or have the patient place *his* fingers upon *your* palpating fingers and follow the motions (Fig. 7-12C); this has the effect of substituting his own fingers to which he is not ticklish.

Direct Tenderness. This finding indicates a part of the abdomen for careful and detailed examination. Tenderness may be caused by localized inflammation of the abdominal wall, the peritoneum, or a viscus. A solid organ may be tender when its capsule is distended. This sign has had wide acceptance, but in a recent study of 120 patients admitted as emergencies with localized abdominal pain, 24 had abdominal tenderness when the underlying muscles were tensed; but only one of these proved at operation to have a detectable intra-abdominal cause [H. Thomson and D. M. A. Francis: Abdominal-Wall Tenderness: A Useful Sign in the Acute Abdomen, *Lancet,* **2:**1053–54, 1977].

Rebound Tenderness (Blumberg's Sign). Press the tips of the approximated fingers gently into the abdominal wall, then *suddenly* withdraw them from contact (Fig. 7-12D). Transient pain after withdrawal of pressure is called *rebound tenderness.* The pain may occur at the site of pressure or remote from it. If the site of inflammation has been previously suspected, it is preferable to press deeply in a spot remote from the suspected region. An alternate and less painful method is the use of *light indirect percussion.* Rebound tenderness is a reliable sign of peritoneal inflammation. Similarly, one may elicit evidence of peritoneal irritation by grasping the patient with both hands at the bony pelvis and vigorously moving the subject from side to side. As the peritoneal surfaces are made to move over each other, pain is reported when inflammation exists.

Jar Tenderness (Markle's Sign). For the ambulatory patient the finding of jar tenderness in the abdomen may prove superior to *rebound tenderness* as a localizing sign of peritoneal irritation. The sign is produced by the *heel-drop jarring test* described by Markle [George B. Markle, IV: A Simple Test for Intraperitoneal Inflammation, *Am J. Surg.*, **125:**721–22, 1973]. With the examiner demonstrating, the patient stands on the floor with straightened knees. He raises his body on his toes, then suddenly relaxes so his heels hit the floor and jar the whole body. The patient is asked for the *presence of* and *location of*

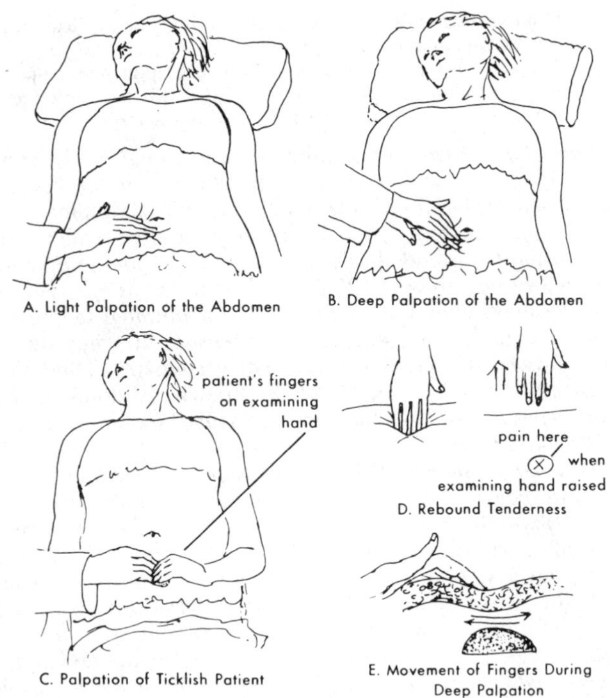

Fig. 7-12. Palpation of the abdomen. **A.** Light palpation. *The palm of the hand rests lightly but firmly upon the abdomen, and the adducted fingers are pressed into the abdominal wall to a depth of about 1 cm. The purpose is to scout the entire abdominal wall for regions of tenderness and increased resistance from muscle spasm or solid masses. Care should be taken to avoid digging into the wall with the tip of the fingers. It should be obvious that the examiner's fingernails should be short.* **B.** Deep palpation. *This can be accomplished with the same technique employed for light palpation, except that the examiner presses more deeply. Another effective method is to reinforce the palpating hand by pressing on the ends of its fingers with the fingers of the other hand. In this situation, the superimposed hand is given the task of exerting all the considerable required pressure while the underlying hand acts solely as the sensor to feel for masses and other signs.* **C.** Palpation of the ticklish abdomen. *In a ticklish person it is often impossible to feel the abdomen without stimulating voluntary*

any resulting abdominal pain. False-positive signs are uncommon. The sign may be elicited when rigid abdominal muscles prevent the palpation necessary to elicit rebound tenderness. Abdominal pain on walking is probably the equivalent of the test.

Clinical Occurrence. Peritoneal irritation of acute appendicitis, cholecystitis, abscess, infarction of abdominal organs, acute diverticulitis, regional ileitis, pelvic inflammation, and other conditions associated with peritonitis and/or intra-abdominal inflammation.

Cutaneous Hyperesthesia. An area of hyperesthetic skin can frequently be demonstrated over an inflamed appendix that has not yet perforated. Either of two methods may be employed (Fig. 7-13A). The point of a pin can be stroked lightly over the skin in parallel lines while watching the patient's face for expression of pain. In the other method, the skin is grasped lightly between thumb and index finger; the fold is gently pulled away from the underlying layers of the wall. This maneuver is painful in hyperesthetic areas. Care should be taken to avoid pinching the skin.

Subcutaneous Crepitus. In medicine, the term *crepitus* is employed not only in its original sense of a crackling sound, but also to a variety of widely differing tactile sensations (crepitant rales, bone crepitus, tendon crepitus, joint crepitus, crepitation of the gut). In the subcutaneous tissue, crepitus is the tactile sensation imparted when gas bubbles in the skin or underlying layers are stroked with the fingers. The bubbles feel like small

---

muscular contraction. This can be overcome if the patient is permitted to place his hand lightly upon your examining hand and follow its movements. This gives the illusion that patient is feeling himself and that never tickles. **D.** Rebound tenderness. *In a region of the abdomen remote from that of suspected tenderness, the hand is pushed deeply into the abdomen, then abruptly withdrawn. Pain is experienced in the affected region from rebound of the tissue. Such tenderness is usually a sign of peritoneal irritation.* **E.** Exploration during palpation. *When the examining hand is palpating the abdomen, especially deeply, the hand is moved in a special manner. The fingers remain relatively fixed to a place on the skin, and the wall of the abdomen is carried with the fingers in a slow gentle to-and-fro motion to distinguish underlying masses and surfaces. The fingers do not glide over the skin but carry the skin with them.*

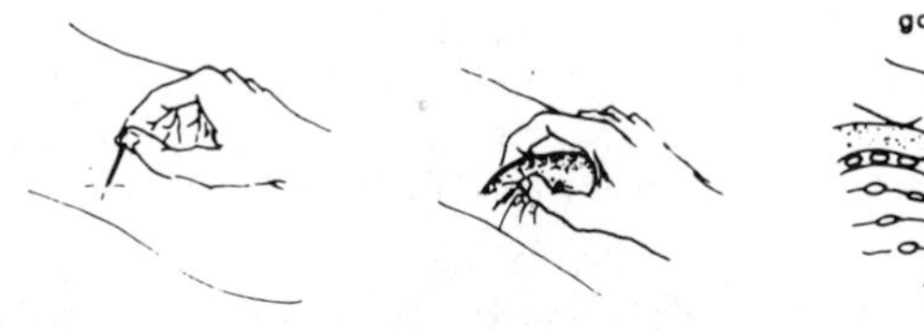

Fig. 7-13. Testing for hyperesthesia and subcutaneous crepitus. **A.** Hyperesthesia. *In one method, the skin is stroked lightly with the point of a pin, and the patient is asked to tell when the sensation of pain is elicited; or the patient's facial expression may be observed for signs of discomfort. In another method, a fold of skin is plucked lightly between thumb and index finger, pulling the fold of skin away from the underlying layers. The maneuver is painful in areas of cutaneous hyperesthesia; care should be taken not to pinch the skin painfully. In acute appendicitis, an area of hyperesthesia is frequently found in the right lower abdominal quadrant; it may involve the whole quadrant or any portion of it. The presence of hyperesthesia in acute appendicitis precedes perforation.* **B.** Subcutaneous crepitus. *When bubbles of air or other gas are present in the subcutaneous tissues or underlying muscle, pressure on the skin produces a peculiar sensation caused by the sliding of bubbles from under the fingers or, in some cases, the bursting of bubbles. Occasionally this may be accompanied by a crackling sound. The presence of subcutaneous crepitus is pathognomonic of subcutaneous emphysema or gas gangrene.*

fluctuant nodules that move freely when the tissue is pressed (Fig. 7-13B). The nodules themselves are not painful or tender. This type of *subcutaneous crepitus* is pathognomic of subcutaneous emphysema or gas gangrene. In subcutaneous emphysema the bubbles contain air that has entered the tissues through operative wounds or from trauma, such as a fractured rib piercing the lung. In gas gangrene anerobic microorganisms growing in the tissues form the gas bubbles. In the latter condition, there are signs of severe generalized infection that distinguish it from the milder emphysema.

Resistance to Palpation: Voluntary Rigidity of Muscle. Increased tone of the muscles of the abdominal wall results from an unrelaxed posture, from chilling by the external environment or the cold hands of the examiner, or from fear of painful manipulation. The rigidity interferes with effective deep palpation. It is distinguished from involuntary rigidity by being abolished with suitable maneuvers. The examination should be made in a warm room or with the patient adequately covered. The examiner's hands should be warm; it may be necessary to wash them in hot water. The patient must rest supine and be comfortable, the head being supported by one or more pillows. Placing a pillow under the knees, causing slight flexion of the thighs, may relax the patient. Have the patient breathe through the wide-open mouth. Conversation with the patient sometimes relaxes him. Reassurance against pain can be imparted with soothing words and a deliberate careful manner of the examiner. When the usual measures fail, the examiner may press hard on the lower sternum with his left hand, while palpating the abdomen with his right. When the patient attempts inspiration against this pressure, he must relax his abdominal muscles.

Resistance to Palpation: **Involuntary Rigidity of Muscle.** Reflex muscle spasm is caused by peritoneal irritation, either *infectious* or *neoplastic.* Persistence of rigidity despite relaxing maneuvers proves it involuntary. Frequently rigidity of this type is unilateral, while voluntary rigidity is symmetric. Pain is elicited when the patient attempts to raise the trunk from the horizontal without using his arms. Involuntarily rigid muscles are not necessarily tender, so the resistance must be distinguished from masses in the abdominal wall. Placing the examining hands symmetrically on the patient's abdomen, in each of the quadrants in turn, and gently and alternately evaluating muscle tenseness on each side reveals location of involuntary guarding when asymmetry is discovered.

Resistance to Palpation: **Abdominal Masses.** If sufficiently large or close to the abdominal wall, masses cause increased resistance to light palpation. The solidity of a mass must be distinguished from muscle spasm. One notes the distribution of the area of resistance, whether it corresponds to an abdominal muscle or resembles the shape of a viscus. If the presence of a mass is established, its location must be determined whether *in the wall* or *in the cavity.* Failure to raise the question of an *intramural* location sometimes results in the erroneous conclusion that all masses are within the cavity. A classic example of a frequently misdiagnosed mass is *hematoma of the abdominal rectus muscle,* mistaken for an intra-abdominal mass. Intramural masses are

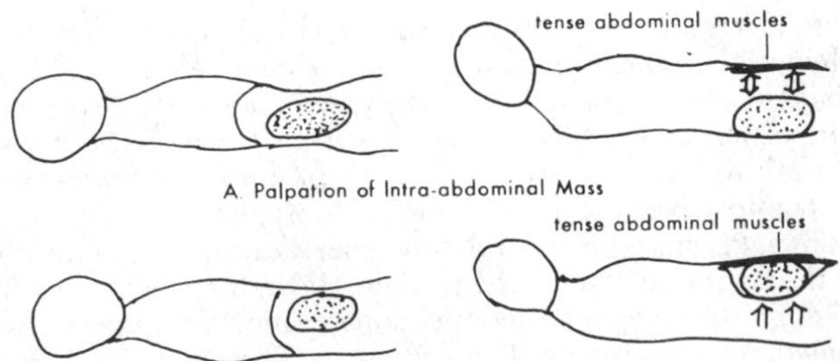

B. Palpation of Mass in Abdominal Wall

Fig. 7-14. Distinction between intramural and intra-abdominal masses. *This problem has been the subject of classic errors in clinical medicine. A mass felt in the abdomen erroneously may be interpreted as intra-abdominal when in fact it is in the abdominal wall. This sounds improbable, but many good clinicians have been tripped up by it. Palpating the mass while the patient raises his head from the pillow will distinguish it. When the abdominal muscles tense, the intra-abdominal mass moves away from the palpating hand, while the intramural mass remains accessible.*

palpable when the abdominal muscles are tensed; masses in the cavity are shielded from palpation in this situation (Fig. 7-14). Light palpation can only determine the presence of a mass and its location; further information must be sought by deep palpation and other procedures.

Deep Abdominal Palpation

METHOD OF DEEP ABDOMINAL PALPATION. **After using light palpation, delve deeper. Pursue the findings from inspection and light palpation; search for deep tenderness and masses not previously suspected.**

Posture of the Patient: **Although most of the abdominal examination is performed with the patient *supine*, do not develop such a fixed routine that you are psychologically unwilling or unable to employ other postures in the search for information. When appropriate, turn the patient from side to side in the *lateral* positions. Sometimes the *knee-elbow* posture yields evidence of masses not otherwise accessible. The *erect* position may be desirable; it is mandatory in the proper examination for some hernias.**

Methods of Palpation: Deep in the abdomen *single-handed palpation* is employed with the palmar surface of the right hand in contact with the wall; the approximated fingers are pressed more deeply than for light palpation (Fig. 7-12B). The hand should be placed so most tactile sensations are received on the pads of the index and long fingers. In addition to a downward motion, the finger pads should cause the abdominal wall to glide over the underlying structures, backward and forward in a range of 4 or 5 cm (Fig. 7-12E). When the mural resistance is strong, or the target deep, *reinforced palpation* is employed. The examining right hand maneuvered as previously described, but the fingers of the left hand press upon the distal phalangeal joints of the right; thus the left hand produces the pressure while the right hand receives the tactile sensations with its muscles relatively passive. When a mass is small, its thickness is determined by grasping it between the thumb and index finger, when large, *bimanual palpation* is employed by placing a hand on each side of the mass. As the technique varies with the situation, it will be described later. When the presence of free fluid in the abdominal cavity prevents access to masses, *ballottement* is helpful. The fingers of the right hand are thrust suddenly and deeply into the abdomen in the region of the suspected mass, whereat the mass may bound upward and touch the tips of the examining fingers; this occurs when the mass is freely movable.

Attributes of Masses: When a mass is discovered, the examiner seeks the organ or tissue whence it arises and the pathologic condition of the affected tissue. Many conclusions may be derived from the attributes of a mass. During the examination, the complete list of qualities must be ascertained and adequately described; forgetting to examine for one may lead to an error in diagnosis. *Location:* Knowing the site of the mass in the abdomen limits the number of possible organs to be considered; e.g., a mass in the left upper quadrant may be only spleen, left kidney, or colon. *Size:* This may give an insight about the pathologic process involved or its extent; e.g., the largest livers result from carcinoma and myelocytic leukemia. *Shape:* Some organs may be identified by their shape, e.g., kidney, spleen, and liver. *Consistency:* The pathologic process may be inferred from the resistance of the mass to pressure; e.g., carcinoma of the liver may be stony hard, the splenic tumor of infection is soft. *Surface:* The smooth surface of a viscus implies diffuse involvement; a nodular liver, for example, suggests neoplastic metastasis, granulomas, or the irregular fibrosis of portal cirrhosis. *Tenderness:* This may be caused by an acute inflammatory process or distention of the capsule of a viscus; e.g., an acutely distended liver is tender, while the liver is not tender in many neoplastic processes or cirrhosis. *Mobility:* A mass that moves with the diaphragm suggests an organ on a pedicle,

mesentery, or ligament; e.g., this attribute is employed to distinguish between peritoneal and retroperitoneal masses. *Pulsatility:* This attribute is difficult to remember; but its importance should be emphasized. Aneurysms have been incised because the examiner forgot to ask himself whether the mass was pulsating.

CAUTION; NO-TOUCH ISOLATION. **At the first suspicion of cancer in the abdomen, Turnbull advises avoidance of any further palpation of the belly until the lymphovascular pedicle of the tumor has been ligated. He believes this precaution may prevent metastases. On his service, as soon as the abdominal mass is found, a strip of adhesive tape is placed on the patient's abdomen bearing the words "Do Not Palpate" [R. B. Turnbull, Jr., *quoted in* Reducing the Toll of Colon and Rectal Cancer, *Med. World News,* pp. 42–49, June 1, 1979].**

Pulseless Femoral Artery (Leriche's Syndrome). Cultivate the habit of palpating the femoral arteries as the *first procedure* in the examination of the abdomen. Diminution or absence of the femoral pulse may be the first sign encountered in a routine examination that leads to the diagnosis of coarctation of the aorta, terminal thrombosis of the aorta (Leriche's syndrome), thrombosis of the common iliac artery, or dissecting aortic aneurysm. Missing this single sign in a physical examination has resulted in completely overlooking these important conditions. When the femoral pulse is diminished or absent, palpate the iliac pulses up to and including the aortic bifurcation. The aorta divides about 2 cm below and slightly to the left of the umbilicus. Lines drawn from the bifurcation to the midpoints of the lines between anterior superior iliac spines and symphysis pubis delineate the course of the iliac arteries; the upper third represents the common iliac, the lower two thirds marks the external iliacs. These vessels may not be palpable in normal persons, but discrepancies in pulsations between the two sides are particularly significant. The significance of an absent or diminished femoral pulse must also be judged by the presence or absence of the pulses distal to the femorals.

PALPATION OF THE LEFT UPPER QUADRANT OF THE ABDOMEN. **Normally, no masses are palpable in this region. To feel a moderately enlarged spleen or left kidney, stand at the right side of the supine patient and employ *bimanual palpation,* with the right hand pushing into the abdomen and the left hand lifting from the back (Fig. 7-15). To accomplish this lay the palm of the *right hand* on the abdomi-**

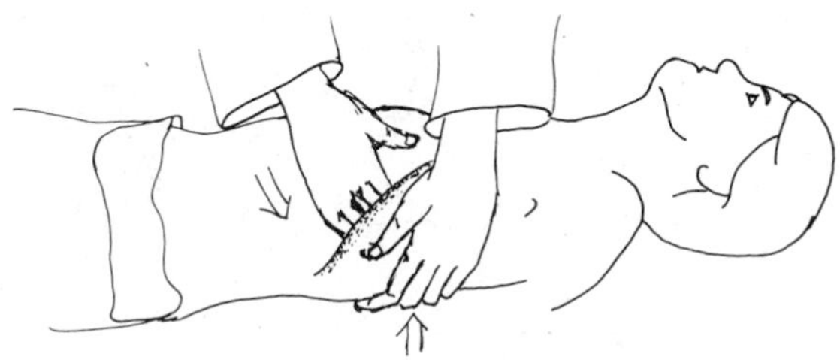

Fig. 7-15. Bimanual palpation of the left upper quadrant. *The right hand is inserted behind the left costal margin in the midaxillary line, and the left hand is placed under the lower thorax so the fingers curl posteriorly under the lower ribs. The patient is asked to take a deep breath; as the height of inspiration is approached, the right hand is thrust more deeply behind the costal margin and upward, while the left hand lifts the posterior thorax in the direction of the arrow. This is repeated several times, the position of the right hand being varied slightly for each trial.*

nal wall in the left upper quadrant and place the tips of the approximated index and middle fingers just inferior to the rib margin in the left anterior axillary line. Place the palm of the *left hand* on the left midaxillary region of the thorax, with the fingers curling posteriorly to support the thoracic wall at the 11th and 12th ribs. Ask the patient to inspire deeply and slowly through the mouth. During inspiration, bring the two hands closer together by *lifting* the posterior wall with the left hand, while gently but firmly *pushing* the approximated fingers of the right hand posteriorly and upward behind the costal margin. If the mutual approach of the two hands coincides properly with inspiration, the descending margin of the enlarged viscus will touch the tips of the right index and middle fingers. If the edge cannot be felt satisfactorily, repeat the procedure with the patient lying partially on his *right side*. The spleen is found more superficial than the left kidney; for the latter, feel more deeply and slightly closer to the midline. Larger masses may be felt without bimanual palpation. The two-handed method is also employed with a type of *ballottement* (Fig. 7-16). Place the hands in the position previously described; *lift* the posterior chest wall with the left hand, but let the right hand passively receive the impulse from the mass that is pushed forward. This maneuver indicates the posterior extent of the mass; kidney usually lies farther back than spleen. Other masses in the left upper quadrant must be examined as circumstances require. With *Middleton's method* for palpating the moderately enlarged spleen, have the patient place his left fist beneath the left

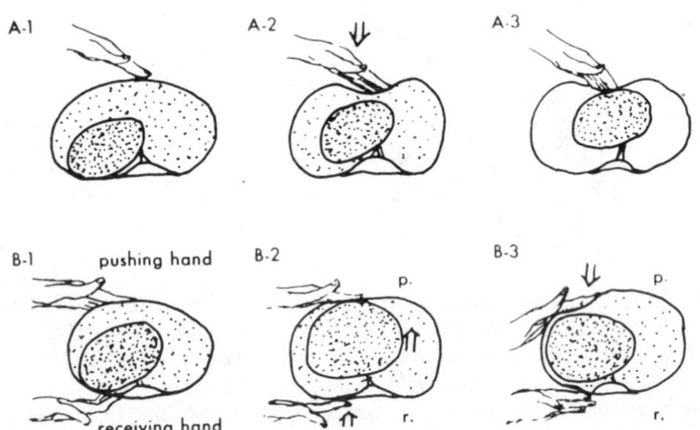

Fig. 7-16. Ballottement of masses in the abdomen. *The term* ballottement *is applied to two somewhat different maneuvers.* **A.** *In using one hand, the approximated fingers are abruptly plunged into the abdomen and held there; a freely movable mass will rebound upward and be felt with the fingers. This is most commonly employed to feel a large liver obscured by free fluid in the abdominal cavity.* **B.** *Bimanual ballottement is used to determine the size of a large mass in the abdomen. One hand* (p.) *pushes the anterior abdominal wall, while the receiving hand* (r.) *palpates the flank to get an estimate of the thickness of the mass.*

thorax and lie on it (Fig. 7-17). Stand on the patient's *left* side, facing his feet, and curl both your hands over the left costal margin so your fingertips are pointing upward behind the ribs. Feel the splenic edge during the patient's deep inspiration.

LUQ Mass: ***Splenomegaly.*** The normal adult spleen lies immediately under the vault of the left diaphragm with its convex surface separated from the thoracic cage by the costophrenic sinus of the pleura that contains lung only during deep inspiration. When normal in size and position, the spleen is never accessible to abdominal palpation (Fig. 7-18). Its long axis lies immediately behind and parallel to the oblique 10th rib in the midaxillary line; its length is about 12 cm (one handbreadth). Its 7-cm width (four fingerbreadths) spreads from the 9th to the 11th ribs. Because of its oblique direction the width determines the vertical extent of the *area of splenic dullness* in the midaxilla. Percussion of this area is a desirable routine;

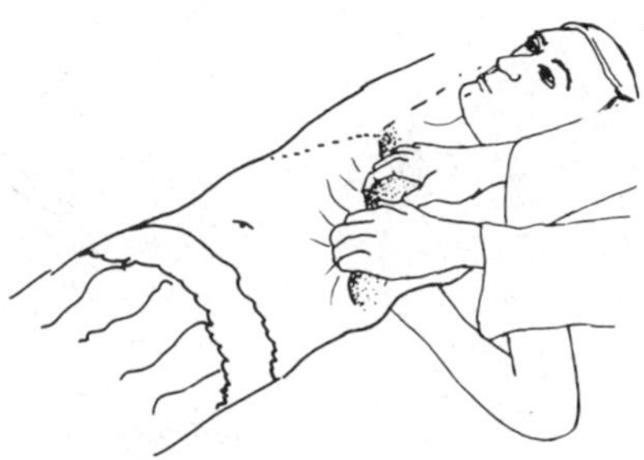

Fig. 7-17. Palpation of the spleen (Middleton's method). *The examiner stands at the patient's left side, facing his feet. The patient's left hand is placed under the left 11th rib so his thorax is elevated somewhat from the table. The examiner curls both hands around the left costal margin so the fingers are up under the ribs. When the patient inspires deeply, the splenic margin is felt on the fingertips.*

when the extent is normal, splenomegaly is almost certainly excluded. Extension of the area of splenic dullness may be caused by fluid in the stomach or feces in the colon, but finding it should prompt the examiner to search more carefully for a large spleen.

Normally, the spleen weighs about 150 gm; some disorders increase its weight to 6000 gm or more. With rare exceptions, the enlarged spleen retains its characteristic shape and markings. Since extension superiorly is blocked by the diaphragm, enlargement displaces the lower pole downward from behind the thoracic cage and along its oblique axis toward the *right* iliac fossa. Although seldom does it cross the midline, the lower pole may reach the pelvis on the left. Acute infections produce moderately enlarged soft spleens with blunted edges; chronic disorders cause firm or hard spleens and sharp edges. The enlarged spleen is not tender except when the peritoneum is inflamed from infection or infarction. During enlargement the characteristic *splenic notch* is retained on the medial edge near the lower pole.

The examiner must examine for splenomegaly with certain circumspection. While uncommon, the spleen has been occasionally ruptured during the overvigorous attempt to identify enlargement. This has occurred most often in the patient with infectious mononucleosis.

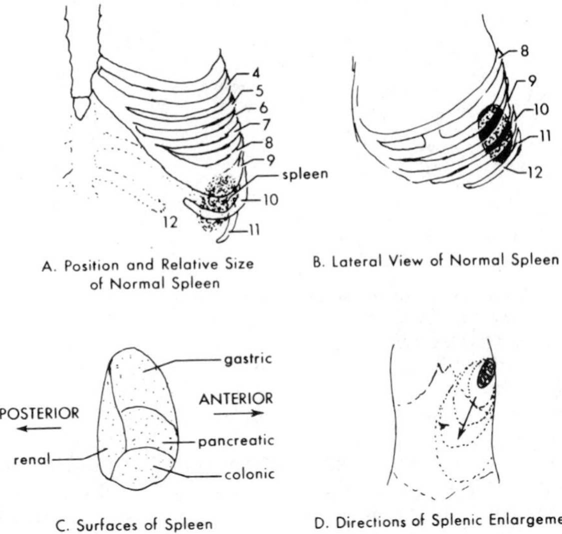

Fig. 7-18. Anatomic relations of the normal and enlarged spleen. **A.** *Position of the normal spleen viewed from the anterior surface of the thorax and abdomen. The area of splenic dullness is in the left posterior axilla and usually does not exceed a vertical distance of more than 8 or 9 cm.* **B.** *Normal spleen from the left lateral view; the spleen lies obliquely with its long axis along the 10th rib, its long borders coinciding with the 9th and 11th ribs.* **C.** *The anterior surface of the spleen is divided into regions touching other viscera.* **D.** *The directions in which the spleen enlarges are indicated by the dotted lines; the long axis of enlargement points downward and obliquely toward the symphysis pubis.*

A common problem is to distinguish between an enlarged spleen and left kidney. This is often difficult; frequently a renal tumor is mistaken for spleen; both organs have the same general shape. The enlarged kidney pushes forward and downward to assume a position approximately similar to an enlarged spleen. The renal tumor is usually thicker than spleen, as demonstrated by bimanual palpation; it also extends farther posteriorly. The spleen may have a sharp edge, a complete distinction; the kidney never has. A fissure on the medial edge would seem to identify the mass as spleen, but lobulation of a renal tumor can closely simulate a splenic notch. Intravenous pyelography, CT scanning, or ultrasonography may be required to make the distinction.

Clinical Occurrence. An etiologic classification for splenomegaly includes infections (bacterial, viral, and protozoal), circulatory disturbances, hemolytic disorders, polycythemia vera, lymphomas, some metabolic disorders, and neoplasm. Adams' classification according to the degree of enlargement is most useful in diagnosis and is presented here in somewhat abridged form. SLIGHT ENLARGEMENT: chronic passive congestion in long-standing cardiac failure, acute malaria, typhoid fever, subacute bacterial endocarditis, other acute and subacute infections, disseminated lupus erythematosus, rheumatoid arthritis, thrombocytopenic purpura, thalassemia minor. MODERATE ENLARGEMENT: rickets, hepatitis, hepatic cirrhosis, lymphoma (including the leukemias), infectious mononucleosis, pernicious anemia, hemolytic anemias, abscesses and infarcts, amyloidosis, schistosomiasis. GREAT ENLARGEMENT: chronic myelocytic leukemia, myelofibrosis, Gaucher's disease, Niemann-Pick's disease, thalassemia major, chronic malaria, congenital syphilis, leishmaniasis, portal vein obstruction.

LUQ Mass: ***Enlarged Left Kidney.*** Each kidney normally weighs about 150 gm, about the weight of the spleen. The long axis is about 11 cm, the width is about 5 cm, and the thickness about 2.5 cm; so the kidney resembles the spleen in size and shape. In the supine position, the bottom of the abdominal cavity is formed by the vertebral column and the two psoas muscles, originating on the 12th thoracic vertebra, diverging as they course downward to form an isosceles triangle (Fig. 7-19). The left kidney lies with its edge and hilum just overlapping the border of the Psoas. The midposterior surface is crossed by the 12th rib. The upper two thirds of the anterior surface of the kidney is overlaid in turn by the spleen, which is mostly lateral and anterior. Although the lower renal pole is considerably inferior to the spleen, the normal-sized left kidney cannot be felt through the abdominal wall. When the kidney enlarges, it is contained posteriorly by the Psoas and the 12th rib; the overriding spleen prevents extension superiorly; it can only push anteriorly and downward. The palpable renal tumor presents a mass, shaped like kidney and spleen, that ballottement shows extends posteriorly farther than the

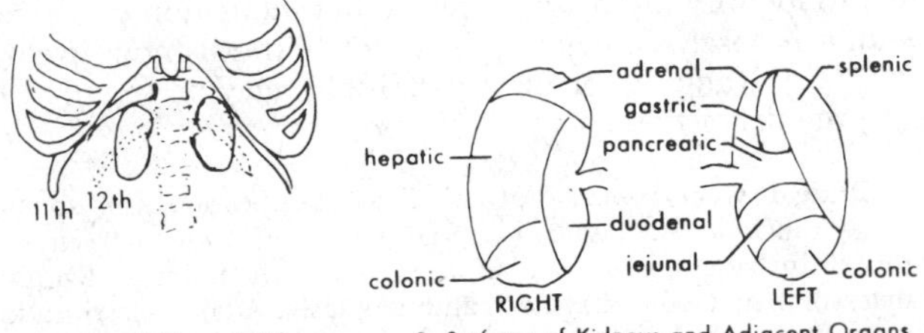

Fig. 7-19. Anatomic relations of the normal kidneys. **A.** *The position of the normal kidneys is indicated, as viewed from the anterior surface of the abdomen. Note the right kidney lying in front of the 12th rib, while the slightly higher left kidney is in front of the 11th and 12th ribs.* **B.** *The anterior surfaces of both kidneys show the regions touched by overlying viscera.*

spleen is usually located. The kidney always lacks the sharp edge the spleen may present because of its retroperitoneal position. A lobulation of the kidney may be mistaken for the splenic notch. More often than the spleen, the surface of the enlarged kidney may be irregular from neoplasm or cysts. A very large mobile renal tumor may assume a position in the midline as well as a huge hydronephrotic kidney that presented precisely in the same location.

Clinical Occurrence. Hydronephrosis, neoplasm, cysts.

Costovertebral Tenderness. This is elicited by palpation with *one finger.* The finger is pressed in a radial direction into the soft tissues enclosed by the *costovertebral angle* between the spine and the 12th rib (Fig. 7-19). Alternatively, the heel of the palm may be used to strike the same point to cause jarring of the surrounding tissues in the area of the kidney. Tenderness in this region indicates inflammation of the kidney or the para-nephric region, as in pyelonephritis.

LUQ Mass: ***Ptotic Left Kidney.*** A displaced normal-sized kidney offers little difficulty in recognition. When it slides from its normal position, it can be readily felt and diagnosed by its shape and size; it may occur in the pelvis.

PALPATION OF THE RIGHT UPPER QUADRANT OF THE ABDOMEN. **The liver, gallbladder, and right kidney are the chief objects of attention**

case is diagnosed in retrospect, after considering other causes of acute diarrhea.

— *Acute Nonbloody Diarrhea:* **Food Intolerance.** When allergic persons eat antigenic foods they may react with nausea and vomiting and diarrhea. The history usually reveals the diagnosis. Causative antigens include seafoods, especially shrimp, rice, and cereal mixes.

Acute Illness After Dining: **Chinese Restaurant Syndrome.** This has been attributed to sensitization to monosodium glutamate, a food additive plentiful in Oriental restaurants. It is characterized by sudden onset 10 to 20 *minutes* after eating of *severe headache, burning sensations,* and *feelings of pressure* about the face, occasionally *chest pain.* Often *prostration, gastric distress,* and *pain* in the axillae, neck, and shoulders develop.

— *Acute Nonbloody Diarrhea:* **Spurious Diarrhea of Fecal Impaction.** Patients may complain of diarrhea; but close questioning discloses the stool volume to be small and the passage attended by much tenesmus and straining. Digital examination encounters masses of impacted feces in the rectum that cannot be evacuated.

— *Acute Nonbloody Diarrhea:* **Cholera.** Infection with *Vibrio cholerae* is encountered in the endemic regions of the world. The incubation period is 1 to 3 days. There are sudden abdominal cramping, vomiting, voluminous watery stools containing flecks of mucus ("rice-water stools"). The toxin, liberated by the organism, stimulates active anion secretion by the mucosal cells. Extreme dehydration and prostration rapidly progress with resulting electrolyte imbalances. The skin is cold, cyanotic, and lacking turgor. Hypotension and tachycardia ensue; death is frequent without prompt rehydration.

— *Acute Bloody Diarrhea:* **Hemorrhage from Posterior Penetrating Duodenal Ulcer with Erosion of Gastroduodenal Artery.** Penetrating duodenal ulcers, if on the posterior wall of the duodenum, erode and cause the gastroduodenal artery to bleed. Hemorrhage may be massive and life threatening. Besides other evidence of hypovolemia due to blood loss, there is a characteristic finding upon auscultation of the abdomen. Due to the cathartic action of the blood in the gastrointestinal tract and the rapid peristalsis caused by this, the sound heard is akin to bubbles of gas percolating through heavy oil.

— *Acute Bloody Diarrhea:* **Staphylococcal Food Poisoning.** From

1 to 6 hours after a meal, the patient is seized with severe cramping abdominal pains, nausea and vomiting, bloody diarrhea, and prostration. The symptoms usually last only a few hours. Frequently large groups of diners are affected. The food has been prepared in advance and stored without proper refrigeration. The staphylococci usually have been introduced from lesions on the skin of food handlers; during storage the organisms produce an enterotoxin.

— *Acute Bloody Diarrhea:* **Poisoning with Heavy Metals or Drugs.** Soon after ingestion of the toxic agent, nausea and vomiting are accompanied by cramping abdominal pains and bloody diarrhea. The heavy metals (such as arsenic, cadmium, copper, or mercury) may be ingested accidentally, or with suicidal or homocidal intent. Arsenic is the favorite of poisoners; let no physician forget that he may be confronted with an attempted murder. The chronic manifestations of heavy metal intoxications are discussed in the larger textbooks.

— *Acute Bloody Diarrhea:* **The Dysenteries.** Dysentery is a diarrhea in which the stools contain *pus* and *blood,* indicating intestinal inflammation. Bacterial causes are *Salmonella paratyphi A* and *B,* and *enteriditis; Shigella dysenteriae, flexneri,* and *sonneri.* Protozoal causes are *Entamoeba histolytica, Giardia lamblia, Trichomonas hominis,* and *Balantidium coli.* The character of the stools and the accompaniment of fever usually distinguish this group from simple gastroenteritis. Although unknown at the time, the duration of dysentery is longer. The protozoa are found by microscopic examination of the stools; bacteria are cultured from the feces. Sigmoidoscopic examination may reveal evidence of ulceration (p. 582).

— *Acute Bloody Diarrhea:* **Ulcerative Colitis.** Although a chronic disease, its onset may be sudden, resembling an acute dysentery. The absence of organisms in the stools and the subsequent course suggest the diagnosis (see p. 583).

— *Chronic Intermittent Diarrhea:* **Irritable Colon.** The patient with this common disorder is usually a nervous, anxious person with a long history of bowel symptoms but without loss of weight. Longer periods of constipation are interspersed by shorter bouts of diarrhea. Often the patient regards the constipation as normal and complains of the diarrhea. Passage of nonbloody mucous is suggestive. During periods of constipation the stools are *scybalous,* described as being like marbles.

— *Chronic Intermittent Diarrhea:* **Hypermotility in Generalized Diseases.** *Thyrotoxicosis:* often the stools are increased in number, but true diarrhea is a sign of a dangerous stage in the disease. *Adrenal cortical insufficiency:* untreated patients may have nausea, vomiting, and diarrhea. *Pernicious anemia:* occasionally an untreated patient has diarrhea that is relieved by drinking dilute hydrochloric acid. *Hypoparathyroidism:* diarrhea is rare; it responds to treatment with vitamin D. *Carcinoid tumor:* the intermittent gastrointestinal symptoms include diarrhea.

— *Chronic Intermittent Diarrhea:* **Chronic Pancreatitis.** Characterized by episodes of abdominal pain and loose, fatty stools, resembling attacks of acute pancreatitis (p. 543), this condition is usually encountered in a patient who is an alcoholic or has cholelithiasis. The stools are soft, frothy, and malodorous; they frequently float on water. *Laboratory Findings.* The serum amylase is usually elevated 8 hours after onset of an episode if there is sufficient functioning exocrine gland to produce enzymes. Fecal fat is elevated. *X-ray Findings.* When present, pancreatic calcification is diagnostic.

— *Chronic Intermittent Diarrhea:* **Fibrocystic Disease.** Although an autosomal recessive disease usually associated with childhood, patients with mild forms are now attaining adult life when the cause of the pancreatic insufficiency is more difficult to diagnose. In adults, the high salt content of sweat is not distinctive, so diagnosis rests upon the occurrence of fibrocystic disease in the family and pancreatic function determinations.

— *Chronic Constant Diarrhea:* **Nontropical Sprue** (Adult Celiac Disease). In this disorder the ingestion of gluten interferes with the absorption of food to cause a chronic malabsorption syndrome with diarrhea and inanition. The stools are soft, frothy, and malodorous from unabsorbed fat. *Laboratory Findings.* Neutral fat in the stools may be seen through the microscope; free fatty acids of the stools are increased. The fasting carotene level of the serum may be low. A macrocytic anemia is common. Prompt discontinuation of toxic glutens, found in wheat, barley, rye, buckwheat, and oats, ought to lead to swift clinical improvement. *X-ray Findings.* The barium meal reveals loss of the fine detail of the intestinal mucosa; instead, the barium is segmented and flocculated, forming puddling in the intestinal loops. Biopsy of the small intestine may be necessary for diagnosis.

— *Chronic Constant Diarrhea:* ***Ulcerative Colitis.*** Progressive inflammation of the colon occurs, with remissions and exacerbations. The cause is unknown. The clinical picture varies from the acute episode resembling dysentery, with fever, abdominal pain, tenesmus, and bloody diarrhea, to mild abdominal pain with formed stools coated with a little blood, and no fever. When symptoms are severe, anorexia produces extreme weight loss. Defecation is often attended by severe abdominal cramps. An association of this disease with the development of carcinoma is well recognized. The longer the duration of symptoms, and the greater the length of colon involved, but not the severity of symptoms, are important in assessing risk of tumor occurrence. *Sigmoidoscopy.* The diagnosis is usually made by inspection of the mucosa. In some patients, inflammation involves only the lower 10–12 cm of rectum, where the mucosa is red, edematous, and extremely friable, so the slightest touch causes bleeding. Often the mucosa of the entire rectosigmoid is covered by a layer of purulent exudate hiding multiple ulcers. *X-ray Findings.* The barium enema may show that the haustral markings are obliterated. In long-standing disease, the lumen is contracted and irregular, the mucosa exhibits multiple irregularities secondary to pseudopolyp formation, ulcerations, and hairline projections from the mucosa. The terminal ileum may be inflamed and dilated, in contrast to the constriction found in regional enteritis. *Distinction:* The disease must be distinguished from Crohn's colitis as well as amebiasis and bacillary infections.

— *Chronic Intermittent Diarrhea:* ***Regional Enteritis*** (Crohn's Disease, Terminal Ileitis). Although frequently limited to the terminal ileum, this disease is a chronic inflammatory disorder that may progress upward throughout the small intestine. Attacks of colicky pain occur in the right lower abdominal quadrant, commonly accompanied by diarrhea. Weight loss may be severe. An acute attack may resemble appendicitis so closely that operation is necessary. Perforations, strictures, and fistulas are common complications. *Sigmoidoscopy.* Although the chief focus of the disease is in the small intestine, frequent complications can be seen: perianal suppuration, anal stricture, stricture at the rectosigmoid junction, nodular submucosal masses. *X-ray Findings.* Barium in the small bowel may show strictures, fistulas, loss of mucosal detail, tubular thickening of the submucosa. A secure diagnosis can be made only at operation and depends upon gross and microscopic examination of the involved bowel.

— *Chronic Intermittent Diarrhea:* ***Tuberculous Enteritis.*** Usually secondary to pulmonary tuberculosis, the ileocecal region may become inflamed. Although asymptomatic in some, many patients have alternating diarrhea and constipation, with occasional cramps in the lower abdomen. The ascending and transverse colon are often involved, occasionally the entire large bowel is affected. Occult blood may be lost in the fecal stream, and a moderate anemia may present as a result. Colonic symptoms are constant diarrhea, and there are severe colicky pains and extreme weight loss. Symptoms such as these, occurring in the patient with known pulmonary tuberculosis or symptoms of such a pulmonary infection, are suggestive. *X-ray Findings.* Barium in the distal small bowel or cecum shows spastic filling defects and hypermotility. *Therapeutic Test.* A positive skin test for tuberculosis and response to appropriate antituberculous therapy may help to establish the diagnosis.

— *Chronic Diarrhea:* ***Colonic Amyloidosis.*** *Secondary* amyloidosis may occur with regional enteritis or ulcerative colitis, when no specific symptoms can be attributed to the amyloid disease. *Primary* amyloidosis of the colon may produce a chronic diarrhea. Biopsy of colonic mucosa is the best diagnostic procedure.

— *Chronic Diarrhea:* ***Whipple's Disease*** (Intestinal Lipodystrophy). This is a progressive wasting disease that can occur at any age, but most commonly in the fourth and fifth decades. Its chief clinical characteristics are polyarthritis, pigmentation of the skin, polyserositis, and the malabsorption syndrome. Lymphadenopathy and fever are frequent. *Laboratory Findings.* Anemia, accelerated erythrocyte sedimentation rate, and occasionally eosinophilia. *X-ray Findings.* The appearance of the small bowel resembles that in sprue, so it is nonspecific. *Biopsy.* Histologic examination is diagnostic; lymph nodes may be excised from the periphery, or epithelium may be removed from the jejunum by the flexible gastroscope.

— *Chronic Diarrhea:* ***Internal Alimentary Fistula.*** A fistula between the proximal and distal parts of the alimentary tract produces *diarrhea* with *undigested food* in the feces. The diarrhea may be *intermittent* and results from the introduction and proliferation of bacteria in the proximal gut. The chronic wasting results in a malabsorption syndrome with weight loss, hypoproteinemia, depletion of body water and electrolytes. *Gastrojejunocolic Fistula.* Usually a complication of a retrocolic gastroenterostomy, a stomal ulcer penetrates the nearby transverse colon. *Fecal belching* and *vomiting* accompany the *diarrhea.* *Cholecystoduodenocolic Fistula.* Rarely, a gallstone erodes through the gallbladder wall into the duodenum, and then through the colonic wall; in this case, the diarrhea is not accompanied by fecal vomiting. These fistulas should be suspected when chronic diarrhea develops after gastric operations, or symptoms of cholelithiasis. Both types of fistula are better demonstrated by barium enema than by giving radiopaque medium by mouth.

▼ *Key Sign:* ***Chronic Diarrhea and Malnutrition*** (Malabsorption Syndrome). The diarrhea is caused by the presence in the stools of undigested fat from food or from unhydrolyzed lactose of ingested milk. The differential diagnosis follows, as summarized from W. A. Olsen: A Practical Approach to Diagnosis of Disorders of Intestinal Absorption, *N. Engl. J. Med.,* **285:**1358–61, 1971.

— *Chronic Diarrhea:* ***Steatorrhea.*** With the presence of undigested fat, as triglycerides in the stools, steatorrhea seems probable when (1) inspection and smell indicate the stools to be frothy, greasy, and foul-smelling, (2) inspection of the stools microscopically shows fat globules stained with Sudan III, (3) the serum carotene is less than 60 mcg per 100 mL (measured for a period of 72 hours during which dietary intake of fat is about 100 gm per day). Malabsorption is proved when the fat content of the stools exceeds 7 gm daily.

— *Chronic Diarrhea:* ***Steatorrhea and/or Vitamin B12 Deficiency (Blind Loop Syndrome).*** When small bowel conditions exist leading to stasis and bacterial overgrowth, the blind or stagnant loop syndrome may develop. The proliferation of bacteria can occur whenever local stasis or recirculation of small bowel content takes place. Such conditions include surgically created blind pouches, enteroenterostomies, long afferent loops, and adhesions. Additionally, strictures, fistulous communications, and small bowel diverticulae must be considered. The condition must be sought when the patient presents with diarrhea, steatorrhea, weight loss, or macrocytic anemia. Since the bacterial overgrowth is responsible for the malabsorption, a short course of antibiotics, like Lincomycin or tetracycline, should lead to demonstrable improvement.

To distinguish between maldigestion and malabsorption as the cause of the steatorrhea, two tests are needed. In the *xylose test* (for absorptive function of the jejunal mucosa) 25 gm of *d*-xylose is taken by mouth with several tumblerfuls of water and the xylose is measured in a 5-hour urine specimen. The normal exceeds 4 gm (the values are falsely low with poor renal function and in patients with ascites; elderly persons also have low values). The *Schilling test* may be employed as an indicator of absorptive function of the ileal mucosa when given with vitamin B_{12} and intrinsic factor, provided the test is made after pretreatment with antibiotics for several days to obviate the interference of bacterial overgrowth in the stools.

— *Chronic Diarrhea and Malnutrition:* ***Steatorrhea from Maldigestion.*** This partial diagnosis is attained when the xylose test and the Schilling test are normal.

Clinical Occurrence. Gastric surgery (history, x-ray examination); pancreatic insufficiency (history, x-ray for pancreatic calcification, glucose tolerance test, secretin stimulation, measurement of carbonate in duodenal fluid); disease of liver and biliary tract; bacterial overgrowth (Schilling test before and several days after antibiotics, x-ray examination of the gastrointestinal tract); Zollinger-Ellison syndrome (gastric secretory test; serum gastrin); drugs (history); ileal disease, as Crohn's disease, diverticula, intra-alimentary fistulas (x-rays of small bowel).

— *Chronic Diarrhea and Malnutrition:* ***Steatorrhea from Malabsorption.*** When the results of the xylose and Schilling tests show disordered absorption, the following should be considered:

Clinical Occurrence. Celiac disease, tropical sprue, Whipple's disease, lymphangiectasis, amyloid disease (all require biopsy of small bowel mucosa), giardial infestations (examination of duodenal contents, stools for flagella).

Intermittent Diarrhea: ***Lactase Deficiency.*** The disaccharide lactose in milk cannot be digested by about 5% of whites and 25% of blacks in America because they lack the enzyme *lactase.* When a person with this deficit ingests milk he promptly gets a *watery diarrhea* and often *abdominal cramps.* As milk is the only common foodstuff containing large quantities of lactose, avoidance leads to prompt resolution and is the treatment of choice. The defect may be demonstrated by a *lactose tolerance test* in which 50 gm of lactose is given orally and blood glucose measurements are made every half-hour for two hours. In normal persons the blood glucose will rise about 20 mg per 100 ml; in those with lactase deficiency the sugar cannot rise.

▼ *Key Sign:* ***Blood in the Feces.*** If it is not vomited, blood in the alimentary tract eventually passes in the feces. Its effect on the appearance of the stools depends upon the volume of blood and its rate of progress through the tract.

— *Black or Tarry Stools:* ***Melena.*** Experiments have shown that swallowing 50 to 60 ml of blood produces a tarry stool. The digestive enzymes convert the hemoglobin to black pigment that gives a *positive guaiac or benzidine test.* Commonly, commercially available guaiac-impregnated slides, such as Hemoccult® or Hematest®, are used. Frequent causes of black stools are:

Clinical Occurrence: SIMULATED MELENA (with negative guaiac test). Charcoal, iron sulfide formed from iron medication, bismuth used in radiographic studies, ingestion of bilberries or black cherries.

CHANGED BLOOD (with positive guaiac test; bleeding usually from duodenum or above). *Swallowed:* from hemoptysis or epistaxis. *Esophagus:* bleeding esophageal varix, ulcer, or neoplasm. *Stomach:* hiatal hernia, gastritis, gastric carcinoma, gastric ulcer. *Duodenum:* duodenal ulcer diverticula or hematobilia. *Small Intestine:* ulcerated Peyer's patches in typhoid fever, embolism of superior mesenteric artery, thrombosis of mesenteric veins, contusions from external trauma, intestinal polyps, duodenal diverticulum.

— *Bloody Red Stools.* Usually the site of hemorrhage is in the colon or below. But a copious hemorrhage higher will pass through undigested.

Clinical Occurrence: RED STOOLS WITH NEGATIVE GUAIAC TEST. Ingestion of large quantities of beets or certain fruits.

RED STOOLS WITH POSITIVE GUAIAC TEST. *Anus* (blood on outside of stool): hemorrhoids, fissure in ano, fistula in ano, prolapse of anus. *Rectum* (blood on outside of stool): polyps, carcinoma, proctitis, injury, ulcers from tuberculosis or syphilis. *Colon:* diverticulosis, diverticulitis, vascular ectasias, carcinoma, polyps, tuberculous ulcer, intussusception, dysentery, acute colitis, ulcerative colitis, actinomycosis, thrombosis of mesenteric veins, embolism of mesenteric artery, poisons (arsenic, phosphorus, mercury), purgatives, fecal impaction, infestation with *Oxyuris vermicularis.* *Ileum:* bleeding from Meckel's diverticulum, intussusception, typhoid fever, thrombosis and embolism of vessels, injury. *Jejunum:* ulceration. *Infections:* cholera, yellow fever, sprue, relapsing fever, leptospirosis. Scurvy. Vitamin K deficiency. Thrombocytopenia. Pseudoxanthoma elasticum.

— *Normally Colored Stools with Positive Guaiac Test ("Occult Blood").* A hemorrhage of small volume from any site in the alimentary tract or the upper respiratory tract may give a positive chemical test for blood without coloring the stool. The source must be sought by esophagram, x-ray examination of the entire alimentary tract, esophagoscopy, gastroscopy, colonoscopy, sigmoidoscopy. The value of complete and direct visualization of the colon, using the flexible colonoscope to identify sources of bleeding is now appreciated to be a diagnostic tool of major importance [R. G. Maxfield and C. M. Maxfield: Colonoscopy as a Primary Diagnostic Procedure in Chronic Gastrointestinal Tract Bleeding. *Arch. Surg.*, **121**:401–3, 1986.].

— *Gastrointestinal Bleeding Associated with Dermal Lesions.* Of the many cases with gastrointestinal bleeding, 90% occur from duodenal ulcer, malignancy, or esophageal varices, but the remaining 10% are associated with dermal lesions having their counterparts in the gastrointestinal tract [S. M. Bluefarb and W. A. Carr: Cutaneous Manifestations Associated with Gastrointestinal Bleeding, *Mod. Med.*, pp. 55–60, Dec. 27, 1971]. We are indebted to the authors for most of the following list of dermal lesions:

Peutz-Jegher Syndrome. Melanin spots on lips, buccal mucosa, and tongue suggest bleeding polypoid lesions in the small intestine.

Hereditary Hemorrhagic Telangiectasia (Rendu-Osler-Weber Disease). Telangiectases on the face, buccal mucosa, and extremities suggest similar lesions in the gastrointestinal tract.

Blue Rubber-Bleb Nevus Syndrome. Cavernous hemangiomas of the skin, especially on the trunk or extremities, suggest similar lesions of the small intestine.

Ehlers-Danlos Syndrome (Cutis Elastica). Hyperelastic skin, hyperreflexible joints, petechiae, easy bleeding of the skin. Also may have intestinal hemorrhage from deficiency of factor IX.

Pseudoxanthoma Elastica. Lax elastic tissue of skin, eye, cardiovascular system, and gastrointestinal tract. Skin contains small, soft yellow-orange papules running parallel to natural skinfolds; also angioid streaks in retina. Disintegration of arteries in the gastrointestinal tract causes hemorrhages.

Neurofibromatosis (von Recklinghausen's Disease). *Café au lait* pigmentation with sessile, pedunculated, or subcutaneous skin fibromas; may develop similar ones in gastrointestinal tract and they may bleed.

Amyloidosis (Either Primary or Secondary with Multiple Myeloma). Wax-colored papules, nodules, tumors, about the face, lips, ears, and upper chest. Often macroglossia. Deposits about blood vessels and in mucosa cause bleeding.

Malignant Atrophic Papulosis (Degos' Disease). Vasculitis of the skin and mucosa. Small red papules on the skin; soon become umbilicated, with porcelain-white depressed centers and dry scale. Border disappears, leaving a white patch. May have acute abdominal pain with vomiting and bleeding; may progress to peritonitis and gangrene.

Dermatomyositis. Nonpitting edema of the face; heliotrope discoloration of the eyelids, erythema over the bony prominences, pigmentation. Skeletal muscles have local and general inflammation; gastrointestinal bleeding lesions are common.

Schoenlein-Henoch Purpura. Symmetric purpura on the buttocks, extensor surfaces of the limbs; angioneurotic edema; gastrointestinal pain with thromboses producing mucosal ulcers and bleeding.

Drug Eruptions. Aspirin causes macular and purpuric lesions of lower limbs. Erosive lesions cause bleeding from gastrointestinal tract. Coumarin may cause petechiae, ecchymoses, and hemorrhagic infarcts in gastrointestinal tract.

Scurvy. Perifollicular hemorrhages, ecchymoses of legs, bleeding gums, loose teeth, gastrointestinal bleeding.

Polycythemia Vera. Purplish red color of skin and mucosa; hemorrhages, spider nevi, rosacea, peptic ulcer.

Lymphoma. Many types produce bleeding lesions in skin and mucosa.

Kaposi's Sarcoma. Usually on skin of feet—becomes symmetric; dark-blue color—nodules and plaques that are hemorrhagic.

Mastocytosis. Brown-red macules; urticaria develops, also cirrhosis of the liver and esophageal varices.

Palmar Varices with Gastric Varices. One case report [W. C. Sherwood: Palmar Varices and Gastrointestinal Bleeding, *Arch. Intern. Med.*, **128:**598–99, 1971].

▼ *Key Sign:* ***Constipation.*** With constipation, the frequency of fecal evacuations is less than normal. But application of this definition to a patient requires knowledge of his individual norm, since human beings exhibit great diversity in their bowel habits. One must ascertain whether the patient's stated norm is actually what he has always lived with in health, or whether his concept of a norm has been established by the folklore that good health requires one "good" bowel movement each day. Many normal persons get along very well with two or three evacuations a week. Probably the only symptom of constipation is the gradual development of a sense of fullness in the abdomen, often delayed for an astonishing length of time.

Failure to conform to the pattern of daily evacuation has caused untold anxiety, headaches, listlessness, and other symptoms. Unfortunately, many physicians and the entire nursing profession have contributed greatly in perpetuating the public alarm and discomfort. Forty years ago, when obsessive bedside care was in its heyday, it took a strong-minded and courageous bed patient to withstand a nurse who appeared at the bedside, stern but beautiful in starched whites, armed with a cathartic or enema can. The sole indication for her attack was a zero on the bedside chart in the little square for yesterday in which the daily bowel movements were recorded. But there is less bullying today. The house officer thoughtfully includes the stereotyped written order "If no B.M. in the P.M., give M.O.M. in the A.M." "Thoughtfully" for himself—not the patient—because he doesn't want to be called at night by a patient who regards the daily bowel movement as one of his constitutional guarantees.

Nevertheless, an actual deceleration in the frequency of bowel movements may be an important clue to several disorders.

— *Acute Constipation: **Intestinal Obstruction.*** This is discussed elsewhere (pp. 556–59).

— *Acute Constipation: **Fecal Impaction.*** The disorder usually occurs in debilitated or dehydrated patients who are bedfast. Often it is initiated by the ingestion of barium for x-ray examination of the gastrointestinal tract. The patient may experience no discomfort and hence does not complain; someone finds that there have been no bowel movements for several days. Or the patient complains of constipation, tenesmus, and inability to defecate. A digital examination of the rectum reveals hard fecal masses that must be removed manually. Occasionally the impacted masses stimulate small watery passages that attract attention to the condition (see Spurious Diarrhea, p. 529). An exception to the typical clinical picture was one patient, a young athletic executive with an irritable colon. After a very busy week with irregular meals and long working hours, he developed a fecal impaction that required manual removal.

— *Chronic Constipation:* ***Irritable Colon*** (Spastic Colon). The most common cause of constipation, this disorder is characterized by longer periods of constipation alternating with shorter bouts of diarrhea (see also p. 530). Either symptom may serve as the entering complaint. The triad of symptoms is (1) longstanding intermittent constipation, (2) scybalous stools, (3) abdominal pain relieved by defecation.

— *Chronic Constipation:* ***Atonic Colon.*** The patient has a long history of constipation, fancied or real, with the habitual daily use of cathartics or enemas. The stools may be alternately voluminous and scanty. Palpation of the abdomen often reveals large fecal masses; stools may be felt in the rectum during digital examination.

— *Chronic Constipation:* ***Megacolon.*** Lifelong constipation with occasional passage of an enormous formed stool suggests megacolon, either from lack of ganglionic cells to innervate the colon proximally from the anal sphincter for varying distances, or from chronic contraction of the anal sphincter. X-ray examination demonstrates colonic dilatation.

— *Chronic Constipation:* ***Carcinoma of Descending Colon.*** A recent onset of constipation associated with cramping abdominal pain after lifelong regular bowel habits suggests the growth of cancer in the descending colon. Digital examination of the rectum including testing for occult fecal blood should be followed by sigmoidoscopic or colonoscopic inspection and barium enema to demonstrate the neoplasm.

— *Chronic Constipation:* ***Miscellaneous Causes.*** Rarer causes are rectal stricture, myxedema, hyperparathyroidism, medication with ganglionic blocking agents, opiates, psychologic depression, Parkinson's disease, cerebral infarction.

▼ *Key Symptom:* ***Acute Abdominal Pain.*** Severe acute abdominal pain heralds a variety of disorders that create a situation known in surgical slang as the *acute abdomen.* The physician pursues the diagnosis with a sense of urgency, because early surgical operation may be lifesaving in some disorders, contraindicated in others. He collects the facts by repeated examinations at the bedside within a few hours, be it day or night. Great reliance is necessarily placed upon symptoms and signs; some assistance is obtained from emergency x-ray examinations; laboratory tests are less important. The common denominator among these conditions is *acuteness* and *pain in the abdomen.*

Pain is frequently the diagnostic key. Relatively few findings may distinguish several conditions. Much importance attaches to the *location* of the pain and tenderness (Fig. 7-27), their *changing position,* their variations in *quality* during the course of observation. For example, the patient with intra-abdominal visceral pain may walk about, but when the viscus perforates causing peritonitis, he lies very still in bed. Hence, previous administration of narcotics handicaps the physician by masking the symptoms and signs. Usually the severity of the symptoms brings the patient to the physician within a few hours of onset, so chronic diseases are not possibilities, although their history must be searched for as possible antecedents for the acute phase. Use the jar test (p. 499) to help decide the presence of peritoneal inflammation.

— *Acute Epigastric Pain:* **Acute Appendicitis (*Early*).** Epigastric pain is the initial symptom in a constant sequence that develops in the course of acute appendicitis. *Diffuse pain* arises in the midline at variable distances between the xiphoid process and the umbilicus; it is not accompanied by tenderness. This pain has been attributed to reflex peristalsis and pyloric spasm. The pain may waken the patient from a sound sleep. Later, classically, *nausea* or *vomiting* occurs. As a third incident, the *pain becomes generalized,* then finally it shifts to the *right lower quadrant.*

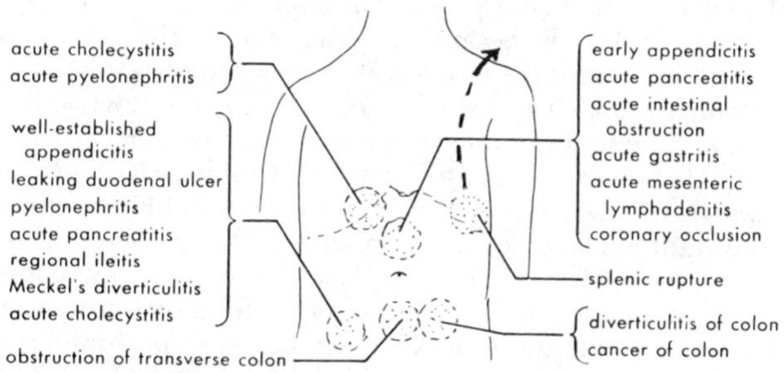

Fig. 7-27. Common locations of acute abdominal pain. *In general the painful spot is also tender, but not always. Note especially that the pain of acute appendicitis is early in the epigastrium, later in the right lower quadrant. Pain in the spleen commonly radiates to the top of the left shoulder. Pains considered in this group are ordinarily constant, in contrast to the intermittent pain of colic.*

Until this localization occurs, the diagnosis of appendicitis cannot be made, and often is not even anticipated. The subsequent course is described under RLQ Pain: Acute Appendicitis (Intermediate) (p. 551).

— *Acute Epigastric Pain:* ***Perforation of Peptic Ulcer.*** The patient may give a long history of dull epigastric pain occurring 3 or 4 hours after meals, relieved by food or alkali; or vague discomfort in the upper abdomen may have been present for only a few days. Occasionally, there are no antecedent symptoms of indigestion. Cope recognizes three stages described here: *Stage of Prostration (Primary Shock).* The patient experiences a *sudden excruciating pain* in the epigastrium and frequently collapses. Soon the pain spreads over the entire abdomen; sometimes it intensifies in the suprapubic region because of the downward flow of gastric contents. The face is *anxious* and *pale gray;* the body is covered with *cold sweat.* The respiratory movements are shallow. *Retching* or *vomiting* occurs. Shock may be manifested by a body temperature of 95° or 96° F (35° or 35.5° C). Hypotension occurs, with systolic measurements under 100 mm Hg. The initial stage may last for a few minutes to several hours. *Stage of Reaction (Masked Peritonitis).* This is but a brief respite for the patient; it may also deceive the inexperienced physician. The blood pressure rises to normal values and the skin becomes warmer. But generalized abdominal pain and tenderness persist, although lessened in intensity. He turns cautiously because of pain; the thighs are flexed for comfort. Boardlike *involuntary rigidity* causes retraction of abdominal muscles and shallow respiratory movements. The pelvic peritoneum is tender when examined rectally. *Free fluid* can be demonstrated in the abdominal cavity. *Gas under the diaphragm* may be evident by a diminished area of liver dullness in the right axilla, or by an x-ray film of the abdomen in the erect position. *Pain on the tops of both shoulders* from irritation of both diaphragms indicates anterior perforation of the stomach; pain on only the right shoulder points to perforation of the pylorus or duodenum. *Stage of Frank Peritonitis.* Soon the classic signs of advanced peritonitis appear. *Ileus* distends the abdomen. *Vomiting* resumes and persists with increased violence. Again the temperature declines to subnormal levels. The entire abdomen is *tender*, but rigidity may lessen in the late stage. The results of dehydration and pain produce the classic *facies hippocratica,* with hollow features and anxious expression. Death usually ensues in 3 days.

— *Acute Epigastric Pain:* ***Limited Perforation of Peptic Ulcer.*** Occasionally the stage of prostration is mild and the pain is limited to the epigastrium because the released gastric contents become walled off to produce a subphrenic abscess; or rarely, the abscess forms in the lesser peritoneal sac. The symptoms and signs of subphrenic abscess then predominate (p. 518).

— *Acute Epigastric Pain:* ***Acute Pancreatitis.*** Without warning, the patient is struck with *excruciating epigastric pain,* severe enough to cause collapse. This is probably caused by stimulation of the adjacent celiac plexus. Later, the pain radiates to one or both *lumbar regions;* sometimes irritation of the phrenic nerve causes *pain in the left shoulder.* Occasionally, the pain spreads over the entire abdomen and especially to the *right lower quadrant.* Characteristically, it is knifelike with a boring quality, going directly through to the back. As the pain is aggravated when the patient is supine, the patient may assume a *sitting* position, leaning forward to lessen the pain. Usually *profound shock* occurs, with lowered body temperature and hypotension. Nearly always, *retching* and *vomiting* are severe; the symptoms are more intense and prolonged than in perforation of the stomach. Frequently one is impressed with the great disparity between the severity of the symptoms and the paucity of abdominal findings. *Epigastric tenderness* is always present. Muscle rigidity is usually *absent;* when present, it is confined to epigastrium. Occasionally one can feel a *tender transverse mass* deep in the epigastrium. Slight *jaundice* may be evident in one or two days. Two or three days after onset, blue or green *ecchymoses* occasionally appear in the flank (Turner's sign) from extravasation of hemolyzed blood and degradation of the hemoglobin. Bluish discoloration of the *umbilicus* (Cullen's sign) may occur from the same cause. Occasionally *glycosuria* is noted as well as hypocalcemia, the severity of which often parallels the degree of pancreatitis. For 6 or 8 hours after onset, the *serum amylase* values may be greatly elevated but this finding is very evanescent; an increase in urinary amylase and especially lipase persists somewhat longer. In addition to biliary calculi and/or pancreatic calcifications, identified as such on abdominal radiographs, a single dilated atonic loop of small bowel, the sentinel loop, representing localized ileus secondary to the inflamed pancreas, may be seen. The diagnosis is confirmed by the finding of a 5% or greater amylase-creatinine urinary clearance ratio. Later, a *pseudocyst* may form in the epigastrium from an accumulation of blood and fluid in the lesser peritoneal sac. *Distinction.* The picture just described may be an isolated episode of acute pancreatitis most often associated with cholecystitis, but, except for the history, it is also indistinguishable from an acute exacerbation of chronic relapsing pancreatitis caused by a heavy continuous intake of ethanol for several years.

Clinical Occurrence. Numerous factors have been listed as causing attacks of acute pancreatitis; clinically the most common are (1) biliary tract disease and (2) excessive alcohol intake. Other causes include hyperlipidemia, pancreatic ductal obstruction, vascular compromise, mumps, drug-induced phenomena.

— *Acute Epigastric Pain:* ***Occlusion of Mesenteric Vessels.*** The superior mesenteric artery or vein is most commonly involved, by either embolism or thrombosis. Arterial occlusion is more likely to produce the typical clinical picture; venous thrombosis is often atypical. Antecedent disease, including a history of recurrent postprandial abdominal pain suggestive of abdominal angina is reported in up to 50% of those with acute thrombotic occlusion; hepatic cirrhosis or severe arteriosclerosis also favors thrombosis. The onset is *sudden* with *acute agonizing pain* between the xiphoid and the umbilicus; slight, if any, relief is afforded by narcotics. This symptom complex occurring in any individual with cause for having mural thrombi in the heart, especially those with rheumatic or atherosclerotic heart disease, must alert the diagnostician to the possibility of embolic disease to the superior mesenteric vessels. Usually, there is a paucity of localizing signs; but occasionally a *tender mass* is palpable in the epigastrium. The temperature becomes subnormal and hypotension accompanies. There is evidence of a severe and profound metabolic acidosis. These events are soon followed by the signs of intestinal obstruction: abdominal distention, ileus, and vomiting. Blood may be passed per rectum. Frequently, there is *hemorrhage* into the peritoneal cavity; needle aspiration of the sanguinous fluid assists in the diagnosis.

— *Acute Epigastric Pain:* ***Dissecting Aneurysm.*** This commonly occurs in middle aged hypertensive black males. It also kills half the patients with the rare mesodermal defect recognized as Marfan's syndrome. Blood extravasates into the media of the aorta, splitting the layers in its downward course. The entrance is usually at the base of the aorta, and in that instance the *pain* begins in the thorax and radiates to the neck and arms; later the pain reaches the abdomen. In some instances, abdominal pain is the initial complaint. This is agonizing to the extent that narcotics do not provide relief. The pain is usually in the epigastrium, causing intense *involuntary rigidity* of the abdominal muscles. The blood pressure is not affected early. Branches of the abdominal aorta may be progressively occluded, so the upper *arterial pulses* on one or both sides are first to disappear. Poor circulation of the spinal cord causes *numbness* and even *hemiplegia.* The electrocardiogram is unaffected, which is important because a real problem is encountered in differentiating acute dissection from acute myocardial infarction. The *disparity in the pulses* may be the most important clue to the diagnosis. (See also p. 245). The disease occurs in pregnancy, arteriosclerosis, myxedema, pseudoxanthoma elasticum. Occasionally dissection is slow and symptomless. Echograms with B-mode display aid in the diagnosis of the abdominal lesion while the angiogram is diagnostic if one identifies splitting or distortion of the contrast column, alternate flow patterns and/or aortic valvular insufficiency.

— *Acute Painless Epigastric Distention:* ***Acute Gastric Dilatation*** (Acute Gastrectasis, Primary Ectasia of Stomach, Arteriomesenteric Ileus, Gastrojejunal Ileus, Acute Paresis of Stomach, Postpartum Dilatation of Stomach, Acute Duodenal Occlusion, Acute Gastrorrhea, Acute Gastric Succhorrhea). The patient, bedridden from some other disorder, becomes *suddenly sicker* and assumes an anxious or apathetic appearance. Often this is accompanied by *vomiting,* sudden *distention* of the upper abdomen, and *hypotension* with a thready pulse. Careful inspection of the abdomen shows a *dilated stomach* filling the epigastrium or reaching to the pelvis. The abdominal mass is *tympanitic* and emits a *succussion splash.* Early, *visible peristalsis* may be present; later, peristaltic sounds are weak or absent, indicating *ileus.* The diagnosis is confirmed by aspiration of the stomach that produces a large volume of fluid. Less dramatic and more chronic cases are frequent and more difficult to diagnose; the only definite sign may be x-ray evidence of delayed gastric emptying. The disorder produces profound imbalances in fluid and electrolytes. The routine use of nasogastric suction following abdominal surgery has remarkably reduced the development of this condition in the postoperative patient. ***Pathophysiology.*** The mechanism is not precisely known; it is attributed to a reflex paralysis of gastric muscles that permits the accumulation of fluid and swallowed air.

Clinical Occurrence. The major provocative factors are the triad of *pain, abdominal trauma,* and bodily *immobilization:* thus 60 to 70% of cases occur postoperatively. A myriad of specific diseases may precipitate this syndrome. Somewhat bizarre is the *cast syndrome,* in which acute gastric dilatation is initiated by the application of a hip spica for the treatment of a bone fracture [M. N. Dorph: The Cast Syndrome, *N. Engl. J. Med.,* **243:**440–42, 1950].

— *Acute RUQ Pain:* ***Acute Cholecystitis.*** The onset is not so sudden as that in perforation or acute intestinal obstruction. *Diffuse pain* develops in the right upper quadrant of the abdomen; occasionally it radiates to the top of the right shoulder. *Vomiting* is slight or moderately severe; it is intensified by the presence of localized peritonitis. *Tenderness* is constant and localized behind the inferior margin of the liver. *Fist percussion* over the liver produces pain, but this sign also occurs in acute hepatitis (Fig. 7-22, p. 515). When the tips of the fingers are held under the right costal margin and the patient is asked to inspire, there is *inspiratory arrest* (Murphy's sign). Friction fremitus and friction rub have been reported over the inflamed viscus [G. G. Nicholas and E. Williams: Friction Rub in Acute Cholecystitis; An Unusual Finding, *J.A.M.A.,* **218:**1945–46, 1971]. The abdominal muscles do not become rigid unless peritonitis is present. As the attack progresses, in approximately one-third of patients, an exquisitely *tender globular mass* may be felt behind the lower border of the liver; though such a finding flies in the face of Courvoisier's law. Rarely the distended gallbladder reaches the right lower quadrant. Moderate fever is usually present with temperatures ranging from 100° to 103° F (37.7° to 39.4° C). When the temperature is greater than 102° F, the diagnosis of acute suppurative cholangitis must be entertained. With inflammation of the cystic duct, the temperature curve is irregular; sometimes most of the day is afebrile, but the evening temperature shoots to 105° F (40.5°

C), accompanied by chills (Charcot's fever). During an attack, studies dependent upon demonstration of concentration of bile within the gallbladder are negative, or demonstrate *nonvisualization*. A past history of food dyscrasias, including fats and foods known to contain cholecystokinins, and/or similar previous attacks in patients with known cholelithiasis is often present. Jaundice may occur if there is an associated choledocholithiasis or as a result of direct involvement of the liver by the adjacent inflamed gallbladder.

— ***Acute RUQ Pain:* Cholelithiasis.** Gallstones cause no symptoms unless a calculus enters the cystic duct to stimulate *colic*, or it perforates the wall of the gallbladder. An attack of colic may be uncomplicated, or it may be associated with acute cholecystitis, when the symptoms of both occur. *Gallstone colic* occurs suddenly in the right upper quadrant and radiates to the inferior border of the right scapula (Fig. 7-28). The pain is severe enough to cause the patient to double up; it comes in paroxysms, with intervening free intervals. During the attack, the right upper quadrant is *rigid;* the muscles are flaccid between pains. If they contain calcium, gallstones can be demonstrated on the plain x-ray film. Calculi in the right upper quadrant

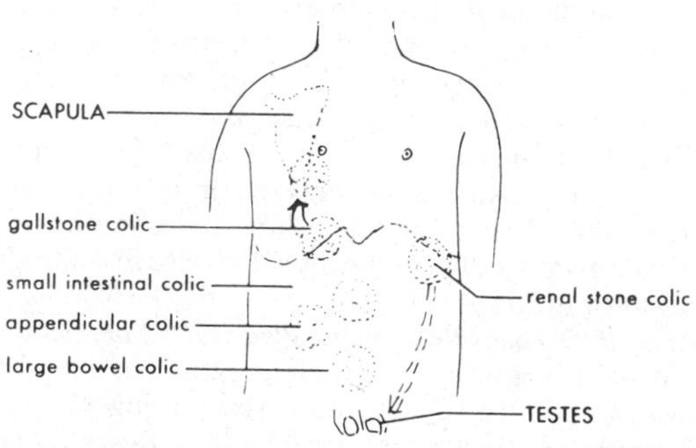

Fig. 7-28. Locations of abdominal colic. *Colic means a special type of pain, notable for its severity and its paroxysmal occurrence. It occurs when a hollow viscus is obstructed and pain results from muscular contractions trying to overcome the impediment. Note especially the radiation of gallstone colic from the right upper quadrant of the abdomen to the angle of the right scapula behind. The colic of renal calculus frequently radiates to the testis on the same side.*

may, however, be in the renal pelvis, and should be differentiated from gallstones. Cholecystograms with opaque medium may show negative shadows of stones if the viscus can concentrate the dye. Ultrasonic examination will visualize gallstones not revealed by the contrast method, giving only 3% false positives, as compared with 3 to 14% with the contrast. CT scans may help.

— *Acute RUQ Pain:* ***Rupture of the Gallbladder.*** The initial picture may be either that of acute cholecystitis or gallstone colic. *Pain* in the right upper quadrant becomes constant and gradually spreads to the remainder of the abdomen. Signs of generalized peritonitis appear, in this case, *bile peritonitis.* This condition is characterized by severe prostration and shock secondary to the chemical irritation caused by the bile. The same picture can be seen following routine cholecystectomy, when, in the postoperative period, the tie or ligature comes off of the cystic duct.

— *Acute RUQ Pain:* ***Leaking Duodenal Ulcer.*** A small perforation of a duodenal ulcer permits slow leakage of contents into the right lumbar region, causing *pain, tenderness,* and *rigidity* in the right upper quadrant. An antecedent history of the pain and peptic ulcer is usually obtainable. There is also *tenderness* in the midline of the epigastrium. X-rays of the upper GI tract reveal the duodenal ulcer. The gastric and duodenal contents can track down into the right lower quadrant and lead to a false diagnosis of appendicitis.

— *Acute RUQ Pain:* ***Acute Hepatitis.*** Usually fever and malaise are present, suggesting a generalized infection. If palpable, the entire liver is *tender,* the edge blunt and smooth. *Fist percussion* over the liver produces pain, as it does also in acute cholecystitis. Jaundice may appear.

— *Acute RUQ Pain:* ***Right-Sided Pleurisy.*** The patient complains of pain in the right upper quadrant of the abdomen, but the examiner can elicit no corresponding tenderness at the inferior border of the liver or behind it. Respiratory movements accentuate the pain, so the patient takes *shallow breaths.* The temperature is usually high, 104° to 105° F (40.0° to 40.5° C). A pleural *friction rub* or signs of pneumonia may be present. An x-ray film of the chest is mandatory in the evaluation of any patient with an acute abdomen, but it may not show any abnormality.

— *Acute RUQ Pain:* ***Right Ureteral Colic.*** The onset is sudden, with *excruciating pain* in the right upper quadrant, radiating to the right flank. The patient *bends double* with agony and may collapse. There is usually more restless, violent movement than with pancreatitis or dissecting aneurysm. Frequently the pain radiates to the right testis, vulva, or groin. *Vomiting* is usually severe. Micturition may produce pain and *bloody urine.* A calculus may be seen in appropriate x-ray films.

— *Acute RUQ Pain:* ***Right Pyelonephritis.*** Acute pyelonephritis produces *pain* in the right upper quadrant, fever of 101° to 104° F (38.3° to 40.0° C), and leukocytosis up to 20,000 per cu mm. At first the pain is quite severe and it may be accompanied by *vomiting. Tenderness* is found in the right upper quadrant, suggesting acute cholecystitis, although the region is not so painful on palpation. Usually, the finding of albumin and leukocytes in the urine clarifies the diagnosis. Occasionally, the urinary signs are absent, raising doubt of the presence of renal disease. Pyelourethrograms may yield characteristic signs. A normal gallbladder will be visualized in the cholecystogram.

— *Acute RUQ Pain:* ***Rupture of the Liver.*** Spontaneous rupture of the liver, as a complication of oral anticoagulant therapy, has been reported [H. Dizadji, R. Hammer, B. Strzyz, and J. Weisenberg: Spontaneous Rupture of the Liver, *Arch. Surg.,* **114:**734–35, 1979]. The association of the development of benign hepatomas and focal nodular adenomas of the liver in young women taking oral contraceptives is well recognized. Such a presentation in conjunction with a history of oral contraceptive use must place the diagnosis of rupture of such lesions high on the list of probabilities. A blow on the abdomen or right lower thorax may not leave external marks of trauma but be sufficient to rupture the liver. Severe *pain* and *tenderness* in the right upper quadrant are the rule. Since there is usually profuse hemorrhage, shock ensues with hypotension, subnormal temperature, and extreme prostration. Rupture of the liver and spleen have been diagnosed by scintigrams with the injection of technetium (Tc 99m sulfur colloid).

— *Acute RUQ Pain:* ***Rupture of Right Kidney.*** Trauma to the right lower thorax, especially from the back, may rupture the kidney. *Pain* and *tenderness* are present in the right upper quadrant and toward the lumbar region. *Hematuria* is obvious, unless the ureter is obstructed by a blood clot that prevents drainage from the affected side. It is generally advisable in all patients being evaluated for multiple trauma that an intravenous pyelogram be obtained in order to identify the fact that two kidneys are present and that there is normal function. Signs of shock may not be prominent because hemorrhage is not profuse or is contained in the retroperitoneum.

— *Acute LUQ Pain:* ***Splenic Infarction.*** The normal spleen is seldom affected; usually the patient has splenomegaly from some hematologic disorder, such as polycythemia vera, sickle-cell anemia, leukemia, or myelofibrosis. The condition also occurs in subacute bacterial endocarditis. Severe sharp *pain* develops in the left upper quadrant, accompanied by rigidity of the regional abdominal muscles. Frequently the pain radiates to the *top of the left shoulder.* Fever and leukocytosis may be present. In a few days, a splenic *friction rub* may be heard and felt from perisplenitis over the infarcted area.

— *Acute LUQ Pain:* ***Splenic Rupture.*** A blow over the left lower thorax or the left upper abdomen may cause rupture of a normal spleen without external signs of trauma. Rarely, the spleen ruptures spontaneously when enlarged from infectious mononucleosis, sepsis, or infarction. Large soft spleens have been ruptured during palpation. Intense *pain* occurs in the left upper quadrant, radiating to the top of the left shoulder (Kehr's sign). Hemorrhage is profuse and signs of shock frequently occur: pallor, subnormal temperature, hypotension.

Pain or *tenderness* in the left upper quadrant and pain radiating to the left shoulder strongly suggest splenic rupture. *Kehr's sign* is reported to occur in 9 out of 10 cases of splenic rupture [A. B. Lowenfels: Kehr's Sign—A Neglected Aid in Rupture of the Spleen, *N. Engl. J. Med.*, **274:**1019, 1966]. The pain may be accentuated by elevating the foot of the bed to increase the contact between free blood in the peritoneal cavity and the phrenic nerve in the diaphragm. The diagnosis of intra-abdominal hemorrhage is made most frequently by peritoneal lavage. The technique first described by Root, *et al.* in 1965, with subsequent minor variations, has become a virtual standard for all emergency treatment centers [H. D. Root, C. W. Hauser, C. R. McKinley, J. W. LaFave, and R. P. Mendola: *Diagnostic Peritoneal Lavage, Surgery,* **57:**633–39, 1965]. The technique must be learned by all the individuals seeing and evaluating traumatized patients. Scintigraphy with Tc 99m colloid is diagnostic; also arteriography [R. N. Bark and M. H. Whaley: The Application of Splenic Arteriography in the Diagnosis of Rupture of the Spleen, *Am. J. Roentgenol.*, **104:**662–67, 1968].

— *Acute LUQ Pain:* ***Left Pyelonephritis.*** Diagnosis should not present the difficulties that arise on the right side (p. 549).

— *Acute LUQ Pain:* ***Left Ureteral Colic.*** See discussion under Right Ureteral Colic, p. 549.

— *Acute LUQ Pain:* ***Rupture of the Left Kidney.*** See discussion under Rupture of Right Kidney, p. 549. In a boy who exhibited signs of slight hemorrhage from rupture of the left kidney, hypertension developed that lasted for two weeks; this was attributed to a hematoma compromising the renal artery and producing the *Goldblatt phenomenon.*

— *Acute RLQ Pain:* **Acute Appendicitis (*Intermediate*).** During the progression of events in the development of acute appendicitis, certain symptoms and signs follow an almost invariable sequence: first, epigastric pain (see p. 541); second, nausea or vomiting; third, shifting of the pain from the epigastrium to the right lower quadrant and the development of deep tenderness there; fourth, fever; fifth, leukocytosis. If the patient presents a different sequence of events, the diagnosis of appendicitis should be questioned. *Deep tenderness* is first demonstrated at the base of the appendix, just below the midpoint of a line between the anterior superior iliac spine and the umbilicus, when the appendix is typically placed. At this stage, the fever is usually between 101° and 103° F (38.3° and 39.4° C), seldom higher. The leukocytosis is polymorphonuclear, with counts between 10,000 and 20,000 per cu mm; higher values suggest perforation. In many cases, one can map out an area of *hyperesthesia* in the right lower quadrant, variable in extent and shape.

The preceding description applies when the appendix is typically placed, lateral to the cecum, or medial and anterior to the ilium. When it lies behind the ilium, or ascends behind the cecum, the deep tenderness is less; vomiting is infrequent. With the appendix in the true pelvis, the right lower quadrant is not tender; but rectal palpation demonstrates tenderness in the peritoneal pouches.

— *Acute RLQ Pain:* **Acute Appendicitis (*with Perforation*).** When the appendix ruptures, the *pain accentuates, vomiting recurs,* the temperature rises still higher, and the leukocytes increase over previous counts. The resulting abscess forms a *tender mass*, although this finding may also be caused by edema and inflammation of the cecum, a phlegmon. Other signs depend somewhat upon the location of the appendix. ***Extrapelvic Appendix.*** When perforation is retrocecal, the back muscles are inflamed and one may elicit *tenderness below the 12th rib on the right.* With the appendix lateral to the cecum, a *mass* is felt, guarded by intense involuntary rigidity of the abdominal muscles. Irritation of the psoas muscle causes the patient to *flex the right thigh* or hold it rigidly extended. The *iliopsoas test* elicits *pain* when the supine patient tries to flex the thigh against the resistance of the examiner's hand (Fig. 7-29A). When the appendix is medial and behind the ilium, an abscess may involve the right ureter, causing *pain on urination* and the presence of white cells in the urine. ***Intrapelvic Appendix.*** When the appendix lies within the true pelvis, *diffuse suprapubic pain* occurs. There is no rigidity of the abdominal muscles. Irritation of the bladder and rectum produces *painful urination* and *tenesmus.* A prime diagnostic sign is the demonstration of a palpable *tender mass* in the peritoneal pouch by rectal examination. The

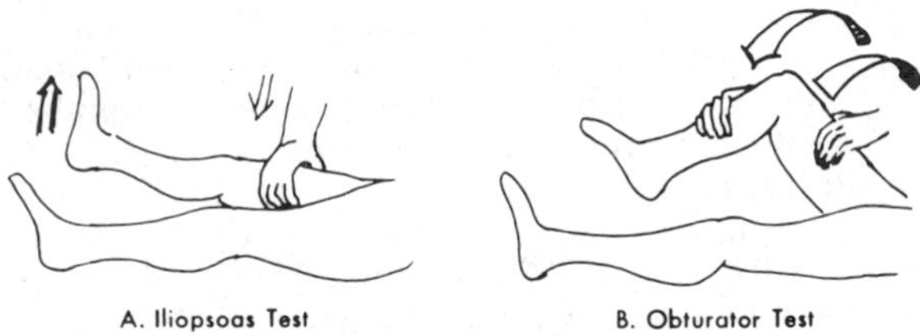

Fig. 7-29. Tests for irritation of the iliopsoas and obturator muscles. *Abscesses in the pelvis may be localized by demonstrating irritation of the more lateral iliopsoas or the medial obturator internus muscles.* **A.** Iliopsoas test. *The supine patient keeps his knee extended and is asked to flex the thigh against the resistance of the examiner's hand. Pain in the pelvis indicates irritation of the iliopsoas.* **B.** Obturator test. *The supine patient flexes the right thigh to 90°. At the patient's right, the examiner immobilizes the ankle with his right hand; with his left hand, he pulls the knee lateralward for external rotation, medialward for internal rotation. The rotation produces pelvic pain from an inflamed muscle. Examination of the left limb requires standing at the patient's left side and reversing procedures.*

abscess may lie in contact with the Obturator internus; the *obturator test* produces suprapubic pain by flexing the thigh and rotating the femur internally and externally (Fig. 7-29B).

— *Acute RLQ Pain:* ***Meckel's Diverticulitis.*** Acute inflammation of Meckel's diverticulum is almost impossible to distinguish from acute appendicitis before operation. The only hint that the diverticulum may be the source of infection is the location of the inflammatory mass somewhat more medial than the usual location of the appendix. The diverticulum is also somewhat more mobile.

— *Acute RLQ Pain:* ***Regional Ileitis*** (Terminal Ileitis, Segmental Ileitis, Crohn's Disease). The first attack of ileitis is almost indistinguishable clinically from acute appendicitis. The single clue favoring ileitis is that *diarrhea usually precedes the attack.* If similar antecedent episodes have occurred, the probability is strong for chronic ileitis with an exacerbation.

— *Acute RLQ Pain:* ***Perforated Duodenal Ulcer.*** The contents from a perforated ulcer drain down the right paracolic gutter into the right iliac fossa, where *pain, tenderness,* and *rigidity* may be pronounced (Fig. 7-30). This raises the question of acute appendicitis. In ulcer, however, some pain and tenderness are likely to persist in the epigastrium, directing attention to a history of ulcer symptoms.

— *Acute LLQ Pain:* ***Colonic Diverticulitis.*** Typically, *pain* and *tenderness* are localized in the left lower quadrant, thus presenting no problem in distinguishing from appendicitis. If the co-

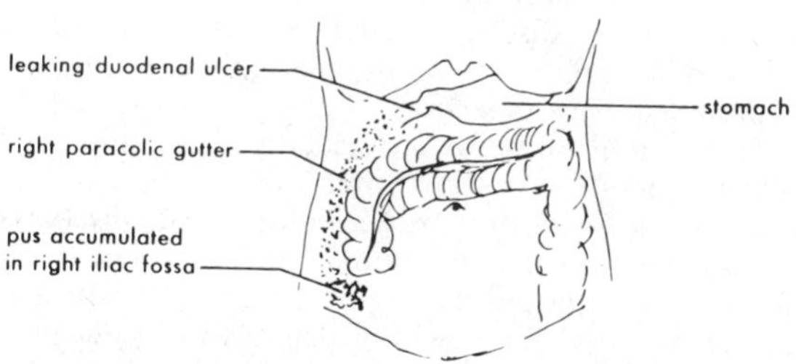

Fig. 7-30. Production of iliac abscess from a leaking duodenal ulcer. *Diagram shows the drainage of the duodenal ulcer down the right paracolic gutter into the right iliac fossa. The path is indicated by stippling.*

lonic loop lies in the pelvis, the condition often cannot be distinguished from pelvic appendicitis before operation. Previous x-ray evidence of diverticula, or a history compatible with diverticulitis would add support to that diagnosis. The differentiation of perforation of a diverticulum or a colonic neoplasm from ruptured appendix, especially when the colonic loop is displaced to the right side, is exceedingly difficult and may, on occasion, only be made at the time of exploration of the abdomen. The absence of the typical sequence of events in acute appendicitis favors other causes of perforation.

— *Acute Suprapubic Pain:* **Rupture of Urinary Bladder.** When the bladder is full of urine, a blow on the abdomen or fracture of the pelvis may cause it to burst. Deceleration automobile injuries, in those wearing seat belts, may also include urinary bladder injuries. Rupture into the peritoneal cavity produces mild peritonitis, as indicated by *pain* and *tenderness* in the suprapubic region. The usual bladder fullness cannot be felt above the prostate in the rectal examination or through the vagina in the female. When the rupture is extraperitoneal, urinary extravasation penetrates the perineum, producing *bogginess* about the rectum and vagina when palpated by rectum. Scrotal swelling may occur: but it is not as consistent or considerable as from extravasation of urine from a severed ureter.

— *Acute Suprapubic Pain:* **Acute Salpingitis.** Sudden fever occurs, with *pain* and *tenderness* in the suprapubic region and often above the inguinal ligaments. The lower abdominal muscles are rigid. Vaginal palpation elicits *pain* in the lateral fornices and adnexa. When the pain is limited to the right side, the condition must be distinguished from acute appendicitis, a difficult task. Usually the onset of salpingitis does not resemble the typical sequence of events in appendicitis (p. 541). The patients have a history of being sexually active, and the acute episode frequently starts just after the cessation of menses. Painful urination and the presence of a vaginal discharge are the most common early symptoms. Finding gonococci in the vaginal secretions favors salpingitis. If a *painful mass* is felt in one or both lateral fornices, the diagnosis of *pyosalpinx with peritonitis* is probable.

— *Acute Suprapubic Pain:* **Rupture of Endometrioma.** Usually this cannot be distinguished from acute salpingitis before operation.

— *Acute Suprapubic Pain:* ***Torsion of Ovarian Cyst Pedicle.*** The cyst may have produced swelling in the suprapubic region that antedated the attack of pain. Sudden *pain* in the region, accompanied by *vomiting,* suggests a twisted pedicle.

Abdominal Pain and Pallor: ***Hemorrhage from Tubal Pregnancy.*** A severe hemorrhage into the abdomen in a previously healthy woman begins with *agonizing pain* and *vomiting* along with abdominal *tenderness.* Signs of *shock* quickly develop, indicated by pallor, prostration, thready pulse, subnormal temperature, and hypotension. The abdomen is *tender* but the walls are often *flaccid;* boardlike rigidity may occur. Sometimes the pain occurs in the suprapubic region, due to the pooling of blood in the pelvis, suggesting pelvic origin; but it may be generalized or in the epigastrium. Later, the abdomen becomes *distended;* signs of *free fluid* may appear. Since rupture of tubal pregnancy usually occurs in the first eight weeks of gestation, menstrual irregularities may have been slight or unnoticed. With subacute hemorrhage, the symptoms are not so severe. The patient may be seen after the first episode has subsided, when hemorrhage has ceased and a clot has formed in the pelvis. She may complain of some suprapubic pain. The clot causes *fullness* of the lower abdomen and gives a *sense of resistance* in palpating the fornices. A definite *mass* of clot or liquid blood may be present in the rectouterine pouch where it can be identified by cul-de-sac puncture, colpotomy, or culdoscopy. Serum or urinary pregnancy tests should be obtained if this diagnosis is entertained. Later, *uterine bleeding* may occur. Rarely, there is a bluish discoloration of the *umbilicus* (Cullen's sign). The severe attack must be distinguished from most other causes of acute abdomen. One must learn to suspect rupture of tubal pregnancy in any fertile woman with acute abdominal pain who has had sexual intercourse within two months.

Abdominal Pain and Pallor: ***Corpus Luteum Hemorrhage.*** Women in the premenopausal age incur the danger of intraabdominal hemorrhage from ruptured corpus luteum when they take anticoagulants. The bleeding may be symptomless, or the classic signs of intra-abdominal hemorrhage may result: lower abdominal colicky pain and rebound tenderness, absence of bowel sounds, the appearance of an adnexal mass, tachycardia, lowering blood pressure, diminishing erythrocyte counts, signs in the ultrasonogram of free fluid (blood) in the peritoneal cavity [M. Waxman and G. J. Baird: Corpus Luteum Hemorrhage, *J.A.M.A.*, **239:**2270–71, 1978]. The corpus luteum cyst is most likely to rupture at about the time of the onset of menses, which helps distinguish it from the symptomatic rupture of the graafian follicle, which normally occurs midcycle and causes the phenomenon of *mittelschmerz*.

Acute Intestinal Obstruction. Pain is almost invariably present from the onset, usually in the epigastrium or near the umbilicus, occasionally suprapubic. The pain is *spasmodic* and colicky from waves of peristalsis attempting to overcome an obstruction. In general, the higher the point of obstruction in the intestine, the more severe the symptoms and signs. *High Small Intestine.* The pain is most intense; the degree of shock greatest. Vomiting is early and severe; fecal vomitus is not produced, because of the location of the obstruction. If the vomitus contains *bile,* the obstruction is beyond the second portion of the duodenum. Abdominal distention appears *late,* and then is limited to the *epigastrium.* Loss of fluids and electrolytes produces *oliguria.* *Low Small Intestine.* The symptoms are less severe, vomiting is delayed, but the vomitus may have a more fecal character. A few hours after onset, *diffuse* abdominal distention occurs, causing a *ladderlike pattern* on the surface. Oliguria is not likely. *Colon.* The pain and shock are less than from obstruction of the small intestine. Vomiting is late and may be fecal. *Constipation* is invariable, but valuable time may be lost in discovering this because the bowel may first empty its contents below the obstruction. An empty rectal ampulla, void of gas, is strong presumptive evidence of colonic obstruction. This is appreciated when a digital rectal examination is done and the mucosal folds collapse around the palpating finger.

Clinical Occurrence. Adhesions from previous surgery within the abdomen are the most common cause of obstruction. Carcinoma in older patients is the next most common, followed by hernias, both inguinal and incisional, as well as internal. Of the other causes, intussusception is most common in infants. The remaining causes, volvulus, gallstones, and inflammatory strictures, contribute only 15% of the cases. Rarely the obstruction is caused by a bezoar [see following item].

Intestinal Obstruction: ***Bezoars.*** These are concretions formed in the gastrointestinal tracts of animals and man, usually formed of hair (*trichobezoar*), plant or fruit fibers (*phytobezoar*), or from medicines (aluminum hydroxide gel, or polystyrene sodium sulfonate)[M. D. Korenman, M. B. Stubbs, and J. C. Fish: Intestinal Obstruction from Medication Bezoars, *J.A.M.A.*, **240:**154–55, 1978].

Obstruction: ***Strangulated Hernia.*** Occlusion of the blood supply of protruding gut or omentum is produced by impingement on a hernial ring. In addition to the symptoms and signs of intestinal obstruction, one finds a *tender painful mass* at the hernial site. The patient usually has knowledge of the antecedent presence of a hernia; suddenly the gut or omentum moves into the hernial sac and becomes trapped, as it were, by virtue of the fact that vascular compromise has led to edema and swelling that does not allow the tissues to return to the abdomen, *incarceration*. The mass becomes painful, vomiting begins. A diagnosis of obturator hernia can only be made by feeling a tender mass per vaginam.

Obstruction with Medial Thigh Pain: ***Obturator Hernia.*** This is the herniation of a segment of small bowel through the obturator foramen of the pubis and ischium. Often only the side of intestine protrudes to form a *Richter's hernia*. In addition to the symptoms of intestinal obstruction and abdominal pain, *pain extends down the medial thigh* to the knee. This pain is augmented by thigh extension, abduction, and external rotation. The preferred position of the thigh is in flexion and external rotation and adduction. Palpation through rectum and vagina may reveal a soft, tender mass in the region of the obturator foramen. The hernia is rarely diagnosed before it has caused intestinal obstruction.

Clinical Occurrence. Usually in thin women over 60 years old.

Obstruction: ***Intussusception.*** This is the commonest cause of intestinal obstruction in infants, where the exciting factor may be trivial, such as a viral infection. In adults, the underlying cause is usually neoplasm in the intestinal wall. Intussusception is the invagination of one segment of gut into the lumen of another part. There are four types: ileum into ileum, ileum into ileocecal valve, ileocecal valve into colon, and colon into colon (Fig. 7-31). The enfolded portion always points *down* the fecal stream. Besides the general symptoms and signs of

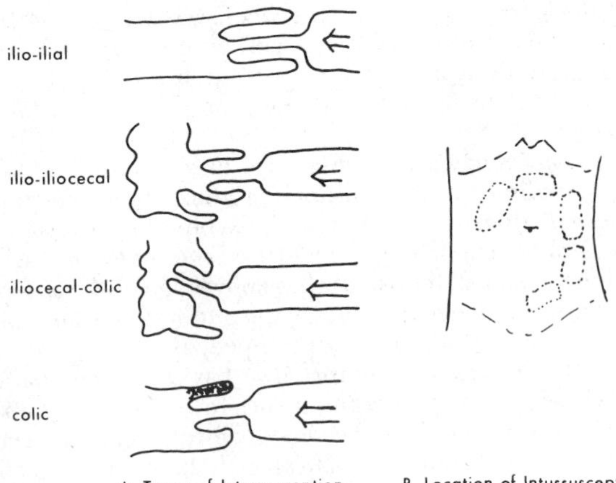

Fig. 7-31. Intussusception. *This is defined as the prolapse of one segment of intestine into another adjoining segment.* **A.** Four types of intussusception. *In all, the enfolding of the lumen is in the direction of fecal flow,as shown by the arrows. In the intracolic type, the stippling indicates a neoplasm that is usually the cause of the telescoping.* **B.** *The usual locations of palpable masses are shown as sausage-shaped outlines, usually in the colon.*

intestinal obstruction, *mucus* and sometimes *blood* are passed from the rectum. The intussusception forms a painful, tender, *sausage-shaped mass* of distinctive size. The lesion can be visualized by ultrasonography, and if one of the latter three types described, which involve the colon, by radiographic contrast study of the colon. Hydrostatic pressure, generated by the study, may be used to reduce the intussusception, thus avoiding surgical intervention.

Obstruction: Colonic Cancer. This is the second most common cause of intestinal obstruction in persons over 50 years of age. Gradually increasing constipation culminates suddenly in the onset of symptoms and signs of low intestinal obstruction. In patients being evaluated for intestinal obstruction by radiographic means, studies of the upper gastrointestinal tract, may occlude. If cancer is suspected in the colon, have the colon examined with a barium enema before giving barium by mouth.

If the obstruction is in the right colon, the cecum suddenly *distends* and forms a *painful rounded mass* in the right lower quadrant. With cancer of the left colon, the descending limb gradually distends, as readily disclosed by palpation and by the plain x-ray film. Tests for fecal blood are commonly positive in persons with colonic neoplasms.

Obstruction: ***Volvulus.*** This is torsion of the gut upon itself, which results in a closed loop obstruction. The site is usually in the cecum or the sigmoid colon and occurs as a result of hypofixation of the bowel, allowing it to rotate upon its mesentery. Distinctive diagnosis is dependent upon identification of a massively distended loop of large bowel, often to enormous proportion, rotating up and out of the pelvis. A *bird beak* cutoff is noted in the barium column of the colon and is pathognomonic. Proctosigmoidoscopy, in the case of sigmoid volvulus, and colonoscopy, in the case of cecal volvulus, may be used both diagnostically and therapeutically.

▼ *Key Symptom:* ***Chronic Abdominal Pain.*** Frequently pain is the symptom that attracts the patient's attention to many chronic abdominal disorders. Lacking pain, the presenting manifestation is often anorexia, nausea, vomiting, constipation, diarrhea, or hemorrhage. Or, unnoticed by the patient, physical examination may reveal ascites or a mass. Chronic disease of a viscus usually produces pain in the same location as that from acute processes (Fig. 7-27); but chronic pain is seldom so severe.

Chronic Abdominal Pain: ***Abdominal Wall Lesions.*** Both laymen and physicians have a remarkable tendency to project pain inward to intra-abdominal structures, when it actually arises from the abdominal wall. It takes a distinct effort to think of disorders of the abdominal wall; this has been the cause of many unnecessary laparotomies.

Clinical Occurrence [After E. D. Palmer: Two Cases of Nonvisceral Abdominal Wall Pain, *AFP*, 1978, p. 115]: SKIN: herpes zoster, infections, burns; MUSCLE: rectus abdominis rupture or hematoma, toxic spasms from spider bites, trichinosis, abscess: HERNIAS: epigastric, hypogastric, inguinal, incisional, Spigelian; BONE: lower rib fracture, slipping rib, xiphoidynia, metastatic lesions, herniated intervertebral disk: CONNECTIVE TISSUE: dermoid tumor, postlaparotomy inflammation; NERVE ROOT: leukemia, lymphoma, arthritis, herpes zoster; URACHUS: abscess, mucinous carcinoma. Rectus abdominis nerve entrapment syndrome.

Abdominal Wall Pain: ***Rectus Abdominis Nerve Entrapment Syndrome.*** Any intercostal nerve from T-7 to T-11 may be entrapped at the lateral border of the rectus sheath after it has traversed it. The pain usually occurs *proximal* to the entrapment site and is characterized by being *increased* when the patient raises the lower limb to tense the rectus muscles. The pain is temporarily relieved by the injection of local anesthetic agent into the trigger region. Entrapment may occur from overuse of the rectus muscles to compensate for instability of the lumbosacral spine, or fibromyositis of the abdominal wall [A. S. Tung, R. Tenicela, and J. Giovannitti: *J.A.M.A.,* **240:**738–39, 1978].

— *Chronic Epigastric Pain:* ***Xiphisternal Arthritis.*** The patient complains of epigastric or retrosternal pain that radiates to the back. Palpation elicits *tenderness* in the xiphisternal joint that reproduces the complaint. Injection of cortisone and lidocaine into the joint gives complete relief. When the xiphoid cartilage is *not palpated* the pain may be mistaken for that of angina pectoris, peptic ulcer, hiatal hernia, or chronic pancreatitis.

— *Chronic Epigastric Pain:* ***Peptic Ulcer.*** *Epitome: epigastric pain, 1 to 4 hours postprandially, with rhythmicity and periodicity; relieved by food, H_2 blockers, and alkali.* The symptoms are essentially similar whether the ulcer be gastric, pyloric, duodenal, or stomal (anastomotic, marginal). The initial cause of the lesion is controversial, but all agree that ulcer pain is produced by the action of gastric HCl in high concentration on inflamed surfaces or breakdown of the normal mucosal barrier to rather more normal amounts of acid. ***The Pain.*** Its attributes (PQRST) are usually diagnostic; *provocation*—fasting, drinking alcohol or coffee; *palliation*—ingestion of food or alkali; *quality*—gnawing, aching, burning, or hunger; *region*—in the epigastrium near the xiphoid, sometimes radiating to the back; *severity*—the pain may vary from mild discomfort to severe; *temporal relations*—when eating habits are regular and adjusted to nocturnal sleep, the pain has *rhythmicity;* it occurs 1 to 4 hours after meals and may awaken the patient between midnight and 2:00 A.M.; the afternoon pain is often the most severe; pain is rare before breakfast. Each episode of steady pain lasts at least 30 minutes, with spontaneous subsidence or persistence until the next meal relieves it. The symptoms also have *periodicity;* most often they occur twice a year, in June and between October and March. The periods last from a few days to several months; often the remissions are spontaneous. The factors inducing a symptomatic period are unknown. *Other Symptoms.* Constipation is frequent; but nausea, vomiting, and water brash are less common. The appetite is normal. *Curling's ulcer* is a special type in which a single or multiple lesions occur near the pylorus a few days after an external body burn; the ulcers may perforate or bleed. *Cushing's ulcer,* results from marked hypersecretion of gastric acid occurring after severe brain injury or following central nervous system surgical procedures. *Physical Signs.* Frequently there is *moderate tenderness* localized to an area about 3 cm in diameter just below the xiphoid. As Moynihan said, "Anamnesis is everything, the physical examination nothing." *Laboratory Findings.* High concentration of free HCl in the gastric juice is the rule in duodenal ulcer disease, less so with gastric ulcers. *X-ray Findings.* Usually an ulcer crater can be seen to confirm the diagnosis; occasionally one must treat the patient for an ulcer when the roentgenologist cannot find it. Upper gastrointestinal endoscopy has come, in many areas, to replace contrast studies to make the diagnosis. An added advantage to endoscopy is the ability to biopsy gastric lesions, which is necessary to differentiate ulcer from carcinoma. At the Mayo Clinic gastroscopic findings differed significantly from x-ray findings in 7 to 35% of cases [A. J. Cameron and B. J. Ott: The Value of Gastroscopy in Clinical Diagnosis, *Mayo Clin. Proc.,* **52:**806–808, 1977]. *Complications.* Hemorrhage, pyloric obstruction, perforation. The occurrence of peptic ulcer and renal calculus should prompt a search for hyperparathyroidism. In diseases of the stomach or duodenum that can be visualized by x-rays, gastroscopy should also be performed.

— *Abdominal Discomfort After Milk Drinking:* ***Lactase Deficiency.*** *Pathophysiology:* Lactose (milk sugar) in the small intestine of humans is hydrolyzed to glucose and galactose by the enzyme *lactase.* In lactase deficiency, either inherent or acquired, the surplus lactose enters the colon unhydrolyzed, only to be metabolized by the intestinal flora to *hydrogen,* CO_2*, and short-chain organic acids.* One cupful of milk thus produces four volumes of *flatus.* *Symptoms:* The metabolites, hydrogen, CO_2, and organic acids, are extremely irritating to the gut, causing *colicky abdominal pains, abdominal distention, borborygmi,* and *watery stools.* ***Laboratory Findings:*** The stools give a positive reaction with the Clinitest for glucose, since lactose is also a reducing substance. An hour after the ingestion of a loading dose of lactose, there is a rapid rise of hydrogen in the breath being tested. [See Editorial: Lactose Malabsorption and Lactose Intolerance, *Lancet,* **2:**831–32, 1979.]

Clinical Occurrence. *Inherent:* some individuals in all races; congenital, with autosomal dominance inheritance. Some Caucasians are homozygous for lactase deficiency after weaning; most nonCaucasians (Blacks, Orientals) are homozygous for lactase deficiency after weaning. *Acquired:* any enteropathy, malabsorption, sensitization to cow's milk, massive small-bowel resection, Whipple's disease, regional enteritis, cystic fibrosis, giardiasis, nonbacterial jejunitis.

— *Chronic Epigastric Pain:* ***Pyloric Obstruction.*** Usually obstruction results from duodenal scarring of peptic ulcer. Pain is not an invariable accompaniment; if present, it ranges from *vague discomfort* to *colicky pain* in the epigastrium, usually *soon after eating.* When vomiting occurs, *food may be rejected* that has been eaten many hours or days before. Bile-stained vomitus excludes the possibility of pyloric obstruction. Palpation of the abdomen may elicit a loud *succussion splash* in the stomach. Gastric aspiration may yield a liter or more of retained contents. Occasionally the condition is practically *symptomless,* and it is found only on x-ray examination of the stomach. When gastric retention is demonstrated, organic stenosis must be distinguished from neuromuscular disturbances causing spasm that subsides in a few days of rigorous treatment for peptic ulcer.

— *Chronic Epigastric Discomfort:* ***Postgastrectomy Syndromes.*** The considerable loss in stomach capacity from subtotal gastrectomy often results in the precipitous entrance of a hypertonic food mixture into the small intestine; this causes complex sequelae that are poorly understood. *Dumping Syndrome.* When a meal has nearly filled the abbreviated stomach, or *within 30 minutes afterward,* the patient experiences *epigastric discomfort* (not pain), weakness, pallor, sweating, nausea (but not vomiting), palpitation, and a feeling of epigastric fullness. *Reclining* often relieves the symptoms. Certain foods, particularly those with high osmotic loads, such as creamed vegetable soups, elicit the syndrome. *Hypoglycemic Syndrome.* More than *two hours after eating,* some symptoms of hypoglycemia appear: sweating, trembling, weakness, hunger, nausea, vomiting. If a 6-hour glucose-tolerance test is performed, giving the sugar by mouth, a period of hyperglycemia is followed by sudden hypoglycemia that is accompanied by the symptoms elicited in the history. The disorder causes weight loss or inability to gain weight, iron deficiency, and a deficit in vitamin B_{12} (after 3 years), with their attendant syndromes.

— *Chronic Epigastric Pain:* **Diaphragmatic (Hiatal) Hernia.** This is described on p. 247.

— *Chronic Epigastric Pain:* **Pancreatitis.** The chronicity is established by a history of repeated similar attacks, any of which seems identical with those of acute pancreatitis (p. 543). As time passes, the acute seizures become more frequent, but there are no symptoms during remissions. In the late stages, the painful attacks are accompanied by symptoms and signs of diabetes and steatorrhea. A palpable pancreatic pseudocyst may develop. *Laboratory Findings.* Fat in the stools, glycosuria. *X-ray Findings.* Calcification in the pancreas may be visible on the x-ray films.

— *Chronic Epigastric Pain:* **Gastric Carcinoma.** Relatively late in the disease *pain* begins. If ulceration is present, the pain may resemble closely that of peptic ulcer (p. 560). Or the pain may be a *steady unremitting ache* in the epigastrium, sometimes radiating to the back. Usually the appearance of the pain will be preceded by anorexia, loss of weight, and weakness; none of these symptoms is characteristic of peptic ulcer. Upper gastrointestinal endoscopy and biopsy distinguishes between the two.

— *Chronic RUQ Pain:* **Chronic Cholecystitis With or Without Calculi.** The pain in the gallbladder region ranges from *continual ill-defined distress* to recurring attacks of *biliary colic.* In the latter type, paroxysms of *colicky pain* occur in the RUQ and often radiate to the *right scapula;* deep inspiration intensifies the pain, causing inspiratory arrest (Murphy's sign, p. 516). Usually *deep tenderness* is localized to a portion of the lower margin of the liver. *Fist percussion tenderness* (p. 515) is usually present during the attack and for several days afterward. Although observable icterus is rare, transient increase in the *serum bilirubin* is common when gallstones have contributed to the attack. *X-ray Findings.*

Cholecystography with dye given orally frequently, but not invariably, results in nonvisualization of the gallbladder. When gallstones contain calcium, they may be seen in the x-ray film without the administration of opaque dye; noncalcified stones may be seen as negative shadows when the dye is given. High resolution real time ultrasonography permits thorough examination of the gallbladder area. Two authors have suggested the technique will replace cholecystography for the diagnosis of cholelithiasis [P. L. Cooperberg and H. J. Burhenne: Real Time Ultrasonography, *New Engl. J. Med.*, **302:**1277–79, 1980.]. A newer approach to the diagnosis of acute biliary disease employs gamma-emitting agents for hepatobiliary scanning. ^{99m}Tc-DISIDA(2,6 diisopropylphenyl-carbamoylmethyl aminodiacetic acid) is rapidly cleared from the blood, excreted by the liver, and appears in the biliary duct system. The gallbladder visualizes when the cystic duct is patent and then appearance of the tracer in the duodenum confirms common duct patency [C. A. Suarez, F. Block, D. Bernstein, A. Sefarini, G. Rodman, and R. Zeppa: The Role of H.I.D.A./P.I.P.I.D.A. Scanning in Diagnosing Cystic Duct Obstruction, *Ann. Surg.*, **191:**391–96, 1980].

— *Chronic RUQ Pain:* ***Hepatic Carcinoma.*** Probably the key to the diagnosis is usually the palpation of a mass in the liver. Occasionally, *nondescript pain* or discomfort is the entering complaint. Often the attendant symptoms are anorexia, loss of weight, and weakness. Seldom does the patient notice the hepatic enlargement until the examiner calls attention to it. The neoplasm may be primarily in the liver, a *hepatoma,* or secondary multiple metastases. The liver is often *stony hard,* a consistency that resembles no other process except hepatic cirrhosis, which is a virtually coexistent condition for hepatic carcinoma in the United States. When a single compact mass is felt in the liver, hepatoma or abscess should be suspected; but hepatoma is more likely to arise among the other nodules of hepatic cirrhosis. Occasionally, a *peritoneal friction rub* or a *bruit* may occur near the mass. Jaundice may be present when neoplasm has obstructed major branches of the biliary tree. A mass in the liver, accompanied by erythrocytosis and normal arterial saturation of oxygen, should suggest hepatoma with ectopic erythropoietin production. Alpha-fetoproteins are elevated in 80% of those with hepatoma and, in Third World countries, serum markers often show evidence of past viral hepatitis. *X-ray Findings.* A scintiscan of the liver after the administration of radioisotopes intravenously may delineate a single or multiple masses of nonfunctioning tissue. Arteriograms often show either neovascularity or a tumor stain in the sinusoidal phase.

— *Chronic Upper Abdominal Pain:* ***Carcinoma of the Pancreas.*** Although the disease may be *painless,* one of three patterns of pain often occurs: *colicky pain,* often in the RUQ; *constant dull pain* in the midepigastrium with *low back pain; paroxysmal periumbilical pain,* radiating widely to chest and back. *Anorexia, vomiting,* and extreme *weight loss* are common. Diarrhea occurs in a few, but constipation is more frequent. *Physical Signs.* Without metastases, there are usually no specific signs. Perhaps the best clue in some cases is the picture of an ill-nourished patient who spends most of his time in a chair, leaning forward to secure some relief from severe back and abdominal pain. When the head of the pancreas is involved, as is most often the case, early *painless persistent jaundice* is the rule. As the tumor enlarges the nearly universal triad of pain, weight loss, and jaundice ensues. The first sign of pancreatic carcinoma may be *superficial migrating thrombophlebitis.* Metastases cause hepatomegaly, distended gallbladder, ascites, and peripheral edema. A mass in the epigastrium is usually a late occurrence. *Laboratory Findings.* No tests are diagnostic. Serum trypsin and exopeptidase may be elevated in either carcinoma or pancreatitis. Radioactive photoscanning and pancreatic angiography may contribute evidence. *X-ray Findings.* Widening of the duodenal loop demonstrated by upper gastrointestinal series may support the diagnosis. Endoscopic retrograde cholangiopancreatography and cytology of pancreatic secretions may be useful. *Diagnosis.* In general, biochemical tests have failed as aids to diagnosis, and the classic x-ray examination of the pancreas was no more successful. But the recent rapid advances in ultrasonography and computed tomography have increased diagnostic accuracy manyfold. Ultrasonography should precede tomography because it is the less expensive of the two procedures [J. R. Malagelada: Pancreatic Cancer. An Overview of Epidemiology, Clinical Presentation, and Diagnosis, *Mayo Clinic Proc.,* **54:**459–67, 1979].

— *Chronic Upper Abdominal Pain:* ***Abdominal Angina*** (Visceral Ischemia Syndrome, Intestinal Ischemia S., Duodenal Compression, Celiac Artery S., Superior Mesenteric Artery S.). This is a type of abdominal pain believed to be provoked by visceral ischemia from lesions in one or more regional arteries. The name *angina* derives from a supposed analogy with angina pectoris in which the pain is thought to be caused by insufficiency of the coronary artery. This visceral ischemia is characterized by a triad of *postprandial pain, anorexia* from fear of eating, and *weight loss*. Usually the pain is in the upper abdomen or the periumbilical region; sometimes it radiates to the back. It is typically intermittent, often coming on 30 minutes after eating, and persisting from 20 minutes to three hours. But many persons notice no relation of the pain to meals and no response to attempted alleviation. *Diarrhea* is fairly frequent; occasionally occult fecal blood is found. Sometimes a *short systolic bruit* is audible in the epigastrium or the umbilical regions. ***X-ray Findings.*** No abnormalities are found in visualizing the gastrointestinal tract with barium. If the clinical course merits surgical operation, aortograms should be obtained; partial or complete occlusion of branches of the celiac or superior mesenteric arteries may be demonstrated along with evidence of an increased collateral circulation. ***Pathophysiology.*** The abdominal pain has been attributed to visceral ischemia, augmented by postprandial congestion. Until recently the proof of the condition was purely anatomic and circumstantial. When a patient with abdominal pain had arteriography showing stenosis or occlusion of an artery in the region and demonstrated greater than a 35 mm Hg gradiant across a stenotic area, the surgeon performed bypass, endarterectomy, or reimplantation procedures. The patient either recovered from pain or his symptoms returned. But the premise that arterial stenosis causes the pain has now been attacked. Recently aortograms with both lateral and posteroanterior views were obtained from 50 patients without abdominal pain [D. C. Levin, and H. A. Baktaxe: High Incidence of Celiac Axis Narrowing in Asymptomatic Individuals, *Am. J. Roentenol. Radium Ther. Nucl. Med.,* **116:**426–29, 1972]. Twelve of the 50 patients had 50% narrowing in the proximal celiac axis. One of the twelve had an abdominal bruit; three had collateral circulation from the superior mesenteric artery. The authors concluded that operation should be undertaken only (1) when other causes of pain had been excluded and (2) when the symptoms were serious and unrelenting. ***Diagno-***

sis. Only made by surgical exploration, measurement of arterial gradiants and flow characteristics, and subsequent therapeutic test.

Clinical Occurrence. Atherosclerosis; compression of the celiac artery by the arcuate ligament of the diaphragm when the artery joins the aorta above the diaphragm; fibromuscular hyperplasia, neoplasia, embolism, polyarteritis nodosa, thromboangiitis obliterans, carcinoid [J. Bricker, L. G. Bartholomew, J. C. Cain, and M. A. Adson: Syndrome of Intestinal Arterial Insufficiency ("Abdominal Angina"), *Arch. Intern. Med.,* **117**:632–38, 1966].

The Rectosigmoid

The rectosigmoid may be thought of as a field of diagnostic examination in the terminal colon, accessible to palpation through the anus and available to inspection through the sigmoidoscope for a distance of about 25 cm, which limits the extent of the region (Fig. 7-32). The limits have been extended beyond this by the flexible fiberoptic instruments. The rectosigmoid region includes the anus, the rectum, and the distal portion of the sigmoid colon that can be reached with the sigmoidoscope. Since the sigmoidoscope is merely a type of speculum, employed in the physician's office or clinic without anesthesia, its use should be considered part of the examination of the abdomen.

Rectosigmoid Examination

METHOD OF RECTOSIGMOID EXAMINATION. **The methods of examination are inspection, with or without specula, and palpation. The patient may be examined in several positions, each with its advantages and disadvantages (Fig. 7-33). The *left lateral prone position* (Sims's position) permits adequate inspection of the perianal region and the anal mucosa with a speculum. Palpation of the anal canal and rectum is feasible. The position is not desirable for digital palpation of the peritoneal contents through the rectum, because masses tend to fall away from the examining finger. It can be employed on a patient who is extremely weak and confined to bed. The *lithotomy position* is probably most used for routine examination where no detailed inspection of the anus is required. Examination in this position is facilitated by having the buttocks raised on an overturned bedpan or pillow. It affords convenience in palpation of the rectum and is necessary to feel the contents of the peritoneal cavity. It**

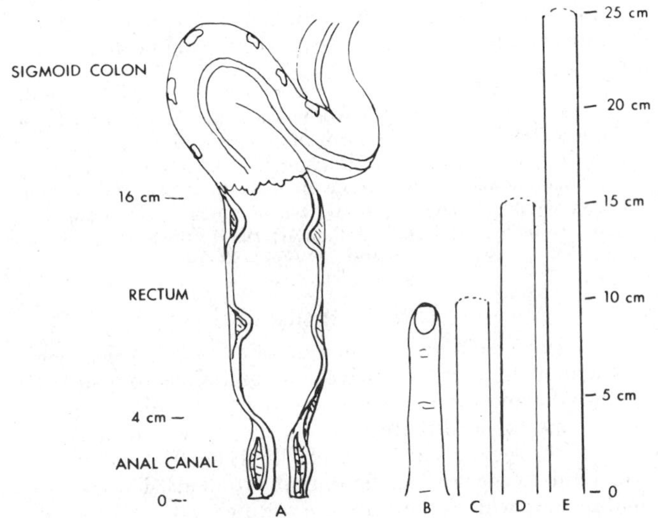

Fig. 7-32. Comparison of lengths of rectosigmoid segments with rigid examining instruments. *All lengths are drawn to scale.* **A.** *The rectosigmoid is shown with the anal canal of 4 cm, the rectum and valves of Houston of 12 cm, and the lower part of the sigmoid colon whose total length is 40 cm.* **B.** *An average index finger, 10 cm long and 22 mm in diameter.* **C.** *A typical anoscope, 9 cm, with an added 1 cm of curved obturator.* **D.** *A proctoscope of 15 cm.* **E.** *Sigmoidoscope of 25 cm. The newer fiberoptic flexible instruments are considerably longer.*

cannot be employed with the specula. Most uncomfortable for the patient, the *knee-chest* or *knee-elbow position* should be reserved for examination with specula, preferably supporting the patient on a special table; but lack of this elegant article should not defer or deter the examination. The *standing position,* with the patient leaning over and resting the trunk on a table, may also be employed for speculum examination and palpation of the rectum.

The Anus

The anal canal, from 2.5 to 4 cm long in the adult, is the terminal part of the colon. The tube is surrounded by two concentric layers of voluntary muscle, the *external* and *internal sphincters.* The external muscle is voluntary, the internal one is involuntary. A small band of the external sphincter overrides

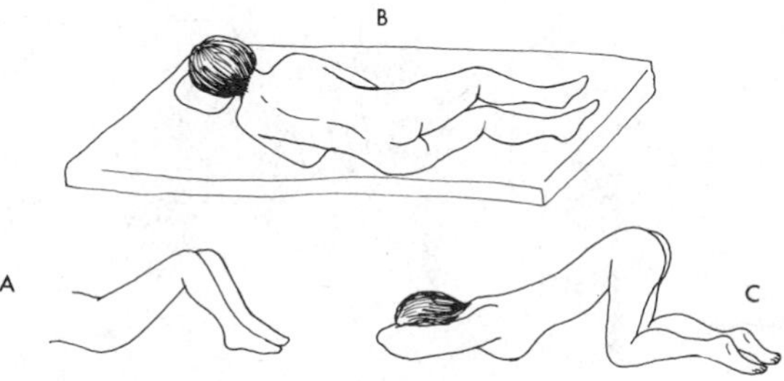

Fig. 7-33. Positions of the patient for rectal examination. **A.** *Modified lithotomy position.* **B.** *Left lateral prone position (Sim's position).* **C.** *The knee-chest position.*

the end of the internal sphincter and thus is felt first by the entering finger, although the name of the muscle refers to its being outside the internal sphincter, rather than to its superficial position in the body. The mucosal lining of the lumen extends slightly outside the sphincter, so the mucocutaneous junction may be exposed to inspection without a speculum. For the structure of the anal mucosa, consult Fig. 7-34. When inserting a finger or speculum, it is important to remember that the anal canal slants obliquely downward and backward, so the axis of entry should point toward the umbilicus.

Examination of the Perineum

INSPECTION OF THE PERINEUM. **In whatever position selected for the patient, the buttocks should be spread wide apart. Inspect the skin of the perineum and perianal region for signs of local inflammation, sinuses, fistulas, and bulges. The mucocutaneous junction may be seen by everting tension on the skin of each side of the anus.**

Pruritus Ani. Although pruritus is a symptom, the signs of chronic itching are evident in the perianal skin containing excoriations and thickening (lichenification). Unfortunate patients affected have a maddening uncontrollable desire to scratch; however, any relief of pain is very short-lived. When the involved skin is moist, the pruritus is usually caused by infection with bacteria or fungi or by pinworms, *Enterobius vermicularis,* in children. When dry, the cause is presumably neurogenic.

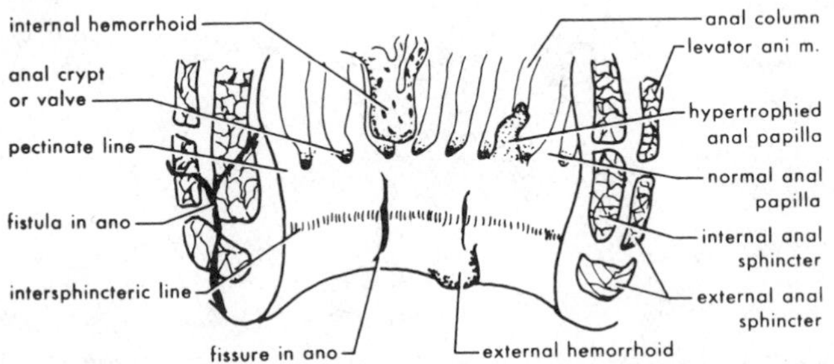

Fig. 7-34. Anatomy of the anal canal. *The diagram shows the interior and cross section of the canal. The anal columns (c. of Morgagni) descend vertically from the rectum and end in anal papillae that fuse to form the pectinate or dentate line; behind are the anal valves (crypts of Morgagni). The cut walls show the internal anal sphincter surrounded by the external sphincter that protrudes distally. The junction between the edges of the two sphincters forms the intersphincteric line. Internal hemorrhoids arise proximal to the pectinate line, external hemorrhoids distally. Two anal fissures are shown, one distal to a resulting hypertrophied papilla. A fistula (black and irregular) drains from an abscess in a rectal crypt (or valve) to the skin near the anus.*

Coccygeal Sinus (Pilonidal Sinus). Rarely a congenital tract extends from the coccyx or sacrum to the perineum where it usually drains to the exterior in the midline posterior to the anus (Fig. 7-35A). The sinus is lined with epithelium and hairs, hence the alternate name of *pilonidal.* When the tract becomes blocked, it may form a tender *dimple* or *bulge* just below the coccyx, or one side, usually the left. Many authors now consider most lesions to be acquired from the embedding of hairs in the skin and underlying tissue, although the associated finding of an increased incidence of spina bifida occulta among patients with the disorder supports the congenital pathogenesis.

Fistula in Ano. A track from an anorectal fissure in the anal canal drains externally through the perianal skin. According to *Salmon's law* (Fig. 7-35), when the fistula is posterior to the anus or more than one inch (2.5 cm) from the anus anteriorly, the abscess is in the posterior anal canal; fistulas draining anterior, closer than one inch to the orifice, come from abscesses in the anterior part of the canal. *Goodsell's rule* simply states

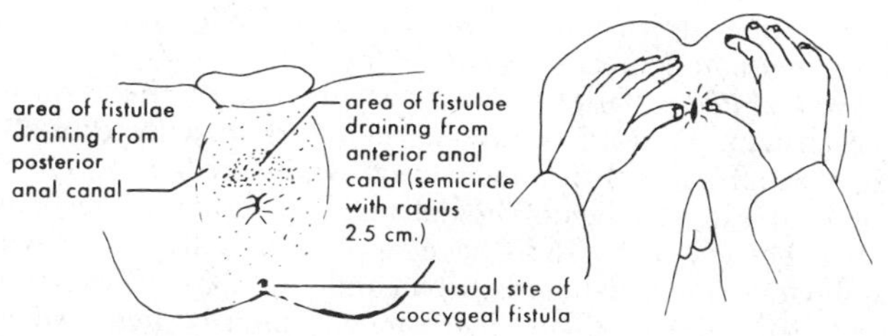

Fig. 7-35. Examination of the perineum. **A.** Fistulae in the perineum. *The heavily stippled semicircular area anterior to the anus, with a radius of 1 inch (2.5 cm), covers the location of fistulae on the skin that may be expected to drain from the anterior surface of the anal canal, according to Salmon's law. Anal fistulae draining to the skin in the lightly stippled area come from abscesses in the posterior surface of the canal. A coccygeal fistula (pilonidal) is usually in the midline, near coccyx or sacrum.* **B.** Retraction of the anus externally. *This illustrates a method of stretching the anal orifice for inspection of a fissure in ano, external hemorrhoids, or prolapsing internal hemorrhoids or polyps.*

that posterior sites drain posterior to a line between the ischial tuberosities; anterior ones drain radially from their points of origin. Gentle palpation around the orifice of the fistula may reveal the course of the track as a subcutaneous cord. Fistulas should not be probed from the exterior, but the source should be sought from the inside through the anoscope.

Fissure in Ano. Early, the lesion appears as a slitlike separation of the superficial anal mucosa, suggesting a longitudinal tear. The extreme pain associated with the condition is due to spasm of the anal sphincter. If the patient complains of pain in the region, do not attempt a digital examination before inspecting the terminal mucosa by retracting the skin on both sides and looking for the fissure posteriorly (Fig. 7-35B). It is an extreme unkindness to the patient to attempt further examination without either analgesics being given, or even an anesthetic. Chronicity leads to the presence of an ulcerating crater with evidence of secondary infection.

External Hemorrhoids. Around the anal orifice, ragged tabs of skin are certainly external hemorrhoids (Fig. 7-34). When inflamed, they are red and tender and sometimes must be distinguished from internal hemorrhoids by following them to their origin below the pectinate line.

Sentinel Pile. Various authors seem to apply this term to two structures. More commonly, it refers to a hyperplastic tag of skin frequently found external to a fissure in ano, resembling an external hemorrhoidal tag; also called *fibrous anal polyp.* The name has also been applied to a hypertrophied anal papilla internal to a fissure in ano (Fig. 7-34). This lesion arises from the pectinate line, while an internal hemorrhoid arises above it.

Rectal Prolapse. When the patient strains, as if to defecate, the rectal mucosa may evert below the sphincter (Fig. 7-36). If the patient complains of this occurrence but the procedure fails to demonstrate, have him squat and strain in the position for defecation. The prolapse may be either *mucosal* or *complete;* in the latter case the sphincters are included.

Internal Hemorrhoids. On straining, internal hemorrhoids may prolapse into view as red masses covered with mucosa (Fig. 7-36). If they cannot be seen in this manner, they must be viewed through the anoscope because nonthrombosed hemorrhoids are not palpable.

Perianal Hematoma. During a bout of acute abdominal pain the occurrence of a perianal hematoma should suggest the dissection and leakage of the abdominal aorta. In a case report, the hematoma appeared two hours after the vessel ruptured. Extravasated blood discolored the perianal skin for a radius

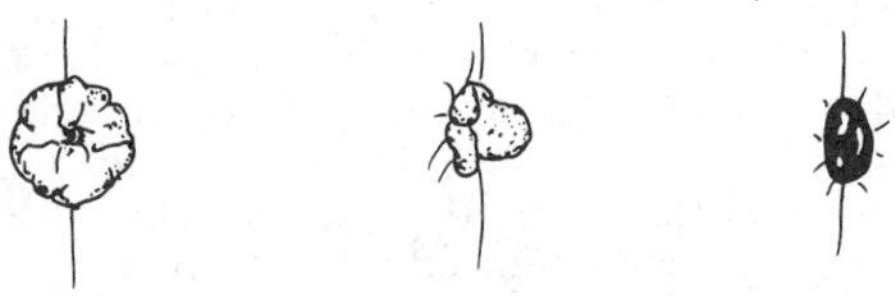

Fig. 7-36. Some external anal findings. **A.** *Rectal prolapse appears as a red doughnut of most rectal mucosa protruding through the anus.* **B.** *Thrombosed external hemorrhoids are semispheric masses of erythematous skin at the mucocutaneous junction with the anus.* **C.** *Internal hemorrhoids are mucosal masses sometimes seen through the retracted anus.* **D.** *Fistulous opening in the skin is accompanied by a papule of hypertrophied skin on the margin of the orifice.*

of 4 to 5 cm. Laparotomy showed a tear in an aneurysm on the posterior wall of the abdominal aorta; the hematoma had spread into the sigmoid mesocolon and between the levatores ani [S. K. Tamvakopoulous, W. P. Corvese, and L. L. Vargas: Perianal Hematoma—Sign of Leakage After Rupture of Aortic Aneurysm, *N. Engl. J. Med.*, **280:**548–49, 1969]. For those whose memories need further help, this might be called the *blackbottom sign.*

▼ ***Key Symptom: Pain in the Perineum.*** Perineal pain accompanies many disorders in the pelvis; but with few exceptions, the diagnosis must be made by the physical examination rather than the history. Many anatomic structures are concerned:

Clinical Occurrence: SKIN: intertrigo, eczema, condyloma. ANAL REGION: thrombosed hemorrhoids, fissure in ano, fistula in ano, anal ulcer, folliculitis, carcinoma. VAGINA: vaginitis, inflammation of Bartholin's glands, cystocele, rectocele, epithelioma. TESTIS: perineal position of undescended testis. URETHRA: injury or rupture, fistula, urethritis, urethral calculus. BLADDER: cystitis, calculus, carcinoma, tuberculosis. PROSTATE: acute prostatitis, abscess, calculus, carcinoma. WITHOUT PHYSICAL SIGNS: proctalgia fugax.

— *Brief Intense Perineal Pain:* ***Proctalgia Fugax*** (*fugax* = fleeting). This is more common in men than women. Often the patient is awakened from a sound sleep with intense pain in the perineum, near the coccyx or within the rectum. The paroxysm attains an agonizing climax in 1–2 minutes, impelling the patient to arise and walk about. The pain subsides rapidly and completely in about 5 minutes. Relief is obtained by pressure on the perineum or an enema of warm water. Occasionally the paroxysm is initiated by straining at stool, prolonged sitting on a hard surface, or ejaculation. The mechanism is attributed to spasm of the Sacrococcygeus or Levator ani muscles.

— *Brief Intense Perineal Pain:* ***Familial Rectal Pain.*** Several families have been studied with an autosomal dominant-gene-transmitted disorder in which the affected persons experience *excruciating pain near the anus* shooting down the legs. The pains last about a minute and are followed by a profound *skin flush* beginning on the buttocks and genitalia, progressing down the posterior aspect of one or both thighs and legs. Most often this pain is initiated by defecation or trauma to the perineum. The onset is during infancy and the affected person develops fear of defecation until he learns to pass feces slowly and gently. Although defecation is the most common triggering stimulus, the pains are occasionally initiated by micturition, rectal and vaginal examinations, coitus, or labor. Some families have associated pains in the eyes or jaws [R. E. Dugan: Familial Rectal Pain, *Lancet,* **1:**854, 1972; T. P. Mann, and J. E. Cree: *Ibid.,* **1:**1016–17, 1972].

ANAL PALPATION. **Cover the exploring index finger with a rubber glove or finger cot. With the patient in the lithotomy position, palpate the perineum gently around the orifice of sinuses and fistulas for subcutaneous cords giving clues to the direction of tracks. Palpate any bulges in the perineal tissue. Then press the finger in the tissue around the anal orifice for tender abscesses, especially searching for ischiorectal abscesses between the anus and the ischial tuberosities. Reassure the patient about the examination and have him breathe deeply through the mouth. Lubricate the tip of the covered examining finger with surgical jelly and place the *pad* of the finger on the anal sphincter (Fig. 7-37). Press gently and slowly until the sphincter relaxes and admits the curve of the pad. Then rotate the pad, admitting the tip of the finger also. Gradually insert the finger as far as possible, directing attention to the tactile sensations along the tract. When inserting the finger, point it in the direction of the umbilicus. Proper manipulation should not be painful unless a fissure in ano or a thrombosed hemorrhoid be present. While the finger passes through the anal canal, a distance of two inches (4 cm), estimate the caliber of the canal and the sphincter tone; feel for *masses.* To feel the abscess causing a fistula, use bidigital palpation between index finger in the canal and the thumb on the skin of the perineum.**

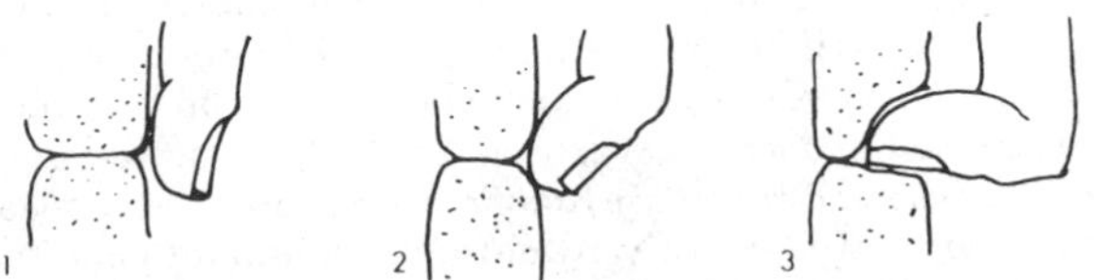

Fig. 7-37. Insertion of the finger into the anus for examination. **(1)** *The pad of the gloved index finger is placed gently over the orifice, until the external sphincter is felt to relax.* **(2)** *Then the tip of the finger is rotated into the axis of the canal and inserted gently.* **(3)** *Finally the finger is pushed farther through the canal. The entire procedure should be slow and gentle. The physician who rushes this procedure should be condemned to have this done to him.*

Ischiorectal Abscess. This may not give visible signs because it is deep-seated. Tenderness on deep palpation between anus and ischial tuberosity locates the site.

Tight Sphincter: ***Apprehension.*** The most common cause of a tight anal sphincter is apprehensiveness of the patient. Some have had previous experience with a rough examination and know that it may be excruciatingly painful. Preliminary verbal assurance from the physician should be supported with appropriate actions by him. Gently and slowly increase the pressure of the finger pad on the sphincter, then insert the tip. When one feels the sphincter tighten, arrest the movement for a minute, leaving the finger in place until the sphincter is felt to relax; then push a little further. The patient will be pleasantly surprised at the lack of pain and consider you more skillful than your predecessor. While the procedure may be uncomfortable, it should not be painful.

Tight Sphincter: ***Fissure in Ano.*** When the sphincter is in spasm that cannot be relaxed by gentleness, suspect a fissure and search through the anoscope, but only after an analgesic or anesthetic has been administered.

Tight Sphincter: ***Anal Stricture.*** When digital insertion is attempted, the tip of the finger is obstructed by dense fibrous bands that narrow the canal. Such strictures most commonly develop secondarily to operative procedures performed upon the anal canal, usually extensive hemorrhoidectomies. This condition is to be distinguished from fibrosis of the sphincters, next discussed.

Tight Sphincter: ***Fibrosis of Anal Muscles.*** The entire canal is narrowed so the finger feels encased in a rigid tube. This is caused by senile fibrosis of the anal muscles, frequently producing the fecal impaction of which the patient complains.

Tight Sphincter: ***Anal Carcinoma.*** This neoplasm is an infrequent cause of narrowing of the anal canal. In its later stages it becomes fungating and readily visible. The squamous cell cancer may cause pruritus and skin changes, which ought to lead to biopsy to confirm the diagnosis.

Relaxed Sphincter: ***Lacerated Anal Muscles.*** Commonly, a deficit in the anal sphincter is the result of perianal laceration during childbirth; occasionally, it is a poor result of operation for fistula in ano. When the anus is retracted by pulling the skin from each side, a dimple is visible in the posterior part of the anal ring. The sphincter feels weak when the finger is inserted.

Relaxed Sphincter: ***Atony of the Muscles.*** Especially in early tabes dorsalis, and occasionally in other lesions of the spinal cord, the sphincter is atonic. The finding should prompt a careful neurologic examination.

Anal Intermuscular Abscess. Abscesses between the muscles of the anus cause agonizing pain during defecation and discomfort during sitting. In *high abscesses* a tender mass is felt just above the anorectal junction. *Low abscesses* are most frequently found with bidigital palpation near the distal end of the anal canal.

ANOSCOPIC EXAMINATION. **The anal canal is not inspected routinely, but the procedure is indicated when external signs, palpable masses in the canal, sphincter spasm, pain, or bleeding direct attention to the region. The anal canal can be viewed only when examined through a speculum. Although the proctoscope or the sigmoidoscope may be used for this purpose, the anoscope is specifically designed for the procedure. The instrument is available in many styles and sizes. Essentially, it is a tube fitted with an obturator whose tip is suitably rounded and conical. The tube is usually about 9 cm long and is available in diameters from 8 to 22 mm, to suit the size of the canal. Operating anoscopes often have a complete or partial longitudinal slit in the cylinder for access to lesions in the canal. The simple diagnostic types are usually not equipped with built-in lights, but depend for illumination on direct light from the outside or reflected light from a head mirror. Plastic disposable anoscopes are available that have the advantages of allowing visualization through the scope walls. *After palpation has demonstrated no obstruction,* anoscopic examination can proceed. The patient is placed in the left lateral prone, the knee-chest or knee-elbow, or the standing position leaning over a table. A good light must be ensured. With the obturator completely filling the tube, the instrument is well lubricated with surgical jelly. The tip of the obturator and its surrounding tube is gently inserted through the sphincter, aiming the instrument at the umbilicus. When the tube is inserted more than 2 inches (5 cm), the obturator is removed and the interior inspected. Slowly the tube is withdrawn, inspecting the walls of the canal as they close behind the receding tip of the tube. The findings are discussed in the order they are likely to appear as the tube is being withdrawn.**

Prolapsed Rectal Polyp. When pedunculated, polyps in the lower rectum may be seen in the anoscope as spheric masses covered with mucosa. Their origin can be seen as definitely in the rectal mucosa.

Internal Hemorrhoids. Irregular globular masses, covered with mucosa, arise above the pectinate line and may prolapse into the anal canal (Fig. 7-34). They are distinguished from external hemorrhoids that arise below the pectinate line and are covered with skin. Their surface is not so regular as that of rectal polyps.

Internal Orifice of Fistula in Ano. Most fistulae in ano arise from abscesses in the anal crypts (crypts of Morgagni), and the internal orifices of their tracks can be found just above the pectinate line, where they may be probed (Fig. 7-35A).

Clinical Occurrence. Single fistulas arise from nonspecific causes. Multiple fistulas are especially found in tuberculous proctitis, regional ileitis, ulcerative colitis, bilharziasis, lymphogranulomatous stricture of the rectum, and colloid carcinoma.

Hypertrophy of Anal Papilla (Sentinel Pile). Enlargement of an anal papilla occurs proximal to the chronic fissure in ano and is sometimes mistaken for an internal hemorrhoid or a rectal polyp. Its origin in the pectinate line should distinguish it (Fig. 7-34).

External Hemorrhoids. These are covered with skin and arise distal to the pectinate line. When they are thrombosed, they feel firm and are very painful to the patient. Their appearance may be purple-red, demonstrating the contained clotted blood. If there is sufficient edema of the overlying skin they may be white in color (Fig. 7-34).

Fissure in Ano. When this lesion cannot be seen externally by everting the anal mucosa, it is definitely diagnosed by anoscopic examination. It appears as a longitudinal laceration of the skin distal to the pectinate line (Fig. 7-34). It usually lies on the posterior surface of the canal. Chronic lesions stimulate hypertrophy of an anal papilla (sentinel pile).

The Rectum

The rectum is a specialized continuation of the colon, about 12 cm long. It begins in the sigmoid colon at the level of the

3rd sacral vertebra and ends at the entrance to the anal canal. Near its distal end it dilates to form the *rectal ampulla.* In the rectum are found four semilunar transverse folds, the *valves of Houston,* some of which are inconstant. Since the combined length of the anal canal and the rectum is about 16 cm, the 10-cm examining finger cannot reach the entire length. The upper two thirds of the rectum is covered by peritoneum. Below that point in the male, the anterior peritoneal surface extends downward as the *rectovesical pouch* to within 7.5 cm of the anal orifice, so it is readily accessible to the average examining finger, 9 or 10 cm in length. In the female, the *rectouterine pouch* extends downward anteriorly to within 5.5 cm of the anal orifice. Within reach of the finger in the rectum of the male are the prostate gland, the seminal vesicles, and the two lower valves of Houston, when present. In the female, the examining finger in the rectum can reach the cervix and fundus uteri, and the two lower rectal valves.

Examination of the Rectum

As discussed elsewhere (p. 522), three distinct and separate purposes are served in examination of the rectum: (1) palpation of the contents of the lower peritoneal cavity, (2) palpation of the adjacent internal genital organs in male and female, (3) examination of the walls of the rectum itself. While these three purposes are accomplished by the examination of one region, it is psychologically important to consider each in its proper setting, as a part of the abdominal examination, as a procedure in the examination of the genital organs, or as a search for intrinsic disease of the rectal wall.

Rectal Palpation. **This is a continuation of palpation of the anal canal; the finger is merely pushed beyond the rectoanal junction, and the walls of the ampulla are felt. After passing the rectoanal ring in the male, the finger encounters on the anterior wall in sequence: the prostate gland (p. 619), the seminal vesicles (p. 621), and the rectovesical pouch (p. 621). Posteriorly is the hollow of the sacrum and the coccyx. The lateral walls are also examined. On the anterior wall of the female, one encounters in sequence: cervix uteri (p. 625), the retroverted fundus uteri (p. 638), and the rectouterine pouch (p. 636). The rectal wall is palpated for masses and narrowing of the lumen.**

Benign Rectal Stricture. A congenital stricture is occasionally encountered as a narrow crescentic fold at the rectal entrance to the anal canal. This marks the imperfect fusion of the hindgut with the proctodeum. According to Bailey, a *fibrous stricture* in the same region is most likely the result of an operation for internal hemorrhoids. A *tubular stricture,* tough and rubbery, may be the result of lymphogranuloma venereum. A *sharply delimited stricture* is usually the result of x-ray or radium therapy for carcinoma.

Carcinoma of the Rectum. Cancer may cause plateau-like, nodular, annular, and cauliflower masses in the rectum. Further information should be sought by direct visualization and biopsy.

Rectal Polyps. Some of these lesions can be palpated, but they must be viewed through the speculum to be recognized.

Edema of the Rectal Wall. Sometimes volvulus of the pelvic colon produces massive edema of the rectal wall that can be readily palpated as extreme bogginess.

Coccygeal Tenderness. When the patient complains of pain in the region of the coccyx, *coccygodynia,* one should test for tenderness and pain in the sacrococcygeal joint. During digital examination of the rectum, place the index finger in the rectum on the anterior surface of the coccyx and press the posterior surface of the bone with the thumb on the skin outside. The bone is moved backward and forward to elicit pain in the joint. The coccyx may be abnormally directed by previous fracture or injury. This most commonly arises following the *humorous* practice of pulling a chair out from under an individual as he is sitting down. The pain can be extreme and may be exacerbated by sitting and upon defecation.

Chordoma of the Sacrum. Causing vague pain and spontaneous bladder or bowel dysfunction, an otherwise generally asymptomatic round and very firm rectal mass, occurs posterior to the rectal wall, where the sacrum ought to be. X-rays reveal a lytic expansile destructive lesion which displaces the rectum anteriorly [T. C. Kaiser, D. J. Pritchard, and K. K. Unni: Clinicopathologic Study of Sacrococcygeal Chordoma, *Cancer,* **54:**2574–78, 1984].

Fecal Impaction. The examining finger in the rectum discovers the lumen to be filled with hard dry masses of feces. These must be removed by breaking up and extracting the pieces with the finger. The symptoms leading to this finding may be vague. The patient may complain of constipation or obstipation; but sometimes there is diarrhea, the fecal stream passing around the impaction to produce incontinence. In debilitated or postoperative conditions, the patient may be merely restless, have fever or anorexia. The administration of barium suspensions as contrast media for x-ray examination is a common cause of impaction. It is for this reason that barium in the gastrointestinal tract is to be eschewed when abdominal surgery is done. The postoperative ileus allows for the maximum extraction of water from the fecal bolus. Patients experiencing the passage of such a barium-containing fecal mass have described the phenomenon as equivalent to giving breech birth to a porcupine.

Pulsatile Rectal Mass: ***Aneurysm of Internal Iliac (Hypogastric) Artery.*** On the back of the sacral portion of the pelvis lies a broad flat band consisting of the lumbosacral trunk and the sacral plexus; the components of the sciatic nerve emerge inferiorly from this plexus. The internal iliac (hypogastric) artery descends over the pelvic brim to lie directly in front of the nerves. An *aneurysm* of the artery can compress the plexus against the sacrum to produce *sciatica;* the dilated artery is felt as a *pulsating mass* during digital examination of the rectum. Three such cases have been reported [E. M. Chapman, R. S. Shaw, and C. S. Kubik: Sciatic Pain from Arteriosclerotic Aneurysm of Pelvic Arteries, *N. Engl. J. Med.*, **271**:1410, 1964].

The Sigmoid Colon

The sigmoid colon extends from the iliac flexure of the descending colon to the rectum. In the pelvis, the sigmoid runs transversely from the left ilium toward the right side of the pelvis. Doubling on itself, it passes leftward toward the midline, thence downward to meet the rectum at the level of the 3rd sacral vertebra, frequently forming a crude S from which the name is derived. The sigmoid colon is about 40 cm long, but the extent to which the lumen is accessible to inspection with a straight tube is limited by the turns in the mobile bowel that can be threaded on the rigid instrument (Fig. 7-38). This length governs the dimension of the sigmoidoscope, which is generally 25 cm long. Of this length 4 cm is taken up by the anal canal, 12 cm by the rectum, leaving

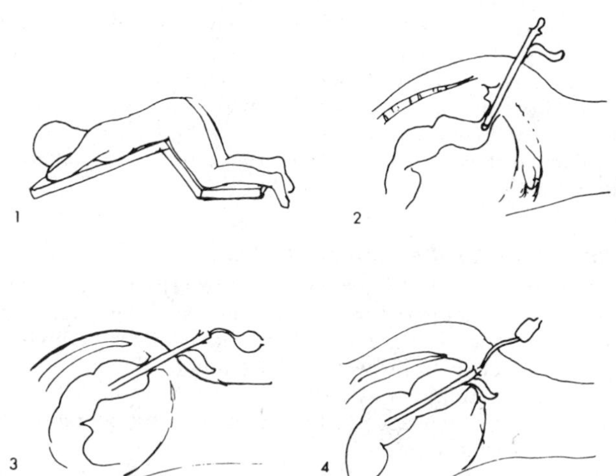

Fig. 7-38. Insertion of the rigid sigmoidoscope. *The patient assumes the knee-chest position, or on a special examining table he lies prone as in* (**1**). *First a digital examination of the anal canal is performed to ensure the absence of an obstructive lesion that would contraindicate passage of an instrument blindly.* (**2**) *The lubricated sigmoidoscope, with obturator in place, is held so the tip is aimed at the umbilicus; the tip of the obturator is pressed gently and slowly through the anal sphincters until the end of the tube is within the rectal ampulla. The obturator is then withdrawn and air is admitted to inflate the rectum; the rectal wall is then inspected. As the tip is inserted farther and moved about, the folds of the valves of Houston are encountered as partial or complete obstructing curtains to farther passage.* (**3**) *Under direct and continuous observation, a little air is pumped into the rectum and the folds are seen to open, almost like an iris diaphragm, pointing the direction for further insertion.* (**4**) *Finally the tube is passed the entire length or an impassible obstruction arrests ingress. The instrument is opened to the atmosphere and slowly withdrawn while the walls of the canal are inspected. If during the examination the "way" is lost, the scope is withdrawn several centimeters and started forward again.*

about 9 cm for the sigmoid colon. Sigmoidoscopic examination is an exceedingly useful aid in diagnosis. It permits inspection of a segment of bowel that is particularly difficult to examine satisfactorily with contrast medium and x-ray procedures. Previously it has been said that 75% of the polyps and carcinoma of the large bowel are within the reach of the instrument. The last two decades have seen an upward and to the right march of carcinomas and their precursors, polyps, so that colonoscopy and contrast studies, especially double contrast barium enemas, have become routine for complete examination and evaluation.

Examination of the Sigmoid Colon

The indications for sigmoidoscopy are (1) when attention is directed to the lower bowel by symptoms of bleeding, pain, constipation, or diarrhea; (2) when evidence of a pathologic process is obtained by inspection of the anus or digital examination of the rectum; (3) as part of a periodic examination of patients in the older age groups for the prevention and early detection of cancer.

METHOD OF SIGMOIDOSCOPIC EXAMINATION. **First make a digital examination of the rectum to *ensure the absence of an obstruction* in the anal canal or the lower rectal ampulla that would make blind insertion of a rigid tube dangerous. If possible, it is often helpful for the patient to have taken an oral cathartic the night before examination. Prepare the rectosigmoid by giving cleansing enemas until the returns are clear. If the patient is strong enough, place him in the knee-chest position on a table or bed. If he is too debilitated, the left lateral prone position (Sims's) is the best compromise (Fig. 7-33). Drape him carefully for minimum exposure of buttocks and genitalia. Before each step in the examination, explain to the patient what you are about to do. With the obturator in place, lubricate the tip of the instrument well with surgical jelly and insert it gently into the anus, aiming the tube in the direction of the patient's umbilicus (Fig. 7-38). Gradually ease the tip of the tube in to a depth of 5 cm (2 inches), when it should be past the anal canal. Withdraw the obturator to permit air at atmospheric pressure to inflate the rectal ampulla. Affix the lens cap to the tube, turn on the light, and inspect the walls of the ampulla. Under direct illumination, gradually push the instrument farther, changing the angle of the tube to pass the folds of the valves of Houston as they are encountered. To assist in this maneuver, cautiously pump air into the tube with the rubber bulb, using the minimum inflation necessary. Manipulate gently enough to avoid pain. At the depth of about 16 cm (6 inches), a sharp turn to the patient's right is usually encountered, marking**

entrance to the sigmoid colon. Attempt to engage the tip of the tube in the lumen of the sigmoid by changing the angle of the instrument, and insert the tube to its full length of 25 cm (10 inches). *Do not force the tube at any time;* better to be satisfied with a lesser distance. When ingress is arrested, gradually withdraw the tube, inspecting the entire circumference of the walls as withdrawal proceeds. During egress, deflate the gut lumen by opening the lens cup to the outside air. Finally, inspect the anal canal as the tube is being withdrawn.

Normal Variations in Rectal Mucosa. Great individual variation occurs in the vascular patterns visible in the rectal mucosa. The appearance varies normally in the same person. Enemas cause temporary hyperemia; the response is greatly accentuated when the enema solution is irritating. Especially in children, sometimes in adults with generalized lymphoid hyperplasia, the rectal walls appear pebbled from enlargement of the lymph follicles in the mucosa. Mucus is a normal secretion of the rectal epithelium, and the quantity is increased by emotional disturbances, inflammation, or sodium biphosphate in commercial enema fluids. A dry sticky bowel, the so-called *proctitis sicca,* results from a paucity of mucus, often encountered in patients with the cathartic habit.

Diffuse Rectal Ulceration: ***Trauma.*** Most frequently this is caused by the use of retention enemas, heated in excess of 105° F (40.5° C), or by enema solutions with concentrations of hydrogen peroxide in excess of 3%. The peroxide produces tenesmus, the passage of mucus, and finally hemorrhage. The amount of damage depends upon the time of exposure and the concentration of the irritant. The mucosa contains patchy areas of denuded epithelium with intervening friable tissue. The diffuse distribution of the lesions and the history of the instillation make the diagnosis.

Diffuse Rectal Ulceration. ***Ulcerative Colitis.*** The findings vary with the chronicity of the disease and its intensity. No signs are pathognomic. Early involvement shows diffuse hyperemia, edema, increased mucus, and a mucosa that bleeds easily when traumatized. A similar appearance occurs in bacillary dysentery. Later, the mucosa is studded with minute yellow abscesses that are discrete and slightly elevated. Still later, the mucosa acquires the granular appearance of pink sandpaper; the slight trauma of wiping with a swab causes bleeding. The edges of the valves of Houston lose their normal sharpness and become rounded (Fig. 7-39C). In advanced stages, scars and contractures are seen. X-ray examination with a barium enema discloses loss of haustral markings and narrowing of the gut lumen. The differentiation between ulcerative colitis and granulomatous disease of the colon goes beyond the scope of this text; however, the two parameters most helpful are distribution of the lesions and an assessment of whether the lesions are transmural or involve the mucosa only.

Rectosigmoid Lesions of Regional Ileitis. Although no rectal lesions are characteristic for the disease, a frequent association is observed with anal abscesses and fistulas, extrarectal abscesses, and ulcer and stricture. Evidence of the disease in the terminal ileum should always be sought when these rectal conditions are encountered.

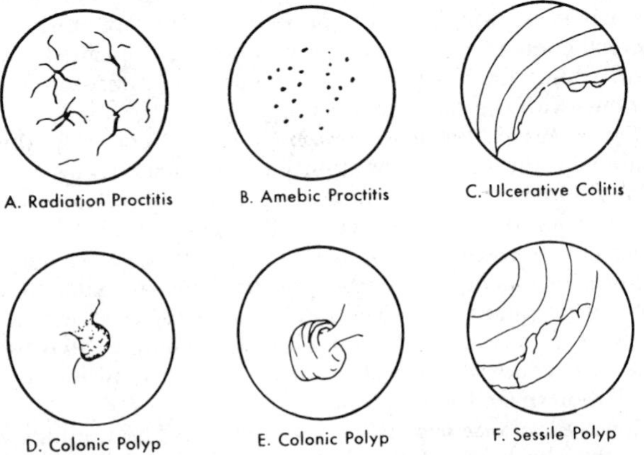

Fig. 7-39. Sigmoidoscope findings I. **A.** Radiation proctitis. *The mucosa contains telangiectatic vessels, plainly visible through thinned membranes.* **B.** Amebic proctitis. *Discrete punched-out small ulcers with umbilicated or raised edges are typical but not diagnostic.* **C.** Ulcerative colitis. *Advanced stage shows irregularity of a fold of the valve of Houston.* **D and E.** Pedunculated polyps. **F.** Sessile polyp.

Diffuse Rectal Ulceration: **Lymphogranuloma Venereum.** This is a venereal disease caused by a rickettsia-like organism *Miyagawanella lymphogranulomatis.* It begins with a transient genital lesion and a rash that quickly clear, leaving chronic progressive involvement of the lymphatics. From the inguinal lymph nodes the rectum becomes involved. Early the rectal mucosa appears red and friable. Later, the lower half of the rectum becomes the site of inflammation, involving the entire wall so the lumen narrows. It is denuded of mucosa and the ulcerations bleed easily. The late result is rectal stricture. The history of bubo and a positive skin test with the Frei antigen make the diagnosis. The blood serum contains complement-fixing antibodies for the Frei antigen.

Discrete Rectal Ulcer: **Trauma.** Abrasions with enema tips or endoscopic instruments are most frequent. The resulting ulcers are usually on the anterior rectal wall from failure to realize that the rectum curves posteriorly from the anus. The ulcer is linear, usually 1 to 2 cm long and 1 to 2 mm wide.

Discrete Rectal Ulcer: **Irradiation.** Commonly this results from the treatment of uterine cancer with radium; hence, the ulcer is usually on the anterior rectal wall, 6 to 10 cm above the pectinate line. The appearance varies from an area of mild hyperemia to a patch of green-gray with a tenacious slough. When scarring occurs, the surface is covered with telangiectases, pathognomonic of irradiation (Fig. 7-39A). Later, strictures may form. The ulcer may erode to form a rectovaginal or rectovesical fistula.

Discrete Rectal Ulcer: **Tuberculosis.** This has raised borders and varies in size and shape. The appearance is not characteristic. It resembles the ulcer of amebiasis and regional ileitis. The diagnosis is inferred by the occurrence of far-advanced tuberculous lesions elsewhere in the body.

Discrete Rectal Ulcer: **Bacillary Dysentery.** Early in the disease, there are no localizing signs except hyperemia, edema, and small hemorrhagic areas, resembling the appearance of ulcerative colitis. When ulcers occur, they are large, flat, and superficial. Jackman compares the appearance to the effect expected from shaving the mucosa with a razor. The ulcers are covered with a gray membrane, easily wiped off. Microscopic examination of the fecal mucus reveals a predominance of polymorphonuclear leukocytes, while protozoal infections stimulate the outpouring of monocytes. Bacteriologic cultures yield *Shigella dysenteriae* or related organisms.

Discrete Rectal Ulcer: ***Amebic Dysentery.*** The early stage looks like a minute polyp, raised, red, 3 to 5 mm in diameter (Fig. 7-39B); the center may be yellow. When the cap of the ulcer is rubbed off, a small depression can be seen. The fully developed ulcer is *punched-out,* with elevated edges. Swabs or scrapings should be taken from the ulcers for microscopic examination for *Entamoeba histolytica.* The punched-out ulcer is said to be pathognomonic, but experienced workers are not willing to be that dogmatic, especially when the disease has been partly treated with antibiotics.

Discrete Rectal Ulcer: ***Carcinoma.*** The general characteristics of a malignant ulcer are its elevated edges and an irregular excavated center (Fig. 7-40). It varies greatly in size and shape. Its appearance is not diagnostic.

Discrete Rectal Ulcer: ***Schistosomiasis.*** Rarely seen in the United States, the ulcers are described as tiny red spots, set in normal mucosa. The accompanying polypoid lesions are granulomas that contain the eggs of *Schistosoma mansoni.*

Discrete Rectal Ulcer: ***Balantidiasis.*** This is a rare cause of ulceration. The ulcers are not characteristic, but they resemble

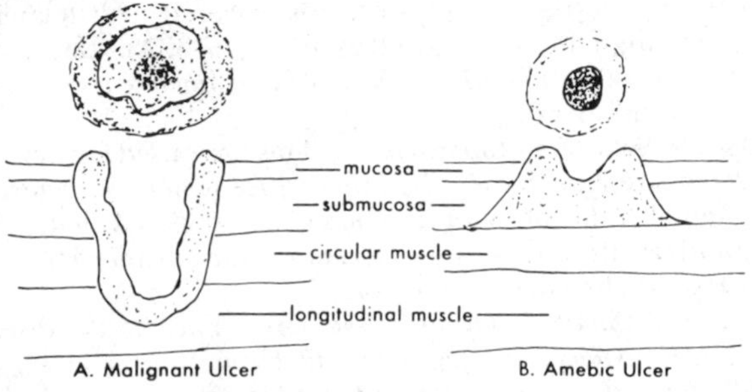

Fig. 7-40. Malignant and amebic ulcers of the colon. **A.** Malignant ulcer. *Section shows the penetration of the ulcer through most layers of the gut, with deep excavation and elevated irregular borders. Above it is the sigmoidoscopic appearance.* **B.** Amebic ulcer. *The abscess arises in the submucosa, pushes above the mucosal surface, and excavates in the center, producing the umbilicated punched-out appearance in the sigmoidoscope, as depicted above.*

the punched-out lesions of amebiasis. The presence of *Entamoeba histolytica* must be excluded, and *Balantidium coli* must be demonstrated, to make a diagnosis.

Rectal Polyps and Carcinoma. Diagnostically, these two lesions are considered together, because most rectal carcinomas are thought by some, denied by others, to arise as polyps and, in the early stage, cannot be distinguished except by pathologic examination. About 50% of both colonic polyps and carcinomas occur within reach of the sigmoidoscope. Polyps and early carcinomas are elevated lesions of the mucosa, either sessile or pedunculated (Fig. 7-39D-F). Polyps may be either single or multiple; when multiple, some may be malignant while others are benign. Either may bleed easily or cause diarrhea. When carcinoma has outgrown its polypoid configuration, it is rarely confused with other lesions because its size and the tendency to ulcerate and produce obstruction are characteristic. The ulcers are deep and irregular, with elevated borders. Multiple polyps may occur in several generations of persons, *familial multiple polyposis.* A rare hereditary type, the *Peutz-Jeghers syndrome,* is the combination of multiple polyps in the small intestine and colon, and melanotic spots in the mucosa of the lips and cheeks, the skin around the external nares and the eyes, and the nails of the fingers and toes. In Gardner's syndrome, a kindred of patients exists who have multiple colonic polyps, indistinguishable from the polyps of those seen in familial polyposis, in conjunction with bone tumors and extra-abdominal desmoid tumors. As these polyps have the same malignant potential as those in familial polyposis, polyps must be sought in persons identified with having the other two portions of the triad; soft tissue and bony tumors. Isolated cases do occur without antecedent family history; however, when a patient is diagnosed, family members ought to be evaluated. A rather new syndrome, *Turcot,* associates malignant tumors of the central nervous system with probably premalignant colon polyps.

Rectal Granuloma. These are rare sessile lesions caused by nonabsorbable surgical sutures, barium entering the bowel wall, the injection of mineral oil in the treatment of internal hemorrhoids, amebiasis, and histoplasmosis.

Intramural Lesion: ***Carcinoid.*** Most often this is present as a submucosal nodule, 2 to 10 mm in diameter, harder than a polyp; it shows through the mucosa with a yellow cast (Fig.

7-41C). When they ulcerate, carcinoids resemble adenocarcinomas. Some secrete serotonin into the systemic venous blood, allowing for the development of the Carcinoid Syndrome, producing nausea and vomiting, diarrhea, periodic flushing of the face, pulmonic stenosis, and tricuspid stenosis and insufficiency.

Intramural Lesion: ***Leiomyoma and Leiomyosarcoma.*** The benign lesions are usually submucosal, firm nodules, about 4 to 5 mm in diameter, that have no distinguishing features (Fig. 7-41D). When the mucosa is eroded off of the surface of these masses, bleeding, which may be brisk, can occur.

Intramural Lesion: ***Benign Lymphoma and Lymphosarcoma.*** Usually these are sessile submucosal lesions, showing through the mucosa with a blue-gray color. The malignant lesions are likely to be multiple, occurring in other parts of the body.

Intramural Lesion: ***Hemangioma.*** The appearance may range

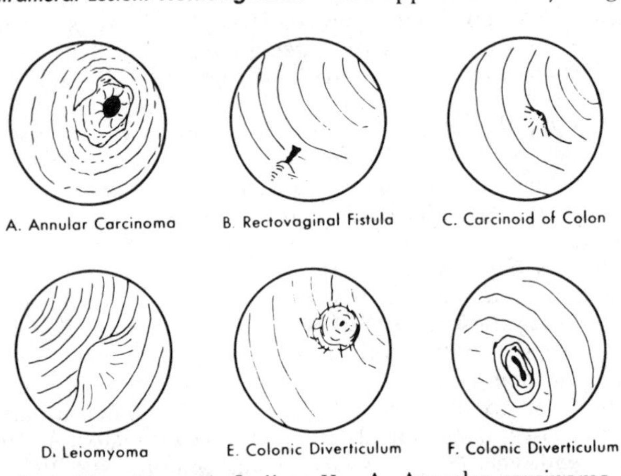

Fig. 7-41. Sigmoidoscopic findings II. **A.** Annular carcinoma of the colon. *A perceptible section of the lumen is narrowed by encircling carcinoma.* **B.** Rectovaginal fistula. *The rectal opening of the fistula is seen in the foreground as a black irregular crevasse.* **C.** Carcinoid of the colon. *A submucosal growth pushes up the epithelium and shows through it as a yellow nodule.* **D.** Leiomyoma of the colon. *This is a large submucosal lesion elevating the overlying epithelium.* **E and F.** Diverticula of the colon. *The orifices of the pouches may be plainly seen. Their lumens may be filled with feces.*

from a compact sessile polypoid mass to a nodular sheath encompassing the entire rectal wall. They are blue or purple. Bleeding from the lesions is frequent; hemorrhage after biopsy is spectacular.

Rectal Stricture. The diagnosis of the anatomic derangement is obvious. The lumen of the rectum is narrowed, frequently requiring the use of small diameter sigmoidoscope. By this means the examiner determines whether the constriction is *tubular,* from diffuse scarring of the wall, or *annular* (Fig. 7-41A), from a localized process. Tubular constriction is caused by lymphogranuloma venereum, ulcerative colitis, hot or caustic enemas. Annular constriction is more likely to be produced by annular carcinoma, radium or x-ray therapy, extirpation or injection of internal hemorrhoids. Ischemic stricture has recently been described following abdominal aortic aneurysm replacement, and has occurred, apparently because of extensive vascular disease, in conjunction with resection of the inferior mesenteric artery [P. R. Jochimsen: Ischemic Proctitis and Stricture Following Aortic Aneurysm: Management by Resection Using a Posterior Approach. *Contemp. Surg.,* **25:**17–20, 1984]. Even though the process is very old, the relationship to lymphogranuloma can be established by the skin test with the Frei antigen and the complement-fixation test with the same agent.

Melanosis Coli. A harmless but spectacular condition is observed in which melanin is deposited in the mucosa from the ileocecal valve to the mucocutaneous junction of the anus. It seems to be associated with the frequent use of cathartics for many months. The mucosa may be light tan, or any darker shade to black, with lymph follicles of the mucosa showing up as yellow dots. The distribution is somewhat mottled. The black coloration may be mistaken for dead bowel.

8

The Genitalia

▼ *Key Symptom:* ***Frequent Urination.*** The adult male bladder holds about 500 mL. An average output of urine in 24 hours is 1200 to 1500 mL; but this volume may be modified by fluid intake, sweating, outside temperature, vomiting, or diarrhea. Although the average adult micturates above five or six times daily, variations occur with fluid output, individual habits, irritation of the genitourinary tract. Normal kidneys excrete less urine during sleep, so most persons are not interrupted to urinate, although some have habitual nocturia. Nocturia also occurs with most disorders causing increased frequency of urination.

Clinical Occurrence: POLYURIA. Excessive fluid intake from habit or alcoholic beverages, which have the action of suppression of the individual's endogenous antidiuretic hormone levels. *Excessive Use of Tea or Coffee:* these drinks contain diuretic xanthines. *Diabetes Mellitus:* glycosuria induces an osmotic diuresis. *Diabetes Insipidus:* a deficit of vasopressin prevents urinary concentration by the kidneys. *Chronic Glomerulonephritis:* the kidneys reach a stage when they are unable to concentrate urine. *Emotional Diuresis:* this is usually temporary. POSTRENAL CAUSES. *Prostatic Obstruction:* with incomplete emptying of the bladder, the residual urine requires but little augmentation to fill the viscus and cause an urge to micturate, so called, overflow incontinence. *Bladder Stone:* bodily movements cause the stones to irritate the bladder, so increased frequency may occur by day but be absent at night. *Carcinoma of Bladder:* distention of the affected bladder wall is painful, so frequency is induced to avoid discomfort. *Infections:* irritations from pyelitis, cystitis, prostatitis, urethritis, salpingitis, appendicitis, renal tuberculosis. *Diminished Bladder Capacity:* tumor or stone in bladder, extrinsic pressure from tumor or gravid uterus, fibrosis of bladder wall. *High Acidity of Urine:* especially encountered in children.

▼ *Key Symptom:* ***Difficult Urination*** **(*Dysuria*).** The patient may complain of *hesitancy* in starting the urinary stream or that unusual *straining* is required to maintain the stream. This is usually attributable to partial obstruction of the urethra or a disturbance in nervous stimulation of the bladder.

Clinical Occurrence: BOTH SEXES. Urethral stricture, calculus in bladder or urethra, blood clot in bladder or urethra, carcinoma of urethra, paralysis of bladder, myelitis, tabes dorsalis, multiple sclerosis, spinal cord tumor, syringomyelia. EXCLUSIVELY MALE. Hyperplasia of prostate, prostatitis, tuberculosis of prostate. EXCLUSIVELY FEMALE. Uterine fibroid, gravid uterus, carcinoma of vaginal wall.

▼ *Key Symptom:* ***Painful Urination.*** Pain in the penis or the female urethra can be distinguished as follows:

Clinical Occurrence: PAIN DURING URINATION. Urethral obstruction, urethritis, meatal ulcer. PAIN AFTER URINATION (usually with a prickly sensation in glans penis). Bladder calculus, cystitis, vesical tuberculosis, prostatitis, seminal vesiculitis.

▼ *Key Sign:* ***Urinary Retention.*** Acute urinary retention in the bladder is usually painful, so it is distinguished from the painless anuria or oliguria. It may develop in the situation where the patient is unable to communicate the nature of his discomfort. One is reminded of the patient in the Surgical Intensive Care Unit, on a respirator following open heart surgery, who was being seen by the consultant psychiatrist because he was uncontrollable even though heavily sedated and having received large quantities of analgesics. It was then found that the Foley catheter was kinked and not properly draining. Correction of this *minor* error, led to complete resolution of the difficulty. But chronic retention develops gradually and is painless; the only symptoms may be frequent urination of small amounts or incontinence. The patient may have a sensation of fullness in the bladder but often this is absent. The condition is discovered when examination of the abdomen discloses a suprapubic swelling that may extend to the umbilicus. Catheterization yields a large volume of urine and the abdominal swelling disappears.

Clinical Occurrence: MECHANICAL OBSTRUCTION OF URETHRA. Urethral stricture, urethral calculus, traumatic rupture of the urethra, prostatic hyperplasia, acute prostatitis, abscess of the prostate, pedunculated bladder tumor. NERVOUS DISORDERS: Urethral spasm after operations in the inguinal region or the perineum, paralysis of the bladder in paraplegia, tabes dorsalis, or myelitis.

▼ *Key Symptoms:* ***Anuria and Oliguria.*** In *oliguria* the 24-hour urinary output is between 50 mL and 400 mL (4–25 mL per hour). The output is 0 to 50 mL in *anuria.* Even with dehydration normal kidneys continue to excrete more than 600 mL daily, so oliguria and anuria indicate dangerous degrees of acute renal dysfunction requiring immediate treatment. Acute renal failure often occurs suddenly and unexpectedly during the care of the patients for another disorder. Usually patients do not complain of lack of urine. So, too often, these ominous signs are discovered by accident after existing for many hours. The attention of physicians and nurses has been directed to the care of injuries, operations, or the course of the primary disease, and anuria may be overlooked unless all attendants are alert in collecting urine specimens. The physician should ensure a hospital routine that will facilitate the discovery of a diminished urinary output. Once the fact of oliguria or anuria has been established, the cause must be determined quickly by considering the many possibilities. Often the cause may be suspected from knowledge of the preexisting disease. When the diagnosis is not clear, urologic examination should be made promptly in a search for postrenal causes that are not evident. The following is a *clinical* classification of causes that is considered more diagnostically useful than the usual pathologic categorizations.

Clinical Occurrence: POSTTRAUMATIC. Hypovolemic shock, crush syndrome, burns, heat prostration, hematoma, or rupture of kidney. POSTOPERATIVE. Aortic resection, cardiotomy, repair of injuries to blood vessels. INSTRUMENTATION. Retrograde pyelography and catheterization of ureters. BLOOD TRANSFUSION. Hemolysis from mishandled or incompatible blood. INTRAVENOUS INFUSIONS. Hyperosmotic solutions of sucrose, glucose, mannitol, dextran. PREGNANCY. Hemorrhage, premature separation of the placenta, preeclampsia, septic abortion. MCARDLE'S DISEASE. DURING ACUTE NEPHRITIS. DURING INFECTIONS. Pyelonephritis, septicemia, pneumococcal pneumonia (during stage of consolidation oliguria often occurs), epidemic hemorrhagic fever, cholera, and dysentery. DURING MALARIA. Blackwater fever, hypersensitivity to quinine, quinacrine

(Atabrine). DRUGS AND POISONS. Heavy metals: mercury (mercuric chloride, organic mercurial diuretics), bismuth, copper, uranium, arsenic, potassium. *Organic solvents:* carbon tetrachloride, tetrachlorethylene. *Polypeptide antibiotics:* bacitracin, ristocetin, neomycin, kanamycin, polymyxin, colistin. *Biologic poisons:* mushrooms, rattlesnake venom. *Methemoglobinemia:* phenacetin and others. *Sulfonamides, Salicylates:* in massive doses. *Miscellaneous:* inorganic phosphorus, carbon monoxide, cresol, DDT, paraldehyde, ethylene, diethylene glycol, potassium chlorate, thallium, phenylbutazone, heroin, urethane. *Ganglion blocking agents.* CARDIAC. Cardiac failure, myocardial infarction. VASCULAR. Renal infarction from emboli after surgery, vena caval thrombosis. DURING HYPERPARATHYROIDISM. Sudden severe hypercalcemia. DURING SICKLE-CELL ANEMIA. Crisis. DURING OTHER DISEASE. Sarcoidosis, disseminated lupus erythematosus, periarteritis nodosa, dermatomyositis, Wegener's granulomatosis, hypersensitivity angiitis. POSTRENAL OBSTRUCTION. One kidney absent or poorly functioning, renal calculi, cysts, tumors obstructing the ureters, obstruction by crystals of uric acid, oxalic acid, cystine, or calcium.

▼ *Key Sign:* ***Discolored Urine.*** Occasionally a male patient describes an abnormal color in his urine, but his characterization of the hue is seldom accurate. Women rarely observe it because their anatomy precludes the inspection of voided urine. Usually discoloration of the urine is discovered by the physician or others handling specimens for examination. Sometimes the abnormal color leads directly to the diagnosis.

Clinical Occurrence: COLORLESS: urine of low concentration from excessive fluid intake, chronic glomerulonephritis, diabetes mellitus, diabetes insipidus. CLOUDY WHITE: phosphates in an alkaline urine (the cloud disappears with the addition of acid), epithelial cells from the lower genitourinary tract (for the urine of males, see Three-Glass Test, p. 598), bacteria, pus, chyle (when the urine is centrifuged chyle remains homogeneously distributed; milk fat added for malingering floats to the top). YELLOW: highly concentrated normal urine, tetracycline, pyridine. ORANGE: urobilinogen, santonin (anthelminthic), phenindione (anticoagulant). ORANGE IN ACID URINE, RED IN ALKALINE: rhubarb (food and purgative), senna (cathartic), aloes (cathartic), Argyrol (silver protein disinfectant). RED: beets, blackberries, aniline dyes from candy, freshly voided hemoglobin or myoglobin, pyridine, porphyrin, uroerythrin deposited on urate crystals, Pyramidon (aminopyrine), phenolphthalein (a cathartic, red in alkaline urine, colorless in acid urine), sulfonal, picric acid, cascara (cathartic), danthron, rifamysin doxorubicin.

BLUE-GREEN: bilirubin (urine with yellow froth), methylene blue, thymol, phenol (small amounts), indigo carmine, indigo blue, indican, acriflavine (the urine fluoresces). BROWN-BLACK: highly concentrated normal urine, bilirubin (with yellow froth), acid hematin (hemoglobin standing in acid urine), methemoglobin, porphyrin, phenol (black in large quantities), cresol, homogentisic acid, tyrosine. BROWN-BLACK AFTER STANDING: porphyrin (changed from exposure to sunlight), melanin (changed from exposure to sunlight), homogentisic acid (changed from bacterial alkalinization of the urine).

▼ *Key Sign:* **Hematuria.** When erythrocytes enter the urine in excessive numbers, the condition is termed *hematuria*. *Gross Hematuria.* This results when the concentration of red blood cells is sufficient to color the urine red. The red color is frequently noticed by the male patient during micturition, and it brings him rather promptly to the physician; but females rarely detect it. The red urine of hematuria must be distinguished from hemoglobinuria and myoglobinuria by the demonstration of erythrocytes in the *freshly voided* urine. In all three cases the urine gives chemical tests for hemoglobin. Spectroscopic examination distinguishes myoglobin from hemoglobin, but it does not differentiate between intracellular and extracellular hemoglobin. Observation of gross hematuria by the male patient may give further diagnostic clues: *Initial hematuria:* a site of hemorrhage in the urethra. *Terminal hematuria:* a small hemorrhage from the trigone region of the bladder. *Total hematuria:* hemorrhage from the kidney or profuse bleeding from the bladder (the presence of erythrocyte casts in the urine proves the hemorrhage comes from the kidneys). *Microscopic Hematuria.* The excess of erythrocytes is not sufficient to alter the normal color of the urine, so the condition is unnoticed by the patient; it is detected by chemical or microscopic examination of the urine. The red blood cells are seen in the microscopic examination of the *freshly voided* urinary sediment and detected by sensitive chemical tests for hemoglobin. Up to 1,000,000 erythrocytes may be passed in the normal urine in 24 hours, so 2 or 3 erythrocytes per high-power microscopic field of a centrifuged sediment may be considered normal.

In most instances, the occurrence of hematuria demands a complete investigation of the genitourinary tract with intravenous pyelography and cystoscopy. But simple bedside observations must suffice when instrumentation of the urethra and other structures is contraindicated, as in urethral infection or hemorrhagic disorders like hemophilia, thrombocytopenia, prothrombin deficiency, and scurvy.

Clinical Occurrence: KIDNEY. *Traumatic:* blow to the kidney, sudden decompression of overfilled bladder. *Malformation:* polycystic disease of the kidneys. *Neoplasms:* benign and malignant tumors. *Vascular:* renal infarction, periarteritis, aneurysms, hemangiomas, Goodpasture's syndrome, intrarenal arteriovenous fistula. *Infectious:* glomerulonephritis, tuberculosis, hydatid disease. *Hematologic:* uremia, hemophilia, thrombocytopenia, prothrombin deficit, anticoagulant therapy, sickle-cell anemia, scurvy. *Drugs and Poisons:* turpentine, phenol, catharides, potassium chlorate, hexamine, sulfonamides, cyclophosphamide. *Systemic Febrile Disease:* malaria, variola, yellow fever, blackwater fever. *Radiation. Gout.* RENAL PELVIS. Hydronephrosis, pyelitis, calculus. URETERS. Neoplasms, calculus, stricture, ureteritis cystica. BLADDER. Neoplasms, cystitis, tuberculosis, *Schistosoma hematobium,* calculus, endometriosis (hemorrhage during menstruation), foreign body, diverticula, Hunner's ulcer, cystitis cystica, varix. PROSTATE. Engorged veins in hyperplastic prostate, chronic prostatis, carcinoma. URETHRA. Acute urethritis, neoplasms, stricture, calculus, rupture, foreign body, diverticulum, polyps. EXERCISE: 50 marathon runners with beginning negative urines were reexamined after the race; 18% had developed hematuria, one with gross hematuria, 8 with urine containing one to three RBCs per high-power field. These cleared up within two days. With the hematuria was proteinuria, one plus [A. J. Siegel, *et al.:* Exercise-Related Hematuria, *J.A.M.A.,* **241:**391–92, 1979].

▼ *Key Sign:* ***Hemoglobinuria.*** The presence of extracellular hemoglobin in the urine is *hemoglobinuria.* Sufficient concentrations of the pigment in the urine produce a red color. The hemoglobin gives positive chemical tests whether intracellular or extracellular, so hemoglobinuria must be distinguished from *hematuria* by the absence of erythrocytes in *freshly voided* urine, as viewed through the microscope. *Myoglobin* in the urine can be differentiated from hemoglobin only by spectroscopic examination. But a concomitant red coloration of the blood plasma suggests hemoglobinuria; the smaller myoglobin molecules are cleared more rapidly from the urine and passed through the glomerular membrane. When hemoglobin enters the plasma by the intravascular rupture of erythrocytes, or by injection into the veins, it is bound to plasma *haptoglobin* that has a normal concentration of 128 ± 25 mg per 100 mL. The large hemoglobin-haptoglobin complex does not pass through the intact glomerulus. When the binding capacity of haptoglobin is exceeded, free hemoglobin passes through the glomerular membrane. In such event, a freshly voided urine specimen usually contains *hemoglobin casts,* large cylindric aggregates of brown masses. Their presence excludes the possibility that hemolysis occurred in the bladder.

Clinical Occurrence: Extravascular Hemolysis. *Hemolysis in Donor's Blood:* hemolyzed by improper storage; hemolyzed by improper heating or freezing; hemolyzed by addition to blood of distilled water, certain concentrations of glucose, or other destructive agents, including following operative procedures utilizing the extracorporeal oxygenator. *Hemolysis in the Bladder:* hematuria with bladder *urine so dilute* as to hemolyze the erythrocytes (less than sp. gr. 1.006); in *transurethral prostatectomy* associated with hemorrhage, distilled water is placed in bladder to hemolyze cells to clear the vision of the cystoscopist (the free hemoglobin is then taken into the circulation through the opened veins). Intravascular Hemolysis. *Pregnancy and the Puerperium. Extensive Burns. Blood Transfusion:* by the action of incompatible agglutinins or hemolysins. *Infarction of the Kidney. Severe Exercise:* in the syndromes of march hemoglobinuria and paralytic hemoglobinuria, and other severe exertion [W. S. Kaden: Traumatic Haemoglobinuria in Congo-Drum Players, *Lancet,* **1:**1341–42, 1970]. *Exposure to Cold:* paroxysmal hemoglobinuria with high-titer "cold" agglutinins, and with the Donath-Landsteiner hemolysins. *During Sleep:* paroxysmal nocturnal hemoglobinuria (Marchiafava-Micheli syndrome). *Infections:* malaria, blackwater fever, typhus fever, gas gangrene, generalized anthrax, yellow fever. *Transurethral Prostatectomy:* in addition to hemolysis in the bladder from the injected distilled water (see Extravascular Hemolysis, *above*), when water is placed in the bladder under pressure, it is forced into the circulation through the open prostatectomy bed, to hemolyze cells in the bloodstream. *Drugs and Poisons:* sulfonamides, quinine, phenylhydrazine. Rarely, numerous chemicals serve as antigens for the production of hemolysins. In persons with a deficiency in glucose-6-phosphate-dehydrogenase (G-6-PD), intravascular hemolysis and hemoglobinuria are caused by the ingestion of primaquine, sulfonamides, sulfones, and other oxidant drugs. *Favism:* the ingestion of the fava bean by persons with G-6-PD deficiency causes hemolysis and hemoglobinuria. *Bites of Poisonous Snakes and Spiders. Intravascular Trauma:* marching, cardiac-valve prostheses, severe aortic regurgitation, microangiopathic (necrotizing arteriolitis in malignant hypertension).

▼ *Key Sign:* ***Myoglobinuria.*** The excretion of myoglobin, released from damaged muscle, colors the urine red and gives chemical tests for hemoglobin. The muscle pigment must be distinguished from the latter by spectroscopic examination. The lack of a red color in a concomitant plasma specimen hints at myoglobin in the urine. The molecular weight of myoglobin is 17,500 compared to 68,000 for hemoglobin. The lighter molecules pass the glomerular membrane rapidly so the plasma is cleared.

Clinical Occurrence: CRUSH SYNDROME: massive crushing and compression injuries to muscle, first described in British air-raid casualties during World War II. THROMBOSIS OF LARGE MUSCLE MASSES. PSEUDOPARALYTIC SYNDROME: a disorder occurring when race horses undergo sudden unusual exercise. The counterpart is rarely encountered in man. SHOCK FROM HIGH-VOLTAGE ELECTRICITY. HAFF DISEASE (from the German: *Königsberg Haff*): an epidemic myoglobinuria encountered in Königsberg, Germany, caused by the ingestion of fish feeding in a lagoon (*Haff*) polluted with industrial wastes. MCARDLE'S DISEASE: a rare disorder with paroxysms of myoglobinuria induced by exercise. It is caused by a deficiency of phosphorylase, inherited as an autosomal recessive gene. POLIOMYELITIS: rarely. HEROIN ADDICTION [see R. W. Richter, Y. B. Challenor, J. Pearson, L. J. Kagen, L. L. Hamilton, and W. H. Ramsey: Acute Myoglobinuria Associated with Heroin Addiction, *J.A.M.A.*, **216:**1172–76, 1971]. MYOGLOBINEMIA WITH HYPOKALEMIA [see D. S. Campion, J. M. Arias, and N. W. Carter: Rhabdomyolysis and Myoglobinuria Associated with Hypokalemia of Renal Tubular Acidosis, *J.A.M.A.*, **220:**967–69, 1972]. INGESTION OF QUAIL. Since Biblical times the ingestion of quail has been known to produce myoglobinuria in some persons [A. G. Billis, S. Kastanakis, H. Giamarellou, and G. K. Daikos: Acute Renal Failure After a Meal of Quail, *Lancet*, **2:**702, 1971].

The Male Genitalia

Inspection and palpation reveal many disorders of the external and internal male organs of generation and the lower urinary tract. A rewarding routine physical examination should employ all those procedures not requiring the special skills of the urologist. The urologist's field is much more comprehensive; he deals with the entire urinary tract in both male and female. He employs special diagnostic instruments and techniques for examination; he is proficient in the surgical and nonsurgical treatment of genitourinary disease. The gynecologist specializes in the diagnosis and treatment of diseases of the female genitalia. A reasonable familiarity with the genital disorders demonstrated by inspection and palpation would seem necessary for any physician who attempts a physical examination.

THREE-GLASS URINE TEST. **When the symptoms or signs suggest inflammation of the male urethra, the three-glass test should be employed before palpation of the penis is performed. The patient is instructed to void into three conical specimen glasses (Fig. 8-1), putting the first-voided urine into I, the midstream specimen into II, and the remainder of the bladder contents into III. Preferably, the examiner should supervise the collection to caution against interrupting the urinary stream when shifting from one glass to another. He should also observe the force and caliber of the urinary stream for evidence of stricture. The physician inspects each glass for a characteristic cloud of pus, for small commalike mucous shreds from the inflamed anterior urethra, and for larger shreds from the posterior urethra. The initial urine (glass I) washes the pus from the anterior urethra; the midstream specimen (glass II) represents the bladder contents; the terminal specimen (glass III) may contain sediment expressed from the prostate and seminal vesicles by peristaltic action of the urethral musculature in stopping the stream; hence the necessity for uninterrupted voiding of the three specimens. The three-glass test is actually part of the physical examination, not a laboratory test. Later, the cause of the cloudiness in the urine**

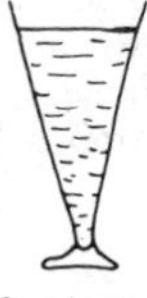

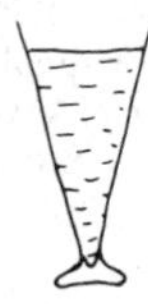

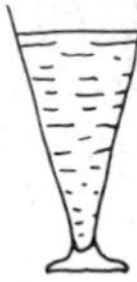

Fig. 8-1. Three-glass urine test. *One voiding of urine is distributed into three specimens as it is being passed from the urethra, so that* **specimen I** *contains the initial portion,* **specimen II** *the midstream portion, and* **specimen III** *the final portion of the bladder contents. Each glass is inspected for the presence of pus and mucous shreds. Particles in the initial specimen only are assumed to come from the urethra. Specimen II is accepted as typical bladder urine. Specimen III may contain pus and mucus expressed from the posterior urethra when peristalsis compresses the prostate and seminal vesicles to stop voiding.*

can be confirmed by microscopic examination and the usual chemical tests may be made on the urine specimens.

Interpretation of the 3-Glass Test (Hinman)

	Glass I	Glass II	Glass III
Acute or subacute urethritis	Cloudy	Clear	Clear
Severe posterior urethritis	Cloudy	Clear or cloudy	Cloudy
Chronic urethritis, anterior	Small comma-shreds	Clear	Clear
Chronic urethritis, posterior	Heavy shreds	Clear	Clear
Chronic urethritis, both	Both shreds	Clear	Clear
Prostatitis	Clear or large shreds	Clear	Large shreds or cloudy
Cystitis, pyelonephritis	Cloudy	Cloudy	Cloudy

The Penis

The shaft of the penis is formed dorsally by two lateral columns of erectile tissue, the *corpora cavernosa penis,* and ventrally by a smaller column of erectile tissue, the *corpus cavernosum urethrae* (corpus spongiosum) containing the urethra (Fig. 8-2). Heavy fibrous tissue binds the three columns into a cylinder. The end of the shaft is surmounted by an obtuse cone of erectile tissue, the *glans penis,* pierced at its top by the *urethral meatus.* The glans forms a shoulder, the *corona,* at its junction with the shaft where there is a slight constriction, the *retroglandular sulcus* or *neck.* A flap of skin, the *prepuce* or *foreskin,* covers the glans. The *frenulum* is a fold of the prepuce that extends ventrally from the urethral meatus to the neck.

METHOD OF PENILE EXAMINATION. **Inspection and palpation distinguish most disorders of the penis. In the adult male, *view* the penis in its usual state, then have the patient *retract the prepuce* from the glans to reveal the size of the preputial orifice and superficial lesions of the corona and retroglandular sulcus. *Palpate* lesions for induration and tenderness. In handling ulcers, *protect* your fingers with a**

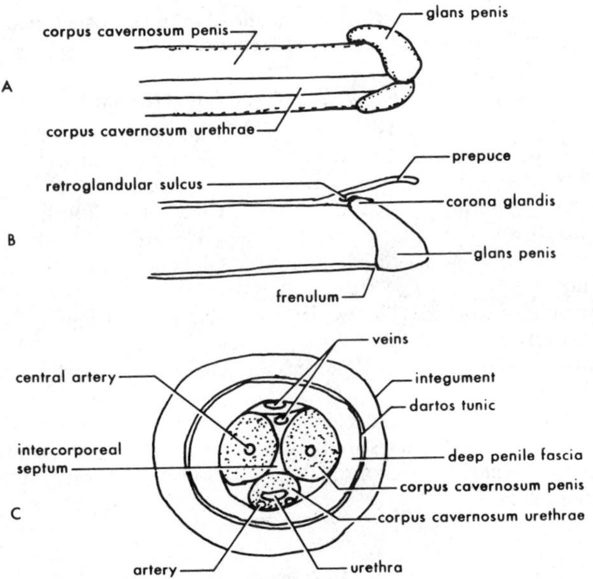

Fig. 8-2. Structure of the penis. *In* **A** *the shaft is diagrammed in its ventrolateral aspect, with integument removed. A sagittal section of the shaft is represented in* **B** *with integument included.* **C** *is a cross section of the shaft.*

rubber glove (*Treponema pallidum* is infective through the unbroken skin). Palpate the length of the shaft, *ventrally* along the corpus cavernosum urethrae from the penoscrotal junction to the meatus, *middorsally* over the intercorporeal septum, and *laterally* over both corpora cavernosa penis, feeling for nodules and plaques. *Compress the glans anteroposteriorly between the thumb and forefinger to open and inspect the terminal urethra. Collect* a drop of urethral discharge for microscopic examination.

Generalized Penile Swelling: ***Edema.*** Fluid accumulates in the loose tissue of the penile integument in anasarca from any cause. Obstruction of the penile veins or inflammation of the penis causes localized edema. Lymphatic obstruction produces elephantiasis.

Generalized Penile Swelling: ***Contusion.*** Especially during erection, trauma to the penis may cause extravasation of blood that is usually painless. In a few days, the skin of the penis and scrotum may be stained blue from degraded hemoglobin.

Generalized Penile Swelling: ***Fracture of the Shaft.*** Severe trauma during erection may rupture one or both corpora cavernosa penis. Severe pain occurs at the time of injury, with immediate subsidence of the erection and temporary relief of pain. Subsequent engorgement from extravasation of blood produces recurrence of pain. *Distinction.* Fracture may not be distinguishable from contusion unless operation is performed.

Penile Ulcer: ***Syphilitic Chancre*** (Hard Chancre, Hunterian Chancre). This is the primary lesion of syphilis, the first manifestation of the disease. The lesion commonly occurs on the corona glandis or the inner leaves of the prepuce, but occasionally on the shaft or the skin of the scrotum. Rarely it is *extragenital,* usually on the lips of the mouth. The chancre begins as a silvery papule that gradually erodes to form a superficial ulcer with a serous discharge containing *Treponema pallidum* (Fig. 8-3A). Since the organisms penetrate the unbroken skin, the lesions should be palpated only through rubber gloves. Early in the evolution, the regional superficial inguinal lymph nodes undergo painless moderate enlargement. The chancre

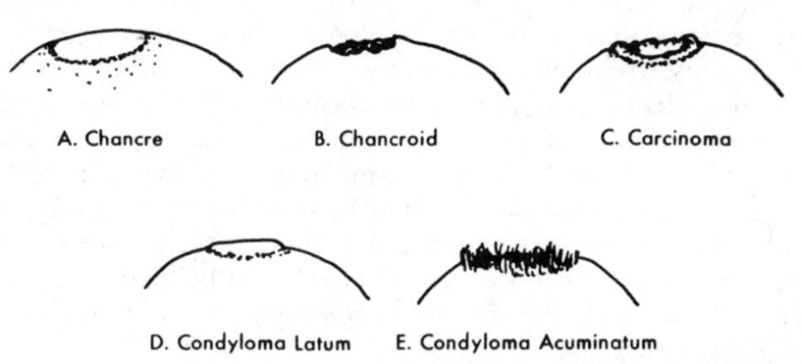

Fig. 8-3. Penile growths. **A.** Chancre. *The border is smooth; there is no necrosis or suppuration. Induration surrounds the lesion so it can be picked up like a disk.* **B.** Chancroid. *The border is irregular, the center necrotic. There is profuse suppuration; induration is absent.* **C.** Ulcerating carcinoma. *The necrotic ulcer may resemble chancroid, but soon the process is surrounded by induration and nodulation.* **D.** Condyloma latum. *This is the flat, nonsuppurating nodule of secondary syphilis.* **E.** Condyloma acuminatum. *The lesions are moist, villous growths that protrude above the skin and undergo secondary ulceration. Acuminate means "pointed."*

is painless, usually single, round or oval, with smooth, slightly raised border. The underlying induration permits the superficial lesion to be lifted as a small disk between the thumb and forefinger. Neither the ulcer nor the lymph nodes suppurate. *Distinction.* The chancre is single, painless, nonsuppurative, with smooth rounded border and indurated base. Physical signs are not conclusive; the diagnosis must be confirmed by demonstrating the *Treponema pallidum* in the serous exudate with the dark-field microscope, since the lesion appears before serologic tests for syphilis become positive. A fluorescein treponema antibody test is available utilizing patients' sera that has been absorbed for cross reactants. This test reacts more quickly for an earlier diagnosis in 20% of those who are VDRL negative.

Penile Ulcer: ***Chancroid*** (Soft Chancre). A suppurative infection caused by the bacillus *Hemophilus ducreyi,* it usually involves the genitalia, although it may be extragenital. The lesion begins as a small red papule that quickly becomes pustular and enlarges to form a punched-out ulcer with undermined edges (Fig. 8-3b). The base is covered with a gray slough, discharging pus profusely. Extensive necrosis ensues and multiple ulcers form. The lesions are quite painful. In a third of the cases, the regional lymph nodes become swollen and tender, the *bubo.* These frequently suppurate. *Distinction.* Multiple nonindurative ulcers cause pain and suppuration. Frequent painful regional lymph nodes, enlarged and suppurating, become adherent to the skin. The organism may be grown out of the bubo, by inoculation on chocolate agar. Staining, gives a typical *school of fish* appearance. While the clinical appearance is quite typical, mixed infections must be excluded by examination of the exudate with the dark-field microscope for the presence of *Treponema pallidum.*

Penile Ulcer: ***Lymphogranuloma Venereum*** (Lymphopathia Venereum, Lymphogranuloma Inguinale). Primarily, this venereal disease involves the lymphatic system. The initial penile lesion, an erosion less than 1 mm in diameter, is frequently overlooked because it is painless and evanescent. It is the site of entry of the causative agent, *Chlamydia trachomatis,* a rickettsialike organism. The organism can be cultured in tissue culture. Occasionally the penile lesion becomes vesicular, papular, or nodular. One or two weeks after the appearance of the primary lesion, the inguinal lymph nodes become swollen and tender; they mat together with areas of softening and reddening of the overlying skin. Multiple small fistulas form, discharging creamy pus or serosanguinous exudate. Healing with much fibrosis occurs over many months. A cicatrizing proctitis may be a late complication. *Distinction.* The late clinical appearance is fairly distinctive. In the early stages, syphilis, chancroid, and herpes progenitalis may have to be excluded. Later, sensitivity to the organism can be demonstrated in 90% of the cases by the intradermal *Frei test*, using a killed suspension of the specific organism, grown on the yolk sac of the chick embryo. The blood serum of the patient also fixes complement with this antigen.

Penile Ulcer: ***Herpes Progenitalis.*** A small group of vesicles surrounded by erythema frequently occurs on the glans or prepuce. The vesicles rupture, producing superficial ulcers that heal in five to seven days. The ulcers may serve as portals of entry for other organisms. *Distinction.* The grouped vesicles or ulcers are fairly characteristic. The evanescence of the lesions soon distinguishes them from other possibilities.

Chronic Penile Ulceration: ***Behcet's Syndrome.*** See p. 893.

Prepuce: ***Phimosis.*** The orifice of the prepuce may be so small that the foreskin cannot be retracted from the glans (Fig. 8-4A). The congenital form results from malformation; the acquired type may be caused by preputial adhesions to the glans as the result of infection. The lips of the prepuce are pallid, striated, and thickened. The narrow orifice may actually obstruct urination. Retained smegma and dirt lead to inflammation and even calculus formation.

Prepuce: ***Paraphimosis.*** A tight foreskin, once retracted, may become edematous, so that it cannot resume its normal position over the glans (Fig. 8-4B). The edema impedes the circulation of the glans so the organ swells. Manual replacement of the prepuce may be attempted: grasp the glans with the left thumb and forefinger, pull on the shaft while massaging the edema of the prepuce and shaft with the surrounding right hand. When the glans is released, the prepuce may slip over it. Surgical incision may be necessary.

Prepuce: ***Preputial Calculus.*** Stones may form in the preputial

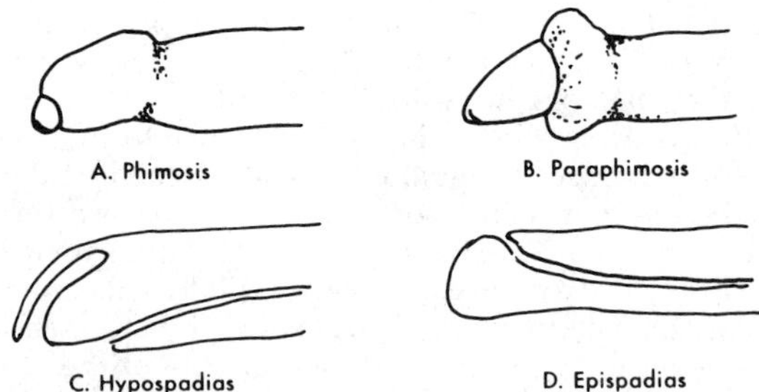

Fig. 8-4. Structural abnormalities of the prepuce (foreskin). **A.** Phimosis. *The preputial orifice is too tight to permit retraction of the foreskin over the glans penis.* **B.** Paraphimosis. *The condition in which a prepuce with small orifice has been retracted from the glans and the lips have impinged on the retroglandular sulcus, preventing return to the normal position. Edema occurs in the prepuce, the skin of the shaft, and the glans.* **C.** Hypospadias. *This is a developmental disturbance in which the meatus of the urethra opens on the underside of the shaft.* **D.** Epispadias. *A developmental anomaly in which the urethra occurs on the dorsal side of the penis.*

sac from the accumulation of dirt and smegma beneath a phimosis, or renal calculi may be passed through the urethra and lodge in the sac.

Glans: ***Condyloma Acuminatum*** (Venereal Wart, Papilloma). This lesion is a villous projection (*acuminata* means "pointed") that may be single or conglomerate (Fig. 8-3E). It occurs on the corona or in the retroglandular sulcus; frequently it is found about the anus. In the presence of moisture, secondary infection produces ulceration. *Distinction.* In its uncomplicated form, the verrucous appearance is quite distinctive. An exuberant growth with much ulceration must be distinguished from carcinoma by biopsy.

Glans: ***Condyloma Latum.*** As the name implies, the growth is flat and warty (Fig. 8-3D). It may occur about the genitalia or anus. It is a secondary syphilid. *Distinction.* The flat appearance is diagnostic. When the lesion has an exuberant growth, it must be distinguished from the acuminate condyloma and carcinoma.

Glans: ***Carcinoma of the Penis.*** Most frequently this lesion occurs after irritation from phimosis, balanitis, or posthitis.

Commonly, the primary lesion involves the dorsal corona; the inner lip of the prepuce is a frequent site. A warty growth develops, ulcerates, and discharges watery pus. Parts of the tumor undergo necrosis and slough (Fig. 8-3C). Metastasis occurs most often to the femoral lymph nodes. *Distinction.* Often the clinical appearance is not sufficiently typical to distinguish from condyloma, so a biopsy is necessary.

Glans: ***Erosive Balanitis.*** The skin of the glans undergoes desquamation and erosion; small ulcers form and become confluent, involving the entire glans. Rarely, this results in gangrene. The identity of the infective organism is unknown.

Meatus: ***Stricture.*** Narrowing of the urethral meatus may be observed after anteroposterior pressure on the glans. It is usually a congenital malformation. Strictures in other portions of the urethra must be demonstrated by the passage of catheters or sounds.

Meatus: ***Papilloma.*** A benign tumor in the meatus may be visible when the orifice gapes from pressure on the glans.

Meatus: ***Urethritis.*** The edges of the meatus may be reddened, edematous, and everted. A variable amount of pus discharges from the urethra. The lymphatic channels in the dorsum of the penis may be tender and palpable. Tender, swollen, palpable lymph nodes develop in the inguinal regions. Micturition and erection may be painful. *Distinction.* The diagnosis is usually obvious by direct inspection and the presence of mucous shreds and pus in the first specimen of the three-glass test. The problem is to determine the causative agent. Thin slide preparations should be stained by Gram's method and a search made for the gram-negative biscuit-shaped diplococci of *Neisseria gonorrhoeae.* Culture methods may be necessary. Nonspecific urethritis is diagnosed by exclusion of gonorrhea. Nonspecific urethritis may constitute a member of the triad, along with conjunctivitis and arthritis, in Reiter's disease; the urethritis frequently appears before the other members.

Meatus: ***Morgagni's Folliculitis.*** The follicles of Morgagni open into the urethra laterally, immediately behind the meatal lips. When the urethral mucosa is inflamed, the mouths of these ducts become prominent, and pus can be seen exuding when the follicles are involved.

Meatus: ***Hypospadias.*** In the fetus the urethral meatus may develop so it occurs on the *ventral* surface of the glans, the shaft, or at the penoscrotal junction (Fig. 8-4C).

Meatus: ***Epispadias.*** Maldevelopment may result in the meatus urethrae opening *dorsally* on the glans, shaft, or at the penoscrotal junction (Fig. 8-4D).

Ventral Shaft: ***Acute Urethritis.*** An acute indurating urethritis, especially as the result of infection from an indwelling catheter, may cause a palpable cord that extends the entire length of the ventral midline of the penis.

Ventral Shaft: ***Urethral Stricture.*** A tunnel stricture of the urethra may cause a palpable cordlike mass in the corpus cavernosum urethrae at the penoscrotal junction. Strictures in other parts of the penile urethra are usually not palpable.

Ventral Shaft: ***Urethral Diverticulum.*** When located at the penoscrotal junction, a diverticulum frequently produces a visible swelling, felt as a soft midline mass.

Ventral Shaft: ***Periurethral Abscess.*** An accumulation of pus in the *midportion* of the penile urethra in Littre's follicle will produce visible swelling.

Ventral Shaft: ***Urethral Carcinoma.*** Occasionally a neoplasm may be felt as an indurated mass in the corpus cavernosum urethrae.

Dorsal Shaft: ***Thrombosis of the Dorsal Vein.*** A thrombus in the dorsal vein of the penis causes a palpable cord, about 1 mm in diameter, in the midline dorsally. This condition is usually secondary to inflammation of the glans.

Dorsal Shaft: ***Varicose Veins.*** Varicosities of the dorsal veins of the penis may be visible and palpable. They may be sufficiently large to require surgical treatment.

Lateral Shaft: ***Cavernositis.*** An irregular hard mass may occur in the lateral or ventral cavernous corpora from inflammation. Priapism and edema usually accompany this condition. Suppuration may occur, with drainage through the skin or the urethra.

Clinical Occurrence. Abscess from trauma or infection. Thrombosis in leukemia, septicemia.

Lateral Shaft: ***Plastic Induration of the Penis*** (Induratio Penis Plastica, Peyronie's Disease, Strabismus Penis). Firm, nontender plaques may be felt laterally in the corpora cavernosa penis or dorsally over the intercorporeal septum. The plaques may be single or multiple; they are not necessarily symmetric. The patient may complain of *curvature of the penis* during erection. ***Pathophysiology.*** This is a chronic disease of unknown cause, characterized by irregular fibrosis of the septum or sheath of the corpus cavernosum penis, extending into the tunica albuginea. It never affects the corpus cavernosum urethrae. It is considered a component of Dupuytren's diathesis along with palmar and solar fibrositis. ***Distinction.*** The findings may resemble those in gumma, scars from trauma, cavernositis, subcutaneous gouty tophi, fibromas, chondromas and carcinoma.

Priapism. Prolonged, persistent, penile erection occurs without sexual desire. The condition is usually painful. ***Pathophysiology.*** Ascending nervous impulses from lesions of the urethra, from direct stimulation of lesions in the spinal cord or nervi erigentes, or from descending impulses from lesions in the cerebrum. Local mechanical causes, such as thrombosis, hemorrhage, neoplasm, or inflammation in the penis. The condition is associated with leukemia and sickle-cell anemia. Surgical manipulation may be required urgently in order to reverse a potentially dangerous situation.

Penile Hypoplasia. Wide variation occurs in the normal size of the penis; the normal range is learned only by the examination of many individuals. Striking discrepancies between the penile size and the age of the patient lead to the inference of hypoplasia or hyperplasia. Penile hypoplasia either is a manifestation of *eunuchoidism* occurring before puberty or is a feature of *intersexuality.* In the latter condition, distinction between a hypoplastic penis with hypospadias and a hyperplastic clitoris may be difficult or impossible without operation and histologic examination of the gonads.

Penile Hyperplasia. This is usually evident only before the age of normal puberty when a discrepancy between size of the organ and age is possible. Commonly, the causes of hyperplasia are tumors of the pineal gland or the hypothalamus, tumors arising from the Leydig cells of the testis, or tumors of the adrenal gland.

Intersexuality. The reader is referred to special works on this subject.

The Scrotum

The scrotum is a pouch formed by a layer of thin rugous *skin* overlying a tightly adherent layer of *dartos tunic,* composed of unstriped muscle fibers and fascia (Fig. 8-5C). The sac hangs from the root of the penis, the left side lower than the right because the left spermatic cord is longer because of the longer column of venous blood; the testicular vein on the left draining into the left renal vein. The skin of the pouch is bisected by a *median raphe* extending from the ventral aspect of the penile shaft, under the entire sac, to the anus. Internally, the two halves of the pouch are separated by a septal fold of dartos tunic. Each half contains a testis with its epididymis and spermatic cord. The scrotal contents slide easily in a *fascial cleft* between the scrotal wall and the covering of the testis and cords. The skin of the scrotum is deeply pigmented and contains large sebaceous follicles that have a tendency to form cysts. The lymph from the scrotum drains to the inguinal lymph nodes but entirely distinct channels lead from the testes to the pelvic nodes. The tone of the dartos muscle determines the size of the scrotum; exposure to external cold shrinks the sac; external heat causes muscle relaxation and enlargement of the pouch. In advanced age, the dartos muscle becomes

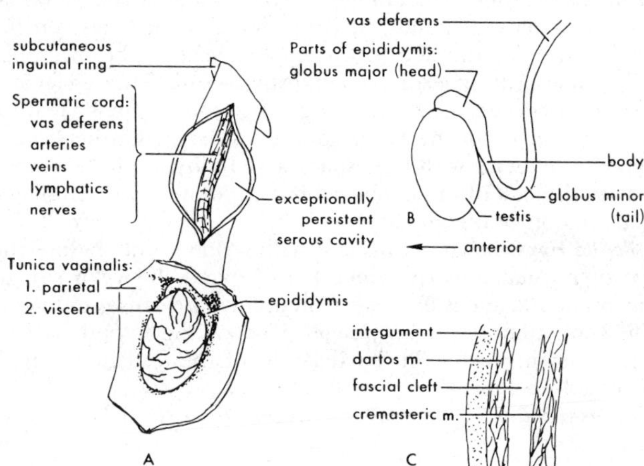

Fig. 8-5. Anatomy of the scrotal layers and epididymis. **A.** *Cavities of the tunica vaginalis are opened anteriorly to show testis and cord.* **B.** *Parts of the epididymis and cord.* **C.** *Layers of the scrotum.*

relatively atonic. The action of the dartos muscles is independent of contractions of the cremasteric muscles.

EXAMINATION OF SCROTAL WALL. **The scrotum is examined by inspection and palpation. Because the rugae are produced by contractions of dartos muscle, the walls should be inspected by spreading the layers between the fingers. Transillumination is readily performed, but it is more informative in examining the scrotal contents.**

Edema of the Scrotum. The thickened wall pits on pressure.

Clinical Occurrence. Cardiac decompensation, nephrosis, portal vein obstruction, and other conditions producing massive edema in the lower half of the trunk. Thrombosis of the pelvic veins. Extravasation of urine. Acute epididymitis. Torsion of the spermatic cord. After paracentesis abdominis, Conn noted the sudden development of edema of the abdominal wall and scrotum. He postulated that the trochar had produced a fistula between the peritoneal cavity and the subcutaneous tissue [H. O. Conn: Sudden Scrotal Edema in Cirrhosis: A Paracentesis Syndrome, *Ann. Intern. Med.*, **74**:943–45, 1971].

Lymphedema of the Scrotum (Elephantiasis Scroti). Obstruction of the inguinal lymphatics from any cause produces edema of the scrotal wall and accumulation of the fluid in the fascial clefts. Most spectacular is the huge scrotum from lymphatic blockage in filariasis, to which the term *elephantiasis* is usually applied.

Sebaceous Cysts of the Scrotum. This is the most common tumor of the wall and is benign. It may be single or multiple. The white contents of the cyst may show through the skin.

Scrotal Hematoma and Laceration. The conditions are evident and cause no difficulty in diagnosis.

Scrotal Gangrene. Necrotizing perineal infections (*Fournier's gangrene*) are polymicrobial, gas-producing, and rapidly progressing. This life-threatening infection of the perineum is caused by mixed organisms, both gram-positive and gram-negative, aerobic and anaerobic, acting in synergism, resulting in subcutaneous vascular thrombosis leading to gangrene of the overlying dermis. Common features include elderly, diabetic patients who present with fever and a toxic appearance, evidence of sepsis and demonstrating necrosis, with crepitus, foul-smelling rapidly advancing lesions of scrotum or labia [P. J.

Kovalcik and J. Jones: Necrotizing Perineal Infections, *Am. Surg.*, **49:**163–66, 1983.]. The condition is life threatening unless antibiotics and wide debridement of all nonviable tissues are instituted promptly.

Scrotal Carcinoma. The neoplasm is similar to those in other areas of skin. They are particularly common in workers in tar and oil, whose clothes cause friction in the scrotal region.

Subcutaneous Emphysema. When subcutaneous emphysema occurs elsewhere in the body, the air may infiltrate the layers of the scrotum (p. 501).

Testis, Epididymis, and Vas Deferens

The testis is a solid ovoid, compressed laterally. The spermatic cord suspends the testis in the scrotum so the long axis of the ovoid is nearly vertical. The upper pole of the smooth testis is capped by the *globus major* or *head* of the epididymis. The *body* of the epididymis forms an elongated inverted cone attached vertically to the posterior surface of the testis. The apex of the cone approaches the lower pole of the testis, where it is called the *globus minor* or *tail* (Fig. 8-5B). It becomes continuous with the *vas deferens* that joins other vessels to form the *spermatic cord.* The spermatic cord consists of the vas deferens, arteries, veins, nerves, and lymphatic vessels, held together by the spermatic fascia. From the testis, the cord extends upward through the fascial cleft of the scrotum, entering the subcutaneous inguinal ring and coursing through the inguinal canal to the abdominal inguinal ring, where its components diverge. In the abdominal cavity, the vas deferens continues backward and downward behind the peritoneum until it lies behind the bladder and anterior to the rectum, joining the duct of the seminal vesicle to become the *ejaculatory duct.* In fetal life, the *saccus vaginalis*, a process of the peritoneum, invades the scrotum, and into this peritoneal pouch the cord descends to assume the adult position. Normally, the funicular (cord) portion of the pouch becomes obliterated, leaving a serous cavity surrounding the testis and epididymis, except for their posterior aspect (Fig. 8-5A). The serous membrane becomes the *tunica vaginalis*, visceral and parietal layers. Abnormal persistence of portions of the saccus vaginalis leads to congenital hernias or funicular hydroceles.

EXAMINATION OF SCROTAL CONTENTS. **Palpation and transillumination distinguish most structures in the scrotal sac. Rarely, auscultation of the scrotum with the stethoscope yields peristaltic sounds from a loop of herniated gut. With swelling of the scrotum, first distinguish between an inguinal hernia and structures normally in the scrotum. After hernia is diagnosed or excluded, examine systematically the structures in the scrotum in the following sequence: (1) testes, (2) tunica vaginalis, (3) epididymis (head, body, and tail), (4) spermatic cord, (5) inguinal lymph nodes. The complete sequence should also be followed in every routine physical examination.**

Scrotal Hernia. Grasp the root of the scrotum between the thumb and forefinger to determine whether the mass extends that high. If the fingers can be inserted above the mass, hernia is excluded. Insert the finger into the subcutaneous inguinal ring and feel for a cough impulse from hernia. Inguinal hernias always descend *in front of the spermatic cord* and testes, so identify these structures and their anatomic relations to the mass (Fig. 8-6M). Transilluminate the mass in a darkened room, or shade the scrotum with a towel, clothing, or bedclothes. With the thumb and forefinger, pull the scrotal wall tightly over the mass. Place the lamp of the flashlight in contact with the posterior wall of the scrotum; shine the light anteriorly through the mass to determine whether the structure is translucent or opaque. Most hernial contents are opaque, although occasionally a gas-filled loop of gut will transmit light. Listen through the stethoscope for peristaltic sounds.

▼ *Key Symptom:* ***Pain in the Testis.*** Pain in the testis is frequently a chief complaint. It may be mild or excruciating. It may emanate from the structure itself or be referred from a remote locus. The principal causes are:

Clinical Occurrence: ACUTE PAIN. *Infectious:* gonorrheal orchitis, bacteremias, urethral instrumentation, mumps, typhoid fever, scarlet fever, influenza. *Urethral Calculus:* either in the urethra or in the prostate. *Trauma:* hematoma or laceration. Gout. Rheumatic fever. Torsion of the spermatic cord. *Hydrocele:* this may develop during some general infectious disease. *Hernia:* incarcerated scrotal hernia may contain intestine. *Referred Pain:* calculus in the upper ureter or renal pelvis, appendicitis. CHRONIC PAIN. *Infectious:* syphilis, tuberculosis, leprosy, brucellosis, glanders, filariasis, bilharziasis. *Neoplasm:* pain usually in later stages. *Hydrocele:* a very large tumor may produce discomfort. *Undescended Testis:* pressure on

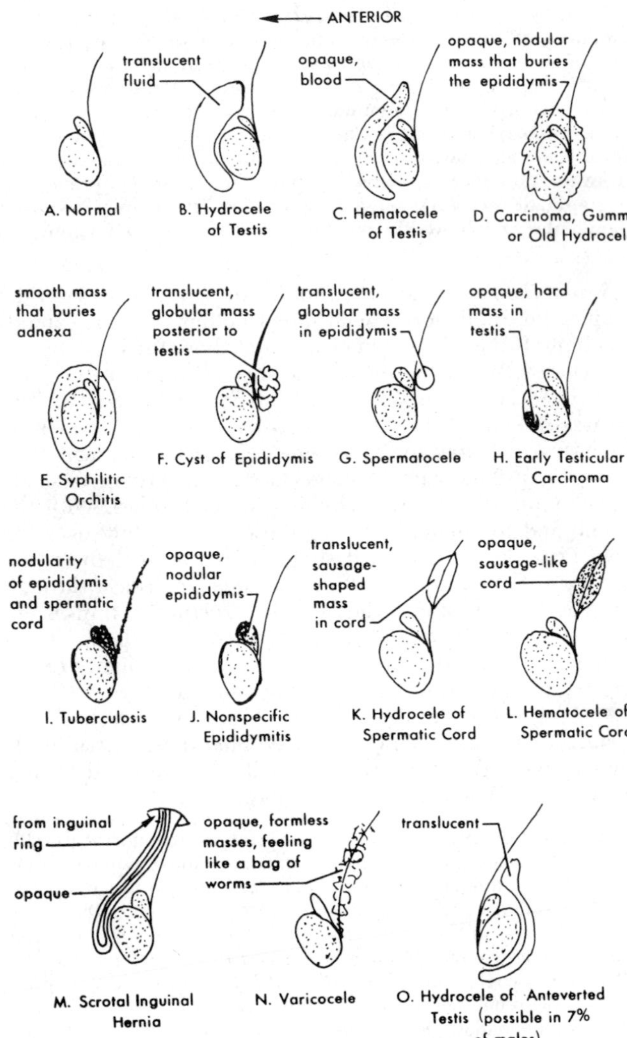

Fig. 8-6. Swellings of the scrotal contents; a diagnostic summary.

the testis when it lies in the inguinal canal. Large varicocele. Carcinoma of lumbar vertebrae or aneurysm in the region stimulating peripheral nerves. *Neuralgia testis:* no organic lesion known.

EXAMINATION OF THE TESTES. **Compare both testes simultaneously by grasping one with each hand, using thumb and forefinger. Determine their size, shape, consistency, and sensitivity to pressure. Even though they feel normal, transilluminate each; one may be atrophied and the normal size attained by a hydrocele.**

Maldescended Testis (Cryptorchism). During fetal development, the descent of the testis may be arrested in the abdomen, in the inguinal canal, or at the puboscrotal junction. Either or both testes may be affected. When the testis remains in the abdomen, it cannot be palpated. In the inguinal canal or at the puboscrotal junction, the testis is palpable, but frequently it is atrophied so the mass is smaller than might be expected. More complicated anomalies of development result in the testis lodging in the perineum near the median raphe of the scrotum, in the femoral canal, or anteriorly and dorsally at the root of the penis. In infants, maldescent must be distinguished from temporary retraction of the testis into the scrotum by contraction of the cremasteric muscles. With the infant undressed, hold him in a squatting position. As the child cries evaluate the scrotum and inguinal canal for the presence of the testicular mass. Bilateral maldescent may result in sterility. A maldescended testis is frequently associated with a congenital inguinal hernia on the same side, as a result of persistence of part of the saccus vaginalis.

Atrophied Testis. The testis may be smaller than normal from maldevelopment. Atrophy may occur after infarction, trauma, orchitis from mumps, syphilis, filariasis, or surgical repair of an inguinal hernia. In a maldescended testis, pressure may produce atrophy.

Testicular Swelling (Nontender): ***Hydrocele.*** Accumulation of serous fluid occurs in the cavity of the tunica vaginalis congenitally or from infection or trauma. Palpation reveals a pear-shaped mass with the smaller pole upward. Pinching the root of the scrotum indicates that the mass does not extend that high. The mass feels smooth and resilient. The testis and epididymis are usually *behind the mass* (Fig. 8-6B), except when *anteversion* is present, and the structures are then anterior (Fig. 8-6O).

Transillumination shows the mass to be *translucent;* it also reveals the opaque shadow of the testis. *Distinction.* The translucency of the hydrocele distinguishes it from the opaque hematocele. Except in anteversion of the testis, the location of the mass in front of the testis distinguishes it from spermatocele that arises from the epididymis and is behind the testis. Hydrocele of the spermatic cord occurs above the testis.

Testicular Swelling (Nontender): ***Hematocele.*** The cavity of the tunica vaginalis may be filled with blood. The swelling resembles that of a hydrocele, but blood is opaque to transillumination (Fig. 8-6C). A history of recent trauma suggests hematocele. Aspiration of the mass may be necessary to distinguish.

Testicular Swelling (Nontender): ***Chylocele.*** In filariasis, opalescent lymph may accumulate in the cavity of the tunica vaginalis. The mass is translucent and distinction from hydrocele can only be made by aspiration of the fluid.

Testicular Swelling (Nontender): ***Tuberculosis.*** A large, hard, nodular mass is produced in the testis by tuberculosis. Palpation does not distinguish it from gumma or neoplasm. Nodular induration of the prostate and seminal vesicles gives presumptive evidence that the testis is involved with the tuberculous process (Fig. 8-6I). Biopsy may be necessary for diagnosis.

Testicular Swelling (Nontender): ***Gumma.*** In tertiary syphilis, a gumma may involve the testis. The organ is enlarged, nontender, indurated, and smooth (Figs. 8-6D and 8-6E). If not enlarged, the testis is harder than normal. The testis loses its normal sensitivity to pressure pain. If serologic tests for syphilis are positive, the inference may be made that the mass is gummatous. A therapeutic test or a biopsy may be indicated for diagnosis.

Testicular Swelling (Nontender): ***Neoplasm.*** Various neoplasms, benign and malignant, that involve the testis can be diagnosed only by biopsy. The testis is usually enlarged, harder than normal, and frequently it contains softer cystic regions (Figs. 8-6D and 8-6H). A carcinomatous testis is heavier than that with orchitis or hydrocele. The presence of metastatic lesions elsewhere is presumptive evidence that a nodule in the testis is neoplastic.

Testicular Swelling (Tender): ***Acute Orchitis.*** Inflammation of one or both testes occurs frequently in mumps, occasionally in other infectious diseases. The gland is swollen, tender, and usually extremely painful. Frequently the inflammation causes acute hydrocele, but the inflammatory edema and the pain of palpation prevent accurate distinction. Often, primary or secondary epididymitis is associated. Orchitis is sometimes confused with torsion of the spermatic cord.

EXAMINATION OF THE EPIDIDYMIS. **Locate each epididymis by palpating the smooth testis to find a vertical ridge of soft nodules beginning at the upper testicular pole and extending to the lower pole. Usually the epididymis is *behind* the testis, but in about 7% of males the structure develops anterior to the testis, *anteversion of the epididymis*. Recognizing the anteversion, the examiner will expect the cavity of the tunica vaginalis to be posterior to the testis. Compare the findings from palpation in both epididymides, in their component segments of head, body, and tail.**

Epididymal Mass: ***Spermatocele.*** Retention cysts of the epididymis, especially in the globus major, contain milky fluid characterized as the color of the second rinsing of the milk bottle. Spermatozoa may be present microscopically. The cysts are usually small but may attain a diameter of 8 or 10 cm. The fluid may be milky or clear; the cyst is usually translucent when transilluminated (Fig. 8-6G).

Epididymal Mass: ***Solid Tumor.*** Opaque masses of the epididymis are rare; when present, they are usually neoplasms. They should be diagnosed by biopsy because they are frequently malignant.

Epididymal Nodularity: ***Syphilis.*** The globus major is usually first involved; then the process extends to the body of the epididymis (Fig. 8-6J). The organ is usually not painful. The cause is inferred from positive serologic tests for syphilis and the presence of syphilitic lesions elsewhere.

Epididymal Nodularity: ***Tuberculosis.*** The body of the epididymis is usually first involved. The hard nodules are not tender. The epididymis becomes adherent to the scrotum, and sinuses may form. The cause is usually inferred from the presence of tuberculosis in other structures.

Epididymal Swelling (Tender): ***Acute Epididymitis.*** Acute infections of the epididymis usually occur from trauma or with infection of other structures in the genitourinary tract. The painful, tender swelling of the epididymis may be accompanied by fever and leukocytosis.

EXAMINATION OF THE SPERMATIC CORD. **Compare both spermatic cords simultaneously by grasping one with each hand at the neck of the scrotum. With the thumb in front and the forefinger behind the scrotum, gently compress the contents of the cord (Fig. 8-7). The normal vas deferens is felt as a distinct hard whipcord; other less definable strands are nerves, arteries, and fibers of cremasteric muscle. The vas may be congenitally absent. Trace the cords down to the testes.**

Thickening of the Vas: ***Deferentitis.*** This is inflammation of the vas deferens. In acute diseases, the vas is tender and swollen. The inflammation is usually an extension from other structures. In chronic inflammation, the vas may be thickened and indurated, with some nodularity (Fig. 8-6I). The finding suggests either tuberculous or syphilitic extension from other parts of the genitourinary tract.

Funicular Mass: ***Hydrocele of the Cord.*** When the saccus vaginalis fails to be obliterated around the spermatic cord, a serous cavity persists. This cavity may become filled with fluid to form a hydrocele. Typically the resulting mass is smooth, resilient, and sausage-shaped; it is located above the testis. The mass transmits transilluminated light (Fig. 8-6K). When no other abnormalities are present, the diagnosis is made by palpation and transillumination. When associated with a hernia, spermatocele, or testicular hydrocele, the distinction may be difficult or impossible without operation. Occasionally there exists a communication between the hydrocele and the peritoneal cavity, so-called *communicating hydrocele.* This is characteristically

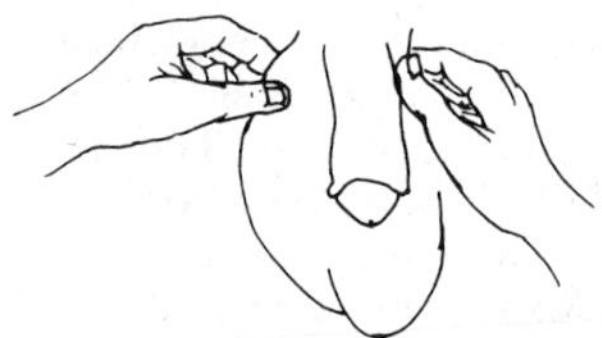

Fig. 8-7. Palpation of the spermatic cords. *Simultaneously each hand grasps a cord between thumb and index finger and the two structures are compared. Normally, the vasa deferentia feel like distinct whipcords; the other components of the cord feel like indefinite strands; they are arteries, veins, vessels, and nerves.*

identified by the variation in size from large to nonexistent, dependent upon the quantity of fluid contained.

Funicular Mass: ***Hematoma of the Cord.*** When trauma causes bleeding around the spermatic cord, a boggy mass may be felt in the region. The mass is opaque to transillumination (Fig. 8-6L). The history of trauma should assist in distinguishing.

Funicular Mass: ***Gumma.*** The granuloma is felt as a solitary mass associated with the spermatic cord. It is opaque to transillumination. Distinction from tuberculoma or neoplasm is made only by finding other signs of syphilis or positive serologic tests.

Funicular Mass: ***Tuberculoma.*** Rarely tuberculosis forms a mass in the cord that is indistinguishable on physical examination from gumma or neoplasm. Finding tuberculous lesions in other structures assists in the interpretation.

Funicular Mass: ***Neoplasm.*** The mass is indistinguishable from gumma or tuberculoma; biopsy is required for diagnosis.

Funicular Mass: ***Varicocele.*** Varicosities of the pampiniform plexus of veins form a soft irregular mass in the scrotum that is rarely mistaken for anything else (Fig. 8-6N). The sensation is usually likened to feeling a bag of worms. The condition occurs predominantly on the *left side;* occasionally it is bilateral; almost never is the right side exclusively involved. The predominance on the left is attributed to the left spermatic vein, which has a larger hydrostatic column of pressure than the right, which empties directly into the vena cava. To distinguish the condition from an indirect inguinal hernia containing omentum, have the patient lie down; place your finger over the subcutaneous inguinal ring. When the patient stands, with your finger in place, the veins refill but the hernia will be held back.

Funicular Mass: ***Torsion of the Cord*** (Testicular Torsion). When the spermatic cord becomes twisted, the arterial blood supply to the testis and its venous and lymphatic drainage are occluded. Venous obstruction occurs first because of the nature of the vessel walls and lower venous pressure as contrasted with arterial wall thickness and arterial pressure. The problem of engorgement is thus compounded. The condition is painful and urgent. It is frequently confused with acute epididymo-orchitis and strangulated scrotal hernia. Palpation reveals a tender, irregular, edematous mass in the scrotum. *Distinction:* Occasionally the twists in the cord can be felt to identify the condition. Five distinguishing features are commonly noted: (1) The testis on the affected side lies higher than normal from the twisting of the cord and the spasm of the cremasteric muscles. (2) Palpation does not distinguish between the testis and the epididymis. In acute epididymo-orchitis, the epididymis can usually be felt separately from the testis. (3) Elevation and support of the scrotum for an hour usually relieve the pain of epididymo-orchitis; it does not ameliorate the pain in torsion (*Prehn's sign*). (4) In torsion, the leg of the involved side is often held in flexion. (5) When a secondary hydrocele is present, the aspirated contents yield serosanguinous fluid from torsion, serous fluid in epididymo-orchitis. Sometimes strangulated hernia cannot be distinguished from torsion without operation.

EXAMINATION OF INGUINAL LYMPH NODES. **In all cases, palpate the lymph nodes in the inguinal and femoral regions. Many apparently normal persons have chronic painless enlargement of nodes in these regions that are diagnostically insignificant. Only the experience of examining many patients yields the criteria by which to judge significant enlargement. Evaluate the patient's hygiene, relative to foot care: how clean the toenails are, presence of athlete's foot or other fungal infections, ingrown toenails; in short, any condition likely to lead to lymphadenopathy secondary to inflammation.**

Lymphadenopathy: ***Syphilis.*** Three to five days after the appearance of a chancre, lymph nodes from the saphenous opening upward become somewhat enlarged, rubbery, and freely movable. The involvement is bilateral, symmetric, and painless.

Lymphadenopathy: ***Chancroid.*** A considerable unilateral enlargement of the inguinal lymph nodes, the *bubo,* occurs early on the side of the genital ulcer. The nodes are tender and frequently suppurate.

Lymphadenopathy: ***Carcinoma.*** Involvement of the inguinal and femoral lymph nodes is frequent in metastasis from carcinoma of the penis.

Lymphadenopathy: ***Lymphogranuloma Venereum.*** Usually the nodes on one side are enlarged. They are not tender. Overlying cutaneous edema develops to distinguish the condition from syphilis.

Lymphadenopathy: Gonorrhea. The regional lymph nodes become moderately enlarged and tender, bilaterally.

The Prostate and Seminal Vesicles

The prostate is a body of gland and muscle, shaped roughly like a truncated cone the size of a chestnut. As it lies in the pelvis, about 2 cm posterior* to the symphysis pubis, the cone is inverted so the base is superior and the apex inferior (Fig. 8-8B and C). The anterior and posterior surfaces are somewhat flattened. The basal surface is directed superiorly and is overlain by the bladder; the apical surface faces inferiorly and rests on the urogenital diaphragm. The *prostatic urethra* pierces the basal or superior surface, slightly anterior to the center, and runs inferiorly in a vertical axis to emerge through the apical or inferior surface of the prostate. The posterior prostatic surface is in close contact with the rectal wall and is the only portion of the prostate accessible to palpation; this surface is slightly convex vertically. A shallow *median furrow* divides all except the upper portion of the posterior surface into a *right* and *left lateral lobe.* Near the superior edge of the posterior surface, i.e., the part farthest from the anus, is a transverse *depression,* made by the *ejaculatory duct* from each side piercing the prostate and converging to enter the urethra. This depression delineates a small portion of the posterior surface posteriorly; this is the *middle lobe* of the prostate. In contact with the posterior wall of the bladder, four radii diverge superiorly from the prostatic base; the medial pair are the *ampullae of the vasa deferentia* and the lateral pair are the *seminal vesicles.* The seminal vesicles are about 7.5 cm long, so the finger in the rectum can reach only their lower portions.

PALPATION OF PROSTATE AND SEMINAL VESICLES RECTALLY. **For this examination, choose between the *lithotomy position,* the *knee-chest position,* the *left lateral prone position* (Sims's), or the *standing elbow-knee position.* Three of these have been considered elsewhere (p. 569). In the last mentioned, the patient stands with legs apart, the trunk flexed on the thighs, and the elbows resting on the knees.**

* In this description the terms *superior* (cephalad), *inferior* (caudad), *anterior* (ventral), and *posterior* (dorsal) are used in their strict anatomic sense and must not be confused with the patient's position during examination.

Palpation of Prostate and Seminal Vesicles Rectally

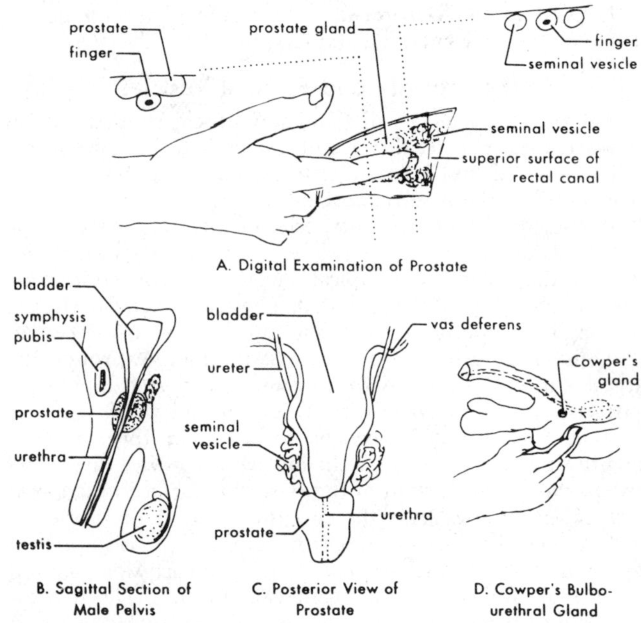

Fig. 8-8. Rectal examination of the male genitalia. **A.** Relations of the examining finger in the rectum to the prostate and seminal vesicles. *The view is from the inferolateral aspect, when the patient is in the lithotomy position. The near section depicts the finger underneath the prostate gland; the other section shows the finger between the two seminal vesicles.* **B.** *This shows a sagittal section of the male penis.* **C.** *A posterior view of the prostate, seminal vesicles, and vasa deferentia.* **D.** Palpation of Cowper's bulbourethral gland. *The diagram shows a sagittal section of the male pelvis in the lithotomy position. The tip of the index finger is in the rectum with the pad facing the anterior rectal wall, between the inferior border of the prostate and the inner edge of the anal canal. The thumb is outside the rectum, pressing the perineum on the medial raphe toward the fingertip. A normal gland is not palpable, but an inflamed one is tender; if it contains pus, it forms a palpable mass, from pea size to hazelnut size, as shown in the round black spot, one gland on each side of the urethra.*

We prefer the lithotomy position because it gives better access to the peritoneal pouches. Whatever the position, the details of the procedure are the same. Cover the examining hand with a rubber glove and lubricate the forefinger with surgical jelly. Place the *pad* or *pulp* of the forefinger on the anal orifice (Fig. 7-37, p. 574) and press gently until the sphincter relaxes, admitting the curve of the pad. Then incline the finger until the *tip* is also inserted. Gradually ease the tip past the anal canal and into the rectal ampulla. Keep the pad of the finger facing the *anterior* rectal wall. As the finger moves cephalad from the anal canal, it encounters the elastic bulging surface of the prostate (Fig. 8-8A). Feel the *median furrow* that separates the *lateral lobes*. When the fingertip reaches the superior edge of the prostate, the median furrow thins out to the flat *middle lobe*. Superior to the prostate, the fingertip reaches the *seminal vesicles* on either side of the midline. Normally, the seminal vesicles are not palpable because they are too soft; only diseased structures can be felt. The anal sphincter is *tight* in acute infections, *relaxed* in prostatic cancer. Determine whether the prostatic *surface* is smooth or nodular; whether the *consistency* is elastic, hard, boggy, soft, or fluctuant; whether the *shape* is rounded or flat; whether the *size* is normal, enlarged, or atrophied; whether *sensitivity* to pressure is abnormal; whether there is normal *mobility* or fixation. Examine each seminal vesicle for *distention, sensitivity, size, consistency, induration,* and *nodules*. Palpate in the region of the *bulbourethral glands of Cowper,* one on each side of the midline just inferior to the caudal border of the prostate. They are normally not palpable; when enlarged, they are felt as rounded masses in the anterior rectal wall. Either clean the patient or provide tissues for it to be accomplished.

Prostatic Enlargement (*Nontender*): ***Benign Hyperplasia.*** When the lateral lobes are involved, they are symmetrically enlarged, elastic to rubbery or firm, and the rectal mucosa can be made to slide over them readily. Hyperplasia of the median lobe may be difficult to detect because the bulk of the lobe may protrude anteriorly to produce urethral obstruction, without being palpable.

Prostatic Enlargement (*Nontender*): ***Carcinoma.*** Frequently this starts as a palpable hard nodule near the posterior surface of the prostate. As it grows, the entire gland may become stony hard, or there may be several hard nodules. The median furrow becomes obliterated. Early spread is often in the direction of the seminal vesicles. A high index of suspicion of cancer exists when these findings prevail.

Prostatic Nodular Induration (Nontender): ***Tuberculosis.*** The nodular indurated prostate is almost always accompanied by nodular induration of one or both seminal vesicles and nodulation of the vas deferens. This pattern strongly suggests tuberculosis. Nodular induration of the prostate can only be the result of carcinoma. If associated tuberculosis cannot be found elsewhere, biopsy is necessary for diagosis.

Prostatic Enlargement (Tender): ***Acute Prostatitis.*** Gentle palpation reveals an enlarged tender prostate, surrounded by edematous tissue. The terminal specimen in the three-glass urine test contains large mucous shreds. Massage of the prostate is contraindicated to obtain fluid for examination.

Chronic Prostatitis. Palpation of the prostate may not reveal distinctive findings. A history suggesting chronic urinary tract infection prompts the three-glass urine test in which the terminal specimen contains large mucous shreds. *Prostatic massage* is accomplished by firmly stroking the posterior surface of the prostate repeatedly from the lateral margins toward the midline, sometimes a painful procedure. The fluid is milked from the urethra and examined in the microscope. In prostatitis, the fluid contains many leukocytes.

Palpable Seminal Vesicle. ***Vesiculitis.*** The normal seminal vesicle is not palpable. When the structure can be felt as a dilated or indurated mass, it is the site of acute or chronic infection. The finger in the rectum may procure fluid for examination by *massaging* the vesicle toward the prostate, then milking the urethra to produce the seminal fluid.

Palpable Cowper's Gland: ***Cowperitis*** (Inflammation of Bulbourethral Gland). Normally the bulbourethral glands are not palpable. When they are inflamed, they are exquisitely tender. In chronic inflammation they enlarge from the size of a pea to that of a hazelnut. The tenderness or mass is readily demonstrated, if the condition is considered and searched for in the proper place. One gland lies on each side of the membranous urethra between the inferior edge of the prostate and the inner border of the anal canal. With the forefinger in the rectum, explore the anterior rectal wall inferior to the prostate and superior to the edge of the anal canal (Fig. 8-8D). At the same time the thumb is held outside on the median raphe of the scrotum just anterior to the anus. The tissue between the thumb and forefinger is compressed to detect tenderness or a mass.

The Female Genitalia

▼ *Key Symptoms:* ***Menstrual Disorders.*** The anterior pituitary gland produces the follicle-stimulating hormone FSH, the luteinizing hormone LH, and the luteotropic hormone LTH. An output of FSH causes the maturation of a graafian follicle in the ovary by growth of its granulosa cells and the formation of follicular fluid. In combination with FSH, the second pituitary hormone, LH, causes the theca interna to secrete estrogen. The mature follicle ruptures through the ovarian surface, releasing the ovum into the peritoneal cavity and thence down the fallopian tube to be implanted in the uterine endometrium. The ruptured follicle in the ovary becomes the corpus luteum, whose cells secrete both estrogen and progesterone under the influence of LH and LTH. If the ovum is not fertilized, the corpus luteum gradually degenerates and scarifies. Ovulation occurs about 2 weeks before menstruation. During the time when estrogen is the primary secretion, the uterine endometrium undergoes proliferation. Later, when the secretion of progesterone predominates, the stimulation of estrogen is inhibited and the endometrium degenerates and sloughs in the menstrual blood. Menstruation usually begins (*menarche*) between the ages of 12 and 15 years in temperate climates, at 9 or 10 years in the tropics. The menopause may occur between the ages of 35 and 50 years.

Thus menstrual disturbances may be caused by disorders of the anterior pituitary gland, the hypothalamus, the thyroid gland, the ovary, or the uterus.

— *Profuse Menstruation:* ***Menorrhagia.*** Usually the menstrual cycle recurs in periods of 27 to 32 days, although some women are normally irregular. The menstrual flow lasts about 5 days. During the entire period the average blood loss is from 60 to 250 mL, most during the first and second day. A menstrual pad is considered filled when it contains 30 to 50 mL of blood. Menorrhagia is the condition in which menstruation persists longer, or the daily volume of flow is greater than normal.

Clinical Occurrence: HORMONAL. Puberty, premenopausal, hypothyroidism. GENITAL. Endometritis, salpingitis, leiomyofibroma, endometrial or cervical polyps, endometriosis. INFECTIOUS. Influenza, typhoid fever, cholera, scarlet fever, malaria, diphtheria, the exanthemata. CIRCULATORY. Congestive cardiac failure, pulmonary hypertension, portal hypertension, essential hypertension, scurvy. HEMATOLOGIC. Coagulation defects (thrombocytopenia, prothrombin deficit, hemophilia), leukemia. EMOTIONAL.

— *Intermenstrual Bleeding:* ***Metrorrhagia.*** Although metrorrhagia is commonly synonymous with intermenstrual bleeding, the term is often used in the absence of menstruation. Some causes of menorrhagia, in more severe form, produce metrorrhagia.

Clinical Occurrence: PREGNANCY. Threatened abortion, ectopic pregnancy, hydatid mole. GENITAL. Benign and malignant neoplasms, cervical erosions, endometriosis, tuberculosis of the uterus. CARDIOVASCULAR. Essential hypertension, scurvy. HEMATOLOGIC. Thrombocytopenia, hemophilia, leukemia. HORMONAL. Dysfunctional uterine bleeding. INFECTIOUS. Pelvic inflammation.

— *Absent Menstruation:* ***Amenorrhea.*** The causes of absence of menstruation are many. Some are given here.

Clinical Occurrence: PHYSIOLOGIC. Before puberty, after the menopause, during pregnancy and lactation. MALFORMATION (also called *primary amenorrhea*). Ovarian agenesis or dysgenesis (Turner's syndrome), uterine agenesis, imperforate hymen (cryptomenorrhea). ACQUIRED (also called *secondary amenorrhea*). *Pituitary:* Simmonds' disease. Sheehan's syndrome, Chiari-Frommel disease. *Thyroid:* hyperthyroidism or hypothyroidism. *Uterus:* radiation or destructive curettage of endometerium, hysterectomy. *Ovary:* oophorectomy, ovarian radiation, polycystic ovaries (Stein-Leventhal syndrome), masculinizing ovarian tumors, chemotherapy. *Metabolic and Nutritional:* diabetes mellitus, malnutrition, anorexia nervosa, obesity, debilitating diseases. *Hematologic:* severe anemia, leukemia, Hodgkin's disease. *Nervous:* emotional disorders, imbecility. *Fevers. Poisoning:* with lead, mercury, morphine, alcohol.

— *Painful Menstruation:* ***Dysmenorrhea.*** The most prominent and most frequent complaint is *severe abdominal cramps* in the suprapubic region. Less severe are accompanying backache and headache. The severity of the pain is doubtless enhanced in some patients by fear. The most common is a *primary* or *intrinsic spastic* condition with no anatomic cause. It may disappear after a pregnancy. Male physicians ought not to disregard the symptom complex without attempting to find relief for the patient. It is now reasonably well understood that the symptoms relate to prostaglandin formation and release from the endometrium. Prostaglandin formation inhibitors or blocking agents can be quite helpful. Other conditions that may cause painful menstruation are endometriosis, uterine retroversion, pelvic neoplasms, and pelvic inflammations.

The Pelvic Examination

Inspection and palpation of the female pelvis reveal many disorders of the reproductive organs, the lower urinary tract, and the lower abdomen. In one sense, the pelvic examination is an extension of abdominal palpation and thus is *mandatory* for every female. Clinical experience is replete with cases in which neglect of the pelvic examination led to serious errors in diagnosis. We believe one deterrent from examining the pelvis routinely is the inconvenience of employing the vaginal speculum. If omission of the speculum would lead to more pelvic examinations, we would compromise for a routine digital examination of the vagina and rectum, reserving inspection through the speculum for cases in which symptoms or palpatory findings demanded more details. Aside from this argument, clinical experience has led to the judgment that routine inspection of the cervix with the Papanicolaou smear is rewarding in detecting early cancer.

METHOD OF VAGINAL EXAMINATION. **Arrange this procedure as the last in the physical examination because it requires special posture, equipment, and attendance of a female assistant who also serves as chaperone. Ask the patient to empty her bladder, disrobe, and assume the lithotomy position on the examining table. Cover her body with a sheet, place her heels in stirrups attached to the table, and wrap the lower corners of the sheet around her legs, leaving considerable slack for the cloth to envelop the thighs and lower abdomen (Fig. 8-9A). Shine a bright light onto the perineum from an examining lamp, a head mirror, or a flashlight. Sit in front of the perineum on a low stool within reach of a side table containing specula, forceps, gauze, rubber gloves, lubricating jelly, and the materials for making slide preparations for the Papanicolaou test and bacteriologic cultures. For a complete examination, the following sequence is suggested: (1) inspection of the vulva, (2) insertion of the vaginal speculum, (3) preparation of slides for cytologic examina-**

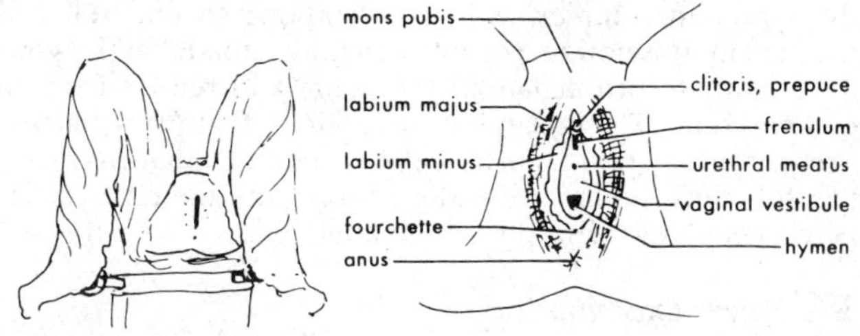

Fig. 8-9. Examination of the vulva. **A.** Draping for pelvic examination. *The patient assumes the lithotomy position with heels placed in stirrups projecting from the end of the examining table. A sheet is spread over the patient so the two lower corners are wrapped about the thighs and legs. The middle of the lower edge of the sheet is slackly draped over the lower abdomen.* **B.** Topographic anatomy of the vulva. *The recessed vestibule contains a relatively small vaginal orifice, surrounded by one of the usual patterns of unruptured hymen. Bordering the vestibule are the two projecting folds of often deeply pigmented skin, the labia minora. Anteriorly, accessory folds of the labia form the prepuce that encloses the clitoris. Lateral to the labia minora are two parallel ridges of skin and fat that form the labium majus on either side of the labia minora.*

tion and bacteriologic tests, (4) inspection of the vaginal walls and cervix, (5) digital bimanual examination of the uterus and adnexa, (6) rectal vaginal examination. When the patient is too weak to be examined on the table, have her assume the lithotomy position in bed and omit examination with the speculum. Reserve the left lateral prone position for patients who have ankylosis of the hips or knees and those who are too weak for the lithotomy position.

The Vulva

The *vulva* or *pudendum* comprises the external genitalia of the female. The symphysis pubis is surmounted anteriorly by a fat pad, the *mons pubis* (Fig. 8-9B). At puberty, the eminence becomes covered with hair that extends onto the skin of the abdomen to form a transverse borderline, the base of an inverted triangle called the *female escutcheon*. This hair distribution contrasts with the *male escutcheon* that describes an upright triangle with the apex near the umbilicus. The *labia majora* are elevated ridges extending inferiorly and posteriorly from the pubic mons nearly to the anus, forming the sides of a lens-shaped figure. They contain fat, blood vessels, nerves, and tissue resembling the dartos tunic in the scrotum. Between the two labia majora are two smaller skin folds, the *labia minora,* that extend posteriorly from the clitoris to be united in front of the anus by a transverse fold, the *frenulum labii* or the *fourchette.* The *clitoris* is the erectile homologue of the penis, composed of two small corpora cavernosa and surrounded by folds of the labia minora, the *preputium clitoridis* and the *frenulum of the clitoris.* The cleft posterior to the clitoris, between the two labia minora, is called the *vestibule.* It is pierced by the *urethral meatus,* about 2.5 cm posterior to the clitoris, and the *vaginal orifice* immediately posterior to the meatus. The vaginal opening is a median split, varying inversely as the size of the hymen. The *hymen* is a thin membrane covering part of the vaginal orifice. Commonly a perforate ring, widest posteriorly, the hymen may be cribriform, fringed, or even imperforate. After rupture, the hymenal remnants heal as caruncles.

INSPECTION OF THE VULVA. **Observe the skin of the perineum for swelling, ulcers, and changes in color. Separate the labia with the thumb and forefinger to inspect the clitoris and vestibule. Examine the urethral meatus for developmental anomalies, discharge, caruncle, neoplasm, and Bartholin abscess. Inspect the vaginal orifice for discharge, gaping of the edges, protrusion of the vaginal walls. Note the state of the hymen.**

Atrophy of the Skin: ***Kraurosis Vulvae.*** The skin is pallid, wrinkled, thinned, inelastic. In advanced stages, there is shrinkage of the integument. The condition occurs in women beyond the menopause; its cause is unknown.

Vulval Ulcers. These may be nonspecific. Venereal disease produces lesions similar to those of the male: chancre, chancroid, granuloma inguinale, lymphogranuloma venereum, herpes progenitalis (see p. 601 ff.).

Diffuse Inflammation: ***Vulvitis.*** The skin is hot, edematous, and red. The condition may result from a vaginitis with an irritating discharge, such as gonorrhea or trichomoniasis.

Vulval Tumor: ***Condyloma.*** Either condyloma acuminatum or latum may occur on the vulva or perianally as they do on the male genitalia (see p. 604).

Vulval Tumor: ***Neoplasm of the Skin.*** This must be distinguished from granulomas and condylomas by appearance and biopsy.

Swelling of the Vulva: ***Lymphedema*** (Elephantiasis Vulvae). Obstruction of the lymphatic channels from any cause may produce edema of the labia and surrounding tissues. Irritation may produce hypertrophy of the labia.

Swelling of a Labium Majus: ***Hematoma.*** A large, painful, bluish swelling of the labium may occur within a few hours after local trauma. Without a history of trauma, the condition may be confused with cellulitis of the vulva.

Swelling of a Labium Majus: ***Labioinguinal Hernia.*** Failure of the peritoneal pouch to obliterate in the fetus may permit a hernia to descend from the abdomen into the labium majus, producing a visible swelling. Its characteristics resemble the scrotal hernia in the male (see p. 611).

Swelling of a Labium Majus: ***Abscess of the Greater Vestibular Gland*** (Vulvovaginal Gland Abscess, Bartholinitis). The gonococcus commonly causes abscesses of this structure. If the abscess is large, the posterior portion of the labium is swollen; the overlying skin is tender, hot, and red. The mass is fluctuant. When the signs of inflammation subside, a cyst may remain. Smaller abscesses of the gland are found only by vaginal examination and will be discussed under that procedure.

Meatus: ***Urethritis.*** A purulent discharge issues from the meatus. This is usually caused by the inflammation from the gonococcus, sometimes from some other organism. Palpation of the anterior vaginal wall, beginning at the cervix and stroking toward the meatus, reveals tenderness and induration along the course of the urethra. Pus may be squeezed from the meatus in this manner. A urethral diverticulum may also produce pus.

Meatus: ***Inflammation of the Periurethral Duct*** (Skenitis). The periurethral duct (Skene's gland) lies on either side of, and posterior to, the female urethra, just inside the meatus. Often it becomes the site of chronic infection in gonorrhea. If inflamed, the mouth of the duct is visible and red, when viewed with the spreading of the meatal lips.

Meatus: ***Urethral Caruncle.*** The papilloma appears as a small red mass in the meatus or the visible portion of the urethra. It usually occurs as a complication of urethritis. It is tender and painful on urination.

Meatus: Prolapse of the Urethra. Slight gaping of the meatus is common in the multipara. In a more severe degree, the urethral mucosa may protrude from the meatus and become tender and inflamed; this often occurs after the menopause.

The Vagina, Uterus, and Adnexa

From its orifice, the *vagina* extends posteriorly into the pelvis, *inclining* about 45° with the horizontal plane of the erect body (Fig. 8-10). Normally, it is a collapsed tube with a posterior* (or inferior) wall, 9 cm long. The tubal ceiling is formed by the shorter anterior vaginal wall (6 to 7.5 cm), extended by the vaginal surface of the cervix uteri in the same plane. Thus, the fundus uteri is almost perpendicular to the plane of the vagina. The recess of the vagina behind the cervix is termed the *posterior fornix;* recesses on either side of the cervix are called *lateral fornices.* The vaginal mucosa is thrown into transverse rugae, separated by furrows of variable depths. Through the vagina, the nulliparous *cervix uteri* appears as a smooth button with its face rounded and pierced by a hole or slit, the *cervical os.* The anterior and posterior lips of the os are usually in contact with the posterior vaginal wall. Dorsal to the posterior vaginal wall lies the rectum; ventral to the anterior vaginal wall are the urethra and bladder. The peritoneal cavity extends inferiorly behind the posterior fornix to form the *rectovaginal pouch* (cul-de-sac of Douglas); its lower part is interposed between the rectum and the cervix.

The *uterus* is a muscular organ, shaped like an inverted pear, flattened anteroposteriorly. It is *inclined* forward, 45° from the horizontal plane of the erect body. From either side of the broad uterine top a *uterine tube* (fallopian tube) extends for about 10 cm, curving laterally and posteriorly in the pelvis. The tubes, suspended by the *mesosalpinx,* form the upper border of the *broad ligament* that spreads to the uterine fundus and the sides of the pelvis. The uterus with the two wings of broad

* Since the axes of the vagina and uterus are approximately equidistant from the vertical and horizontal planes of the erect body, their surfaces can be described with reference to either plane. Hereafter, *anterior* and *posterior,* instead of *superior* and *inferior,* are employed to designate these structures with axes at 45°.

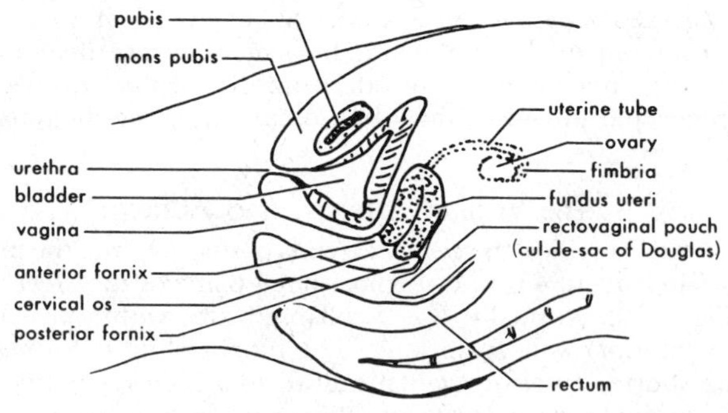

A. Sagittal Section of Female Pelvis

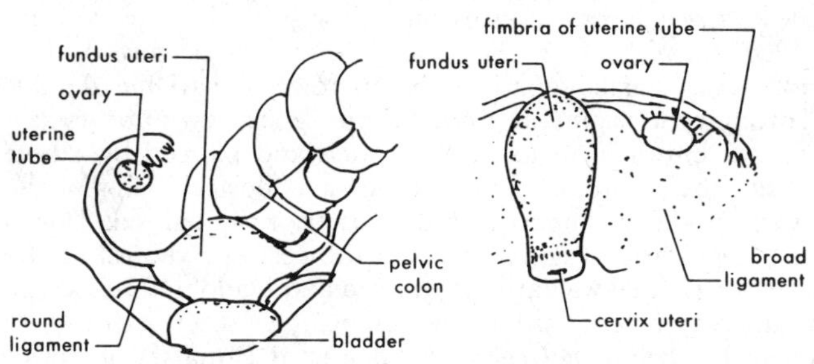

B. Pelvis from Above and in Front

C. Posterior View of Uterine Structures

Fig. 8-10. Anatomy of the uterus and adnexa. **A.** Diagram of a sagittal section of the female pelvis. *Note the 45° slope of the vagina with the vertical axis of the body, and the axis of the uterus perpendicular to the vaginal axis. The lips of the cervix uteri are shown to be in the same plane as the anterior vaginal wall that is shorter than the posterior wall. Note the relation of the rectovaginal pouch (cul-de-sac of Douglas) to the anterior rectal wall; hence, its accessibility to an examining finger in the rectum. With the fundus uteri in the normal position, note its inaccessibility to a rectal examining finger and the closeness of the top of the fundus to palpation from the lower abdomen.* **B.** View of the pelvis from above and in front. *Note how the round ligament curves anteriorly and the uterine tubes curve posteriorly.* **C.** Posterior view of the uterus and broad ligaments, spread out. *Note the suspension of the ovary near the fimbriated end of the uterine tube. The uterine tube forms the upper border of the broad ligament.*

ligament forms a transverse septum dividing the pelvis into an anterior and posterior fossa. On the posterior surface of the broad ligament the ovaries are suspended by short ligaments near the uterine tubes. Each ovary lies medial and below the fimbriated end of its tube.

VAGINAL INSPECTION PER SPECULUM. **Separation of the walls by a speculum permits vaginal inspection, the acquisition of epithelium for cytologic examination, the making of biopsies, and the collection of materials for bacteriologic tests. Insertion of the unlubricated speculum *should precede* the digital examination of the vagina because the presence of lubricating jelly on the cellular specimens interferes with the Papanicolaou stain. Select a clean bivalve speculum of suitable size and ensure its proper temperature by immersing it in warm water and drying it. With the *left* hand, grasp the handle and close the blades of the speculum. Retract the vaginal wall by pressing posteriorly on the fourchette with the *right* forefinger (Fig. 8-11A). Insert the closed blades into the vaginal orifice, with their width held *vertically,* until their tips reach the upper vagina. Then turn**

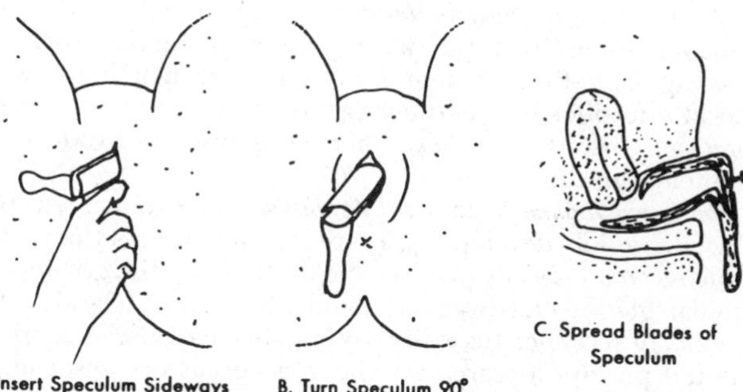

Fig. 8-11. Use of the vaginal speculum. *The introitus is retracted posteriorly, with the index finger of the right hand* (**A**). *The closed blades of the vaginal speculum are inserted in the vagina with the widths of the blades vertical. When the closed blades of the speculum have been well inserted, their widths are rotated to a transverse position* (**B**) *and the blades separated and locked open. A sagittal section* (**C**) *shows the open blades of the speculum in proper position with the upper shorter blade lifting the vault of the vagina to expose the cervix uteri on the anterior vaginal wall.*

the widths of the blades to a *transverse* position (Fig. 8-11B), separate the blades, and lock them open with the set screw. Illuminate the vaginal cavity with a head mirror or other suitable light. Move the speculum handle so the blade tips seek to expose the cervix uteri (Fig. 8-11C). Make slide preparations for the Papanicolaou test by wiping the lips of the cervical os with a cotton-tipped applicator or an Ayres spatula. Roll the cotton tip on a glass slide, place the slide in a fixative solution. If the cervical os is obscured by discharge, gently sponge it with gauze held in the foreceps. When indicated, inoculate bacteriologic cultures from the exudate. *Inspect the cervix* for color, lacerations, ulcers, and new growths. *Inspect the cervical os* for size, shape, color, discharge, and polyps. *Inspect the vaginal walls* by rotating the speculum to expose all the cavity. Look for abnormal redness or blueness of the mucosa. Determine whether a discharge exudes from the walls or from the cervical os. Finally, carefully withdraw the speculum.

Bluish Vagina: ***Cyanosis.*** The mucosa may be cyanotic in pregnancy (Chadwick's sign) or from a pelvic tumor. The generalized cyanosis of congestive cardiac failure is also visible in the mucosal lining.

Reddened Vagina: ***Simple Vaginitis.*** Diffuse reddening of the mucosa results from the decomposition of retained urine in the vagina, hot douches, or a foreign body, such as a pessary. Local infections result from organisms carried in by douches or other means. Some exanthematous diseases produce enanthemas in the mucosa.

Reddened Vagina: ***Gonorrheal Vaginitis.*** The gonococcus produces a rapidly developing, severe inflammation of the vaginal mucosa that typically involves the urethra and the greater vestibular glands (vulvovaginal glands, Bartholin's glands). The history of recent coitus with no other obvious cause for vaginitis should prompt a search for the gonococcus organism in the discharge.

Reddened Vagina: ***Trichomonas Vaginitis.*** The protozoan *Trichomonas vaginalis* produces a reddened mucosa, studded with small hemorrhagic spots. The resulting discharge is yellow, frequently foamy. The condition is distinguished from gonorrheal vaginitis by its failure to inflame the urethra and greater vestibular glands. In a more chronic stage, the vaginal mucosa contains scattered red papules, giving a granular appearance. The diagnosis may readily be made by suspending a bit of discharge in isotonic saline solution, making a hanging drop of the suspension, and finding the parasites by microscopic examination.

Reddened Vagina: **Adhesive Vaginitis** (Atrophic Vaginitis). The mucosa contains abraded patches and adhesions that bleed easily. Frequently, a bloody discharge results. The condition is postmenopausal.

Reddened Vagina: **Other Types of Vaginitis.** In *aphthous vaginitis,* superficial white patches with inflammatory bases stud the mucosa. The appearance resembles thrush in the mouth that is caused by the same fungus, *Candida albicans;* the spores and mycelial threads may be seen in the wet smear. *Diphtheritic vaginitis* is rare; it is characterized by a membrane similar to that in the pharynx.

Vaginal Ulcers. The same types that occur on the vulva may involve the vaginal mucosa (see p. 627).

Vaginal Neoplasm. New growths in the vaginal mucosa may be primary or secondary to carcinoma of the uterus, rectum, bladder, or the external genitalia.

Cervix: **Laceration.** During labor the cervix nearly always sustains some laceration (Fig. 8-13A, p. 639). Commonly the tear is transverse and *bilateral;* occasionally the laceration is *unilateral,* or multiple tears produce a *stellate* lesion. Recently torn edges appear raw. In a few weeks, healing leaves scarred fissures or notches. The cleft lips of the cervix may become *everted;* healing may be incomplete, causing an area of *erosion.*

Cervix: **Cyanosis** (Chadwick's Sign). Bluish discoloration of the cervix is a sign of early pregnancy. It also occurs in tumors of the pelvis and in congestive cardiac failure.

Cervical Discharge: **Endocervicitis.** A mucopurulent or purulent discharge emerges from the cervical os (Fig. 8-13A, p. 639). The cervical lips are usually inflamed and eroded. The absence of tenderness of the fundus uteri indicates that the inflammation is limited to the cervical canal. The condition may be acute and is usually caused by gonorrhea or puerperal infection; a chronic form accompanies repeated pregnancies.

Cervical Discharge: **Endometritis.** The appearance of the cervix is similar to that in endocervicitis, but tenderness of the fundus indicates involvement of the endometrium.

Cervical Erosion. Superficial inflammation of the cervix, without ulceration, is usually the result of a discharge from the os. Inspection alone cannot distinguish erosion from carcinoma in situ and invasive carcinoma.

Cervical Ulcer. There is a loss of epithelium and sloughing of underlying tissue. This may result from the abrasion of a pessary. Specific causes are chancroid, syphilis, tuberculosis, and carcinoma. Biopsy is indicated when tests for microbial diseases are negative.

Cervical Hypertrophy. The lips of the cervix may enlarge and elongate. This most frequently occurs in the nullipara of less than 35 years. The cause is unknown. *Distinction:* In hypertrophy the fundus retains its normal position; the cervix is also prominent in uterine prolapse, but the fundus descends toward the vaginal orifice. The cervix retains its normal contour in hypertrophy, whereas neoplasm distorts the proportions.

Cervical Polyp. A soft, bright red, benign tumor, usually pedunculated, often emerges from the cervical os (Fig. 8-13A). It may cause discharge and bleeding.

Cervical Cysts. Occlusion of glands in the cervical mucosa causes retention cysts called *nabothian follicles* that are visible with the use of the vaginal speculum.

Cervical Carcinoma. A *chronic ulcer* of the cervix with *induration* is the early sign of carcinoma. Frequently a bloody discharge follows straining or coitus. These findings should prompt cytologic examination by the Papanicolaou technique; if this leaves doubt, biopsy should be made. In the later stages, extensive ulceration, induration, and nodulation make the diagnosis obvious.

BIMANUAL PELVIC EXAMINATION. **Skillful examiners advise the habitual use of the same hand for vaginal palpation: whether it be the right or the left is a matter of personal preference. Many gynecologists palpate the vagina with the left hand and handle instruments with the right. The invariable use of the same hand in the bimanual examination permits each hand to become accustomed to its role, and the sense of touch is educated for the objects encountered. In the following directions, the *right* hand is arbitrarily assigned to the vagina and the *left* hand is employed to palpate the abdomen. If obstruction from a persistent hymen or a constricted vagina does not interfere, employ two fingers for insertion in the vagina. Place the gloved *right* hand in the *gynecologic position:* index and middle fingers straight and close together, thumb widely abducted, fourth and fifth fingers folded into the palm. Lubricate the straight fingers** with jelly. Spread the labia with the *left* thumb and forefinger to avoid the discomfort of pulling pubic hair into the vagina. Insert the two lubricated fingers in the vaginal cavity with the hand supine so the finger pads face the anterior vaginal wall (Fig. 8-12A). Examine each structure systematically. *Vaginal wall:* Feel for tenderness of inflammation; induration from scars, granulomas, and neoplasm; strictures of the walls; adhesions (do not confuse with the normal transverse rugae). *Base of bladder:* Palpate the midline of the anterior vaginal wall, halfway between the introitus and the cervix, for tenderness and induration produced by cystitis and neoplasm of the blad-

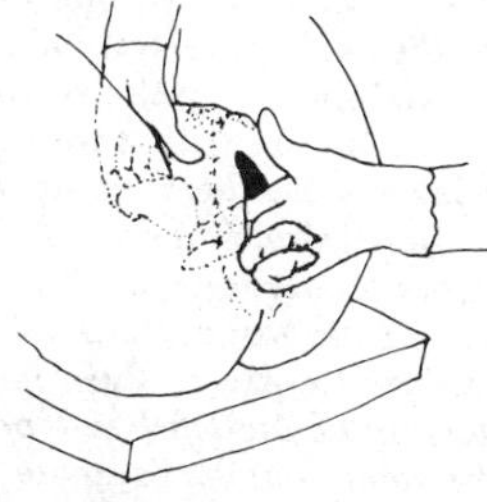

A. Bimanual Pelvic Examination

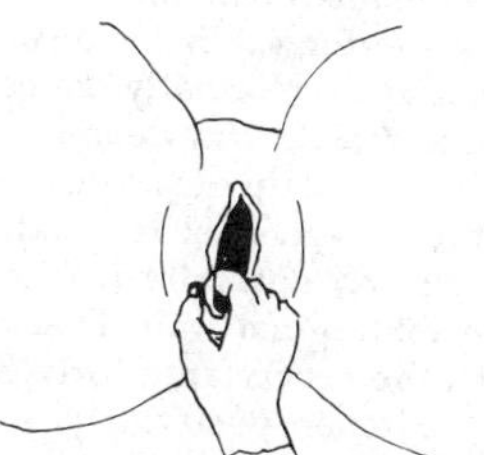

B. Palpating Bartholin's Gland (vulvovaginal gland)

Fig. 8-12. Bimanual pelvic examination. **A.** Palpation of the uterus. *The index and long fingers of the right hand are inserted in the vagina so the tips of the fingers are facing anteriorly and touching the cervix uteri. The fingers of the left hand are pressed deep into the abdomen, above the mons pubis, and are pushing the top of the uterine fundus downward and forward, to be felt by the two vaginal fingers. The adnexa are examined similarly, except the vaginal fingers are placed to the side of the uterus and the abdominal fingers are pushed into the belly at a point 2 inches (5 cm) medial to the anterior superior iliac spine. The attempt is made to approximate the tips of the two examining hands. The abdominal fingers are pulled inferiorly to push the tube and ovary into the tips of the vaginal fingers. The examiner is prompted to make a habit of always using the same hands for the same positions in the examination. Most right-handed persons use the right hand in the vagina. But gynecologists frequently use the left hand in the vagina so the right hand is free for the use of instruments.* **B.** Palpation of the greater vestibular gland (Bartholin's gland). *The index finger is inserted in the vagina near the posterior extent of the introitus. The thumb of the same hand is pressed outside on the corresponding portion of the labium majus and the finger and thumb are approximated to feel an abscess or induration in Bartholin's gland.*

der. *Urethra:* Palpate the midline of the anterior vaginal wall near the introitus for tenderness and induration in the urethra. *Greater vestibular glands* (vulvovaginal glands or Bartholin's glands): With the forefinger inside the vagina and the thumb opposite and outside on the posterior part of the labium majus, feel the inner wall for abscess or tenderness (Fig. 8-12B). Then evert that part of the vaginal mucosa to look for a red spot or pus marking the opening of an inflamed duct. The normal glands and ducts cannot be seen or felt. *Pelvic floor:* Note the size of the introitus. With the examining fingers facing posteriorly, press the pelvic floor inferiorly and posteriorly to determine the resistance or relaxation. Have the patient strain as if to defecate and note bulging of the vaginal wall through the introitus. *Rectum:* Note the distortions of the anal sphincter. Palpate the posterior vaginal wall for tenderness and masses in the rectum. *Cervix uteri:* Normally the cervix feels like a button with a rounded face and a central depression; its consistency has been compared to that of the tip of the nose. Palpate the shape, size, and consistency of the cervix. Feel for nodules and ulcers. Determine the axis of the cervix; normally it faces posteriorly in the same plane as the anterior vaginal wall. *Fundus uteri:* With the fingers in the vagina, push the cervix anteriorly, while the fingers of the *left* hand press the abdomen posteriorly, just above the mons pubis. Estimate the size of the fundus, its axis, and characterize any nodules that may be present. *Adnexa:* Place the vaginal fingers on one side of the cervix and push their tips superiorly and posteriorly as far as possible. With the fingers of the *left* hand, locate a point on the same side of the abdomen about 2 inches (5 cm) medially from the anterior superior iliac spine. Push the abdominal fingers deep so their tips approach the vaginal fingers. This should bring the approximated hands *back* of the uterine tubes and ovaries. If the structures are not felt at that point, move the fingertips of both hands inferiorly toward the pubis, so that the adnexa pass between the two hands. Exert abdominal pressure gently, but deeply, pressing the two hands a little closer each time the patient expires, so muscle spasm will not be stimulated. The role of the abdominal hand should be to displace the structure, while the vaginal hand feels them. *The normal ovary and tube are usually not palpable.* When the normal tube is felt, it is about 4 mm in diameter, about half the size of a common pencil. It has the consistency of a piece of rubber tubing. The normal ovary is about 4 cm by 2 cm by 8 mm; the lateral face is, therefore, about the size of the distal phalanx of the examiner's thumb, but the thickness of the ovary is about half that of the digit. The ovary is soft and naturally tender to palpation. Note significant enlargements, abnormal tenderness, and characterize other masses or induration.

Vaginal Tenderness: ***Vaginitis.*** Tenderness of the walls and a discharge from the introitus may be the first signs of vaginitis encountered, if a speculum examination has not been performed (see discussion p. 632).

Greater Vestibular Glands: ***Bartholinitis.*** Inflammation of these glands (also called *vulvovaginal glands, Bartholin's glands*) must be searched for whenever a vaginitis exists, or when a mass is found in the labium majus. The glands are particularly involved in gonorrhea. Tenderness or a mass is found in the vaginal wall, near the posterior portion of the vaginal orifice, on either side (Fig. 8-12B). The normal glands are not palpable and their ducts are not divisible. Inflammation causes a red spot in the mucosa at the site of the ductal orifice, and pus may be expressed from it.

Rectovaginal Fistula. A fistual from rectum to vagina is usually suggested by the history of fecal contamination of the vagina. The mouth of the fistula may be palpable as a small patch of induration in the posterior wall of the vagina. Otherwise the opening should be searched for through the vaginal speculum. Such a communication usually follows a difficult delivery with tearing of the perineal body or after radiation or extensive perineal surgery for malignancy.

Pelvic Floor: ***Enlarged Introitus.*** When the hymen is ruptured, the vaginal orifice normally admits the examiner's two fingers. When three fingers are accommodated, the introitus is definitely enlarged, usually indicating some degree of pelvic relaxation from childbirth.

Pelvic Floor: ***Colpocele*** (Vaginal Prolapse). Redundant walls of the vagina, either anterior or posterior, may protrude through the vaginal orifice. If the walls are not accompanied by bladder or rectum, the condition is termed a *colpocele.*

Pelvic Floor: ***Cystocele*** (Vesicle Prolapse). When the patient stands, or strains while supine on the table, a portion of the bladder, covered by vaginal mucosa, emerges from the introitus as a soft spheric tumor (Fig. 8-13B). This finding indicates pelvic laceration during childbirth.

Pelvic Floor: ***Rectocele*** (Rectal Prolapse). Standing or under strain, a portion of the rectum, covered by vaginal mucosa, protrudes from the introitus (Fig. 8-13B). This is evidence of pelvic laceration during childbirth.

Pelvic Floor: ***Uterine Prolapse.*** The uterus lies lower than nor-

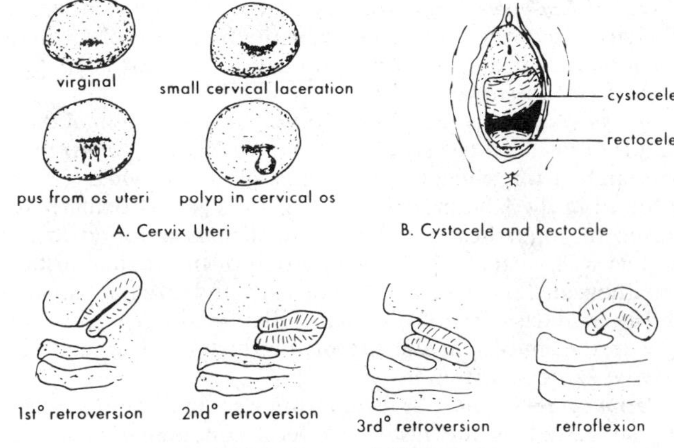

Fig. 8-13. Some pelvic findings. **A.** Lesions of the cervix uteri. *In normal persons the cervical os has several patterns, one of which is shown here. The lacerations of childbirth leave various scars. Pus or a polyp may be seen coming out from the os.* **B.** Cystocele and rectocele. *When the patient is asked to strain as if to defecate, the introitus widens and an anterior bulging may develop from above (cystocele) or below (rectocele). The bulges may be small, or the organ may protrude at all times and becomes nearly completely exteriorized.* **C.** Uterine displacements. *If the axis of the uterus remains straight and the whole organ is tilted, it is called retroversion; if the axis of the uterus is bent, the condition is called retroflexion. In 1st-degree retroversions, the axis is tipped slightly posteriorly and the cervix maintains its normal relation to the fundus; the fundus is still forward enough so it cannot be felt in the posterior fornix or rectum. 2nd-degree retroversion: the axis of the fundus coincides with that of the vagina; the plane of the cervix is transverse to the vagina; the fundus can be felt in the posterior fornix and the rectum. 3rd-degree retroversion: the axis of the fundus and cervix is in the direction of the spine and the plane of the cervix faces the anterior wall of the vagina. The fundus encroaches upon the rectum. In retroflexion the plane of the cervix is felt in the normal position but the fundus is palpable through the posterior fornix and rectum.*

mal in the vaginal cavity, or it may protrude from the introitus, cervix most inferior. Trauma related to repeated childbirth is the most important etiologic factor for the development of the preceding four conditions, which are manifestations of vaginal relaxation. Occasionally, however, the defects must be considered as congenital, as they do occur in the nulliparous patient. Symptoms, usually volunteered by the patient, consist of description of their "insides coming out."

Cervix: ***Softening.*** The cervix becomes softer than normal during the first trimester of pregnancy, which serves as one of the early signs of the condition.

Cervix: ***Masses.*** A cervical polyp may be felt as a small soft tumor emerging from the cervical os. The nature can be determined by viewing it through the vaginal speculum. A hard mass in one lip of the cervix suggests a neoplasm and requires a biopsy.

Cervix: ***Lacerations.*** Healed lacerations of the cervix leave notches or fissures in the surface of the cervix that can be felt with the finger (for the patterns of lacerations, see p. 638).

Mass Replacing the Cervix: ***Uterine Inversion.*** A large mass in the vagina can be palpated upward to the expected location of the cervix, but neither the cervix nor the fundus uteri can be felt in its normal location. The mass may bleed easily or slough, because its surface is endometrium. This must be distinguished from massive cervical neoplasm and submucous myoma.

Uterus: ***Softening*** (Hegar's Sign). During the first trimester of pregnancy the fundus uteri softens at the junction of the cervix with the body. This change in consistency is easily palpable; sometimes the contrast between fundus and isthmus is so pronounced that the cervix seems to separate from the fundus. The softening of the uterine isthmus is regarded as a reliable sign of early pregnancy.

Uterine Tenderness: ***Endometritis.*** Tenderness of the body of the uterus and the presence of a discharge issuing from the os establish the diagnosis of endometritis. This is distinguished from a cervicitis because, in the latter, the discharge is not accompanied by uterine tenderness. Usually infection of the endometrium is caused by gonorrhea, sepsis from childbirth or abortion.

Uterus: ***Displacement.*** Commonly the displacement is posterior. *Retroversion* is displacement of both fundus and cervix in a common axis; when freely movable, it is symptomless and present in 25% of normal women; when fixed, it suggests endometriosis. *Retroflexion* is posterior displacement of the fundus, but the cervix retains its normal axis, so that the fundus is bent upon the cervix (Fig. 8-13C). In *first-degree retroversion,* the fundus is tipped slightly backward so that it is out of reach of the vaginal finger. In *second-degree retroversion* the axes of uterus and vagina coincide, so that the posterior surface of the fundus is felt extending superiorly behind the cervix. In *third-degree retroversion* the fundus is so far posterior that its posterior surface cannot be felt slanting in the direction of the spinal column. In retroflexion, the cervix is in its normal axis, but the fundus can be felt posterior to the cervix. *Lateral displacement* of the uterus is frequently caused by adhesions or masses in the adnexa.

Uterine Enlargement: ***Pregnancy.*** Generalized uterine enlargement in a woman of fecund age should suggest the possibility of pregnancy. In the first few months of pregnancy, the gravid uterus has no distinguishing palpable shape or size. Other symptoms and signs of pregnancy should be sought: morning sickness, engorgement of the breasts, amenorrhea, cyanosis of the vaginal and cervical mucosa (Chadwick's sign), softening of the cervix, softening of the uterine fundus (Hegar's sign). The urine should be submitted for the Pregnosis urinary pregnancy test, or chorionic gonadotropin (beta subunit)-quantitative serum test. In large tumors arising from the pelvis, the gravid uterus must be distinguished from ovarian cysts by feeling the fetal parts and hearing the fetal heartbeat. The size of the tumor can be compared with the height of the uterus at various stages of pregnancy: 3 months—at the pubis; 6 months—at the umbilicus, 9 months—at the xiphoid.

Uterine Enlargement: ***Leiomyofibroma*** (Fibroid). Hard painless nodules, frequently multiple, are firmly attached to the fundus. The nodules and the fundus move freely together. An asymmetric gravid uterus is sometimes mistaken for a uterine fibroid in a woman of fecund age. Fibroids are more common in Blacks than in Caucasians.

Uterine Enlargement: ***Neoplasm of the Fundus.*** Carcinoma and sarcoma of the fundus produce more or less generalized enlargement. An associated bloody discharge prompts curettage of the uterine canal revealing the diagnosis.

Tubal Mass: ***Salpingitis.*** With acute gonorrheal inflammation, the uterine tubes are tender and frequently surrounded by purulent exudate that obscures the separate structures in the adnexa. Movement of the uterus and cervix is extremely painful. (For more discussion, see p. 554.) In more chronic stages, the exudate and fibrosis around the tubes feel like an unyielding mass, termed a *frozen pelvis*. As the result of sealing a tube at both ends by inflammation, the tube may be filled with fluid and feel like a sausage-shaped mass, termed a *hydrosalpinx*, or pus, *pyosalpinx*.

Tubal Mass: **Ectopic Pregnancy.** Occasionally a slight enlargement of the uterine tube may be felt that ultimately proves to be a tubal pregnancy. Experienced clinicians believe that irregular vaginal bleeding and pelvic pain indicate ectopic pregnancy until excluded. A bloody vaginal discharge may indicate that the tube has ruptured. Softening of the cervix and fundus occurs with tubal pregnancy, as well as in intrauterine pregnancy, but movement of uterus and cervix is painful. Occasionally a bulging mass is felt in the rectovaginal pouch from a pelvic hematoma.

Tubal Mass: **Tuberculosis.** Ordinarily tuberculosis cannot be distinguished by physical examination from other types of inflammation causing chronic salpingitis. Usually the specific diagnosis is made at operation. The palpable evidence of chronic salpingitis, with absence of signs of uterine infection, strongly suggests tuberculosis.

Pelvic Mass: **Endometriosis.** In this condition, aberrant islands of endometrium become implanted in the ovaries, posterior surface of uterus, sigmoid colon, and uterosacral ligaments. Nodular masses surrounded with fibrosis may be felt. Frequently the ovaries are enlarged. The uterus is fixed and painful on movement; masses are tender when palpated. The history yields symptoms of dysmenorrhea, pains in the abdomen and sacral region, accentuated during menstruation.

Solid Ovarian Mass: **Oophoritis.** Although inflammation of an ovary causes it to enlarge, the change in size is usually not detected by palpation because the same inflammatory process involves the uterine tubes, so that the component structures in the mass cannot be recognized.

Solid Ovarian Mass: **Neoplasm.** A variety of benign and malignant neoplasms may involve the ovaries that can only be distinguished by operation.

Solid Ovarian Mass: **Endometriosis.** Enlargement of the ovaries is frequently encountered in endometriosis (above).

Fluctuant Ovarian Mass: Cyst. A fluctuant nontender spheroidal mass may be felt in the region of the ovary. When the mass is relatively small, the palpatory evidence is diagnostic. When the cyst so enlarges that it emerges from the pelvis and into the abdomen, no distinctive pelvic signs are present and the mass must be distinguished from other possibilities in the abdominal cavity (see p. 520).

RECTOABDOMINAL EXAMINATION IN THE FEMALE. **After digital examination of the vagina has been completed, insert the forefinger of the gloved right hand into the anal canal, as described in Fig. 7-37 (p. 574). Palpate the anal canal for the intrinsic lesions previously described. Then, using the left hand to press upon the lower abdomen as in the bimanual vaginal examination, palpate the genitalia through the rectum. Test the anal sphincter for evidence of lacerations from childbirth. Through the anterior rectal wall, locate the cervix uteri. Attempt to feel the fundus uteri through the rectum; this may be the only route by which a retroverted or retroflexed uterus is palpable. Push the finger to its highest extent and palpate the anterior rectal wall in the region of the peritoneal rectovaginal pouch (cul-de-sac of Douglas) (Fig. 8-10). Feel for a prolapsed ovary, for metastatic masses from abdominal carcinoma, for a tender accumulation of pus or blood. Thickening of the rectovaginal septum or parametrium occurs from spread of cervical carcinoma, puerperal infection, and abortions. Ordinarily the female genitalia are felt much more satisfactorily through the vagina than per rectum. In the virgin, however, vaginal palpation may not be feasible, and enough may be learned by rectal examination to make diagnoses or exclude them.**

Anal Laceration. A complete laceration of the anus is evident by the appearance of the part. The edges may not be approximated; if they are, they form an irregular line rather than a depression with puckered borders. Palpation reveals weakness of the sphincter. This condition is usually the result of an extensive pelvic laceration from childbirth. When the Sphincter ani is involved the condition is termed a *third-degree* laceration.

Uterine Retroversion. The uterine fundus is felt through the anterior rectal wall when it cannot be palpated per vaginam.

Rectovaginal Fistula. Since this lesion is frequently the result of radiation therapy, the rectal wall may be indurated from scar tissue. As has been previously noted, the fistula should be looked for from the vaginal side.

Neoplasm. Extension of neoplasm from the uterus may be felt in the rectum.

Masses in the Rectovaginal Pouch. These may be a prolapsed ovary, a loop of bowel, carcinoma of the colon, a rectal shelf (see p. 525), an accumulation of pus or blood from abdominal lesions.

9

The Spine and Extremities

The musculoskeletal system has three major functional components: the bones, the muscles, and the nerves supplying the muscles. Tendons, ligaments and joints complete the system. Any diagnostic examination involves overlap of the arbitrary divisions between internal medicine, surgery, neurology, and orthopedics. Most examiners follow a routine in which anatomic regions are examined in a sequence dictated by the mechanical convenience of the doctor and patient, rather than a logical exploration of physiologic systems. Any attempt to present diagnostic findings as they are encountered in an anatomic region necessitates considerable cross reference to the examination of the nervous and the cardiovascular systems.

Diseases of Bone

▼ *Key Symptom:* ***Bone Pain.*** Pain in the bones is often the only symptom of osseous disease; it may be accompanied by *localized tenderness* and *swelling.* Characteristically, bone pain is *worse at night;* often it is intensified by movement or weight-bearing. Bone pain may be referred to the nearest joint. When pain is near a joint, careful examination for the exact location of the tender locus often distinguishes between articular and bone pain. Squeezing the overlying muscles between thumb and index finger should exclude *tender muscles* as the source of pain. The occurrence of bone pain should prompt x-ray examination of the bones of the region.

Clinical Occurrence: ACUTE PAIN. Fractures, tendon ruptures, ligament avulsions, osteomyelitis. CHRONIC PAIN. *Infections:* Brodie's abscess (localized staphylococcal infection of the metaphysis of a long bone), untreated syphilis enduring more than 3 years, syphilitic osteoperiostitis, tuberculosis of bone. *Neoplastic:* osteosarcoma, multiple myeloma, giant-cell tumor, primary reticulum-cell sarcoma, Ewing's tumor, eosinophilic granuloma of bone, carcinomatous metastases to bone, fibrosarcoma, chondrosarcoma. *Hyperparathyroidism:* osteitis fibrosa cystica generalisata (von Recklinghausen's disease of bone). *Metabolic:* osteoporosis, osteomalacia. *Miscellaneous:* osteitis deformans (Paget's disease of bone), hypertrophic osteoarthropathy, bone infarction (in hemoglobin S and C diseases, Legg-Perthes' disease of the femoral head, and Osgood-Schlatter's disease of the tibial tuberosity).

Disseminated Diseases of Bone

Disseminated diseases of bone pose special problems in diagnostication because they cause few or no symptoms. The attention of the physician is usually attracted to the bones by *bone pain* or *tenderness, bone deformities,* the occurrence of *spontaneous* or *pathologic fractures,* or chance findings in the *x-ray films* taken for other purposes. Frequently the osseous deformities are distinctive on physical examination. When x-ray signs are not specific, the diagnosis is usually established by determinations of serum calcium, phosphorus, alkaline and acid phosphatase, and the urinary excretion of calcium.

Osteoporosis. Increased resorption of bony cortex from disuse, lack of sufficient intake of building materials, or excessive loss of mineral constituents from the body is the usual cause. Cortical deficiency is especially severe in the vertebrae and pelvic bones. *Bone pain* occurs with fracture; kyphosis is the only physical sign. *Complication.* Spontaneous or pathologic fracture. *Distinction.* X-ray films disclose increased radiolucence of bone with loss of fine trabeculation; these findings also occur in osteomalacia, hyperparathyroidism, metastatic carcinoma, and multiple myeloma. Osteoporosis is distinctive among these by having normal concentrations of serum calcium, phosphorus, and alkaline phosphatase.

Clinical Occurrence: Senility, postmenopausal estrogen deficit, atrophy of disuse, malnutrition, deficit of vitamin C, Cushing's syndrome, eunuchoidism, therapy with adrenal corticosteroids, hyperthyroidism, renal insufficiency, and the prolonged administration of heparin.

Osteogenesis Imperfecta (Brittle Bones, Fragilitas Ossium, Osteopsathyrosis, Hypoplasia of Mesenchyme). Persons with this disorder are born with a deficit in osseous matrix as the result of an autosomal dominant gene of varying penetrance. In all affected individuals the bones are harder and more brittle than normal, so *spontaneous* or *pathologic fractures* are common. The fractures are sometimes *painless*. Several eponymic categories are based on the association of this condition with other mesenchymal defects; one commonly emphasized is the *blue sclerae*. The bony defect produces *short stature;* a *deformed skull* is often present. *Hypermobility of joints* is common. *Distinction.* X-ray films show generalized radiolucence of bone, suggesting osteoporosis; but the *epiphyses are normal.* The normal values for serum calcium, phosphorus, and alkaline phosphatase exclude other causes.

Rickets. A deficit of vitamin D before epiphyseal closure in childhood results in inadequate calcification of cartilage and new bone. Clinically, the condition is characterized by *restlessness, frequent crying, excessive sweating.* The muscles become *atonic.* Softening of bone produces *craniotabes, Parrot's bosses, rachitic rosary, Harrison's grooves, thoracic kyphosis* or *lordosis, genu valgum* or *varum, contracted pelvis.* With the sole exception of the rosary, all deformities are permanent stigmas of childhood disease. *Distinction.* The physical signs of active rickets are quite diagnostic when present. The x-ray findings are usually distinctive. Serum concentrations of calcium and phosphorus are subnormal; the serum alkaline phosphatase is elevated.

Osteomalacia. A condition chemically similar to rickets, it occurs after the epiphyses are closed and results from deficits of calcium or phosphorus in a variety of conditions, preventing calcification of newly formed bony matrix. The early stages yield no symptoms or signs. Later, *bone pain* from fractures and *tenderness* occur; *low back pain* and striking *muscle weakness* are common. Low blood calcium may produce spontaneous *carpopedal spasm* of tetany, with *Chvostek's sign* and *Trousseau's sign.* *Complications.* Spontaneous or pathologic fractures. *Distinction.* Increased radiolucence of bone occurs as in osteoporosis, osteitis fibrosa cystica, metastatic carcinoma, and multiple myeloma. Osteomalacia is distinguished by a normal or low serum calcium, low phosphorus, and high alkaline phosphatase. Low urinary output of calcium indicates insufficient intake; a high output results from abnormal mineral losses.

Clinical Occurrence. Decreased intestinal absorption or dietary lack of calcium or vitamin D; excessive loss in the feces from pancreatic disease, sprue; increased urinary calcium excretion from renal tubular acidosis, Fanconi's syndrome, or essential hypercalciuria; rapid deposition of calcium and phosphorus in the tissues after ablation of the parathyroid glands or in spontaneous hyperparathyroidism.

Osteitis Deformans (Paget's Disease of Bone). A disease in adults of unknown cause is characterized by increased destruction of bone balanced by a rapid growth of new bone with imperfect architecture. *Bone pain* is inconstant, seldom severe. With the exception of the hands and feet, any bones may be involved. The skin over affected bones may be *warmer* than normal. The classic osseous deformities are *increased girth of the calvarium, thoracic kyphosis, genu varum, shortening of the spine* by flattening of the vertebrae to give the appearance of *disproportionately long arms*. *Complications.* Spontaneous or pathologic fractures, single or multiple osteogenic sarcomas in sites of osteitis, increased blood flow through the spongy bone producing the dynamic effect of an arteriovenous fistula leading to cardiac failure. *Distinction.* X-ray films show exaggerated distorted trabeculations of bone. The serum calcium and phosphorus values are normal, the alkaline phosphatase is elevated. Occasionally, the x-ray appearance closely resembles that produced by metastatic carcinoma from the prostate gland, but the serum acid phosphatase is elevated in the latter; it is normal in Paget's disease.

Hyperparathyroidism, Primary: ***Osteitis Fibrosa Cystica Generalisata*** (Recklinghausen's Disease). Accelerated production of parathyroid hormone causes the rate of bone destruction to exceed new bone formation; osseous rarefaction occurs. Cysts are formed in the skull and long bones when the cause is a parathyroid tumor; they do not occur when the condition is secondary to chronic nephritis. The disease is symptomless for a long time; late *bone tenderness,* muscle weakness, and waddling gait may occur. The bone cysts cause visible and palpable *swellings;* a cyst of the jaw is often mistaken for epulis. The coincidence of peptic ulcer and renal calculus should prompt a search for hyperparathyroidism. **Complication.** Spontaneous or pathologic fracture. **Distinction.** X-ray films, especially of the long finger, show generalized radiolucence of bone, with loss of trabeculation; the appearance of bone cysts is distinctive; pathognomonic is a jagged feathery border in the subperiosteal layer of the phalanges. In primary hyperparathyroidism, the serum calcium is elevated, the phosphorus is low; in chronic nephritis, the calcium concentration is normal or low, the phosphorus high. Both conditions have elevation of the serum alkaline phosphatase. The x-ray and biochemical findings distinguish the condition from osteoporosis and osteomalacia, which also display osseous radiolucence.

Fibrous Dysplasia of Bone (Osteitis Fibrosa Cystica Disseminata). The cause of this disease is unknown. The architecture of one or more bones is distorted by fibrosis; the cranium and long bones are especially involved. Usually symptomless, the disease is manifest by *bowing* of the affected long bones. The skin often contains *melanotic spots* with jagged borders. In young girls, *precocious puberty* may occur. **Distinction.** X-ray films show signs similar to osteoporosis and osteomalacia in the involved bones, but there is no generalized radiolucence. Concentrations of serum calcium and phosphorus are normal; the serum alkaline phosphatase is elevated only when bone involvement is extensive.

Dyschondroplasia: ***Hereditary Multiple Exostoses.*** The hereditary disease is characterized by exostoses arising from the bony cortex, deforming the metaphyseal region of some long bones. Involvement is usually bilateral but not symmetric. The ulna may be shortened, producing *ulnar deviation* of the hand. *Valgus deformities* of the ankle are common. The only symptom may be *mechanical interference in a joint.* **Distinction.** The appearance of the exostoses is typical in x-ray films.

Dyschondroplasia: ***Ollier's Disease (Multiple Enchondromas).*** This is probably a *congenital* disease of unknown cause; otherwise it closely resembles hereditary deforming chondrodysplasia. When associated with hemangiomas, it is known as *Maffucci's syndrome.*

Achondroplasia (Chondrodystrophia Foetalis). Beginning in fetal life, this skeletal disease is frequently hereditary, although sporadic cases occur. In individuals surviving intrauterine life, there is a disturbance in the growth of cartilage and endochondrial bone that produces the classic *achondroplastic dwarf,* having a normal, healthy life-span. The *stature is foreshortened* considerably by the small lower limbs supporting a relatively large trunk, so the central point of the figure is near the xiphoid process where normally it is at the symphysis pubis. The humeri and femora are relatively shorter than the forearms and legs. The diminutive figure is surmounted by a *large brachycephalic head.* Other stigmas are *saddle nose, thick lips, protruding tongue, high arched palate, trident hands* (short thick fingers diverging from the bases like spokes of a wheel), *restricted extension of the elbows, thoracic kyphosis, tilted pelvis.* **Distinction.** The physical signs are diagnostic. X-ray films show characteristic signs, although seldom needed for diagnosis. No biochemical abnormalities are known.

Marfan's Syndrome (Arachnodactyly). This is a congenital disease, frequently inherited as an autosomal dominant, but sporadic cases occur. It affects the development of bone, ligaments, tendons, arterial walls, and supporting structures in the heart and eyes. Many persons show only a few stigmas, but the complete syndrome presents a striking portrait. The long slender phalanges, *spider fingers,* have given the name *arachnodactyly* to the disease; the term is misleading because some patients with Marfan's syndrome lack the sign. The skull is long and narrow, the palate high and arched. The long bones are thin and elongated so the *finger-to-finger span* with the spread-out arms exceeds the body height. Thoracic deformities may be either *pectus excavatum* (funnel breast) or *pectus carinatum* (pigeon breast). The spine may exhibit *fused vertebrae* or *spina bifida.* Weakness of joints permits *hyperextension* (double-jointedness), *dislocations, kyphoscoliosis, pes planus* or *pes cavus.* The ears may be long and pointed, *satyr ear.* Weakness of the supporting structures of the eye produces elongation of the globe (*myopia*), *retinal detachment, lenticular dislocation, blue sclerae.* Degeneration of the elastic media causes *aneurysms* of the aorta and pulmonary artery; rupture of these with *dissection* is a common cause of early death. Deformities of the cardiac valve cusps are sites for *subacute bacterial endocarditis.* The foramen ovale may remain *patent.* **Distinction.** The combination of several of the deformities assures the diagnosis. In the incomplete syndrome, the diagnosis is supported by finding increased urinary excretion of hydroxyproline.

Hypertrophic Osteoarthropathy. Occurring in a wide variety of conditions, this syndromic tetrad of unknown cause consists of (1) clubbing of the fingers, (2) new osseous formation in the periosteum of the long bones, (3) swelling and pains in the joints, (4) autonomic disturbances of the hands and feet, such as flushing, sweating, and blanching. The earliest sign is *clubbing of the fingers,* often the only component of the tetrad to appear (see Clubbing of the Fingers, p. 689). With progressive osseous changes mild *bone pain* may occur. *Swelling* and *pain in the joints* may become severe. In advanced cases, *sweating* and *flushing* of the hands and feet may alternate with *Raynaud's phenomenon.* **Distinction.** The diagnosis is assured when clubbing of the fingers is evident. Excessive enlargement of the hands and an elevated serum phosphorus may suggest acromegaly, which must be excluded by absence of other bony changes associated with hyperpituitarism.

Clinical Occurrence. *Pulmonary disease,* as benign or malignant neoplasm, lung abscess or bronchiectasis, tuberculosis, intrathoracic aneurysm, and pulmonary emphysema. *Cardiac disease,* especially cyanotic congenital heart disease, subacute bacterial endocarditis. *Hepatic disease,* as cirrhosis, amyloidosis, and liver abscess. *Gastrointestinal disease,* as neoplasms, chronic dysentery, steatorrhea, ulcerative colitis, and regional ileitis. Secondary polycythemia. Myxedema. Pregnancy. Dysproteinemia.

Carcinomatous Metastasis to Bone. The condition may be discovered by the appearance of a *localized swelling* or *pain* in a bone; often it is found by chance x-ray visualization of the bones or the occurrence of a pathologic fracture.

Clinical Occurrence. The most frequent sites of the primary lesion are breast, stomach, thyroid gland, prostate gland, kidney, and bronchus.

Multiple Myeloma. The plasma cells of the bone marrow undergo malignant changes causing invasive destruction of bone, anemia, and the production of abnormal plasma proteins. The complaints may be so vague that for a long time the patient may be considered psychoneurotic. The most common definite symptom is *bone pain,* either localized or general. In its absence, the presenting complaints may be referable to either the *anemia* or a *pathologic fracture.* **Distinction.** In a general hospital, perhaps the correct diagnosis is most often suggested by the roentgenologist, who notices characteristic punched-out areas in the bones on films taken for other purposes; these findings most often occur in the skull. But frequently, the x-ray films show merely generalized osseous radiolucence. Either this finding or the anemia should prompt bone marrow aspiration, which usually shows the pathognomonic cytologic picture. The presence of Bence Jones protein in a fresh specimen of urine in half the cases is diagnostic; but usually it is not found on routine urinalysis, it must be searched for with special tests. The first indication of an abnormal plasma protein may be finding an accelerated erythrocyte sedimentation rate; in the absence of an obvious infection, this should lead to tests of the plasma proteins, revealing hyperglobulinemia and a specific myeloma protein migrating homogeneously between the regions of gamma and beta globulins. As an example, we once saw a patient who was admitted to the hospital for a fracture, not recognized as pathologic. The surgeon noticed an anemia and ordered a blood transfusion. In crossmatching the patient's blood, intense rouleaux interfered with the test; this suggested tests of serum proteins, and hyperglobulinemia was found. More x-ray films of bones showed punched-out areas. The appearance of the bone marrow was diagnostic for multiple myeloma.

Localized Disorders of Bone

Fractures: General Physical Signs. Expose the injured part for examination, using gentleness and care to *minimize movement* that is painful and dangerous. Cut or slit clothing from the part rather than move the bones. Unavoidable movement often reveals *abnormal mobility* and *bone crepitus,* two distinctive signs of fracture, but signs one does not deliberately try to elicit. Unlike sprain or soft-tissue injury, *loss of function* usually occurs in the part, the patient's voluntary act to avoid pain. The *position of an injured limb* is sometimes diagnostically significant. *Deformities* as diagnostic signs are discussed in the regional examination. Localized *bone tenderness* indicates the site of the fracture. *Shortening of a long bone* may be the crucial sign of an impacted fracture; methods of measurement are described later on. Although an inconstant accompaniment of fracture, *primary shock* must be recognized and treated. Late inconstant signs are *fracture blisters,* blebs containing serum or blood usually distal to the fracture of a leg or ankle; *ecchymoses,* occurring hours or days after a fracture; *swelling from callus,* appearing several weeks after a fracture, sometimes the only diagnostic sign of greenstick fracture. ***Greenstick Fracture.*** Commonly in children, one side of the bone is broken, the other merely bent. Deformity and crepitus are absent, pain is slight. Localized *bone tenderness* may be the only immediate clue; the late manifestation is *callus formation.* ***Separated Epiphysis.*** This occurs in the adolescent and the physical signs are the same as with complete fracture or a slipped capital femoral epiphysis. ***Compound or Open Fracture.*** A complete fracture in which a bone fragment pierces the skin or mucosa. ***Impacted Fracture.*** One bone fragment is driven firmly into the other. There is *little pain* on movement and *no crepitus.* The contour of the bone may be altered, and measurements disclose *shortening* of a long bone.

Spontaneous or Pathologic Fracture. This is a complete fracture that occurs with trauma insufficient to break a normal bone. Since the judgment of amount of trauma is difficult and diseased bone may be subjected to much trauma, spontaneous fractures are sometimes mistaken for traumatic fractures. X-ray signs of generalized or local bone disease will frequently distinguish. Sometimes spontaneous fractures are less painful than those of healthy bone.

Clinical Occurrence. Osteomalacia, osteoporosis, osteitis deformans, osteitis fibrosa, cystica generalisata, multiple myeloma, fragilitas ossium, primary and metastatic neoplasms in bone.

Fractures: ***Fat Embolism.*** *Pathophysiology:* Usually after trauma, and especially after fractures, fat globules appear in the veins and act as emboli to the lungs and other tissues. Embolism begins rather slowly and attains a maximum in about 48 hours. The source of the fat droplets is in dispute. One theory views the fat as merely pouring into the veins from disrupted fat-containing tissues; another explanation assumes the release of some substance that alters the fat emulsion in the plasma. As support for the latter belief is the observation that intravascular coagulation occurs coincident with thrombocytopenia. Open fractures furnish less emboli than closed fractures. Long bones, pelvis, and ribs furnish more emboli; sternum and clavicle furnish less.

The timing of important fracture complications is summarized in the old maxim, *2nd hour—shock, 2nd day—fat embolism, 2nd week—pulmonary embolism.* The onset of fat embolism is sudden, with *restlessness* and vague *pain in the chest. Dyspnea* and *cyanosis* are common from pulmonary involvement; some purulent sputum may be produced, devoid of blood but occasionally containing diagnostic *fat droplets. Fever* occurs, often in excess of 101° F (38.3° C), with a disproportionately high pulse rate. Within a few minutes cerebral symptoms and signs appear; they are extremely variable; *delirium* and *coma* indicate a grave prognosis. On the second or third day, *petechiae* appear over the shoulders and chest, in the conjunctivae and retinae. *Drowsiness* with *oliguria* is almost pathognomonic; occasionally *fat droplets in the urine or cerebrospinal fluid* clinch the diagnosis. The mortality is between 20 and 30%. ***Laboratory Findings.*** Test of G. W. Nice for fat in plasma: (1) draw 5 to 10 mL blood and centrifugate, (2) pipet the supernatant plasma off and mix it with oil red stain, and shake, (3) refrigerate plasma for a few minutes; fat globules float to top and can be counted in the hemocytometer (*J. Kansas Med. Soc.*, **73:**441–43, 1972). Other tests: thrombocytopenia; anemia; hypocalcemia; fat droplets in stained frozen clots; elevated serum lipase; lipuria (let large specimen of urine stand in refrigerator for 6 hours and then stain drop of supernatant with Sudan III and examine in microscope). Look for "snowstorm" infiltrate in lung fields of chest x-ray films. [For extended discussion see H. R. Gossing and T. A. Donohue: The Fat Embolism Syndrome, *J.A.M.A.*, **241:**2740–42, 1979.]

Clinical Occurrence [H. Gong, Jr.: Fat Embolism. *Postgrad. Med.*, **62:**40–48, 1977]. Trauma (especially fractures and burns), abdominal surgery, cardiac massage, extracorporeal circulation, poisoning, chronic alcoholism, diabetes mellitus, sickle-cell anemia, infections, collagen vascular diseases, eclampsia, overhydration.

Acute Osteomyelitis. Bacteria from superficial infections are carried in the blood and lodge in the terminal capillary loops of the metaphyseal cortex, causing a purulent necrosing process that emerges to the periosteum. The infection usually occurs in childhood; staphylococci are the chief offenders. The onset is usually sudden with *fever* and *pain.* If the patient is old enough, he may be able to *point to the painful site,* although the pain may be referred to the nearest joint. Inspection frequently discloses localized *swelling* and *redness* of the overlying skin. Passing the fingers lightly over the skin may demonstrate an area of *increased warmth.* Light percussion on the bone with the fingertips frequently discovers the site of *tenderness.* Failing with this method, firm pressure with the forefinger should begin in a normal region and be repeated, moving toward the suspected site until the point of maximum tenderness is found. On the tibia, a pencil may be rolled between the two hands along the subcutaneous bony surface, exerting pressure to elicit tenderness. *Limited motion* in the nearest joint and occasionally *joint effusion* give a clue to the location. The initial infection is in the metaphysis, near but not involving the epiphysis. ***Distinction.*** The diagnosis is made exclusively with the clinical findings; x-ray examination is seldom helpful in the initial phase. In rheumatic fever, the maximum tenderness is in the joint line, rather than near it as in osteomyelitis; tenderness in rheumatic fever is above and below the joint, while the tender site in osteomyelitis is in only one direction from the joint line. The tenderness in suppurative arthritis is also above and below the joint, while tenderness is on one side only in osteomyelitis with joint effusion. Sometimes deep cellulitis cannot be distinguished clinically from osteomyelitis. The pain of anterior poliomyelitis is found throughout the muscle mass. The painful nodules of erythema nodosum can be freely moved over the bone.

Chronic Osteomyelitis. After the acute phase, the purulent discharge from the necrosing bone breaks through the periosteum and drains through *sinuses* in the skin. The circulation of the cortex becomes impaired, producing islands of dead bone, *sequestra.* A sequestrum may be surrounded by new bone, the *involucrum,* and be absorbed or discharged through the sinus; usually surgical removal is required. Continuing necrosis of bone and retention of sequestra cause persistence of the sinus. The sinal orifice is characterized by *exuberant granulation tissue* (proud flesh). ***Distinction.*** The presence of a chronic sinus, surrounded by proud flesh, and x-ray evidence of bone necrosis are diagnostic.

Bony Swellings. The swelling is detected by inspection and palpation, but the signs are rarely diagnostic. X-ray findings may be distinctive, but biopsy is often indicated. The *location* of the swelling in the long bone may be distinctive. Hamilton Bailey formulated the following diagnostic aids: (1) Swelling in all diameters of the bulbous end of a long bone is caused by giant-cell tumor. (2) Swelling on one aspect of a bone, near the epiphyseal line, is an epiphyseal exostosis. (3) Swelling in all diameters, beginning at the metaphysis and extending toward the center of gravity, may be Brodie's abscess, osteoid osteoma, or osteosarcoma. (4) Swelling in all diameters, at the center of gravity, may be Ewing's tumor, eosinophilic granuloma, or bone cyst. (5) Think of the possibility that any localized bone tumor may be metastatic from a distant primary; so complete examination is indicated.

Bony Nodules (Occupational). Repeated trauma to a limited region of soft tissue and underlying bone during work or sport may cause bosses of the bones with overlying calluses. Among these are *surfer's knots,* on the dorsa of the feet, from weight-bearing with the dorsa in contact with the surfboard as the patient sits crosslegged [D. W. Gelfand: Surfer's Knots, *J.A.M.A.,* **197:**149, 1966]; painter's bosses, on the subcutaneous surface of the tibia at the junction of the upper and middle thirds, result from standing on a ladder and resting the tibiae against the next higher rung [G. E. Ehrlich: Painter's Bosses, *Arch. Intern. Med.,* **116:**776, 1965].

Diseases of Joints

The Arthritides

Many classifications of joint diseases have been devised, some quite formidable, none entirely satisfactory. Since they are grouped according to cause, they are not directly applicable to the problems in diagnostication; the cause is frequently unknown until the diagnosis is made. Most clinicians approach the patient by comparing his findings with prototypes of the more common diseases of joints; if the comparison is not close, they search for more distinctive findings. Descriptions of these prototypal entities follow.

▼ *Key Symptom:* ***Pain in the Joints.*** Because of the frequency of arthritis, pain in the joints is a common entering complaint.

The *location* of the pain, its *severity*, and its *duration* are important clues to the diagnosis. Aside from the various types of arthritis, the causes of joint pains are few.

Clinical Occurrence: ARTHRITIDES: acute and chronic. HEMARTHROSIS: traumatic, with or without hemophilia or other bleeding disorders. HYDRARTHROSIS: synovitis from any cause (the pain is caused by pressure from movement or weight-bearing). BONE FRACTURE: the fracture extends into the joint. TORN INTRACAPSULAR CARTILAGE.

GENERAL EXAMINATION OF JOINTS. **Examine all joints systematically from head to foot or in reverse sequence. Place the patient so the joint to be examined is supported at rest with the least pain and muscle spasm. Compare symmetric joints when one of a pair is involved. Observe *joint deformity* from swelling, subluxation, contracture, or ankylosis. Note the *size* and *contour* of the joint compared with your previous exact knowledge of the location of the joint capsule. Inspect the *color* of the overlying skin; feel the skin for its *temperature*. Palpate gently to locate areas of *tenderness* in the skin, muscles, bursae, ligaments, tendons, fat pads, and joint capsule. Palpate the *synovial membrane:* the normal one is not palpable; a *thickened synovium* feels "doughy" or "boggy" in the region of soft tissue that is normally undistinguished. Test the joint cavity for *fluctuation* by pressing a lateral bulge with the fingers of one hand while the fingers of the receiving hand rest upon the opposite bulge; fluid in the joint cavity will displace the receiving fingers. Fluctuation may be in the joint cavity or in a bursa; the borders and other anatomic relations will distinguish which. Test *range of motion* in the joint by anchoring one member with your hand and directing the patient to move the other member (*active motion*). Test *passive motion* by anchoring one member with one of your hands while the other hand moves the other member gently to the limit. Palpate to determine whether the limitation of motion is from *muscle spasm*, *fibrositic gelling* that improves with repeated movement, *effusion* in the joint cavity, *locking* from loose bodies in the joint, *fibrosis* ("soft arrest"), *bony ankylosis* ("hard arrest"). Palpate over the joint for *crepitus* on motion.**

Acute Monarticular: ***Suppurative Arthritis.*** Usually one joint is involved during the course of an infection whose primary symptoms and signs are in parts of the body remote from the joint. Inflammation of the joint often begins suddenly with *chills* and *fever*. The joint *swells* rapidly; it is *painful* and *tender*. The overlying skin is *red* and *warm*. The swelling becomes *fluctuant*, indicating fluid in the synovial cavity. Aspiration of the cavity discloses *pus;* bacteriologic cultures of the purulent exudate yield the causative organism.

Clinical Occurrence. Commonly during diseases caused by streptococci, staphylococci, meningococci, and gonococci. *Rarely* as a complication of brucellosis, typhoid fever, glanders, blastomycosis, granuloma inguinale, infections with *Haemophilus influenzae,* and others.

Acute Monarticular: ***Early Gout.*** A history of several similar episodes is often diagnostic, so the initial attack presents the chief problem. Frequently the patient is awakened by mild *burning, tingling, numbness,* or *warmth* in a joint. The site rapidly *swells* and becomes excruciatingly *tender,* intolerant of the pressure of the bedclothes. Typically the overlying skin becomes *red* or *violaceous.* Often there are *malaise, headache, fever,* and *tachycardia.* Leukocytosis and accelerated erythrocyte sedimentation are present. Untreated, the attack lasts for one or two weeks. In over half the cases, the metatarsophalangeal joint of the great toe is affected, when the ancient term *podagra* can be applied. Other sites are the instep, ankle, heel, elbow, or hand. *Bilateral* or *migratory* joint involvement, which sometimes occurs, excludes cellulitis, fracture, and suppurative arthritis. The attacks may be triggered by trauma, surgical operation, exposure to cold, changes in atmospheric pressure, acute infections, overindulgence in food or alcoholic beverages, the injection of foreign protein, the administration of diuretics, uricosuric agents, antileukemic drugs, epinephrine, ergotamine, liver extract. (See p. 665 for *Tophaceous Gout.*) *Distinction.* During the attack, the blood uric acid level is elevated (the value is not significant unless the blood urea nitrogen is normal). Relief of the symptoms and signs within two days after administration of colchicine is diagnostic; cortisone and phenylbutazone also relieve.

Secondary Gout. Besides the classic inherited gout are certain other conditions with hyperuricemia and inflamed joints, either from overproduction of uric acid or poor urinary excretion. *Overproduction* polycythemia vera, chronic granulocytic leukemia, therapy with cytolytic drugs. *Renal Retention of Urates.* Lactaciduria in glycogen-storage diseases, beta-hydroxybutyraturia from high-fat diet or starvation, diuretics, salicylates, and chronic lead poisoning (saturnine gout) [G. V.

Ball and L. B. Sorensen: Pathogenesis of Hyperuricemia in Saturnine Gout, *N. Engl. J. Med.,* **280:**1202, 1969].

Acute Monarticular: ***Pseudogout*** (Articular Chondrocalcinosis, Calcium Pyrophosphate Dihydrate Deposition Disease). This disorder presents to the clinician as an acute arthritis having marked similarity to true gout. Often the patient has had multiple episodes. The attack *begins abruptly* with extremely *painful swelling* and *heat* usually in a single joint, occasionally in two or more. The knee is most commonly affected, the wrist is next. The symptoms and signs are intense for two to four days, then they gradually subside during the next two weeks. Fever usually accompanies the inflammation (100° to 103° F) (37.8° to 39.4° C). *Pathophysiology.* Apparently the deposition of crystals of calcium pyrophosphate dihydrate in the synovial fluid triggers the inflammation. The cause of the deposition is unknown; the concentration of calcium is normal is tissues and serum. Some writers believe the disease to be hereditary. The condition is often associated with mild diabetes mellitus, hyperparathyroidism, or essential hypertension. *Laboratory Findings.* Blood counts are normal but the erythrocyte sedimentation rate is acclerated. Tests for latex fixation and antinuclear antibodies are negative. The serum calcium and alkaline phosphatase are normal. The serum uric acid blood levels are not elevated. *X-ray Findings.* Chondrocalcinosis appears as multiple punctate calcium deposits arranged linearly in the cartilage, most often of the wrist and symphysis pubis. Hyaline cartilage calcification appears as thin lines of punctate deposits that parallel underlying bone. *Synovial Fluid.* The fluid is usually copious and turbid, with poor viscosity. Leukocyte counts are reported as 50,000 to 75,000 per cu mm with 95% polymorphonuclears. The quality of the mucin is considered "good." Crystals of calcium pyrophosphate dihydrate are present within and outside the cells. They are described as 3 to 15 mμ long parallelopiped rods or rhomboids, with weak birefringence, positive in the polarizing microscope with a first-order red plate compensator. The presence of these crystals is diagnostic. *Distinction.* Besides the crystals in the synovial fluid pseudogout fails to respond to the administration of colchicine. There is also dramatic relief from pain with the aspiration of the synovial fluid [M. Skinner and A. C. Cohen: Calcium Pyrophosphate Dihydrate Crystal Deposition Disease, *Arch. Intern. Med.*, **123:**636–44, 1969].

Chronic Monarticular: ***Tuberculous Arthritis.*** Occurring usually in a patient between the ages of 9 and 30 years, there is *chronic swelling* of a single joint, with only *moderate pain.* Joint *effusion* may be present with *thickening of the synovium.* Most commonly affected are the hips, spine, and knees. Painless regional lymphadenopathy is usually found. *Distinction.* X-ray films may show destruction of contiguous bone or loss of cartilages. Cultures of the joint fluid yield tubercle bacilli; biopsy of the synovium may be necessary.

Chronic Monarticular: ***Gummatous Arthritis.*** Clinically, this may be identical with tuberculous arthritis; positive serologic tests for syphilis make the distinction.

Acute Migratory: ***Rheumatic Fever.*** This disease is a delayed inflammatory reaction of mesenchymal tissue following infection with group A hemolytic streptococci. The classic picture of a moderately severe case begins from one to four weeks after streptococcal pharyngitis, with gradual onset of *malaise, increased fatigability,* and *anorexia.* Either slight or high *fever* is usually present. An early manifestation is often *epistaxis.* At the onset, a single large joint becomes *painful,* exquisitely *tender,* and *swollen;* the overlying skin is *red* and *hot. Fluid often forms* in the joint cavity; when aspirated, it is found to be turbid from leukocytes, but cultures remain sterile. With the fever and signs of illness persisting, the signs of joint inflammation spontaneously subside in a few days, to appear in another joint, and later another, a *migratory* arthritis. *Precordial pain* or discomfort suggests cardiac involvement; the signs may range from tachycardia to muffled heart sounds, cardiac enlargement, systolic murmurs, pericardial friction rub, gallop rhythm. Electrocardiographic evidence of myocardial involvement may be present. With intensification of the disease, *subcutaneous rheumatic nodules* may appear as firm, nontender masses over the joint prominences and tendon sheaths of the limbs, scalp, and spine. They are loosely attached to the underlying tissue; when numerous, their distribution tends to be symmetric. The appearance of the nodule often presages severe cardiac involvement. Two distinct types of skin lesions may be associated with rheumatic fever; neither is pathognomonic.

Erythema marginatum or *circinatum* is characterized by coalescing circular erythematous areas over the trunk and extremities, migratory and transitory, changing within the hour. Less common, *erythema nodosum* is manifest by *dull red, exquisitely tender nodules,* about 1 cm in diameter, mostly over the anterior aspects of the legs, seldom above the knees. They are often mistaken for abscesses, but they never suppurate. A crop of lesions involutes in a few days, to be followed by another crop. The involuting lesion discolors the skin as a hematoma would. *Distinction.* The typical clinical picture is fairly distinctive; there are no diagnostic laboratory tests. Anti-streptolysin-O titers are significantly high in 85% of cases; but this is merely evidence of recent streptococcal infection; it does not prove the presence of rheumatic fever. The disease is protean in its clinical manifestations. Joint involvement may be so mild that pain is unaccompanied by physical signs of inflammation. The arthritis may be monarticular or polyarticular, instead of migratory, so months of observation may be required to distinguish from rheumatoid arthritis; involvement of the temporomandibular joint often occurs in rheumatoid arthritis, practically never in rheumatic fever. Rheumatic fever leaves no residual joint deformity. Early, the inflammation of a single joint with effusion requires distinction from suppurative arthritis by proving the fluid to be sterile.

Acute Migratory: ***Gonococcal Arthritis.*** An infectious arthritis is the most common extragenital complication of gonorrhea. One to four weeks after the beginning of the urethritis, inflammation may suddenly occur in the knees, wrists, and ankles, although other joints may be affected. The most common pattern is a *migratory* arthritis, resembling the first few weeks of classic acute rheumatic fever. Small amounts of thin fluid may accumulate in joint cavities from which organisms are difficult to isolate. In other cases *suppurative arthritis* develops with inflammation of a single joint and production of purulent exudate in which the gonococcus can be stained or cultured. Some patients follow a third pattern, indistinguishable clinically from rheumatoid arthritis. *Tenosynovitis* in the hands, wrists, or feet is more common in gonorrhea than in arthritis from any other cause. *Distinction.* The diagnosis may not be easy; the gonococcus is difficult to culture; gonorrheal infection in the female genitalia may not be obvious. Resemblance to Reiter's syndrome (nonspecific urethritis, arthritis, and conjunctivitis) may be close, since catarrhal conjunctivitis is present in 10% of patients with gonorrhea. The gonococcal complement-fixation test is diagnostic *when the titer rises* during the course of the disease.

Inflammatory Polyarthritis: **Rheumatoid Arthritis.** A disease of unknown cause, it is characterized by proliferative inflammation of the body's connective tissue, especially the articular synovia. Granulation tissue from the proliferating synovia penetrates the joint cavity in tonguelike projections, called *pannus,* that undergo fibrosis and cause ankylosis. Usually the smaller articulations are involved, often symmetrically. The onset may be insidious; the first symptoms are *stiffness* or *pain on motion* of the joints. Early, the involvement may be *migratory;* finally one or more joints become *swollen, painful,* and *tender.* Low-grade *fever* is often present. When the onset is sudden, pain and swelling often occur simultaneously in several joints, with high fever and prostration. An involved interphalangeal joint becomes *fusiform* from fluid in the joint cavity (fluctuant) or thickening of the joint capsule (more than normal thickness of tissue over bone). *Tenderness* is confined to the region of the capsule. Early, joint *motion is limited* by pain or fluid, later by fibrosis or muscle shortening. The overlying skin becomes *shiny* with disappearance of the normal fine linear furrows of the epidermis; picking up a fold of skin reveals it to be *thinner* than normal. *Atrophy of adjacent muscles* is rapid and disproportionately severe for the disuse. Although remissions may occur, the disease is usually progressive over a period of several years. Finally, complete fixation of the joint, *ankylosis,* results. *Subluxations* are frequent; lateral deflection and subluxation of the metacarpophalangeal joints produce characteristic *ulnar deviation.* Low-grade tenosynovitis is manifest as *fluctuant swelling of the tendon sheaths.* In 20 to 30% of cases, subcutaneous *rheumatic nodules* develop, similar to those in rheumatic fever. Found over joint prominences and tendon sheaths, they are painless, firm, and freely movable over bones. *Pleural effusion* or *pulmonary nodules* may accompany or antedate the joint involvement. *Distinction.* There is no specific diagnostic laboratory test. A *rheumatoid factor* can be demonstrated in the plasma by the latex or bentonite tests in 70 to 95% of the cases, but the reaction is not entirely specific. Frequently the clinical course must be observed over many months before the disease can be distinguished from rheumatic fever. In the early stages, migratory arthritis is common to both. Reiter's syndrome can closely resemble rheumatoid arthritis until the appearance of a urethritis or a conjunctivitis. An initial single inflamed joint may suggest suppurative arthritis, until aspiration of joint fluid excludes the presence of organisms. An episode of acute gout may be suggested, but normal blood uric acid and lack of response to colchicine make it improbable. The pleural and synovial fluid in rheumatoid arthritis is characterized by glucose content of less than 10 mg/100 mL, a fact that is helpful in diagnosis. Rheumatoid arthritis frequently involves the temporomandibular joint to distinguish it from rheumatic fever.

Inflammatory Polyarthritis: **Variants of Rheumatoid Arthritis.** Several apparent clinical entities are tentatively considered to be variants of rheumatoid arthritis. *Felty's syndrome* is the triad of rheumatoid arthritis, splenomegaly, and leukopenia; many clinicians now regard this as long-standing rheumatoid arthritis complicated by hypersplenism. *Juvenile rheumatoid arthritis* (Still's disease) is rheumatoid arthritis modified by the conditions of childhood. Cardiac complications are more common than in adults; frequently enlargement of the lymph nodes, liver, and spleen occurs; disturbed bone growth causes skeletal deformities. Arthritis occurs in *agammaglobulinemia* in 25% of the cases. *Palindromic rheumatism* presents multiple afebrile attacks of polyarthritis lasting for only 2 or 3 days, leaving no residua. *Sjögren's syndrome* is diagnosed when two of the triad are present: keratoconjunctivitis sicca, xerostomia, and rheumatoid arthritis. *Ankylosing spondylitis* (Marie-Strümpell-Bechterew disease) is a chronic progressive arthritis of the spine and pelvis, leading to complete ankylosis; in 20% of the cases there is accompanying rheumatoid arthritis of limbs. *Psoriatic arthritis* develops in some persons with long-standing psoriasis. In most cases the joint disease is indistinguishable from rheumatoid arthritis; but in a few there is an added destructive process in the terminal phalanges that is diagnostic in x-ray films. *Reiter's syndrome* is the triad of rheumatoid arthritis, nonspecific urethritis, and conjunctivitis.

Chronic Polyarthritis: **Systemic Lupus Erythematosus (*SLE*).** This is a chronic inflammatory disease involving many systems. The cause is unknown. *Lupus,* the Latin word for wolf, was applied because the malar erythema on the cheeks of patients resembled the coloring of a wolf's face. No one symptom or sign is pathognomonic of the disorder: rather a cluster of attributes presents the picture. The three most common symptoms or signs are *constitutional symptoms of fatigue or fevers* (80–90% of cases), *arthritis or arthralgias* (90%), *skin rashes* (50–60%) [A. D. Steinberg: Systemic Lupus Erythematosus, In *Cecil Textbook of Medicine*, 17th ed., 1985, Philadelphia, W.B. Saunders Co., p. 1924.]. *Musculoskeletal System:* pains in the joints and inflammation resembling rheumatoid arthritis. *Mucocutaneous:* the "butterfly rash" is a maculopapular scaly erythematous process forming the "wings" of the butterfly on each malar prominence with the "trunk" of the insect on the bridge of the nose; it is more intense after exposure to sunlight. In addition, there are skin atrophy, telangiectasia and mucosal ulcers. *Kidneys:* acute nephritis or nephrotic syndrome. *Cardiovascular:* endocarditis, pericarditis, and myocarditis occur in about one third of patients. *Pulmonary:* pleurisy with effusion and *friction rub;* often associated with pulmonary infiltrations are shown by x-ray films. *Nervous system:* personality disorders, psychoses, seizures and peripheral neuropathies. *Gastrointestinal: anorexia, nausea, loss of weight; passive congestion of the liver* with *hepatomegaly. Reticuloendothelial System:* spleen and lymph nodes enlarged. *Laboratory Findings:* anemia, thrombocytopenia; elevated ESR; false-positive test for syphilis, circulating anticoagulant, antinuclear antibodies, anti-DNA, anti-Sm, and reduced hemolytic complement in active disease. Criteria for classification of systemic lupus erythematosus were revised in 1982 [E. M. Tan, A. S. Cohen, J. F. Fries, et al.: The 1982 Revised Criteria for the Classification of Systemic Lupus Erythematosus, *Arthritis Rheum.*, **25:**1271–77, 1982.].

Vasculitis with Rheumatoid Arthritis (For classification and pathophysiology see p. 465). *Involved Vessels:* small cutaneous vessels, synovium, and rheumatoid nodules. The arteritis occurs when the rheumatoid arthritis becomes severe. Also may be involved: the arterioles, the intermediate arteries, and large veins.

Inflammatory Polyarthritis: **Arthropathy of Iron Storage Disease.** Some authors have reported that the onset of an apparent chronic rheumatoid arthritis turned out to be the beginning of iron storage disorder [U. M. Seffar, V. L. Fornasier, and I. H. Fox: Arthropathy as the Major Clinical Indicator of Occult Iron Storage Disease, *J.A.M.A.*, **238:**1825–28, 1977].

Inflammatory Polyarthritis: **Arthritic Manifestations of Specific Diseases.** Joint inflammation with temporary resemblance to rheumatic fever or rheumatoid arthritis is a transient episode in many specific diseases, most of them infectious. The distinguishing signs of the specific disease usually lead to the diagnosis, so confusion with the nonspecific forms is brief.

Clinical Occurrence. *Typhoid fever* is occasionally complicated by polyarthritis or spondylitis. *Salmonella infections* infrequently present transient polyarthritis. *Drug reactions* and *serum sickness* often exhibit pain and swelling of joints. *Subacute bacterial endocarditis* is frequently accompanied by polyarthritis. *Intestinal lipodystrophy* (Whipple's disease) is often preceded for many years by rheumatoid arthritis. Rarely, mumps is complicated by polyarthritis that occurs about six weeks after the parotitis. *Epidemic pleurodynia* is sometimes associated with pain and swelling in the joints. *Rubella* (German measles) rarely exhibits mild joint pain and swelling. *Ulcerative colitis* occasionally is accompanied by rheumatoid arthritis; in a few cases, a monarticular arthritis ("toxic arthritis") waxes and wanes with the colonic symptoms. *Regional ileitis* rarely induces a spondylitis. *Erythema multiforme* often exhibits arthralgia, occasionally polyarticular arthritis. *Erythema nodosum* in three quarters of the cases shows some joint involvement. *Behçet's disease* occasionally is complicated by polyarthritis. *Brucellosis* may be complicated by polyarthritis, spondylitis, or even suppurative arthritis. *Secondary syphilis* often has transient swelling of the joints. *Acute leukemia* not infrequently produces an arthritis resembling rheumatic fever. *Mycotic infections* (coccidioidomycosis, histoplasmosis, blastomycosis, cryptococcosis, actinomycosis) often exhibit polyarthritis.

Noninflammatory Polyarticular: **Osteoarthritis** (Hypertrophic or Degenerative Joint Disease). *Clinical signs* of inflammation are relatively slight. The wear and tear on joints, accumulated from many years of skeletal movements and probably other factors, produce degeneration of articular cartilages. Thus exposed, the bone ends rub directly on each other so their surfaces become worn and polished. The joint capsules are little affected, so adhesions are not formed, and although joint motion is restricted, *ankylosis does not result.* The bony margins proliferate to form spurs, lipping, and exostoses. With each passing year the disease progresses; symptoms and signs are first noticed in middle age, in some persons sooner than others. The weight-bearing joints are most affected, but excessive wear from unusual occupations or postural defects accentuates the process in single joints. Great individual variation is noted in the symptoms, unrelated to the objective signs of joint disease. In most patients, the joints are *painless,* but a few complain bitterly. The most common symptom is *stiffness after rest;* this disappears with a little movement. The patient may note *grating during motion.* The *range of motion is normal;* there is no ankylosis. Enlargement of the terminal interphalangeal joints of the fingers, *Heberden's nodes,* is frequently encountered. Occasionally, *painless effusion* occurs, especially in the knee. *Special Forms. Osteoarthritis of the hip* (malum coxae senilis) is destruction of the hip joint, frequently disabling. *Osteoarthritis of the spine* (hypertrophic spondylitis) produces much lipping and many spurs around the vertebral bodies, probably associated with regeneration of intervertebral disks. Variable stiffening and pain result. The osteoarthritis of *acromegaly* is caused by overgrowth of bone and cartilage. Osteoarthritis in *alkaptonuria* (ochronosis) results from excessive pigment deposits in the joints. The osteoarthritis in *hemophilia and allied conditions* follows the organization of repeated hematomas with calcification.

Noninflammatory Polyarticular: **Tophaceous Gout.** Clinical signs of inflammation are relatively slight. After years of episodes of acute gouty arthritis, when the output of uric acid can no longer compensate for the rate of production, crystals of sodium urate are deposited in the tissues as *gouty tophi.* In the joints, they erode cartilage and bone; acting as foreign bodies, they stimulate low-grade inflammatory processes that extrude the tophi through the skin in *sinuses.* The masses of urates and cartilaginous degeneration produce *painless nonfunctional* joints with *grotesque nodular swellings.*

Painless Monarticular: **Neurogenic Arthropathy** (Charcot's Joint). Loss of painful or proprioceptive sensations in a joint permits excessive traumatization. Repeated injuries cause successively *three stages of articular damage:* hydrarthrosis, joint degeneration, new-bone formation in the joint. In any stage, the diagnostic clue is the *absence of pain with movement* that would ordinarily be painful with sensory abnormalities in the involved limb. In the initial stage, *hydrarthrosis* is the only anatomic finding. Later additions are *subluxation* and *hypermobility* of the joint. Finally, the joint capsule becomes *enlarged* and *hard* from new bone. Crepitus is pronounced; *painless deformities* may be bizarre. The condition is usually *monarticular*. Finding an anesthetic joint derangement calls for tests of tendon reflexes, pupillary reactions, temperature sensation, and glucose in the urine.

Clinical Occurrence. Tabes dorsalis (knee most commonly involved; hip, ankle, lower spine, less frequently). Diabetes mellitus (tarsal and metatarsal joint most commonly, ankle occasionally, knee rarely). Syringomyelia (usually joints of the upper limbs). Repeated injections of a joint with adrenal corticosteroids (the only condition without neural deficit).

Painless Bilateral Knee Effusions: ***Arthritis of Congenital Syphilis*** (Clutton's Joints). At puberty a child with congenital syphilis may develop *painless* bilateral effusions in the knee joints.

Episodic Painless Effusions of the Knees: ***Intermittent Hydrarthrosis.*** The patient experiences episodes of painless swelling and joint effusion in one or both knees, with no constitutional symptoms. The episodes recur over a number of years. Frequently the periodicity is remarkably precise, with an average duration of 3 to 5 days and intermissions averaging 7 to 11 days. The cause is unknown; occasionally the condition presages the onset of rheumatoid arthritis.

Neoplasms of Joints. Rarely joints are the sites of neoplasm, benign or malignant. *Persistent painless swelling* without definite trauma is usually an indication for biopsy. The occurrence of *bloody joint effusion* without trauma also requires prompt histologic examination.

Painless Nodules Near Joints or Tendons. Several diseases produce painless nodules in joint capsules, tendons, ligaments, or in the surrounding connective tissue. *Subcutaneous nodules of rheumatic fever* are freely movable and occur especially over bony prominences or tendons. *Subcutaneous nodules of rheumatoid arthritis* and *systemic lupus erythematosus* are usually over bony prominences and loosely attached to articular capsules; they are also found in the periosteum or the deeper layers of the skin. *Gouty tophi,* although usually collected in bursas, are also formed in the Achilles tendon and the cartilage of the ear. *Xanthomas of essential hypercholesterolemia* occur in tendons of the hands and in the Achilles tendon and patellar tendon;

their presence is diagnostic. *Juxta-articular nodes* (*Jeanselme's nodules*) occur near joints in syphilis, yaws, and other treponemal diseases.

***Nontender Fluctuant Swelling Near Joints and Tendons:* Synovial Cysts.** These are either bursae and tendon sheaths distended by fluid or *protrusion cysts* from joint capsules herniated by hydrostatic pressure. All are *nontender* and *fluctuant.* The protrusion cysts usually *collapse under pressure.* Radiograms of the spaces injected with contrast media depict connections with joint cavities. *Synovial cysts* usually occur in the course of *rheumatoid arthritis;* sometimes they antedate the more usual symptoms and signs by several years. Palmer writes that in the *hands* protrusion cysts usually occur on the dorsal aspects of the proximal interphalangeal joints. When cysts arise from the extensor sheaths of the *wrists* they cause oval swellings in the dorsum of the hand. In this region the synovial cysts are often called *ganglions.* The olecranon bursa of the *elbow* is frequently distended. Involvement of the *shoulder joint* produces a globular swelling. In the *ankle,* either the retrocalcaneal or the retroachilles bursa may be affected and must be distinguished from subcutaneous edema and fat pads about the joints. The protrusion cyst of the *knee* is well-recognized under the eponym *Baker's cyst* or *popliteal cyst* (p. 758). The fluid in synovial cysts ranges from clear yellow with low cell count to opalescent with many cells and rice bodies.

Noises in Joints. Moving joints may emit several types of sounds that prompt medical consultation. The knees or hips especially may produce *creaking;* this usually results from gross loss of cartilage that permits the rubbing together of apposing bone ends. *Joint crepitus* is a grating sound whose vibrations may also be palpated. It is produced by the roughened surfaces of synovia rubbing together in osteoarthritis, rheumatoid arthritis, acromegaly, and scleroderma. The exact mechanism is not understood, but its presence does not indicate serious joint disease. Some persons have apparently normal joints that *crackle* under certain conditions. This noise has been reproduced experimentally. Increasing traction is applied to a metacarpophalangeal joint to cause slow separation; in some persons a bubble of carbon dioxide will form in the synovial fluid. Further separation causes sudden collapse of the bubble with the production of noise; the joint space containing fluid and gas suddenly expands. When traction is discontinued, it takes about 15 minutes for the gas to resorb and the joint to return to normal size, when the procedure can be repeated.

Disorders of Muscles

▼ *Key Symptom:* ***Muscle Pain.*** Pain in the muscles is distinguished from articular or neuritic pain by eliciting moderate *tenderness* when a muscle mass is squeezed between the examiner's thumb and index finger. With experience, one can learn to detect the unusual *hardness* of a muscle due to tonic contraction. Both muscular and articular pains are intensified by movement. Neuritic pain is associated with tenderness over the nerve trunk and intensification of the pain in the distribution of its branches. But chronic neuritic pain also stimulates secondary tonic muscle contractions. Some causes of muscle pain are listed.

Clinical Occurrence: ACUTE PAIN. *Traumatic:* muscle strain, hematoma of muscle. *Acute Febrile Infections:* malaria, rubella, influenza, rheumatic fever, epidemic pleurodynia (Bornholm disease, devil's grip), dengue, rat-bite fever, trichinosis. *Hyponatremia:* dehydration, diuresis, malabsorption. *Myoglobinopathies:* McArdle's disease (paroxysmal myoglobinuria), march myoglobinuria (march gangrene). CHRONIC PAIN. *Traumatic:* chronic muscle strain, tonic contractions (such as tension headaches). *Arthritides:* rheumatoid arthritis, osteoarthritis. *Collagen Diseases:* dermatomyositis, systemic lupus erythematosus, polyarteritis nodosa. *Metabolic:* hypoparathyroidism. Polymyalgia rheumatica, disseminated candidiasis.

— *Myalgia with Trigger Point:* ***Myofascial Syndrome.*** Many patients seek medical consultation for chronic recurrent pain in the distribution of one or more muscles. The pain may be lancinating, aching, boring, or a feeling of muscular stiffness. Often the patient relates the onset to some specific trauma. *Physical Findings.* The involved muscles may or may not be in *spasm,* but the distinguishing feature is the presence of one or more *trigger points.*

The examiner should palpate the entire region carefully with firm pressure of the fingertips. Often the trigger point is discovered some distance from the *referred pain area.* ***Pathophysiology.*** Pains from the muscles and tendons at the trigger areas are believed to bombard the brain constantly, whence impulses are sent through afferent spinal pathways to cause muscle spasms and diminished blood flow; these, in turn, cause more pain impulses. *Distinction.* The diagnosis is confirmed when the pain dramatically disappears a few minutes after intramuscular injection of the primary trigger point with 1 to 5 mL of 1% solution of lidocaine or procaine with a short 23- or 24-gauge needle.

— *Nocturnal Pain:* ***Musculoskeletal Night Pains.*** Certain chronic disorders of the musculoskeletal system manifest *pain with nocturnal exacerbation.* Often the occurrence of such pain is of diagnostic and therapeutic importance [F. D. Hart, R. T. Taylor, and E. C. Huskisson: Pain at Night, *Lancet,* **1:** 881–84, 1970. H. H. G. Eastcott: Pain at Night, *Lancet,* **1:** 1056–57, 1970].

Clinical Occurrence. Rheumatoid arthritis, ankylosing spondylitis, polymyalgia rheumatica, degenerative joint disease (osteoarthritis), periarthritis of the shoulder, gout, carpal-tunnel syndrome, metastatic disease of bone, night cramps, ischemic peripheral vascular disease.

Pains in Neck, Trunk, and Arms: ***Polymyalgia Rheumatica*** (Polymyalgia Arteritica, Myalgic Syndrome of the Aged, Senile Arthritis, Anarthritic Rheumatoid Disease, Periarthrosis Humeroscapularis, Pseudopolyarthrite Rhizomelique). This belongs to the large group of segmental necrotizing vasculitides and is often associated with the other giant-cell manifestations of temporal arteritis and carotid arteritis (see p. 465 for classification). *Age and Sex:* usually the 5th or 6th decade with slight preference for women. *Involved Vessels:* intermediate and large arteries. *Symptoms: pain and stiffness of muscles* of neck, shoulders, back, and thorax. Although spontaneously painful, the muscles are *seldom very tender;* the stiffness is relieved by motion. The only distinguishing laboratory finding is an *elevated erythrocyte sedimentation rate* (*ESR*). *Therapeutic Test:* symptoms promptly relieved with steroids. Biopsy sometimes necessary. Ten more years of clinical experience since publication of the early descriptions have added more features to the clinical picture and also have raised doubts whether this is a distinct disease or a variant of rheumatoid arthritis in elderly women. The association with giant-cell arteritis has been confirmed and the frequent occurrence of carpal tunnel syndrome noted.

A curious high frequency of sternoclavicular swelling and tenderness has been encountered.

Muscle Atrophy. Loss of muscle substance occurs from *disuse* or from damage to *muscle tissue* or motor *nerves*. Since atrophy is slow to develop, the neurogenic causes are found in the list of chronic continuing paralyses. The physical sign of atrophy is loss of muscle mass.

Muscle Contracture. Fibrosis of muscle produces permanent shortening. The condition may result from muscle *disuse*, prolonged *ischemia* leading to necrosis of muscle fibers, or *inflammatory processes* as in dermatomyositis. The physical signs of contracture are that the muscle is reduced to a hard cord, smaller in diameter than normal; the shortened muscle does not permit full movement about the joint, a condition to be distinguished from ankylosis of the joint.

Muscle Hypertrophy. Increase in muscle volume is usually the result of exercise and conditioning. It may also occur in hypothyroidism, congenital myotonia, congenital athetosis with feeblemindedness, familial muscular dystrophy and focal myositis.

Masses in Muscle. To prove that a mass is intramuscular, with the muscle relaxed the mass must be freely movable transversely to the long axis; tensing the muscle must limit the transverse mobility. A mass may result from rupture of a muscle, herniation of a muscle through its sheath, intramuscular hemorrhage, neoplasm, localized myositis ossificans.

Abnormal Muscle Movements. Consult pp. 790–95.

The Upper Limb

In the examination, this anatomic region includes the structures of the neck, shoulder girdle, upper arm, forearm, hand. When neither abnormal movements nor gross anatomic changes are evident at a glance, the physician usually begins with a detailed examination of the hands and works upward, the sequence used here.

▼ *Key Symptom:* ***Pain in the Upper Arm, Forearm, and Hand.*** When pain is sharply localized in an extremity, the diagnosis is relatively simple. But often the pain is more or less diffuse throughout the upper limb, so an anatomic classification of causes is useful.

Clinical Occurrence: SHARPLY LOCALIZED PAIN. Arthritis, bursitis, bone fracture, tendon rupture, tenosynovitis, cellulitis, muscle strain, neoplasm, polymyalgia rheumatica, embolism, claudication. DIFFUSE PAIN. *Vertebral:* herniated cervical intervertebral disk, fracture-dislocation, spondylitis, Pott's disease, neoplasm of bone. *Spinal cord:* syringomyelia, tumor, radiculitis, meningitis of cord. *Retrograde pain:* from carpal tunnel syndrome. *Generalized:* from shoulder-hand syndrome. *Referred pain:* angina pectoris (medial aspects of arms and volar aspects of forearms in 1st dermatome).

The Hand

The hand includes the carpal, metacarpal, and phalangeal bones, their joints, and the covering soft tissues. Abnormalities in *size* and *disproportions* in parts are usually caused by bone growth. The *postures* of the hand result from pain, unusual muscle pull, or joint disorders; usually growth is normal. Notice the sex difference: in the male the ring finger is longer than the index finger; the female index finger is usually longer than her ring finger.

Enlargement of One Hand: ***Hemihypertrophy and Local Gigantism.*** An entire side of the body may be enlarged in a congenital deformity known as *hemihypertrophy. Local gigantism* is often the result of a congenital arteriovenous fistula of the upper limb. In either case, the hand is perfectly proportioned.

Dwarfing of One Hand: ***Unilateral Atrophy.*** A hand may be the site of congenital atrophy, cause unknown.

Large Hands: ***Acromegaly and Gigantism.*** The hands enlarge from overgrowth of bone and soft tissues, stimulated by an excess of somatotropic hormone, usually from an eosinophilic adenoma of the anterior pituitary gland. When the condition occurs before the epiphyses close, the enlarged skeleton is perfectly proportioned and the condition is termed *gigantism.* When growth occurs after epiphyseal closure, the skeletal pattern is called *acromegaly,* in which the hands, feet, face, head, and soft tissues are enlarged. The bones of the hands are perfectly proportioned, but soft-tissue overgrowth increases the finger girth, making them ponderous, a *paw hand* or *spade hand.* Acromegalic arthritis is frequently present (see p. 665). X-ray films of the finger tufts and sella turcica are frequently distinctive.

Large Hands: ***Hypertrophic Osteoarthropathy.*** All dimensions of the hands are increased, as in acromegaly, but the condition is invariably accompanied by extreme clubbing of the fingers and parrot-beak nails (see pp. 689 and 691).

Small Hands: ***Acromicria.*** Diminutive hands usually result from congenital anomalies of obscure cause.

Long Slender Hands: ***Spider Fingers*** (Arachnodactyly, Marfan's Syndrome). All the long bones of the hands are slender and elongated, often with hyperextensible joints (Fig. 9-1B). But the condition must be distinguished from some normal persons who are tall and have proportionately long digits. The hands in Marfan's syndrome may show a positive *thumb sign* (Steinberg's s.). When the fingers are clenched over the thumb, the end of the thumb protrudes beyond the ulnar margin of the hand [A. S. Parker and H. F. Hare: Arachnodactyly, *Radiology*, **45**:220–26, 1945]. Another diagnostic assist is the *wrist sign* in which the patient encircles his own wrist with his thumb and little finger proximal to the styloid process of the ulna. In normal persons the encircling digits scarcely touch, but in arachnodactyly they may overlap by 1 to 2 cm [B. Walker and J. L. Murdock: The Wrist Sign. A Useful Physical Finding

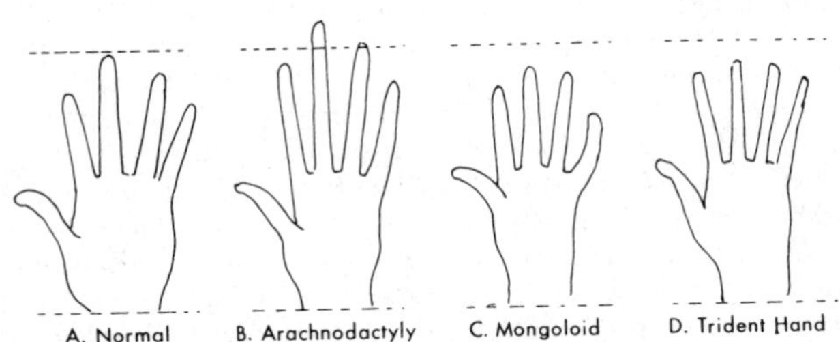

Fig. 9-1. Congenitally disproportionate hands. **A.** *A sketch of a normal hand is drawn to scale to be compared with the abnormalities. It should be noted that in practically all normal male hands the ring finger is longer than the index finger; most women have longer index fingers, although a few exceptions occur.* **B.** Arachnodactyly. *A synonym is "spider fingers." These occur in Marfan's syndrome. The fingers are remarkable for their length and slenderness; the joints are abnormally hyperextensible.* **C.** Mongolism or Down's syndrome. *The digits are short and the little finger often has a peculiar radialward curve.* **D.** Trident hand. *This occurs in achondroplasia. The fingers are short and almost equal in length; the index and middle fingers are widely separated.*

in the Marfan Syndrome, *Arch. Intern. Med.*, **126**:267–77, 1970]. The positive sign results from the combination of long digits and narrow wrist. Neither the thumb sign nor the wrist sign is absolute proof of Marfan's syndrome.

Long Slender Hands: ***Eunuchoidism.*** These may be similar to the spider fingers in Marfan's syndrome.

Short Thick Hands: ***Cretinism.*** The hands are short, thick, and fat. The radius may be shortened.

Short Thick Hands: ***Mongolism.*** The hands are short and thick; the thumb diverges from nearer the wrist than normal; the little finger is *curved* (Fig. 9-1C).

Divergent Fingers: ***Trident Hands.*** A characteristic of achondroplasia, the fingers approach *uniform length* and *radiate* from the hand like the spokes in a wheel with a fat hub (Fig. 9-1D).

Rudimentary Hand: ***Club Hand.*** A developmental anomaly, stunted or normal fingers are mounted on a stub of indeterminate shape (Fig. 9-2A).

Position of Anatomic Rest. In inflammations of the hand, the parts are held in the position to ease the pain, with fingers and thumb flexed, the index finger less bent than the others (Fig. 9-2C).

Malposture: ***Ulnar Deviation or Drift.*** Most common in rheumatoid arthritis, the phalanges are deflected toward the ulnar side from subluxations of the metacarpophalangeal joints (Fig. 9-2B).

Malposture: ***Clawhand.*** The claw is formed by hyperextension of the metacarpophalangeal joints and flexion of the interphalangeal articulations (Fig. 9-2D). This occurs from the predominant pull of the Extensor communis digitorum and the Flexor digitorum against weak or paralyzed interosseus and lumbrical muscles. Paralysis may result from brachial plexus or ulnar nerve injuries, syringomyelia, the muscular atrophies, or acute poliomyelitis.

Malposture: ***Ape Hand.*** The thumb is held in extension by its inability to flex (Fig. 9-2E). This may occur in syringomyelia, progressive muscular atrophy, amyotrophic lateral sclerosis.

Malposture: ***Carpal Spasm*** (Accoucheur's Hand, Obstetrician's Hand). The characteristic position occurs in tetany (Fig. 9-2F). The thumb is flexed into the palm; the wrist and metacarpophalangeal joints are also flexed, while the interphalangeal

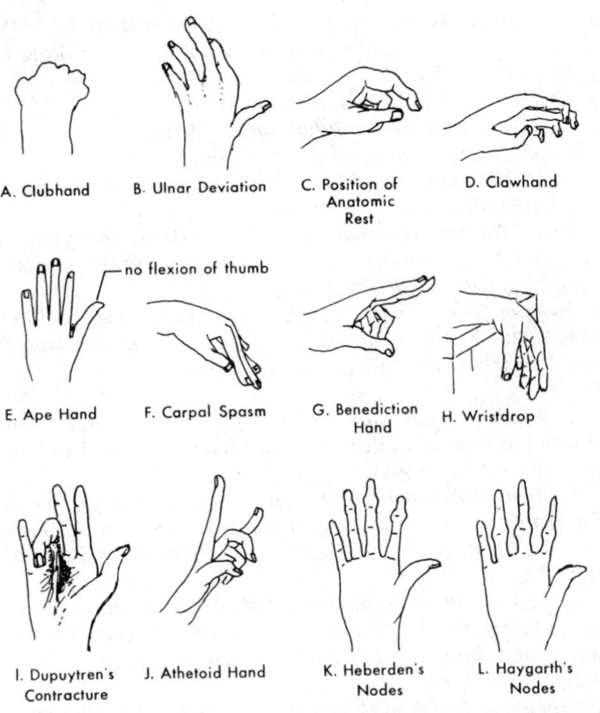

Fig. 9-2. Mostly acquired deformities of the hand. **A.** Club hand. *This is a congenital lesion in which the hand development is rudimentary; the stub may be surmounted by rudimentary or normal digits.* **B.** Ulnar deviation. *Also called "ulnar drift." It is a posture of the hand that develops during rheumatoid arthritis and is primarily due to muscle atrophy and the muscle pull on subluxated joints.* **C.** Position of anatomic rest. *The position is assumed in the normally developed hand with deep-seated infection. The fingers are partially flexed, the index finger less than the others.* **D.** Clawhand. *There is hyperextension of the metacarpophalangeal joints and flexion of the interphalangeal joint. It results from brachial plexus injuries, syringomyelia, and other lesions of the median and ulnar nerves.* **E.** Ape hand. *The thumb is held in extension because it cannot be flexed. This occurs in syringomyelia, amyotrophic lateral sclerosis, and progressive muscular atrophy.* **F.** Carpal spasm. *This is also called "obstetrician's hand" or "accoucheur's hand" because it somewhat resembles the position of the physician's*

joints are hyperextended and the fingers are adducted in the shape of a cone. The spasm is involuntary and usually painless (see p. 783).

Malposture: **Benediction Hand** (Preacher's Hand). The ring and little fingers are flexed while the other digits move normally and may be extended to produce the posture (Fig. 9-2G). This occurs in ulnar nerve palsy and syringomyelia.

Malposture: ***Wristdrop.*** When the pronated hand is held horizontally without support from beneath, it may drop from the wrist from weakness of the extensors (Fig. 9-2H). The common causes are radial nerve palsy, poliomyelitis, or poisoning from lead, arsenic, or alcohol.

Malposture: ***Athetoid Hand.*** A grotesque pattern is seen in athetosis in which involuntary muscle spasms produce simulta-

---

hand in making a pelvic examination. The thumb is flexed on the palm, the wrist and proximal digital joints are flexed, while the middle and distal joints are extended, with fingers adducted. All the musculature is rigid. This posture occurs in tetany; when present, it is involuntary and cannot be altered by the patient. **G.** Benediction hand. *This posture results from the inability to extend the ring finger and the little finger because of ulnar palsy or syringomyelia. It is named from the ecclesiastical gesture of pronouncing benediction.* **H.** Wristdrop. *This results from weakness of the extensors of the wrist; it is best shown by supporting the wrist and demonstrating the inability to extend the hand against the pull of gravity. It occurs in radial nerve palsy; in poisoning from lead, arsenic, or alcohol, and in poliomyelitis.* **I.** Dupuytren's contracture. *Named after a surgeon, whose name is always pronounced in the French manner, this is a chronic fibrotic process of the palmar fascia in one or both hands, with resulting contracture involving the ring finger and sometimes the little finger. The process is seen and felt as a tough ridge in the palm. It is often hereditary. It may be associated with a similar process in the soles and a fibrotic process in the corpora cavernosa of the penis, which has the separate name of Peyronie's disease.* **J.** Athetoid hand. *The hand involuntarily assumes postures with some fingers flexed and some extended; these change rapidly; the figure shows only one.* **K.** Heberden's nodes. *There are irregular bony enlargements of the distal interphalangeal joints of the index, long, and ring fingers; they are larger in the dominant hand. They are inherited, especially in women, but they can occur in single joints from repeated trauma, as in baseball finger. They are regarded as a form of osteoarthritis.* **L.** Haygarth's nodes. *The spindle-shaped enlargements of the middle interphalangeal joints occur in rheumatoid arthritis.*

neous flexion of some digits and hyperextension of others (Fig. 9-2J).

Malposture: ***Dupuytren's Contracture*** (Palmar Fibrosis). This disorder usually begins after the age of 40 years as a small *painless nodule* that can be palpated in the palmar aponeurosis near the base of the digit. The nodule remains inconspicuous to the patient until it extends to form a *plaque* or *band* adhering to the palmar fascia and producing *retraction* and *dimpling* of the palmar skin. One or both hands may be involved. The ring finger is most often affected, but others may be included in order of diminishing frequency: the little, the long, the index, and the thumb. Retraction of the fascia forces the affected finger into *partial flexion* (Fig. 9-2I). Palpation of the palm reveals a *hard cord* over the tendon. Passive extension of the finger raises the cord taut where it can be readily seen. If this thickening and hyalinization of collagen fibers in the aponeurosis progress, a *painless contracture* of the digit results that may require surgical correction. The contracture, named after the French surgeon Baron Guillaume Dupuytren, is considered by some writers as the prototypical manifestation of *Dupuytren's disease.* Less common manifestations, occurring singly or in combination, are *plantar fibrosis* (Ledderhose's syndrome), *knuckle pads, plastic induration of the penis* (Peyronie's disease, strabismus penis), *fibrosis of the male breast* (fibrosis mammae virilis). About 40% of the patients have affected kin; only white persons are susceptible. Men are twice as often affected as women. The manifestations are particularly common in persons with alcoholic cirrhosis of the liver, epilepsy, or diabetes mellitus; the cause for these associations is unknown [for more details *see* J. Pojer, M. Radivojevic, and T. F. Williams: Dupuytren's Disease, *Arch. Intern. Med.,* **129:**561–66, 1972] [Editorial: The Puzzle of Dupuytren's Contracture, *Lancet,* **2:**170–71, 1972].

Malposture: **Volkmann's Ischemic Contracture (Late Stage).** The *fingers are held in flexion* by shortening of the fibrotic bellies of the digital flexors in the forearm. Since the flexor tendons are free to move in their sheaths, *slight extension* of the fingers is permitted with passive motion of the fingertips when the wrist is held in flexion. This distinguishes it from Dupuytren's contracture and adhesions of flexor tendons to their sheaths; both prevent any extension. In Volkmann's contracture, the fibrosis of muscle is the end result of ischemic necrosis from occlusion of the arteries by (1) a tight cast near the elbow, (2) a tight bandage or tourniquet on the upper arm, (3) arterial injury from a supracondylar fracture of the humerus, (4) arterial embolism, or (5) intense arterial spasm from injections into its lumen. ***Ischemic Stage:*** Early recognition at this stage may prevent damage leading to contracture. The onset of ischemia is indicated by the *five p's:* pain, puffiness, pallor, pulselessness, and paralysis. Passive extension of the fingers produces *pain in the forearm.* The fingers may be *cyanotic;* they are often *edematous.* The radial pulse is usually *impalpable.* The skin over the hands is *cool.*

Dorsum of the Hand

Interosseus Muscle Atrophy. Atrophy of the interossei is indicated by sunken soft tissues between the extensor tendons on the dorsum (Fig. 9-3A). This can be seen and palpated.

Painless Swelling of the Dorsum. The most common cause of edema of the dorsum of the hand is an infection in the *palmar* fascia; since the tissues are looser on the back of the hand, the lymph accumulates there from the dense palm. *Unilateral edema* may also occur from occlusion of the venous or lymphatic drainage of the upper arm. *Bilateral edema* can occur from congestive cardiac failure or obstruction of the superior vena cava.

Painful Dorsal Swelling: ***Dorsal Abscess.*** There are edema, localized tenderness, induration, sometimes redness on the dorsum. Fluctuation may not be present.

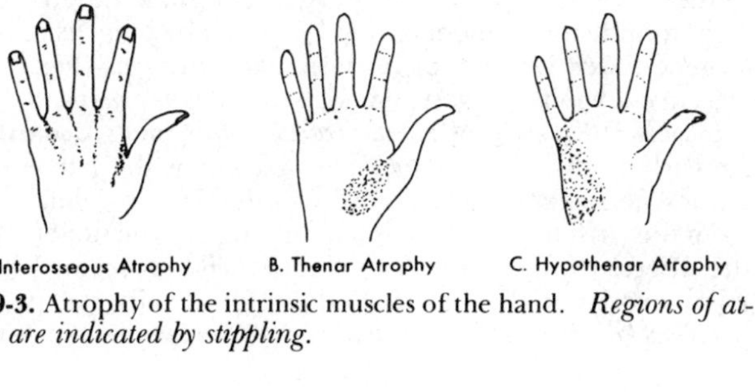

A. Interosseous Atrophy B. Thenar Atrophy C. Hypothenar Atrophy

Fig. 9-3. Atrophy of the intrinsic muscles of the hand. *Regions of atrophy are indicated by stippling.*

The Palm

Yellow Palms: **Carotenoderma.** This is the yellow color imparted to the skin by carotene. The pigment is concentrated in the stratum corneum that is thickest in the *palms* and *soles.* The pigment is excreted in the sebum; since the sebaceous glands are thickest on the *forehead* and *nasolabial folds,* these areas are often stained by excessive pigment secretion. The yellow color is distinguished from bile pigments in the tissues that are distributed *uniformly,* including coloration of the sclerae and thin skin. Excessive carotene excretion occurs in normal persons from chronic ingestion of large quantities of carrots, squash, oranges, peaches, apricots, and leafy vegetables. Since carotene is converted to vitamin A in the liver with the assistance of thyroid hormone, carotenoderma occurs in hepatic disease and myxedema.

Granular Palms: **Hyperkeratoses.** Palpation of the palms with the fingertips calls attention to rough granular excrescenses in the horny layer. Perhaps the most common cause of hyperkeratosis in the palms is *chronic arsenic poisoning.* Shaking hands with a patient may provide the first clue that arsenic is present. A rare cause is an autosomal dominant disease, *hyperkeratosis (tylosis) palmaris et plantaris.*

Thenar Atrophy. The bulk of the thenar eminence is formed by the bellies of Opponens pollicis, Abductor pollicis brevis, and Flexor pollicis brevis. Diminution in size of the eminence may accompany general atrophy of all intrinsic hand muscles (Fig. 9-3B). Localized atrophy suggests a lesion of the *median nerve.*

Hypothenar Atrophy. The hypothenar eminence is formed by the bellies of Palmaris brevis, Abductor digiti quinti, Flexor digiti quinti, and Opponens digiti quinti. The bulge is reduced in generalized atrophy of intrinsic hand muscles (Fig. 9-3C). Selective atrophy suggests damage to the *ulnar nerve.*

Localized Thickening of Palmar Fascia: **Dupuytren's Contracture.** An early finding, *antedating the contracture,* is the palpation of a thick nontender nodular cord or ridge in the palmar fascia from the wrist toward the base of the ring or little finger. When the affected fingers are extended, a *dimple* is formed in the palm overlying the flexor tendon (for details see p. 676).

Painful Palmar Swelling: **Infection of the Web Space.** Early there are fever and malaise. Diffuse *pain* is felt in the hand, with *dorsal edema.* When localization has occurred, the two involved *fingers are separated* by swelling at their bases. The skin over the web, both back and front, is *reddened.* Maximal *tenderness* is located on the palmar surface near the base of the involved finger (Fig. 9-4A).

Painful Palmar Swelling: ***Infection of the Thenar Space.*** The affected *thenar eminence is swollen* when compared to its mate. The distal phalanx of the thumb may be flexed, but extension is *not resisted,* in contradistinction to the finding in tenosynovitis of the Flexor pollicis longus.

Painful Palmar Swelling: ***Deep Abscess of the Palm.*** In addition to severe *dorsal edema,* the *concavity of the palm is obliterated,* or even elevated; the raised area is *tender.*

Painful Palmar Swelling: ***Abscess of the Ulnar Bursa.*** There are *dorsal edema* and *fullness on the ulnar side of the palm* (Fig. 9-4A). The point of maximum *tenderness* is halfway between the lunate and the fifth metacarpophalangeal joint.

Painful Palmar Swelling: ***Abscess of the Radial Bursa.*** The *distal thenar phalanx is rigidly flexed.* There are *tenderness* and *swelling* over the sheath of the Flexor pollicis longus (Fig. 9-4A).

Painful Palmar and Digital Swelling: ***Acute Suppurative Tenosynovitis.*** *Throbbing pain* may begin in a finger and progress toward the palm. *Dorsal edema* appears. The entire finger *swells.* The

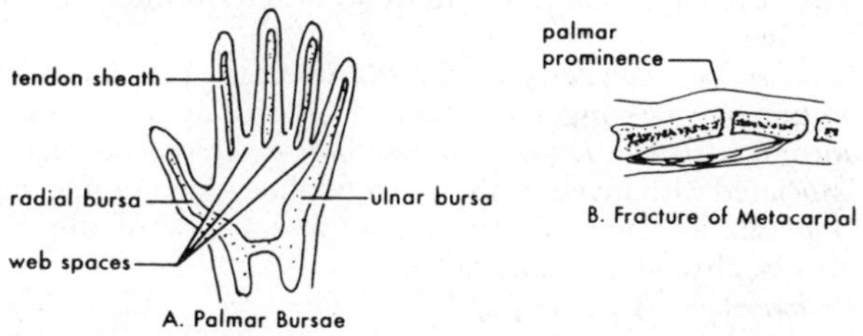

Fig. 9-4. Swellings of the hand. **A.** Palmar bursae. *The locations of the bursae are indicated by stippling. Note the tendon sheaths ending proximately near the palmar crease; there is a connection between the radial and ulnar bursa. The radial bursa is continuous from the thumb to the region of the thenar eminence. The web spaces are indicated as sites of abscesses.* **B.** Fracture of a metacarpal bone. *Diagram shows displacement of the fragments into the palm where an abnormal prominence may be noted.*

affected finger is held in the posture of rest, *slightly flexed;* the patient *cannot move the finger.* Even gentle passive extension of *adjacent* fingers is *painful,* so the examiner should not attempt to test the affected finger. To find the point of maximum tenderness, have the patient rest the supinated hand on a table. Test for tenderness by gently palpating with the blunt end of an applicator or tongue depressor. If the point is located at the proximal end of the tendon sheath of the index, middle, or ring finger, *involvement of the sheath* is certain. If there is no localization, the sheath may have ruptured.

Painful Palmar Swelling: ***Fracture of a Metacarpal Bone.*** In a complete fracture, the fragments of the metacarpal bone are bowed into the palm to produce a *painful prominence* (Fig. 9-4B). The prominence may be obscured by soft-tissue swelling, but dorsal palpation will yield localized tenderness at the end of the fragment. In *spiral fracture of a metacarpal,* clenching the fist shows loss of prominence in the corresponding knuckle. *Bennett's fracture* is an oblique break through the base of the first metacarpal with frequent subluxation of the joint. The thumb is *semiflexed,* and it *cannot be opposed* to the ring or little finger. The fist cannot be clenched.

The Fingers

Some affections of the fingers have been included in consideration of the entire hand; the more localized disorders are discussed here.

Malformation: ***Polydactyly*** (Supernumerary Fingers). The condition may be congenital, familial, or associated with certain syndromes. In the *Laurence-Moon-Biedl syndrome,* polydactyly is associated with juvenile obesity, retinal degeneration, genital hypoplasia, and mental retardation; about 80% of the cases of this syndrome are familial.

Malformation: ***Syndactyly*** (Webbed Fingers). This is a congenital or hereditary deformity. The web may be formed only of soft tissue between the fingers, or the web may cover fused bones. Scar tissue from burns may form an acquired web.

FUNCTIONAL TESTS OF FINGERS. **The fingers are named *thumb, index, long, ring,* and *little.* The phalangeal joints are termed *distal, middle,* and *proximal;* the first two are interphalangeal, the third is**

metacarpophalangeal. The aspects of the fingers are *dorsal* and *volar*, the latter is on the same face as the palm. The functional assessment of the joints is illustrated in Fig. 9-5. The normal limits of motion are indicated by zones with indefinite borders to emphasize individual variation and changes from aging. The testing of muscles is described on p. 789.

Painless Nodules on Distal Finger Joints: ***Heberden's Nodes.*** On one or more fingers, except the thumb, the *distal joints* are enlarged by *hard nodules,* 2 to 3 mm in diameter, one on either side of the dorsal midline (Fig. 9-2K). The nodules are *painless;* motion is *unlimited.* They are more pronounced on the dominant hand. Involvement of several joints is more common in women in whom they appear at the menopausal age. The condition in women is usually hereditary. The process is a localized osteoarthritis; its appearance does not presage the development of a generalized distribution. A single joint is more commonly involved in men, this the result of trauma. A good example of traumatic involvement is the *baseball finger* when the joint has been injured by blows on the fingertip.

Fusiform Polyarticular Swellings: ***Rheumatoid Arthritis*** (Haygarth's Nodes). The *middle* and *proximal* finger joints are usually affected (Fig. 9-2L). The joint profile is *fusiform,* in contrast to the nodularity of Heberden's nodes. This is the classic lesion of rheumatoid arthritis in which the primary inflammatory process involves the periarticular tissue. *Pain* and *tenderness* vary greatly, depending upon the activity of the inflammation. The joint capsule is *thickened; fluid* in the joint cavity often contributes to the increased girth. During an acute episode, the overlying skin may be *warm* and *flushed.* In a more chronic state, the skin is *thinned* and *shiny,* with absence of the normal linear epidermal furrows. In the joints *limitation of motion* is common, varying from slight to *ankylosis.*

Fusiform Monarticular Swelling: ***Tuberculous Dactylitis.*** Usually a single interphalangeal joint is involved, although polyarticular disease is not uncommon. A *fusiform swelling* envelops the joint, causing gradually increasing *pain, tenderness,* and *skin flushing.* The condition may progress to form an abscess. Chronic progression of unremitting inflammation in a single joint suggests tuberculous infection rather than rheumatoid arthritis.

Fusiform Monarticular Swelling: ***Syphilitic Dactylitis.*** The appear-

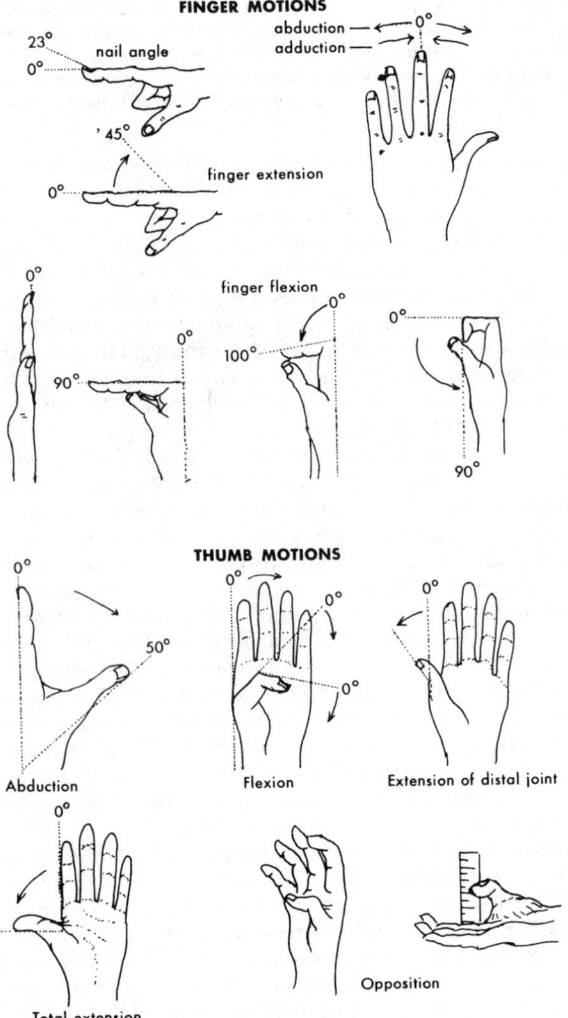

Fig. 9-5. Motions of fingers and thumb.

ance of the joint resembles tuberculous infection; but frequently it is distinguished by being *completely painless.* Ultimately *sinuses* may form in the inflamed site.

Fusiform Monarticular Swelling: **Sprain of an Interphalangeal Joint.** A painful fusiform joint swelling may persist for several months. In most cases there is a history of trauma.

Localized Swelling over a Joint: **Ganglion of a Digit.** A ganglion is a cyst resulting from myxomatous degeneration of a joint capsule. In the finger it usually occurs on the *volar aspect,* rarely on the dorsum. A *small tense nodule* appears over an interphalangeal joint; frequently it is mistaken for a sesamoid bone. It may be so tense that it feels *bony hard;* usually it is not fluctuant. Pressure may elicit *slight tenderness.* Often there is slight *transverse mobility.* Large ganglia are *translucent.* X-ray films exclude sesamoid bone by the absence of calcification.

Flexion Deformity of Distal Finger Joint: **Mallet Finger.** The terminal phalanx of the finger is permanently flexed at the distal joint; it cannot be voluntarily extended (Fig. 9-6A). This is caused by rupture of the extensor tendon that inserts on the terminal phalanx or fracture of the distal phalanx.

Flexion Deformity of the Middle Finger Joint: **Typewriter Finger** (Buttonhole Rupture). The finger is permanently flexed at its *middle joint* and lacks voluntary extension (Fig. 9-6B). It results from rupture of the extensor tendon inserting on the middle phalanx. Further flexion of the middle joint may produce a palpable or audible diagnostic *click,* as the lateral slips of the distal extensor tendons diverge and slip laterally over the head of the proximal digit, hence, *buttonhole rupture.*

Flexion Deformity of the Thumb: **Saluting Hand.** This is approximately the position of the hand in an American military salute (Fig. 9-6C). The thumb is limply flexed in the palm and cannot be voluntarily extended because of rupture of the tendon of the Extensor pollicis longus. The tendon is often worn through by moving over the fragments of a Colles' fracture; rupture may occur from three weeks to four months after the fracture has been set.

Painful Extension Snap of Finger: **Trigger Finger.** Either the middle or ring finger is usually involved (Fig. 9-6D). Flexion of the finger feels normal; but reextension is accompanied by a

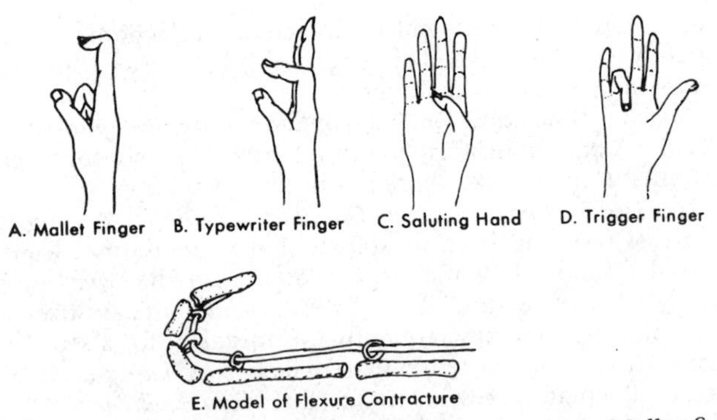

Fig. 9-6. Acquired flexion deformities of the fingers. **A.** Mallet finger. *Rupture of the extensor tendon at its insertion on the terminal phalanx causes a permanent flexion deformity at the distal interphalangeal point.* **B.** Typewriter finger. *There is permanent flexion of the proximal interphalangeal joint from rupture of the extensor tendon inserting on the middle phalanx, giving a position similar to that employed when using a typewriter.* **C.** Saluting hand. *This posture results from rupture of the extensor pollicis longus, so the thumb is held in permanent flexion in the palm.* **D.** Trigger finger. *The long or ring finger moves into flexion painlessly, but attempted extension is temporarily impeded; finally, extension is accomplished with a painful snap.* **E.** Diagnosis of flexure contractures of the hand. *Apparent contractures can occur from muscle atrophy or adhesions in the tendon sheath. With sheath adhesions, passive motion of the tendon is nil. If the condition is caused by muscle shortening, there is always enough play so slight motion of the tendon through its sheath can be demonstrated.*

painful snap that the patient sometimes refers to the dorsum of the hand. For an unknown cause, a nodular thickening forms in the long flexor tendon opposite the metacarpal head. In the position of extension, the nodule lies within the tendon sheath; during flexion it is pulled out of the proximal end of the sheath by the powerful flexor muscles, without pain or snap. But during reextension, the constricted mouth of the sheath momentarily resists the pull of the weaker extensor muscles for reentry of the nodule. Entry is suddenly achieved with a painful jerk.

Contracture of a Flexor Tendon: ***Tendon Adhesions or Tendon Shortening.*** Adhesions between a tendon and its sheath are caused by suppurative tenosynovitis or Dupuytren's contracture. Fibrotic shortening of the tendon without synovial adhesions occur in Volkmann's ischemic contracture. Distinction between the two mechanisms can be made with the wrist *flexed.* Grasp the tip of the flexed finger and pull it in the direction of extension. With the slack provided by wrist flexion, the shortened tendon permits *partial extension;* adhesions to the sheath or palmar fascia entirely *prevent extension* (Fig. 9-6E).

Flexion Deformity from Tight Skin: ***Sclerodactyly.*** In the acrosclerotic type of scleroderma, the skin and underlying tissues may become contracted and fibrosed to a degree in which the condition must be distinguished from muscle contracture or rheumatoid arthritis. Movements of the digits are inhibited by the tight envelope, but there is *no ankylosis* or *swelling of joints.* All digits are usually involved. Raynaud's phenomenon may be associated; calcinosis of the skin is often present. Areas in other parts are usually involved in the sclerodermatous process with thickening, stiffening, hyperpigmentation, and limited motion. Opening the mouth and respiratory movements may be limited.

Digital Infection: ***Paronychia.*** The skin over the mantle of the nail and the lateral nail folds is *swollen, reddened, painful,* and *tender* (Fig. 9-7A). When pus is *over* the nail, light palpation over the inflamed area provokes *exquisite pain.* Pain from pressure *on the nail* indicates subungual abscess, between nail plate and periosteum.

Digital Infection: ***Abscess of the Apical Space.*** Usually after a puncture wound beneath the nail, the distal quarter of nail bed becomes *extremely painful* without much swelling (Fig. 9-7B). The nail bed shows *red* through the plate. Maximum *tenderness* is proximal to the free edge of the plate, in contradistinction to a felon that produces tenderness at the fingertip. The epitrochlear lymph node may become *swollen* and *tender.* When the abscess ruptures, drainage is at the free edge of the nail plate.

Digital Infection: ***Abscess of the Terminal Pulp Space*** (Felon). Inflammation of the terminal finger pad is confined by tough fascia attached to the periosteum (Fig. 9-7C). The onset is heralded by *swelling* of the fingertip and *dull pain.* The pain gradually heightens and becomes *throbbing. Tenderness* is intense. The presence of pus is indicated by *induration* of the

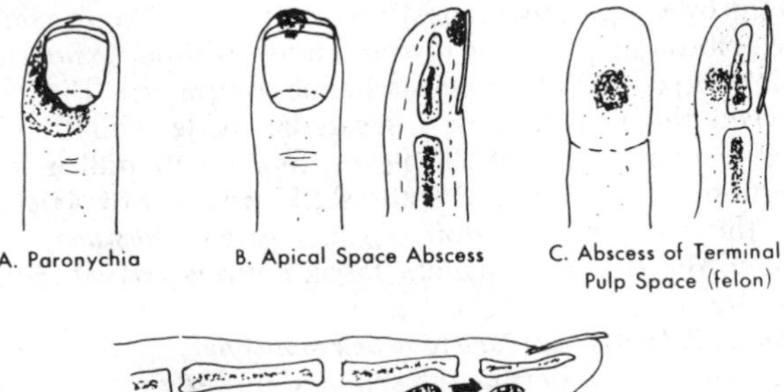

Fig. 9-7. Common locations for abscesses in the fingers. **A.** Paronychia. *An abscess often forms in a nail fold or mantle. The soft tissue is swollen, red, and very painful.* **B.** Abscess of the apical spaces. *The apical space is located in the nail bed near the free margin of the nail plate.* **C.** Abscess of the terminal pulp space (felon). *The pus accumulates in the dense compartmented fibrous tissue that is adherent to the periosteum. The stippled region on the volar surface represents the site of rupture through the skin.* **D.** Abscess of the volar spaces. *The stippled regions are the sites of abscesses; the arrows point the direction of burrowing to reach the flexor creases of the finger. The target spots for the arrows are the points at which the abscesses drain through the skin.*

pulp and *loss of resilience.* The great pressure in the confined space may cause the abscess to burst through the volar surface of the finger pad, or it may produce osteomyelitis.

Digital Infection: ***Abscess of the Middle Volar Pulp Space.*** The finger is held in *partial flexion* to reduce the pain. A *painful, tender swelling* occurs on the volar aspect of the finger between the distal and middle joints (Fig. 9-7D). The symptoms resemble those of the felon. Osteomyelitis may occur, or the abscess may burst after burrowing to the *distal* flexor crease.

Digital Infection: ***Abscess of the Proximal Volar Pulp Space.*** An abscess forms on the volar aspect between the middle and proximal joints (Fig. 9-7D). The symptoms and signs are similar to those in the middle space, except the infection burrows *proximally* to involve the web space.

Specific Digital Ulcer: **Chronic Paronychia.** Chronic ulceration of the nail mantle and lateral folds occurs in occupations requiring frequent immersion of the hands in water or contaminated oil. The ulcers are indolent; abscess formation is rare.

Specific Digital Ulcer: **Verruca Necrogenica** (Pathologist's Wart, Butcher's Wart). A *bluish red patch* appears on the skin; later it becomes papillomatous and *warty; pus* may exude from the tissues. The lesion results from inoculation with *Mycobacterium tuberculosis.* The pathologist is infected at the autopsy; butchers and packing-house workers handle infected meat. Usually, the lesions are indolent with no constitutional symptoms, but one packing-house worker had a necrotic ulcer on the finger, epitrochlear and axillary lymphadenopathy, pleural effusion, and high fever, from infection with a bovine strain of the tubercle bacillus.

Specific Digital Ulcer: **Tularemia** (Rabbit Fever). A common prelude is experienced by the hunter who skins a rabbit and punctures his finger with a bone fragment. A rather benign-looking ulcer appears in the wound, with surrounding erythema, but little pain. *Satellite buboes* develop and may suppurate. Often there are malaise and fever. The causative organism proves to be *Pasteurella tularensis,* which produces a fatal disease of rabbits and other game animals. Man may be infected by direct contact of the hands, as a hunter or butcher. The disease may also be transmitted by the bite of an infected wood tick, *Dermacentor andersoni.*

Specific Digital Ulcer: **Chancre.** This is an extragenital primary lesion of syphilis. A *painless elevated ulcer* appears on the finger. The underlying induration is peculiarly *discoid,* so it can be picked up like a small coin. Painless nonsuppurating swelling of a regional lymph node follows. The lesion may be encountered in physicians, dentists, and midwives, who contract it by examining patients.

Specific Digital Ulcer: **Erysipeloid.** A localized dermal infection of the fingers or hands, it produces an area of *swollen, slightly tender, violaceous* skin, defined by sharp borders, rarely extending above the wrist. The inflammation resolves in a few days, leaving pigmentation. The disease is probably caused by *Erysipelothrix rhusiopathiae,* acquired by handling infected mammals and fish.

Nodules in the Finger Web: **Barber's Pilonidal Sinus.** Short hair shafts may penetrate the skin of the finger webs and produce inflammation. One or more *nodules* may be felt in the soft skin; they are drained by sinuses, seen as *black dots* between the fingers.

Digital Fractures and Dislocations. Since the phalanges are subcutaneous, fractures and dislocations offer no particular difficulties in diagnosis. The physical signs of *tenderness* and *deformity* are sufficient to indicate the lesion to anyone with a knowledge of anatomy.

Circulatory Disorders in the Fingers. These are discussed under the examination of the cardiovascular system (see pp. 417–36).

The Fingernails

The astute diagnostician always examines the fingernails. With the exception of the eye, there is no region of comparable size in the body in which so many physical signs of generalized disease can be found. The nails continue to grow throughout life at a measurable rate, providing a horny record of brief or prolonged disturbances of nutrition. They also serve as windows through which to view capillary changes associated with constitutional disease.

The *nail plate* is a horny semitransparent rectangle, convex in both dimensions, with a smaller radius of curvature transversely than longitudinally (Fig. 9-8). The nail plate rests upon and adheres to the *nail bed,* a layer of modified skin on the dorsal aspect of the terminal phalanx. The bed is studded with small longitudinal ridges containing a rich capillary network, showing through the nail plate as a pink surface. Roughly the proximal third of the nail bed is composed of partially cornified cells containing granules of keratohyalin; this specialized layer is the *matrix,* where new nail is made and added to the nail plate, forcing it distally. The matrix is viewed through the nail plate as the white *lunula.* The proximal part of the nail plate, buried in a dermal pouch, is the *root;* the distal part not adherent to the bed is the *free edge;* the *body* is the intervening portion. The dermal lip of the pouch is called the *mantle;* it terminates in a sharp cornified rim, the *cuticle.* The sides of the nail plate are buried in *lateral nail folds* of skin and cuticle.

Throughout life the nail plate grows continuously by elonga-

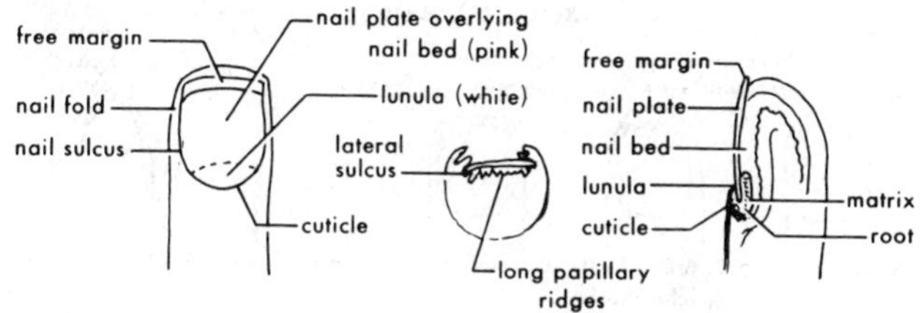

Fig. 9-8. Anatomy of the fingernail. *The nail plate is formed by the cells of the matrix and extruded distally to the free margin where the plate separates from the nail bed. The lunula marks the extent of the matrix under the nail plate.*

tion from the root. The average time for growing a new nail is about 6 months; it grows faster in youth than in old age. Most changes in the fingernails have accompanying counterparts in the toenails, but signs in the latter are not so evident.

Absence of Nails. As a congenital anomaly, the nails may fail to develop; sometimes this defect is associated with ichthyosis. A traumatized nail may be shed; damage to the matrix prevents regrowth.

Irregular Short Nails: **Bitten Nails.** The free edge of the nail plate may be absent from the nervous habit of biting the nails (Fig. 9-9A). This is a revealing clue to the person's affect.

Square Round Nail Plates: **Acromegaly and Cretinism.** Disproportionate growth may produce nail plates more wide than long.

Long Narrow Nail Plates: **Eunuchoidism and Hypopituitarism.** The nails are longer and narrower than usual; they may simulate those in Marfan's syndrome.

Brittle Nail Plates: **Onychorrhexis.** The cut edges of the various keratin layers may be laminated and present a steplike appearance. Borders may be frayed and torn (Fig. 9-9B). Many times the cause is not evident; the condition may be associated with malnutrition, iron deficiency, thyrotoxicosis, or calcium deficit.

Friable Nail Plates: **X-ray Irradiation.** The edges may be frayed, the growth stunted. They are often softened (Fig. 9-9D).

▼ *Key Sign:* **Clubbing of the Fingers.** This condition has intrigued physicians since the time of Hippocrates because of its unknown mechanism and its association with many serious constitutional disorders. Efforts to discover the mechanism

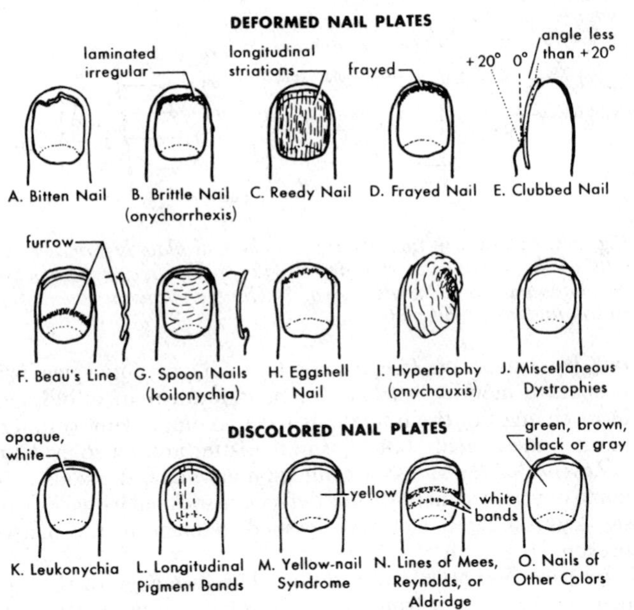

Fig. 9-9. Diagnosis of fingernail lesions I. *Many, but not all, nail lesions have been assembled here to simplify the diagnosis. More lesions are being described from time to time. In many cases, before the chart can be used, it is necessary to know whether the lesion is in the nail plate or in the nail bed. The distinction can usually be made by noting whether the abnormal color is changed by pressure on the nail plate.*

have so far failed; a popular hypothesis ascribes it to hypoxia, but this does not explain its presence in many entities.

— *Convex Nail Plates:* ***Clubbing of the Nails, Without Periostosis*** (Watch-Crystal Nails, Hippocratic Nails, Parrot-Beak Nails, Serpent-Head Nails, Drumstick Fingers). The affection is usually *painless* and *bilateral,* although rarely it has occurred on one hand secondary to aortic aneurysm or arteriovenous fistula of the subclavian artery. The thumbs and index fingers are usually first involved, later the other fingers and toes. Clubbing is reversible when the cause is removed.

There are only *two diagnostic signs,* floating nails and alterations in the unguophalangeal angle; these persist through all stages of the disorder. Both signs result from proliferation of the tissue between the nail plate and the bone.

Floating nail can be demonstrated by pressing the mantle with the tip of your finger and finding the plate root to be *resilient* and *springy* (Fig. 9-9E). With pressure the plate sinks toward the bone; with release of pressure, the plate springs away from the bone. The sensation may be accurately simulated with your own nail. With your right index finger, press the mantle of the nail on your left middle finger; you will find the plate rests snugly against the bone; there is no movement. Now oppose your left thumb to the free edge of the nail just tested and press the edge hard in such direction as to accentuate the slight natural convexity of the plate. While the nail is thus under tension, test its mantle again with your right index finger; you will find the plate root to be separated from the bone by tension so it sinks with pressure and springs back when released.

Obliteration of the unguophalangeal angle is noted by inspection of the profile of the terminal digit. Normally (Fig. 9-10), the angle between the nail plate and the proximal part of the digit is 160° *or less:* a restatement of this dimension that is easier to estimate is, the nail makes an angle of 20° *or more* with the *projected line* of the digit. When clubbing occurs, subungual proliferation causes *diminution* in this 20° angle (or with the other method of measurement, an *increase* in the 160° angle) (Fig. 9-11); the angle may be entirely obliterated so the digit and plate lie in a straight line (an angle of 0° or 180°). Further progress may form an angle exceeding 180° (Fig. 9-11). Before the lesion has advanced very far, the profile shows the *outline of the plate root* in the mantle. Many physicians do not realize the promptness with which this proliferative reaction occurs. We have noted the floating nail and the change from the normal angle 10 days after a tonsillectomy that induced a lung abscess.

Convexity of the nail appears later than the two chief signs; it is not necessarily distinctive of clubbing because it occurs in other conditions; clubbing may occur without curving of the nail. Usually in clubbing, a month or so after the occurrence of the floating nail and the alteration of the nail angle, a *transverse ridge* in the plate comes to view from beneath the mantle. The ridge marks the change from the distal normal curve to

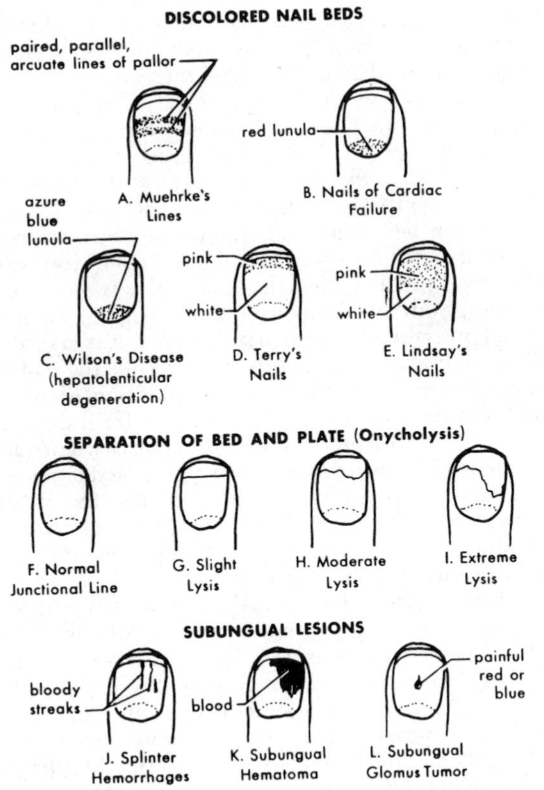

Fig. 9-10. Diagnosis of fingernail lesions II.

the proximal nail with a new curve of smaller radius. An opportunity to follow the progress is occasionally afforded by a patient with subacute bacterial endocarditis. When first seen after a duration of 3 months, a transition ridge is already visible (Fig. 9-11). After successful treatment of the infection, a second ridge appears, this one marking the transition between distal abnormal curvature and proximal normal profile. In a case with the process over 6 months old, an entire nail with an abnormally convex profile is formed; this condition is best

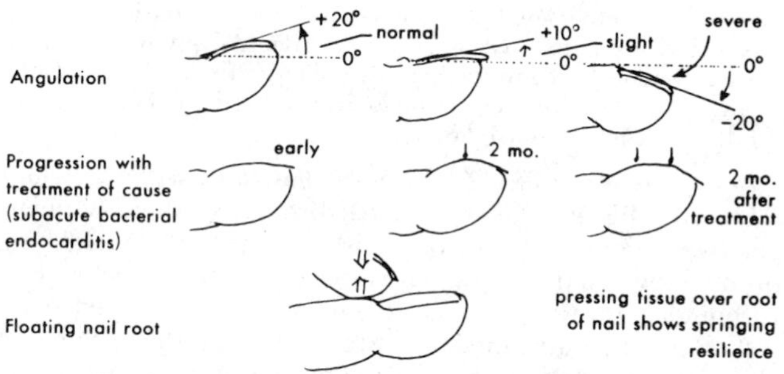

Fig. 9-11. Characteristics of clubbed nails. *There are three principal signs of clubbing of the fingers:* (**1**) *angulation: the normal nail plate makes an angle of 20° or more dorsalward with the axis of the finger; diminution in the angle is evidence of beginning clubbing;* (**2**) *curvature of the nail: the normal curve is on a very long radius; the clubbed fingers describe a curve with a much shorter radius;* (**3**) *floating nail root: pressing the portion of the nail plate covered with skin reveals a springiness that is abnomal.*

described as the *watch-crystal nail.* In a still older process, when the soft tissue and terminal phalanx have become thickened and the convexity of the nail plate is extreme with bulbous fingers, the more appropriate terms are *drumstick fingers, parrot's beak,* or *serpent's head.* In the literal sense, the term *clubbing of the fingers* should be reserved for a late stage; unfortunately usage applies it to the general process in all stages from the first sign of floating nail. *Distinction:* The floating nails and alteration of the unguophalangeal angle distinguish clubbing from all other conditions, such as convexity of the nails in certain occupations, inherited forms, Heberden's nodes, the acromegalic hand, chronic paronychia, rheumatoid arthritis. X-ray films do not assist, except in the late stage when fraying of the phalangeal tufts occurs.

Clinical Occurrence. PULMONARY DISEASE is the most common cause, such as bronchiectasis, lung abscess, pulmonary tuberculosis with cavitation, pulmonary emphysema, lung neoplasm including carcinoma and lymphoma. *Cardiovascular disease* ranks second, such as cyanotic congenital heart disease, subacute bacterial endocarditis, secondary polycythemia. A *miscellaneous group* includes hepatic cirrhosis, chronic obstructive jaundice, thyrotoxicosis, and a familial type. Rarely other conditions seem to have induced the lesion. Clubbing has been reported as occurring after the production of an arteriovenous fistula for dialysis [D. E. Leb and J. K. Sharma: Clubbing Secondary to Arteriovenous Fistula Used for Hemodialysis, *J.A.M.A.*, **240:**142–43, 1978].

— *Convex Nail Plates:* ***Clubbing of the Nails with Periostosis*** (Hypertrophic Pulmonary Osteoarthropathy, Marie-Bamberger Syndrome). This disorder is characterized by clubbing of the fingers and periosteal new-bone formation (see p. 689). Although many writers conceive it as merely an enhanced manifestation of the same unknown process that produces clubbing alone, others prefer to restrict the term *hypertrophic pulmonary osteoarthropathy* to cases with periosteal proliferation. An inherited disorder, *pachydermoperiostosis,* is characterized by clubbing of the fingers, periostosis, thickening and oiliness of the skin, and hyperhidrosis of the hands and feet. It is transmitted as an autosomal dominant [D. L. Rimoin: Pachydermoperiostosis (Idiopathic Clubbing and Periostosis), *N. Engl. J. Med.*, **272:**923, 1965].

Longitudinal Ridging in Nail Plate: ***Reedy Nail.*** An exaggeration of the normal, the cause is unknown; it has been attributed to many conditions, but the diagnostic significance is meager (Fig. 9-9C).

Transverse Furrow in Nail Plate: ***Beau's Line.*** The matrix may form a transverse indentation in the nail plate during a severe illness. As the nail elongates, the furrow moves into view from beneath the mantle, progresses distally, and is finally pared off (Fig. 9-9F).

Concave Nail Plate: ***Spoon Nails*** (Koilonychia). The natural convexity is replaced by concave nails in saucer form (Fig. 9-9G). Often the nail plate is thinned. The condition is most often encountered in hypochromic anemias and iron deficiency. Rarely, it occurs in rheumatic fever, lichen planus, and syphilis.

Concave Nail Plate: ***Eggshell Nails.*** The nail plate is thinned and its free edge is curved sharply outward from the digit (Fig. 9-9H). The cause is obscure; it has sometimes been ascribed to vitamin A deficit.

Hypertrophy of the Nail Plates: ***Onychauxis.*** The nail plate becomes greatly thickened by piling up of irregular keratin layers

(Fig. 9-9I). The cause is unknown; it may be familial or the result of chronic fungal infections.

Dystrophy of the Nail Plates: Under this head are grouped many ill-defined changes with opacities, furrowing, ridging, pitting, splitting, fraying, all testaments to poor nutrition of the nails (Fig. 9-9J). They are encountered in chronic infections of the nails, lesions of the nerves supplying the limb, vascular deficits of the extremity, the collagen diseases.

White Nail Plates: ***Partial Leukonychia.*** Irregular white areas in the nail plates are common and are not diagnostically significant.

White Nail Plates: ***Total Leukonychia.*** The nail plates are completely chalky white (Fig. 9-9K). The condition is inherited as a dominant character with varying penetrance. [See colored photographs, J. F. Harrington: *Arch. Intern. Med.,* **114:**301, 1964, or P. D. Samman: *The Nails in Disease,* 3rd ed. William Heinemann Medical Books, Ltd., London, 1978, p. 54.]

Transverse White Banded Nail Plates: ***Lines of Mees, Reynolds, or Aldrich.*** The nail plates contain transverse white bands that are laid down during a generalized illness or poisoning. The formation ceases with recovery, producing a white band that moves distally with growth of the nail plate (Fig. 9-9N). Some conditions in which the lines have been seen are poisoning with arsenic, thallium, fluoride; infectious fevers including malaria and pneumonia; other illnesses such as renal insufficiency, cardiac failure, myocardial infarction, Hodgkin's disease, sickle-cell anemia. The bands are probably evidence of a lesser degree of injury than Beau's lines.

Yellow Nail Plates: ***Yellow-Nail Syndrome.*** The nail plates become yellow or yellow-green; they thicken and grow more slowly (Fig. 9-9M). Excessive transverse curvature may occur associated with deficiency in cuticle and nailfold. Occasionally there are ridging and onycholysis. The disorder results from impeded lymphatic circulation; often it antedates lymphedema of the face and legs. [See colored photograph, P. D. Samman: *The Nails in Disease,* 3rd ed. William Heinemann Medical Books, Ltd., London, 1978, p. 54.]

Discolored Nail Plates: ***Miscellaneous Varieties.*** Various drugs, infections, and stains occasionally color the nail plates (Fig. 9-9O). *Blue-Green:* infection with *Pseudomonas. Brown-Yellow:*

ingestion of phenindione. *Brown or Black:* fungal infections, fluorosis, quinacrine. *Blue-Gray:* argyria.

Transverse Brown Nail Bands: ***Daunorubicin Therapy.*** Transverse bands of varying colors have been reported during chemotherapy. Usually a number of drugs are being given so it is difficult to ascribe the color to a single one [M. de Marini, A. Hendricks, and G. Stolzner: Nail Pigmentation with Daunorubicin, *Ann. Intern. Med.,* **89:**516–17, 1978] [D. W. Nixon: Alterations in Nail Pigment with Cancer Chemotherapy, *Arch. Intern. Med.,* **136:**1117–18, 1976].

White Proximal Nail Beds: ***Terry's Nails.*** The proximal 80% or more of the nail bed is *white* (Fig. 9-10D), leaving a distal band of normal pink [R. Terry: *Lancet,* **1:**757, 1954]. The mechanism is unknown. The nail findings are associated with hepatic cirrhosis.

White Proximal Nail Beds: ***Half-and-Half Nail*** (Lindsay's Nails). Somewhat similar in appearance to Terry's nails, the proximal 40–80% of the nail beds is *white,* but the distal portion is *red, pink,* or *brown* (Fig. 9-10E). The colored portion is sharply demarcated, usually by a curved line parallel to the free edge of the nail plates. Constriction of the venous return deepens the color of the distal portion, but only a slight pink is induced in the proximal bed. Of 25 patients with these nails, 21 had azotemia, 2 had minor degrees of renal disease, and 1 had no perceptible renal lesion [P. G. Lindsay: *Arch. Intern. Med.,* **119:**583, 1967].

White Banded Nail Beds: ***Muehrcke's Lines in Hypoalbuminemia.*** Paired narrow arcuate bands of pallor, parallel to the lunulae, appear in the nail beds (Fig. 9-10A). They occur during periods of hypoalbuminemia (less than 2.0 gm per 100 mL) and resolve when the deficit has been corrected. Since they are not in the nail plates, they do not move distally with nail growth [R. C. Muehrcke: *Br. Med. J.,* **1:**1327, 1956].

Red Half-Moons in Nail Beds: ***Nails of Cardiac Failure.*** The lunulae are *red* instead of the normal white (Fig. 9-10B). They are associated with cardiac failure [R. Terry: *Lancet,* **2:**842, 1954].

Azure Half-Moons in Nail Beds: ***Nails of Hepatolenticular Degeneration (Wilson's Disease).*** The lunulae are colored *light blue* (Fig. 9-10C). [See colored photograph, A. G. Bearn and V. A. McKusick: *J.A.M.A.,* **166:**904, 1958, and reprinted in

French's Index of Differential Diagnosis, 9th ed. The Williams & Wilkins Co., Baltimore, 1967, p. 288.]

Separation of the Nail: **Onycholysis.** The nail plate separates at its free edge from the nail bed. Normally the line of adhesion of plate to bed is a smooth curve (Fig. 9-10F). Separation often occurs in *thyrotoxicosis* where the earliest stage is conversion of the curved adhesion to a *straight line.* Later, this adhesion line dips proximally into the nail bed as a *jagged projection* that gathers dirt because it is inaccessible to cleaning. Frequently, this stage resembles the lesion from running a splinter under the nail; only the history can distinguish. Onycholysis may also occur in eczematoid dermatitis, psoriasis, and mycotic diseases of the nails.

Subungual Hemorrhages: **Splinter Hemorrhages.** *Linear red* hemorrhages occur in the nail bed, running from the free margin proximally for several millimeters (Fig. 9-10J). They are most common in subacute bacterial endocarditis and trichinosis. More recent observations have shown a high incidence in persons engaging in manual labor.

Subungual Hemorrhages: **Traumatic.** Trauma produces hemorrhages in the nail beds; the diagnosis is obvious.

Subungual Pigmentation: **Ungual Melanoma.** A rare location for malignant melanoma (2.5% of melanomas), but more common than glomus tumor, ungual melanoma is most frequently found under the nails of the thumb or great toe. Its characteristic sign is Hutchinson's melanotic whitlow with leaching of melanin from under the nail to its border and into the paronychial area.

Painful Red or Violet Subungual Spot: **Glomus Tumor.** Tumors arise from the glomus bodies throughout the tissues; they are especially common in the nail bed where they are *exquisitely painful;* they are not painful elsewhere. A glomus tumor is seen through the nail plate as a *round, red* or *violet spot.* The appearance resembles a hemangioma, but the latter is *not* tender or painful. Diagnosis is important because surgical excision is required for relief of pain.

Hemorrhages on Hands and Feet: **Janeway's Spots.** These are erythematous or hemorrhagic, macular or nodular lesions in the skin, only a few millimeters in diameter. They may occur in the palms, soles, or in the distal parts of the finger pads. Although painless and nontender, they may ulcerate. Crops appear for a few hours to several days. Most writers consider them as hallmarks of bacterial endocarditis or mycotic aneurysm. The causative organisms have been isolated from the lesions. [See colored photograph, D. F. Cross and J. B. Ellis: *Arch. Intern. Med.*, **118:**588, 1966.]

The Wrist

The region of the wrist includes the radiocarpal joint, the eight carpal bones in two parallel rows, and the overlying tendons. The *radiocarpal joint* is the articulation of a concave with a convex surface (Fig. 9-12). The proximal concave surface is formed by the distal end of the *radius* and the adjacent triangular *articular disk* that caps the distal end of the *ulna*. The distal convex surface consists of the curving sides of three carpal bones of the proximal row, from the radial to the ulnar side, the *navicular,* the *lunate,* and the *triangular*. The *pisiform* does not participate, since it lies on the volar aspect of the triquetrum. Of the carpal bones, the navicular is most commonly fractured, since the radius has wider contact with it than with the lunate, and the forces transmitted from the ulna to the triangular are cushioned by the articular disk. The *major synovial cavity* lies between the concave and convex surfaces; a *minor cavity* separates the distal end of the ulna and the articular disk, extending proximally between radius and ulna.

Knowledge of the topography is necessary to examination of the wrist (Fig. 9-13). *Volar Aspect of the Wrist.* The *Pisiform bone* can be palpated as a bony prominence on the ulnar side, just distal to the palmar crease and proximal to the base of the hypothenar eminence. The outlines of four tendons can

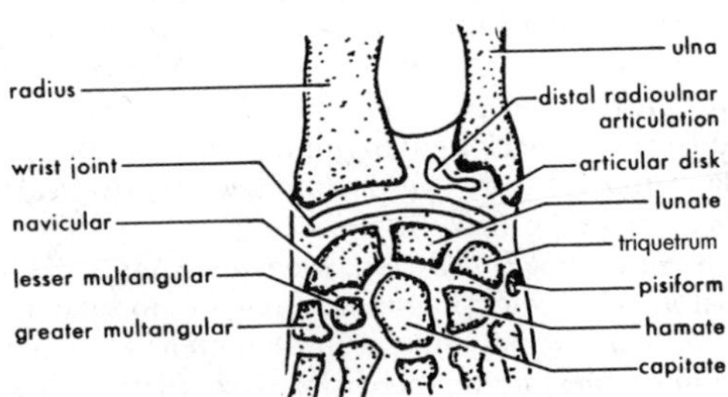

Fig. 9-12. Bones of the wrist.

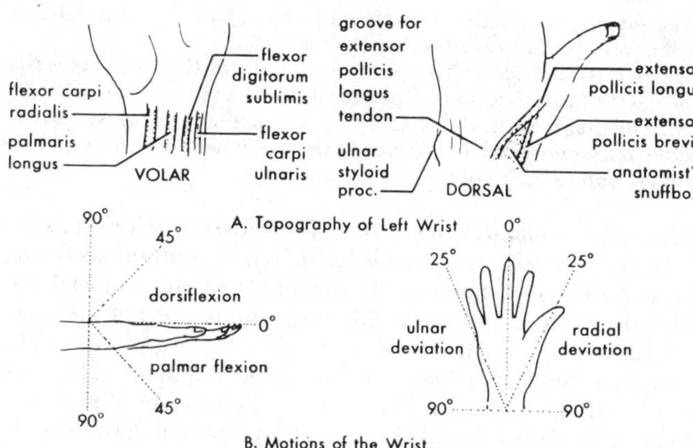

Fig. 9-13. The wrist. **A.** Topography of the wrist joint. **B.** Motions of the wrist joint.

usually be seen. With the digits slightly flexed and muscles tensed, three tendons are apparent in most persons; from ulnar to radial side, they are the *Flexor carpi ulnaris, Palmaris longus,* and *Flexor carpi radialis.* The Palmaris longus is absent in about 10% of persons. With the fist clenched hard, the tendon of the *Flexor digitorum sublimis* also appears between the Flexor carpi ulnaris and the Palmaris longus. *Dorsal Aspect of the Wrist.* The most conspicuous prominence is the *ulnar styloid process.* Extension of the thumb accentuates the borders of the *anatomist's snuffbox,* a recess formed by the more prominent *Extensor pollicis longus* and radially by the less pronounced *Extensor pollicis brevis.* In the intervening hollow can be felt the *radial artery* and the *radial styloid process.* On the ulnar side of the Extensor pollicis longus tendon is a prominence formed by the articular margin of the radius, called the *dorsal radial tubercle* (Lister's tubercle); this marks the ulnar lip of the tendon's groove.

Examination of the Wrist. **Inspect and palpate the wrist for *swelling, tenderness,* and *deformities*. Seek *weakness* and *atrophy* in the muscles of the forearm that supply the hand. If one wrist is involved, measure the *circumference* of each forearm at several corresponding levels from the ulnar styloid processes. Palpate the moving**

wrist for *crepitus;* with the stethoscope *auscultate* the volar surface of the joint for *fine crepitus* that cannot be felt.

Testing Wrist Motion: **The primary motions of the wrist are *extension-flexion* (dorsiflexion and palmar flexion) and *radial-ulnar deviation.* The diagrams in Fig. 9-13 depict the methods of measurement. When only one wrist is affected, compare it with the other, since average values vary with age.**

Fusiform Swelling of the Wrist. The causes are distinguished by physical signs. *periarticular Edema.* The subcutaneous tissues around the joint, but outside the limits of the synovial sac, pit with pressure. *Capsular Thickening.* The regions of the synovial sac and joint capsule feel doughy. *Fluid in the Joint.* The region of the synovial sac is bulging and fluctuant. The fluid may be effusion, pus, or blood, to be distinguished by aspiration. *Bony Enlargement.* The shape by palpation distinguishes between osteophytes at the joint margins, local neoplasm of bone, or generalized acromegalic hyperplasia.

DIAGNOSTIC ASPIRATION OF THE WRIST JOINT. ***Materials:*** **soap, water, alcohol, and skin antiseptic. Sterile equipment should consist of towels, rubber gloves, 1% procaine hydrochloride solution, two 24-gauge needles (1½ inches long) for procaine, two aspirating needles of 18 gauge (2 inches long) with short bevels, a 5-mL syringe for procaine, a 25- or 50-mL syringe for aspiration, gauze bandages, adhesive tape, specimen tubes, and measuring glass. *Technique:* Have the patient's forearm resting prone on a table so the hand hangs over the edge to flex the wrist. Cleanse the dorsal aspect of the wrist with soap and water, alcohol, and antiseptic solution; dry with sterile sponges. Drape the site of injection with sterile towels. Palpate the edge of the dorsal radial tubercle (Lister's) on the ulnar side of the Extensor pollicis longus tendon. Infiltrate the skin and subcutaneous tissue with procaine solution, using the small needle and small syringe. With the 18-gauge needle attached to the larger syringe, insert the needle perpendicular to the skin at a point just distal to the dorsal radial tubercle. If the needle goes easily to a depth of 1 to 2 cm, it is probably in the joint cavity. Aspirate the desired fluid, withdraw the needle and apply a sterile dressing. In most instances, gross inspection is sufficient to distinguish synovial fluid, pus, or blood. A cell count may be required on cloudy fluid; cultures may be made.**

Painful Swelling or Limited Motion of the Wrist: **Chronic Arthritis.** With active inflammation, there is *fusiform enlargement* of the wrist joint, accompanied by variable degrees of *pain* and *tenderness.* The overlying skin may be *warm* and *reddened.* In rheumatoid or gonococcal arthritis there is frequently *limited motion.* Normal mobility is usually observed with osteoarthritis, but *crepitus* is frequent in the joint. The joint is swollen *without increased heat* in tuberculous arthritis; early *sinus* formation occurs.

Painful Swelling in the Anatomist's Snuffbox: **Acute Nonsuppurative Tenosynovitis.** *Pain* is experienced in the region of the snuffbox; a *sausagelike swelling,* about $1\frac{1}{2}$ inches (4 cm) long (Fig. 9-14C), involves the tendon sheath of the Extensor pollicis brevis and Abductor pollicis longus, at the radial border of the hollow. When the tendons are moved, *crepitus* can be felt over the sheath. The cause is usually trauma, although inflammation can be produced by gout or gonococcal infection.

Chronic Pain in the Anatomist's Snuffbox: **Chronic Stenosing Tenosynovitis** (DeQuervain's Disease). The tendon sheath of the Extensor pollicis brevis is *painful.* In long-standing cases, one or two *swellings,* the size of orange seeds, are palpable in the snuffbox near the radial styloid process. *Crepitus* is absent. A

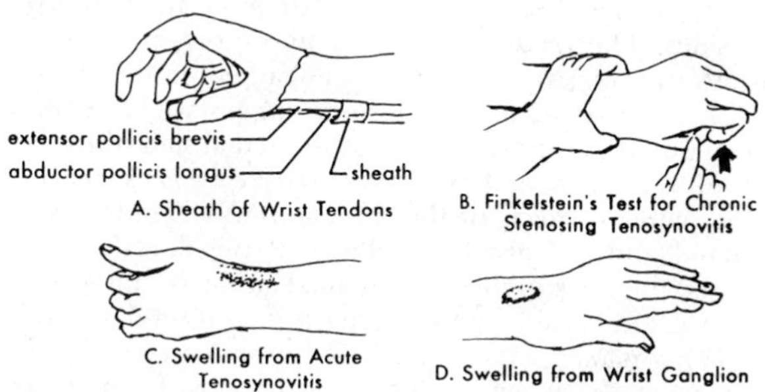

Fig. 9-14. Some disorders of the wrist. **A.** Sheaths of the wrist tendons. *This shows the sheath, which swells to obstruct the motion of the tendons of extensor pollicis brevis and abductor pollicis longus in chronic stenosing tenosynovitis.* **B.** Finkelstein's test for tenosynovitis. *The patient clenches his fist upon his thumb; the examiner pushes the base of the flexed thumb forcefully toward the ulna to elicit pain in the radial styloid process.* **C.** Swelling from acute nonsuppurative tenosynovitis. **D.** Frequent site of ganglion of the wrist. *The swelling is painless and sometimes translucent.*

chronic inflammation involves all layers of the tendon sheath. There are four signs: (1) When the fist is clenched over the flexed thumb, forceful ulnar deviation of the hand by the examiner elicits *pain* at the radial styloid process (*Finkelstein's test,* Fig. 9-14B). (2) The pain from the maneuver may be transmitted down the thumb or toward the elbow. (3) Passive extension of the thumb is painless. (4) *Tenderness* extends from the radial styloid process proximally for ½ inch (1.3 cm).

Localized Painless Swelling on the Dorsum: ***Ganglion.*** A cyst from myxomatous degeneration of the capsule of the joint most frequently occurs on the dorsum of the naviculolunate joint (Fig. 9-14D). The swelling is *round, sessile,* and *tense;* it is *translucent.* Flexion of the wrist brings it into prominence; extension obscures it.

Numbness, Tingling, and Pain in the Hand: ***Carpal Tunnel Syndrome*** (Compression Neuropathy of the Median Nerve in the Carpal Tunnel). The patient complains of attacks of *numbness* and *tingling* of the hand, particularly *at night.* There may be associated *pain,* limited to the hand or running up the forearm. Ultimately, there are progressive *weakness* and *awkwardness* in the finer movements of the fingers. The condition is most common in middle-aged women; it may be unilateral or on both sides. The median nerve is compressed in the channel beneath the volar transverse carpal ligament in the wrist (Fig. 9-15). *Distinction:* Once the history suggests it, the physical signs should be sought. *Atrophy* of the radial half of the *thenar eminence* occurs in half the cases. *Hyperesthesia* is distributed on the palmar aspects of the three and a half radial digits of the hand and the distal two thirds of the dorsal aspects of the same fingers supplied by the median nerve. Light percussion on the radial side of the Palmaris longus tendon produces a *tingling sensation* (Tinel's sign). The *appearance* or *exacerbation* of symptoms is caused by flexion of the wrist for 60 seconds; extension gives *relief.* Or, have the patient approximate the palmar surfaces of his hands so the wrists are forcefully dorsiflexed and the fingers extended. Measurement of nerve conduction will yield diagnosis when physical signs are negative.

Clinical Occurrence: Trauma from excessive flexion of the wrist. Impingement upon the carpal tunnel by arthritis, sarcoidosis, amyloid deposits, gouty tophi, acromegalic hyperplasia, or the soft-tissue

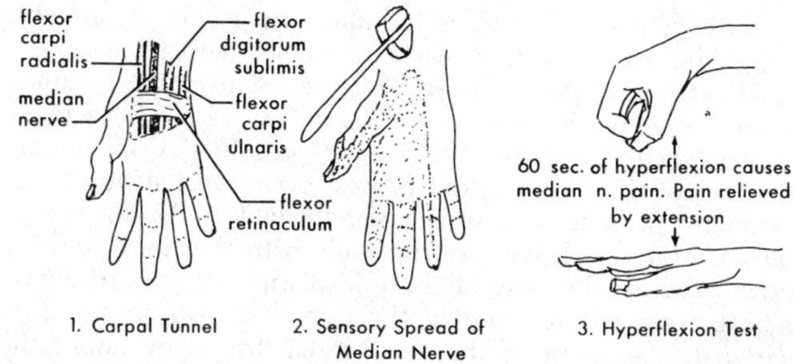

Fig. 9-15. Carpal tunnel syndrome. **1.** *The flexor retinaculum in the wrist compresses the median nerve to produce hyperesthesia in the radial 3½ digits.* **2.** *Percussion on the radial side of the palmaris longus tendon produces tingling in the 3½ digital region (Tinel's sign).* **3.** *Hyperflexion of the wrist for 60 seconds may produce pain in the median nerve distribution; this is relieved by extension of the wrist.*

swelling in pregnancy or myxedema. Inheritance has been reported in one family [R. G. Gray, M. J. Poppo, and N. L. Gottlieb: Primary Familial Bilateral Carpal Tunnel Syndrome, *Ann. Intern. Med.*, **91**:37–40, 1970].

The Forearm

The radius and ulna are practically subcutaneous so they can be palpated throughout their extent. The dorsal muscle mass is formed by the extensors of the hand, the volar mass by the flexors. Both the radial and ulnar arterial pulses are palpable above the wrist (see p. 421). The motions of the forearm are pronation and supination (Fig. 9-16).

Smooth Curvatures of Bones: ***Diseases of Osseous Growth.***

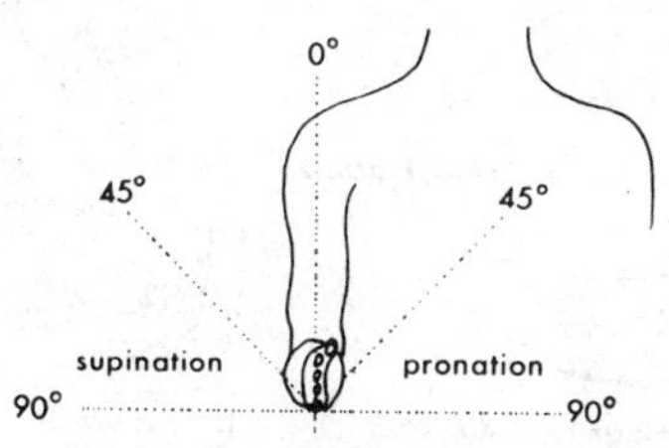

Fig. 9-16. Forearm motion.

Smooth curves of the radius and ulnar are usually attributable to syphilis, rickets, osteomalacia, or osteitis deformans.

Silver-Fork Deformity: ***Colles' Fracture.*** The most common cause is a fall on the outstretched hand. The radius is fractured within 1 inch (2.5 cm) of its distal end (Fig. 9-17A). Concomitant fracture of the ulnar styloid process occurs in half the cases. When the pronated arm is laid upon the table, its profile resembles a dinner fork lying horizontally with the tines pointing downward, so the base of the tines forms an upward curve. The corresponding *hump* in the fractured arm occurs from *dorsal* displacement of the distal radial fragment, above the wrist. To exclude a hump from soft-tissue swelling, palpate the volar aspect of the radius and compare it with its uninjured mate; the normal anterior convexity of the shaft is obliterated below the fracture.

Reversed Silver-Fork Deformity: ***Smith's Fracture*** (Reversed Colles' Fracture). Like Colles' fracture, this is a break of the distal end of the radius; but the distal fragment is displaced *volarward*, making a deformity somewhat resembling the horizontal silver fork with its tines pointing upward (Fig. 9-17B). The fracture usually results from a blow or fall on the hyperflexed hand.

Dorsal Angulation of the Wrist: ***Madelung's Deformity.*** The pronated hand presents a profile in which the wrist is deformed by a sharp protrusion upward (dorsally) of the lower ulna (Fig. 9-17C). This is caused by a dorsal subluxation of the distal end of the ulna, usually in an adolescent girl.

Pain and Tenderness in the Bony Shafts: ***Radial and Ulnar Fractures.*** In fractures of the *ulnar shaft*, the bone is well splinted by

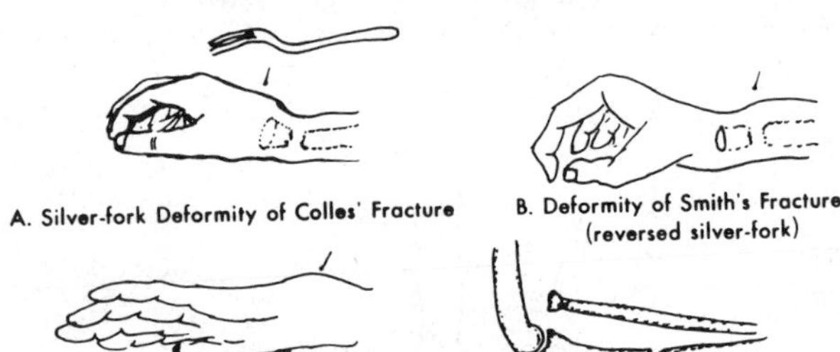

A. Silver-fork Deformity of Colles' Fracture

B. Deformity of Smith's Fracture (reversed silver-fork)

C. Madelung's Deformity of the Wrist

D. Fracture of Ulnar Shaft

Fig. 9-17. Traumatic deformities of the forearm.

the radius, so displacement and deformity are rare (Fig. 9-17D); the only physical signs may be *localized tenderness* and *swelling*. Especially in children, ulnar fractures are frequently accompanied by volar dislocation of the radial head (Monteggia's fracture-dislocation); this permits considerable *bowing* of the fractured ulna. Fractured *radial shaft* presents variable degrees of *bowing*, especially with concomitant dislocation of the lower radioulnar joint.

Painful Angular Deformity: **Fractures of Both Forearm Bones.** Greenstick fractures produce little deformity, but combined complete fractures of radius and ulna present easily recognizable distortions.

The Elbow

There are two articulations in the elbow. The *humeroulnar joint* is hinged (ginglymus), formed by the semilunar notch of the ulnar *olecranon process* embracing and moving around the transverse drum of the spool-shaped *trochlea* in the distal

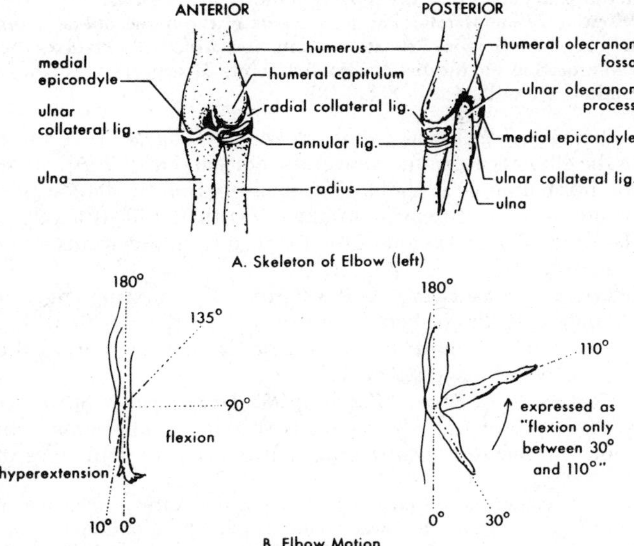

Fig. 9-18. Skeleton and motions of the elbow.

humeral end (Fig. 9-18A). When the elbow is in full extension, the olecranon process fits into the olecranon fossa of the humerus, just above the trochlea. The trochlea occupies the middle third of the lower humeral end; immediately lateral is a hemispheric eminence, the *capitulum,* upon which a cupshaped depression in the radial head pivots and glides to form the *humeroradial joint.* The radial head is a squat cylinder whose sides rotate in the *annular ligament* during pronation and supination of the forearm.

In a topographic view from the back (Fig. 9-19A), the *flexed* elbow presents three bony prominences of an *inverted equilateral triangle;* the two basal points are the *medial* and *lateral epicondyles* of the humerus; the tip of the *olecranon process* forms the apex. During full *extension* the three points form a *straight line.*

EXAMINATION OF THE ELBOW. **Inspect and palpate the region for *tenderness, swelling, deformities,* and *atrophy.* Swellings are more common on the extensor surface. Rheumatoid nodules are often found in the olecranon bursa and distally in the ulnar region. With the stethoscope, auscultate the moving joint for *fine crepitus.***

***Testing Elbow Motion:* The movements of the humeroulnar joint are extension-flexion. Pronation-supination principally involves the humeroradial and the distal radioulnar joints. Measurements of these motions are indicated in Fig. 9-18B.**

Deformity of the Elbow: ***Cubitus Valgus.**** The carrying angle of the elbow is accentuated over the normal (Fig. 9-20A). Since the normal angle is about 170°, measured on the lateral side of the arm and forearm, an angle less than 170° is a valgus deformity; the deviation of the forearm from the arm is more than 10°.

Deformity of the Elbow: ***Cubitus Varus.*** The carrying angle of the elbow is diminished from the normal (Fig. 9-20A); that is, the angle is more than 170°, or the deviation from the line of the arm is less than 10°.

Swelling of the Elbow: ***Effusion in the Elbow Joint.*** Since the synovial sac of the elbow joint is very loose, distention with fluid produces *fluctuant bulging* posteriorly, on both sides of

* To remember the meaning of valgus and varus: *valgus* means "out," *varus* means "in." *Valgus* and *out* each have one more letter than the opposite *varus* and *in.* The terms apply to deviation from the midline of the long bone *distal* to the involved joint.

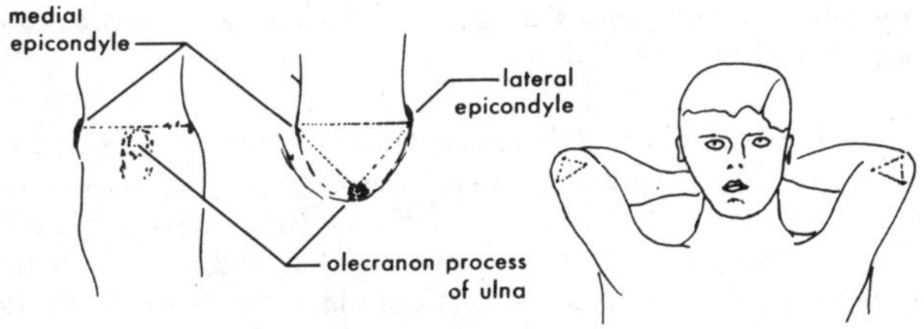

Fig. 9-19. Topographic relations of the elbow. *In extension the ulnar olecranon process lies on a straight line between the medial and the lateral epicondyles of the elbow. In flexion, the olecranon process moves downward to produce an inverted equilateral triangle between the three bony prominences. In examining the elbow after trauma, any distortion of this triangle points to a fracture involving one or more of its points.*

the olecranon process and the attached Triceps brachii tendon, and anteriorly in the antecubital fossa (Fig. 9-20B). Since the posterior swelling is nearer the surface, it is more accessible to palpation. The elbow is held in *semiflexion* to accommodate maximal fluid volume. Careful note of the borders of the sac in Fig. 9-20B will assist in distinguishing whether the fluid is in the joint cavity or in the olecranon bursa. Fluid in the bursa causes a bulging that *overlies* the olecranon process. The joint cavity may be distended by synovial fluid, pus, or blood, distinguished by aspiration.

Diagnostic Aspiration of the Elbow Joint. **Use the same materials and general technique as in aspiration of the wrist joint (p. 700). A convenient position of the elbow is full extension so the synovial sac is compressed to produce maximum bulging posteriorly. Pointing**

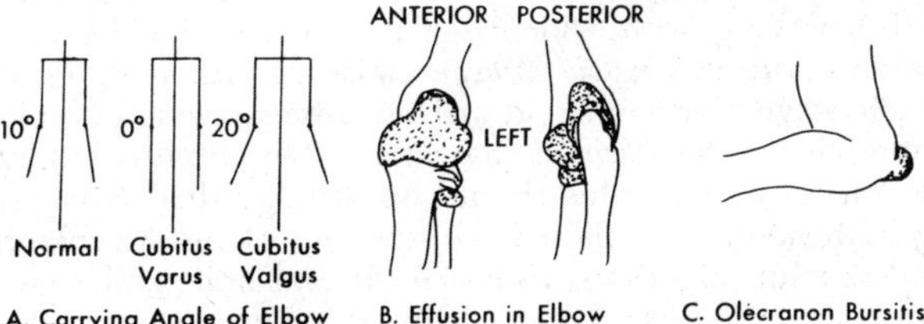

Fig. 9-20. Disorders of the intact elbow.

the needle medially, insert it lateral to the olecranon process and just proximal to the radial head.

Swelling of the Elbow: ***Olecranon Bursitis*** (Miner's Elbow, Student's Elbow). Trauma, inflammation, or gout may produce an accumulation of fluid in the *olecranon bursa*, a subcutaneous space overlying the olecranon process (Fig. 9-20C). The swelling is *fluctuant.* The location of the bulge readily distinguishes it from swelling on the sides of the olecranon process caused by fluid in the cavity of the joint.

Antecubital Pain and Tenderness: ***Bicipital Bursitis.*** A bursa beneath the Biceps brachii tendon may become inflamed from repeated trauma, as in pitching a ball. There is no swelling. Localized *tenderness* is present at the insertion of the tendon; the *pain is accentuated* by flexion and supination.

Lateral Elbow Pain: ***Radiohumeral Bursitis*** (Tennis Elbow). There is *throbbing pain* in the lateral aspect of the elbow, accentuated by extension of the wrist, as in lifting small objects. Paradoxically, lifting heavy objects is *painless* when flexion of the wrist is not involved. Palpation discloses *tenderness* over the lateral epicondyle or distally near the radial head where the extensors of the head are attached. In *Cozen's test* the patient is asked to keep his fist clenched while extending the wrist; grasp his forearm with your left hand while your right pulls his hand toward flexion against the patient's resistance; this causes *pain* at the lateral epicondyle, reproducing the patient's symptom. In *Mill's maneuver* have the elbow held in extension with the wrist flexed; when you forcefully pronate the forearm against the patient's resistance, the characteristic epicondylar *pain* is elicited.

Arthritis of the Elbow. Any type of arthritis may involve the *elbow joint* (see pp. 655–67). *Suppurative arthritis* produces painful swelling, with evidence of pus in the joint. *Rheumatic fever* and *acute rheumatoid arthritis* cause painful swelling; the chronic stage of rheumatoid arthritis often results in limited joint motion. *Osteoarthritis* is characterized by crepitus, but little pain on movement; this should be distinguished from *loose body* in the joint when there is a history of locking. An enlarged painless joint, suggesting osteoarthritis but unilateral, may be *neurogenic arthropathy* (Charcot's joint); when encountered in the elbow, syringomyelia is the most likely cause.

Posttraumatic Elbow Pain: ***Subluxation of the Radial Head.*** This lesion usually occurs in children (the "pulled elbow"). There is no deformity of the elbow. *Tenderness* is maximum near the radial head. Flexion-extension elicits *pain;* but pronation and supination are painless.

Posttraumatic Elbow Pain: ***Fracture of the Radial Head.*** Usually this is incurred in a fall on the outstretched hand. Swelling is minimal. There is no deformity of the elbow; the bony equilateral triangle is normal. Flexion and extension are painless, but there is severe *restriction* of pronation-supination and the radial head is *tender.*

Posttraumatic Elbow Pain: ***Fracture of the Olecranon Process.*** Pronounced *swelling* results, particularly around the dorsum of the elbow. The olecranon process is *tender.* When the fracture is complete, the patient *cannot extend* the flexed forearm (Fig. 9-21A). The *altitude* of the bony equilateral triangle may be diminished.

Posttraumatic Elbow Pain: ***Humeral Supracondylar Fracture.*** The injury is usually caused by falling on the outstretched hand; it is commonly seen in persons under 10 years of age. Usually the distal fragment is *displaced posteriorly,* so the angulation of the elbow is *unusually prominent* (Fig. 9-21B). The forearm is

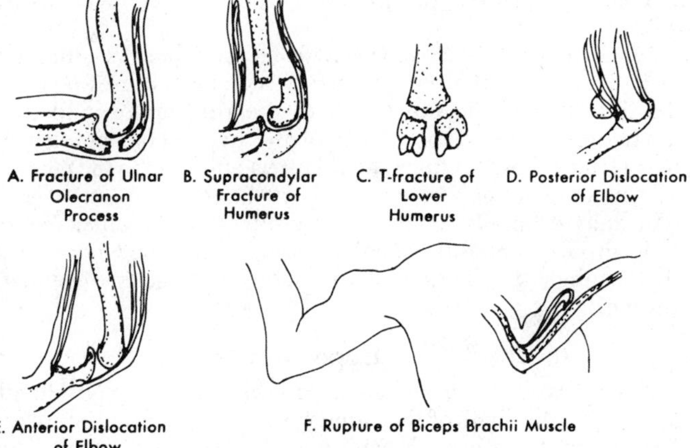

Fig. 9-21. Fractures and dislocations about the elbow.

supported with the other hand. The elbow's bony equilateral triangle is intact. *Tenderness* and *swelling* are present at the fracture site. *Avoid moving the fragments* to prevent injury to the antecubital structures. Seek the early signs of Volkmann's contracture and median nerve injury by *palpating the radial pulse* and *testing sensation* in the radial three and a half digits (see p. 676 for Volkmann's contracture). In the uncommon *anterior* displacement of the distal fragment, the signs may be less distinctive and require x-ray examination.

Posttraumatic Elbow Pain: ***Lower T-Shaped Humeral Fracture.*** A blow on the elbow may result in the humeral shaft being driven between the two condyles, producing *widening* of the elbow (Fig. 9-21C). Without separation of the condyles, *crepitus* of the fragments occurs with the lightest palpation. Swelling may obscure the *distortion* of the bony equilateral triangle, but blood in the joint cavity produces *fluctuation* and *bulging* on both sides of the olecranon process.

Posttraumatic Elbow Pain: ***Dislocation of the Elbow.*** Falling on the outstretched hand usually causes a *posterior* dislocation (Fig. 9-21D). The olecranon process is *unusually prominent.* The arm assumes an attitude of *40° of flexion;* the joint is *immovable,* actively or passively. The forearm is *not supported* by the opposite hand. The altitude of the bony triangle is *shortened* or *abolished.* The last two features distinguish it from supracondylar fracture.

Pain in Ulnar Side of Hand: ***Ulnar Tunnel Syndrome.*** Compression or injury in the ulnar nerve at the elbow causes *pain* in the little finger, the ulnar half of the ring finger, and the ulnar side of the palm. *Atrophy* of the hypothenar eminence may result. These findings should direct attention to the elbow. The ulnar nerve may be stretched or injured by a *cubitus valgus* deformity or an old elbow fracture. Press on the ulnar nerve in its groove behind the median epicondyle; if *tingling* occurs, in the ulnar distribution of the hand, it suggests the ulnar drome.

The Upper Arm

For convenience in examination, this region is considered to include the shaft of the humerus and its covering muscles, principally the Biceps brachii and the Triceps brachii. The proximal end of the bone is included in the examination of the shoulder, the distal end with the elbow.

Bicipital Humps: ***Rupture of the Biceps Brachii.*** The profile of the Biceps may be marred by a single hump or two humps in tandem. *One hump* is the result of rupture of the *tendon* or *sheath* of the muscle (Fig. 9-21F). Rupture of the *belly* causes *two humps.* Traumatic rupture occurs suddenly from lifting excessive weight, hence a history of the event will be available. Insidious rupture may not furnish a historic episode; this should suggest degeneration of the bicipital long head tendon in the shoulder joint, often osteoarthritic. Rupture of the long head tendon is commonest; forearm flexion is *weak.* Rupture of the muscle sheath may not greatly impair strength.

Painful Immobility of the Upper Arm: ***Fracture of the Humeral Shaft.*** In either type, the upper arm is *useless,* so it is *held* in the opposite hand. In *transverse fracture,* usually caused by a direct blow, there is unmistakable *angular deformity.* In *spiral fracture,* commonly from a fall on the hand, deformity may not occur. Lacking deformity, gently palpate with the fingertips the lateral and medial aspects of the humerus for local *tenderness* and *swelling.* Only as a last resort, grasp the elbow with your right hand and attempt *careful lateral elevation* of the humerus, while your left hand holds the upper part of the bone fast. With fracture, this maneuver discloses *mobility* and *crepitus.* In all cases of fractured humerus, feel the *radial arterial pulse* and test for *radial nerve injury.* Test the motor function of the nerve by having the patient flex the elbow with the forearm pronated and look for *wrist drop.* Anesthesia on the *radial dorsum of the hand* is evidence of sensory loss of the radial nerve.

The Shoulder Joint and Girdle

For examination, the shoulder girdle includes the scapulohumeral joint, the clavicle, and the scapula, and their ligamentous connections. The shoulder joint is a ball-and-socket (enarthrodial) articulation with the hemispheric *humeral head* fitting into the shallow *scapular glenoid cavity* (Fig. 9-22). The two articulating surfaces are enclosed by opposite ends of a short tube of *articular capsule.* Forming a rigid guard or fender above the joint is an arched superstructure of an anterior scapular projection, the *coracoid process,* and a posterior scapular process,

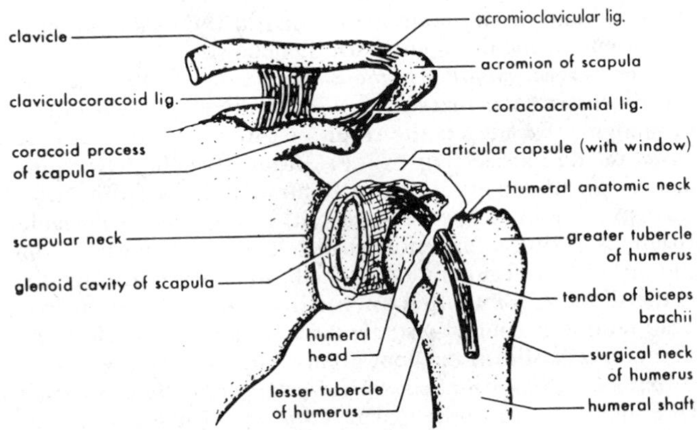

Fig. 9-22. Anatomy of the shoulder joint. *The anterior window in the joint capsule exposes the inner attachment of the biceps brachii muscle.*

the *acromion.* These are connected by the intervening *coracoacromial ligament.* This arch is surmounted by a second, made up of the *clavicle,* connected to the acromion by the *superior acromioclavicular ligament,* and to the underlying coracoid process by the *coracoclavicular ligament.* From its origin within the tubular capsule, and *tendon* of the long head of the Biceps brachii emerges anteriorly through a capsular opening between the *greater* and *lesser tubercles* of the humeral head. The joint capsule is lined by a synovial membrane with a prolongation forming a tubular sheath for the bicipital tendon; the sheath follows the tendon distally to the surgical neck of the humerus.

Apposition of joint surfaces is accomplished entirely by muscle pull; the joint capsule is very loose, so it exerts little tension except in extreme positions. The shoulder joint enjoys great freedom of motion from the shallowness of the glenoid cavity and the lack of restraining ligaments; but this also makes it vulnerable to frequent dislocation. The scapula is held to the thoracic wall entirely by muscle pull; its wing glides freely over the thoracic muscles from which it is separated by bursae. Scapular movements add greatly to the mobility of the upper limb; in examination, scapular motion must be distinguished from movements of the scapulohumeral joint. It is helpful to realize that in the entire mass of shoulder girdle, the single ligament-bone connection with the axial skeleton is the *sterno-clavicular joint;* the linkage is from sternum to clavicle, to coracoid and acromion of the scapula, to glenoid process.

The principal bony landmarks of the shoulder joint form a right-angled triangle: the tip of the *coracoid,* the *greater tubercle* of the humeral head, and the *acromion.* The right angle is at the greater tubercle (Fig. 9-23A). The acromion is easily *seen* and *felt* at the end of the clavicle. The coracoid must be palpated near the anterior border of the deltoid muscle on a horizontal line with the greater tubercle.

▼ ***Key Symptom:* Pain in the Shoulder.** Frequently pain in the shoulder is a chief complaint, and the patient finds difficulty in localizing it more sharply until the clinician makes a physical examination. But the diagnostician often receives important clues when he insists on eliciting the attributes of the pain

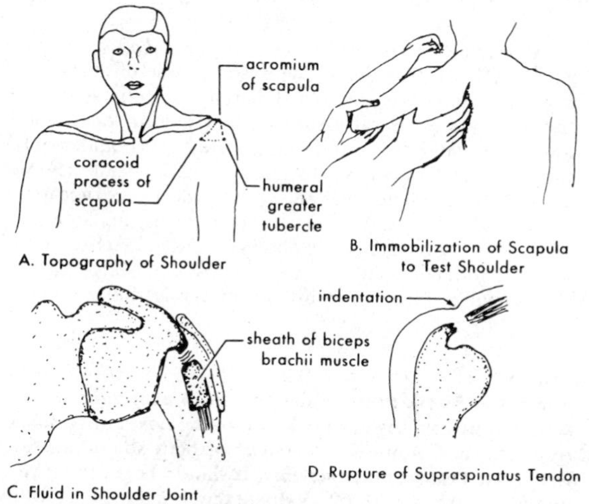

Fig. 9-23. Examination of the shoulder joint. **A.** Topography of the shoulder. *The bony prominences of the humeral greater tubercle and the coracoid and acromial processes of the scapula form a right-angled triangle.* **B.** Immobilization of the scapula to test shoulder motion. **C.** Fluid in the shoulder joint. *The heavily stippled structures are the joint capsules distended with fluid.* **D.** Rupture of supraspinatus tendon.

(PQRST): provocative and palliative circumstances, the quality of the pain, the precise anatomic region, the severity, and the timing. Both in history taking and in the physical examination it is helpful to consider a list of conditions arranged in an anatomic classification.

Clinical Occurrence: PAIN FROM SHOULDER STRUCTURES. *Shoulder Joint:* arthritis of shoulder, effusion into the joint capsule. *Tendons:* Supraspinatus tendinitis, rupture of Supraspinatus tendon (partial or complete), rupture of long tendon of Biceps brachii, bicipital tenosynovitis. *Muscles:* muscle strain, fibrositis, myositis, hematoma, rupture of muscle (complete or incomplete), polymyalgia rheumatica. *Bones:* fractures of humeral neck, scapular neck, clavicle; subluxations of humeral head, acromioclavicular joint, sternoclavicular joint. *Nerves:* compression in the superior thoracic aperture by cervical rib, Scalenus anticus muscle (Scalenus anticus syndrome), 1st rib and clavicle (costoclavicular syndrome); shoulder-hand syndrome. *Vascular:* aneurysm of the subclavian artery of arch of aorta.

PAIN REFERRED TO THE SHOULDER. *Cardiovascular:* angina pectoris (to either or both shoulders), aneurysm at base of aorta. *Pleura:* irritation of pleura of central part of diaphragm from pleurisy, pneumonia; irritation of apical pleura by tuberculosis, pneumothorax, or carcinoma (Pancoast's syndrome). *Spleen* (left shoulder only): infarction, rupture. *Subphrenic:* abscess, leaking peptic ulcer. *Stomach and Duodenum:* flatulence, gastritis, peptic ulcer, gastric carcinoma. *Liver and Gallbladder:* cholelithiasis, cholecystitis, hepatitis, hepatic cirrhosis or carcinoma, hepatic abscess. *Pancreas:* chronic inflammation, carcinoma, calculus, or cyst. *Nerves:* hemiplegia, herpes zoster, brachiitis, caries or neoplasm of cervicothoracic vertebrae, spinal cord tumor.

PRELIMINARY INSPECTION AND PALPATION OF THE SHOULDER JOINT. **Have the patient strip to the waist and sit in a straight chair while you stand behind and tower over him looking down upon his shoulders from above. Compare the *contour* of both shoulders for *local muscle atrophy*. Test *scapular mobility;* it should begin to move when elevation of the arm attains 60°. Palpate the *scapular spine*, following it forward to the acromion. Feel the *subdeltoid bursa* lying just beneath the deltoid muscle. Feel the greater tuberosity of the humerus, where the tendons of the supraspinatus, infraspinatus, and teres minor insert to form the *rotator cuff*. Feel for defects or tenderness in the cuff. Feel the *acromioclavicular joint;* the clavicle should rotate as the shoulder is raised. Feel the groove between greater and lesser tuberosities where the *biceps brachii tendon* lies; test for tenderness** in its sheath. Feel the *sternoclavicular joint* for enlargement or tenderness. Feel the lesser tuberosity for a *defect* in subscapularis muscle.

Inspect the shoulder anteriorly and the scapula posteriorly for *deformities* and *muscle atrophy,* realizing that nearly everyone carries one shoulder higher than the other. Seek *tenderness* in the sternoclavicular joint, the acromioclavicular joint, the clavicular shaft, and the scapula. Auscultate the joints for *fine crepitus.* To test the *mobility* of the shoulder joint, stand at the patient's *side* to glance either anteriorly or posteriorly and to manipulate from both aspects. Test the unaffected shoulder first and compare the affected side with it. *Active motion:* For *elevation,* grasp the scapular wing and hold it fast to the thorax with one hand while the patient's arm is still resting at his side (Fig. 9-23B). With your other hand, raise his arm laterally by the elbow and let him complete the motion as far as possible, with the scapula fixed. For *adduction,* rest the fingers of one hand on the top of his shoulder with your thumb behind fixing his scapula; with your other hand, lead the patient's flexed elbow across the front of his chest and let him move it as far as he can to place his flexed wrist over his shoulder. For *outward rotation,* fix the scapula as for adduction; grasp the patient's wrist with your free hand, flex his elbow at about 90° and lead his arm laterally and let him move it as far as possible toward the coronal plane of the trunk. For *inward rotation,* ask the patient to put his hand behind his back and his hand as high as possible up his spine. *Passive Motion:* When there is a deficit in active motion, use the same holds as for active motion; gently pull the arm in the desired direction toward the normal limit. In addition, test the *Supraspinatus tendon* and the *subacromial bursa* from behind by placing your hand over the shoulder so your index finger palpates the tendon just behind its attachment on the greater tubercle of the humeral head, and your middle finger palpates the subacromial bursa. With your far hand on his flexed elbow, move the arm backward and forward a few times to detect *crepitus* or *Tenderness* at the two points. *Axillary Examination:* Place your fingers in the axilla with the pulps facing laterally; palpate the humeral head and the lateral aspect of the glenoid synovial sac.

MEASUREMENTS OF SHOULDER MOTION. **Imagine the shoulder joint as the center of a sphere, marked as a terrestrial globe with a north and south pole and meridians (Fig. 9-24). Then a parasagittal plane through the shoulder joint describes an anterior meridian on the sphere's surface that is designated as *0° of abduction;* those meridians lateral to it mark degrees of *abduction;* those medial to it are degrees of *adduction.* When the arm hangs at the patient's side, it is in *0° of elevation and 0° of abduction.* The arm can be lifted from the south**

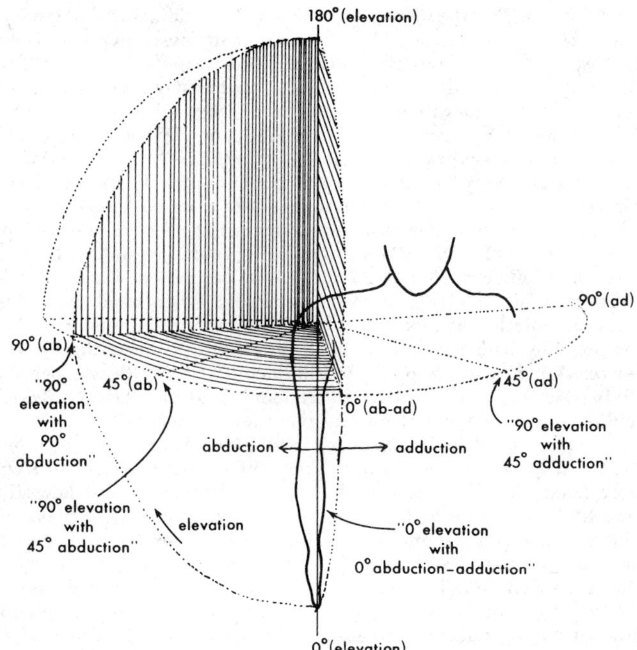

Fig. 9-24. Motion at the shoulder. *There has been much confusion in terminology about shoulder motion, so the one presented has been adopted by many because it leaves no room for misinterpretation. Elevation is a movement of the arm along any meridian, measured from position 0° at the south pole. Elevation along the meridian in the parasagittal plane passing through the shoulder joint is with 0° abduction-adduction. Movement medial to this is adduction, movement lateral to the plane is abduction. When the arm is elevated in any other meridian than the parasagittal one, the motion is expressed as "30° elevation in 48° abduction" or "70° elevation in 90° abduction."*

pole to the north pole,or from *0° to 180° of elevation*. But in elevating, the arm must follow in a meridian that designates abduction or adduction. If the arm is raised directly forward of the shoulder to the horizontal, the position is *90° of elevation with 0° of abduction*. When the arm is raised laterally to the horizontal, the position is *90° of elevation with 90° of abduction*. If, however, the arm is raised

to the horizontal in a meridian medial to *0°*, the position is *90° of elevation with perhaps 20° of adduction. Outward* and *inward rotation* may be performed with the upper arm at the side in *0° of elevation with 0° of abduction,* or the motion may be carried out along one of the meridians of abduction-adduction.

AUSCULTATION OF BONY CONDUCTION THROUGH THE SHOULDER. The olecranon-manubrium percussion sign proved useful in evaluating 96 patients with anterior shoulder dislocations, clavicular fractures, and humeral fractures in which there were no false positive errors and a 15% false negative error. Place the bell of the stethoscope over the manubrium with the patient's elbows flexed at 90° and percuss the olecranon. Normally, with no disruption of bony conduction, sequential percussion of both sides will produce equal crisp sounds. When dislocation or fracture disrupts bony conduction, the affected side will be duller in pitch and intensity [S. L. Adams: Clinical Use of the Olecranon-Manubrium Percussion Sign in Shoulder Trauma, *Ann. Emerg. Med.* 15:658, 1986.].

ASPIRATION OF THE SHOULDER JOINT. Fluid rarely accumulates in the shoulder joint. When it does, the capsule bulges anteriorly, presenting a fluctuant swelling just medial to the humeral head (Fig. 9-23C). This is the point to insert the aspirating needle, using the materials and general technique described for aspirating the wrist joint (p. 700).

Arm Elevation at 90° of Abduction: ***Distinctive Deficits.*** Certain diagnostic clues are disclosed by observing the patient while he slowly *elevates* the arm from 0° toward 180° at 90° of abduction, that is, raising the arm in the coronal plane of the trunk (Fig. 9-25). *Full motion,* from 0° to 180° of elevation, is good evidence of lack of serious injury to shoulder joint and girdle. *Pain* between 60° and 120° of elevation, with the remainder of the arc painless, points to partial rupture of the Supraspinatus tendon or chronic supraspinatus tendinitis. *Minimal elevation* and *support* of the arm with the opposite hand point to fracture, dislocation, or complete rupture of the Supraspinatus; in the latter case, all passive motions of the joint are normal. *Pain* throughout the range of elevation indicates arthritis. Descriptions of these conditions follow.

Pain Between 60° and 120° of Arm Elevation at 90° Abduction: ***Partial Rupture of the Supraspinatus Tendon.*** The tendon is torn incompletely; the rotator cuff is intact. *Pain* is referred to the

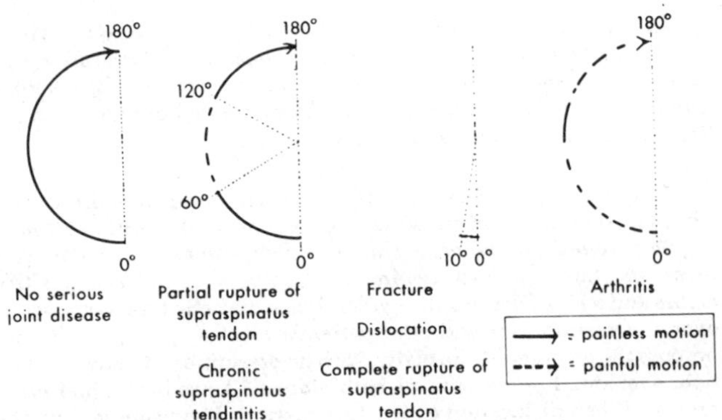

Fig. 9-25. Causes of pain and limited motion with elevation of the arm in 90° of abduction.

insertion of the deltoid muscle, but there is no tenderness at that point; sometimes the pain extends down the arm to the elbow or beyond. *Active attempts* to elevate the arm, at 90° abduction, are painless in the range of 0° to 60°, where *excruciating pain* inhibits further elevation; nor will pain permit *passive motion* beyond that point. *Tenderness* is elicited just beneath the acromial tip or in the notch between greater and lesser humeral tubercles. *Distinction.* At the onset, the condition can be distinguished from supraspinatus tendinitis only by the history of trauma and resistance to external rotation.

Pain Between 60° and 120° of Arm Elevation at 90° Abduction: **Supraspinatus Tendinitis.** *Acute Supraspinatus Tendinitis with Calcification.* In a person 25 to 45 years of age, a *dull ache* develops in the shoulder without antecedent trauma. The *pain* steadily worsens and may be excruciating. Elevation of the arm is particularly *painful;* the range from 0° to 60° is painless. *Tenderness* is pronounced beneath the acromial tip. X-ray films occasionally show calcium deposits in the tendon. The pain subsides spontaneously and permanently within a few days. *Chronic Supraspinatus Tendinitis.* The patient is usually between 45 and 60 years old. Without preceding trauma, *dull pain* develops in the shoulder. *Elevation* of the arm, at 90° of abduction, is *diagnostic.* The movement is painless from 0° to 60° of elevation; at the latter angle the patient feels a *jerk* and *agonizing pain* at the insertion of the deltoid muscle; but this spot is completely lacking in tenderness. Totally unsuspected by the patient, pronounced *tenderness* can be elicited in the notch between the greater and lesser tubercles of the humeral head, or beneath the acromial tip. There, *crepitus* may also be present with motions of the Supraspinatus. Lying on the shoulder produces pain that prevents sleeping on the affected side for months. The condition usually subsides spontaneously in 6 months.

Minimal Arm Elevation and Support with Opposite Hand: **Complete Rupture of the Supraspinatus Tendon.** This usually occurs between the ages of 55 and 65 years. There is some accompanying tearing of the *rotator cuff*, composed of the tendons of the Infraspinatus, Subscapularis, and Teres minor. *Active elevation* can proceed to less than 40°; he finds it impossible to lift further, but *passive motion* to 180° is *free* and *painless*. There is resistance to external rotation when the arm is held at the side with elbow flexed. After 3 weeks, *atrophy* of the Supraspinatus and Infraspinatus occurs. As the arm is moved forward, one can palpate a *jerk, fine crepitus*, and an *indentation* in the subacromial region between the greater and lesser humeral tubercles (Fig. 9-23D).

Pain in the Shoulder: **Coracoiditis.** Repeated acute or chronic stresses may produce inflammation of the tip of the coracoid process at the origin of the short head of the biceps brachii and the coracobrachialis muscles. *Diagnosis:* The history of trauma with pain and tenderness at the tip of the coracoid process, relieved by the injection at that site of local anesthetic, confirms the diagnosis. Further confirmation consists in reproducing the pain by flexing the elbow, resisting supination of the forearm, adduction and external rotation of the humerus, resisting forward flexion of the shoulder, resisting adduction of the flexed shoulder.

Shoulder Pain: **Tear of Rotator Cuff.** Shoulder pain occurs when the arm is in abduction where the tear strikes the coracoacromial ligament. The arm can be passively abducted, but the shoulder is weak. As the region of pain is approached, the shoulder weakens and drops abruptly. Shoulder motion is mostly with the scapula. Atrophy of the cuff muscles may be palpated (composed of supraspinatus, infraspinatus, and teres minor).

Minimal Arm Elevation with Support of Opposite Hand: **Shoulder**

Dislocation. Usually the humeral head is displaced *anteriorly* and slightly *medially,* to a position *under* the coracoid process, from its normal lateral location immediately below the acromial tip and behind the coracoid (Fig. 9-26A). Thus, the bony shoulder triangle is *disrupted.* The shoulder profile is *flattened* by recession of the humeral head from its normal position; flattening can also be caused by atrophy of the Deltoideus. Palpation of the upper third of the Deltoideus discloses the *bony hardness* of the humeral head in the normally soft belly. In the *ruler test of Hamilton,* a straight edge can rest simultaneously on the *acromial tip* and the *lateral epicondyle* of the elbow; normally, the humeral head obtrudes. The test is also positive in displacement from fracture of the femoral neck. Useful in obese pa-

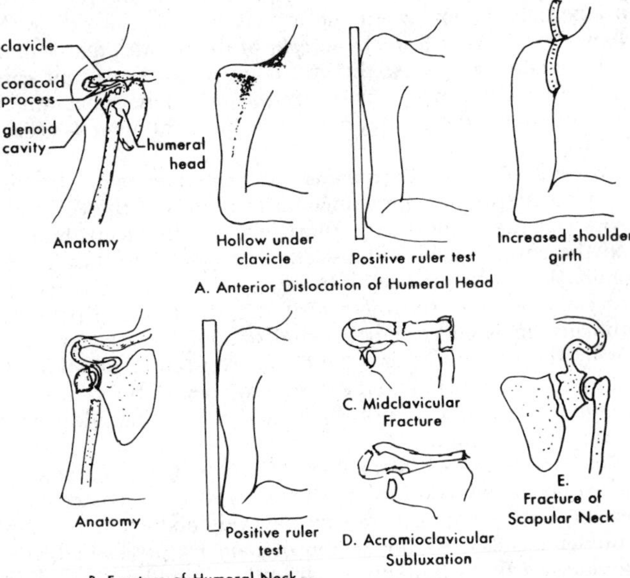

Fig. 9-26. Traumatic disorders of the shoulder. **A.** Anterior dislocation of the humeral head. **B.** Fracture of the humeral neck. **C.** Midclavicular fracture. **D.** Acromioclavicular subluxation. **E.** Fracture of the scapular neck.

tients, *Calloway's test* consists in measuring the girth of the two shoulder joints. A tape measure is looped through the axilla and the girth measured at the acromial tip; the *girth* of the affected joint is increased. In *Dugas' test,* the patient *cannot adduct* the arm sufficiently to place his hand on the opposite shoulder. ***Posterior Dislocation.*** In this rare occurrence, the humeral head may be felt in the back, under the spine of the scapula near the base of the acromial process; the condition is not always disclosed by an anteroposterior x-ray film. ***Injuries from Shoulder Dislocation.*** Damage to the *axillary nerve* causes paralysis and atrophy of the Deltoideus. *Rupture* of the Supraspinatus tendon may occur. Associated *fracture* of the humeral neck or *avulsion* of the greater humeral tubercle is common. *Feel the pulses* of the arm to detect compression of the axillary vessels.

Minimal Arm Elevation and Support with Opposite Hand: Humeral Neck Fracture. Usually this results from a fall on the outstretched hand. *Pain* is present in the shoulder, with *immobility* of the arm, supported by the opposite hand. Viewed laterally, the profile may show an *anterior angular deformity* (Fig. 9-26B). The axillary aspect of the arm, or the thoracic wall, may contain *ecchymoses. Rotate* the arm gently, while palpating the humeral head; if not impacted, the head *will not move* with the shaft, confirming the diagnosis. When displacement is present, the *ruler test of Hamilton* (see above) may be positive; a straight edge can simultaneously touch the acromial tip and the lateral epicondyle. If a break cannot be proved, consider *impacted fracture* and measure the distance from acromial tip to epicondyle on the two sides; the impacted side should be shorter.

Minimal Arm Elevation and Support with Opposite Hand: Clavicular Fracture. Fractures of the center of the shaft are most common. They are readily diagnosed by inspection and palpation, since the fragments are usually *displaced* (Fig. 9-26C). Greenstick or impacted fractures may be detected by *tenderness* and *swelling.*

Minimal Arm Elevation and Support with Opposite Hand: Acromioclavicular Subluxation. There is *pain* in the shoulder with reluctance to elevate the arm that is supported by the opposite hand. Inspection may disclose *elevation* of the distal clavicular end. Have the patient place the hand of the affected side on the opposite shoulder and lean forward; press firmly upon the distal end of the clavicle; the end of the bone *springs downward* and the maneuver is *painful* (Fig. 9-26D).

Minimal Arm Elevation and Support with Opposite Hand: ***Sternoclavicular Subluxation.*** Forward dislocation and subluxation, the more common injury, cause *painful clicking* in the joint region with elevation of the arm at 0° abduction. The deformity is usually obvious to inspection. The rarer backward dislocation exhibits a *hollow* where normally the clavicular head protrudes. If the mediastinum is invaded, dyspnea and cyanosis occur.

Minimal Arm Elevation and Support with Opposite Hand: ***Scapular Fracture.*** There is *pain* in the shoulder that prevents elevation of the arm (Fig. 9-26E). To examine, sit at the patient's affected side. At his left side, place your left forearm under his left forearm for support and palpate his shoulder with your right hand. Now elevate his forearm in 90° of abduction and feel *crepitus* in the joint, strongly suggesting fracture of the scapular neck when the clavicle is intact.

Restriction of All Shoulder Motions: ***Arthritis.*** All types of arthritis occasionally involve the shoulder. In the early stages of inflammatory processes, motions are inhibited by *pain;* later, *adhesions* form to restrict motion. *Effusion* into the joint capsule is relatively rare. Osteoarthritis is revealed by crepitus in the joint; motion is not limited. With chronically limited motion, generalized muscle *atrophy* occurs.

Restriction of All Shoulder Motions: ***Frozen Shoulder.*** This curious disease of unknown cause occurs in men between 50 and 60 years, about 10 years younger in women. Subacute inflammation of the entire rotator cuff develops. At onset, *pain* may resemble that of partial rupture of the Supraspinatus. But the pain *intensifies* to prevent the patient's sleeping on the affected side. Progressive *limitation of motion* ensues until complete ankylosis *abates* the pain. There is concomitant muscle *atrophy*. After many months, the disorder may completely subside with restoration to normal.

Pain in Deltoid Muscle: ***Subdeltoid Bursitis*** (Subacromial Bursitis). Formerly regarded as a clinical entity, inflammation of the subdeltoid bursa is now considered as a complication of partial or complete rupture of the Supraspinatus tendon. The symptoms and signs have been described under that topic (p. 718).

Pain at Pectoralis Major Insertion: ***Bicipital Tenosynovitis.*** A day or so after excessive use of the Biceps brachii, *pain* develops near the insertion of the Pectoralis major on the humerus; the pain may shoot down the arm. Shoulder motions are somewhat *limited,* especially elevation of the arm with 90° of abduction. Actually, there is inflammation of the tendon sheath of the Biceps where it emerges anteriorly from the capsule of the shoulder joint. To diagnose, have the patient *flex* his elbow to 90° and *pronate* his forearm. Grasp his hand and ask him to *supinate* against your resistance. When the maneuver produces *pain* in the anteromedial aspect of the shoulder, it is a positive *Yergason's sign.*

Painful Nodules in Shoulder Muscles: ***Fibrositis.*** A single muscle or group of muscles about the shoulder may be *painful* on arising; exercise abolishes the pain. Small *trigger nodules* may be palpated on the surface of the muscle, attributed by some writers to fatty hernias within the muscle mass that become edematous and cause muscle spasm. There is some doubt that this is a clinical entity.

Shoulder-Pad Sign of Amyloidosis. Case reports have reemphasized bilateral swelling of the shoulder joints as a conspicuous sign of amyloid disease [G. A. Katz, J. P. Peters, C. M. Pearson, and W. S. Adams: The Shoulder-Pad Sign—A Diagnostic Feature of Amyloid Arthropathy, *N. Engl. J. Med.,* **288:**354–55, 1973]. The periarticular swellings feel hard and rubbery; their appearance suggests the shoulder pads worn in playing American football. Besides the involvement of other joints, associated features may be subcutaneous nodules and carpal-tunnel syndrome. The diagnosis is proved by biopsy of the periarticular mass. Other observers report that aspirated fluid from such pads do not contain inflammatory elements, but instead, they found kappa M-component and fragments staining with Congo red, and having green refringence [D. A. Gordon, M. A. Ogryzls, W. Pruzanski, and H. A. Little: Shoulder Pads in Amyloid Arthropathy, *N. Engl. J. Med.,* **288:**1080, 1973].

Winged Scapula: ***Paralysis of the Long Thoracic Nerve.*** Ask the patient to stand and push with his hands against a wall while you observe his scapulae (Fig. 9-27A). Paralysis of the Serratus anterior permits its scapula to be separated posteriorly from

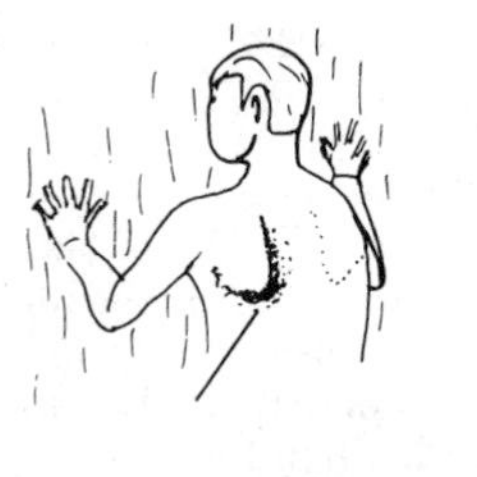

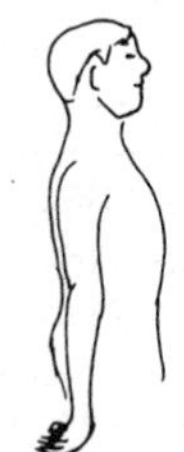

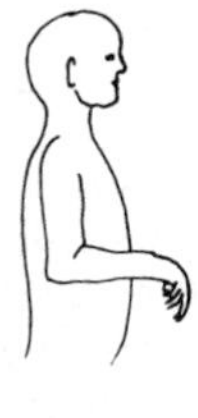

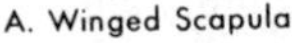

A. Winged Scapula B. Flail Arm C. Spastic Arm

Fig. 9-27. Disorders of the intact shoulder. **A.** Winged scapula. *When the patient faces a wall and pushes his hands against it, the scapulae are held to the thorax by the serratus anterior muscles. Paralysis of a long thoracic nerve permits the involved scapula to protrude posteriorly in this test so it forms a winged scapula.* **B.** Flail arm. *The arm hangs limply at the side with palm posterior and fingers partially flexed. This occurs from extensive injury of the brachial plexus or poliomyelitis.* **C.** Spastic arm. *The arm assumes flexion at the elbow with the upper arm at 0° elevation, flexion at the wrist and fingers, with slight adduction of the humerus; the forearm is in pronation.*

the thoracic wall, a *winged scapula.* The injury is caused to the long thoracic nerve by stretching during heavy lifting or from severance during mastectomy.

Winged Scapula: Sprengel's Deformity. This is a congenital condition with unilateral or bilateral winged scapulae. It is sometimes associated with a short webbed neck.

Widespread Involvements of the Upper Limb

Fail Arm. After injuries to the brachial plexus or poliomyelitis, the arm may hang limply at the side with the flexed palm facing backward, as the English say, "like a policeman taking a tip" (Fig. 9-27B).

Spastic Arm. After hemiplegia, the arm may be carried at 0° elevation with flexion of the elbow, wrist, and fingers (Fig. 9-27C).

Disorders of the Superior Thoracic Aperture. These are discussed with the cardiovascular system (pp. 429–32).

The Spine

The Cervical Spine

For convenience in examination, the cervical spine may be considered apart from the remainder of the spinal column (Fig. 9-28A). Usually there are seven cervical vertebrae of which three are specialized: C-1 is the *atlas* (bearing a globe like its namesake the Greek god); C-2 is the *axis* about which the atlas rotates; C-7 is the *vertebra prominens*. *Nodding* and *lifting* the head occur chiefly at the atlanto-occipital joint. *Flexion* and *extension* involve C-3 to C-7. The midcervical vertebrae permit *lateral bending*. *Rotation* occurs chiefly at the atlantoaxial joint. For measurements of motions see Fig. 9-28B.

▼ *Key Symptom:* ***Backache.*** In common usage *backache* refers to the spinal region inferior to the 7th cervical vertebra, while the neck is considered separately. Many causes of backache are listed as follows:

ACUTE. *Bones:* fractures, dislocations. *Cartilages:* herniated intervertebral disk. *Joints:* acute localized arthritis from specific microorganisms, arthritis associated with acute generalized infectious diseases, acutely torn or avulsed ligaments. *Muscles:* acute muscle strain, acute myositis, hematoma. *Nerves:* after myelography, subarachnoid hemorrhage, poliomyelitis, tetanus. *Referred Pain:* angina pectoris, acute retrocecal appendicitis, acute pancreatitis, acute cholecystitis, gallstone colic, pneumothorax, pleurisy, dissecting aortic aneurysm.

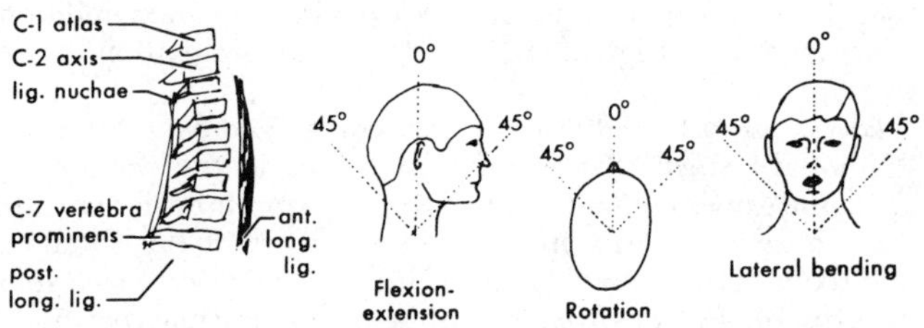

Fig. 9-28. Anatomy and motions of the cervical spine. **A.** The skeleton of the cervical spine. **B.** Motions of the cervical spine.

CHRONIC. *Bones:* osteoporosis, osteomalacia, Pott's disease (tuberculous spondylitis), osteitis of syphilis and Paget's disease (osteitis deformans), primary or secondary neoplasm of bone, spina bifida. *Cartilage:* herniated intervertebral disk. *Joints:* ankylosing spondylitis (Marie-Strümpell-Becterew disease), osteoarthritis. *Muscles:* chronic muscle strain, fibrositis. *Nerves:* syringomyelia. *Referred Pain:* esophageal carcinoma, peptic ulcer, chronic pancreatitis, pancreatic carcinoma, hypernephroma, hepatomegaly from any cause, spinal cord tumor, aortic aneurysm.

EXAMINATION OF THE CERVICAL SPINE. **Have the patient seated. View the neck from the front, sides, and back for *deformities* and unusual *posture*. Ask the patient to *point* to the site of his pain. Test *active motions* of the neck with the instructions: "chin to chest," "chin to right and left shoulder," "ear to right and left shoulder," and "head back." With the flat of the hand, palpate the paravertebral muscles for the hardening of *muscle spasm*. Test for *tenderness* of the spinous processes by palpation and by percussion with the finger or rubber hammer. With your stethoscope auscultate the moving joints for *crepitus*.**

Torticollis (Wryneck). This is described on p. 206.

Pain in the Neck: ***Nuchal Headache.*** Commencing unilaterally in the occipital region, in a few hours *dull pain* moves to the back of the eye, where it may reside for hours or days; the pain may become *throbbing*. Careful detailed palpation of the posterior cervical muscles may disclose one or more *trigger points* that reproduce the pain, although the muscle itself is not tender. The pain may be *reproduced* or *accentuated* by pressing on the vertex of the skull when the neck is bent laterally. Passive extension of the neck may *relieve* the pain. *Distinction.* The physical signs in the neck distinguish the condition from migraine, trigeminal neuralgia, and brain tumor. See also pp. 63–75.

Pain in the Neck and Shoulder: ***Pancoast's Syndrome*** (Superior Pulmonary Sulcus Syndrome). A tumor in the pulmonary apex, the upper mediastinum, or the superior thoracic aperture may cause *severe pain* in the posterior part of the shoulder and axilla, often shooting down the arm. *Acroparesthesia* may be present. *Paresis* or *atrophy* of arm muscles may occur. In addition to neck and shoulder pain, the complete syndrome includes the early development of *Horner's syndrome* (unilateral miosis, ptosis of the eyelid, absence of sweating on the affected side of the face and neck). *Distinction.* It must be distinguished from rupture of the Supraspinatus tendon, cervical spondylitis, and peripheral neuritis, by demonstration of a tumor in the lung apex or neck.

Pain in the Neck and Shoulder: ***Cervical Spondylosis*** (Cervical Osteoarthritis). The term *spondylosis* is preferred to describe the complications from degeneration of the vertebrae and their intervertebral disks, with traumatic rupture or degeneration of the nucleus pulposus. Osteophytes forming about the degenerating tissue may encroach upon the intervertebral foramina or protrude into the spinal cord. *Pain* is usually present in the neck and frequently extends to the shoulder, the occipital scalp, or down the arm. *Numbness* and *tingling* of the hands are frequent, but muscle atrophy is rare. Active and passive motions of the neck may be painless, but they often produce *crepitus* to be heard by the patient, palpated and auscultated by the examiner. The bicipital tendon reflex is frequently *diminished* or *absent.* With the patient's head held in extension by the examiner, coughing may *reproduce the pain.* *Distinction.* The x-ray findings are diagnostic for degenerative disease of the cervical spine, but the same findings are present in most persons beyond 50 years. Attribution of the symptoms to spondylosis depends upon exclusion of other causes, such as incomplete rupture of the Supraspinatus, Pancoast's syndrome of shoulder pain, and peripheral neuritis.

Attacks of Nuchal Rigidity with Arm Pain: ***Cervical Syndrome.*** Usually the onset is preceded by minor trauma, such as stretching the arms. *Painful spasm* of the neck muscles causes temporary *torticollis,* with the head *tilted away* from the painful side. Sharp shooting *pains* spread slowly down the shoulder, the lateral aspect of the upper arm, and the radial aspect of the forearm, to the wrist. When the hand is occasionally involved, there are *tingling* and *numbness* in the thumb, index and middle fingers. The neck muscles are *rigid* on the affected side. *Tenderness* is often present in the Trapezius, Brachioradialis, Pectoralis major, and the forearm extensors. The *biceps* and *triceps jerks* are frequently diminished or absent. Symptom-free *intervals* occur.

Clinical Occurrence. Commonly, the cause is narrowing of intervertebral foramina or compression of nerve roots by osteophytes.

Uncommonly, the lesion is caused by protrusion of an intervertebral disk.

Stiff Neck, with or without Pain: ***Tuberculous Spondylitis*** (Cervical Pott's Diseases). The neck is held *stiffly;* spontaneous rotation of the head is absent. There may be *pain* in the neck, but often it is painless. When seated, the patient may *support his head* with his hands (*Rust's sign*). An abscess of the cervical vertebra may point to the retropharyngeal space. The diagnosis of tuberculous bone disease is usually made by x-ray signs.

Posttraumatic Neck Pain and Headache: ***Whiplash Cervical Injury*** (Extension Cervical Injury). Sudden forceful hyperextension of the neck, with flexion recoil, commonly occurs to a rider in an automobile that is struck from behind (Fig. 9-29). The ligamentum nuchae is ruptured; rarely the spine of C-7 is fractured also. *Posterior neck pain* develops slowly over hours or days. Succeeding nerve-root irritation incites *spasm* of the neck muscles and *torticollis. Occipital headache* develops, sometimes with *blurring of vision.* The chin is turned *toward* the painful side of the neck. Palpation over the lower cervical spinous processes elicits *tenderness.* An effusion with *soft crepitus* can sometimes be felt over the lower part of the ligamentum nuchae. The *biceps jerk* is frequently *diminished* or *absent* on one or both sides. Occasionally, the pupil is *dilated* on the affected side.

Posttraumatic Neck Pain: ***Fracture of a Spinous Process.*** Vertebrae near the cervicothoracic junction are usually involved in this fracture because their spinous processes are long and thin;

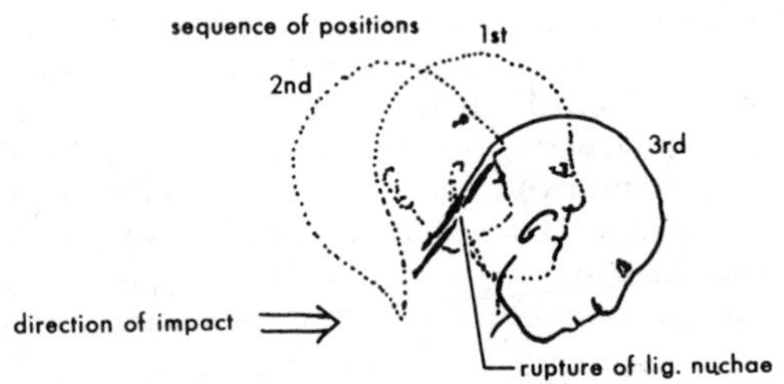

Fig. 9-29. Extension injury (or whiplash) of the cervical spine. *Violent impact from behind produces rapid translation between three sequential positions, causing rupture of the ligamentum nuchae.*

they break readily from a direct blow or from violent muscular contraction, such as raising a heavy load with a shovel. *Sudden severe pain* extends from the neck to the shoulder, *accentuated* by flexion and rotation of the neck. Over the fracture site, *tenderness* is exquisite. Sometimes the fractured process is *mobile* laterally, and motion causes *crepitus.*

Posttraumatic Neck Pain: ***Flexion Fracture of the Neck.*** Usually C-5 is fractured by hyperflexion of the neck, such as incurred when a diver strikes his head on the bottom. If the patient survives immediate death or quadriplegia, he can walk *without supporting his head* with his hands. Pain *restricts* all motions of the neck. The spinous process of the affected vertebra is *tender;* it may be somewhat *prominent.*

Posttraumatic Neck Pain: ***Partial Dislocation from Hyperextension.*** A fall or blow on the forehead may hyperextend the neck to rupture the anterior longitudinal ligament. There is intense *pain* in the neck. One spinous process may seem more *prominent.* Paraplegia frequently occurs. X-ray examination is required for diagnosis.

Posttraumatic Neck Pain: ***Fracture of the Atlas (C-1).*** If immediate death does not result, the patient *supports his head* with his hands; he is *unable to nod* the head. There is severe *occipital headache.* X-ray diagnosis should not be entirely relied upon to exclude fracture.

Posttraumatic Neck Pain: ***Fracture of the Odontoid Process.*** Usually from a diving accident, the lesion frequently causes immediate death from injury to the brainstem. The surviving patient can walk *without supporting the head* with his hands. The diagnostic sign: *He cannot rotate the head.* If the clinical diagnosis is not made *immediately* and the neck *completely immobilized,* sudden death is the rule. There is no time before immobilization for x-ray examination.

Thoracolumbar Spine and Pelvis

Below the neck, the vertebral column normally consists of 12 thoracic (dorsal) vertebrae, 5 lumbar vertebrae, and a fused mass of variously separated 5 sacral and 4 coccygeal vertebrae, articulated with the pelvic bones. Viewed laterally, the vertebral column presents four curves to be carefully noted (Fig. 9-30A). Least pronounced is the *cervical curve,* which is convex forward, beginning at C-2 and ending at T-2. The *thoracic curve* is concave

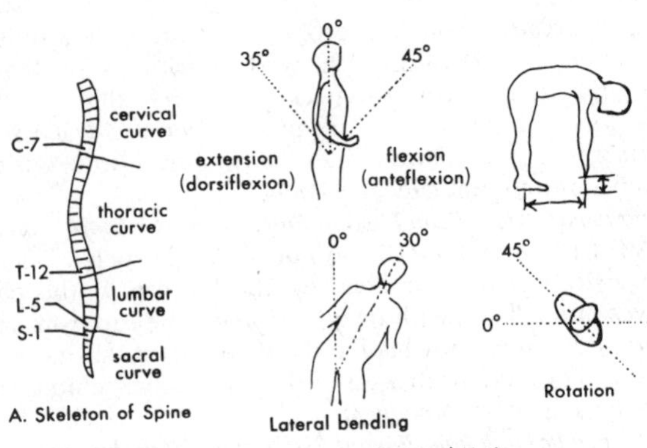

Fig. 9-30. Skeleton and motions of the entire spine.

forward, beginning at T-2 and ending at T-12. The *lumbar curve,* more pronounced in the female, is convex forward, from T-12 to the lumbosacral joint. The *pelvic curve,* concave forward and downward, extends from the lumbosacral joint to the tip of the coccyx. The spinal motions are *flexion-extension, lateral bending,* and *rotation.* For methods of measurement, see Fig. 9-30B.

GENERAL EXAMINATION OF THE THORACOLUMBAR SPINE AND PELVIS. ***With the Patient Standing:*** **A man should be completely undressed, although he may retain his undershorts. A woman's clothes should be replaced by a short-sleeved examining gown that ties in back so it may be opened to reveal the spine. Note gross *deformity,* muscle *atrophy,* local *swelling.* Inspect the spinal profile for abnormal *curvature.* View the back for *lateral deviations* of the spine. If the spinal processes are hidden by muscle or fat, palpate each and *mark it* with a dash from a skin pencil; the resulting broken line will disclose any deviations from the midline. When lateral deviation is present, have the patient *lean forward,* and inspect from behind the upward bulges of the muscle masses beside the spine; in structural scoliosis, one lumbar mass will be *higher* than the other (Fig. 9-31). Curvature or deviation may also result from muscle spasm or disease of ligaments or joints. Palpate for *tenderness.* Feel with the flat of the hand for *hardened muscles* from spasm. Have the patient tense the glutei to reveal *atrophy.* Percuss each spinous process with finger or rubber hammer to elicit *tenderness.* Have the patient walk and note his *gait.***

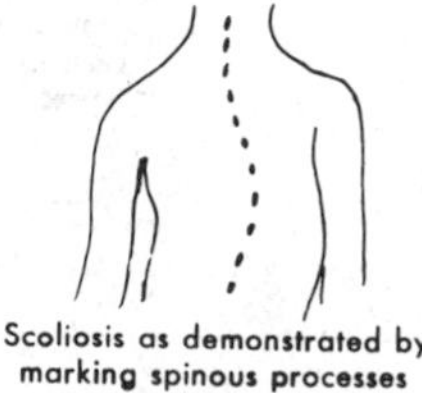

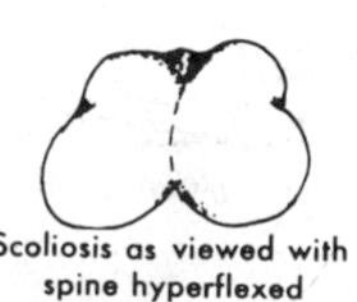

Fig. 9-31. Structural scoliosis. *Inspection of the flexed spine from behind shows the unequal elevation of the two erector spini masses of muscle.*

Get him to hop on alternate feet to find muscle *weakness* and *pain*. Direct the patient to *flex, extend,* and *laterally bend* the spine without assistance. *Test rotation* by grasping the hips while he turns first one shoulder, then the other. Palpate for *tenderness* and for hardened muscles of spasm any region that emits pain.

With the Patient Supine: Have the patient lie face upward on a hard examining table; the head may be pillowed and the knees slightly flexed for comfort. Make the *straight-leg—raising test* (Fig. 9-32A) by grasping the ankle, with the knee held in extension, and lifting the lower limb to determine range of flexion in the hip joint. Note the location of elicited pain, especially contralateral radiation indicating nerve-root compression. With the straight limb elevated at a little less than complete flexion, *dorsiflex the foot* for aggravation of pain. *An alternative test* is to gradually extend the flexed knee, with the finger pressing upon the tibial nerve in the popliteal fossa; this produces pain if there is irritation of the lower lumbar nerve root. Perform *Patrick's test* for external rotation of the hip joint (Fig. 9-32B) by passively flexing the knee to a right angle and placing the foot on the opposite patella; then pull the flexed knee lateralward as far as the hip joint permits. Normal performance (negative Patrick's sign) excludes symptomatic disease of the hip joint. In *Graenslen's test* of the sacroiliac joint (Fig. 6-32C), have the patient hold the knee of his affected side with both his hands, flexing the knee and the hip to fix the lumbar spine against the table; then hyperextend the other thigh by pushing it downward over the side of the table; an affected sacroiliac joint will emit *pain* from this maneuver.

With the Patient Prone: Request the patient to turn from the supine to the prone position, and note the amount of guarding used as an indication of the *severity* of his pain. Place a pillow between the table and his pelvis for comfort. Note whether the muscle spasm and spinal deformity, observed while erect, *persist* in the prone position. Reexamine for areas of *tenderness* and *deformity*. A stepwise

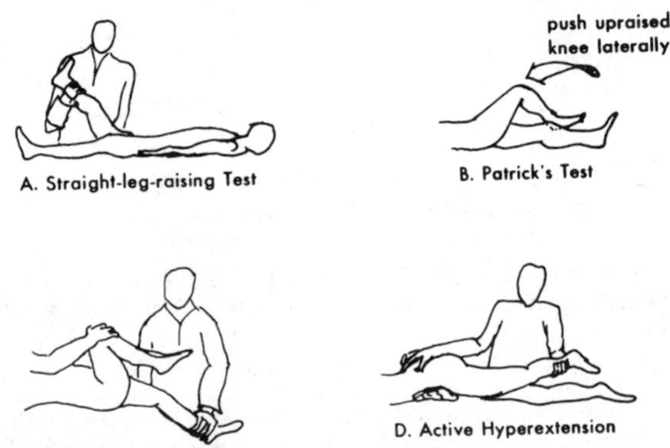

Fig. 9-32. Tests of the hip joint. **A.** Straight-leg–raising test. *To test the range of hip flexion the examiner lifts the supine patient's lower limb when the knee is held in extension.* **B.** Patrick's test. *Lateral rotation of the hip is assessed by having the knee flexed and the foot of that leg placed upon the opposite patella. The examiner then pushes the flexed knee lateralward to rotate the head of the femur outward.* **C.** Passive hyperextension of the thigh (Graenslen's test). *The supine patient flexes his knee and femur on the affected side and holds the knee with his hands to eliminate lumbar lordosis. The examiner then hyperextends the unaffected thigh by letting it sink over the side of the table. In disease of the sacroiliac joint, the maneuver evokes pain in that place.* **D.** Active hyperextension. *With the patient prone and his abdomen resting upon a pillow, the patient lifts his spine against the resistance offered by the examiner's hand; sacroiliac disease evinces pain.*

deformity between L-5 and S-1 indicates spondylolisthesis. With the heel of the hand, press along the spinous processes; *pain from light pressure* suggests approximating spines with an intervening bursa; *pain from deep pressure* occurs with involvement of intervertebral facets or disks. Active hyperextension (Fig. 9-32D) may aggravate the pain when the patient attempts to *lift his spine* against the resistance of the examiner's hand held in the lumbar region. Look for diminished tendon reflexes and atrophy of muscle masses in the lower limb as evidence of nerve injury in the back.

Dorsal Protrusion from Spine: ***Spina Bifida Cystica.*** Failure in fusion of the neural arch of a vertebra is *spina bifida.* In *spina bifida occulta,* there is no protrusion of the meninges; the only external manifestation may be a *dimple* in the skin, a patch of *hair,* or a lipomatous *nevus.* When the meninges form a sac protruding through the defective arch, it is a *meningocele* (Fig. 9-33A). The sac is *covered by healthy skin;* the local swelling is filled with spinal fluid, so it is *fluctuant* and *translucent.* When the sac contains spinal cord or cauda equina, it is termed a *myelomeningocele;* the overlying skin is frequently *defective* and transillumination may show cord or nerve fibers. Transmission of pressure from the open fontanelle to the meningocele proves the communication to be wide. Sometimes a *sinus* leads from a spina bifida occulta to the skin of the sacral region, a *congenital sacrococcygeal sinus,* often mistaken for a pilonidal sinus.

Lateral Deviation of the Spine: ***Scoliosis.*** Lateral deviation with a *single curve* is usually postural, as proved by its disappearance in extreme spinal flexion. An S-*shaped* or other *complex curve* may be compensatory or structural (Fig. 9-33B). *Compensatory scoliosis* occurs with torticollis, thoracoplasty, congenital dislocation of the hip, and shortened lower limb. *Structural scoliosis* occurs in congenital deformities, paralysis of back or abdominal muscles, and in other unexplained conditions. (For the effects of scloiosis on the thorax, see p. 277. See also Fig. 9-31.

Forward Spinal Curvature: ***Kyphosis.*** The forward concavity of the thoracic curve is accentuated, producing a hunchback (Fig. 9-33B). A *smooth curve* results from faulty posture, rigid kyphosis of adolescence (Scheuermann's disease), ankylosing spondylitis,

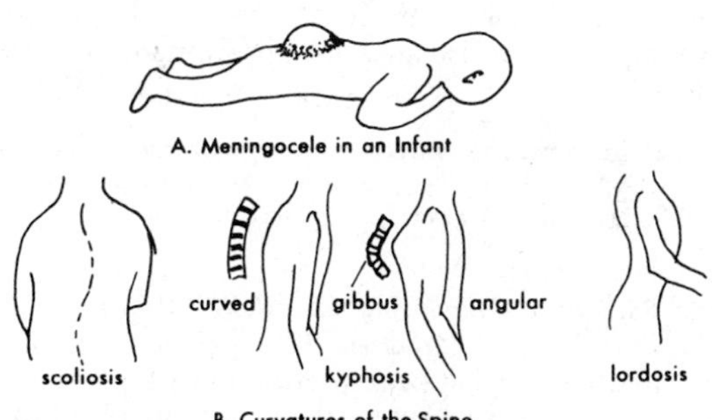

Fig. 9-33. Spinal disorders. **A.** Meningocele. **B.** Curvatures of the spine.

osteitis deformans (Paget's disease of bone), senile osteoporosis (dowager's hump), and senile kyphosis (dorsum rotundum). Of these, only the curve of faulty posture disappears with spinal flexion. An *angular curve* is also called a *gibbus;* it is caused by the collapse of the bodies of one or more contiguous vertebrae from compression fracture, metastatic carcinoma, or infectious spondylitis. (For the effect of kyphosis on the thorax, see p. 275).

Backward Spinal Curvature: ***Lordosis.*** The normal posterior concavity of the lumbar curve is accentuated (Fig. 9-33B). This may be to counterbalance a protuberant abdomen in advanced pregnancy, obesity, rickets, or cretinism. It compensates for other spinal deformities in spondylolisthesis, thoracic kyphosis, flexion contracture of the hip joint, congenital hip dislocation, coxa vara, shortening of the Achilles tendons. (For the resulting thoracic deformities, see p. 276).

Pain in the Spine: ***Infectious Spondylitis.*** At the site of the lesion *pain* and *tenderness* of the spinous vertebral processes are usually present, although not invariably in tuberculosis. Often there is accompanying *spasm* of the Sacrospinalis. The pain may be *referred* along a spinal nerve to be mistaken for appendicitis, pleurisy, or sciatica, *if the back is not examined.* Collapse of the vertebral body causes a *gibbus;* paraplegia may result. *Psoas abscess,* classic in tuberculosis, may form along the sheath of the Psoas and point beneath the inguinal ligament. Pain in the spine may be localized by having the patient jump and land on his heels, *heel-landing test.* *Distinction.* The diagnosis of spondylitis is usually confirmed by the x-ray findings. The causative organism is isolated by appropriate bacteriologic methods.

Clinical Occurrence. Infections with pyogenic organisms, such as hemolytic *Staphylococcus aureus,* are most common. Tuberculosis, typhoid fever, brucellosis, coccidioidomycosis, actinomycosis are rare causes.

Chronic Back Pain: ***Ankylosing Spondylitis*** (Marie-Strümpell-Bechterew Syndrome). *Prodrome:* Nonspecific symptoms often begin in childhood and appear intermittently for 5 or 10 years. Episodes of acute or subacute arthritis may involve hip, knee, shoulder, sternoclavicular, or manubriosternal joints, prompting a transient diagnosis of Still's disease. At this age there is little hint of the ultimate mature pattern. **Mature Symptoms:** In the late teens or early twenties attention gradually centers on the spine. *Pain* and *morning stiffness* are felt in the lumbar region and hips. Slowly the process ascends the lumbar and thoracic spine; the cervical region may be involved late. The symptoms fluctuate between remissions and exacerbations. **Physical Signs:** *Tenderness* is found over the involved joints. The spine loses its *flexibility;* the normal lumbar lordosis is straightened. Spinal *rotation* and *lateral bending* are impaired. Iridocyclitis occurs in one fifth of the cases. A unique type of *aortic regurgitation* occasionally develops. **Laboratory Findings:** The rheumatoid factor is generally absent from the blood. **X-ray Findings:** Diagnostic signs are bilateral sclerosis of subchondral bone, blurred sacroiliac joints, fusion of sacrum and ilium, calcification of intervertebral disks and ligaments. **Extra-articular Associations:** nongranulomatous anterior uveitis, pleuropulmonary lesions (apical fibrobullous disease, pleural effusion, pleural thickening, aspergillosis of the lung), aortic regurgitation, cardiac conductive abnormalities, thickening of the aortic valve wall and sinuses, amyloidosis, high incidence of HLA-B27 antigen [H. B. Luthra: Extra-articular Manifestations of Ankylosing Spondylitis, *Mayo Clin. Proc.*, **52:**655–56, 1977].

Clinical Occurrence. Idiopathic, psoriasis, segmental ileitis (Crohn's disease), ulcerative colitis, Reiter's disease, intestinal lipodystrophy (Whipple's disease).

Low Back Pain with Spinal Indentation: Spondylolisthesis. Usually L-5 slips forward on S-1 (Fig. 9-34A) because of fracture or degeneration of the articular processes of the neural arch; occasionally, a defect of the lamina may be inherited. If symptoms occur, there is usually *low back pain,* often referred to the coccyx or the lateral aspect of the leg (L-5 dermatome, see pp. 828–31). Inspection frequently discloses a *transverse loin crease* in the back. Palpation of the lumbar region reveals a *deep recession* of the spinous process of L-5. There is *restricted flexion* of the lower spine. X-ray findings confirm the diagnosis.

Low Back Pain: Prolapsed Intervertebral Disk (Fig. 9-34B). The onset of low back pain may be *gradual;* or the pain may occur *suddenly,* with or without *sciatica;* occasionally, sciatica is the

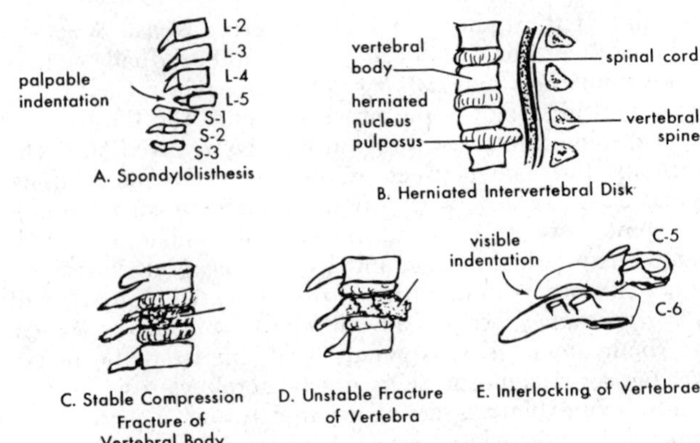

Fig. 9-34. Lesions of a single vertebra. **A.** Spondylolisthesis. **B.** Herniated intervertebral disk. **C.** Stable compression fracture of a vertebra. **D.** Unstable compression fracture of a vertebra. **E.** Interlocking or subluxation of vertebrae.

presenting symptom. Sciatic pain begins in the buttock, but soon radiates to the thigh; in severe cases, the pain involves the leg, usually the lateral aspect, and some or all of the toes rm (dermatomes L-4 to S-3, see pp. 828–31). Coughing, sneezing, or the Valsalva maneuver *accentuates* the pain. Herniated disk is attended by symptom-free remissions; continuous back pain is usually caused by some other lesion.

EXAMINATION FOR HERNIATED DISK. ***Examination Standing:*** **The patient stands with the spine *flexed*, frequently with concomitant *lateral deviation* toward the affected side. Active *flexion* and *extension* of the spine are *limited*, but *lateral bending* and *rotation* are little affected. Local *deep tenderness* is usually present 2 inches (5 cm) lateral to the midline, more pronounced on the affected side. *Muscle spasm* is most severe over the ipsilateral Sacrospinalis. *Examination Prone:* Look for muscle rigidity, areas of tenderness, tender fibrositic nodules, and trigger points. With sciatica, test the ankle jerks; they are lost with nerve irritation, regardless of cause. Test spinal *extension;* it is diminished with prolapsed disk and spondylitis. *Examination Supine:* Measure the lower limbs (p. 745) to exclude deformities of the hip joint. In sciatica, test for *toe-drop*, especially of the great** toe. With the straight-leg–raising test, record the angle at which pain is experienced; then repeat the maneuver, dorsiflexing the foot sharply, as the painful angle is approached, to stretch the sciatic nerve and test its irritability. In rigid adolescent kyphosis, flexion in this test is limited to about 60°. Pain occurs at less than 40° when there is actual impingement of a prolapsed disk; when pain occurs only at much greater angles, the sensitivity of the nerve may be from other causes. Check sensation for the dermatome level involved. *Reverse Straight-Leg–Raising Test for Intervertebral Disk.* [See R. C. Gardner: New Test for Intervertebral Disk Disease, *Ann. Intern. Med.*, 75:480–81, 1971.] With the patient still lying *prone* and his knee flexed maximally on the thigh, the normal person complains of quadriceps tightness in the *anterior thigh.* But with true disk disease, the pain is felt *in the back* or in the *sciatic distribution* on the affected side. This pain is evoked by the root tightening over the involved disk, while abdominal compression increases the pressure in the subarachnoid space. The author found the test to be negative in neurotic patients. *Crossed-Straight-Leg–Raising Test:* This is considered by some writers to be pathognomonic of herniated disk. Have the patient with low back pain and unilateral sciatic pain lie supine and lift the unaffected limb with the knee held straight. In the presence of herniated disk this maneuver will exacerbate the pain in the affected limb and also cause sciatic pain in the hitherto unaffected limb [W. R. Hudgins: *N. Engl. J Med.*, 297:1127, 1977; J. M. Sherwin: *N. Engl. J. Med.*, 298:1285, 1978].

Posttraumatic Middle Back Pain: **Stable Compression Fracture of Vertebral Body** (with Intact Spinal Ligaments). Usually the thoracic or lumbar vertebrae are fractured by trauma that crushes their bodies, such as forceful hyperflexion of the spine, falling and landing on the feet or buttocks, or a downward blow on the shoulders (Fig. 9-34C). *Pain* and *tenderness* at the fracture site may be mild, or even absent for weeks, so fracture may not be suspected until an x-ray film is taken. Occasionally, slight *kyphosis* is present.

Posttraumatic Middle Back Pain: **Unstable Compression Fracture of Vertebral Body** (with Torn Spinal Ligaments) (Fig. 9-34D). Rupture of the interspinal and supraspinal ligaments, accompanying the compression fracture, permits the articular facets of two adjacent vertebrae to slide apart; on recoil, they may *interlock* (Fig. 9-34E). This dangerous condition should be diagnosed clinically by palpating a *gap between two spinous* *processes,* to be distinguished from fracture-dislocation by x-ray films.

Posttraumatic Low Back Pain: **Fracture of a Transverse Process.** Usually the transverse process of a lumbar vertebra is fractured from violent contraction of the attached muscles. If caused by a direct blow, repeated searches for *blood in the urine* are required to exclude a concomitant ruptured kidney. There is *severe pain* in the lumbar region, with intense *muscle spasm.* The spinous processes are *not tender.* Only x-ray films can make the diagnosis.

Posttraumatic Low Back Pain: **Fracture of a Lamina.** This usually occurs in the lumbar vertebrae. *Pain* and *tenderness* are present. The diagnosis is only possible in the x-ray films.

Posttraumatic Back Pain: **Fracture-Dislocation of Vertebrae.** Violent hyperflexion of the spine, in addition to fracturing the vertebrae, may tear the supporting ligaments, permitting vertebral dislocation and consequent damage to the spinal cord. This complication should be suspected when the palpating finger finds a *gap between two spinous processes.* X-ray examination is needed to distinguish the condition from unstable compression fracture.

TESTING FOR TENDERNESS OF THE SACROILIAC JOINT. **Have the patient seated with his back toward you. Locate the sacroiliac joints by the *dimples* in the overlying skin. If dimples are lacking, place your thumbs on the *iliac crests* with your hands around his trunk (Fig. 9-35); follow the crests medially with your thumbs to locate the *posterior superior iliac spines;* move your thumbs one fingerbreadth medial to the spines for the area of the joints most accessible to palpation. With your thumbs in place, have the patient bend forward slowly, and press deeply along the joint clefts to elicit tenderness.**

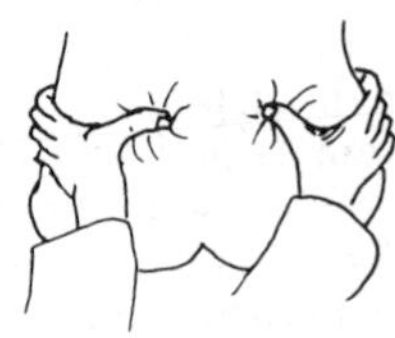

Fig. 9-35. Palpation of the sacroiliac joints.

Sacroiliac Pain: **Sacroiliac Strain.** Strain or postpartum relaxation of the ligaments about the joint is followed by inflammation. The patient complains of *pain* in the joint or in one of the reference areas, the inguinal region, the upper outer quadrant of the buttock, or the posterolateral aspect of the thigh (dermatomes L-4, L-5, S-1, see pp. 828–31). The pain is *accentuated* by spinal rotation, but not by extension or flexion. The sacroiliac joint is *tender.* The tendon reflexes in the lower limbs are normal.

Sacroiliac Pain: **Sacroiliac Arthritis.** There is *painful stiffness* in the joint on arising; *pain* may be referred to the upper outer quadrant of the buttock, the inguinal region, or the posterolateral aspect of the thigh. Sometimes there is a *limp.* Spinal rotation *accentuates* pain. The joint is *tender.*

Clinical Occurrence. Reiter's syndrome, ankylosing spondylitis, or unassociated with other conditions.

Sacroiliac Pain: **Tuberculous Arthritis.** Frequently there is *pain* in the lower midline of the spine, in the inguinal region, or sometimes in the sciatic distribution. Although the abscess is extra-articular, joint *pain* and *tenderness* are intense. The abscess may burst and drain through the skin over the joint, posteriorly, or in the inguinal region along the Iliopsoas.

Lumbosacral Pain: **Lumbosacral Strain.** Usually the patient is a woman, between 25 and 50 years of age, who complains of *aching pain* near L-5 or S-1; the pain may radiate forward or to the lateral aspect of the thigh. Flexing the back *accentuates* the pain. Standing or sitting, the profile shows *increased concavity* of the lumbar curve; motion of the spine is usually accompanied by some *muscle spasm.* Spinal flexion is slightly *limited.* The patient cannot lie flat *without flexing* the knees and hips to relieve pain. The straight-leg–raising test is negative except that *lumbosacral pain* occurs at extreme flexion. Have the patient lie prone with the pelvis resting on four pillows to separate the spinous processes. In this position, palpation of the supraspinous ligament reveals *tenderness* above or below the spine of L-5; sometimes a *depression* is found at that site.

Lumbosacral Pain: **Various Causes.** In many instances, the symptoms closely resemble those of lumbosacral strain, but most physical signs of strain are absent or equivocal, so other causes should be sought.

Clinical Occurrence: Pregnancy, pelvic tumor, prostatitis, prostatic carcinoma, Reiter's syndrome, functional backache.

Low Back Pain: ***Pointing Test for Malingering.*** Low back pain is a favorite complaint of malingerers. One method of exposure is *Magnuson's test.* When the patient indicates a painful spot in the lower back, it is marked with a skin pencil. As a diversion, the examiner proceeds with tests elsewhere in the body; later, he again palpates the back and elicits a *different* painful site. The patient with organic disease identifies the same point each time.

The Lower Limb

The Hip Joint and Thigh

In the diagnostic examination, the hip joint and thigh are considered together. The straight femoral axis slants medialward toward the knee. The *greater trochanter* of the femur presents a lateral body mass, palpable through the thigh muscles (Fig. 9-36A). On the medial side and a little distal is the *lesser trochanter,* smaller in size and inaccessible to palpation. Arising between the trochanters, the *femoral neck* slants proximally and medially, forming an angle with the straight femoral axis of 120° to 160° (greatest in children, about 127° in adults). It follows that increase in the angle produces lateral deviation of the femoral shaft, *coxa valga;* decrease in the angle deviates the shaft medially, *coxa vara.* The neck is surmounted by the globular *femoral head* that fits into the cupped *acetabulum* of the hip bone, forming a ball-and-socket joint. This joint permits flexion-extension, abduction-adduction, rotation in extension (inward and outward), and rotation in flexion (inward and outward). For measurements see Fig. 9-36C. An important topographic relationship is defined by *Nélaton's line,* extending from the anterior superior iliac spine to the ischial tuberosity. With the *thigh flexed,* the line passes through the tip of the greater trochanter, but an upward deviation of 1 cm is considered normal (Fig. 9-36B).

▼ *Key Symptom:* ***Pain in the Hip, Thigh, or Leg.*** Pain in the lower extremity frequently presents the problem of distinguishing between the primary lesion and painful structures resulting from the redistribution of weight bearing to favor the original

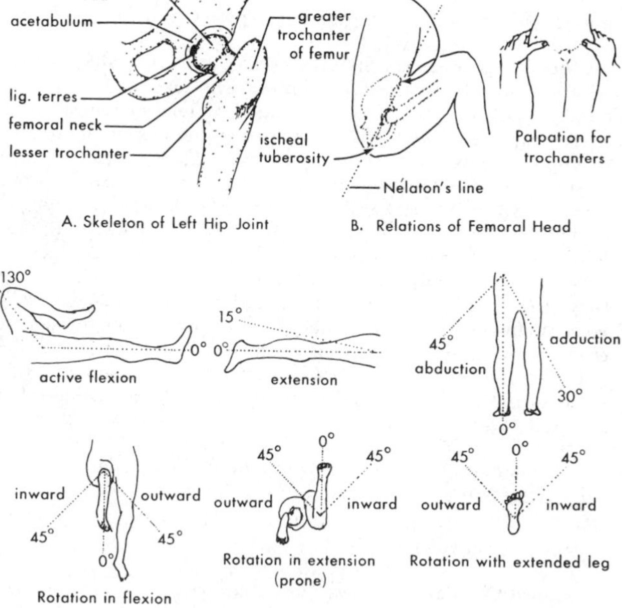

Fig. 9-36. Anatomy and motions of the hip joint. **A.** Skeleton of the left hip joint. **B.** Relations of the femoral head. *The femoral greater trochanter lies on Nélaton's line between the anterior superior iliac spine and the ischial tuberosity. The relative positions of the femoral heads with respect to the trochanters can be compared on the two sides as illustrated. The thumbs are placed upon the anterior superior iliac spines, while the fingers rest upon the greater trochanters of the femora. Small disparities in distance are readily detected.* **C.** Motions of the hip joint.

disorder. For example, limping on a chronically painful foot causes muscle strain throughout the pelvis and both lower limbs. In many cases one identifies the painful structure by precise localization of the tenderness together with movements of the limb that produce accentuation of the pain. Palpation may demonstrate discontinuity of structures, dislocations, crepitus in bones or tendon sheaths, abscesses, neoplasms. An anatomic classification for diagnostic purposes follows.

Clinical Occurrence: SHARPLY LOCALIZED PAIN: *Muscles:* muscle strain, myoischemia, cellulitis, fibrositis, herniation of fat through muscle sheath, bursitis, infarction of muscle. *Tendons:* tenosynovitis, tendon rupture. *Joints:* arthritis, herniated intervertebral disk, dislocations, subluxations, spondylolisthesis. *Bones:* fractures, neoplasms, osteomyelitis, osteoporosis, osteomalacia. *Arteries:* thrombosis, embolism, arteritis. *Veins:* thrombosis, thrombophlebitis.

PAIN DISTRIBUTED BY LUMBOSACRAL OR PELVIC NERVES. *Intrinsic Lesions:* direct trauma, neuritis, tabes dorsalis, neoplasms (especially neurofibromas), peripheral neuritis, postherpetic neuralgia. *Compression or Invasion:* by abscesses, granulomas, neoplasms, dislocations, subluxations, spondylolisthesis, aneurysms, meningeal hemorrhage (compressing the cauda equina), hydatid cyst, herniated intervertebral disk. *Referred Pain:* special attention should be devoted to the fact that lesions in the hip joint sometimes produce *pain in the knee.*

— *Sacral Pain:* ***Lesions of the Cauda Equina.*** Pain may be localized to the *sacral region,* but the overlying skin may be *anesthetic.* Frequent accompaniments are *bladder* symptoms, relaxation of *anal sphincter,* and *impotence.*

Clinical Occurrence. *Compression:* herniated intervertebral disk with posterior protrusion, hydatid cyst, neoplasms. *Intrinsic Lesions:* neurofibroma or other neoplasm, hemorrhage or infection of the meninges, intrathecal injections.

— *Pain in Buttock and Posterior Thigh:* ***Sciatica.*** This is pain in the distribution of the sciatic nerve. The discomfort is felt in the buttock, the posterior thigh, the posterolateral aspect of the leg, and around the lateral malleolus to the lateral dorsum of the foot and the entire sole. When the nerve is *directly* involved, paresthesias are felt in the same distribution. Pain and paresthesias are *intensified by coughing* or *straining at defecation.* The nerve trunk is *tender* when palpated externally at the sciatic notch or when felt on the lateral wall of the rectum during a digital examination. Pain is also elicited by *stretching* the nerve when the leg is extended while the thigh is flexed (*Lasègue's sign or straight-leg raising*). Rectal examination should always be made to elicit nerve tenderness and find masses impinging on the trunk. A *pulsating rectal mass associated with sciatica* should suggest aneurysm of the internal iliac or common iliac artery compressing the nerve (p. 580).

Clinical Occurrence. Sciatica may be produced by all the disorders listed as causes of localized pain in the lower limb. But the great majority of the cases can be attributed to herniated intervertebral disk, spondylosis, or sacroiliac disease.

— *Pain in the Buttock:* ***Ischiogluteal Bursitis*** (Weaver's Bottom). It is well to recall this ancient but seldom-mentioned ailment [R. Swartout, and E. L. Compere: Ischiogluteal Bursitis. The Pain in the Arse, *J.A.M.A.*, **227**:551–52, 1974]. *Symptoms.* The onset is sudden with exquisite, unrelenting *pain in the buttock.* The pain may be spontaneous or provoked by riding a tractor or on other vibrating poorly cushioned seat. The pain persists all night; the patient rolls and tosses in a vain attempt to find comfortable posture. Mild analgesics give no relief. The pain is *aggravated by sitting,* but a hard seat is preferable to a soft one. *Coughing* induces pain down the posterior aspect of the thigh to the knee. Often the patient needs assistance with dressing and undressing. *Physical Signs.* The patient looks haggard from lack of sleep. He stands and walks with a *list toward the affected side;* the stride on his affected side is *shortened* and he *circumducts that foot* when walking. To stand on *tiptoe* is painfully impossible. Watch the patient get onto the examining table; he sits with his *affected buttock carefully elevated,* and to lie down he supports his pelvis with the hand on the unaffected side, suggesting sciatic nerve irritation. *A very tender ischial tuberosity is a cardinal sign.* When supine, the straight-leg–raising test causes *pain at 40°* elevation from the table (Lasègue's sign). *Patrick's fabere sign* is present and causes severe pain (in this test the heel of the affected side is placed on the contralateral patella and the ipsilateral knee is pushed outward to rotate the hip laterally). Although very painful, a rectal examination in the supine position is necessary, where one palpates a region of *tender, bulging, doughy tissue* in the lateral rectal wall. *Laboratory Findings.* Not diagnostic. *Pathophysiology.* When the patient stands, the gluteal muscles cover the ischial tuberosities, but when sitting the muscles slide upward and expose tuberosities to outside pressure through only intervening skin and fibrous tissue. Long sitting on a hard surface with the thighs somewhat hyperflexed will cause irritation of the bursa (its presence is inconstant). Certain occupations involving this posture tend to induce the disorder, as indicated by the ancient name derived from Chaucer's weaver [R. F. Buchan: Weaver's Bottom, *J.A.M.A.*, **228**:567–68, 1974]. *Distinction.* Pain in the buttock suggests herniated intervertebral disk, thrombophlebitis, spinal cord tumor, lumbosacral disease, sacroiliac disease, spondylolisthesis, spasm of the piriformis muscle [P. R. Trommer: Letter, *J.A.M.A.*, **228**:566, 1974]. Patients with herniated disk and lumbosacral disease lie quietly and lack Patrick's fabere sign, both contrasting with ischiogluteal bursitis. In spinal cord tumor, percussion over the spine aggravates the pain. X-ray films show spondylolisthesis.

Clinical Occurrence. Chronic trauma to bursa; a complication of gout [C. R. Anderson: Weaver's Bottom, *J.A.M.A.*, **228**:565, 1974].

— *Pain in the Thighs:* ***Bacteremia.*** Bilaterally painful or tender anterior thighs were prominent presenting symptoms in 4 patients ranging in age from 22 to 37 years who subsequently were proved to have bacteremia with *Neisseria meningitidis, Staphylococcus aureus* (2), and *Streptobacillus moniliformis.* Other patients observed, but not examined as intensively, had anterior thigh pain or tenderness with bacteremia from *Streptococcus pneumoniae, Streptococcus pyogenes, Klebsiella pneumoniae, Escherichia coli,* and *Pseudomonas aeruginosa.* The discomfort disappeared rapidly after administration of appropriate antibiotics. The authors stress that the myalgias suggest bacteremia only if they are localized and bilateral. Physical examination reveals only tenderness and biopsies have not been made. The mechanism and frequency of occurrence are unknown, but the authors suggest that the symptom, when present, may be helpful to encourage the prompt initiation of antibiotics after blood cultures are obtained [Louria, D. B., et al.: Anterior Thigh Pain or Tenderness: A Diagnostically Useful Manifestation of Bacteremia. *Arch. Intern. Med.*, **145**:657–58, 1985.].

— *Pain in the Calves:* ***Intermittent Claudication.*** The Latin *claudicatio* means limping or lameness. The patient limps from *pain* or *weakness* in the calf or foot. There are *no symptoms at rest.* But after walking a certain fixed distance, he experiences pain or weakness in the calf muscles of one or both legs. If he stops walking, symptoms subside within a few minutes, permitting him to resume walking for another similar distance without symptoms. When he continues walking despite symptoms, muscle cramps are likely to occur; occasionally the pain subsides while walking. ***Physical Signs.*** In the affected limb pulsations are *diminished* or *absent* in the popliteal, dorsalis pedis, and posterior tibial arteries, and also occasionally in the femoral artery. Each patient has a fairly constant fixed distance of locomotion that produces pain. The distance is shortened by progressive narrowing of the arterial caliber or by diminution of oxygen-carrying capacity of the blood from anemia or oligocythemia. ***Pathophysiology.*** The caliber of arterial lumens in the legs is sufficient for the resting muscles. But during locomotion the increased circulatory demands of the muscles cannot be met, and unknown metabolites accumulate and cause pain, as in angina pectoris. The arterial caliber determines the fixed distance of symptomless walking. Anemia increases the deficit by loss of oxygen-carrying capacity; in polycythemia the increased viscosity of the blood slows the flow rate.

Clinical Occurrence. Atherosclerosis of the arteries in the legs, thrombosis, embolism, thromboangiitis obliterans, premature calcification of arteries in pseudoxanthoma elasticum.

— *Unilateral Claudication in the Young:* ***Popliteal Artery Entrapment Syndrome.*** The patient is not old enough to have atherosclerosis. He develops *unilateral claudication,* with absence of or diminished pulses in the ipsilateral popliteal and dorsalis pedis arteries. The arteriogram shows clearly a congenital anomaly in which the popliteal artery is entrapped by the medial head of the gastrocnemius muscle [G. R. Turner, W. G. Gosney, W. Ellingson, and M. Gaspar: Popliteal Artery Entrapment Syndrome, *J.A.M.A.,* **208:**692–93, 1969].

EXAMINATION OF THE HIP AND THIGH. ***With the Patient Erect:*** **The patient should be stripped from the waist down, although a woman may be permitted to wear a G string, covering the perineum but not the buttocks. Look for abnormalities of *gait;* swinging the limb from the lumbar spine suggests ankylosis; the *waddling gait* is typical in bilateral hip dislocation; the *gluteal gait* (Trendelenburg gait), with the trunk listing to the affected side with each step, suggests unilateral hip dislocation; the *painful gait* is not distinctive. With the patient standing still, look for a *list* to one side, *asymmetry* of the buttocks and other muscle masses, *scars,* and *sinuses.***

Sites of Pain: Have the patient *point* to the site of pain. An affected hip joint commonly causes pain in the inguinal region or in the buttocks posterior to the greater trochanter. Most misleading, pain from the hip joint may be felt *only in the knee;* this has led to many diagnostic errors.

Lateral Tilting of the Pelvis: Sit in front of the standing patient, with your thumbs on the anterior superior iliac spines, and ascertain whether the interspinous line is horizontal.

Lateral tilting results either from adduction of one thigh or from actual shortening of the limb. Next, ascertain the distance between the greater trochanters and the anterior superior iliac spines: with your middle fingers, find the tips of the greater trochanters and palpate the distances to the spines; small disparities can be detected in this manner. If one trochanter is higher, place books or blocks under the foot of the shorter limb until the pelvis is horizontal; this provides an accurate measurement of shortening.

With the Patient Lying: Have the patient lie on a hard examining table. All the following tests are made in the supine position, except that for extension.

Test for Rotation with Extension: This motion should be tested first because it is gentlest; if painful, all other maneuvers should be carried out cautiously, or modified. With the patient *supine,* place a hand on each side of the lower thigh and rock it from side to side, watching the patella or the foot for the range of rotation (Fig. 9-37A). Alternatively, the foot may be rocked from side to side.

Test for Rotation with Flexion: With the patient *supine,* flex the knee and hip to right angles, then move the knee from side to side.

Test for Abduction: Have the patient lying *supine* with both legs together. Place a hand on his iliac crest and grasp his ankle with your other; gradually abduct his thigh until you feel the pelvis move, and note angle attained.

Test for Adduction: With each of your hands, grasp an ankle of the *supine* patient, holding one leg down in extension while you move the other thigh across it; note the angular deviation from the neutral position; normally the thigh should cross the other midthigh.

Test for Flexion: With the patient *supine,* place your supinated hand under his lumbar spine; flex his *unaffected* thigh until his spine presses your underlying hand against the table to indicate that lordosis has been overcome; then flex the affected thigh to note any deficit in motion (Fig. 9-37C). When the test discloses diminution in flexion masked by lumbar lordosis, it is called *Hugh Owen Thomas' sign.*

Test for Extension: With the patient *prone,* steady his pelvis with one hand, while you raise his limb posteriorly by grasping his ankle with the other; normal extension is about 15°.

The Anvil Test: If other maneuvers have not been painful, raise

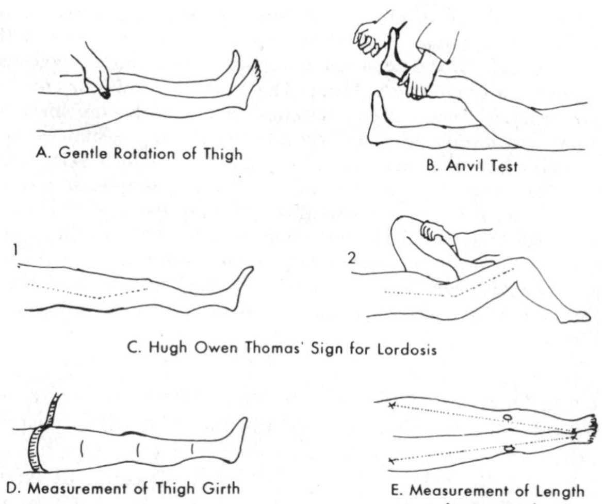

Fig. 9-37. Tests of the hip joint and thigh. **A.** Gentle rotation of thigh. **B.** Anvil test. **C.** Hugh Owen Thomas' sign for lumbar lordosis. *Flexion of the unaffected hip presses the lumbar spine against the table. If flexion of the hip is shown to be impaired by this method of eliminating lumbar lordosis, it is a positive Hugh Owen Thomas' sign.* **D.** Measurement of the girth of the thigh. *Mark similar levels on both limbs, measured down from the anterior superior iliac spines. Measure the girth at each level.* **E.** Measurement of length of limbs. *Have the two limbs approximated, or in the same relative positions from the midline. Measure from the anterior superior iliac spine to the medial malleolus, with the tape running medial to the patella.*

the limb of the supine patient from the table, with the knee in extension, and strike the calcaneus with your fist, using a moderate blow in the direction of the hip joint (Fig. 9-37B). This may elicit pain in early disease of the joint.

Direct Palpation of the Hip Joint: **Facing the patient, examine his left hip with your right hand, and his right with your left. Hook your fingers about the greater trochanter with your thumb placed on the anterior superior iliac spine. With your thumb, follow the inguinal ligament medially until you feel the pulsating femoral artery; then move your thumb just below the inguinal ligament and lateral to the artery; this should bring your thumb over the small portion of the femoral head that is extra-acetabular. Exert increas-**

ingly firm pressure to elicit *pain* from arthritis. Rock the femur gently, to feel *crepitus*. If the head *does not move,* fracture of the neck is probable. If the head *cannot be felt,* dislocation is suggested.

Measurement of the Lower Limbs: **The girth of the thighs and legs is ascertained by measuring the circumferences with a tape measure at symmetric levels, predetermined by measuring distances from the anterior superior iliac spine and marking with a skin pencil (Fig. 9-37D). The *length* of the lower limbs is measured in straight lines from the anterior superior iliac spines to the medial malleoli of the tibiae (Fig. 9-37E). Care should be taken to have the tape in a straight line running medial to the patellae. Both extremities should lie exactly equidistant from the midline. If one limb cannot be placed in normal position, its opposite should be measured in a similar position.**

Painless Limping: ***Dislocation of the Hip.*** When congenital, the condition is frequently unnoticed until walking discloses a *limp* or other *abnormal gait.* *Before Walking.* A child who has not begun to walk at 18 months should be suspected of having congenital hip dislocation. The buttocks and perineum may be unusually *broad; adductor folds* may be present on the medial aspects of the thighs. Examination shows *inability to abduct* the thighs to 80° in flexion. Pathognomonic for subluxation is *Ortolani's jerk sign,* in which the baby is supine on the table. Stand at its head and grasp the thighs in your hands. Fix the opposite side of the pelvis to the table by encircling the thigh with your hand so the thumb presses along the subcutaneous aspect of the tibia. On the side to be tested, grasp the thigh with your hand so your thumb is on the medial aspect, just below the inguinal fold, and your fingers are over the trochanteric region. While slowly abducting the thigh, push downward on the flexed knee with your thumb and pull upward with your fingers near the trochanter, until you feel a *click* as the femoral head engages the acetabulum. *In Childhood and Adolescence.* Note a *female contour* to the pelvis (both sexes have male contour at this age), and the *prominence* of the buttocks and abdomen. Seek a *gluteal* or *Trendelenburg gait* in which the hip lurches *upward* and the shoulder dips *downward* on the weightbearing side. Test for *shortening of the thigh* by having the patient supine and inspecting from the foot of the table while the knees and thighs are flexed; one knee will be higher than the other in unilateral disease. Have the patient undressed and standing while you inspect the buttocks. Ask the patient to stand on one leg; normally, the free buttock is raised when the pelvis tilts (Fig. 9-38A). In *Trendelenburg's sign,* the free buttock *falls* because the muscles are not strong enough to sustain position when the femur is not engaged in the acetabulum. The sign is also positive in affections of the glutei, in fracture of the femoral head, and in severe degrees of coxa vara. ***In Adults.*** In addition to the childhood signs, there are *hip pain* and *premature osteoarthritis* of the affected joint. ***Pathologic Dislocation.*** Hip dislocation may occur from infections of the joint, spastic paralysis, poliomyelitis, and spina bifida.

Painless Limping: ***Osteochondrosis*** (Legg-Calvé-Perthes' Disease). Aseptic necrosis of bone results in collapse and mushrooming of the femoral head. It may be unilateral or on both sides. The cause is unknown: it usually occurs in children, but sometimes persists in adults. Usually it begins with a *painless limp.* Early, all motions of the hip are slightly *impaired.* Later, there is severe *limitation* of abduction and inward rotation with flexion. Muscle *atrophy* and slight *shortening* of the limb are common. The *waddling gait* suggests dislocation of the hip. The x-ray findings are diagnostic. The affected joints later become the site of osteoarthritis.

Pain in the Hip: ***Acute Suppurative Arthritis of the Hip.*** Usually,

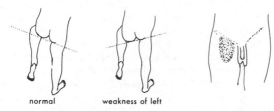

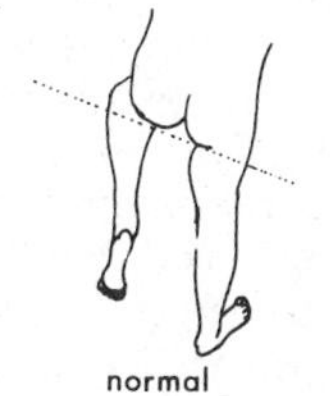

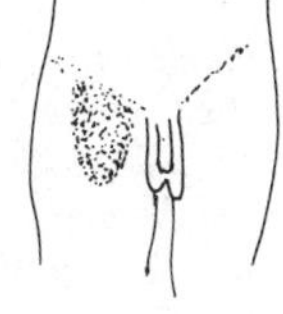

normal   weakness of left

A. Trendelenburg's Sign (sagging of unsupported buttock)

B. Subinguinal Painless Swelling

Fig. 9-38. Lesions of the hip and groin. **A.** Trendelenburg's sign. *When the patient stands on one foot, the unsupported buttock normally rises; the buttock falls in dislocation of the hip, weakness of the gluteal muscles, or paralysis.* **B.** Subinguinal painless swelling. *Swelling below the inguinal ligament may be either a psoas abscess or an effusion in the psoas bursa. Absence of an accompanying mass in the psoas fossa above the ligament excludes psoas abscess.*

there are *pain in the hip, fever, leukocytosis,* and *prostration.* All motion of the hip is painful. Sometimes *fluctuation* can be felt in the joint capsule. Do not forget that pain may be referred *only to the knee.* Pain in the knee should always prompt examination of the *hip.* Early diagnosis is *urgent* because the joint cartilage may be irreparably damaged in a few days, if proper drainage is not provided promptly.

Pain in the Hip: ***Tuberculous Arthritis.*** The onset is insidious with the appearance of a *limp.* Pain in the hip or thigh may occur only after exertion, subsiding with rest. There is early flexion of the hip masked by lumbar lordosis, as detected by *Hugh Owen Thomas' sign* (p. 746). The thigh may be held in slight *abduction* and *lateral rotation,* to best accommodate the joint effusion. When the fluid absorbs, the posture changes to *flexion, adduction,* and *inward rotation.* Finally, erosion of the joint causes shortening of the limb.

Pain in the Hip: ***Slipped Epiphysis of the Femoral Head.*** A *limp* with *hip pain* develops during adolescence, usually in boys who are either obese or unusually tall and thin. The distinguishing feature is *painful limitation of inward rotation* when thigh and knee are both flexed. This may be succeeded by *shortening* and *outward rotation* from anterosuperior displacement of the femoral neck.

Pain in the Hip: ***Osteoarthritis*** (Malum Coxae Senilis). Occasionally painless, the chief symptom is usually *boring pain* in the joint; it may be referred to the back or the knees. Early there is *stiffness* after rest, disappearing with exercise. The patient may be unaware of the *limp.* Separation of the thighs is restricted by pain; later, walking is *curtailed* from the discomfort. In unilateral disease, the thigh is held in *adduction,* with *eversion* of the foot; the pelvis is *tilted upward* on the affected side. None of these signs is evident in bilateral disease. In either case, passive motion is restricted in all directions. Capsular swelling from thickening and effusion may be *palpable.* Motion of the joint causes palpable and auscultatable *crepitus.*

Pain in the Hip: ***Fibrous Ankylosis of the Hip.*** The joint is apparently immobile, but *pain* distinguishes the condition from painless bony ankylosis. Usually there is *slight motion,* as detected by placing one hand on the anterior superior iliac spine while rocking the femur from abduction to adduction. There is complete immobility in bony ankylosis.

Painless Mass in the Femoral Triangle: ***Psoas Abscess.*** This is usually the result of osseous tuberculosis. A *painless mass* appears beneath the inguinal ligament in a conical form (Fig. 9-38B). Palpation discloses a similar swelling in the iliac fossa, to distinguish it from effusion in the Psoas bursa.

Painless Mass in the Femoral Triangle: ***Psoas Bursitis.*** Occasionally associated with osteoarthritis of the hip, an effusion develops in the Psoas bursa. There is conical swelling beneath the inguinal ligament that is so tense that it is not fluctuant (Fig. 9-38B). The absence of a mass in the iliac fossa excludes Psoas abscess.

Posttraumatic Hip Pain: ***Traumatic Dislocation of the Hip.*** While the patient is sitting, a blow on the knee may drive the femoral head *posteriorly* out of its socket, frequently fracturing the rim of the acetabulum (Fig. 9-39A). The *pain* is severe and constant in the inguinal region and thigh. The thigh lies in *extreme inward rotation, adduction,* and slight *flexion* (Fig. 9-39B). Only the foot can be actively moved. The greater trochanter is abnormally *prominent,* while palpation beneath the inguinal ligament for the femoral head yields instead an *indentation.* Passive rotation of the femur is *absent.* The limb is *shortened* about 2 inches (5cm). The rare *anterior dislocation* occurs from landing on the feet in a fall. The joint is *fixed* in *abduction, outward rotation,*

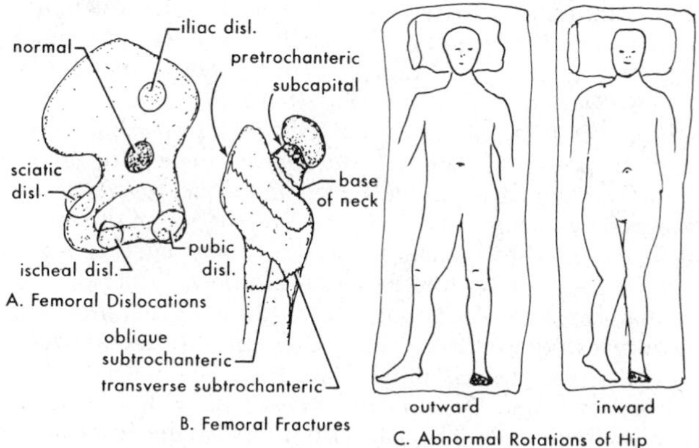

Fig. 9-39. Femoral dislocations and fractures.

and slight *flexion* (Fig. 9-39C). There is no shortening of the limb, because the head is impaled anteriorly in the iliofemoral ligament.

Posttraumatic Hip Pain: ***Fracture of the Femoral Neck.*** Usually with a fall, the femoral neck may be fractured below the capsule, *low fracture,* or within the capsule, *high fracture* (Fig. 9-39C). In the extracapsular break, the femur rests in abnormal *outward rotation* of about 90° and there is shortening; in an intracapsular fracture the joint capsule *restrains* rotation to about 45° and swelling of the upper thigh is considerable. If the patient can lift the foot off the bed, the fracture is *impacted.* In impacted fractures, the patient can sometimes walk with little pain, so the break is unsuspected; but passive rotation of the thigh will usually yield some pain.

Posttraumatic Hip Pain: ***Avulsion Fracture of the Lesser Trochanter.*** This usually occurs in muscular young men. The sitting patient cannot flex the thigh (Ludloff's sign).

Posttraumatic Thigh Pain: ***Fracture of the Femoral Shaft.*** This is usually attended with great shock because of blood loss; careful observation by the physician is required. The thigh is *rotated externally,* often with obvious grotesque deformity.

Swelling of the Thigh. Minimal herniations and exostoses are *painless;* bone tumors *cause pain.*

The Knee

For examination, the region of the knee includes the femorotibial and tibiofibular joints, the patella, the adjacent segments of the femur, tibia, and fibula, their ligaments, menisci, and muscles. Viewed from below (Fig. 9-40), the articular surface of the lower femoral end is shaped like a horseshoe with its open end posterior. The two anteroposterior legs of the shoe are formed by nearly parallel *lateral* and *medial femoral condyles,* separated by the *intercondyloid fossa.* The surface of the anterior bow is indented by a shallow median groove curving upward over the anterior femur, the *patellar surface.* Superior to the articular surfaces of the condyles are the medial and lateral epicondyles. Viewed from above, the upper tibial end presents two lateral oval facets, almost flat, the *medial* and *lateral tibial condyles,* separated by an *intercondyloid fossa* with anterior and posterior segments. The lateral borders of the fossa are the raised rims of the condyles, the *intercondyloid eminences.* On

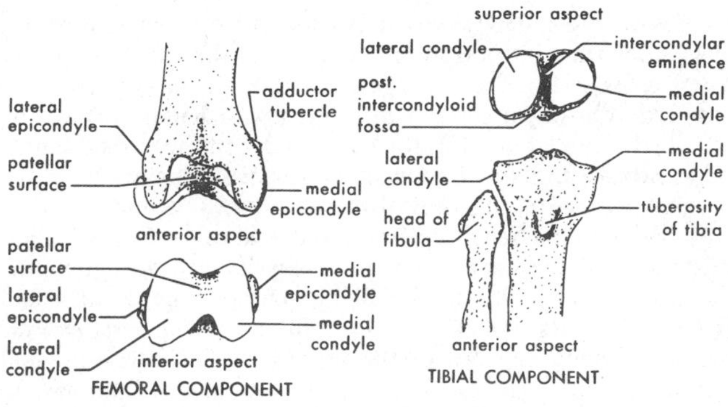

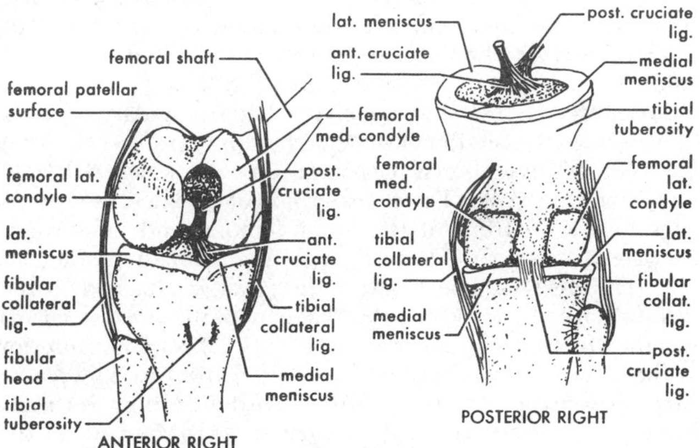

Fig. 9-40. Articular surfaces and ligaments of the right knee.

the anterior tibial surface, slightly below the point, is a midline eminence, the *tibial tuberosity*.

The knee joint is triarticular, with a medial and a lateral condyloid articulation and an anterior joint where the patella glides over the femur. The femoral condyles may be likened to two thick disks, with their edges resting upon the almost flat tibial condyles. The small radius of curvature of the disks presents little apposing surface with the tibia in any position.

The *lateral* and *medial menisci* are flattened crescents of fibrocartilage that rim the peripheral borders of the tibial condyles. Their cross sections are wedge-shaped, with the thickest part outward. This arrangement deepens the articular surfaces of the tibial condyles and fills the space between the curved femoral condyles and the flatter tibial surface. The menisci are covered with smooth synovial membranes. The ends of their crescents are attached in the intercondyloid fossa. The principal internal bands are the anterior and posterior cruciate ligaments, named for the positions of their attachments *on the tibia* and from their courses in crossing each other. The *anterior cruciate ligament* begins in front of the anterior tibial intercondyloid eminence and passes upward, backward, and *lateralward,* to be fixed to the back of the lateral femoral condyle (remember: *anterior to lateral,* A-L). The *posterior cruciate ligament,* attached to the posterior intercondyloid fossa, passes upward, forward, and *medialward,* to be fixed to the front of the medial femoral condyle (remember: *posterior to medial,* P-M).

Considered a sesamoid bone, the flat triangular *patella* is embedded in the tendon of the Quadriceps femoris. The distal extension of this tendon is the *patellar ligament,* attached distally to the tibial tuberosity. During extension of the knee, the patella rides loosely in front of the lower femoral end; in flexion, the patella apposes the lateral part of the medial femoral condyle (Fig. 9-41A). The head of the *fibula* is attached to the *lateral* tibial condyle by an arthrodial joint of the *articular capsule* and the anterior and posterior ligaments. This joint is inferior to the knee joint and entirely separated from it. The *fibular collateral ligament* is a strong fibrous cord ascending vertically from the lateral aspect of the fibular head to the back of the

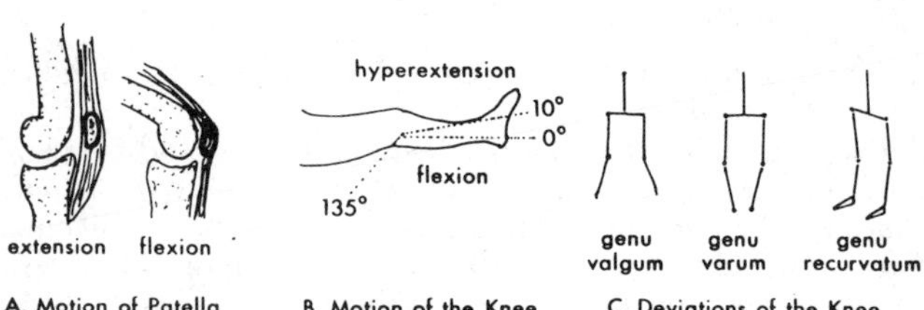

Fig. 9-41. Motions and deviations of the knee.

lateral femoral condyle. Its opposite is the *tibial collateral ligament* ascending from the medial aspect of the medial tibial condyle to the lateral aspect of the medial femoral condyle.

The *articular capsule* of the knee joint is a complex of fibrous sheets reinforced by bands from the muscle tendons around the joint. It forms a single sac that envelops the articular surfaces of both pairs of condyles. It is lined by a synovial membrane forming the largest joint cavity in the body. A precise knowledge of the extent of this sac is diagnostically important. At the femorotibial apposition the sac lines the articular capsule. A large *suprapatellar pouch* of the sac ascends anteriorly, first between the patella and the anterior aspect of the femur, then into a bursa between the Quadriceps tendon and a fat pad in front of the femur.

The principal *bursae of the knee joint* are of diagnostic interest: (1) a bursa lying between the skin and the patella, (2) a smaller bursa interposed between the patellar ligament and the infrapatellar fat pad, (3) a bursa between the skin and the tibial tuberosity, (4) the largest, lying between the Quadriceps tendon and the femur.

The normal movements of the knee are flexion and extension. Hyperextension is an unnatural motion. For measurements, see Fig. 9-41B.

GENERAL EXAMINATION OF THE KNEE. **Have the legs and thighs uncovered, and the patient standing. Inspect the knee region for *deformities, swelling,* and *muscle atrophy.* Note the *position* of the patella. Supplement inspection with palpation of abnormalities. Test swellings for *fluctuance* in the standing and reclining positions. Search for points of *tenderness.* Palpate for *doughy enlargement* and *obliteration of bony landmarks* indicating thickening of the synovium. With the patient supine, test for range of *flexion* and *extension;* test for abnormal *lateral mobility* of the knee. With a history of *pain* in the knee or *locking,* test for internal disorders of the knee joint, as described under a special heading.**

Painless Unilateral Knee Deformity: ***Neurogenic Arthropathy*** (Charcot's Joint) (Fig. 9-42C). When this is encountered, consider the gross painless deformity of Charcot's joint; see p. 665.

Knee Deformity: ***Genu Varum*** (Bowleg). The legs deviate *toward* the midline so the knees are farther apart than normally when the medial malleoli are approximated (Fig. 9-41C). The

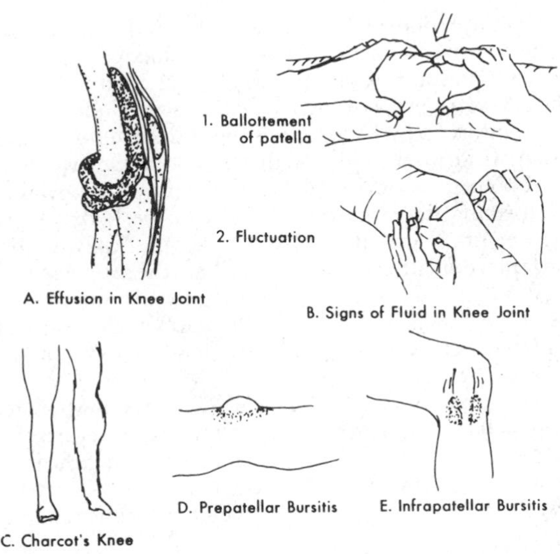

Fig. 9-42. Swellings of the knee and their diagnosis.

deformity is measured by having the patient supine with the medial malleoli together; the distance between the medial aspects of the two knees is measured. The patient usually walks with the feet turned inward.

Clinical Occurrence. Rickets affecting the upper tibial and lower femoral epiphyses, osteitis deformans (Paget's disease of bone), and occupational, as in cowboys and jockeys.

Knee Deformity: ***Genu Valgum*** (Knock-Knee) There is *lateral deviation* of the leg from the midline, usually bilateral (Fig. 9-41C). The most common cause is more prominent development of the medial femoral condyles; occasionally, laxity of ligaments of the knee is responsible. The amount of deviation is measured with the patient standing and the knees approximated; the distance between the medial malleoli is measured.

Knee Deformity: ***Genu Recurvatum.*** The knees are fixed in *hyperextension* with little ability to flex (Fig. 9-41C). This is a congenital deformity, usually from contracture of the Quadriceps femoris. The patellae are small or absent.

Anterior Knee Cyst: ***Fluid in the Knee Joint (Synovial Fluid, Pus, or Blood).*** An excess of synovial fluid in the knee joint is usually termed an *effusion* or *hydrarthrosis;* blood in the joint cavity is *hemarthrosis;* the presence of pus indicates *suppurative arthritis,* the term *pyarthrosis* is seldom used. The physical signs are the same for all; the joint contents can be *ascertained* only by diagnostic aspiration. *Moderate Amounts of Fluid.* Find *swelling above* and *on both sides* of the patella in the suprapatellar pouch of the joint sac, obliterating the natural hollows in these regions. The swelling may assume the shape of a horseshoe around the patella (Fig. 9-42A). Have the patient lie supine with the knees extended. Look for a bulge just inferior to the patella. Test for *patellar ballottement, patellar tap,* or *floating patella,* by encircling the suprapatellar region of the thigh with a hand that compresses the sides and anterior portion, while the fingers of the other hand push the patella sharply against the femur (Fig. 9-42B). If fluid is present in sufficient quantity to elevate the patella from the femur, the bone will sink under pressure and strike the femur with a *palpable tap.* *Large Amount of Fluid.* Test for *cross fluctuation* by placing the receiving hand in the suprapatellar region while the pressing hand squeezes the swelling on either side of the patellar ligament below the patella. The presence of fluctuation indicates communication with the region above, excluding swelling in the prepatellar bursa. *Small Amounts of Fluid.* Compress the swelling in one of the obliterated hollows beside the patellar ligament; watch the hollow slowly refill.

Clinical Occurrence. *Effusion of synovial fluid* is commonly caused by trauma, rheumatoid arthritis, osteoarthritis, gout, villous synovitis, articular chondrocalcinosis (pseudogout), serum sickness, intermittent hydrarthrosis. *Hemarthrosis* is usually attributable to trauma, coagulation deficit, or neoplasm. *Purulent joint fluid* is the mark of suppurative arthritis.

DIAGNOSTIC ASPIRATION OF THE KNEE JOINT. **Using the materials and general procedures described for aspiration of the wrist joint (p. 700), have the patient lying supine with the knee extended. Insert the needle at a point 1 to 2 cm medial to the inner border of the patella. Point it lateralward and posteriorly to go well under the patella.**

Anterior Knee Cyst: ***Prepatellar Bursitis*** (Housemaid's Knee). A *fluctuant swelling* occurs subcutaneously over the lower half of the patella and the upper half of the patellar ligament, the distribution of the prepatellar bursa (Fig. 9-42D). *Distinction.* The distribution differs from fluid in the joint cavity that produces swelling on either side of the patella and the patellar ligament, and the Quadriceps tendon.

Clinical Occurrence. Any occupation that produces chronic trauma to the tissue overlying the patella. Rarely tuberculosis causes an infection in which the effusion contains melon-seed bodies.

Anterior Knee Cyst: ***Infrapatellar Bursitis*** (Clergyman's Knee). A swelling occurs on both sides of the patellar ligament, near the tibial tuberosity, the position of the infrapatellar bursa (Fig. 9-42E). *Fluctuation* can be demonstrated from one side of the ligament to the other.

Clinical Occurrence. Repeated trauma to the region of the tibial tuberosity, incurred in a variety of occupations, such as roofers, floor-layers, and painters.

Anterior Knee Swelling. ***Liposynovitis Infrapatellaris*** (Hoffa's Disease). The infrapatellar fat pad becomes inflamed, causing *tenderness* and *swelling* on both sides of the patellar ligament. The tenderness and lack of fluctuance distinguish it from a cystic mass.

Popliteal Cyst: ***Popliteal Abscess.*** The *swelling* may be minimal; instead, there is *tender induration* in the popliteal fossa. The knee is held in partial *flexion* to relieve pain; extension is *painful. Fluctuation* is late in appearance. Examine the foot for the source of infection.

Popliteal Cyst: ***Semimembranosus Bursitis.*** Fluid accumulates in the bursa between the head of the Gastrocnemius and the tendon of the Semimembranosus, forming the upper medial border of the diamond-shaped popliteal fossa (Fig. 9-43). Extension of the knee, as in standing, causes *tensing* of the bursa; flexion *relaxes* it. Fluctuation is difficult to demonstrate. The swelling may be *translucent.*

Popliteal Cyst: ***Morrant Baker's Cyst.*** In contrast to the Semimembranosus bursitis, this cyst is in the *midline* of the fossa, at or below the femorotibial junction (Fig. 9-43). It *protrudes* when the knee is extended and is *not visible* with flexion, unless it is very large. The best view can be obtained by inspection of the fossa when the patient is standing. Sometimes, *dull pain*

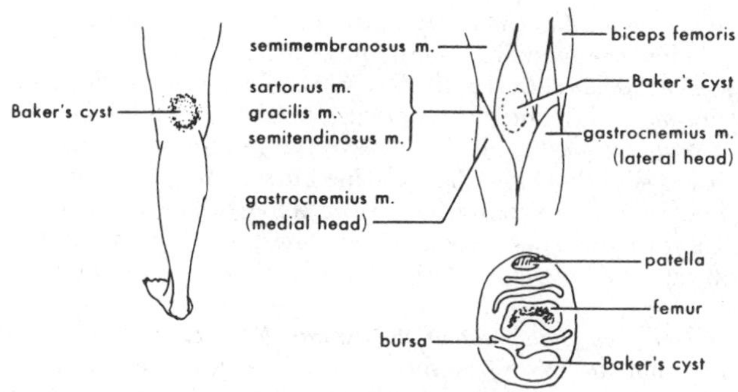

Fig. 9-43. Popliteal fossa.

is produced. The cyst is a pressure diverticulum of the synovial sac protruding through the joint capsule of the knee. If the communication is patent, gradual steady pressure on the sac forces some fluid back into the joint cavity, temporarily *reducing* the swelling. The swelling may be *translucent.* It is often a complication of rheumatoid arthritis; it may compress popliteal vessels. The diagnosis is confirmed and detailed by ultrasonography and air arthrography, if contrast media in the joint is contraindicated. *Distinction:* If the artery is still patent, *forced extension of the knee* or *strong dorsiflexion of the foot* will obliterate the pedal pulse. Femoral arteriography will indicate the aberrant course of the artery [L. K. Mark *et al.:* Popliteal Artery Entrapment Syndrome. *J.A.M.A.,* **240:**464–66, 1978].

Popliteal Cyst: **Neuromyxofibroma.** This resembles an enlarged bursa, except that it is *tender* and the pain radiates *down to the foot,* indicating involvement of the common peroneal or the lateral popliteal nerve.

Popliteal Cyst: **Popliteal Aneurysm.** This feels like a cyst. Unless conscious effort is made to find it, the examiner *may not realize that the swelling is pulsatile.* The dilatation may be arteriosclerotic or syphilitic.

Medial Knee Cyst: **Anserine Bursitis.** The *bursa anserina* lies deep to the tendons of the Sartorius, Gracilis, and Semitendinosus that form the *pes anserina* or goose's foot, and superficial to the tibial collateral ligament (Fig. 9-43). Fluid in this space produces a *fluctuant swelling* on the medial aspect of the knee, just below the medial femoral epicondyle.

Medial Knee Cyst: ***Cyst of the Medial Meniscus.*** A developmental anomaly of the medial meniscus, the cyst protrudes medially as a *fluctuant swelling* at the level of the femorotibial junction, so it lies slightly below the anserine bursa. The cyst may point either anterior or posterior to the tibial collateral ligament. Flexion of the knee makes it *more prominent.* The swelling is oval with the long axis *transverse. Dull pain* may result on standing.

Lateral Knee Cyst: ***Cyst of the Lateral Meniscus.*** The cyst is congenital, occurring at the femorotibial junction, posterior to the fibular collateral ligament. Flexion accentuates the *transverse fluctuant swelling.* It may be *painful.* Occasionally, it protrudes in the popliteal fossa.

Posttraumatic Pain near the Patella: ***Rupture of the Rectus Femoris Muscle.*** The muscle fibers of the Rectus femoris separate from the tendon well above the patella. The knee is held in *semiflexion.* The normal mass of muscle *cannot be felt* in the suprapatellar region. Later, torn fibers contract into a *lump* that enlarges when the patient tenses the thigh muscles; a *hollow* is felt distal to the lump.

Posttraumatic Patellar Pain: ***Transverse Patellar Fracture.*** Frequently there is separation of the bone fragments, so the joint is *semiflexed* and active *extension is impossible* (Fig. 9-44A). To determine separation, run the thumbnail down the subcutane-

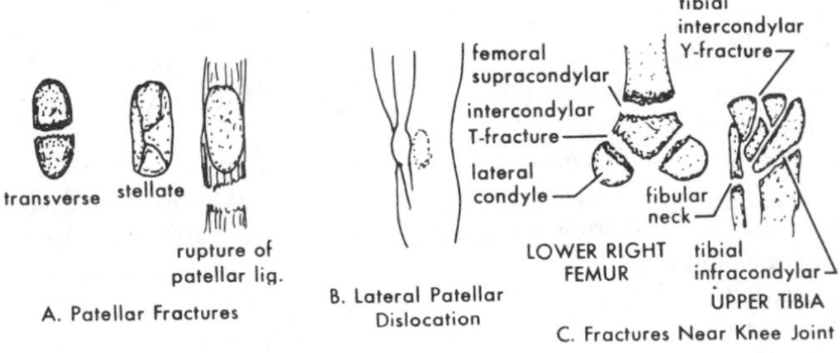

Fig. 9-44. Fractures in the knee region.

ous surface of the patella to feel a *crevice: Hemarthrosis* always occurs.

***Posttraumatic Patellar Pain:* Stellate Patellar Fracture.** This occurs from a direct blow. The fragments are not separated (Fig. 9-44A). The knee is *semiflexed;* active extension is possible but *painful.* Palpation of the patella with the thumbnail discloses *no crevice.*

***Posttraumatic Patellar Pain:* Rupture of the Patellar Ligament.** The pathognomonic sign is an *upward shift of the patella.* When the swelling subsides, the ruptured ligament may be palpated (Fig. 9-44A). Concomitant *avulsion of the tibial tuberosity,* as in Osgood-Schlatter's disease, is distinguished by *tenderness* in that prominence.

***Patellar Pain:* Chondromalacia Patellae.** Usually in women, degeneration of the articular surface of the patella occurs from unknown cause. Attacks of *pain* are precipitated by kneeling; often slight *effusion* occurs. Joint motion is painless. Pressing the patella against the condyles elicits *tenderness.* Patellar *crepitus* may be demonstrated with motion.

***Sudden Collapse with Locking Knee:* Recurrent Patellar Dislocation.** This usually occurs in women. The knee suddenly *gives way* with *sudden pain* and subsequent *swelling.* The patella is *displaced laterally* (Fig. 9-44B). Between attacks, the diagnosis must be made from the history. Quadriceps *atrophy* may occur. One can demonstrate *increased lateral mobility* of the patella.

***Posttraumatic Knee Pain:* Femoral Supracondylar Fracture.** A direct blow above the patella may produce a fracture 1 to 2 inches (2.5 to 5 cm) above the femoral condyles (Fig. 9-44C). Active motion of the knee is *impossible.* Much *tenderness* and *swelling* occur just above the patella. Displacement is usually absent. If displacement occurs, the distal fragment is pulled backward by the Gastrocnemius; *palpate the pulses* of the dorsalis pedis and the posterior tibial arteries for evidence of damage to the soft structures.

***Posttraumatic Knee Pain:* Femoral Condylar Fracture.** One condyle may be displaced upward, or the two may be separated by a T-fracture (Fig. 9-44C). The knee is *widened,* or the *upward displacement* of the condyle is obvious.

***Posttraumatic Knee Pain:* Tibial Infracondylar Fracture.** A fall with the knee extended and bent medially may cause fracture of one or both tibial condyles below the joint (Fig. 9-44C). There are *pain, swelling,* and *hemarthrosis.* A *valgus deformity* may result. Occasionally, a concomitant *fracture of the fibular head* is found.

Examination of the Ligaments of the Knee Joint. **This procedure is indicated when the cause of joint pain or locking has not been disclosed by the general examination just discussed. *History:* Ask the patient to *point* to the site of pain. Obtain a detailed account of *antecedent trauma.* Secure exact information about the *motions causing locking;* ask for a demonstration of the *position of fixation* during locking (true locking occurs at 170° of knee extension); ascertain whether unlocking was *sudden* or gradual as in muscle spasm. *Inspection:* Examine the patient supine on the table. Note evidence of joint *effusion* and muscle *atrophy. Palpation:* Feel the knee joint carefully for *point tenderness.* Palpate the *surface* of the patella and under its borders; then push the patella aside and palpate the underlying femorotibial *junction.* During joint motion, feel for a *click with pain.* A painless click is relatively unimportant; it may be caused by a tendon slipping over an eminence. *Active Motion:* Test the range of extension and flexion. *Passive Motion:* Test the range of extension and flexion. *Passive Motion:* Test extension and flexion, realizing that joint effusion limits motion. Immediately after injury, muscle spasm and swelling may seriously interfere with adequate examination, so keep the joint motionless for a day or two an reexamine.**

McMurray's Test **(Fig. 9-45A): With the patient *supine* on the table, grasp his knee with one hand so your fingers press the medial and lateral aspects of the joint, and grasp his heel with the other so the plantar surface of the foot rests along your wrist and forearm. First, *flex his knee* until the heel nearly *touches the buttock.* Next, rotate the foot *laterally* to test the posterior half of the medial meniscus. With the foot in continual lateral rotation, *bring the leg up* so the knee makes a right angle. If a *click* is felt or heard during the *extending* motion, and the patient recognizes it as the sensation preceding pain or locking, the medial meniscus is torn.**

Apley's Grinding Test **(Fig. 9-45B): Have the patient lie *prone* on a low couch, about 2 feet (60 cm) high, with his affected limb next to the examining side. Grasp the foot with both your hands and *flex* the knee to 90°. Then rotate the foot *laterally;* this should cause little discomfort. Next, rest your knee on his hamstrings to *fix* the femur, and pull the leg to *further flexion* while the foot is held in lateral rotation. *Pain* on this further flexion indicates a lesion of the *tibial collateral ligament.* Then compress the tibial condyles**

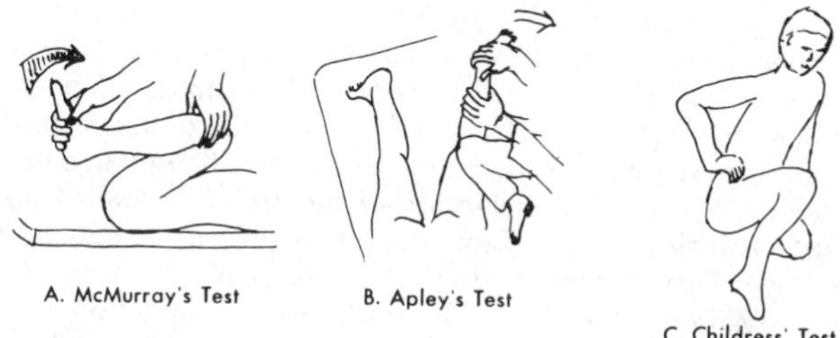

Fig. 9-45. Tests for rupture of the medial meniscus. **A.** McMurray's test. *Have the patient supine and stand at his affected side. Place one hand on his foot, the other on the affected knee. Flex the knee until the heel nearly touches the buttock. Then rotate the foot laterally to test the posterior half of the meniscus. Then with his foot still in lateral rotation, extend the knee to 90°, feeling and listening for a click that would indicate a torn ligament.* **B.** Apley's test. *Have the patient prone with the affected knee near the examiner. Grasp the foot and flex the knee to 90°, then rotate the foot laterally. Holding this position, place your knee on his hamstrings to fix the femur against the table, and pull the knee to greater flexion; if pain is produced, the tibial collateral ligament is torn. Compress the tibial condyles on the femoral condyles with the weight of your body on the plantar surface of his foot; this maneuver produces pain when the medial meniscus is torn.* **C.** Childress' test. *Have the patient squat on his toes and waddle from one foot to the other. Complete flexion cannot be attained when the posterior horn of the medial meniscus is torn.*

onto the femoral condyles by forcing your body weight onto the plantar surface of the foot, still in lateral rotation. Pain from this maneuver indicates tear of the *medial meniscus*.

CHILDRESS' DUCK-WADDLE TEST **(Fig. 9-45C). This is strenuous and is reserved for athletes. Have the patient *squat* and *waddle on his toes,* swinging from side to side. With rupture of the posterior horn of the meniscus, complete flexion *cannot be attained;* the maneuver elicits *pain* or *clicking* in the posteromedial portion of the joint.**

Medial Knee Tenderness: ***Rupture of the Medial Meniscus.*** The meniscus is usually injured when the knee is twisted *medially* while *flexed* and *weight-bearing.* The cartilage may be split longitudinally, or either anterior or posterior horn may be torn. But most commonly, there is a *bucket-handle tear* in which the horns remain attached while the curved portion is torn from its fixation on the tibial surface, so the loop is free to move laterally *into* the joint. *Locking* may occur. The most constant sign is *tenderness* over the tibial collateral ligament at the level of the joint line, when the knee is *flexed*. Tearing of the posterior horn causes tenderness *posterior* to the tibial collateral ligament.

Medial Knee Tenderness: ***Rupture of the Tibial Collateral Ligament.*** Injuries of the ligament occur from *valgus bending* of the knee. Usually the femoral attachment is torn; less often is the tibial end detached. The midportion is attached to the medial meniscus, so its injuries are properly associated with rupture of that cartilage. *Incomplete Rupture.* *Pain* in the region is severe, but function is not completely lost and movement is resumed in a few hours. The region of the ligament is *tender* and somewhat *swollen*. Lateral mobility is lacking, although attempts to elicit it evoke *pain* at the site. *Complete Rupture.* In addition to *pain* and *swelling* at the site, palpation may disclose a movable fragment of bone at the ligamentous attachment. *Slight lateral mobility* of the knee joint is often present; *pronounced mobility* indicates accompanying rupture of the anterior cruciate ligament.

TEST FOR LATERAL MOBILITY OF THE KNEE JOINT **(Fig. 9-46): Have the patient supine, and the knee in full extension, with the hip slightly flexed. Let an assistant steady the thigh with both hands while you grasp the ankle and rock the leg from side to side. The resulting motion should be compared with the normal side, which is preferably tested first. *An alternate method* is to have the patient seated while you stand. Grasp the ankle with one hand, lifting the leg to full extension; hold the knee with your other hand supinated so your fingers curl around into the popliteal fossa. Brace the back of the**

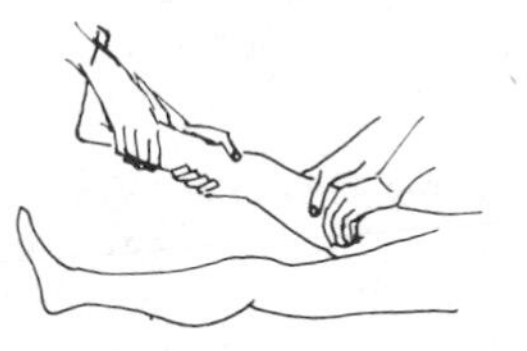

Assisted test for lateral stability of the knee

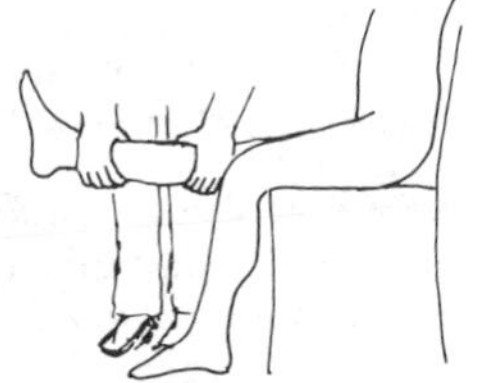

Unassisted test for lateral stability

Fig. 9-46. Tests for lateral stability of the knee joint.

supine hand against your knee while you pull the leg laterally against it. The movement should be compared with the unaffected side.

Lateral Knee Tenderness: ***Rupture of the Lateral Meniscus.*** The trauma may be so slight as to escape attention. *Pain* in the knee joint may be on the lateral aspect, but paradoxically it is often on the *medial* side. *Tenderness* is found on the lateral side over the femorotibial junction. *McMurray's* and *Apley's tests* are positive when the procedures are modified by producing *inward rotation of the foot* instead of outward rotation (p. 762). Locking of the joint is uncommon.

Lateral Knee Tenderness: ***Rupture of the Fibular Collateral Ligament.*** The injury is produced by *varus bending of the knee* and is uncommon. Usually the fibular attachment is torn; the head of the fibula may also be avulsed. *Tenderness* is found on the lateral aspect of the knee between the lateral femoral epicondyle and the fibular head. With complete severance, *the ends may be palpated. Crepitus* may be elicited to indicate avulsion of the fibular head. Slight *lateral mobility* of the knee joint may be present. A frequent complication is *damage to the common peroneal nerve,* so test movements of the anterior and lateral muscles of the leg and the short extensors of the toes.

Knee Pain, Recurrent Locking: ***Loose Body in the Joint.*** A history of intermittent joint *pain* with recurrent *effusions* or *locking* should suggest a loose body in the joint cavity. *Crepitus* may be present; rarely, the examiner may be able to palpate a mass. X-ray films usually disclose the body that is either a chip of bone from a fracture, an osteophyte from osteoarthritis, or a flake of bone in *osteochondritis dissecans.*

Instability of the Knee Joint: ***Rupture of the Anterior Cruciate Ligament.*** Violent injury to the knee joint often ruptures the anterior cruciate ligament. *Early Stage.* At the time of injury, there is great *pain,* followed by *hemarthrosis.* The joint is held in slight *flexion.* The diagnosis cannot usually be made until swelling subsides or the blood is aspirated from the joint. *Later Stage.* The principal symptom is *instability of the knee* in walking down stairs.

DRAWER SIGN **(Fig. 9-47A). This indicates anterior instability of the knee joint. Have the patient lie supine and flex the affected knee to a right angle. Sit on the patient's foot to *fix* it. With both**

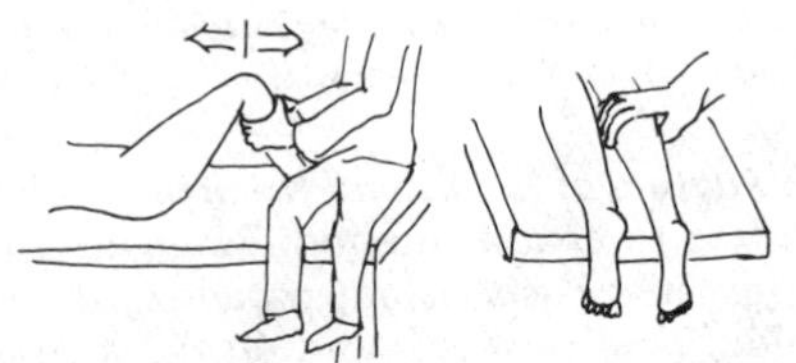

A. Drawer Sign for Torn Cruciate Lig. B. Examination for Ruptured Achilles Tendon

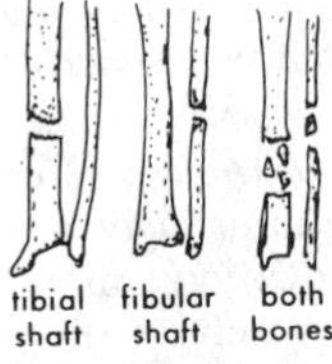

C. Fractures of Lower Tibia & Fibula

Fig. 9-47. Traumatic lesions of knee and ankle. **A.** Drawer sign for torn cruciate ligament. *The supine patient flexes his knee and rests his foot flat on the table. The examiner sits on the foot to anchor it. Then he pulls the head of the tibia toward himself to test the anterior cruciate ligament; forward motion of more than 1 cm is positive. Pushing the knee backward tests the posterior cruciate ligament.* **B.** Examination for ruptured Achilles tendon. *The prone patient hangs his feet over the end of the table. Inspection shows less natural plantar flexion on the side of rupture. Simmonds' test: Squeeze the calf muscles transversely; a normal or partially ruptured tendon will produce plantar flexion; complete rupture will not respond.* **C.** Fractures of tibia and fibula.

your hands, grasp the upper part of the leg with your fingers in the popliteal fossa and *pull* the head of the tibia toward you so it glides on the femoral condyles. Forward movement of more than 1 cm is a *positive anterior drawer sign*, indicating rupture of the anterior cruciate ligament. Always compare the motion of the unaffected knee. Excessive forward play should suggest an accompanying rupture of the tibial collateral ligament.

Instability of the Knee Joint: ***Rupture of the Posterior Cruciate Ligament.*** The injury usually results from a direct blow on the head of the tibia while the knee is flexed. The signs are similar to injury of the anterior cruciate ligament, except there is a positive *posterior* drawer sign. In this case, the sign is elicited by *pushing* the tibial head backward on the femoral condyles (see preceding item).

Chronic Arthritis of the Knee. Acute inflammation may be rheumatic fever or rheumatoid arthritis. The chronic stage may be rheumatoid arthritis, with accompanying limitation of motion and muscle atrophy. Chronic swelling with crepitus suggests either osteoarthritis or gout.

Vascular Disorders of the Leg. These are described on pp. 420–25.

The Leg

Posttraumatic Midcalf Pain: ***Soleus Tear.*** Trauma causing extreme *dorsiflexion* of the foot may tear the Soleus muscle. This produces severe *pain* and *tenderness* in the midcalf, since the Soleus underlies the Gastrocnemius.

Posttraumatic Ankle Pain: ***Rupture of the Achilles Tendon.*** The injury is usually incurred when the body weight is forcefully applied to the ball of the foot in *plantar flexion.* Complete rupture usually occurs about 2 inches (5 cm) above the calcaneal insertion of the tendon. There is sudden excruciating *pain* in the region. Attempts at limping are thwarted by severe pain. Examine the patient in the *prone* position, with the feet hanging over the end of the table (Fig. 9-47B). The foot on the affected side is held in *less plantar flexion* than its mate. The distal portion of the affected tendon seems *thicker* and *less stretched.* In complete rupture, a *gap* can be felt in the tendon; the calf muscles are contracted to form a visible *lump.* Passive dorsiflexion is *excessive.* *Simmonds' Test.* With the legs in the previously described position, squeeze the calf muscles transversely; plantar flexion of the foot results normally or with incomplete rupture; the motion is absent when the tendon is severed completely.

Posttraumatic Anterior Leg Pain: ***Fracture of the Tibial Shaft.*** The injury may be a fall on the leg or a *direct* blow to the anterior tibia (Fig. 9-47C). *Pain* is severe, and the leg *cannot bear weight.* If the skin is unbroken, palpation discloses *localized tenderness* at the fracture site. Rolling a pencil over the subcutaneous aspect of the tibia will also discover local tenderness.

Posttraumatic Anterior Leg Pain: ***Fracture of the Fibular Shaft.*** A *direct* blow on the anterolateral aspect of the leg is the most common cause (Fig. 9-47C). Usually the patient *can walk.* There is pain in the anterior leg. Normally, compressing the tibia and fibula together will cause the fibula to bend inward, *springing the fibula;* this is absent in complete fracture and the maneuver causes *pain* at the fracture site.

Posttraumatic Leg Pain: ***Fracture of Both Tibia and Fibula.*** This injury is the most common cause of compound fracture (Fig. 9-47C). Frequently the foot is *turned outward* in obvious deformity; further manipulation should be avoided, but *always palpate* the dorsalis pedis pulse for evidence of arterial damage. Lacking obvious deformity, ascertain whether the normal *straight* *line* is present between the medial aspect of the great toe, the medial malleolus, and the medial patellar border.

Abrupt Calf Pain: ***Tear of Gastrocnemius*** (Tennis Leg). Violent motion with a combination of extension and dorsiflexion of the ankle may cause a sudden sensation like a *blow* to the posterior calf, sometimes accompanied by an *audible snap.* The next step elicits intense pain in the posteromedial midcalf. Collapse or fainting often results; the person cannot walk without help. *Physical Signs. Local tenderness* and a *palpable defect* in the medial belly of the gastrocnemius. Within a few hours swelling obscures the defect for a few days. The power of *plantar flexion is diminished;* muscle tone is absent in the medial head of gastrocnemius for a few weeks. Several days later, ecchymoses extend from the medial calf to the heel and ankle. Some ankle *edema* may form [A. I. Froimson: Tennis Leg, *J.A.M.A.,* **209:**415–16, 1969].

Clinical Occurrence. In middle-aged persons during the following activities: serving a tennis ball or attempting to strike it while stretching sideways; stepping down from a curb or stepladder; slowly running or jogging.

Postexercise Tibial Pain: ***Stress Fracture of the Tibia.*** An incomplete cortical fracture of the tibia results from repeated strenuous use of the leg by athletes, dancers, soldiers, and others. A gradual onset of *dull aching pain* occurs within shortening intervals after exercise. The pain may persist with hours of rest. *Localized tenderness* over the tibia can be demonstrated, frequently along the medial subcutaneous border. *Pain* at the fracture site may be induced by *springing the tibia:* with the patient supine, place one hand on his knee and the other on his heel; pull the tibia laterally against your knee as a fulcrum. The diagnosis rests upon physical signs; x-ray films are frequently negative.

Postexercise Anterior Leg Pain: ***March Gangrene*** (Anterior Tibial Compartment Syndrome). Several hours after unusually strenuous leg exercise, *stiffness followed by pain* occurs in the anterior tibial muscular compartment. The region becomes *swollen, tender,* and *warm.* If these findings do not suggest the diagnosis *promptly,* so that the fascial sheath is incised, gangrene of the muscles results.

Postexercise Subpatellar Pain: ***Osteochondritis of Tibial Tubercle***

(*Osgood-Schlatter's Disease*). This a traction injury in adolescents in which the tibial tubercle is partly avulsed. The site gives rise to *pain after exercise*. A *tender mass* is felt and seen at the attachment of the patellar tendon.

Thickened Achilles Tendon. The thickening is more evident to palpation when the foot is dorsiflexed. The difference between the two tendons can be confirmed by lateral x-ray films of the heels in which the tendon shadows are obvious. The upper range of variation in the diameters of the pair of normal tendons is about 2 cm.

Clinical Occurrence. Xanthomata, rheumatoid nodules, repaired rupture of a tendon, acromegaly, tuberous xanthomatosis without hyperlipidemia.

The Ankle Joint

The ankle joint is a hinged articulation (ginglymus) between the tibia and the talus (astragalus) of the foot. The upper articular surface of the talus, the *trochlea*, is shaped like a pulley with a transverse axis, so the flat sides face medialward and lateralward (Fig. 9-48). The upper curvature of the pulley

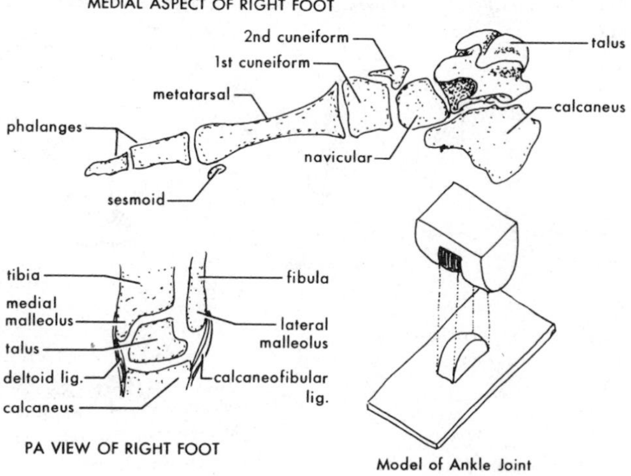

Fig. 9-48. Skeleton of the ankle joint.

articulates with a flat surface at the lower end of the tibia. At the sides of the tibial flat surface are downward projections, the *medial malleolus* of the tibia and the *lateral malleolus* of the fibula; these serve as the sides of a mortise articulating with the flat surfaces of the pulley holding it in place. During motions of the ankle, the tibial flat surface rides along the curved side of the pulley, thus changing the angle between leg and foot. The lower ends of the tibia and fibula are bound together by strong bands of the *anterior* and *posterior tibiofibular ligaments.* The medial malleolus is attached below to the talus by a triangular band, the *deltoid ligament,* that also joins the calcaneus. The lateral malleolus is attached below to the talus and the calcaneus by the *calcaneofibular ligament* and the *anterior* and *posterior talofibular ligaments.* The joint capsule surrounds the articulation and is lined with synovial membrane.

The motions of the angle joint are *dorsiflexion* (extension) and *plantar flexion* (flexion) (Fig. 9-49B). The only bony landmarks are the *lateral* and *medial malleoli;* the lateral is lower than the medial (remember: LL).

EXAMINATION OF THE ANKLE JOINT. **Have the patient supine on a table. Inspect the ankle joint for *pitting edema* and *swelling* of the joint. Test *dorsiflexion* and *plantar flexion* by grasping the heel firmly**

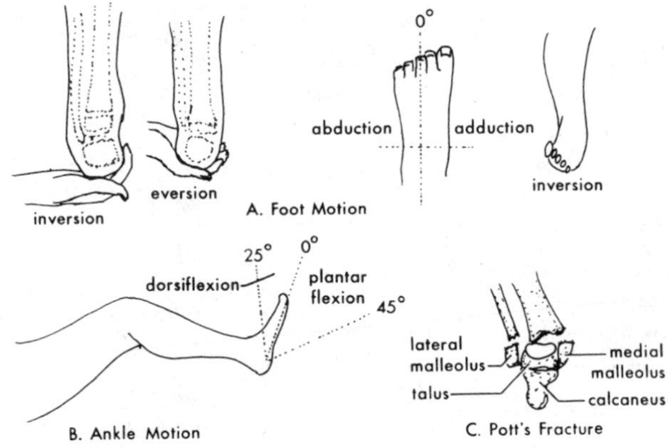

Fig. 9-49. Motions and fractures of the ankle.

with your *left* hand to immobilize the subtalar joints, while your *right* hand grasps the midfoot and moves only the talocrural joint.

Swelling of the Ankles: ***Subcutaneous Edema.*** This pits with pressure (see p. 336 for discussion).

Swelling of the Ankle Joint: ***Effusion into the Joint.*** The foot is held in slight *dorsiflexion* and *inversion.* The distended joint produces *bulging* beneath the extensor tendons, near the talotibial junction and in front of the lateral and medial malleolar ligaments.

Posttraumatic Lateral Ankle Pain: ***Rupture of the Joint Capsule.*** Forceful *plantar flexion* with eversion of the foot may break the anterolateral portion of the articular capsule. *Pain* and *tenderness* occur just anterior to the lateral malleolar ligaments (calcaneofibular and talofibular). A *hematoma* in the site rapidly appears, accompanied by some edema.

Posttraumatic Lateral Ankle Pain: ***Rupture of the Calcaneofibular Ligament.*** This results from *forced inversion* of the foot. The *tenderness* is anterior and inferior to the lateral malleolus; in a Pott's fracture, the lateral malleolus itself is tender. With *complete rupture,* careful passive inversion of the foot demonstrates *tilting* of the talus.

Posttraumatic Medial Ankle Pain: ***Rupture of the Deltoid Ligament.*** The ligament is so strong that it rarely breaks except as a complication of Pott's fracture-subluxation.

Posttraumatic Lateral Ankle Pain: ***Pott's Fracture-Subluxation.*** Usually from forced *eversion* of the foot, the fibula is fractured $1\frac{3}{4}$ inches (4.3 cm) above the malleolar tip (Fig. 9-49C). Often there is some *lateral* and *posterior displacement* of the talus. The *pain* is greatest near the lower end of the fibula. The patient *cannot stand or walk.* There is *no active motion* of the ankle. The intermalleolar distance is *greater* on the affected side. The dorsum of the foot may be *shortened.* When the fracture is incurred by landing on the feet, Pott's fracture may be complicated by an upward pushing of the talus that tears the lateral ligaments, called *Dupuytren's fracture;* the distance from malleolus to sole is *shortened.*

Pain or Click During Dorsiflexion with Eversion: ***Recurrent Slipping of Peroneal Tendons.*** The tendons of Peroneus longus and brevis curve behind and under the lateral malleolus, held in a groove by the *superior peroneal retinaculum,* a ligamentous band. Relaxation of the retinaculum may permit slipping of the tendons during dorsiflexion with eversion. *Pain* or *click* occurs with the slipping; but they are easily replaced, so the examiner must rely on the history.

Pain on Inversion of the Foot: ***Chronic Stenosing Tenosynovitis of the Peroneal Tendon Sheath.*** This causes *pain only on inversion* of the foot. *Tenderness* and *swelling* occur in the sheath behind and below the lateral malleolus.

The Foot

EXAMINATION OF THE FOOT. **Have the patient remove shoes and stockings or socks. Inspect the shoes for *uneven wear;* the well-functioning foot wears down the *lateral edge* of heel and sole; fair function of the foot wears heel and sole *evenly;* the poorly functioning foot wears the *medial* side and *tilts* the vertical heel seam in a *valgus* direction. Have the patient stand while you look for *deformities,* the *height* of the pedal arches, and *alignment* (a plumb line hanging from the midpatella should point between the 1st and 2nd metatarsal bones). Have the patient *point* to the site of pain; palpate the site for *tenderness.* With the patient supine, look for *cutaneous* lesions. Test *motion* by supporting the heel with the supine hand and grasp the foot with the other hand, to move it in *dorsiflexion, plantar flexion, eversion,* and *inversion* (Fig. 9-49A).**

The Entire Foot

Pedal Deformity: ***Talipes*** (Fig. 9-50). The five principal varieties are *talipes varus* (inversion), *talipes valgus* (eversion), *talipes equinus* (plantar flexion), *talipes calcaneus* (dorsiflexion), and *talipes* or *pes cavus* (hollowing the instep). Combined deformities are *talipes equinovarus* (clubfoot), *talipes equinovalgus, talipes calcaneovarus,* and *talipes calcaneovalgus.* The diagnosis is usually made by inspection.

Pedal Deformity: ***Pes Planus*** (Flatfoot) (Fig. 9-50). In this condition, one or more of the pedal arches are lowered. A functional classification includes *relaxed flatfoot,* in which the arch is lowered only while bearing weight; *rigid flatfoot,* caused by bony or fibrous ankylosis; *spasmodic flatfoot,* from contraction of the Peronei; *transverse flatfoot,* from flattening of the transverse arch.

EXAMINATION FOR FLATFOOT. **Have the patient stand with the feet parallel and separated by about 4 inches (10 cm). Note the height of the *medial longitudinal arch;* if flattened, ascertain whether it re-**

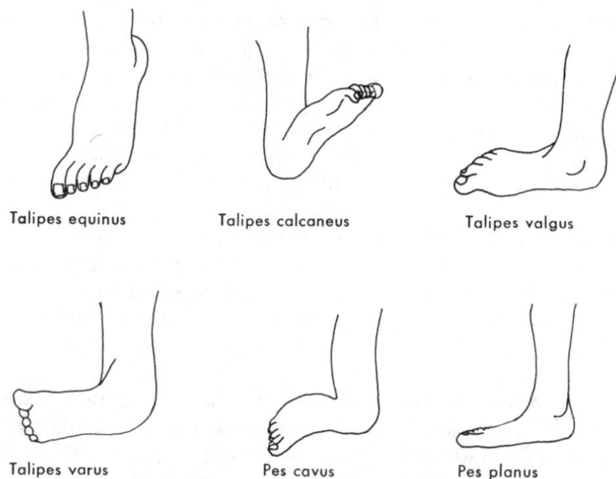

Fig. 9-50. Deformities of the foot.

sumes normal shape when weight is removed. Have him stand on his heels to test strength of the anterior leg muscles. Test for *shortening* of the Achilles tendon by dorsiflexion in the supine position. Test *inversion,* limited by spasm of the Peronei. *Test eversion,* limited in rigid flatfoot.

Cutaneous Lesions

Thickening of Thin Skin: ***Hard Corn*** (Heloma Durum). Undue pressure on thin skin, especially that covering the toes, produces a conical structure of keratin pointing into the dermis where it causes *pain.* It has a central core that can be seen when the top is pared away.

Thickening of Thin Skin: ***Soft Corn*** (Heloma Mollis). This is a corn on an interdigital surface that undergoes maceration from moisture and infection. It is quite *painful.*

Thickening of the sole: ***Callus.*** An area of Thickened skin develops in the sole as a protection against repeated pressure. It usually occurs under the metatarsal heads and the heel. Abnormal locations are clues to unusual distributions of weight. Calluses are *infrequently painful.*

Sharply Circumscribed Thickening of the Sole: **Plantar Wart** (*Verruca Pedis*). This is a warty growth caused by a virus infection. The verrucous nature may not be apparent because it is overlaid with callus. The lesions are frequently multiple. Through the sole they appear as *dark pearls; black spots* of hemorrhage may be apparent. *Pruritus is frequent.* Weight-bearing causes *pain.* Direct pressure does not yield tenderness, but pinching from the sides is *painful.*

Ulcer of the Sole: **Perforating Neurotrophic Ulcer.** A punched-out indolent painless ulcer occurs under a metatarsal head, in the pulp of the toe, or on a heel. It is often the result of peripheral neuritis in diabetes mellitus or a spinal cord lesion.

The Heel

Posttraumatic Heel Pain: **Calcaneal Fracture.** Landing on the heel from a fall may cause fracture of the calcaneus (os calcis) (Fig. 9-51A). The heel appears *broader* than normal from the back; the hollows beneath the malleoli are *obliterated. Tenderness* is maximal in the calcaneus near the insertion of the Achilles tendon. Palpation below the malleolus discloses the sides of the calcaneus to be *flush* with the malleolus, rather than indented. All motions of the ankle are *restricted* by pain. A *hematoma* forms in the sole of the heel.

Pain in the Heel: **Retrocalcaneal Bursitis.** The bursa between the Achilles tendon and the calcaneus may be inflamed so there are *pain, swelling,* and *tenderness* near the tendinous insertion (Fig. 9-51B). The lesion is incurred by wearing high-heeled shoes or stiff-backed boots.

Pain in the Heel: **Infracalcaneal Bursitis.** (Policeman's Heel). This is the result of excessive walking; the patient is usually obese. *Pain* is present in the ball of the heel. *Tenderness* occurs over the tuberosity of the calcaneus (Fig. 9-51B).

Pain in the Heel: **Infection of the Calcaneal Fat Pad.** Strong fibrous bands extend from the plantar fascia to the skin; their interstices are filled with fat. Infection is compartmented by the fibrous bulwarks. Inflammation in the unyielding tissue causes *intense pain.* The region is too *tender* to permit weight bearing. Usually edema accumulates around the ankle; *fluctuation* occasionally is present.

Pain in the Heel: **Arthritis.** This is difficult to diagnose unless

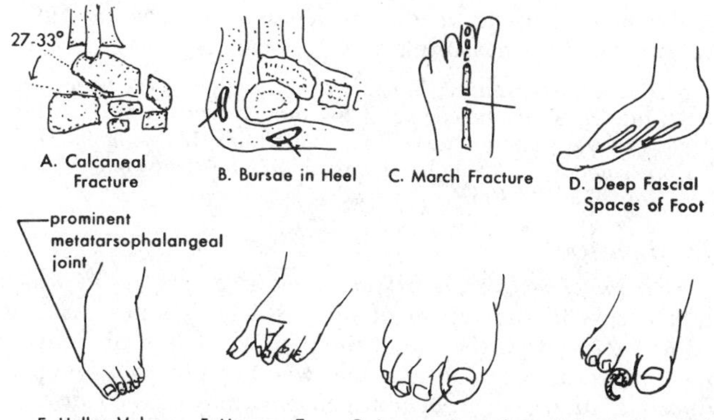

Fig. 9-51. Lesions of the foot. **A.** Calcaneal fracture. *The normal rise given by the bone is lost so the malleolus is closer to the floor. The heel is broadened.* **B.** Bursae in the heel. **C.** March fracture of a metatarsal bone. **D.** Deep fascial spaces of the foot. **E.** Hallux valgus. *This deformity shows lateral deviation of the great toe, with prominence of the 1st metatarsophalangeal joint.* **F.** Hammer toe. *The second toe is always affected. There is permanent flexion of the proximal interphalangeal point.* **G.** Ingrown toenail. *This always affects the great toe. Usually the lateral edge of the nail plate grows into the nail fold and produces a painful ulcer.* **H.** Ram's horn nail. *This is an overgrowth of the toenail with great thickening and torsion.*

other joints are also involved. There is disagreement as to whether *calcaneal spurs* cause pain.

Pain in the Heel: Tarsal-Tunnel Syndrome. The tarsal tunnel is behind and inferior to the medial malleolus of the tibia. Its bony floor is roofed by the flexor retinaculum (lancinate ligament) extending from the medial malleolus to the calcaneus. Through the tunnel pass several tendons and the posterior tibial nerve, which divides into the calcaneal nerve to the skin of the heel, the medial plantar nerve to the skin and muscles on the medial aspect of the sole, and the lateral plantar nerve to the lateral portion of the sole. Compression of the nerves in the tunnel causes *numbness, burning pain,* or *paresthesias* in portions of the sole. *Paresis* or *paralysis* of some small muscles of the foot may occur. Occasionally a *tender area* may be palpated at the margin of the medial malleolus. The diagnosis must be confirmed by measuring nerve velocities.

Clinical Occurrence. Fracture or dislocation of the bones near the tunnel, traumatic edema of the tunnel, tenosynovitis, chronic stasis of the posterior tibial vein, foot strain [J. Goodgold, H. P. Kopell, and N. I. Spielholz: The Tarsal-Tunnel Syndrome, *N. Engl. J. Med.*, **273:**742, 1965].

The Forefoot

Metatarsal Pain: ***Metatarsalgia.*** This is a *symptom* in which *pain* occurs in the region of the metatarsal bones. Ask the patient to *point out* the site of the pain with a pencil. Squeeze the foot transversely to ascertain whether the pain is reproduced. Flatfoot, corns, or fibroneuroma may be the cause.

Metatarsal Pain: ***Metatarsal Stress Fracture*** (March Fracture). Excessive walking or standing may cause a fracture of the metatarsal shaft (Fig. 9-51C). *Pain* develops *gradually. Muscle cramps* and slight *swelling* may occur. Motion of the corresponding toe is *painful.*

Metatarsal Pain: ***Infection in the Interdigital Space.*** Puncture of the sole may cause infection of one of the four interdigital subcutaneous spaces. The resulting abscess may remain under the sole, or it may point between the two metatarsals to the dorsum of the foot, forming a collar-stud abscess. Walking produces *pain* between the metatarsals. *Tenderness* is localized to the interdigital space. *Swelling of the dorsum* occurs when the abscess has penetrated through the thickness of the foot.

Pain in the Instep: ***Infection in the Deep Fascial Spaces.*** The central plantar space has four compartmented levels between the sole and the pedal arch (Fig. 9-51D). Infection of the spaces occurs from direct puncture or backward extension from an interdigital space. The diagnostic couple is *tenderness in the instep* and *dorsal edema.* The curve of the instep becomes *obliterated.*

Translucent Swelling on the Dorsum: ***Ganglion.*** This is a cyst arising from a tarsal joint capsule or an exterior tendon.

Contracture of Plantar Fascia: ***Ledderhose's Syndrome.*** The palmar fascia becomes thickened, but it is usually symptomless. It may occur unilaterally or on both sides; occasionally it is associated with Dupuytren's contracture of the palms and Peyronie's syndrome (strabismus penis) (pp. 676 and 606).

The Toes

Lateral Deviation of the Great Toe: **Hallux Valgus.** Lateral deviation of the great toe produces abnormal prominence of the 1st metatarsophalangeal joint (Fig. 9-51E). The 2nd toe may overlap the 1st, or it may be a hammer toe. The great toe retains good motion. *Pain* is caused by accompanying hammer toe, an inflamed bursa over the prominent metatarsophalangeal joint (*bunion*), or metatarsalgia from transverse flatfoot (splay foot).

Stiffened Great Toe: **Hallux Rigidus.** Chronic arthritis or epiphysitis of the 1st metatarsophalangeal joint from injury or wearing short shoes may cause *ankylosis,* usually in extension; occasionally there is fixation in the more awkward flexion. Flexion is present *only* in the interphalangeal joint. *Pain* in the joint occurs in walking and climbing. Osteophytes may cause *palpable irregularity* on the joint edges.

Fixation of Smaller Toe in Flexion: **Hammer Toe.** Usually the 2nd toe is involved. The proximal joint is *fixed in dorsiflexion,* the middle joint is fixed in *plantar flexion,* while the distal joint is *freely* movable (Fig. 9-51F). A corn or inflamed bursa frequently occurs on the prominent joint. The condition is usually bilateral; it often accompanies hallux valgus.

Shortened 5th Toe: **Absence of Middle Phalanx.** This is a frequent developmental anomaly.

Overlapping of 5th Toe: A frequent anomaly, this may be sufficiently awkward to cause symptoms.

Painful Swelling of a Toe: **Fractured Phalanx.** No matter how trivial the trauma seems, consider the possibility that the bone has been fractured. A physician consulted one of us after injecting himself with penicillin for 2 weeks because he thought he had a refractory infection of the toe. Imagine his chagrin when an x-ray film disclosed a fracture?

Painful Swelling of the Great Toe: **Gout.** This is the classic lesion of early gout, described on p. 657.

The Toenails

The toenails undergo the same changes as the fingernails, but most of the signs are less pronounced. But painful lesions are accentuated by weight-bearing; the fingernails have no similar irritant. Certain lesions of the toenails need special mention.

Subungual Pain: **Ingrown Toenail** (Onychocryptosis). Usually the lateral nail fold of the great toe is affected. Excessive transverse growth of the nail plate causes the lateral edge to lacerate the nail fold. An *ulcer* is formed and maintained by repeated trauma and infection (Fig. 9-51G). Weight-bearing is painless, but any pressure on the nail plate, as from shoe or sock, elicits *tenderness.* Exuberant granulation tissue may form in the nail fold.

Subungual Pain: **Subungual Exostosis.** The great toe is usually involved. An exostosis arises from the dorsal surface of the distal phalanx to penetrate the distal half of the nail bed, and subsequently the nail plate itself. Early, a painless *discoloration* under the nail is visible; later, the nail is pushed upward and split. The protruding surface becomes covered with granulations that form *painful ulcers.*

Subungual Pain: **Glomus Tumor.** This is similar to the painful lesion under the fingernail (p. 697), except that the toenail is subjected to more trauma; hence the pain is more of a discomfort.

Overgrowth of the Toenail: **Ram's Horn Nail** (Onychogryposis). The nail becomes *thickened, conical,* and *curved,* like a ram's horn; it may assume grotesque shape and size (Fig. 9-51H).

BRIEF EXAMINATION FOR SKELETAL INJURIES. **This is recommended for the rapid examination of injured but conscious persons to uncover skeletal lesions not specifically complained of [*adapted from* A. J. Neufeld: A 10-Minute Exam to Pinpoint Skeletal Injuries, *Consultant,* pp. 57–59, Nov., 1972]. This examination should be undertaken after emergencies have been cared for.**

Head: **Have the patient *open and close his mouth* and *bite down* when your fingertips are on the *masseter muscles;* if no pain is elicited, the facial bones are not affected. Palpate the *zygomatic arch* and *nose* for tenderness. Palpate the *scalp* for bruises and lumps. With your hands press from opposite *sides of his head* for the pain of a skull fracture.**

Neck: **Have him *roll his head* gently from side to side while your fingers palpate the *neck muscles* for tenderness or spasm. Ask him to *lift his head* while you place your hand under it; ask him to *push down* with his head to estimate his strength and discomfort.**

Chest: **Ask him to *take a deep breath;* if this is painful, place your hands on opposite sides of his chest and *squeeze* to locate the point of tenderness of a rib fracture.**

Spine: With the patient supine, slip your hand under his back, *lift his chest* slightly, and run your fingers over the *spinous processes* for tenderness and angulation.

Arms and Hands: Have the patient move his *arms, hands,* and *fingers,* in succession and through full range. *Twist each finger* for phalangeal and metacarpal injuries. *Shake hands,* both right and left, and ask him to *twist his arm,* with elbow both straight and flexed. Performance of these motions, with normal strength and painlessly, excludes injuries of hand, wrist, forearm, elbow, arm, shoulder, clavicle, and scapula.

Legs and Feet: Ask him to *move first one leg,* then the other, through full range. *Twist each toe.* Have him *stretch his legs* flat on the table. *Press his feet together* and have him *rotate* them laterally against your resistance. If he employs normal strength without pain, you have excluded injuries of legs and pelvis.

Pelvis: This may be further examined by *compression medially* with a hand on each ilium or hip joint. Place your clenched fist between his knees and ask him to *squeeze* it; lack of pain excludes fractures of pelvis and femora.

10

The Neuropsychiatric Examination

In the routine physical examination, most clinicians test the components of the nervous system piecemeal as they elicit the history and examine the body by regions. The patient's speech and behavior may betray the presence of many abnormalities of cerebral function. When examining the head, the physician usually tests some of, if not all, the cranial nerves. Muscular strength is often evident by inspection of the gait and other movements. A representative selection of deep reflexes is elicited. When clues to malfunction of the nervous system are encountered, a more complete and systematic neurologic examination supplements the routine.

The first objective of the systematic neurologic examination is to discover all behavioral, sensory, motor, and coordinative deficits. After a complete inventory, the clinician deduces the site of the lesion by utilizing certain physiologic and anatomic facts, some of which are:

Item. When the deficits involve intellect, memory, or higher brain function, the lesion involves the cerebral hemisphere.

Item. When the deficits include impairment of consciousness, the brainstem is involved.

Item. When early central paralysis can be excluded, paralysis with loss of the appropriate deep reflexes indicates a lower motor neuron lesion interrupting the reflex arc. This may reflect disease of the nerve root or spinal cord (level of motor neuron).

Item. Paralysis with an accentuated deep reflex indicates an upper motor neuron lesion. This may reflect disease of the hemisphere, brainstem, or spinal cord.

Item. In the spinal cord, the ascending tracts for discrimination sense decussate at the medullary level, but the tracts for pain and temperature sense cross over where they enter the cord, which produces dissociation in sensory abnormalities and differences in sides between motor and sensory phenomena.

Item. Like the tracts for discriminative sense, the descending motor tracts decussate at the medullary level. Paralysis is contralateral to lesions above the medulla and ipsilateral below.

Item. A lower motor neuron paralysis accompanied by anesthesia in the appropriate region usually indicates a peripheral nerve problem, since many nerves carry both motor and sensory fibers; sometimes spinal root or segmental cord lesions cause similar signs.

Item. Muscle atrophy with fasciculation results from a lower motor neuron lesion; without fasciculation, atrophy is often attributable to intrinsic muscle disease.

The Cranial Nerves

The 12 pairs of cranial nerves emerge from the brain and pass through foramina in the base of the skull.

Olfactory Nerve (1st Cranial)

The olfactory mucosa lining the upper third of the nasal septum and the superior nasal concha contains the receptors and ganglion cells. Their fibers converge into about 20 branches that pierce the cribriform plate of the ethmoid bone and consolidate to form the olfactory tract.

TESTING SMELL. **Ensure the patency of the nasal passages. Have the patient close his eyes; test each nostril separately while the other is occluded. Ask the patient to identify familiar odors, such as tobacco, coffee, cloves, and peppermint. Noxious substances, such as ammonia, should not be used because they also stimulate receptors of the trigeminal nerve and give a false positive response.**

Optic Nerve (2nd Cranial)

The structure of the optic nerve, chiasm, and tract is discussed on p. 92.

TESTING THE RETINA. **Use suitable tests for vision, depending upon the patient's acuity and ability to cooperate (p. 124). Examine the fundi with the ophthalmoscope (p. 112). Test the visual fields by the confrontation method (p. 80); perimetry may be required for more accurate and detailed information.**

Oculomotor Nerve (3rd Cranial)

This is the motor nerve to five extrinsic eye muscles: Levator palpebrae superioris, medial rectus, superior rectus, inferior rectus, and inferior oblique. Its nucleus lies in the floor of the cerebral aqueduct subdivided into a part for each muscle. After emergence from the brain, the nerve proceeds between the superior cerebellar and posterior cerebral arteries, then lateral and forward to the posterior clinoid process, then along the lateral wall of the cavernous sinus, to enter the orbit through the superior orbital fissure. Unilateral complete paralysis is usually caused by intracranial pressure or aneurysm with spontaneous subarachnoid hemorrhage. Pupillary sparing oculomotor nerve palsy may be a complication of diabetes mellitus.

TESTING FOR OCULOMOTOR PARALYSIS. See p. 90.

Trochlear Nerve (4th Cranial)

The superior oblique runs through the trochlea or pulley which imparts the name to the motor nerve. The trochlear nucleus lies in the floor of the cerebral aqueduct, where it follows a circuitous course around the superior cerebellar and cerebral peduncles, to pierce the free border of the tentorium cerebelli near the posterior clinoid process. It proceeds forward in the lateral wall of the cavernous sinus and passes through the superior orbital fissure to enter the substance of the superior oblique muscle.

TESTING FOR TROCHLEAR PARALYSIS. See p. 88.

Trigeminal Nerve (5th Cranial)

The largest cranial nerve, its *sensory* root supplies the superficial and deep structures of the head and face; its *motor root* innervates the muscles of mastication. The sensory root arises in the trigeminal ganglion, lying at the petrous apex of the temporal bone; the fibers pass backward to enter the pons where one part ends in a nucleus and the other portion descends through the pons and medulla to the substantia gelatinosa. Going forward, the 1st division, or *ophthalmic branch,* of the trigeminal emerges from the trigeminal ganglion, giving fibers to the cornea, ciliary body, conjunctiva, the nasal cavity and sinuses, the skin of the eyebrows, forehead, and nose. The 2nd division or *maxillary branch,* supplies sensory fibers to the skin of the side of the nose, the lower eyelid, and the upper lip. The 3rd division, or *mandibular branch,* is mixed; its sensory fibers supply the skin of the temporal region, the auricula, the lower lip, the lower face, the mucosa of the anterior two thirds of the tongue, the mandibular gums and teeth; its motor root innervates the muscles of mastication: Masseter, Temporalis, internal and external Pterygoid. Irritative lesions of the motor root may cause spasm or trismus. Irritation of the sensory root results in tic douloureux.

TESTING THE TRIGEMINAL NERVE. ***Motor Division:*** **Look for tremor of the lips, involuntary chewing movements, and trismus (spasm of the masticatory muscles). Test the pairs of temporal and masseter muscles by palpating symmetric regions while the patient clenches the teeth; compare muscle tension on the two sides (Fig. 10-1A). The mouth cannot be closed tightly in bilateral paralysis. Have the patient open his mouth; in unilateral paralysis, the mandible *deviates toward* the weak side, indicated by the vertical misalignment of the upper and lower medial incisors. *Sensory Division:* With the patient's eyes closed, test tactile perception of the facial skin by asking him to indicate when you touch him with a shred of gauze (Fig. 10-1B). Test sense of touch in the oral mucosa by stroking with a wooden applicator. Test pain sensibility of the skin and mucosa with pin pricks. When pain sensitivity is lost, test for temperature perception by touching with test tubes of warm and cold water. In each test, compare symmetric points; map out areas of abnormal sensation in detail. The jaw jerk tests both the motor and sensory components of the trigeminal nerve. Test the corneal reflex by having the patient look upward while you gently touch the cornea (not the conjunctiva) with a small shred of gauze; this induces blinking normally. The corneal reflex tests both the trigeminal and facial nerves. It is a bilateral reflex testing the 5th and 7th cranial nerves on the side stimulated and the 7th consensually. With an afferent (5th) lesion,**

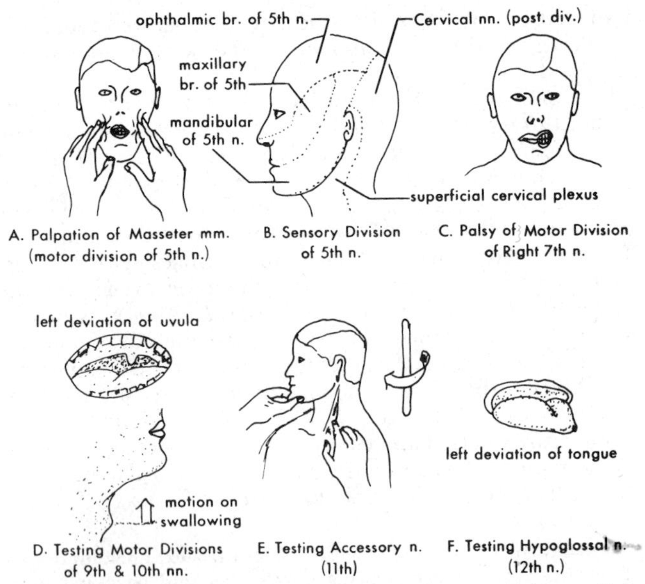

Fig. 10-1. Testing some cranial nerves. **A.** Motor division of the 5th (trigeminal) nerve. *Palpate the masseter muscles with the finger-tips while the patient clenches his teeth; disparity in tension of the two muscles indicates paralysis on the weak side, if and when the teeth are aligned naturally, or a tongue blade is inserted to correct a malalignment. If there is malalignment of the incisors when the mouth is opened, paralysis of the pterygoid muscle on the weak side is indicated.* **B.** Sensory division of the 5th (trigeminal). *The three branches of the sensory trigeminal are opthalmic, maxillary, and mandibular, as indicated by the areas.* **C.** Motor division of the 7th (facial). *When the patient opens his mouth to show his clenched teeth, only the unparalyzed side of the face retracts; the cheek muscles form creases on the normal side; the eyelid partially closes. The paralyzed side remains smooth with eyelid open.* **D.** Motor division of the 9th (glossopharyngeal) and 10th (vagus) nerves. *When the patient opens the mouth and says "ah," the uvula deviates toward the strong side. Upon swallowing the larynx normally elevates, as indicated by the motion of the thyroid cartilage in the neck (Adam's apple); it does not rise in bilateral paralysis.* **E.** The accessory (11th) nerve. *The patient is asked to rotate his head toward the midline against the resistance of the examiner's hand; the other examining hand palpates*

both sides will be depressed. With an efferent (7th) lesion, the direct reflex is lost, and the consensual is preserved.

Abducens Nerve (6th Cranial)

The abducens is the motor nerve to the lateral rectus. Its nucleus lies beneath the facial colliculus. The nerve runs below the posterior clinoid process, through the cavernous sinus and the superior orbital fissure, to enter the substance of the lateral rectus muscle. ***Structures in the Cavernous Sinus:*** The 3rd, 4th, 5th (ophthalmic and maxillary divisions), and 6th cranial nerves and the internal carotid artery. Injury is likely from infection around the midbrain, fractures of the orbit or petrous portion of the temporal bone, aneurysm of the internal carotid artery, mastoiditis, or intracranial pressure.

TESTING FOR ABDUCENS PARALYSIS. See p. 88.

Facial Nerve (7th Cranial)

The facial nerve contains motor, autonomic, and sensory fibers. It supplies *motor fibers* to the muscles of the scalp, face, and auricula, as well as to the Buccinator, Platysma, Stapedius, Stylohyoideus, and the posterior belly of the Digastricus. Autonomic motor fibers run through the chorda tympani nerve, a branch of the facial, to cause vasodilatation and secretion in the submaxillary and sublingual salivary glands. *Sensory fibers* furnish the organs of taste on the anterior two thirds of the tongue and sensation to the ear canal and behind the ear. The cause of peripheral palsies of the facial nerve is usually unknown; they occasionally occur in poliomyelitis, amyotrophic lateral sclerosis, syringomyelia, multiple sclerosis, tumors, infectious polyneuritis (Guillain-Barré syndrome), syphilis. The most common isolated facial nerve lesion is *Bell's palsy*.

TESTING THE FACIAL NERVE. ***Motor:*** **Inspect the face in repose for evidence of flaccid paralysis (Bell's palsy). Have the patient perform seven different motions to demonstrate the paralyzed side and**

---

the degree of tension in the sternocleidomastoid muscle. The trapezius can likewise be tested for paralysis. **F.** The 12th (hypoglossal) nerve. *The protruding tongue deviates to the paralyzed side; muscle atrophy may also be present. Occasionally deviation of the tongue results from an upper motor neuron lesion.*

whether caused by a *lower motor neuron* (LMN) lesion, or an *upper motor neuron* (UMN) lesion. In general, UMN lesions do not affect the upper lid or forehead; the paralysis of the mouth is overcome by motions responding to emotion. (1) *Face in repose:* Shallow nasolabial folds in both UMN and LMN; palpebral fissure widened in LMN. (2) *Elevation of eyebrow:* Elevation of the eyebrow and wrinkling of the forehead absent in LMN, present in UMN. (3) *Frowning:* Lowering of eyebrow absent in LMN, present in UMN. (4) *Tight closing of the eyes:* Absent in LMN, with unclosed eye upturned (Bell's phenomenon), an associated movement (p. 91), lid closed normally in UMN. When the eyes are tightly closed, weakness of one upper lid might be detected by forcing the lids open with the thumb. (5) *Showing teeth:* The mouth does not elevate in either UMN or LMN (Fig. 10-1C). (6) *Whistling and puffing cheeks:* Absent in both UMN and LMN. (7) *A natural smile:* The mouth does not elevate in LMN; a symmetric smile may occur in UMN. Fine *tremors* of the lips occur in diffuse brain disease. The face is expressionless, the *masklike facies,* in paralysis agitans. A *tic* is a repetitive movement of a group of facial muscles (see p. 791). *Sensory* (*Taste*): Test with sugar, vinegar (dilute acetic acid), quinine, and table salt. Write the words "sweet," "sour," "bitter," and "salty" on a piece of paper so the patient can point out his sensations. Hold the protruded tongue in gauze and touch successively each side of the anterior two thirds of the lingual dorsum with the test substance on an applicator. Have the tongue rinsed well with water between tests. Sensation about the ear can also be tested with a pin.

Repeated Bell's Palsy: **Melkersson's Syndrome.** This is a triad of *scrotal tongue* (lingua plicata) with repeated attacks of *Bell's palsy* and painless nonpitting *facial edema.* The cause is unknown [J. M. Streeto and F. B. Watters: Melkersson's Syndrome, *N. Engl. J. Med.,* **271**:308, 1965].

Acoustic Nerve (8th Cranial)

The 8th nerve is a relatively short trunk consisting of the *cochlear* and *vestibular nerves;* both are sensory, but morphologically and functionally distinct. Beginning in different nuclei, the two sets of fibers join a single trunk entering the internal auditory meatus. The cochlear nerve supplies the organ of Corti while the vestibular nerve furnishes sensory endings for the semicircular ducts.

TESTING THE ACOUSTIC NERVE. ***Cochlear Portion:*** **The tests for hearing are described on p. 191.** ***Vestibular Portion.*** **Note spontaneous nystagmus; use labyrinthine tests described on p. 193.**

Glossopharyngeal Nerve (9th Cranial)

The nerve contains sensory, motor, and autonomic fibers. It supplies the sensory organs for pain, touch, and temperature in the mucosa of the pharynx, fauces, and palatine tonsil; in addition, it is the nerve of taste for the posterior third of the tongue. Somatic motor fibers travel through both the glossopharyngeal and the vagus to innervate the muscles of the pharynx. The trunk emerges from the medulla, passes through the jugular foramen of the skull with the vagus and accessory nerves. It follows the internal carotid artery and curves under the styloid process, then goes forward to the pharynx.

TESTING THE GLOSSOPHARYNGEAL NERVE. **This is tested with the vagus nerve.**

Vagus Nerve (10th Cranial)

Most extensive of the cranial nerves, the vagus carries motor, sensory, and autonomic fibers to the neck, thorax, and abdomen. In the jugular fossa its branches are the pharyngeal, the superior laryngeal, the recurrent laryngeal, and the superior cardiac; the thoracic branches are the inferior cardiac, the anterior and posterior bronchials, and the esophageal; in the abdomen are the gastric, the celiac, and the hepatic.

TESTING OF THE GLOSSOPHARYNGEAL AND VAGUS NERVES. ***Pharynx:*** **Have the patient open his mouth and say "ah," noting whether the uvula elevates. Absence of elevation indicates bilateral paralysis; in unilateral elevation, the uvula deviates** ***toward the strong side*** **(Fig. 10-1D). Note whether the faucial pillars converge equally. Test the gag reflex by touching the back of the tongue with a tongue blade. Test the pharyngeal mucosa for areas of anesthesia by touching with an applicator and pricking with a pin.** ***Larynx:*** **Watch the laryngeal contours in the neck to ascertain whether they rise with swallowing (Fig. 10-1D). Test further by having the patient swallow some water; paralysis may cause regurgitation. Note hoarseness for unilateral vocal cord paralysis, or dyspnea and inspiratory stridor for bilateral involvement. Make an indirect examination of the vocal cords, as on p. 167.**

Accessory Nerve (11th Cranial)

The accessory nerve (formerly the *spinal accessory*) is motor to the Trapezius and the Sternocleidomastoid. It arises in the medulla the upper cervical cord and passes through the foramen magnum; emerging from the skull through the jugular foramen, it runs backward near the jugular vein, and descends to the upper part of the Sternocleidomastoid, which it pierces and supplies; thence it proceeds to the posterior triangle of the neck to supply the upper portion of the Trapezius.

TESTING OF THE ACCESSORY NERVE. **Palpate the upper borders of the Trapezii while the patient raises his shoulders against the resistance of your hands. Test the Sternocleidomastoideus by having the patient turn his head to one side and attempt to bring his chin back to the midline against the resistance of your hand (Fig. 10-1E). Note the strength of rotation and the prominence of the tensed muscles in the neck.**

Hypoglossal Nerve (12th Cranial)

The hypoglossal is the motor nerve to the tongue. It arises in the medulla, passes through the hypoglossal canal beside the foramen magnum, courses downward with the internal carotid artery, the jugular vein, and the vagus nerve, then curves forward behind the mandible to the lingual root.

TESTING OF THE HYPOGLOSSAL NERVE. **When the tongue protrudes, look for tremors and other involuntary movements. Note atrophy of one lateral muscle mass and fasciculations. When one side is paralyzed, the tongue deviates *toward the weak side* (Fig. 10-1F). Test muscle strength by having the patient push the tongue against the cheek while your hand resists from the outside. Test lingual speech by having the patient repeat such words as "round the rugged rock the ragged rascal ran" and "third riding artillery brigade."**

Motor Functions

The functions of the motor system depend upon the anatomic state of the muscles and the condition of their motor nerves. Joint motion must be tested to assess muscle movements, so orthopedic and neurologic examinations overlap and are interdependent.

Muscle Atrophy. Whenever possible, compare symmetric muscle masses. The circumferences of the two counterparts are compared at the same level. When bilateral atrophy is suspected, the examiner must evaluate the findings from his knowledge of normal anatomy and the individual variations encountered in his experience with many persons.

Muscle Tone. Resistance to passive motion discloses abnormalities in muscle tone. The examiner learns the feel of normal resistance with which he may compare the findings in the patient. In testing tonus, the patient is told to relax; compliance is assessed by evaluating his attitude and testing when his attention is diverted. Lifting a limb from the bed and watching it fall discloses its tonus. When the patient sits on the edge of the examining table, the freedom with which the legs swing indicates tonus. In *cogwheel rigidity* the increased tonus of the limb is released by degrees, so passive motion is jerky. In *upper motor neuron paralysis,* tonus of the stretched muscles is increased, *spasticity*. When a limb is moved against spastic muscles, the resistance may suddenly cease, giving a *clasp-knife effect*. Long-continued spasticity results in fibrosing muscles and shortening, *contracture*. Spasticity results from upper motor neuron lesions. Hypotonia occurs with lower motor neuron injury, such as poliomyelitis, a root syndrome, peripheral neuritis; it is also encountered in cerebellar and other central lesions. Extrapyramidal lesions, as paralysis agitans, produce hypertonia.

Muscle Strength. First, let the patient actively move the muscle (Fig. 10-2). When motion is accomplished, have him contract the muscle while you pull against it; or have the patient move

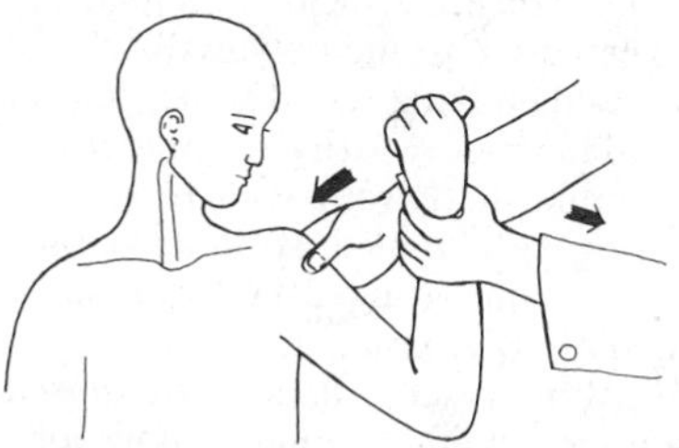

Fig. 10-2. Testing muscle strength. *Either the examiner pulls against the tensed muscles of the patient, or the patient is required to act against the resistance of the examiner.*

against your resistance. If he cannot move a limb in the usual manner, lay the extremity on the table or bed and have the patient move it in a direction unaffected by gravity. The use of an arbitrary scale is desirable for recording muscle strength;

Grading of Muscle Strength (Oxford Scale)

Grade 0	No movement
Grade 1	A flicker or trace of movement without joint motion
Grade 2	Partially moves body part with gravity eliminated
Grade 3	Completely moves body part against gravity
Grade 4	Completely moves body part against gravity and some resistance
Grade 5	Normal

Abnormal Muscle Movements

Most abnormal movements of muscle are responses of normal contractile tissue to abnormal nervous stimuli, so they are properly included in the neurologic examination. But the signs are frequently encountered in an appraisal of the musculoskeletal system by anatomic regions.

Paralysis of Muscles. This is defined as loss or diminution in motor power of muscle from affections of motor nerves or muscle fibers. The following categories are diagnostically useful: *Continued Muscle Paralysis. Acute:* trauma to nerves, poliomyelitis, Guillain Barre, spinal cord trauma, polyneuropathy (in porphyria, beriberi), severe myasthenia gravis, polymyositis, dermatomyositis, stroke. *Chronic:* progressive muscular dystrophy, cord degeneration of pernicious anemia, diabetic neuropathy, multiple sclerosis, chronic polymyositis, progressive muscular atrophy and related conditions, peroneal muscular atrophy, amyloid polyneuropathy, chronic nutritional neuropathy, chronic plumbism, thyrotoxic myopathy. *Episodic Paralysis.* Myasthenia gravis, familial periodic paralysis, hereditary adynamia, paramyotonia congenita, hyperpotassemia and hypopotassemia, acute thyrotoxic myopathy.

Tremors. Involuntary contractions of muscle groups produce oscillating movements at one or more joints. The amplitude may be either fine or coarse; the rate either rapid or slow. Movements may be rhythmic or irregular. *All tremors* *disappear during sleep. Fine rapid tremor* may occur in anxiety states, but is is most typical in thyrotoxicosis, chronic alcoholism, and dementia paralytica. *Rest tremor* is classically associated with Parkinson's syndrome in which it is coarse, alternating, rather slow, maximal when the muscles are at rest; it is partially or completely abolished by voluntary movements. The alternation of the fingers is often characterized as a "pill-rolling tremor." The senile or familial tremor also occurs at rest, but it is augmented by voluntary movements. *Action* or *intention tremor* occurs in multiple sclerosis and cerebellar disease in which voluntary movements initiate and sustain a slow oscillation of wide amplitude.

Cogwheel Rigidity. On passive motion of a limb, the examiner feels muscular resistance as a series of jerks alternating with periods of arrest. This phenomenon is a special expression of the rest tremor in paralysis agitans. It disappears during sleep.

Tics. Normal movements of muscle groups, such as grimacing, winking, shoulder shrugging, are repeated at inappropriate times. The reaction is stereotyped for the individual. Some consider them psychogenic because they are abolished by diverting the patient's attention. They disappear during sleep.

Choreiform Movements. Rapid, purposeless, jerky, asynchronous movements involve various parts of the body. Although some are spontaneous, many are initiated and all are accentuated by voluntary acts, as in extending the arms or walking. They commonly occur in both Sydenham's and Huntington's chorea; in the latter, the movements are coarser and more bizarre. They disappear with sleep.

Athetoid Movements. In contrast to choreiform movements, these are slower and writhing, resembling the actions of a worm or snake. The distal parts of the limb are more active than the proximal. Grimaces are more deliberate than in chorea. The grotesque *athetoid hand* is produced by flexion of some digits with others extended. They disappear with sleep. The mechanism of production is not understood, but the movements are frequently associated with diseases around the basal ganglion.

Hemiballismus. One side of the body is involved by sustained, violent, involuntary flinging movements of the limbs.

These result from a lesion in the contralateral subthalamic nucleus of Luys, usually secondary to stroke. They disappear with sleep.

Myoclonus. A single sudden jerk, or a short series, occurring in slow or rapid succession, may be so powerful as to throw the patient to the floor.

Myotonia. The muscles continue in contraction after a voluntary or reflex act has ceased. Recovery from contraction induced by a reflex hammer is prolonged. After shaking hands, the fingers reluctantly relax. When the fingers are flexed on the supinated palm, attempted extension is slow and difficult. The slow relaxation from a tendon jerk, exhibited in myxedema, has been attributed to myotonia, but this is disputed. The movement is typical of myotonia congenita and myotonia atrophica.

Tetany. The threshold of muscular excitability is lowered so involuntary spasms occur, either painless or painful. The contracting muscles feel rigid and unyielding. Spasm may be preceded by numbness and tingling in the lips and limbs. Contractions of the hands and feet are termed collectively *carpopedal spasm* (see p. 673). In carpal spasm the wrist is flexed; flexion at the metacarpophalangeal joints is combined with extension of the interphalangeal joints; the hyperextended fingers are also adducted to form a cone; the thumb is flexed upon the palm. This presents a diagnostic posture called *obstetrician's hand* or *accoucheur's hand.* In *latent tetany* carpal spasm may be induced by occluding the brachial artery for three minutes with an inflated sphygmomanometer cuff; successful induction by this maneuver is called *Trousseau's sign.* Tapping the facial nerve against the bone just anterior to the ear produces ipsilateral contraction of facial muscles; this is *Chvostek's sign.* It is uniformly present in latent tetany, but rudimentary reactions occur in some normal persons. In *spontaneous tetany* most body muscles are involved to produce *laryngeal stridor, tonic* and *clonic convulsions, epileptiform seizures,* even death.

Clinical Occurrence. Parathyroid deficit. Hyperventilation. Calcium deprivation or loss in other diseases. Deficit or loss of body magnesium.

Tetanus. This disease is caused by the action of the toxin of *Clostridium tetani* on myoneural junctions. A single muscle or many groups become rigid with *sustained tonic spasm,* hence the term *lockjaw.* Loud noises, bright lights, or pain induce *superimposed violent convulsions.* The condition should not be confused with tetany, which it resembles only in name.

Jacksonian Seizures. This is an episodic disorder. An attack often begins with twitching of the muscles in a single region of the body. The twitches become more violent with increasing amplitude; the disturbance spreads to contiguous muscle groups until the entire ipsilateral side may be involved in clonic contractions. The seizure may stop at any stage of its spread, or the contralateral side may be affected to produce a generalized attack. Consciousness is usually retained, except when the attack is generalized. Usually the seizures are caused by a focal lesion in the motor cortex supplying the muscles initially involved in the progression.

Epileptic Seizures. ***Major Motor*** (grand mal). There may or may not be a warning. Several hours or days before the attack *prodromata* may be noted with feelings of strangeness, dreamy states, increased irritability, lethargy or euphoria, ravenous appetite (*bulimia*), feelings of impending disaster, headaches, or other symptoms. The *aura* is the first part of the attack, and the patient learns its foreboding significance. He often experiences vague epigastric sensations; nausea or hunger may occur; palpitation, vertigo, or sensations in the head are sometimes noted. Any aura or focal seizure reflects focal brain disease. Consciousness is lost suddenly and simultaneously with the *epileptic cry* from sudden expulsion of air through the glottis. The patient is helpless and falls wherever he may be, often incurring injuries. *Tonic spasm* of all muscles occurs; it may be so violent as to fracture bones. *Breathing ceases* from spasm of the thoracic muscles; *cyanosis* may be deep. Suddenly, the tonic state subsides, followed by *clonic movements* that increase in strength with repetition; then, these movements cease. *Foaming at the mouth* results from forced expulsion of air and saliva. Clonic movements of the jaws cause *biting* of the lateral aspect of the tongue and lips. Frequently there is *involuntary defecation* and *urination.* Consciousness usually returns in a few minutes or hours, frequently followed by lapsing into a deep sleep. Patients often complain of headache or confusion afterwards. They may have stiff or sore muscles. ***Absence*** (petit mal). An episode consists of a sudden transitory *diminution* or *loss of consciousness* with no abnormal muscle movements. The attack usually lasts from several to 90 seconds, during which the patient's *widely opened, staring eyes* are almost diagnostic when seen by the examiner. Full consciousness is rapidly and completely restored. Injuries may result from the momentary lapse, but there is no loss of postural tone. The patient is vaguely aware that he has "missed something." ***Partial Complex*** (psychomotor). Often an aura of abnormal psychic event; olfactory, visual, or gustatory disturbances, or even phenomena such as *deja vu,* can initiate the attack. The attack may last from a few minutes to a few hours. Sudden but subtle loss of higher levels of consciousness occur in which the patient is unaware of what transpires, but he retains motor functions and ability to react in automatic fashion. He may respond to questions, but his answers disclose his lack of understanding; this may be *the only objective clue.* Repetitive aimless movements, which are often stereotyped, may be reported. Patients generally do not become violent or assaultive during an attack. Only occasionally are there tonic muscle spasms of the limbs. Amnesia for the attack is partial or complete. This condition should prompt a search for a focal lesion in the temporal lobe.

Myoedema. In some persons, a light tap of a reflex hammer upon the belly of a superficial muscle causes a localized contraction forming a *visible ridge* that persists for 5 to 8 seconds. This is conceded to be a manifestation of muscular irritability, so "myoedema" is a misnomer. The Deltoideus or Pectoralis is usually the muscle tested. In the century or so that this phenomenon has been recognized, various attempts have been made to find satisfactory correlation with disease processes. The sign was not a reliable indicator of serum albumin concentration.

Fasciculations. Twitching may be observed in a resting muscle from spontaneous firing of motor units or bundles of fibers. *Coarse* twitches are often caused by exposure to cold, fatigue, or other conditions; their import is not serious. *Fine* twitchings must be carefully sought because they are not powerful enough to move a joint or a part. They should be sought when the patient is resting. In the presence of muscle atrophy or weakness, their presence is attributable to progressive denervation of muscle. *Fibrillations* are twitches of individual muscle fibers;

they are invisible, but can be demonstrated by electromyography.

Flapping Tremor of Hands and Feet: ***Liver Flap*** (Asterixis). Have the patient elevate his arms to 90° in 0° abduction, with hands pronated and fingers spread. At the wrists and interphalangeal joints, there are *jerky alternations of extension* and flexion. Two or three per second, in cycles of a few seconds separated by rest periods of one or two seconds. The fingers *deviate laterally* and exhibit a *fine tremor.* When the leg of the supine patient is elevated and the foot dorsiflexed, a similar tremor occurs at the ankle. Or have the wrists dorsiflexed; after a short wait the hands will flap up and down. For the obtunded patient, an alternate test is to nduce him to squeeze two of the physician's fingers; with asterixis, the examiner can feel the patient's fingers alternately clenching and unclenching. Asterixis can also be demonstrated with the tongue, elbows, eyelids, and fingers [S. J. Winawer: Foot and Other Flaps, *N. Engl. J. Med.,* **289:**1256, 1973].

Clinical Occurrence. Hepatic failure on the verge of coma, cerebrovascular disease, uremia, severe pulmonary insufficiency.

Movements from Specific Muscles and Nerves

It is frequently desirable to identify the muscles and nerves involved in a deficit of bodily movement. The following is a compilation of the principal muscle movements, their causative muscles, and their innervation (in parentheses).

Eyebrow, elevation: Frontalis (7th cranial from inferior pons).

Eyebrow, depression downward and inward, wrinkling of the forehead: Corrugator (7th cranial from inferior pons).

Upper eyelid, elevation: Levator palpebrae superioris (3rd cranial from upper midbrain).

Eyelids, closing, wrinkling of forehead, compression of lacrimal sac: Orbicularis oculi (7th cranial from inferior pons).

* *Eyeball, elevation and adduction:* Superior rectus (3rd cranial from upper midbrain).

**Eyeball, elevation and outward rotation:* Inferior oblique (3rd cranial from upper midbrain).

**Eyeball, depression and rotation downward and inward:* Inferior rectus (3rd cranial from upper midbrain).

**Eyeball, depression and rotation downward and outward:* Superior oblique (4th cranial from midbrain).

**Eyeball, adduction:* Medial rectus (3rd cranial from upper midbrain).

**Eyeball, abduction:* Lateral rectus (6th cranial from inferior pons).

Pupil, constriction: Ciliary (3rd cranial and parasympathetic from upper midbrain).

Lips, retraction: Zygomatic (7th cranial from inferior pons).

Lips, protrusion: Orbicularis oris (7th cranial from inferior pons).

Mouth, opening: Mylohyoid (5th cranial from pons), Digastricus (7th cranial from pons).

Mandible, elevation and retraction: Masseter and Temporalis (5th cranial from midpons).

Mandible, elevation and protrusion: Pterygoid (5th cranial from midpons).

Pharynx, palatine elevation and pharyngeal constriction: Levator veli palatini and Pharyngeal constrictor (9th and 10th cranial from medulla).

Tongue, depression and protrusion: Genioglossus (12th cranial from medulla).

Neck, rotation of the head: Sternocleidomastoid and Trapezius (11th cranial from medulla and upper cervical cord).

Neck, flexion: Rectus capitis anterior (C-1 to C-3).

Neck, extension, and rotation of the head: Splenius capitis et cervicis (C-1 to C-4).

Neck, lateral bending: Rectus capitis lateralis (C-1 to C-4 and suboccipital nerve).

Spine, flexion: Rectus abdominis (T-8 to T-12).

* *Ophthalmologic Interpretation of Muscle Action:* The items marked with asterisks constitute the actions of the oculorotatory muscles, as assigned by the anatomists and some neurologists. Sharply divergent interpretations are furnished by the ophthalmologists on the basis of clinical findings. The direction of movements of the eyes is a result of the actions of synergists and antagonists producing six *cardinal positions of gaze,* corresponding to the six extraocular muscles. Paralysis of a single muscle results in the inability of the eye to attain its cardinal position, which, in four of the six muscles, does not correspond to the prediction of the anatomists (see Fig. 10-3).

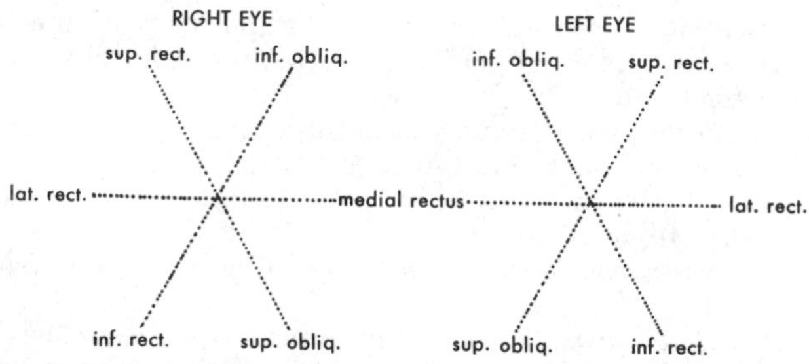

Fig. 10-3. The cardinal positions of gaze. *Each of the six positions is the result of synergists and antagonists acting with a specific muscle. Paralysis of the specific muscle prevents the eye from attaining the cardinal position for the muscle.*

Spine, extension: Thoracic and lumbar intercostals (thoracic nerves from T-2 to L-1).

Spine, extension and rotation: Semispinalis (thoracic nerves from T-4 to T-12).

Spine, extension and lateral bending: Quadratus lumborum (lumbar plexus from T-10 to L-2).

Ribs, elevation and depression: Scaleni and Intercostal (cervical and thoracic nerves from C-4 to T-12).

Diaphragm, elevation and depression: the diaphragmatic muscles (phrenic nerve from C-3 to C-4).

Arm, elevation: Supraspinatus (suprascapular nerve from C-5 to C-6), upper Trapezius (11th cranial from C-3 to C-4).

Arm, elevation and rotation: Deltoid (axillary nerve from C-5 to C-6).

Arm, depression and adduction: middle Pectoralis major (anterior thoracic nerve from C-5 to T-1).

Scapula, rotation and extension of neck: upper Trapezius (11th cranial from C-3 to C-4).

Scapula, retraction with shoulder elevation: middle and lower Trapezius (11th cranial from C-3 to C-4).

Scapula, elevation and retraction: Rhomboids (dorsal scapular nerve from C-5).

Ribs, elevation: Serratus posterior superior (from T-1 to T-4).

Arm, depression and medial rotation: Subscapularis (subscapular nerve from C-5 to C-7), Teres major (thoracodorsal nerves from C-5 to C-7).

Arms, depression and lateral rotation: Infraspinatus (suprascapular nerve from C-5 to C-6).

Elbow, flexion: Biceps brachii, Brachialis (musculocutaneous nerve from C-5 to C-6).

Elbow, extension: Triceps brachii (radial nerve from C-7 to T-1).

Elbow, supination: Biceps brachii (musculocutaneous nerve from C-5 to C-6), Brachioradialis (radial nerve from C-5 to C-6).

Elbow, supination and elbow flexion: Brachioradialis (radial nerve from C-5 to C-6).

Elbow, pronation: Pronator teres (median nerve from C-6 to C-7).

Wrist, extension and adduction: Extensor carpi ulnaris (radial nerve from C-7 to C-8).

Wrist, extension and abduction of hand: Extensor carpi radialis longus (radial nerve from C-6 to C-7).

Wrist, extension of the hand: Extensor digitorum communis (radial nerve from C-7 to C-8).

Wrist, flexion and abduction: Flexor carpi radialis (median nerve from C-7 to C-8).

Wrist, flexion and adduction: Flexor carpi ulnaris (ulnar nerve from C-7 to C-8).

Thumb, adduction and opposition: Adductor pollicis longus (ulnar nerve C-8 to T-1).

Thumb, abduction and extension: Abductor pollicis longus and brevis (median and radial and [posterior interosseous nerves] from C-7 to C-8).

Thumb, extension of distal phalanx: Extensor pollicis longus (radial nerve from C-7 to C-8).

Thumb, extension of proximal phalanx: Extensor pollicis brevis (radial nerve from C-7 to C-8).

Thumb, flexion of distal phalanx: Flexor pollicis longus (median nerve from C-7 to T-1).

Thumb, flexion of proximal phalanx: Flexor pollicis longus and brevis (median nerve from C-7 to T-1).

Thumb, flexion and opposition: Opponens pollicis (median nerve from C-8 to T-1).

Fingers, flexion and adduction of little finger: Opponens digiti minimi (ulnar nerve from C-8 to T-1).

Fingers, adduction of four fingers: Palmar interossei (ulnar nerve from C-8 to T-1).

Fingers, abduction of four fingers: Dorsal interossei (ulnar nerve from C-8 to T-1).

Fingers, extension of hand: Extensor digitorum communis (radial nerve from C-7 to C-8).

Fingers, flexion of hand: Palmar interossei (interosseous nerves from C-7 to T-1), Lumbricales (ulnar and median nerves from C-7 to T-1).

Fingers, extension of interphalangeal joints: Interossei palmaris and Lumbricales (interosseous nerve; median and ulnar nerves from C-7 to T-1).

Fingers, flexion of the distal phalanges: Flexor digitorum profundus (median and ulnar nerves from C-7 to T-1).

Fingers, flexion of middle phalanges: Flexor digitorum sublimis (median nerve from C-7 to T-1).

Abdomen, compression with flexion of trunk: Rectus abdominis (lower thoracic nerves from T-6 to L-1).

Abdomen, flexion of abdominal wall obliquely: Obliquus abdominis externus (lower thoracic nerves from T-6 to L-1).

Hip, flexion: Iliacus (femoral nerve), Psoas (L-2 to L-3), Sartorius (femoral nerve from L-2 to L-3).

Hip, extension: Gluteus maximus (inferior gluteal nerve from L-4 or S-2), Adductor magnus (sciatic nerve and obturator nerve from L-5 to S-2).

Hip, abduction: Gluteus medius (superior gluteal nerve from L-4 to S-1), Gluteus maximus (inferior gluteal nerve from L-4 to S-2).

Hip, adduction: Adductor magnus (sciatic and obturator nerves from L-5 to S-2).

Hip, outward rotation: Gluteus maximus (inferior gluteal nerve from L-4 to S-2), Obturator internus (branches from S-1 to S-3).

Hip, inward rotation: Psoas (branches from L-2 to L-3).

Knee, flexion: Biceps femoris, Semitendinosus, Semimembranosus, Gastrocnemius (all through sciatic nerve from L-5 to S-2).

Knee, extension: Quadriceps femoris (femoral nerve from L-2 to L-4).

Ankle, plantar flexion: Gastrocnemius (Tibial nerve from L-5 to S-2).
Ankle, dorsiflexion: Anterior tibial (Deep peroneal nerve from L-4 to S-1).
Ankle, inversion: Posterior tibial (Tibial nerve from L-5 to S-1).
Ankle, eversion: Peroneus longus (Superficial peroneal nerve from L-4 to S-1).
Great toe, dorsiflexion: Extensor hallucis longus and brevis (Superficial peroneal nerve from L-4 to S-1).

Some Peripheral Nerve Palsies, Chiefly Motor

Horner's Syndrome. A lesion of the cervical sympathetic chain produces the following signs on the ipsilateral side: (1) partial ptosis of the upper eyelid, (2) constriction of the pupil, *miosis,* that does not dilate when the skin on the back of the neck is pinched, (3) absence of sweating on the forehead and face of the affected side when the lesion is in certain sites (Fig. 10-4A). Contrary to some statements, enophthalmos does not occur; the ptosis merely gives an illusion of recession for the eyeball. If damage to the sympathetics occurs early in life, pigmentation of the iris may be affected; e.g., the affected iris may remain blue when the other changes to brown.

Clinical Occurrence. Occurs on the ipsilateral side with mediastinal tumor; has been reported with spontaneous pneumothorax; brainstem stroke.

Flail Arm: ***Erb-Duchenne Paralysis.*** Lower motor neuron paralysis of the brachial plexus may occur from forceful depression of the shoulder during birth, or a blow on the shoulder later in life. The arm hangs limply with the fingers flexed and turned posteriorly, a *flail arm* (p. 724). With partial recovery, motions of the elbow and hand may be regained. The biceps reflex is lost; there is muscle wasting.

Clawhand: ***Klumpke's Paralysis.*** A lower motor neuron lesion of the brachial plexus may be acquired at birth or later. Paralysis of the intrinsic hand muscles results in the clawhand (p. 673). Sensation on the ulnar aspect of the arm, forearm, and hand may be lost.

Weak Lateral Elevation of the Arm: ***Axillary Nerve Paralysis.*** This may be caused by neuritis, fracture of the humeral neck, disloca-

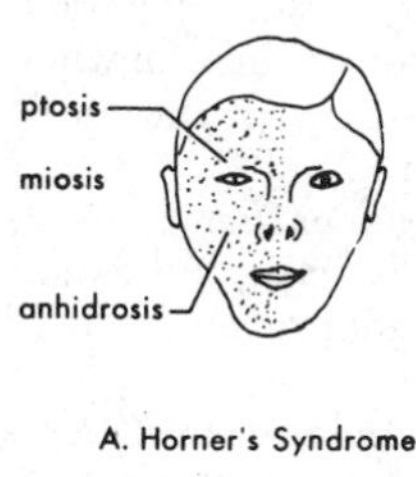

A. Horner's Syndrome

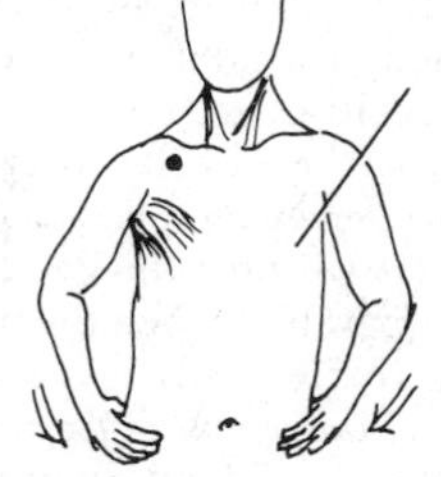

B. Paralysis of Pectoralis Major

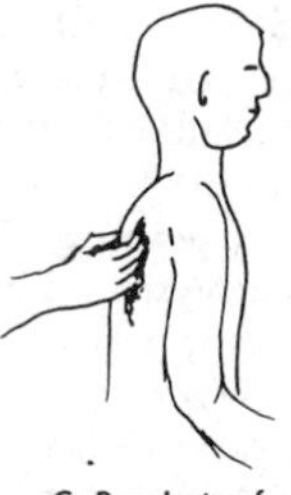

C. Paralysis of Latissimus Dorsi

Fig. 10-4. Nerve lesions of the upper trunk. **A.** Horner's syndrome. *Injury to the superior cervical sympathetic ganglion on one side causes ipsilateral ptosis of the eyelid, miosis, and anhidrosis of the face.* **B.** Paralysis of the pectoralis major muscle. *Injury to the anterior thoracic nerve causes paralysis of the pectoralis major and minor muscles. When the patient is asked to press his hands down on his hips, the normal pectoralis muscle is tensed but the paralyzed one is not.* **C.** Paralysis of the latissimus dorsi muscle. *The examiner grasps the latissimus muscles in his hands and asks the patient to cough. A paralyzed muscle does not tense with coughing.*

tion of the shoulder, or occasionally by scapular fracture. The Deltoid is paralyzed with resultant atrophy. Elevation of the arm in 90° of abduction is impossible. A patch of sensory loss on the lateral aspect of the shoulder is often found.

Shoulder Weakness: ***Dorsal Scapular Nerve Paralysis.*** The nerve supplies the Rhomboids that elevate and retract the scapula. These muscles ascend obliquely from the medial border of the scapula to the spinous processes of the upper thoracic vertebrae. Although covered by the Trapezius, they may be palpated through this superficial muscle when the shoulders are drawn backward; comparison of the two sides may disclose unilateral palsy.

Shoulder Weakness: ***Suprascapular Nerve Paralysis.*** The nerve supplies the Supraspinatus and the Infraspinatus. Paralysis prevents (1) scratching of the back of the head, (2) turning a doorknob with the arm outstretched, (3) completing a line of writing without moving the paper to the left (when the patient is right-handed). Atrophy of these muscles may be palpated as unusual depressions above and below the scapular spine.

Weak Elbow Flexion: ***Musculocutaneous Nerve Paralysis.*** The

Biceps brachii and Brachialis are supplied by this nerve. Paralysis can usually be demonstrated by inspection of the arm when the elbow is flexed against resistance. A small area of anesthesia occurs on the volar surface of the forearm.

Weak Abduction and Depression of the Arm: **Anterior Thoracic Nerve Paralysis.** This nerve supplies the Pectoralis major and minor. Inspection discloses paralysis when the patient presses the hand down upon his hip (Fig. 10-4B).

Weak Abduction and Depression of the Arm: **Thoracodorsal Nerve Paralysis.** The Latissimus dorsi is supplied by this nerve. To demonstrate palsy, grasp the posterior axillary fold of muscle, just below the scapular angle, and have the patient cough; the normal muscle tenses (Fig. 10-4C).

Shoulder Weakness: **Long Thoracic Nerve Paralysis.** The nerve supplies the Serratus anterior that holds the scapula to the thorax. Paralysis produces a *winged scapula* (p. 723) when the patient pushes the hand forward against a wall.

Incomplete Extension of Wrist and Fingers: **Radial Nerve Paralysis.** In its spiral course around the humerus, this nerve is exposed to injury from fracture of the shaft. The radial nerve is often compressed during its course around the spiral groove of the humerus (Saturday night palsy). *Motor Loss.* Injury in the axilla causes paralysis of the Triceps brachii, Anconeus, Brachioradialis, and Extensor carpi radialis longus; a lesion at the level of the upper third of the humerus spares the Triceps; damage between the humeral upper third and 5 cm above the elbow also spares the Brachioradialis; innervation of the extensors of the wrist may be injured at a lower level. Any lesion involving the Extensor carpi radialis longus prevents fixation at the wrist in grasping, thus producing a *wrist drop* (p. 675) (Fig. 10-5A). Paralysis of the Extensor digitorum communis prevents extension of the wrist and fingers; there is thumb and finger drop. When the deep branch of the radial nerve is injured, *radial deviation of the wrist* may occur without wrist drop. *Sensory Loss.* Anesthesia on the dorsum of the hand extends from the radial border to the dorsum of the 5th metacarpal; the dorsum of the thumb is involved, but the other fingers are spared (Fig. 10-5B). The distribution of anesthesia is quite irregular but usually includes dorsum of thumb to first phalanx and web.

Incomplete Flexion of Thumb and Fingers: **Median Nerve Paraly-**

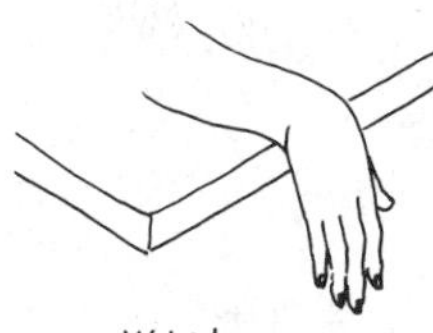

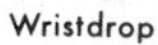

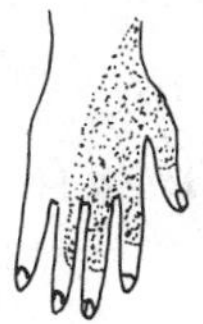

Fig. 10-5. Radial nerve paralysis. *The extensors of the wrist are paralyzed, so the hand droops when it is placed at the end of the table with no support; this sign is called "wristdrop." The region of anesthesia includes the dorsal aspect of the radial 3½ digits (stippled areas).*

sis. The nerve is most exposed to trauma in the antecubital fossa. It supplies the flexors of the wrists, digits, and pronators of the forearm; Pronator teres, Pronator quadratus, Flexor carpi radialis, Flexor digitorum sublimis, Flexor digitorum profundus (except the 4th and 5th digits), Flexor pollicis brevis, Flexor pollicis longus, Opponens pollicis, Lumbrical, Abductor pollicis longus and brevis. All these muscles are innervated below the level of the elbow. The usual site of median nerve entrapment is at the carpal tunnel (See Carpal Tunnel Syndrome, p. 702).

TESTING THE MEDIAN NERVE. ***Ochsner's test*** **(Fig. 10-6A): Have the patient clasp his hands firmly together; the index finger cannot flex when the innervation of the Flexor digitorum sublimis has been injured any place below the antecubital fossa.** ***Flexion of the Thumb*** **(Fig. 10-6B): Hold the patient's first metacarpophalangeal joint with your thumb and index fingers so the metacarpal bone is extended; ask the patient to bend the thumb; failure indicates paralysis of the Flexor pollicis longus, innervated by the volar interosseous that branches from the median nerve in the middle third of the forearm.** ***Abduction of Thumb:*** **Test the action of the Abductor pollicis brevis, innervated exclusively by the median nerve, to distinguish from certain low-level paralysis of the ulnar nerve: (1)** ***Wartenberg's oriental prayer position*** **(Fig. 10-6C). Have the patient extend and adduct the four fingers of each hand, with thumbs extended; have him raise the two hands in front of his face so they are side by side in the same plane, with thumbs and index fingers touching tip to tip; paralysis of the Abductor pollicis brevis prevents full range of thumb abduction, so thumbs do not coincide when index fingers touch. (2)** ***Pen-touching test*** **(Fig. 10-6D). Have the patient rest his supinated hand on the table; hold his fingers flat by resting your fist upon**

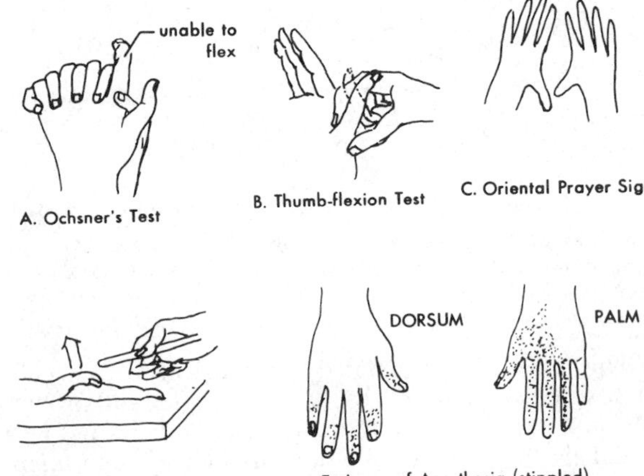

Fig. 10-6. Median nerve paralysis. **A.** Ochsner's test. *The patient clasps his hands but he cannot flex the index finger on the paralyzed side.* **B.** Thumb-flexion test. *The examiner grasps the patient's hand so his thumb and index finger fix the patient's thumb at the proximal joint; then the patient cannot flex the distal joint of his thumb.* **C.** Wartenberg's oriental prayer sign. *The patient is asked to hold his hands with thumbs extended and fingers abducted in front of his face, with palms outward and tips of index fingers touching; paralysis prevents extension of the thumb so its tip cannot reach its mate.* **D.** Pen-touching test. *The supinated hand is laid on the table and a pen or pencil is held horizontally over the thumb. The thumb cannot abduct to touch the object when the median nerve is paralyzed.* **E.** The area of anesthesia. *This includes the radial 3½ digits of the palmar aspect and folds over the tips to the dorsal aspect where it covers the distal phalanges of the same digits (stippled regions).*

them; with your thumb and index finger hold a pen or pencil horizontal above his thumb and ask him to raise his thumb to touch the object in a plane of 90° with the table. This tests his ability to abduct the thumb. ***Sensory Loss:*** **When the nerve lesion is in the wrist, the sensory loss on the palmar surface is restricted to the distal two thirds of the three and a half radial digits (Fig. 10-6E). Tinel's sign (p. 702) is often useful.**

Adductor Weakness of Fingers: ***Ulnar Nerve Paralysis.*** The ulnar nerve is most vulnerable near the elbow where it curves posteriorly around the medial epicondyle. The chief motor disability from palsy is loss of the finer intrinsic motions of the hand, as may be inferred from a list of innervated muscles: Adductor pollicis, Flexor carpi ulnaris, Interosseus palmaris and dorsalis, Flexor pollicis brevis, Opponens digiti minimi, Flexor digitorum profundus (in part). In paralysis of the nerve, inspection will show an *abduction deformity of the little finger* from paralysis of the Interossei, *interosseous muscle atrophy*, and *partial clawhand* from flexion deformity of the middle and distal interphalangeal joints of the ring and little fingers.

TESTING THE ULNAR NERVE. ***Motor Loss:*** **Weakness in adduction of the fingers results from** ***paralysis of the Interosseus palmaris;*** **this may be demonstrated by pulling a sheet of paper from between the patient's extended and adducted fingers to assess the pressure exerted by the sides of his fingers (Fig. 10-7A).** ***Paralysis of the Adductor policis*** **can be tested by asking the patient to grip opposite edges of a folded newspaper between thumbs on top and index fingers underneath. Have him pull each hand toward its nearest paper edge. The thumb, with an inadequate adductor, becomes** ***flexed*** **at its interphalangeal joint from involuntary action of the Flexor pollicis longus, innervated by the median nerve (Fig. 10-7B). In lesions at or below the elbow, test for** ***paralysis of the Flexor carpi ulnaris*** **by having the patient's supinated hand lie on the table. Hold all digits but the little finger flat against the table. Have him abduct his little finger maximally; if there is no paralysis, the tensed tendon may be seen to stand out in the wrist, or it will be palpable (Fig. 10-7C).** ***Sensory Loss:*** **An area of anesthesia covers the one and a half ulnar digits and the corresponding region of the palm. A similar distribution occurs on the dorsal aspect, except when the nerve lesion is at the wrist so the area is constricted to the distal half of the little finger (Fig. 10-7D).**

EXCLUSION TEST FOR MAJOR NERVE INJURY IN THE UPPER LIMB. **Normal sensibility to pinprick in the tips of the index and little fingers** ***excludes major injury to the median and ulnar nerves.*** **Normal ability to extend the thumb and fingers** ***excludes injury of the radial nerve*** **(Fig. 10-8).**

The Sciatic Nerve. Anatomically, the sciatic is two distinct nerves, the *tibial* and *common peroneal*, usually in a single sheath, but functionally quite different; occasionally their trunks are separated. Clinically, it is useful to consider the two components

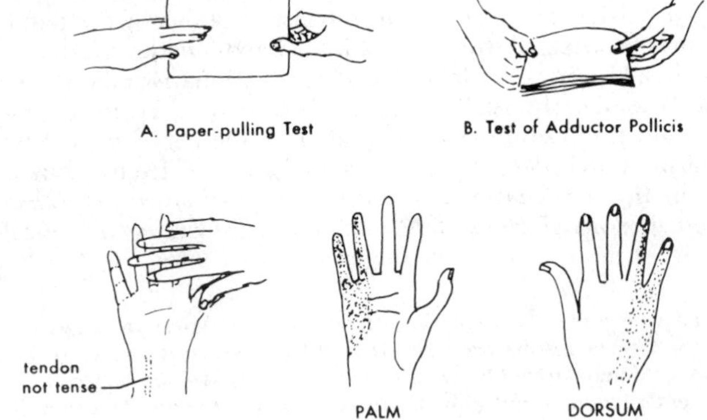

C. Flexor Tendon Test D. Areas of Anesthesia (stippled)

Fig. 10-7. Ulnar nerve paralysis. **A.** Paper-pulling test. *This tests the adductors of the fingers by having the patient hold a piece of paper between two adducted fingers; the examiner pulls the paper to test the strength of compression exerted by the adductors.* **B.** Adductor pollicis test. *The patient grasps the opposite sides of a newspaper or small magazine with his thumbs and index fingers. In ulnar paralysis, the thumb cannot exert enough pressure in adduction, so it flexes involuntarily from action of the flexor pollicis longus.* **C.** Test of flexor carpi ulnaris. *The supinated hand is held upon the table with only the little finger free; the patient attempts to flex the free finger, but the paralyzed tendon in the wrist does not tense.* **D.** Area of anesthesia. *The ulnar 1 ½ digits on both aspects of the hand (stippled).*

as distinct, although their juxtaposition often results in combined lesions.

▼ *Key Symptom:* ***Sciatica.*** Pain from the sciatic nerve is termed *sciatica.* It is described as *burning* or *aching.* Its distribution is typical; beginning in the buttocks it radiates downward in the posterior thigh and the posterolateral aspect of the calf; sometimes it extends around the lateral malleolus of the ankle and the outer aspect of the foot. The pain is *intensified* by coughing, sneezing, laughing, or the straining of defecation. Nerve *tenderness* may be elicited by pressing the fingers into the sciatic notch of the ilium. Sciatic pain can be induced in the affected nerve by *stretching;* with the patient supine and

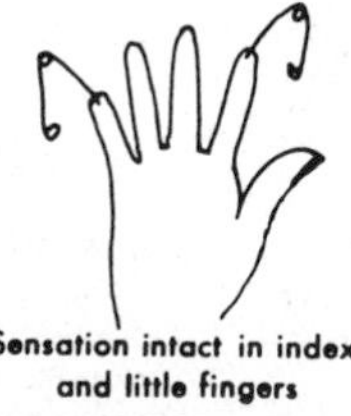

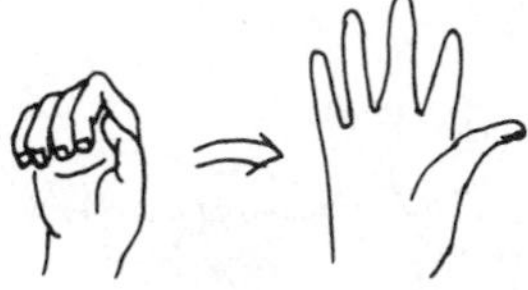

Fig. 10-8. Exclusion test for major nerve injury in the upper limb (Hamilton Bailey). *Sensation is intact in the palmar tips of the index and little fingers; extension of the digits of the hand is unimpaired.*

his thigh and leg both flexed to 90°, the leg is then extended without changing the position of thigh.

Clinical Occurrence. *Lesions of the Cauda Equina:* neuroma, hemorrhage into the meninges, postherpetic neuralgia. *Lesions of the Sacral Plexus and Nerve:* neurofibroma and other neoplasms, diabetic neuritis, polyarteritis nodosa, penetrating lesions. *Lesions of Bone:* osteoarthritis of the spine, spondylitis (tuberculous and other infections), spondylosis, spondylolisthesis, dislocation-fracture. *Lesions of Cartilage:* herniation of intervertebral disk. *Lesions of Arteries:* aneurysm of the internal iliac artery (p. 580). *Lesions of Soft Tissues:* fibrositis, fat herniation, gluteal bursitis, trauma to nerve.

Acquired Calcaneovalgus: ***Tibial Nerve Palsy*** (a Sciatic Component). This is the *motor nerve* to the Gastrocnemius group and intrinsic muscles in the sole of the foot; it is *sensory* to the skin of the sole. Paralysis of the tibial nerve causes a *calcaneovalgus* deformity by the unopposed action of the dorsiflexors and evertors of the foot (Fig. 10-9A). Plantar flexion and inversion of the foot are weak; the *ankle jerk* is absent. The sole is *anesthetic,* thus vulnerable to trophic ulcers (Fig. 10-9A).

Acquired Equinovarus: ***Common Peroneal Nerve Palsy*** (a Sciatic Component). This is the *motor nerve* to the muscles of the anterior and lateral compartments of the leg and the short extensors of the toes; it is *sensory* to the dorsum of the foot and ankle. Peroneal paralysis causes an *equinovarus* deformity with inability to dorsiflex the foot and toes, a *foot drop* (Fig. 10-9B). An area of *anesthesia* covers the dorsum of the foot and sometimes extends up the lateral side of the leg (Fig. 10-9B). Where it winds around the fibular head, the nerve trunk may be rolled under the fingers; this maneuver elicits

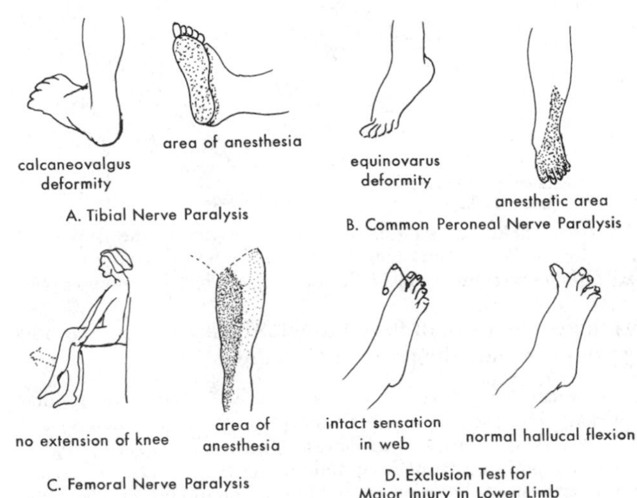

Fig. 10-9. Nerve lesions of the lower limb. **A.** Tibial nerve paralysis. *The foot assumes the posture of calcaneovalgus from paralysis of the plantar flexors. The sole of the foot is anesthetic (stippled region).* **B.** Common peroneal nerve paralysis. *The foot assumes the position of equinovarus; it cannot be dorsiflexed—a foot drop. The dorsum of the foot and frequently the lateral aspect of the leg are anesthetic (stippled region).* **C.** Femoral nerve paralysis. *The knee cannot be extended, as when the patient tries when sitting. The region of anesthesia covers the major portion of the anterior thigh and medial aspect of the leg.* **D.** Exclusion test for major nerve injury in lower limb (Hamilton Bailey). *Sensation is intact in the web between the great toe and second toe; extension (dorsiflexion) of the great toe is normally performed.*

extreme *tenderness* when neuritis is present; there is little tenderness in tabes.

Complete Paralysis of the Foot: ***Combined Tibial and Common Peroneal Palsy*** (Complete Sciatic Paralysis.) All muscles below the knee are paralyzed. An area of anesthesia extends over the sole and dorsum of the foot and up the lateral aspect of the leg.

Lack of Knee Extension: ***Femoral Nerve Palsy.*** This is the motor nerve for the Quadriceps femoris, so the patient cannot walk, and standing is unstable. Extension of the knee is impossible

(Fig. 10-9C). Anesthesia is widespread over the anteromedial aspect of the thigh, knee, leg, and the medial aspect of the foot.

The Reflexes

The simplest of reflex arcs is utilized for the stretch reflex. Its components are a muscle cell, a sensory and a motor neuron. The *afferent limb* of the arc is the sensory neuron whose cell is in the dorsal root ganglion; its dendrite extends to the muscle cell, its axon penetrates the gray matter of the cord. Within the muscle cell, the dendrite ends in a muscle spindle, the specialized *receptor organ*. Stretching the muscle evokes an afferent impulse from receptor to dorsal ganglion, thence by the axon into the cord's gray matter. The impulse passes a synapse between the axon and the dendrite of the motor cell in the gray matter of the anterior horn. The elements of the motor cell constitute the *efferent limb* of the arc. The impulse passes by way of the motor axon through the anterior spinal root and the nerve to the muscle, where the *effector organ*, the muscle fiber, is stimulated to contract.

Most reflex arcs are more complex but are extensions of the basic two-neuron unit (Fig. 10-10). The afferent and efferent neurons may be separated by intervening *connector* neurons at the same spinal level or at widely different levels, so afferent and efferent impulses travel up and down the cord for considerable distances.

The integrity of the reflex arc is broken by malfunction of any of its elements: receptor organ, sensory nerve, dorsal ganglion, spinal gray matter, anterior spinal root, motor nerve, motor end-plate, or effector organ. The physical sign of an

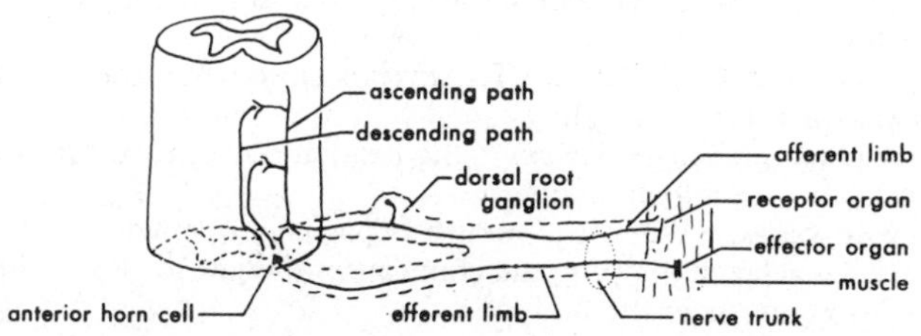

Fig. 10-10. Components of a spinal reflex arc.

interrupted reflex arc is a diminished or absent reflex. When a descending motor pathway (the pyramidal tract) in the cord is injured at a level higher than the reflex arc, normal inhibition from higher centers is lost, as indicated by a hyperactive reflex.

An important feature of the neurologic examination is the assessment of reflex arcs at known levels of the brainstem and spinal cord. The findings permit certain inferences. A normal reflex response (1) attests the integrity of every element in the reflex arc and (2) indicates the proper functioning of the motor tracts descending from levels higher than the reflex center. A diminished or absent reflex indicates malfunction of one or more components of the arc, or absence of facilitatory influences from above. Since the levels of the reflex centers are known, the findings from a systematic inventory may be employed in localizing a lesion.

In the routine examination, the clinician usually tests a few reflex arcs, representative of various levels in the cord and brainstem. When an abnormality is encountered, its lesion is pinpointed by testing more arcs.

Brainstem Reflexes

Many of these are tested in the routine examination of the cranial nerves. The findings are only valuable when the level of the reflex center is known.

Direct Pupillary Reaction to Light. The iris *constricts* when bright light is shone upon the retina.

Consensual Pupillary Reaction to Light. Stimulation of one retina with light causes *contralateral constriction* of the pupil, as well as a homolateral response.

Ciliospinal Reflex. Pinching the skin of the back of the neck causes pupillary dilatation.

Corneal Reflex. Touching the cornea causes blinking of the eyelids.

Orbicularis Oculi Reflex. The eyelids close when the retina is exposed to bright light.

Auditocephalogyric Reflex. The head and eyes turn toward the source of a loud sound.

Jaw Reflex. When the mouth is partially opened and the muscles relaxed, tapping the chin causes the jaw to close. The reflex center is in the midpons.

Gag Reflex. Gagging occurs when the pharynx is stroked. The reflex center is in the medulla.

The Deep Reflexes

These are misnamed *deep tendon reflexes* (DTR): actually they are stretching reflexes in which the muscles are suddenly stretched by a sudden tap with the finger or rubber hammer.

General Principles for Eliciting Deep Reflexes. **Strike a *sudden blow* with the finger or rubber hammer. The desirable point for the blow is over the *tendon of insertion* of a muscle. The muscle should be slightly *stretched* by the position of the limb, or by pressure on the tendon from the examiner's thumb when it is to be struck. The limb should be *relaxed;* when held tensely, the muscles may be relaxed by *reinforcement*. This is accomplished in various ways, such as having the patient concentrate on a voluntary act, as pulling on his interlocked fingers, clenching the fists, or pulling on the table or bed. The following is an arbitrary method of grading.**

Grade 0	0	Absent
Grade 1	+	Diminished but present
Grade 2	++	Normal
Grade 3	+++	Hyperactive
Grade 4	++++	Hyperactive with clonus

Reflex Center at C-5 to T-1: ***Pectoralis Reflex*** (Medial and lateral anterior thoracic nerves). Have the patient elevate the arm about 10° in 90° of abduction (Fig. 10-11A). Place the fingers of your left hand upon the patient's shoulder with your thumb extended downward to press firmly upon the tendon of the Pectoralis major. With the rubber hammer *strike your thumb* a blow directed slightly upward toward the patient's axilla. The muscle contraction can be seen or felt.

Reflex Center at C-5 to C-6: ***Biceps Reflex*** (Musculocutaneous nerve). Arrange the elbow at about 90° of flexion with the arm slightly pronated. Grasp the elbow with your left hand so the fingers are behind it and your abducted thumb presses in Biceps brachii tendon (Fig. 10-11B). *Strike your thumb* a series of blows with the rubber hammer, varying your thumb pressure with each blow until the most satisfactory response is obtained. The normal reflex is elbow flexion.

Reflex Center at C-5 to C-6: ***Brachioradialis Reflex*** (Radial

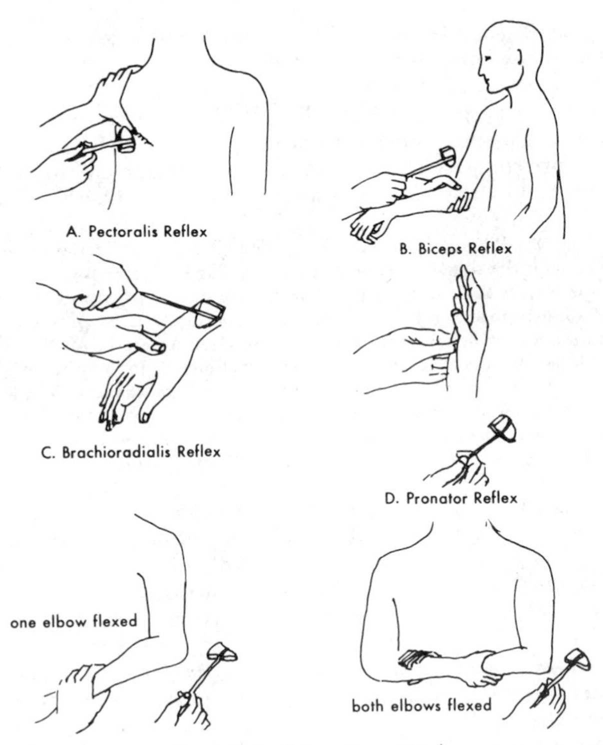

Fig. 10-11. Deep reflexes—I. **A.** Pectoralis reflex. *The examiner places his hand on the patient's shoulder with the extended thumb resting firmly on the tendon of the pectoralis major. His thumb is tapped with a blow from the rubber hammer directed upward. Normally, the muscle contraction can be seen and felt.* **B.** Biceps brachii reflex. *Have the patient's forearm flexed and partially pronated, and his elbow resting in your left hand with your thumb on the biceps brachii tendon. Strike your thumb a series of blows, varying the compression of your thumb on the tendon so optimal responses can be obtained. The normal response is flexion of the elbow.* **C.** Brachioradialis reflex. *Grasp the patient's relaxed and pronated hand with your left hand and tap the forearm directly, just above the styloid process of the radius. The normal response is elbow flexion and forearm supination.* **D.** Pronator reflex. *Suspend the patient's forearm by his hand and tap directly the distal end*

nerve). Grasp the patient's wrist with your left hand and hold his forearm relaxed in partial pronation (Fig. 10-11C). With a vertical stroke, tap the forearm *directly*, just above the radial styloid process. The normal response is elbow flexion and supination of the forearm.

Reflex Center at C-5 to T-1: ***Scapulohumeral Reflex*** (Dorsal scapular nerve). Tap the medial border of the scapula *directly* near its angle. The normal response is scapular retraction. In the prone position, this motion results mostly from contraction of the *Rhomboidei.*

Reflex Center at C-6 to C-7: ***Pronator Reflex*** (Median nerve). Grasp the patient's hand and hold it vertically so the wrist is suspended (Fig. 10-11D). From the medial side, strike the distal end of the radius *directly* with a horizontal blow. The normal response is pronation of the forearm. *Alternate Method.* Strike the distal end of the ulna *directly* with a blow mediad.

Reflex Center at C-7 to C-8: ***Triceps Reflex*** (Radial nerve). Grasp the patient's wrist with your left hand and pull his arm across his chest so the elbow is flexed about 90° and the forearm is partially pronated (Fig. 10-11E). Tap the Triceps brachii tendon *directly* just above the olecranon process. The normal response is elbow extension. *Alternate Method.* Have the patient flex both elbows, bringing his arms parallel across his chest (Fig. 10-11E). Have each hand grasp the other forearm. Reinforcement can be obtained by having him grasp harder and extending the elbow slightly. *Paradoxical Reflex.* With lesions at C-7 to C-8, the elbow may not extend; instead, *flexion* may occur from the higher innervation of the forearm flexors.

Reflex Center at T-8 to T-9: ***Upper Abdominal Muscle Reflex.*** Tap the muscles *directly* near their insertions on the costal margins and xiphoid process (Fig. 10-12A).

---

of the radius with a horizontal blow, using the blunt end of your hammer. The response is pronation of the forearm. **E.** Triceps brachii reflex. *There are two alternative positions. In one the patient's wrist is grasped and his elbow is flexed. The tendon of the triceps is tapped directly just above the olecranon process. The normal response is extension of the elbow. The alternative is to have the patient fold his arms and grasp his forearms with his hands. The triceps tendon is tapped directly. Reinforcement can be obtained by having him tighten the grasp on his arms.*

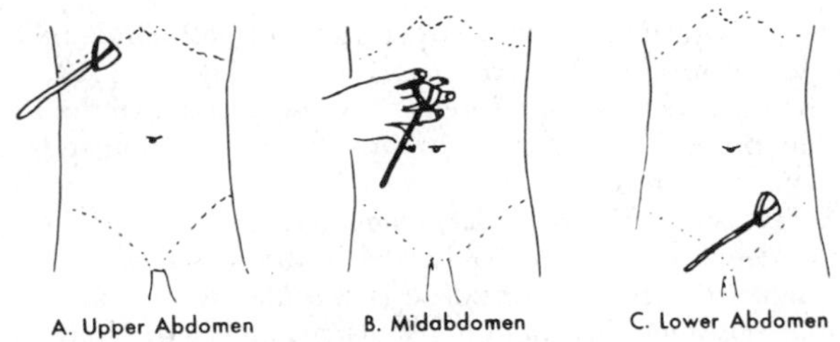

Fig. 10-12. Abdominal muscle reflexes. **A.** Upper abdomen. *Tap the abdominal muscles directly with the reflex hammer, near their attachments to the costal margin.* **B.** Midabdomen. *Place your finger or a double tongue blade upon the muscles and tap the pleximeter.* **C.** Lower abdomen. *Tap directly the lower abdominal muscles at their attachments near the symphysis pubis.*

Reflex Center at T-9 to T-10: ***Middle Abdominal Muscle Reflex.*** Stimulate the muscles of the midabdomen by *tapping an overlaid finger* or doubled tongue blades (Fig. 10-12B).

Reflex Center at T-11 to T-12: ***Lower Abdominal Muscles.*** Tap the muscle insertions *directly,* near the symphysis pubis (Fig. 10-12C).

Reflex Center at L-2 to L-4: ***Quadriceps Reflex*** (Femoral nerve). Several methods are available; select the most convenient. *Legs Dangling* (Fig. 10-13A). Have the patient sit on a table or high bed to permit free swinging of the legs. Tap the patellar tendon *directly* (the tendon is distal to the patella). Normally, extension of the knee occurs and contraction of the Quadriceps femoris may be palpated. *Feet on the Floor* (Fig. 10-13B). The patient sits on a chair or low bed. Have the knee slightly extended from a right angle by moving the foot forward on the floor; have the toes curled in *plantar flexion.*

Tap the patellar tendon *directly;* the normal response is contraction of the Quadriceps, but the foot may also kick. *Lying Supine* (Fig. 10-13C). With your hand under the popliteal fossa, lift the knee from the table. Tap the patellar tendon *directly.* *Lying Supine* (Fig. 10-13D). Grasp the foot, flexing the hip and knee; rotate the knee outward and dorsiflex the foot; tap the patellar tendon *directly.* *Lying Supine* (Fig. 10-13E). With the knee extended and the limb lying on the table, push the patellar tendon distad with your index finger on the insertion of the

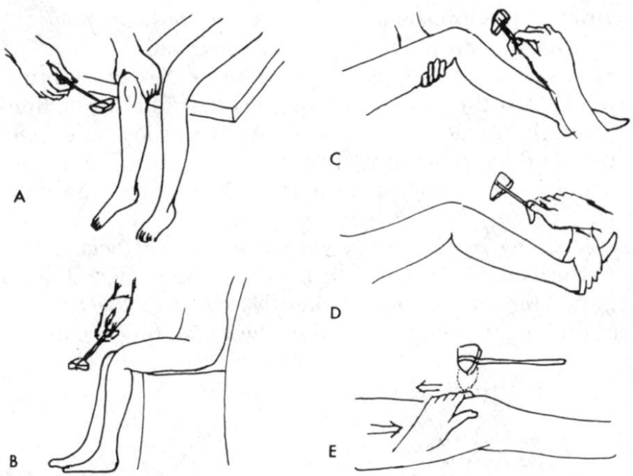

Fig. 10-13. Knee jerk (alternative positions). **A.** With the patient's legs dangling. *Grasp the lower thigh with your left hand while your right delivers a hammer tap on the patellar tendon, just below the patella. The normal response is extension of the knee.* **B.** Sitting. *When the patient sits in a chair with feet on the floor, have him advance his foot slightly. Holding the lower thigh with your left hand direct a hammer blow with your right hand to the patellar tendon.* **C.** With the patient supine. *Flex his knee slightly with your left hand under his popliteal fossa and his muscles relaxed. Strike the patellar tendon directly with hammer in your right hand.* **D.** With the supine patient. *Grasp his foot with your left hand and dorsiflex it while flexing the knee and rotating the hip outward; using your other hand, strike the patellar tendon directly.* **E.** With the supine patient and his knee extended. *Place your left index finger transversely along the proximal border of the patella and push the bone distad; tap your index finger from above downward. The normal response is elevation of the patella and contraction of the quadriceps muscle.*

Quadriceps tendon. Tap downward *on the index finger.* The muscle contraction pulls the patella proximad.

Reflex Center at L-2 to L-4: Adductor Reflex (Obturator nerve). With the patient supine, arrange the lower limb to rest in slight abduction (Fig. 10-14A). Tap the tendon *directly* on the Adductor magnus, just proximal to its insertion on the medial epicondyle of the femur. Normally, the thigh adducts.

Reflex Center at L-4 to S-2: Hamstring Reflex (Sciatic nerve). Have the patient supine with hips and knees flexed at about 90°, and the thighs rotated slightly outward. Place your left hand under the popliteal fossa so the index finger compresses

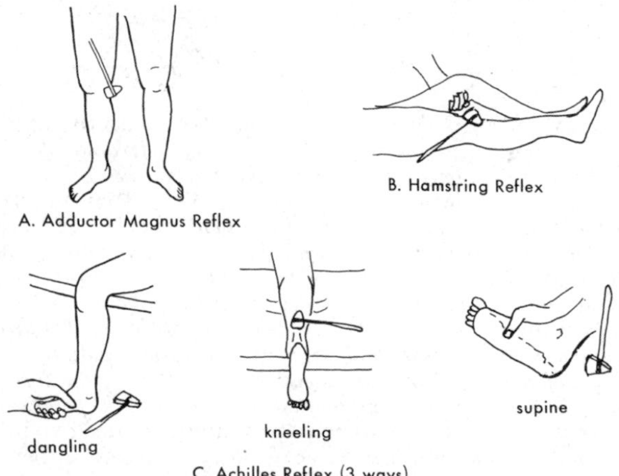

Fig. 10-14. Deep reflexes—II. **A.** Adductor magnus reflex. *Abduct the lower limbs slightly. Tap the tendon of the adductor magnus above its insertion in the medial epicondyle of the femur. The normal response is adduction of the thigh.* **B.** Hamstring reflex. *With the patient supine and his knee flexed about 90°, place your left hand under the popliteal fossa and curl your finger so it compresses the hamstring tendons on the inner aspect of the lower thigh; tap your finger. The normal response is flexion of the knee and contraction of the medial muscle mass of the posterior thigh.* **C.** Achilles reflex (3 ways). Leg dangling. *Grasp the foot and dorsiflex it to tense the tendon; tap the tendon directly with the broad edge of the hammer. Plantar flexion of the foot normally occurs.* Kneeling. Supine.

the *medial hamstring tendon* (a bundle of tendons from Semitendinosus, Semimembranosus, Gracilus, Sartorius) (Fig. 10-14B). Tap your finger. The normal response is flexion of the knee and contraction of the medial mass of hamstring muscles. *Alternate Method.* In the similar manner, with your finger compress the *lateral* hamstring tendon just proximal to the fibular head; tap your finger. The normal response is contraction of the lateral hamstring mass (Biceps femoris) and flexion of the knee.

Reflex Center at L-5 to S-2: ***Achilles Reflex*** (Tibial nerve). Legs dangling (Fig. 10-14C). With your left hand, grasp the foot and pull it in dorsiflexion; find the degree of stretching of the Achilles tendon that produces the optimal response. Tap the tendon *directly.* The normal response is contraction of the Gastrocnemius and plantar flexion of the foot. *Kneeling* (Fig. 10-14C). Have the patient kneel with the feet hanging over the edge of a chair, table, or bed. Tap the tendon *directly,* with your left hand dorsiflexing the foot for optimal stretching of the tendon. Plantar flexion of the foot is the normal response. *Supine* (Fig. 10-14C). Partially flex the hip and knee; rotate the knee outward as far as comfort permits. With your left hand, grasp the foot and pull it in dorsiflexion. Tap the Achilles tendon *directly.* The normal response is plantar flexion.

The Superficial Reflexes

These have reflex arcs whose receptor organs are in the skin, rather than in muscle fibers. Their adequate stimulus is stroking, scratching, or touching. The superficial reflexes are lost in disease of the pyramidal tract.

Reflex Center at T-5 to T-8: ***Upper Abdominal Skin Reflex.*** Have the patient supine and relaxed, with the arms at the sides and knees slightly flexed. Use a fingernail, wooden applicator tip, the end of a split tongue blade, or the blunted handle of a reflex hammer for an instrument. Stroke the skin over the lower thoracic cage, from the midaxillary line toward the midline (Fig. 10-15A). Watch for ipsilateral contraction of the muscles in the epigastric abdominal wall. When the muscle contractions cannot be seen, observe the *umbilical deviation* toward the stimulated side. In very obese persons, retract the umbilicus toward the opposite side to feel it pull toward the side of stimulation.

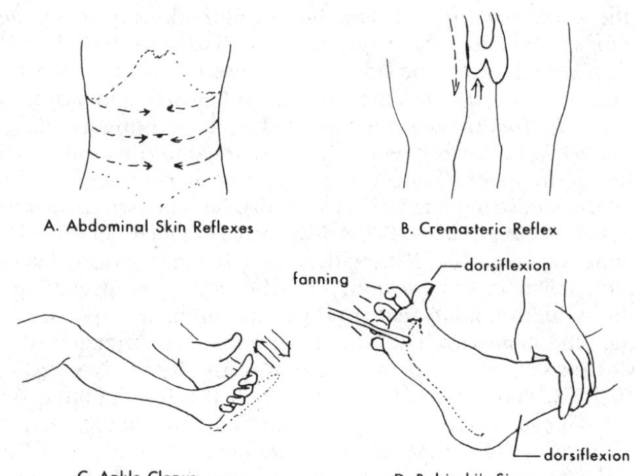

Fig. 10-15. Skin reflexes and pyramidal tract signs. **A.** Abdominal skin reflexes. *Stroke the skin lightly in the upper, middle, and lower abdomen, as indicated by the broken lines. The normal response is contraction of the muscles that pull the umbilicus and the midline to the stimulated side.* **B.** Cremasteric reflex. *In the male, stroke the skin lightly downward in the direction indicated by the broken line. The normal response is prompt elevation of the testis on the same side. A slow tortuous movement results from contraction of the dartos fascia, but this is not the sought-for reflex.* **C.** Ankle clonus. *With the patient supine, lift the knee in slight flexion with the muscles relaxed. Grasp the foot and jerk it into dorsiflexion, then hold it under slight tension in that direction. In a positive response, the foot reacts with a number of cycles of alternating dorsiflexion and plantar flexion. The motion may die in a few cycles (unsustained clonus), or it may persist as long as the tension is held (sustained clonus).* **D.** Babinski's sign. *With a blunt instrument, stroke the sole of the foot along a path indicated by the broken line. Normally, this stimulus produces plantar flexion of the great toe and the smaller toe. In disease of the pyramidal tract, this reflex results, with some or all of four components: dorsiflexion of the great toe, fanning of all toes, dorsiflexion of the ankle, flexion of the knee and thigh.*

Reflex Center at T-9 to T-11: ***Midabdominal Skin Reflex.*** Make similar strokes from the flank toward the midline at the umbilical level.

Reflex Center at T-11 to T-12: ***Lower Abdominal Skin Reflex.***

Make similar strokes from the crests of the ilia toward the midline of the hypogastrium.

Reflex Center at L-1 to L-2: Cremasteric Reflex. In males, stroke the inner aspect of the thigh from the pubis distad (Fig. 10-15B). Normally, this causes contraction of the Cremaster with *prompt* elevation of the testis on the ipsilateral side. A *slow* and *irregular rise* of the testis results from muscular contraction in the dartos tunic and *is not* the reflex response.

Reflex Center at L-4 to S-2: Plantar Reflex. Scratch the sole near its lateral aspect, from the heel toward the toes. Normally, this produces plantar flexion of the toes; often the entire foot responds with plantar flexion.

Reflex Center at L-1 to L-2: Superficial Anal Reflex. Stroke the skin or mucosa of the perianal region. Normally, the external and anal sphincter contracts.

Abnormal Reflexes in Pyramidal Tract Disease

Altered Normal Reflexes. A lesion of the pyramidal tract almost invariably causes complete *suppression* of the normal superficial reflexes caudal to the level of the lesion. On the contrary, the deep reflexes are *hyperactive,* except during the stage of spinal shock, when they are absent.

Muscle Clonus. A hyperactive reflex may produce *clonus,* an abnormal response of the stretch reflex from release of central inhibitions of the reflex arc. Clonus is a rhythmic contraction of muscles initiated by stretching. Clonus may be *unsustained,* lasting for only a few jerks despite continued stretching; or it may be sustained, persisting as long as stretching is applied. *Ankle Clonus (Gastrocnemius Clonus).* This is most commonly encountered. With the knee flexed, grasp the foot and dorsiflex it; rhythmic contractions of the Gastrocnemius and Soleus cause the foot to alternate between dorsiflexion and plantar flexion (Fig. 10-15C). *Patellar Clonus (Quadriceps Clonus).* With the patient supine and the relaxed lower limb extended, grasp the patella and push it quickly distad. The patella will jerk up and down from the rhythmic contractions of the Quadriceps femoris. *Wrist Clonus (Finger Flexor Clonus).* Grasp the patient's fingers and forcibly hyperextend the wrist. The wrist will rhythmically alternate between flexion and extension.

Babinski's Sign. Grasp the ankle with your left hand. With a blunt point and moderate pressure, stroke the sole near its lateral border, from the heel toward the ball, where the course should curve mediad to follow the bases of the toes (Fig. 10-15D). For the blunt point, use a wooden applicator tip, the end of a split wooden tongue blade, or the dull handle end on some reflex hammers; the stimulus *should not be painful.* The complete reflex is (1) dorsiflexion of the great toe, (2) fanning of all toes, (3) dorsiflexion of the ankle, (4) flexion and withdrawal of the knee and hip. Partially developed responses will be encountered, such as only dorsiflexion of the great toe, failure of the small toes to abduct or fan, fanning of small toes without hallucal dorsiflexion. *These partial responses are all pathognomonic* of different degrees of pyramidal disease; so their details of response should be accurately recorded. Alternate methods of eliciting Babinski's reflex have been described as eponymic signs. In *Oppenheim's sign,* hallucal dorsiflexion is elicited with pressure applied by the thumb and index finger, or by the knuckles, to the subcutaneous surface of the tibia. The pressure stroke should begin at the upper two thirds of the bone and be carried distad to ankle. In *Chaddock's sign,* the stimulus is a scratch with a dull point. The path of stimulation should curve around the lateral malleolus of the ankle, then along the lateral aspect of the dorsum of the foot.

Hoffmann's Sign. Have the patient present his pronated hand with fingers extended and relaxed, to be held in your hand. Support his extended middle finger by your right index finger held transversely under his distal interphalangeal joint crease (Fig. 10-16B). With your thumb, press his fingernail to flex the terminal digit and stretch his flexor. The abnormal reflex is flexion and adduction of the thumb; the other fingers may also flex. When the reflex is present bilaterally, it is abnormal but not diagnostic. Unilateral occurrence suggests pyramidal tract disease, especially when accompanied by other signs.

Mayer's Reflex. Have the patient present his supinated hand to you with the thumb relaxed and abducted (Fig. 10-16C). Grasp his ring finger and firmly flex the metacarpophalangeal joint. The normal response is adduction and apposition of the thumb; the *response is absent* in pyramidal tract disease. This is a reliable diagnostic sign.

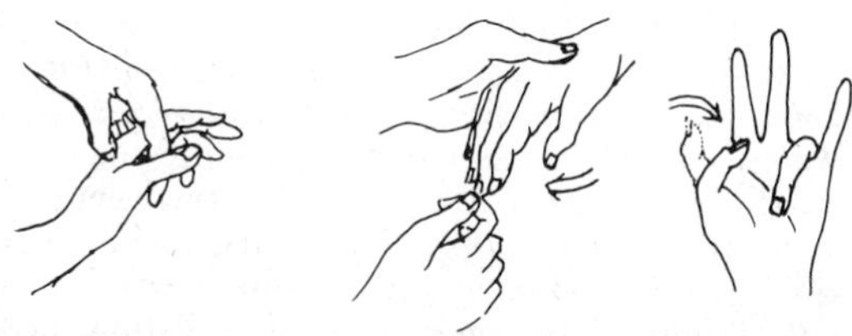

Fig. 10-16. Some pathologic reflexes. **A.** Grasp reflex. *With your index finger, stroke the patient's palm as he grasps your finger. In lesions of the premotor cortex, he may be unable to release his grasp.* **B.** Hoffmann's sign. *Hold the patient's hand relaxed and pronated. Place your index finger under the distal interphalangeal joint of the long finger and flex the terminal phalanx with your thumb. In pyramidal tract disease, the patient's thumb may flex and adduct.* **C.** Mayer's reflex. *Have the patient present his relaxed supinated hand to you. Firmly flex the ring finger at its proximal joint. The normal response is adduction and flexion of the thumb. Absence of this occurs in pyramidal tract disease.*

Primitive Reflexes

All of these signs may represent frontal lobe disease.

Grasp Reflex. Stroke the patient's palm so he grasps your index finger between his thumb and index finger (Fig. 10-16A). When the grasp reflex is present, he cannot release the fingers when he tries. This is a normal response in young infants; later in life, lesions of the premotor cortex may uncover the reflex as a pathologic finding.

Palmomental (Radovici's Sign). Vigorous scratching or pricking of the thenar eminence causes ipsilateral contraction of the muscles of the chin. This occurs in pyramidal tract disease, increased intracranial pressure, latent tetany, and certain other nervous disorders.

Snout/Suck Reflexes. Scratching or gentle percussion of the upper lip may induce a puckering or sucking movement.

Spinal Automatisms

When the central inhibitions of reflexes are lost in severe disease of the spinal cord or brain.

Spinal Reflex Reactions. In extensive lesions of the cord or midbrain, painful stimulation of a limb may produce ipsilateral flexion of both upper and lower extremities, called *ipsilateral mass flexion reflex, spinal withdrawal,* or *shortening reflex.*

Mass Reflex. A transverse lesion of the cord may produce *flexion followed by extension* of the limbs below the level of lesion. In complete transection, *only flexion* occurs, accompanied by contractions of the abdominal wall, incontinence of urine and feces, and autonomic responses, such as sweating, flushing, and pilomotor activity. This complex is termed *mass reflex.* Involuntary urination may be stimulated by stroking the skin of the thighs and abdomen, *automatic bladder. Priapism* and seminal ejaculation may be induced by similar mechanisms. In the *crossed extensor reflex,* flexion of one limb may be associated with extension of its counterpart. In some cases, the *extensor thrust reaction* is encountered; pressure on the sole causes extension of the leg; when the leg is placed in flexion, scratching on the skin of the thigh induces extension of the leg. Painful stimulation of an arm or chest may result in abduction and outward rotation of the shoulder.

Associated Movements

Associated movements are involuntary motor patterns, more complex than reflexes, that normally accompany voluntary acts, such as swinging the arms while walking, facial movements of expression, motions accompanying coughing and yawning. Frequently, these are lost in disease of the pyramidal tract or the basal ganglion. The patient with paralysis agitans walks without swinging his arms; characteristically, he has a masklike face devoid of all emotional expression. The hemiplegic patient carries the affected arm in adduction, with the elbow flexed, the forearm pronated, and the wrist flexed. The paretic arm may involuntarily mimic the voluntary movements of its normal counterpart, *contralateral associated movement.*

Signs of Meningeal Irritation

Meningitis, meningismus, subarachnoid hemorrhage, posterior fossa tumors, and the results of increased intracranial pressure cause abnormal spasms of various muscle groups, which are apparent as special physical signs.

Nuchal Rigidity. The patient cannot place the chin upon his chest. Passive flexion of the neck is limited by involuntary muscle spasm. Testing the passive flexion induces involuntary hip flexion (Brudzinski's sign).

Spinal Rigidity. Movements of the spine are limited by spasms of the Erector spinae. In extreme cases, the spinal muscles are in tetanic contraction, producing rigid hyperextension of the entire spine; the head is forced backward, the trunk thrust forward; the condition is termed *opisthotonos*.

Kernig's Sign. With the patient supine, passively flex the hip to 90° while the knee is flexed at about 90° (Fig. 10-17A). With the hip kept in flexion, attempts to extend the knee produce *pain in the hamstrings* and *resistance* to further extension. This is a reliable sign of meningeal irritation; but it may occur with herniated disk or tumors of the cauda equina.

Brudzinski's Sign. With the patient supine and the limbs extended, passively flex the neck; this produces *flexion of the hips,* a sign of meningeal irritation (Fig. 10-17B).

Coordination

A precise voluntary movement around a joint requires a graded increase of tone in the *agonist,* or prime mover, with a corresponding graded decrease in the tone of the *antagonist.* Other muscles must act to fix the joint with proper tension. The total integration of these movements is called *coordination,* partially mediated through efferent and afferent tracts of the cerebellum. The vestibular apparatus and the cerebral cortex

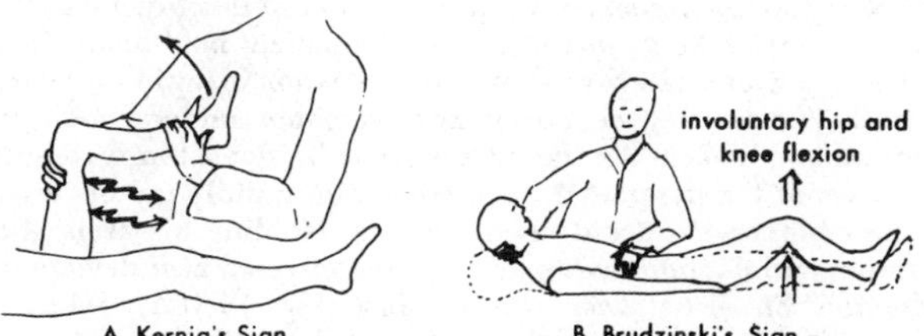

Fig. 10-17. Two signs of meningeal irritation. **A.** Kernig's sign. *With the patient supine, flex the hip and knee each to about 90°. With the hip immobile, attempt to extend the knee. In meningeal irritation, this attempt is resisted and causes pain in the hamstring muscles.* **B.** Brudzinski's sign. *Place the patient supine and hold the thorax down upon the bed. Attempt to flex the neck. In meningeal irritation, this maneuver causes involuntary flexion of the hips.*

also participate in many acts. The perfect execution of skilled acts is *eupraxia;* loss of previous ability in performance is *apraxia.* This reflects a higher brain disturbance in converting an idea into a skilled act.

Equilibration involves the proper functions of the proprioceptive mechanisms, the vestibular apparatus, and the cerebellum. Loss of coordination in maintaining proper posture is *ataxia.* If the patient is incoordinate lying down, he has *static ataxia;* if the condition is only evident on standing or moving, it is *kinetic ataxia.*

TESTING OF STATION (EQUILIBRATORY COORDINATION). ***Position of the Feet:*** **Ataxia from spinocerebellar disease is less when the patient stands on a broad base, the feet widely apart.** ***With Eyes Open or Closed:*** **Cerebellar ataxia is not ameliorated by visual orientation; but the ataxia from posterior column disease involves disordered proprioceptive sensations and** ***only appears,*** **or** ***is worsened,*** **when the eyes are closed (see Romberg's sign, p. 194).** ***Direction of Falling:*** **In disease of the** ***lateral lobe*** **of the cerebellum, falling is** ***toward*** **the affected side; frontal lobe lesions cause falling to the** ***opposite*** **side; lesions of the midline or vermis of the cerebellum may cause falling** ***indiscriminately,*** **depending entirely upon the initial stance of the patient.**

TESTING OF DIADOCHOKINESIA. **Normal coordination includes the ability to arrest one motor impulse and substitute its opposite. Loss of this ability is** ***dysdiadochokinesia,*** **characteristic of cerebellar disease. Many simple tests may be employed to test this function.** ***Alternating Movements*** **(Fig. 10-18A): Have the patient hold his forearms vertically and alternate pronation and supination in rapid succession. In cerebellar disease, the movements overshoot, undershoot, or are irregular and inaccurate; the motions may be slowed or incomplete in disease of the pyramidal tract. Have him rapidly tap his fingers on the table, or close and open the fists. Holding his arms at 90° elevation and 0° abduction may show the affected arm deviating in abduction.** ***Stewart-Holmes Rebound Sign*** **(Fig. 10-18A): While the patient clenches his fist, with elbow flexed and forearm pronated, grasp his fist from above and pull strongly to extend his elbow; then suddenly release your grip and the forearm may rebound in several cycles of extension-flexion, or the patient may strike himself if not guarded.**

TESTING FOR DYSSYNERGIA AND DYSMETRIA. ***Finger-to-Nose Test:*** **With the patient's** ***eyes open,*** **have him partially extend his elbow**

and, in a wide arc, rapidly bring the tip of the index finger to the tip of his nose (Fig. 10-18B). In cerebellar disease, this action is attended by an *action tremor.* When the maneuver is performed with the *eyes closed,* the sense of position in the shoulder and elbow is tested. In a variant of this maneuver, have the patient make wide arcs with both arms to approximate the tips of his index fingers in front of him. *Heel-to-Knee Test:* With the patient supine and the lower limbs resting in extension, ask him to raise one heel and place it upon the opposite knee, then slide the heel down the subcutaneous aspect of the tibia (Fig. 10-18C). The moving foot should be dorsiflexed, and the motion should be performed slowly and accurately. In *cerebellar disease,* the arc of the heel to the knee is *jerky* and *wavering,* the *knee* is frequently *overshot,* and the slide down the shin is accompanied by an *action tremor.* In *posterior column disease,* the heel may have difficulty finding the knee, but the ride down the shin weaves from side to side, or the heel may fall off altogether.

TESTING SKILLED ACTS. **To inspect his handwriting, have the patient write sentences on paper. Test his skill at buttoning and unbuttoning his coat or shirt. Let him pick up pins or thread a needle. Test his skill at cutting figures out of paper with scissors.**

TESTING THE VESTIBULAR APPARATUS. **Past pointing and other tests are described on pp. 193–94.**

The Gait

The gait is influenced by the rate, rhythm, and the character of the movements employed in walking. In assessing the neurologic significance of the gait, painful and restrictive conditions of the joints, muscles, and other structures must be excluded.

Ataxia: ***Cerebellar Disease.*** The ataxia produces a staggering, wavering, and lurching walk that is not benefited by the patient's view of his surroundings. With a lesion in the mid-cerebellum, movements are in *all directions.* When a cerebellar lobe is involved, staggering and falling are *toward* the affected side. The ataxia is somewhat steadied by standing or walking *on a wide base,* i.e., with the legs far apart. Ataxia secondary to vestibular disease may appear similar.

Ataxia: ***Posterior Column Disease.*** In the tabes dorsalis, the posterior column of the cord is affected, so proprioceptive impulses are defective; thus, the ataxia is much greater *with the eyes closed.* The feet are lifted too high; frequently they

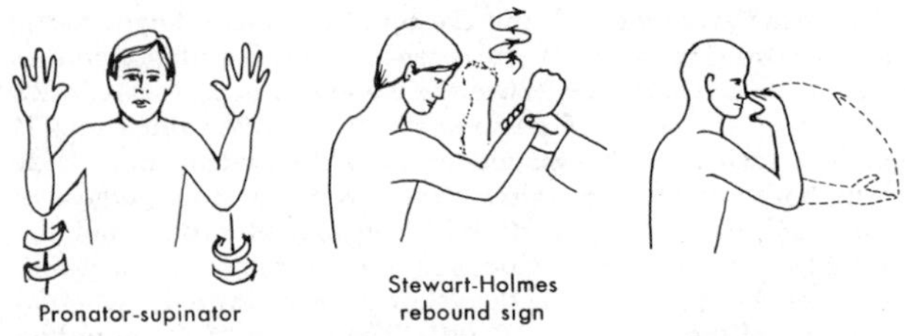

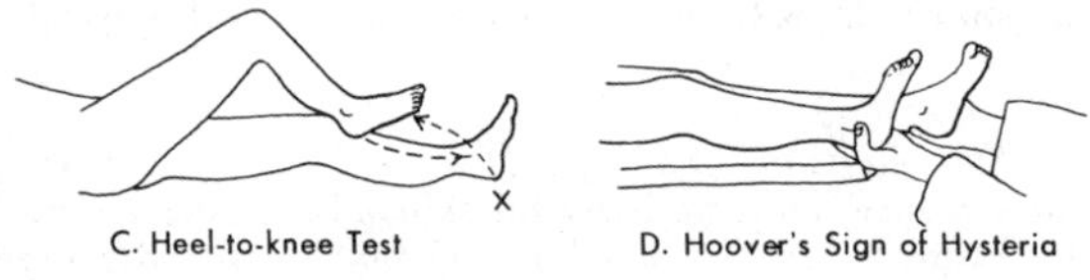

Fig. 10-18. Test for cerebellar disease **A.** Tests for diadochokinesia. *The ability to perform alternating movements may be tested by having the patient hold the forearms vertically; he is then required to quickly alternate pronation and supination in the vertical position. In cerebellar disease the movements overshoot, undershoot, or become grossly confused. Another method is the Stewart-Holmes rebound test in which the patient is requested to flex his biceps brachii muscle by pulling against the wrist held by the examiner. While in full pulling, the examiner suddenly releases the wrist and the patient's arm rebounds with much overshooting; the examiner must guard against the patient hurting himself. There may be several alternating motions to the rebound. This test is positive in cerebellar disease.* **B.** Finger-to-nose test. *With the eyes open, the patient is asked to extend his elbow, then quickly bring his index finger in a wide arc from the dependent position to his nose. With cerebellar disease, this motion is accompanied by an action tremor. When performed with the eyes closed, inaccuracy indicates loss of sense of position.* **C.** Heel-to-knee tests. *With the patient supine and his legs extended, have him lift one heel, place it upon the opposite knee, and glide the heel down the subcutaneous aspect of the tibia. In cerebellar disease, the path of the heel to the knee is shaky, jerky, and frequently overshoots the target, despite the fact that the patient has full view of the movements. The glide down the shin is attended by an action tremor. With the eyes closed, the motions are inaccurate in posterior spinal column disease; frequently*

are set down with excessive force. The patient fixes his eyes where he is walking to compensate for loss of proprioception. Ataxia due to peripheral nerve sensory loss may look similar.

Steppage Gait: ***Foot Drop.*** When the dorsiflexors of the foot are paralyzed, the patient slaps the foot down in walking. To compensate for the toe drop, he must raise the thigh excessively, as if he were walking upstairs.

Clinical Occurrence. Unilateral toe drop usually results from injury of the peroneal nerve. Bilateral paralysis may occur from poliomyelitis, lesions of the cauda equina, or the peroneal atrophy in Charcot-Marie-Tooth disease.

Hemiplegic Gait: ***Spastic Gait.*** The patient walks with the spastic arm (p. 724), while the affected lower limb is extended at the hip, knee, and ankle; the foot is inverted. In walking, the patient may swing the thigh in a lateral arc or push the inverted foot along the floor.

Spastic Gait: ***Scissors Gait.*** In paraplegia with adductor spasm, the knees are pulled together so the body must sway laterally away from the stepping limb to clear the floor.

Festinating Gait: ***Parkinsonian Gait.*** The trunk and neck are held rigidly and flexed; the patient acts as if he were about to fall forward. The associated movements of swinging the arms are lost. The steps are short and shuffling; they become faster in an attempt to avoid falling (festination).

Clownish Gait: ***Huntington's Chorea.*** Walking is attended by grotesque movements caused by the interposition of purposeless involuntary acts.

Waddling Gait: ***Muscular Dystrophy.*** The patient walks with a broad base. The thighs are thrown forward by twisting the pelvis to compensate for the weak quadriceps muscles. A similar gait is employed by those with bilateral dislocations of the hips.

---

the heel slides off the shin; but action tremor is absent. **D.** Hoover's sign of hysteria. *This distinguishes hysterical paralysis of the lower limb from one with an organic cause. Take a position at the foot of the supine patient. Cradle each of his heels in one of your palms and rest your hands upon the table. Have the patient attempt to raise the affected limb. In organic disease, the associated movement causes the unaffected heel to press downward; in hysteria the associated movement is absent.*

Bizarre Gait: ***Hysteria.*** Grotesque movements may be employed in walking when the patient has hysteria; paraplegia and other diseases must be excluded. In this instance, try *Hoover's sign,* depending upon the absence of a normal associated movement. Have the patient supine, stand at the foot of the table, and place a palm under each heel; ask him to raise the affected limb (Fig. 10-18D). In neither organic disease nor hysteria will the leg be raised; but in organic disease, the associated movement of pressing down with the unaffected heel will still be present; it is absent in hysteria. The sign is helpful only when the patient has, or claims to have, *complete* paralysis of one leg.

Leg Discomfort Relieved by Walking: ***Restless Legs Syndrome*** (Ekbom's Syndrome). The patient complains of *leg discomfort at rest.* The sensation may be aching, drawing, pulling, prickling, restlessness, formication, or completely nondescript. Always bilateral, the sensations are *relieved by walking* or massage. There are no pertinent physical findings. Patients with the syndrome have a high incidence of depression, anxiety, or unusual stress. The cause and treatment are unknown.

Sensory Functions

A complete assessment of sensory functions is not made in the routine physical examination. But the history of localized pain, numbness, or tingling or the finding of motor deficits calls for a detailed sensory examination.

The prerequisites for sensory assessment are (1) detailed knowledge of segmental and peripheral nerve distribution in the skin by reference to such charts as Figs. 10-19 and 10-20, (2) a lucid sensorium and adequate attention on the part of the patient to secure his cooperation, and (3) a graphic record of the distribution of sensory deficits. The diagram may be used for immediate comparison on retesting, because several examinations for sensation should always be performed. Disparities in two examinations may point to deception by the patient, so every effort should be made to trick him by varying the order.

The detailed examination of the cranial nerves includes testing of the special senses and the cutaneous sensibility of the head. For the remainder of the body, the distribution of sensibility for cutaneous pain, touch, pressure, position, and vibration

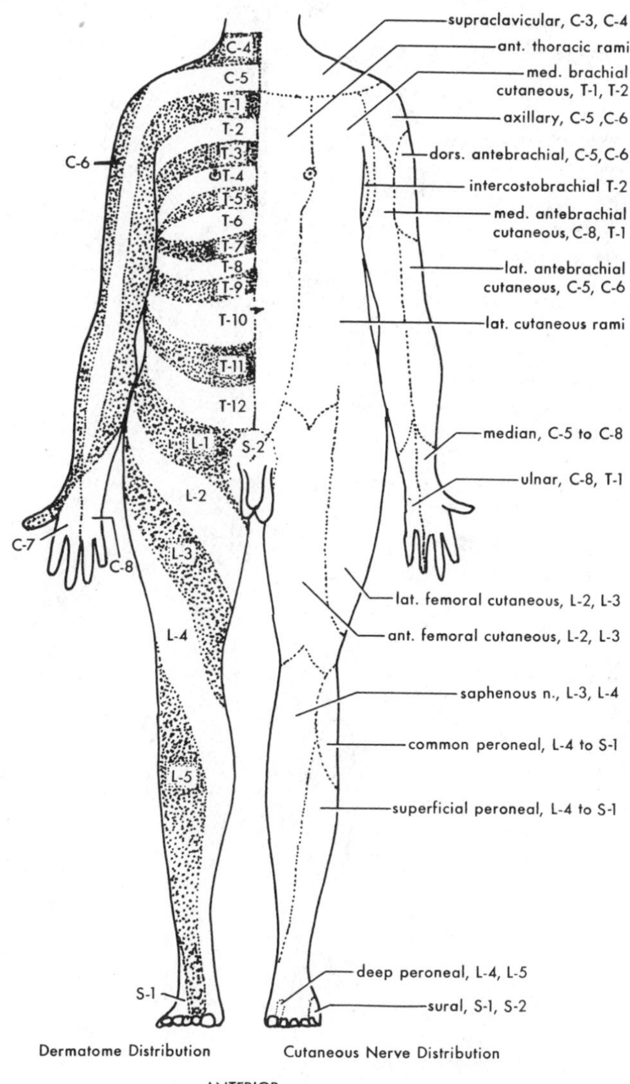

Fig. 10-19. Cutaneous sensation in the anterior aspect of the body.

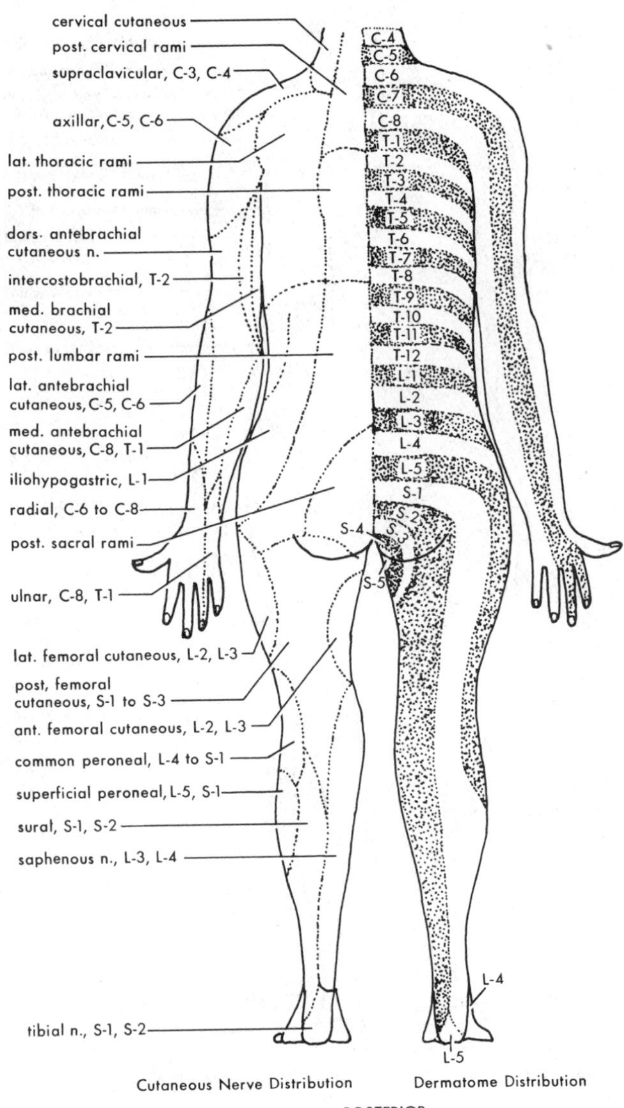
cervical cutaneous
post. cervical rami
supraclavicular, C-3, C-4
axillar, C-5, C-6
lat. thoracic rami
post. thoracic rami
dors. antebrachial cutaneous n.
intercostobrachial, T-2
med. brachial cutaneous, T-2
post. lumbar rami
lat. antebrachial cutaneous, C-5, C-6
med. antebrachial cutaneous, C-8, T-1
iliohypogastric, L-1
radial, C-6 to C-8
post. sacral rami
ulnar, C-8, T-1
lat. femoral cutaneous, L-2, L-3
post, femoral cutaneous, S-1 to S-3
ant. femoral cutaneous, L-2, L-3
common peroneal, L-4 to S-1
superficial peroneal, L-5, S-1
sural, S-1, S-2
saphenous n., L-3, L-4
tibial n., S-1, S-2
C-4
C-5
C-6
C-7
C-8
T-1
T-2
T-3
T-4
T-5
T-6
T-7
T-8
T-9
T-10
T-11
T-12
L-1
L-2
L-3
L-4
L-5
S-1
S-2
S-3
S-4
S-5
L-4
L-5
Cutaneous Nerve Distribution
Dermatome Distribution
POSTERIOR

Fig. 10-20. Cutaneous sensation in the posterior aspect of the body.

should be evaluated. When a deficit in the pain sense is encountered, the sensibility for temperature should also be tested. When an area of altered cutaneous sensibility is found, the borders should be marked with a skin pencil and a diagram should be made in the patient's record.

TESTING PAIN SENSE. ***Superficial Pain:*** **Have the patient close his eyes and indicate whenever he feels a pinprick. The stimulus may be the point of a common pin, held lightly between your thumb and index finger so that the pin slides slightly with each pressure. If there is doubt about the response, mix *sharp* and *dull* stimuli from the point and head of the pin. Perhaps better, use the point and the dull guard end of an open safety pin (Fig. 10-21A). Compare symmetric zones with the same degree of pressure. In mapping the borders of a deficient area, run the stroke from nonsensitive to sensitive skin, having the patient indicate where the sensation changes. Sensibility to pain may be *normal, reduced* (hypalgesia), *absent* (analgesia), or *increased* (hyperalgesia). *Deep Pain:* Test for *deep* or *protopathic pain* by pressure on the eyeballs, the testes, the nerve trunks, and the tendons. For example, in *Abadie's sign* for tabes dorsalis the normal pressure tenderness of the Achilles tendon is lost.**

TESTING TEMPERATURE SENSE. **When the pain sense is impaired, test for sensibility to temperature; the pathways for both senses are closely associated. Have the patient close his eyes, test for "cold" perception by blowing on the patient's skin through your *pursed lips;* in testing for "warmth" perception, blow upon the skin through your *widespread lips,* asking him to distinguish between hot and cold. Temperature discrimination is lost in syringomyelia while tactile sense is retained.**

TESTING TACTILE SENSE. **When his eyes are closed, stroke the patient's skin with a shred of gauze, comparing symmetric points and having him indicate when you touch him. If you suspect that he is using his eyes, make sham tests near but not touching the skin. Grade the results as *normal, anesthetic, hypesthetic,* and *hyperesthetic.* Hysteria may be revealed in outlining the borders of an area of "anesthesia," by stimulating from the center to the border in a zigzagging line that seems to confuse the patient and results in disparities between successive tests.**

Tactile Extinction Test: **In parietal lobe disease, the patient may perceive touch accurately when the stimulation is applied to symmetric points *consecutively;* if the points are stimulated *simultaneously,* he does not perceive on the affected side.**

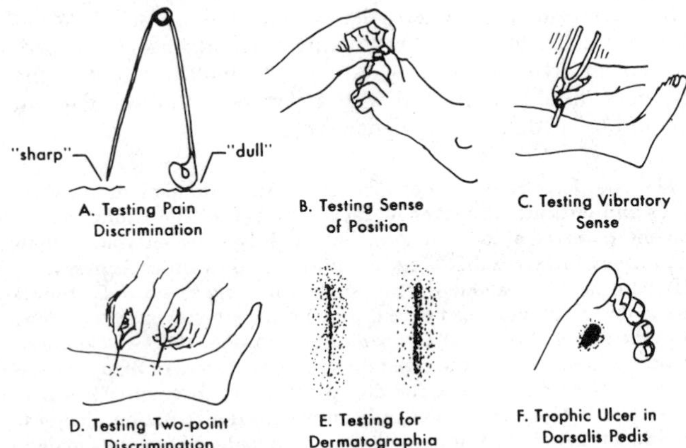

Fig. 10-21. Methods of testing sensory phenomena and others. **A.** Use of safety pin to test pain discrimination in the skin. **B.** Testing sense of position in the toes. *With your thumb and index finger, grasp the lateral and medial sides of a toe to flex or extend it. With the patient's eyes closed, he is asked to indicate the position of the toe. Avoid pressure on the dorsal or plantar surfaces of the digit that might furnish a clue.* **C.** Testing vibratory sense. *Set the tuning fork in vibration and place the end of the handle on a bony surface; ask the patient to indicate when the vibration ceases. Then transfer the handle to the dorsum of your own wrist to test for any residual vibration. Make sham tests by stopping the forks with your fingers before touching the patient.* **D.** Testing two-point discrimination. *Prick the skin simultaneously with two pins, separated by various distances, to determine the minimal separation required to be perceived as two points.* **E.** Testing for dermatographism. *Stroke the skin with a blunt object; the normal response is a pale line along the path of stimulation, the "white line." The abnormal responses are a "red line" in which the area becomes bright red, and then extends with red mottling. In a more exaggerated response the red line develops a wheal that becomes raised, edematous, pale.* **F.** Trophic plantar ulcer in tabes dorsalis.

TESTING PROPRIOCEPTIVE SENSE. ***Position Sense:*** **With the patient's eyes closed, grasp his finger on the sides; extend or flex it and ask him to state its position (Fig. 10-21B). Similarly, test the sense of position in his toes; move his heel and ask him to point to it. Shielded from his view, displace one lower limb and request him to place the counterpart in a symmetric position.**

Pressure Sense: Test the patient's ability to discriminate between objects of different weights by placing them in his palms. Test the ability to distinguish between pressures from the head of a pin and the tip of your finger. Press over the joints and subcutaneous aspects of bones for perception of pressure.

Vibratory Sense (Pallesthesia): Place the handle of a vibrating tuning fork over bony prominences, such as the clavicles, the epicondyles of the elbows, the styloid processes of the radii, the carpi, the knuckles, the epicondyles of the femora, the subcutaneous aspects of the tibiae, the malleoli of the ankles (Fig. 10-21C). Compare symmetric points. When the patient indicates that the vibration of the fork has ceased, place the handle on your own wrist to detect any persistence of vibration. Make sham tests by setting the fork in vibration and unobtrusively stopping it with your finger before applying the handle to the patient. Pallesthesia diminishes with aging, posterior column disease, and peripheral neuropathy.

TESTING HIGHER INTEGRATIVE FUNCTIONS. *Stereognosis:* Test the ability to distinguish forms by placing objects in the patient's hands while his eyes are closed. Present for his identification coins, jackknives, pencils, glass, wood, stone, metal, cloth, and other familiar articles. *Astereognosis* occurs in cortical disease; sensory perception should have been previously demonstrated as normal.

Two-Point Discrimination: Test the ability to distinguish the separation of two simultaneous pinpricks (Fig. 10-21D). By separating two pinpoints with various distances, find the distance at which he perceives them as two points rather than as one. Test and compare symmetric regions. The normal distance varies in different parts of the body, from 1 mm on the tongue, 2–8 mm on the fingertip, 40 mm on the chest and forearm, 75 mm on the upper thigh and upper arm.

Perception of Figures on the Skin (Graphesthesia): Tell the patient whether you will write numerals or letters. Then, with his eyes closed, trace a figure from the announced category upon the skin of the trunk, palm, or dorsum of the hand. Use a blunt point. The figures should be at least 4 cm high. Ask the patient to identify them.

Autonomic Nervous System

Temperature Regulation. Some instances of *hyperthermia* occur from lesions of the hypothalamus or high cervical cord: *hypothermia* is encountered in insulin shock and myxedema, although the role of the autonomics in the latter condition is doubtful.

Vasomotor Disorders. Peripheral vasospasm with pallor and cyanosis occurs locally in Raynaud's phenomenon (p. 432), vasodilatation is evident in erythromelalgia (p. 908), *Dermatographia* is an autonomic reflex stimulated by stroking the skin. Normally, light scratching produces a *white line* limited to the skin area touched. In an exaggerated response, there is a *bright red line* that becomes cyanotic (Fig. 10-21E). In certain persons, a *red mottled flare* develops by lateral extension of the red line. From this a *wheal* may emerge projecting 1–2 mm above the skin level (Fig. 10-21E). In such cases, writing on the skin with a dull point results in embossed letters, giving the name to the condition. Although of great theoretic interest, the finding is of little diagnostic significance.

Perspiration. Localized areas of sweating may occur in syringomyelia, peripheral nerve injury, or neuropathy. *Anhidrosis* is a component of Horner's syndrome (p. 83).

Trophic Disturbances. Trophic changes in the skin occur in peripheral neuropathy, tabes dorsalis, syringomyelia, and Raynaud's disease. The skin becomes shiny, smooth, thin, and dry. Painless *trophic ulcers* develop in the denervated soles of the feet in peripheral neuritis, tabes dorsalis, diabetes, and syringomyelia (Fig. 10-21F). The *neuropathic arthropathy* of Charcot's joints results from trophic disorders of the articular structures; the loss of pain sensations permits excessive trauma and degeneration that present the bizarre painless deformities (p. 665).

Pilomotor Reactions. Scratching the midaxillary skin produces pilomotor erection (goose flesh). The normal response is abolished below the level of a transverse cord lesion. An exaggerated reaction may occur on the affected side in hemiplegia.

Blood Pressure Regulation. Orthostatic hypotension is common with autonomic nervous system diseases and should be sought.

Bladder/Bowel Function. Patients with autonomic nervous system diseases often have incontinence or symptoms from loss of control of bladder and bowel function. These complaints should be sought and further investigated.

Impaired Consciousness

Disturbances of consciousness may be classified partially according to degree. *Lethargy* is drowsiness caused by a condition other than normal sleep. In *confusion* attention is dulled, perception is impaired, memory is defective, and the general awareness of surroundings is limited. In *delirium* confusion is accompanied by hallucinations, often causing violent emotional responses. *Stupor* is a somnolent state during which the patient may be momentarily aroused by questions or painful stimuli; the reflexes are usually preserved. The deepest state of unconsciousness is *coma* in which the patient lies motionless, unresponsive to stimuli, with the deep and superficial reflexes lost, and urinary incontinence. A brief loss of consciousness is *syncope* and presents a different group of diagnostic problems from those suggested by coma.

▼ *Key Symptoms:* **Syncope.** The patient usually complains of "weak spells," "lightheadedness," or "blackouts," without any meaningful qualification. Significant historical details must be sought by careful and searching interrogation of both *patient and witnesses.* The *prototype* of a syncopal attack has three stages: **Prodromal Stage.** This brief period usually begins in the *erect position.* Suddenly the patient feels weak and unsteady; yawning, dimming of vision, nausea and vomiting, and sweating are common. The face becomes *pale* or *ashen gray.* If he reclines promptly the attack may be aborted. **Syncopal Stage** (muscle weakness and impaired consciousness). He falls to the floor from *muscle weakness,* but usually the action is not abrupt, so *no injuries* are incurred. He may be *mentally confused* but still hear voices and dimly see his surroundings; or there is *complete unconsciousness.* This stage may last for a few seconds to half an hour. Usually the muscles are utterly *flaccid* and *motionless;* sometimes there are a few *clonic jerks* of arms and face but seldom a tonic-clonic convulsion. Urinary or fecal *incontinence* is rare. The skin appears strikingly *pale* or *cyanotic;* the pulse is *weak* or absent. *Bradycardia* (or tachycardia from ectopic cardiac rhythm) is accompanied by arterial *hypotension* and extremely *shallow quiet breathing.* **Recovery Stage** (muscle weakness with lucid sensorium). In the horizontal position, the face gradually suffuses with pink, the blood pressure rises, the pulse becomes palpable and accelerated, the breathing deepens and quickens, the eyelids flutter. He awakes with *immediate awareness* of his surroundings. But *muscle weakness persists* for some time; so attempts to rise prematurely will induce another attack. **Pathophysiology.** Syncope occurs during *transient* diminution of the cerebral circulation or changes in the composition of the blood, as in *hypoglycemia* or *hypocapnea.* Impaired circulation of the brain may occur from ineffective cardiac action (myocardial insufficiency or dysrhythmias), loss of peripheral resistance in the vascular tree, or from vascular reflexes. In the erect position consciousness is lost when the mean arterial pressure declines to 20–30 mm Hg, or when the heart stops for 4–5 seconds. In the horizontal position more extreme conditions can be tolerated. *Diagnosis. First Step—Distinction Between Syncope and Akinetic Epilepsy:* Common features in akinetic epilepsy, rare in syncope, are lack of pallor, sudden onset without prodrome, injury from falling, tonic convulsions with upturned eyes, urinary or fecal incontinence, postictal mental confusion with headache and drowsiness. Although most of these features occur occasionally with syncope, their sparsity and the absence of EEG findings are distinctive in most cases. *Second Step—Distinction Among Various Types of Syncope:* The different types of syncope exhibit variations from the prototype in their prodromes and in the accompanying cardiovascular signs described in the following items:

— *Prototypal:* ***Vasopressor Syncope*** (Vasovagal Syncope, The Common Faint). The attack is induced in healthy persons by fear, anxiety, or pain. A hot environment facilitates the onset by producing vasodilatation. Fatigue, illness, or hunger increases the susceptibility. The patient can usually supply a history of the prodrome that is diagnostic. Recovery follows assumption of the horizontal position. ***Pathophysiology.*** The onset is heralded by generalized vasodilatation, especially in the peripheral muscles where no baroreceptor reflex operates to increase cardiac output. The absence of muscular activity produces cerebral ischemia.

— *No Pallor, Normal Pulse Rate:* ***Orthostatic or Postural Syncope.*** Normally in the erect position, pooling of the blood in the lower limbs is prevented by vasoconstriction mediated through the autonomic nervous system. When this compensatory mechanism is blocked, blood is pooled in the legs and arterial hypotension results. Distinctive features are *absence of prodrome, normal heart rate,* and *absence of pallor and sweating.* Recovery occurs in the horizontal position.

Clinical Occurrence. *Drugs:* treatment of hypertension with vasodilators or ganglionic blocking agents. *Debility:* in patients who have been bedridden for a long time. *Varicosities:* pooling of blood in large varicosities or plexuses. *Soldiers at Attention:* standing motionless for a long time precludes muscular contractions that normally pump blood from the legs. *Neuropathies:* peripheral neuritis in diabetes mellitus and tabes dorsalis. *Operations:* extensive sympathectomies for hypertension. *Defective Postural Reflexes:* encountered in some otherwise apparently normal persons. *Severe Anemia.*

— *No Pallor, Normal Pulse Rate:* **Hysterical Syncope.** This is the swoon of young women with strong emotions. It usually occurs in the presence of witnesses. The fall is graceful and harmless. The skin color, heart rate, and blood pressure are all *normal.* Either the patient lies motionless or makes uninhibited resisting movements.

— *No Prodrome, Any Position:* **Adams-Stokes Syndrome.** The attacks of unconsciousness occur when cardiac asystole lasts more than 5 seconds in the vertical position, or 10 seconds in the horizontal. Usually asystole results during the transition from a partial to a complete heart block, or from the onset of paroxysmal tachycardia or ventricular fibrillation. When the heart rhythm is regular and the rate less than 40 a minute, heart block can be distinguished from sinus bradycardia by the variation in intensity of the first heart sounds (p. 367). An ECG may be required for confirmation. In this form of syncope, there is no prodrome; it occurs in any position.

— *After Breathing-Holding or Instrumentation:* **Cardiac Standstill with Syncope.** Rarely, stimulation of the vagus may occur from instrumentation of the pleura ("pleural shock") or bronchus, or by dilatation of an esophageal diverticulum or the duodenum. The standstill may be temporary or permanent.

— *With Exertion:* **Syncope with Valvular Heart Disease.** Exertion may induce typical syncope in a patient with aortic stenosis. More rarely, it occurs with aortic regurgitation, myocardial infarction, or pulmonary hypertension.

— *With Head Movements:* **Carotid Sinus Syncope.** Usually this occurs in patients over 60 years old with hypertension or occlusion of one carotid artery. *Rotation of the head* or wearing a *tight collar* induces syncope. The vagal stimulation may result in one of three responses: (1) sinoatrial block, (2) hypotension without bradycardia, or (3) syncope with *normal* pulse rate and blood pressure. *Diagnosis.* The condition is suspected from the history of relation to certain motions. Circumstantial proof is furnished when an attack is reproduced by massaging the carotid sinus. Before stimulation is attempted, ascertain *whether both carotid arteries are pulsating*. The maneuver is dangerous when one artery is occluded. Both carotids should never be stimulated *simultaneously*. To stimulate, massage the cartoid sinus *gently* so as not to occlude the vessel. Occlusion during the maneuver has produced cerebral infarction and death.

— *Prodromal Paresthesias:* ***Hyperventilation Syncope.*** Before the attack, the patient is anxious or emotionally upset. He is not conscious of hyperventilation but feels tightness in the chest or suffocation. The prodrome is usually attended by *numbness* and *tingling* of arms and face; sometimes *carpopedal spasms* occur (p. 673). Loss of consciousness may be prolonged compared to most other types of syncope; the impairment may be partial. *Pathophysiology.* Hyperventilation results in hypocapnea; this induces diminished cerebral blood flow. The anoxia leads to vasodilatation in the muscles. *Diagnosis.* The proof is in the reproduction of the symptoms by having the patient forcefully overventilate. Rebreathing into a paper bag will arrest the attack and demonstrate a method of self-treatment.

— *During Coughing:* ***Cough Syncope*** (Tussive Syncope). Severe paroxysms of coughing, laughing, or vomiting may induce an attack of syncope, usually in men, rarely in women. The history of the onset is usually diagnostic. The mechanism is disputed: either compression of the cerebrum by transmission of increased intrathoracic pressure to the cerebrospinal fluid, or reduction of cardiac output by the Valsalva maneuver.

— *During Urination:* ***Micturition Syncope.*** Particularly in a patient with peripheral vasodilatation from a warm bed, voiding a large volume may cause syncope. Similarly, the rapid decompression of an overfilled bladder by catheterization, or the removal of large volumes of ascitic fluid, may cause syncope.

— *Related to Meals:* ***Hypoglycemic Syncope.*** The prodrome usually resembles the prototype, but the syncopal stage is frequently prolonged, loss of consciousness is usually incomplete. Rather, there is muscle weakness with mental confusion. *Diagnosis.* The blood sugar is usually below 30 mg per 100 mL; the symptoms are relieved by the intravenous administration of glucose or the hypodermic injection of epinephrine.

Clinical Occurrence. (1) After an overdose of insulin, (2) in alimentary glycosuria, an attack several hours after a rich carbohydrate meal, (3) with subtotal gastrectomy, a half-hour after a carbohydrate meal, (4) with an islet-cell tumor of the pancreas, after exercise while fasting.

Transient Ischemic Attacks (TIA). These are important precursors of a major cerebral infarction. TIA result from a failure of perfusion due to hemodynamic causes or can be produced by microembolism. Small collections of fibrin and platelets float to the brain and produce focal neurologic symptoms. The symptoms reflect the area of ischemic brain. TIA are reversible; events usually last 5–20 minutes. CAROTID ARTERY TIA: Contralateral weakness, clumsiness or numbness of the hand, hand and face, or entire half of the body; dysarthria; aphasia; amaurosis fugax with ipsilateral monocular visual loss (which can be complete blindness, sector visual loss, transient scene blur or fog). VERTEBROBASILAR ARTERY TIA: Binocular visual disturbance or loss; vertigo; dysarthria; ataxia; unilateral or bilateral weakness or numbness; drop attacks (sudden loss of postural tone, collapse without loss of consciousness). Diplopia, syncope, transient confusion or paraparesis are uncommon symptoms of TIA. Neurologic signs are usually absent between attacks. Carotid bruits or retinal emboli may be found. The differential diagnosis of TIA includes convulsions, syncope, migraine, focal cerebral masses, such as subdural hematomas, cardiac diseases, and labyrinthine disorders. ***Prognosis:*** The correct diagnosis of TIA is important because it is a clear indication of impending serious cerebral artery thrombosis. It should prompt precise evaluation of the cerebral arteries by arteriography for possible surgical correction or medical treatment.

▼ *Key Sign:* ***Coma.*** Coma is a state of prolonged unconsciousness. The examination of the patient requires a special approach because he cannot give a history, and cooperation is poor or absent. When the medical student or house officer is first confronted with this situation, he is inclined to be baffled and disconcerted; but experience soon demonstrates that pursuit of a logical procedure leads rapidly to a correct diagnosis in most cases. The examination should be begun with the following classification of causes clearly in mind.

Clinical Occurrence: NO FOCAL SIGNS; NORMAL SPINAL FLUID. *Drugs or poisons:* alcohol, barbiturates, bromides, chloral, opiates, other sedatives, carbon monoxide, gasoline fumes, arsenic, lead, acetylsalicylic acid, carbon dioxide narcosis. *Metabolic Disorders:* uremia, hepatic coma, diabetic acidosis, hypoglycemia, Addison's disease, myxedema coma, hypoparathyroidism, hyponatremia, porphyria, heat stroke, hypoxia. *Systemic Infections:* pneumonia, typhoid fever, septicemia, scarlet fever, measles, smallpox, meningococcal meningitis (Waterhouse-Friderichsen's syndrome), malaria. *Circulatory Collapse:* from any cause, including cardiac decompensation. *Epilepsy. Hypertensive Encephalopathy and Eclampsia. Hyperthermia and Hypothermia:* including myxedema coma. NO FOCAL SIGNS; ERYTHROCYTES OR LEUKOCYTES IN SPINAL FLUID. *Meningeal Irritation:* subarachnoid hemorrhage, acute bacterial meningitis, some viral meningitides, acute hemorrhagic leukoencephalitis. FOCAL SIGNS; VARIOUS SPINAL FLUID FINDINGS. Cerebral hemorrhage, cerebral infarction (from thrombosis or embolism), epidural or subdural hemorrhage, brain contusion, brain tumor, thrombophlebitis, some viral meningitides.

To distinguish hemispheric from posterior fossa or diffuse metabolic lesions of the brain, the neurologic examination evaluates level of consciousness, pupils, extraocular movements, motor signs, corneal reflexes, respiratory pattern, fundi, and meningeal signs. The neurologic examination usually yields clues pointing to a localized lesion. The general examination may disclose signs of diseases that produce either local cerebral lesions or diffuse disorders of the brain. The lumbar puncture gives evidence of increased intracranial pressure, hemorrhage, or infection. Routine hematologic tests reveal anemia, leukemia, lead stippling of the erythrocytes, malarial parasites. Urinalysis shows evidence of nephritis, diabetes, porphyria. Blood chemical tests will discover an elevated urea nitrogen, abnormal levels of serum sodium, calcium, phosphorus, and glucose.

In formulating a diagnosis, two axioms should be followed: (1) *Finding one clue to the cause of coma does not prove the cause.* A comatose patient with the odor of alcohol on his breath may have sustained a head injury while intoxicated. A man injured in an automobile wreck may have had an antecedent cerebral thrombosis that led to the accident. A stoker in a hot engine room may have coma from cerebral malaria rather than heat stroke. An unconscious patient with a few sedative tablets at the bedside may have taken the drug for symptoms of meningitis or brain tumor. (2) *A complete neurologic examination is insufficient; the other systems of the body must also be assessed.* Finding atrial fibrillation raises the possibility of cerebral embolism. The retinae may contain signs of diabetes or nephritis. The evidence of hypertension may be helpful. Demonstration of a consolidated lung suggests lobar pneumonia as the cause of coma. In many cases, routine examination of the abdomen has discovered a distended bladder, which led to a diagnosis of uremia from prostatic obstruction.

HISTORY ABOUT THE COMATOSE PATIENT. **Interview the relatives, acquaintances, attendants, or police officers who discovered the patient. *Circumstances of Discovery:* How was the patient found? Were there any drugs or poisons nearby? Were the surroundings such as to suggest poisoning from carbon monoxide or gasoline fumes? Was there evidence of trauma? What was known about his antecedent intake of food and fluids? Who prepared his food? What were his symptoms and actions before the onset of coma? Did he have pain, diarrhea, or vomiting? *Past History:* Was he known to have epilepsy, diabetes, hypertension, alcohol or drug addiction? Did he have suicidal tendencies; was he ever hospitalized in a mental institution? Was he known to be taking medicines? Had there ever been operations for malignancy?**

PHYSICAL EXAMINATION OF THE COMATOSE PATIENT. ***General Inspection:* Note his *posture*. Look for *tremors* or *muscle jerks*. Inspect the respiratory movements for bradypnea, tachypnea, Kussmaul breathing, Cheyne-Stokes breathing (p. 280).**

***Color:* Look for pallor, icterus, the cyanosis of methemoglobinemia, the cherry-red color of carbon monoxide hemoglobin.**

***Scalp and Skull:* Look for contusions, lacerations, gunshot wounds; palpate for depressed skull fractures.**

***Eyes:* Lift the eyelids and let them close; lagging of one lid suggests hemiplegia. The patient with hysteria *resists* opening by closing the lids tighter, a revealing response. In coma the eyes remain *fixed* or *oscillate slowly from side to side;* oscillation is lacking in hysteria in which the eyes may wander but fix momentarily. *Conjugate deviation* of the eyeballs is *toward* the affected side in destructive lesions of the frontal lobe, *away* from the affected side in irritative lesions. The presence of extraocular muscle palsies assists in localizing a lesion in the skull. *Bilateral widely dilated pupils* occur in profound post-traumatic shock, massive cerebral hemorrhage, encephalitis, poisoning with atropine-like drugs, and the end stages of brain tumor. *Bilateral pinpoint pupils* suggest morphine poisoning or a pontine**

hemorrhage. A unilateral unreactive pupil indicates a rapidly expanding lesion on the ipsilateral side, as in subdural or middle meningeal hemorrhage or brain tumor. Examine the ocular fundi for the exudates and hemorrhages of diabetes and nephritis, the choked disks of increased intracranial pressure.

Facial Muscles: Asymmetry of the face may indicate hemiplegia. The mouth droops on the affected side, the cheek puffs out with each expiration. Painful pressure on the supraorbital notch causes the mouth to grimace in an asymmetric pattern to reveal the weak side.

Oral Cavity: Examine the tongue for lacerations from biting during a convulsive seizure. Look for a diphtheritic membrane, other signs of pharyngitis, or ulceration or discoloration from poisons.

Breath: Smell the breath for acetone, ammonia, alcohol or its successor aldehydes, paraldehyde, and other odors (p. 148).

Ears: Look for pus, spinal fluid, or blood emerging from the external acoustic meatus.

Neck: Test for nuchal rigidity, Kernig's sign, and Brudzinski's sign, for evidence of meningeal irritation.

Limbs: Test each limb successively for flaccidity by lifting it and letting it fall to the bed. If any muscle tone is retained, a difference in the two sides indicates a hemiplegia. The reflexes on the paralyzed side are absent during the stage of spinal shock, but in deep coma all reflexes are lost. In deep coma, Babinski's reflex is present bilaterally, so it cannot be employed to localize a lesion. If some reflexes are retained, a difference in the two sides is significant.

Sensory Examination: In semicoma, only the responses to painful stimuli can be evaluated. The patient will show defensive reactions when pricked in sensitive areas, but no response is forthcoming when analgesic regions are stimulated. If the stimulated region is sensitive, but paralyzed, a defense or withdrawal movement may occur on the opposite side; the facial expression will indicate pain. Deep pressure sense should be tested by compression of the Achilles tendon, the testis, and the supraorbital notch.

Patients lacking certain brainstem reflexes, like pupillary or corneal reflexes, during the first examination in hypoxic coma following cardiopulmonary resuscitation are unlikely to recover. Confused speech, orienting eye movements, normal oculocephalic or oculovestibular responses, and obedience to commands at 1 day, however, predicted a 50% chance of regaining independence [D. E. Levy, et al.: Predicting Outcome from Hypoxic-Ischemic Coma, *J.A.M.A.*, 253:1420–26, 1985.].

LABORATORY EXAMINATION OF THE COMATOSE PATIENT. *Urine:* The findings of particular significance are protein, glucose, acetone, porphyrins, phenol, pus, and blood.

Blood: Some pertinent findings are anemia, leukemia, malarial parasites, stippled erythrocytes (lead).

Blood Chemical Tests: Blood glucose, urea nitrogen, and carbon dioxide content should be done almost routinely. If indicated, many others may be pertinent; serum sodium, calcium, phosphorus, total serum thyroxine, bromides, barbiturates, and salicylates.

Spinal Fluid: The spinal fluid pressure is revealing. The fluid should be examined for xanthochromia, erythrocytes, leukocytes, lymphocytes, protein content, bacteria, and fungi. A VDRL test should be performed on the spinal fluid.

Electroencephalography: Symmetric slow activity may occur with metabolic encephalopathy with focal slowing localized to the side of a structural supratentorial lesion.

DIAGNOSTIC IMAGING OF THE COMATOSE PATIENT. *X-ray:* Radiographs of the skull will reveal skull fractures, bony neoplasms, and lateral deviations of the pineal body that indicate unilateral lesions. Whenever possible, an x-ray film of the chest should also be taken because it may reveal an unsuspected pneumonia or neoplasm. Carcinoma of the lung frequently metastasizes to the brain. *CT:* Scans demonstrate hemorrhage, infarction, subdural hematoma, abscess, hydrocephalus, or tumor. *MRI:* Structural lesions that may cause coma may be revealed with MRI scanning.

Hepatic Coma. This presents four features; only the last is distinctive: (1) *altered mental state,* varying from slight loss of memory to confusion, slurred speech, paranoia, and agitation; (2) *EEG changes,* the waves show the nonspecific slowing and increase in amplitude also encountered in uremia, hypoglycemia, and CO_2 narcosis; (3) *asterixis,* also present in cerebrovascular disease, uremia, severe pulmonary insufficiency; and (4) *fetor hepaticus,* smelling something like old wine, acetone, or new-mown hay; if present, it is distinctive of hepatic coma. Elevated ammonia values in the arterial blood support the diagnosis when specimens are properly collected.

Chronic Alcoholism. This is a compulsive behavioral disorder of imbibing ethyl alcohol *repeatedly* in biologically damaging quantities and *repeatedly,* creating circumstances that are physically damaging and socially degrading to the drinker and others. It is a common ailment; one writer warns that if the physician is not diagnosing chronic alcoholism in at least one of 25 patients seen, the history-taking lacks skill [R. Bates: The Hidden Alcoholic, *Diagnosis:* March–Apr., pp. 22–27, 1979].

Positive responses to the CAGE questions should raise the index of suspicion for chronic alcoholism. CAGE is an acronym to help the physician recall questions focusing on Cutting down, Annoyance by criticism, Guilty feeling, and Eye openers [J. A. Ewing: Detecting Alcoholism. The CAGE Questionaire, *J.A.M.A.*, **252:**1905–07, 1984.]. The diagnostic essential is to secure the details of behavior *repeatedly damaging* to the drinker's health and reputation. Such behavior is socially stigmatized and the patient is reluctant to reveal it to the physician, using all sorts of subterfuges and untruths to conceal it. To circumvent this, the diagnostician must resort to many probing stratagems to uncover the facts. Often the questioning must be oblique instead of blunt. Details are sought that are pertinent to the diagnosis but not recognizable to the patient as being associated with alcoholism. The interrogator searches for many items bearing upon the patient's background, as suggested in the following categories: *Past History:* accidents involving the patient, suicidal attempts, gastrectomy for bleeding gastritis, tuberculosis, pancreatitis. *Family History:* parent dying of cirrhosis of the liver or suicide, parent lost to patient before his/her 15th year of age, alcoholic parent. *Social History:* dropping out of school, belonging to lower socioeconomic group, having parent who is American Indian (40% male alcoholics), Black (10–20% male alcoholics), following an occupation below the patient's level of intelligence or education. *Sex of Patient:* alcoholism commoner in males, in unmarried or divorced persons, in homosexuals. *Race and Religion:* alcoholism *uncommon* in Jews, Moslems, Adventists, Christian Scientists, Chinese, Greeks, Italians. *Personal Behavioral History:* excesses in use of coffee, tea, tobacco; many serious accidents in home, at work, and in automobiles. *Veracity:* purposely or not, the alcoholic grossly underestimates his alcoholic intake (it is revealing to ask the longest time the patient has purposefully gone without a drink; a nonalcoholic has no reason to abstain). After one or two initial experiences the nonalcoholic learns to regulate his/her drinking to avoid severe intoxication and hangovers; the times of drinking are appropriate, and the actions under the influence of alcohol are benign; the alcoholic's conduct is the opposite. The diagnosis of alcoholism is almost certain if, under reasonable questioning, the patient becomes hostile and defensive. Any diagnostic symptoms and signs of alcoholism arise from the complications of the disorder. *Pertinent Physical Signs in a Symptomless Person:* vascular spiders on the skin, hepatomegaly, wrist drop, alcohol or aldehyde on the breath. *Laboratory Findings:* hyperlipemia, SGOT slightly elevated, hypoglycemia during drunkenness; slight hyperuricemia: elevated blood alcohol. *Complications of Alcoholism* [From D. Y. Graham: Guide to the Evaluation of the Alcoholic Patient, *Hosp. Med.*, Jan., pp. 71–88, 1978]: *Withdrawal Syndrome:* tremulousness, delirium tremens (psychomotor agitation, hallucinations with animal subjects) with onset 2 to 3 days after cessation of drinking. *Withdrawal Seizures ("Whiskey Fits," "Rum Fits")*: short-lived grand mal seizures occurring 48 hours after cessation of drinking. *Wernicke-Korsakoff Syndrome:* this is a combination of Wernicke's encephalopathic syndrome (a thiamine-deficiency with dementia) and Korsakoff's syndrome in which there is loss of memory and confabulation). *Peripheral Neuropathies:* often accompanied by wristdrop and painful tender nerve trunks. Toxic amblyopia. Alcoholic cerebellar degeneration. Fatty liver. Muscle wasting. Acute relapsing pancreatitis. Malnutrition and malabsorption. *Cardiomyopathy and myopathy:* depression of bone marrow. Bleeding from esophageal varices, peptic ulcer, and acute gastritis.

▼ *Key Symptom:* ***Dementia.*** The patient is a picture of chronic illness. He is usually *disinterested* and *apathetic,* without reaching a lower level of consciousness. He exhibits only traces of joy or sorrow, most often sadness. Flashes of irritability are interspersed but they are short-lived. The *memory is impaired.* He tends to return to the same complaint every few minutes (perseveration). Bodily movements are *slowed.* Speech is *slurred.* Neurologic examination may be normal, but intelligence is *impaired.* *Distinction:* the condition may resemble a depression, but later the more intensive and consistent changes of affect exclude depression from consideration. Objective memory loss is greater in dementia.

Clinical Occurrence: PARENCHYMATOUS CEREBRAL DISEASE: Alzheimer's disease, Pick's disease, senile dementia. METABOLIC DISORDERS: myxedema, Wilson's disease, chronic liver disease; severe hypertension, multiple infarct dementia; hypoxia, anoxia, hydrocephalus with normal pressure. DEFICIENCY DISEASES: vitamin B_1 deficiency, pellagra, folate deficiency, vitamin B_{12} deficiency. TOXINS AND DRUGS: alcohol, sedatives, tranquilizer.

BRAIN: brain tumors and metastatic cancer, subdural hematoma from trauma. INFECTIONS: CNS syphilis, fungal meningitis, slow virus meningitis.

— *Dementia:* ***C. Wernicke's Encephalopathic Syndrome*** (Presbyophrenia, Cerebral Beriberi, Gayet-Wernicke Hemorrhagic Encephalopathy, Superior Hemorrhagic Polioencephalopathy Syndrome). The usual causes are alcoholism and beriberi; in either case a deficiency of vitamin B_1 (thiamine). There is generalized deterioration of the intellect, often with the development of a *Korsakoff's psychosis* (*amnesia, confusion, confabulation, delirium tremens*). Evidence of cranial nerve involvement consists of horizontal and vertical *nystagmus, ptosis, paresis* of the *external rectus* ocular muscles and *conjugate gaze.* Neuritis of peripheral nerves causes *ataxia of stance and gait.* The administration of B_1 relieves the ocular impairment and the ataxia, but it does not improve the disorder of mentation.

Clinical Occurrence: chronic alcoholism, beriberi, malnutrition, cachexia, thyrotoxicosis, hemodialysis, hyperemesis gravidarum [Editorial: Wernicke's Preventable Encephalopathy, *Lancet,* **1:**1122–23, 1979].

— *Dementia:* ***Alzheimer's Presenile Dementia*** (Alzheimer's Sclerosis or Disease). Beginning in the 4th or 5th decade of life, there is progressive rapid mental deterioration with amnesia, aphasia, agnosia, cortical blindness, followed by disordered pyramidal and extrapyramidal functions.

Psychiatric Diagnosis

Psychiatric Disorders: Organic, Nonorganic, or Both?

The teaching and practice of medicine are highly biased toward the diagnosis of organic diseases rather than psychiatric or nonorganic disorders. Not only do the physical examination, x-ray procedures, and laboratory tests appeal to the physician's urge for purposeful motions and the acquisition of facts through his senses of touch, sight, and hearing, but they may also impress the patient. In most circles it is considered more respectable to have an organic disease than a psychiatric disorder. Also, the treatments of organic diseases are better defined and the results more decisive.

For many reasons, the physician assumes the patient to have

an organic disease until proven otherwise. After organic disease has been excluded, the diagnosis of nonorganic disease is made by exclusion. This precedence is necessary for the health of the patient. If the patient has cardiac failure, it must be treated before psychiatric therapy can be given; otherwise the latter treatment might not be possible.

The distinction between organic disease and a nonorganic disorder is often difficult to make because the symptoms in the psychiatric disorder are often referred to an anatomic region or a physiologic function. For example, a patient with uncontrolled diabetes mellitus may have abdominal pain and a depression; the cause of the pain cannot be determined until a therapeutic test of treating the diabetes to see whether the pain is relieved.

Strategy of Psychiatric Diagnosis

As the physician is taking the history from the patient, relative, or attendant, in a search for clues to organic disease, symptoms suggestive of psychiatric disorders may emerge, or the clinician may observe some abnormal behavior that leads the doctor to hypothesize a psychiatric disorder, *in addition to* or *instead of* organic disease. These phrases are very important because the erroneous tendency is to reason only for one or the other instead of both.

In making psychiatric diagnoses, our impression is that the physician tends to follow the method of matching whole images (the *Gestalt method*) in which the sum total of the patient's attributes are matched with the various patterns of entities in the field of psychiatry. The descriptions of several such patterns follow:

Vagueness, Incongruity: ***Ambulatory Schizophrenia.*** This is a mild type of schizophrenia in which the symptoms are subtle enough to make diagnosis difficult. The physical appearance is usually normal. The patient's response to questions are vague statements that seem slightly irrelevant. Alverez termed them *patients who could not answer questions* [*quoted by* M. H. Hollander in *Basic Psychiatry for Primary Care Physicians*, H. S. Abrams, editor, 1979. Boston, Little, Brown and Co.]. A direct question elicits a sentence beginning with a slight irrelevance but progresses to more inappropriateness and trails off into vagueness. The symptoms are frequently bizarre. Hollander's patient described a sensation "just like I had a hole running from my chest to my back and air blowing through it and causing pain."

The more severe grade of schizophrenia can be recognized by the presence of *the four As* (ambivalence, autistic [self-centered] thinking, inappropriate affect, and antisocial behavior).

Persecutory or Grandiose Delusions: ***Paranoid Reaction.*** During the history-taking the patient's reasoning, mood, and appearance are normal. But sooner or later in the dialogue, the patient reveals in secretive fashion a *delusion of persecution* [*delusion* = a false belief that cannot be corrected by reason; it is logically founded but cannot be corrected by evidence of the patient's own senses. *Illusion* = a false or misinterpreted but real sensory impression. *Hallucination* = a sensory impression of a nonexistent object]. He seems to reason logically up to a certain point, but the significance of some innocent and trivial incident is misinterpreted as evidence of hostility toward the patient. Thereafter a chain of events is incorporated as a conspiracy, despite all proof to the contrary. For example, the senior author saw a lonely widow of middle age who had bought a condominium in Florida where she lived for a short time when a group of men moved into the floor below her. They held noisy parties where rock music was played (this type of music had a bad connotation for the patient). She decided that they were homosexuals "because homosexuals play rock music." She knew the parties were orgies "because they were attended by homosexuals." She complained to the police who told her they could do nothing. Thereafter she thought the subjects of the report gave her menacing glances whenever they met, so she feared for her life. She sold her condominium and moved from Florida to Iowa and took an apartment in a small city. Within a few weeks she thought she saw some of her old "enemies" on the streets of the city and around her apartment house. When the author attempted to reassure her that she was physically well and pointed out that other physicians in other cities had also given her similar reports, she was not comforted because she knew "the medical profession was a national conspiracy that transmitted information about patients nationwide." The author recalls another woman who held an important state office by appointment from the governor. She complained of vague malaise and pains that had come on since she had been noticing night noises outside her apartment door in the residence hotel where she lived. She concluded that these noises were being made by political enemies of the governor who were trying to kill her by blowing poison gas in the keyhole. These patients have their symptoms for many years; they hold fast to their erroneous conclusions regardless of any proof to the contrary; they are litigious; they are numerous.

Clinical Occurrence: Pure paranoia is rare but a paranoid syndrome is encountered in the following disorders: schizophrenia, affective disorders (manic-depressive), personality disorders, temporal lobe epilepsy, brain tumors, hypertensive encephalopathy, uremia, pellagra, Wilson's disease, acute intermittent porphyria, paresis, Addison's disease, Cushing's syndrome [T. C. Manschreck and M. Petri: The Paranoid Syndrome, *Lancet,* **2**:251–52, 1978].

Indecisiveness, Insomnia, Despondency: **Depression.** One of the most common psychiatric disorders encountered by physicians in all types of practice, depressions are often misdiagnosed as being organic disease because the symptoms may be referred to any part of the body. On the first history-taking the patient may deny the distinctive symptoms, and only by repeated questioning are the revealing diagnostic clues uncovered. If the patient does not give a satisfactory history, question the relatives, friends, acquaintances, and attendants. *Sleep disturbance* is one of the most common and most prominent symptoms. *Insomnia* coincides with the onset of the depression. *Despondency* (a feeling of sadness for several consecutive days) is typical. *Increasing irritability, indecision, inability to initiate action,* and *emotional lability* (weeping with little or no provocation) are frequent symptoms. Later, there may be *anorexia* and *weight loss.* The examiner notes *psychomotor retardation* (slow body movements, halting and monotonous speech). A curious symptom is *internal trembling* (felt by the patient but invisible to the doctor). Because any anatomic site may be referred to, depression masquerades under all sorts of organic diagnoses. Frequently the patients entertain thoughts of suicide, but they seldom volunteer this. The mortality from this disorder is from self-destruction, and the physician has a duty to warn the relatives of this. Very often the organic symptoms cannot be separated from those due to the depression—a therapeutic test may help to separate the two. The diagnostic difference between an anxiety state and depression is that the latter has the principal symptoms mentioned earlier.

Muscle Tenseness, Tachycardia, Sweating, Undue Fatigue: ***Anxiety State.*** The patient complains of *cardiac palpitation,* or *tremulousness, sweating,* and undue *fatigue.* These accompany many other symptoms referred to anatomic sites or physiologic functions. He/she is *oversolicitous* about minor discomforts. Repeated questioning is often required to discover that the symptoms began when the patient's son was arrested for peddling drugs, or the daughter became pregnant without benefit of clergy, or the woman was quarrelling with her mother-in-law, or the husband was drinking too much or going with another woman, or the business was going bankrupt, or the patient's relative or friend had developed cancer and he/she was having the same symptoms. The psychiatrists recognize several *defense mechanisms* that operate in anxiety states: (1) *Denial.* The patient denies the existence of disease in him/herself or in the close family, therefore declines treatment and rarely consults the physician. (2) *Regression.* The patient becomes "childish" and requires excessive care because he/she wants to return to happier times to avoid confrontation with current facts. (3) *Displacement.* The patient becomes angry at the situation, but expresses the anger at the performance of the doctor, nurse, or other attendants. (4) *Projection.* The patient attributes to others the guilty feelings that arise from the sickness in order to escape self-blame. (5) *Sublimation.* The patient's emotions are attributed to some socially acceptable cause, such as the weather, old age, or acts of God.

Emotional Immaturity: ***Hysterical Personality.*** Very often the patient is an attractive flirtatious woman who is very *self-centered.* Her dialogue is *shallow,* dealing exclusively with inconsequential subjects. She is dramatically emotional, easily shifting from laughter to tears. She has little respect for facts, but is governed by hastily derived opinions. She uses her sexual attraction for gaining her own ends. She demands constant attention; denied that, she throws tantrums. She consults the doctor for trivial complaints.

▼ *Key Symptom:* **Delirium** (Acute Brain Syndrome, Toxic Psychosis, Cerebral Insufficiency Syndrome, Metabolic Encephalopathy. Exogenous Brain Disease). This is a symptom complex characterized by *sudden onset, marked variability* from time to time and from person to person, *reversible involvement* of the cerebrum, the reticular system, and the autonomic system. The chief features are *lowered level of consciousness* (from dimming to coma); *disorientation* (for time and place); *illusions* (misinterpreted sensory impressions); *hallucinations, mostly visual* (perceptions without sensory stimuli); *wandering and fragmented thoughts; delusions,* often paranoid; *shortened memory* for recent events; *emotions blunted* or *exaggerated; bodily movements abnormal* (nonspecific restlessness, specific asterixis); *specific multifocal myoclonus* (arrhythmic, asymmetric, repetitive muscle contractions); *autonomic* dysfunctions (nausea and vomiting, constipation, diarrhea, incontinence of urine and feces); *cardiovascular* (flushing, pallor, sweating, palpitations, tachycardia, fever). *Distinction.* From schizophrenia (latter has bizarre disorientations, is relatively unemotional, has persecutory delusions, has auditory hallucinations, lacks asterixis and multifocal myoclonus). From hysteria (latter usually has disorientation to persons; hallucinations are rare, memory is good; lacks myoclonus and asterixis).

Clinical Occurrence [*After* C. E. Wells: *Basic Psychiatry for the Primary Care Physician.* H. S. Abram, editor, 1979, Boston, Little, Brown and Co.]: *Drugs* (sedatives, tranquilizers, alcohol, steroids, salicylates, digitalis, alkaloids); *poisons* (heavy metals, carbon monoxide); *cerebral disease* (seizures, trauma, infections, subarachnoid hemorrhage); *endocrine* (insulin reactions, myxedema, hypoparathyroidism, adrenal and pituitary insufficiency); *liver disease* (encephalopathy): *kidney* (uremia); *lungs* (carbon dioxide narcosis, hypoxia); *cardiovascular* (cardiac failure, dysrhythmias, hypertension); *vitamin deficiencies* (pernicious anemia, folate deficiency, thiamine deficiency); *electrolyte imbalances; postoperative states;* miscellaneous *infectious diseases with fever.* (Some persons are more prone to delirium than others; children and old persons are especially susceptible.)

The Signs of Death

Death is an obvious fact of life; most adult human beings have either witnessed it or can make reasonably accurate diagnoses of it. But occasional cases prove too complicated for the layman's signs. One of the horror stories in medical history is the probably apocryphal episode in the life of Vesalius. In 1564, during the height of his European fame as an anatomist, he was appointed physician to Philip II of Spain. He is said to have conducted an autopsy in Madrid on a young nobleman who had been his patient. According to the custom of the time, this was carried out before a large crowd of citizens. When the thorax of the body was opened, the heart was seen to be beating. The doctor was compelled to leave Spain hastily. Probably such experiences have made it necessary to have physicians pronounce the death of patients.

Biologic death is the cessation of function of all bodily tissues. But in the process of dying different tissues deteriorate at varying rates, so a precise endpoint is difficult to determine. For ordinary purposes it is conclusive to recognize the cessation of the "vital signs" (cardiac activity, respirations, and maintained body temperature). But these indicators have proved inadequate in dealing with near-drowning, for example, when unconsciousness, apnea, and imperceptible heartbeat persist for some time after rescue. Different criteria are also required for patients receiving mechanical respiration and cardiac pacing.

DEATH EXAMINATION (FOR MOST PATIENTS). **CARDIAC ACTIVITY: *palpate for pulsations* in the carotid arteries; *auscultate the precordium* for heart sounds (if in doubt, get an ECG).** RESPIRATORY ACTIVITY: ***place the chestpiece* of your stethoscope over the patient's mouth and listen for breath sounds; *hold a cold mirror* in the region of the breath stream to detect a deposit of water vapor.** NEUROLOGIC FUNCTION: ***call to the patient* to test mentation; *retract the eyelids* to observe the fixed dilated pupils of death; *rotate the head* from side to side to ascertain whether the eye position compensates for a fixed target or the eyes remain fixed in their orbits (doll's eyes); *press the sternum and squeeze the Achilles tendons* to test deep pain perception; *lift and let fall* the limbs to test for muscle tone.**

SUPPLEMENTARY DEATH EXAMINATION (ESPECIALLY FOR NEAR-DROWNING AND PATIENTS WITH MECHANICAL VENTILATORS AND PACEMAKERS). **The Harvard Criteria for Brain Death prescribe: (1) absence of responsivity and receptivity, (2) absence of spontaneous movement in respiration and reflex activity, (3) an isoelectric EEG, or (4) abnormal angiogram in which no cerebral perfusion is demonstrated, or (5) abnormal nuclear medicine brain scan in which no cerebral perfusion is demonstrated.**

Part II: Laboratory Data

(Chap. 11)

Here the reader will find the normal and pathologic values for routine hematologic and blood chemical tests delivered by autoanalyzers (Technicon), and automatic blood counting apparatus, commonly in the form of "profiles," as SMA 12/60, SMA 6/60, and CBC (Sequential Multiple Analyzer, 12 or 6 constituents per minute, and Complete Blood Count). The catchwords in boldface are the objects of the tests. They are followed by rather lengthy lists of diseases and disorders in which the datum may occur.

Special tests, as distinguished from routine ones, are not within the scope of this book.

11

Laboratory Values as Clues

This chapter contains the values resulting from tests routinely performed in obtaining "chemical profiles" and "hematologic profiles" by the AutoAnalyzer (Technicon) and blood counting machines. Information that can be derived from examining the blood film and performing a urinalysis has been included with the recognition that the physician should know what to request from his office or hospital laboratory technicians and how to interpret their reports [R. Belsey, D. Baer, and D. Sewell: Laboratory Test Analysis Near the Patient, *J.A.M.A.*, **255:**775–86, 1986.].

To display the lengthy lists of disorders and diseases suggested by an abnormal finding, we have chosen to follow an arbitrary series of categories that we hope will assist as an mnemonic aid. The first part of the list is in anatomic order from head to foot; other following categories are in nonanatomic sequence. The virtue, if any, is that the hurried reader can always expect to find items in the same relative order.

The decision as to which tests, if any, should be obtained routinely can be debated forever. Certainly, the prevalence of the disease in the population seeking medical care should affect their selection [H. C. Sox: Probability Theory in the Use of Diagnostic Tests, *Ann. Int. Med.*, **104:**60–66, 1986.]. The fact is, however, that certain profiles of tests have become very popular because they have permitted physicians to diagnose common disorders before they produce symptoms and signs and progress to irreversible tissue damage. Because of their popularity, these profiles of tests have become relatively inexpensive in the United States. In addition to assisting in the diagnosis, recorded test results help to numerically quantitate the degree of abnormality as "objective findings" for insurance forms and, more importantly, as indicators of response to treatment. The contemporary physician who reports that his patient's pallor diminished while receiving vitamin B_{12} shots, without test results documenting a diagnosis of pernicious anemia and its response to therapy, stresses his credibility in peer review. Tests within profiles will undoubtedly change, but all tests, routine or special, should be justified and selected as those most likely to provide useful information about the patient's problem.

Ranges of normal values are presented for purposes of illustration only. Because each clinical laboratory determines its own normal ranges, those we have listed are not intended to be definitive. Many organizations, including the AMA, have supported the proposal of the American National Metric Council to convert units of measurement to Système International (SI) units. For the reader's convenience, we have included values with SI units in parentheses following the conventional units [G. D. Lundberg, C. Iverson, and G. Radulescu: Now Read This: The SI Units Are Here, *J.A.M.A.*, **255:**2329–39, 1986.].

Most of the normal values for blood tests were adopted from The Normal Reference Values, *N. Engl. J. Med.*, **314:**49, 1986.

Blood Chemistries

alkaline phosphatase, serum. *Pathophysiology:* This includes a number of cellular enzymes that hydrolyze phosphate esters; they are named from their optimum activity in alkaline media. High concentrations of the enzymes occur in the blood during periods of rapid growth, either physiologic or pathologic, and from cellular injury. The enzymes are normally plentiful in hepatic parenchyma, osteoblasts, intestinal mucosa, placental cells, and renal epithelium. Abnormally rapid growth or cell destruction will augment the blood concentration of these enzymes.

Normal Concentration: 30–120 U/L (same).

Increased Concentration: *Physiologic* (high in newborn, declining to puberty; rising every decade after 60 years of age); *bone* (osteitis fibrosa cystica, Paget's disease, osteoblastic bone tumors, metastatic carcinoma in bone, osteogenesis imperfecta, familial osteectasis, myeloma, osteomalacia, rickets, acromegaly, polyostotic fibrous dysplasia); *muscle* (strenuous exercise, clonic and tonic seizures, tissue necrosis); *brain* (cerebral damage); *thyroid* (hyperthyroidism [effect on bone] subacute thyroiditis); *parathyroids* (sometimes hyperparathyroidism [effect on bone]); *heart* (myocardial infarction); *lungs* (sometimes pulmonary infarction); *kidneys* (renal infarction); *liver* (metastatic tumors, abscesses, cysts, parasitic infestations, amyloid, tuberculosis, sarcoid, leukemia); *biliary system* (common duct obstruction from stone or carcinoma, cholangiolar obstruction from hepatitis); *pancreas* (pancreatitis, diabetes mellitus); *stomach* (peptic ulcer); *bowel* (intestinal obstruction, ulcerative colitis, regional enteritis); *genital* (last half of pregnancy); *blood* (pernicious anemia, and other hemolytic anemias); neoplasia (carcinoma of prostate); *infections* (infectious mononucleosis); *chemical imbalances* (hyperphosphatasia); *intake/output* (dehydration, rapid loss of weight); *drugs* (chloropropamide, ergosterol, sometimes intravenous injection of albumin); *technical error* (dehydration of blood specimen).

Decreased Concentration: *Bone* (osteoporosis); *thyroid* (hypothyroidism); *bowel* (celiac disease); *intake/output* (excess ingestion of vitamin D, deficit of vitamin C [scurvy], malnutrition); *chemical imbalances* (uremia, hypophosphatasia, milk-alkali syndrome of Burnett); *blood* (half the patients with pernicious anemia); *technical errors* (use of oxalate in blood collection).

aspartate aminotransferase, serum (see glutamate-oxaloacetate transferase, serum SGOT, and ***transaminase, serum SGOT).***

bicarbonate, total serum (CO_2 content). *Pathophysiology:* Mol. wt. 61. A negative ion with monovalence, CO_2 is formed by cell metabolism and diffused through the body fluids as ionized bicarbonate (HCO_3^-). About one fifth of the total blood bicarbonate is in the form of carbamino hemoglobin. The carbonates are major buffers, along with hemoglobin, phosphates, and free amino and carbonyl groups.

Normal Concentration: 24–30 mEq/L (24–30 mmol/L) [in venous blood serum].

Increased Concentration (hypercapnia): *Thyroid* (severe hypothyroidism); *kidneys* (hyperaldosteronism); *adrenals* (Cushing's disease); *chemical imbalance* (respiratory acidosis, metabolic alkalosis); *drugs* (diuretics).

Decreased Concentration (hypocapnia): *kidneys* (renal failure); *adrenals* (Addison's disease); *intake/output* (diarrhea, starvation); *chemical imbalance* (respiratory alkalosis, metabolic acidosis, diabetic ketosis).

bilirubin, total serum. *Pathophysiology:* Unconjugated bilirubin is manufactured in the reticuloendothelial system with four pyrrole nuclei of heme. It is insoluble in water until conjugated in the liver with glucuronic acid. Four fifths or more is derived from the catabolism of the heme from aging erythrocytes. The water-soluble conjugated bilirubin is normally excreted in the bile. It is bound to the plasma proteins; when the level exceeds 0.4 mg/dL, the water-soluble form appears in the urine.

Normal Concentration: 0.1–1.0 mg/dL (2–18 μmol/L).

Increased Concentration (hyperbilirubinemia): *lungs* (pulmonary infarction); *biliary system* (diseases of the liver, acute cholecystitis, obstructive jaundice, Gilbert's disease, Dubin-Johnson disease); *gastrointestinal tract* (bleeding into it); *blood* (intravascular hemolysis, large hematoma); *infections* (infectious mononucleosis); *poison* (alcohol).

Decreased Concentration (hypobilirubinemia): nonhemolytic anemia and hypoalbuminemia.

calcium, serum (Ca^{++}). *Pathophysiology:* At. wt. 40. About 99% of the body calcium is in the form of insoluble phosphate and carbonate supporting the collagen matrix of the bones. It is in equilibrium with a small amount in the extracellular fluid. The amount varies with the rate of absorption of Ca^{++} from the small intestine and the resorption rate in the glomeruli. Clinically the body Ca is present in three forms: *ionized* or *free* Ca that is physiologically active, *protein-bound* or *nondiffusible,* most of which is loosely bound to plasma albumin, and *complexed* or *complex-bound* that forms relatively soluble fractions complexed with carbonates, citrates, or phosphates. Parathormone (PTH) accelerates release of Ca^{++} and PO_4^{---} from bone with increased excretion of urinary PO_4^{---}; it also converts vitamin D to a more active form. Thyrocalcitonin inhibits bone resorption and decreases serum Ca and PO_4 in the extracellular fluids; in turn this reduces membrane permeability.

Normal Concentration: 8.5–10.5 mg/dL (2.1–2.6 mmol/L). (varies with chemical method).

Increased Concentration (Hypercalcemia): *Bone* (tumor metastatic to bone, lymphoma, multiple myeloma, osteoporosis, immobilization of young persons, Paget's disease); *thyroid* (sometimes hyperthyroidism, sometimes hypothyroidism); *parathyroids* (primary hyperparathyroidism [hyperplasia, adenoma, or cancer hormone]); *adrenals* (sometimes Cushing's disease, sometimes Addison's disease); *genital* (sometimes carcinoma of prostate); *blood* (lymphoma, myeloma, leukemia); *intake/output* (excessive intake of vitamin D); *chemical imbalances* (milk-alkali syndrome of Burnett, hypercalcemia in infants, infantile hypophosphatasia, hyperproteinemia [sarcoidosis, multiple myeloma]); *drugs* (thiazide diuretics); *poisons* (berylliosis); *technical error* (use of cork-stoppered tubes for collection of blood specimens).

Decreased Concentration (Hypocalcemia): *Bone* (osteomalacia, rickets); *thyroid* (hypothyroidism); *parathyroids* (hypoparathyroidism [postthyroidectomy, idiopathic or pseudohypoparathyroidism]); *kidneys* (renal disease with uremia); *pancreas* (acute pancreatitis with much fat necrosis); *genital* (late pregnancy, prostatic carcinoma); *intake/output* (excessive fluid intake, malabsorption of calcium and vitamin D from jaundice, lack of intake of Ca and vitamin D); *chemical imbalances* (hypoproteinemia [cachexia, nephrosis, celiac disease, cystic fibrosis of the pancreas]); *drugs* (antacids), corticosteroids.

chloride, serum (Cl^-). *Pathophysiology:* At. wt. 35.5. The principal anion in the extracellular fluid is Cl^-, balanced by Na^+; anions present in smaller quantities are HCO_3^- and HPO_4^{--}. The cations of lesser amounts are K^+, Ca^{++}, and Mg^{++}. By contrast, in the cellular fluid the chief anions are HPO_4^{--} and SO_4^{--}, balanced by K^+ and Mg^{++}. The quantity of Cl^- is usually proportionate to Na^+, except when there is selective loss of Cl^- in the HCl of vomited gastric juice, or when HCO_3^- is retained in the breath, or when certain diuretics cause disproportionate losses of Na^+ or Cl^-.

Normal Concentration: 100–106 mEq/L (100–106 mmol/L).

Increased Concentration (Hyperchloremia): *Brain* (cerebral damage); *parathyroids* (hyperparathyroidism); *kidneys* (renal tubular acidosis, acute renal failure); *pancreas* (diabetes mellitus); *intake/output* (diabetes insipidus, dehydration); *chemical imbalances* (respiratory alkalosis, metabolic acidosis); *drugs* (diamox, ammonium salts, salicylates); *technical error* (bromide in blood gives false test for Cl^-)

Decreased Concentration (Hypochloremia): *Lungs* (pulmonary emphysema); *heart* (congestive cardiac failure); *stomach* (pyloric obstruction); *bowels* (steatorrhea); *pancreas* (diabetic acidosis); *kidneys* (primary aldosteronism); *adrenals* (Addison's disease); *liver* (cirrhosis); *intake/output* (sweating, diarrhea, malabsorption); *drugs* (diuretics).

cholesterol, serum. *Pathophysiology:* This is one of the plasma lipids that also include triglycerides, phospholipids, and free fatty acids. They are all insoluble in water and are carried in the circulation by four types of lipoproteins as vehicles. Of the four, the low-density lipoproteins (LDL) carry the most cholesterol. Much of the cholesterol comes from the diet, but some is synthesized by the liver, skin, and other organs. Cholesterol is essential to every body cell, and it is a precursor to adrenal steroids, gonadal steroids, and bile salts.

Normal Concentration: 160–240 mg/dL (< 6.35 mmol/L). [varies with method].

Increased Concentration (Hypercholesterolemia): *Thyroid* (hypothyroidism); *kidneys* (nephrosis, chronic nephritis, renal vein thrombosis, amyloidosis, systemic lupus erythematosus [SLE], periarteritis, diabetic glomerulosclerosis); *liver and biliary system* (biliary obstruction [gallstone, carcinoma, cholangiolitic cirrhosis], von Gierke's disease); *pancreas* (diabetes mellitus, sometimes pancreatitis, total pancreatectomy); *intake/output* (dehydration); *chemical imbalances* (idiopathic hypercholesterolemia, lipodystrophy); *poisons* (alcohol).

Decreased Concentration (Hypocholesterolemia): *Thyroid* (hyperthyroidism); *liver* (severe cellular damage); *intake/output* (malnutrition, starvation); *chemical imbalances* (uremia, steatorrhea, Tangier disease); *malignant neoplasms; blood* (pernicious anemia, other hemolytic anemias, hypochromic anemias); *drugs* (cortisone, ACTH).

creatine phosphokinase, serum (CPK). *Pathophysiology:* This enzyme catalyzes the transfer of high energy phosphate between creatine and phosphocreatine, and between ADP and ATP. Principal concentrations of it are found in cardiac and skeletal muscle, and in the brain. Erythrocytes lack this enzyme so autolyzed serum specimens are acceptable for testing.

Normal Concentration: Males: 5–55 mU/mL; females: 5–35 mU/mL (same).

Increased Concentration: *Muscle* (severe exercise, muscle spasms, clonic and tonic seizures, muscle trauma [crush syndrome, postoperatively for about 5 days, electroshock for defibrillation, muscle necrosis and atrophy, intramuscular injections for 48 hours, polymyositis, progressive muscular dystrophy]); *brain* (2 days after cerebral infarction and lasting for 14 days); *thyroid* (hypothyroidism); *heart* (myocardial infarction, dissecting aneurysm); *pancreas* (pancreatitis); *genital* (parturition and last few weeks of pregnancy); *blood* (megaloblastic anemia); *drugs* (salicylates); *poison* (alcohol).

Decreased Concentration: Early pregnancy, drug interference, pancreatitis.

creatinine, serum. *Pathophysiology:* Mol. wt. 113. This is an organic acid resulting from the metabolism of creatine in the muscles. It is distributed throughout the body water. Creatine is formed in the liver and pancreas from arginine and glycine; it is taken up by muscle tissue and converted to creatine phosphate, catalyzed by the enzyme CPK. The creatine decomposes to creatinine at a rate of 1 or 2% per day. Creatinine is cleared from the blood by the glomerular filtration and is not resorbed. Urinary excretion of creatinine thus becomes an accurate indicator of renal function.

Normal Concentration: 0.6–1.5 mg/dL (53–133 μmol/L).

Increased Concentration: *Skin and muscle* (burns, high fevers, cachexia, acromegaly, gigantism); *kidneys* (azotemia, inadequate blood flow to the kidneys [heart failure, dehydration], ureterocolostomy with urinary resorption); *liver* (hepatic insufficiency); *pancreas* (pancreatitis with cholecystitis); *bowel* (blood in the gut); *blood* (plasma cell myeloma); *intake/output* (ingestion of roast beef with excess of creatinine, excessive intake of protein, diarrhea, steatorrhea, vomiting); *chemical imbalances* (alkali-milk syndrome of Burnett); *drugs* (corticosteroids, thiazide diuresis).

Decreased Concentration: None significant.

BUN/Creatinine Ratio Greater Than 10:1: Excessive protein intake, blood in the gut, excessive tissue destruction (cachexia, burns, fever, corticosteroid therapy); postrenal obstruction, inadequate renal circulation (heart failure, dehydration, shock).

BUN/Creatinine Ratio Less Than 10:1: Low protein intake, multiple dialyses, severe diarrhea or vomiting, hepatic insufficiency.

glucose, serum. *Pathophysiology:* Mol. wt. 180. This is the principal body sugar, a 6-carbon monosaccharide. It permeates all body water; the serum level remains fairly constant during fasting; there is a moderate rise after the ingestion of food. The liver cells transform other carbohydrates to glucose. Surpluses of this sugar are converted to glycogen for hepatic storage, or they form fat that is deposited throughout the body. Peripheral utilization of glucose by the tissues depends upon having the proper amounts of insulin. After an average meal, the normal person experiences a blood sugar rise to approximately 180 mg/dL serum; this returns to normal fasting levels within 2 hours. Higher glucose levels in the blood result from either failure to utilize it or the ingestion of superfluous quantities. When the blood concentration of glucose becomes high, the renal threshold is exceeded and glucose is excreted in the urine (glycosuria). The normal renal threshold occurs with a serum glucose of 160–190 mg/dL. This may be higher in a damaged kidney.

Normal Concentration: 70–110 mg/dL (3.9–5.6 mmol/L).

Increased Concentration (hyperglycemia): *Bone and muscle* (acromegaly, gigantism); *brain* (Wernicke's syndrome, subarachnoid hemorrhage, hypothalamic lesions convulsions); *thyroid* (hyperthyroidism); *heart* (myocardial infarction); *lungs* (asthma, pneumonia, pulmonary embolism); *stomach* (bleeding peptic ulcer); *bowel* (regional enteritis, ulcerative colitis); *liver* (hemochromatosis, cholecystitis); *kidneys* (nephritis, renal failure); *adrenals* (Cushing's disease, increased adrenalin, ACTH, pheochromocytoma, stress); *pancreas* (diabetes mellitus, pancreatitis, hypoglycemia); *blood* (hemolytic anemia); *genital* (toxemia of pregnancy); *malignant neoplasm; intake/output* dehydration, malnutrition.

Decreased Concentration (hypoglycemia): *Brain* (hypopituitarism, hypothalamic lesions); *thyroid* (hypothyroidism); *stomach* (postgastrectomy dumping syndrome, gastroenterostomy, carcinoma); *pancreas* (pancreatitis, islet tumor, hypoplasia, diabetes mellitus sometimes); *liver* (glycogen deficiency, hepatitis, cirrhosis, primary or secondary carcinoma); *adrenals* (carcinoma, Addison's disease, medullary unresponsiveness); *neoplasms; chemical imbalances* (von Gierke's disease, galactosuria, maple syrup urine disease, fructose intolerance, leucine sensitivity); malnutrition.

glutamate-oxaloacetate transaminase, serum (SGOT) (synonyms: aspartate aminotransferase, serum, and transaminase, serum SGOT). *Pathophysiology:* This enzyme catalyzes the transfer of the amino groups from aspartate to glutamate and oxaloacetate, involving it in both amino acid metabolism and gluconeogenesis. It is concentrated mostly in the cells of heart, liver, muscle, and kidney; lesser amounts are in pancreas, spleen, lung, brain, and erythrocytes. Tissue injury releases the enzyme into the extracellular fluids, but not necessarily in amounts proportionate to the injury.

Normal Concentration: 0–35 u/L (same).

Increased Concentration: *Muscle* (severe exercise, clonic and tonic seizures, crushing or burning or necrosis of muscle, inflammation from intramuscular injections, polymyositis, muscle dystrophy, rhabdomyolysis); *bone* (neoplastic metastasis, myeloma, Paget's disease); *brain* (cerebral infarction, cerebral neoplasm); *heart* (myocardial infarction—onset after 18 hours, peak in 2 days); *lungs* (pulmonary infections); *kidneys* (myoglobinemia, infarction, azotemia); *liver* (necrosis, cirrhosis, viral hepatitis, cholecystitis, administration of opiates in presence of biliary disease); *pancreas* (pancreatitis, diabetes mellitus); *stomach* (peptic ulcer); *bowel* (regional ileitis, ulcerative colitis); *blood* (hemolytic diseases including pernicious anemia, rhabdomyolysis); *intake/output* (dehydration); *drugs* (salicylates); *poisons* (alcohol); *technical error* (false positive from prostaphilin, polycillin, opiates, erythromycin, dehydration of blood specimen, dust contamination from laboratory).

Decreased Concentration: beriberi, severe liver disease, chronic dialysis, uremia, pregnancy, pyridoxine deficiency, ketoacidosis.

iron, serum (Fe^{++}). *Pathophysiology:* At. wt. 56. The body contains about 3–4 g of this inorganic element essential for hemoglobinization of erythrocytes. Its deficiency represents one of the most common disorders in the world. Approximately 1 mg of iron is absorbed and excreted each day.

Most of the iron circulates in erythrocyte hemoglobin (1.0 mg/1.0 mL packed erythrocytes), with the rest bound to ferritin in stores (approximately 1.0 g), in myoglobin, and with a small fraction incorporated into respiratory enzymes and other sites. Bound to transferrin, radioiron is cleared from the plasma in 60–120 minutes, with 80–90% incorporated into new circulating erythrocytes over the subsequent 2 weeks. The serum concentration of iron decreases by 50–100 μg/dL, with the diurnal acceleration of erythropoiesis in the afternoon, so the times sequential specimens are obtained should be uniform if trends are to be followed.

Normal Concentration: males 80–180 μg/dL (14–32 μmol/L); females 60–160 μg/dL (11–29 μmol/L).

Increased Concentration (Hyperferremia): *Intestinal tract* (excessive absorption [iron therapy, dietary excess, idiopathic hemochromatosis]); *liver* (acute hepatic necrosis, some cases of cirrhosis); *blood* (hemolytic anemia, repeated blood transfusions); *bone marrow* (aplastic anemia, thalassemia, pernicious anemia).

Decreased Concentration (Hypoferremia): *Blood* (iron deficiency anemia, repeated phlebotomy, intravascular hemolysis with hemoglobinuria [paroxysmal nocturnal hemoglobinuria, march hemoglobinuria, prosthetic heart valves]; anemia of chronic disorders [tuberculosis, osteomyelitis, rheumatoid arthritis, cancer]); *lungs* (intrapulmonary hemorrhage in idiopathic pulmonary hemosiderosis); *gastrointestinal tract* (diminished absorption [decreased ingestion, pica, postgastrectomy], chronic bleeding [peptic ulcer disease, gastritis, polyps, ulcerative colitis, colonic carcinoma]); *genitourinary tract* (menorrhagia, iron loss to fetus during gestation, chronic hematuria, loss of transferrin in proteinuria of nephrosis).

iron-binding capacity, serum total (TIBC). The TIBC mainly reflects transferrin and, with the serum iron, may help distinguish between anemias of iron deficiency and those of chronic disorders.

Normal Capacity: 250–460 μg/dL (45–82 μmol/L).

Increased Capacity: *Blood* (iron deficiency anemia, acute or chronic blood loss), *liver* (hepatitis), *genitourinary tract* (late pregnancy).

Decreased Capacity: *Blood* (anemias of chronic disorders

[infections, inflammations, and cancer], thalassemia), *gastrointestinal tract and liver* (hemochromatosis, cirrhosis), *genitourinary tract* (nephrosis).

ferritin, serum: Mol. wt. 680,000. As the major iron-storage protein in the body, it reflects iron stored in the reticuloendothelial system.

Normal Concentration: 18–300 ng/mL (18–300 μg/L).

Increased Concentration: *Blood* (excessive body iron stores from transfusion hemosiderosis, anemias of chronic disorders, leukemias, Hodgkin's disease), *gastrointestinal tract and liver* (excess dietary iron, transfusion hemosiderosis, hemochromatosis).

Decreased Concentration: Iron deficiency anemia (0–18 μg/L).

Increased Concentration: Hemochromatosis >400 ng/L (>160 nmol/L).

lactic dehydrogenase, serum (LDH). *Pathophysiology:* Mol. wt. 140,000. This enzyme catalyzes the oxidation of lactate to pyruvate reversibly. It is found in all tissues so an elevation of the blood level is a nonspecific indicator of tissue damage.

Normal Concentration: 50–150 U/L (same).

Increased Concentration: *Muscle* (necrosis, polymyositis in 25% of cases, muscular dystrophy in 10% of cases, dermatomyositis, progressive muscular dystrophy, myotonic dystrophy [but CPK is more specific for muscle than LDH]); *bone* (carcinomatous metastasis); *brain* (cerebral damage); *thyroid* (hypothyroidism); *heart* (acute myocardial infarction [begins within 10–12 hours, peaks at 48–72 hours, prolonged elevation for 10–14 days—long after CPK and SGOT have returned to normal]); combination myocardial infarction and congestive failure (increase in LDH and LDH_5, but LDH isoenzyme normal in cardiac failure alone); insertion of prosthetic heart valve; cardiovascular surgery; *lungs* (pulmonary embolism or infarction); *kidneys* (renal infarction) high LDH with normal or slight increase in SGOT; *liver* (hepatitis with jaundice, common bile duct obstruction); *bowel* (intestinal obstruction, sprue); *blood* (untreated pernicious anemia, also in other hemolytic anemias, 50% of cases of lymphoma and leukemia); *infections* (infectious mononucleosis); *malignant neoplasm* (50% of cases); *poisons* (alcohol).

Decreased Concentration: X-irradiation; ingestion of clofibrate.

phosphate, serum inorganic (HPO_4^{--}). *Pathophysiology:* This term includes the inorganic phosphorus of ionized HPO_4^{--} and $H_2PO_4^-$ in equilibrium in the serum; only 10–20% is protein-bound. P furnishes the element for synthesizing nucleotides, phospholipids, and the high-energy ATP. When the energy demands are great for glycolysis, the serum inorganic P is decreased.

Normal Concentration: 3.0–4.5 mg/dL (1.0–1.5 mmol/L).

Increased Concentration (hyperphosphatemia): *Bone* (healing fractures, some multiple myelomas, Paget's disease, osteolytic metastases, osteomalacia, acromegaly, rickets); *muscle* (necrosis); *parathyroids* (hypoparathyroidism); *adrenals* (Addison's disease); *liver* (acute yellow atrophy); *bowel* (high intestinal obstruction); *blood* (myelocytic leukemia); *infections* (sepsis); *congenital* (Fanconi's disease); *chemical imbalances* (milk-alkali syndrome of Burkett, rickets, respiratory alkalosis, excess of vitamin K); sarcoidosis.

Decreased Concentration (hypophosphatemia): *Parathyroids* (hyperparathyroidism); *kidneys* (renal tubular defects [Fanconi's syndrome]); *pancreas* (diabetes mellitus); *congenital* (primary hypophosphatemia); *intake/output* (anorexia, vomiting, diarrhea, lack of vitamin D, hyperalimentation in refeeding after starvation, malnutrition); *chemical imbalances* (gout, ketoacidosis, respiratory alkalosis, hypokalemia, hypomagnesemia, primary hyperphosphatemia); *drugs* (intravenous glucose, anabolic steroids, androgens, epinephrine, glucagon, insulin, salicylates, phosphorus-binding antacids, diuretic drugs); *poison* (alcohol).

potassium, serum (K^+, L, kalium). *Pathophysiology:* At. wt. 39. This is the predominant cation in the cellular fluid, while sodium predominates in the extracellular fluids. About 90% of the exchangeable K^+ is within the cells, less than 1% is in the normal serum. So small shifts of K^+ from the cells cause relatively large changes in the smaller serum compartment. Changes in serum concentration of K^+ produce profound effects on nerve excitation, muscle contraction, and in myocardial potential. Since the concentration of K^+ in the erythrocytes is about 18 times as great as that in the serum, hemolysis raises the serum K considerably.

Normal Concentration: 3.5–5.0 mEq/L (3.5–5.0 mmol/L).

Increased Concentration (hyperkalemia). (*Note:* high levels of serum K^+ pose great danger of producing cardiac arrest): *Muscle* (status epilepticus, periodic paralysis, tissue necrosis); *stomach* (hemorrhage from peptic ulcer); *bowel* (hemorrhage into the gut); *kidneys* (renal failure with oliguria or anuria, aldosteronism); *adrenals* (Addison's disease, deficit in renin-angiotensin-aldosterone system); *blood* (accumulation of blood in extracellular spaces, *in vivo* clotting); *intake/output* (dehydration, urinary obstruction, excessive oral intake of K^+ as drug or in food [fruit juices, soft drinks, oranges, peaches, bananas, tomatoes, high-protein diet]); *chemical imbalances* (acidosis, inappropriate antidiuretic hormone ADH, respiratory acidosis); *drugs and therapy* (spironolactone [aldosterone antagonist], triamterene [retains K^+], hemolyzed transfused blood); *technical error* (hemolysis in performing venipuncture or intentional clotting in collecting blood specimens).

Decreased Concentration (hypokalemia) (almost always associated with depletion of K^+ in total body water). *Stomach* (loss of K^+ from vomiting, gastric suction, postgastrectomy dumping syndrome, gastric atony); *bowel* (villous adenoma, colonic cancer, laxative abuse, Zollinger-Ellison syndrome, adynamic ileus); *pancreas* (diabetes mellitus); *kidneys* (polyuria, renal injury, salt-losing nephritis, ureterosigmoidostomy with urinary reabsorption); *adrenals* (Cushing's syndrome); *chemical imbalances (metabolic alkalosis* [from diuresis, primary aldosteronism, pseudoaldosteronism], *metabolic acidosis* [from renal tubular acidosis, diuresis phase of tubular necrosis, chronic pyelonephritis, diuresis after release of urinary obstruction]); *intake/output* (malabsorption and malnutrition); *drugs* (estrogens, salicylates, corticosteroids).

protein, total serum. This is determined as a fraction containing serum albumin and the serum globulins; the fibrinogen was discarded in the clot that separated from the plasma to form the serum specimen. The quantity of the total serum protein, minus the albumin fraction, gives an estimate of the serum globulins.

Normal Concentration: 6–8 g/dL (60–80 g/L).

Increased Concentration (hyperproteinemia): water depletion, multiple myeloma, macroglobulinemia, and sarcoidosis.

Decreased Concentration (hypoproteinemia): *Lymph nodes* (Hodgkin's disease); *heart* (congestive cardiac failure); *stomach* (peptic ulcer); *bowel* (ulcerative colitis); *biliary tract* (acute cholecystitis); *kidneys* (nephrosis, chronic glomerulo- nephritis); *liver* (cirrhosis, viral hepatitis).

—**albumin, serum.** This serum fraction is determined directly by the Autoanalyzer.

Pathophysiology. Mol. wt. about 65,000 daltons. Normally this fraction comprises more than half the total serum protein. Because its molecular weight is low compared to that of the globulins (between 44,000 and 435,000), its smaller molecules exert 80% of osmotic pressure of the plasma. So the concentration of the serum albumin controls the passage of water through the cell membranes by osmosis. In addition, (1) serum albumin serves as a protein store for the body that can be utilized when a deficit develops, (2) it serves as a solvent for fatty acids and bile salts, and (3) it serves as a transport vehicle by loosely binding hormones, amino acids, drugs, and metals.

Normal Concentration: 4.0–6.0 g/dL (40–60 g/L).

Increased Concentration (hyperalbuminemia): No significant correlation with diseases.

Decreased Concentration (hypoalbuminemia): *Bone* (multiple myeloma); *lymph nodes* (Hodgkin's disease); *heart* (congestive cardiac failure); *stomach* (peptic ulcer); *bowel* (ulcerative colitis, protein-losing enteropathies); *liver* (cirrhosis, viral hepatitis); *biliary tract* (acute cholecystitis); *pancreas* (diabetes mellitus); *kidneys* (nephrosis, chronic glomerulonephritis); *blood* (lymphocytic leukemia, myelocytic leukemia, macroglobulinemia, analbuminemia); *collagen diseases* (lupus erythematosus, polyarteritis, rheumatoid arthritis, rheumatic fever); stress, hypersensitivity; *drugs* (estrogens); malnutrition.

—**globulins, serum** (calculated from SMA 12/60). The difference between the values for total serum protein and for serum albumin, as measured by the Autoanalyzer, is assumed to be serum globulins, the plasma fibrinogen being discarded in the clot in preparing the serum specimen. When the globulin level is increased, an analysis of the group of globulins is indicated to identify each component. This is accomplished by *electrophoresis*.

—**globulins, serum** (by electrophoresis). A solution of the serum is added to a medium that is electrified to serve as an electric field. The medium may be filter paper, certain liquids, cellulose acetate, starch block, agar gel, or acrylamide gel. In an electric field the various proteins migrate, each at its own rate, depending on its molecular weight. Each protein may be recognized by its mobility. A specimen of blood plasma subjected to electrophoresis will be found to contain proteins that migrate in several *zones* according to their mobility rates. These zones have been named with Greek small letters; the proteins are named for the zone in which they are found: *alpha-O* (α_0) (for albumin), *alpha-1* (α_1), *alpha-2* (α_2), *beta* (β), *gamma* (γ), and *phi* (ϕ) (for fibrinogen).

Alpha-1* (α_1) *globulin (includes antitrypsin, oromucil, some cortisol-binding globulin). ***Increased Concentration:*** lymph nodes (Hodgkin's disease); *stomach* (peptic ulcer); *bowel* ulcerative colitis); *liver* (cirrhosis); *neoplasm* (metastatic carcinoma); *intake/output* (protein-losing enteropathy); hypersensitivity, stress. ***Decreased Concentration:*** viral hepatitis.

Alpha-2* (α_2) *globulin (includes macroglobulins, haptoglobin, HS glycoprotein, ceruloplasmin, and some immunoglobulins). ***Increased Concentration:*** *lymph nodes* (Hodgkin's disease); *stomach* (peptic ulcer); *bowel* (ulcerative colitis); *liver* (cirrhosis), kidneys (nephrosis, chronic glomerulonephritis); *collagen diseases* (systemic lupus erythematosis, polyarteritis nodosa, rheumatoid arthritis); *neoplasm* (metastatic carcinoma); *intake/output* (protein-losing enteropathies. ***Decreased Concentration:*** *liver* (cirrhosis, viral hepatitis).

Beta* (β) *globulin (includes transferrin, C_3, C_4, hemopexin, some immunoglobulins). ***Increased Concentration:*** *collagen diseases* (rheumatoid arthritis, rheumatic fever); *chemical imbalance* (analbuminemia). ***Decreased Concentration:*** *kidneys* (nephrosis); *blood* (lymphocytic leukemia); *neoplasm* (metastatic carcinoma).

Gamma* (γ) *globulins (include all the immunoglobulins). ***Increasaed Concentration:*** *liver* (cirrhosis); *blood* (myelocytic leukemia); *collagen diseases* (lupus erythematosus, rheumatoid arthritis); *chemical imbalance* (analbuminemia). ***Decreased Concentration:*** *kidneys* (nephrosis); *blood* (lymphocytic leukemia, hypogammaglobulinemia); *intake/output* (protein-losing enteropathies).

Monoclonal Gamma Globulins (recognized in the electrophoresis records by a *sharp and narrow* spike in the gamma region). This is inferred to be the result of proteins of unmixed nature from a single cell line. Such a result calls for further identification in immunoelectrophoresis. *Occurrence:* multiple myeloma, macroglobulinemia, malignancy, benign idiopathic.

Polyclonal Gamma Globulins (recognized in the electrophoresis records by a *broad-based pattern* in the gamma zone). The inference indicates the presence of abnormal proteins from many lines of cells. *Occurrence:* hepatic cirrhosis, diffuse skin diseases, hyperglobulinemic purpura.

—***gammopathies*** (by immunoelectrophoresis). This group of disorders is characterized by the proliferation of one or more of the five human immunoglobulins, IgG, IgA, IgM, IgD, and IgE, normally present in human serum. Their molecular structures differ among them by the possession of various combinations of two out of five *heavy chains* (H-chains) and various coupled two *light chains* (L-chains). The heavy chains are named with small Greek letters, corresponding to the large Arabic capitals of the immunoglobulins: α, β, γ, δ, ϵ; the light chains are called; κ and λ. The five immunoglobulins can be identified by *immunoelectrophoresis.* In this procedure regular electrophoresis is modified by the addition to the medium of specific antibodies.

Immunoglobulin IgG. Mol. wt. 160,000 daltons. This is the smallest molecule of the immunoglobulins and the only one that can pass the placental membranes; therefore, it serves as protection for the newborn until the child's own globulins can be generated. In the adult the immunoglobulin seems to participate in all immune reactions including the isoantibodies for antigen C, D, and E. *Normal Concentration:* 500–1200 mg/dL (5.00–12.00 g/L). *Increased Concentration: bone* (myeloma); *lungs* (pulmonary tuberculosis); *liver* (hepatitis, cirrhosis); *collagen diseases* (systemic lupus erythematosus, rheumatoid arthritis). *Decreased Concentration: lymph nodes* (lymphoid aplasia); *kidneys* (nephrosis); *blood* (agammaglobulinemia, dysgammaglobulinemia, heavy-chain disease, IgA myeloma, macroglobulinemia, chronic lymphocytic leukemia).

Immunoglobulin IgA. Mol. wt. 170,000 daltons. This globulin is especially involved in the protection against viral infections.

It has the added feature of an *excretory form* with a molecular weight of 400,000 daltons, found in colostrum, saliva, tears, bronchial secretions, gastrointestinal secretions, and nasal discharges. It has a special action against viruses of influenza, poliomyelitis, adenoviral diseases, and rhinoviruses. *Normal Concentration:* 50–350 mg/dL (0.50–3.50 g/L). *Increased Concentration:* *liver* (cirrhosis); *blood* (IgA myeloma); *infections; collagen diseases* (systemic lupus erythrmatosus, rheumatoid arthritis); *congenital* (Wiskott-Aldrich syndrome); sarcoidosis. *Decreased Concentration:* normal in some persons; *kidneys* (nephrosis); *congenital* (hereditary telangiectasia, lymphoid aplasia); collagen disease (Still's disease, systemic lupus erythematosus); *liver* (cirrhosis); *blood* (type III dysgammaglobulinemia, agammaglobulinemia, heavy-chain disease, acute lymphocytic lèukemia, chronic lymphocytic leukemia, chronic myelocytic leukemia).

Immunoglobulin IgM. Mol. wt. 900,000 daltons. This is the largest molecule of the immunoglobulins. It is most often elicited during a primary antibody response. The rheumatoid factor and the isoantibodies anti-A and anti-B belong mostly to this class. *Normal Concentration:* 30–230 mg/dL (0.30–2.30 g/L). *Increased Concentration:* *liver* (hepatitis, biliary cirrhosis); *collagen disease* (rheumatoid arthritis, systemic lupus erythematosus); *blood* (macroglobulinemia); trypanosomiasis.

Immunoglobulin IgD. Mol. wt. 185,000 daltons. There is no known specific activity for this protein. *Normal Concentration:* <6 mg/dL (<60 mg/L). *Increased Concentration:* chronic infections, IgD myeloma.

Immunoglobulin IgE. Mol. wt. 200,000 daltons. This protein is involved in atopic reactions. *Normal Concentration:* 20–1000 ng/mL (20–1000 μg/L). *Increased Concentration:* extrinsic asthma (60% of cases); hay fever (30% of cases); atopic eczema, parasitic infestations, IgE myeloma.

—heavy-chain disease. This is a disease characterized by excessive production of proteins with heavy chains. In the electrophoresis they occur as a sharp peak in the beta or gamma region. Immunoelectrophoresis shows marked decrease in the normal IgG, IgA, and IgM.

sodium, serum (Na^+, *L. natrium*). *Pathophysiology:* At. wt. 23. This is the predominant cation in the extracellular fluid, including plasma. Together with Cl^- it makes a major contribution to the osmotic pressure of the serum. Water diffuses between the cellular compartment containing K^+ and the extracellular compartment containing Na^+. The concentration of Na^+ is in equilibrium with K^+ and total body water. Loss of Na^+ is frequently accompanied by an equivalent amount of water (as an isotonic solution), so normal levels of serum Na^+ do not exclude the possibility of water shifts. Thus, a careful history of water intake and output may be necessary to interpret the meaning of the value for serum Na^+.

Normal Concentration: 135–145 mEq/L (135–145 mmol/L).

Increased Concentration (hypernatremia): *Brain* (thalamic lesions); *parathyroids* (hyperparathyroidism); *kidneys* (aldosteronism); *intake/output* (water loss greater than Na loss [vomiting, sweating, hyperpnea, diarrhea], diuresis ([diabetes insipidus, diabetes mellitus, diuretic drugs, diuretic phase of acute tubular necrosis, diuresis after relief of urinary obstruction], excessive Na^+ intake); *chemical imbalances* (hypercalcemia, hypokalemic nephropathy); *drugs* (corticosteroids).

Decreased Concentration (hyponatremia): *Heart* (serum dilution from congestive cardiac failure); *kidneys* (serum dilution from salt-losing nephritis, or nephritis); *liver* (dilution from cirrhosis with ascites); *adrenals* (Addison's disease); *intake/output (fluid loss* [vomiting, sweating, diarrhea, diuresis]), *malnutrition, chemical imbalance* (inappropriate antidiuretic hormone); *spuriously normal serum osmolality* (hyperlipidemia, hyperglycemia [reciprocal decrease of serum Na^+ by 3 mEq/L for every increase of glucose level of 100 mg/dL]).

transaminase, serum (*synonyms:* ***glutamate-oxaloacetate, serum SGOT,*** *which see, and* ***aspartate aminotransferase***).

urea-nitrogen (blood urea nitrogen, BUN, Urea-N). *Pathophysiology:* Mol. wt. 60. Urea is the nitrogenous end product of protein metabolism. It permeates all body water and is excreted in the urine. The traditional method of expression is as urea-nitrogen that is approximately half the weight of urea. The serum level of urea-N results from a balance between the rate of amino acid substrate presented to the liver, the rate of synthesis of urea by the liver, and the rate of urinary excretion of urea. Protein breakdown is accentuated by high-protein diets, blood in the gastrointestinal tract, increased metabolism of tissue, and inhibition of anabolism by corticosteroid drugs.

Normal Concentration: 8–25 mg/dL (2.9–8.9 mmol/L).

Increased Concentration (azotemia): *Thyroid* (increased catabolism in hyperthyroidism); *heart* (myocardial infarction); *kidneys* (impaired renal function, reduced blood flow to the kidneys in congestive cardiac failure, postrenal obstruction); *bowel* (hemorrhage into the gut); *input/output* (salt and water loss [vomiting, sweating, diarrhea, diuresis, lack of drinking water]).

Decreased Concentration: *Muscle* (acromegaly); *kidneys* (nephrosis sometimes); *liver* (liver failure, hepatitis); *genital* (late pregnancy); *intake/output* (low-protein high-carbohydrate diet, intravenous feedings exclusively, celiac disease).

Wallach: BUN 6–8 mg/dL is frequently the result of dehydration: 10–20 mg/dL usually indicates normal renal function; 50–150 mg/dL usually from seriously impaired renal function.

uric acid, serum. *Pathophysiology:* Mol. wt. 169. Uric acid is the end product of purine metabolism. The substrates, phosphoribosylpyrophosphate (PRPP), glutamine, glycine, and aspartic acid, are converted to inosinic acid. This latter, in turn, plus adenylic and guanylic acids are transformed by hypoxanthine-guanine phosphoribosyl transferase (HGPRTase) to form hypoxanthine. This is further transformed to uric acid by action of xanthine oxidase. Normally uric acid is produced at the rate of 10 mg/kg/day in a healthy adult. The body pool is about 1200 mg, distributed to the body water. *Increased synthesis* of nucleic acid breakdown results in the increased uric acid production. Uric acid leaves the body by two routes; through the renal glomeruli, and by bacterial catabolism of uric acid in the gut. Renal excretion of uric acid is increased by expansion of body fluids (by salt or osmotic diuresis), and by vasoconstriction (from angiotensin or norepinephrine infusions). Excretion of uric acid is decreased by dehydration or diuretics.

Normal Concentration: 3.0–7.0 mg/dL (0.18–0.42 mmol/L).

Increased Concentration (hyperuricemia) (*N. B. High values for uric acid are among the most common abnormalities encountered in routine testing, according to Hall and Halfman. This probably accounts for the much too frequent diagnosis of gout. The serum uric acid is elevated in 90% of the cases of gouty arthritis, but the same elevation is noted in 25% of the cases of acute nongouty arthritis and in 25% of relatives of gouty patients. The diagnosis of gout should not be made without the symptoms and signs of the disease*). *Skin* (about half the patients with psoriasis); *thyroid* (hypothyroidism); *parathyroids* (hypoparathyroidism, primary hyperparathyroidism); *lungs* (resolving pneumonia); *kidneys* (renal failure, polycystic kidneys); *genital* (toxemia of pregnancy); *blood* (increased destruction of nucleoproteins [leukemia, multiple myeloma, polycythemia vera, lymphoma], other disseminated neoplasias, hemolytic anemias, sickle-cell anemia); *neoplasms* (metastasis); *cogenital or familial* (Wilson's disease, Fanconi's disease, von Gierke's disease, Down's syndrome); *therapy* (irradiation, cancer therapy, thiazides, other diuretics, small doses of salicylates); *intake/output* (high-protein—low-calorie diet, high nuclear diet [sweetbreads, liver], starvation); *chemical imbalance* (gout, relatives of gouty patients, calcinosis universalis, diabetic ketosis); *poisons* (acute alcoholism, lead poisoning, berylliosis); certain normal *populations* (Blackfoot and Pima Indians, Filipinos, New Zealand Maoris); sarcoidosis. ***Decreased Concentration*** (hypouricemia): *Bone* (acromegaly); *kidneys* (xanthinuria, healthy adults with Dalmatian-dog mutation [isolated defect in tubular transport of uric acid]; *bowel* (celiac disease); *blood* (pernicious anemia in relapse); *congenital* (Fanconi's syndrome, Wilson's disease); *neoplasms* (carcinoma, Hodgkin's disease); *drugs* (ACTH, glyceryl guaicolate, x-ray contrast media).

Hematologic Data

blood film examination. A blood film, prepared or available in the office, nursing unit, or outclinic laboratory, provides the physician with an opportunity of immediately evaluating clues from the history and physical examination, and of personally confirming results of electronic counters in central laboratories requiring hours to days for reporting. Examples of information to be obtained will be given with encouragement to consult standard textbooks of hematology for comprehensive treatment of the subject. Appreciate that cellular morphology may vary depending upon the technique, stain, and location on the blood smear. Select an area for examination where the erythrocytes are close but do not touch each other.

Erythrocyte Morphology: Evaluate color, size, shape, and contents. *Macrocytes* (reticulocytosis, liver disease, megaloblastic anemia); *hypochromic microcytes* (defects in hemoglobin synthesis [iron deficiency, thalassemias, sickle cell disease, and other hemoglobinopathies]); *spherocytes* (hereditary spherocytosis); *schistocytes* (disseminated intravascular coagulation, thrombotic thrombocytopenic purpura, vasculitis, thrombotic microangiopathy, prosthetic heart valves); *tear drop or dacryocytes* (extramedullary hemopoiesis, myelophthisic anemia); *erythroblasts* (extramedullary hemopoiesis, myelophthisic anemia, severe hemolytic anemia, erythroleukemia); *Howell-Jolly bodies* (postsplenectomy, megaloblastic anemia); *basophilic stippling* (lead poisoning, hemolytic disease); *malaria and Bartonella parasites.*

Leukocyte Morphology: Confirm the report of the electronic enumeration and differential leukocyte count. *Toxic granulation of Neutrophils and Metamyelocytes* (bacterial infections); *giant cytoplasmic granules* (Chediak-Higashi syndrome); *bilobed neutrophils* (Pelger-Huet anomaly); *hypersegmented neutrophils* (pernicious anemia, vitamin B_{12} deficiency, folate deficiency, myeloproliferative diseases); *myeloblasts, promyelocytes, myelocytes* (depending upon the number and appearance of immature cells, consider [acute myeloblastic leukemia, acute promyelocytic leukemia, chronic myelocytic leukemia, myelofibrosis, polycythemia vera]); *atypical lymphocytes* (viral infections); *large granular lymphocytes* (natural killer cells of T-gamma lymphoproliferative disease); *lymphoblasts* (acute lymphoblastic leukemia, prolymphocytic leukemia, malignant lymphoma, chronic lymphocytic leukemia, infectious mononucleosis); *plasmablasts* (multiple myeloma).

Platelet Morphology: Confirm the electronic enumeration of the platelet count. In oil immersion fields of 1000× magnification, where the erythrocytes are close but not touching, expect to count 15–20 platelets per field in normal blood films. Scan the sides of the smear for clumps of platelets that may have been counted inaccurately by instrument. *Megathrombocytes* (platelets greater than 2.5 microns in diameter may be increased in conditions of accelerated platelet production, compensating for increased destruction, B_{12} deficiency, folate deficiency, myeloproliferative diseases, Bernard-Soulier syndrome).

erythrocyte measurements (counts, hemoglobin content, and hematocrit). *Normal Values: Counts* 4.2–6.2 × 10^6/μL. *Hematocrit:* males: 42–52%; females: 37–47%; *Hemoglobin:* males: 14–18 g/dL; females: 12–16 g/dL.

erythrocytic indices. These values are all calculated from the counts, hemoglobin content, and hematocrit. The normal ranges are as follows:

$$\textit{Mean Corpuscular Volume (MVC)} = \frac{\text{Hct} \times 10}{\text{RBC in millions}} = 82 - 92\ \mu\text{m}^3.$$

$$\textit{Mean Corpuscular Hemoglobin Concentration (MCHC)} = \frac{\text{Hgb in g/dL} \times 100}{\text{Hct}} = 32 - 36\%$$

$$\textit{Mean Corpuscular Hemoglobin (MCH)} = \frac{\text{Hgb in g/dL} \times 10}{\text{RBC in millions}} = 27 - 31\ \text{pg/cell}.$$

high RBC counts. *Muscle* (burns [contracted blood volume]); *heart* (venous-arterial shunt [right-to-left shunt]); *lungs* (hypoxic diseases); *liver* (hepatoma); *kidneys* (renal cyst or carcinoma); *blood* (contracted blood volume [dehydration, burns, shock], hemoglobinopathies [carboxyhemoglobinemia, sulfhemoglobinemia], polycythemia vera and secondary); *genital* (3rd to 9th month of pregnancy and to 3rd week postpartum, ruptured ectopic pregnancy); *intake/output* (diarrhea, profuse sweating, fluid deprivation]); *chemical imbalance* (diabetic acidosis, high-altitude hypoxia); *drugs* (androgens, diuretics).

low RBC counts. *Heart* (congestive cardiac failure); *kidneys* (renal failure, oliguria); *genital* (pregnancy [expanded plasma volume]); *blood* (macrocytic anemias [pernicious anemia, folate deficiency, refractory anemia, hemolysis or bleeding], normocytic normochromic anemias [bone marrow failure, acute hemorrhage, hemolysis, chronic disease, infections, renal failure, liver disease], microcytic hypochromic anemias

[Fe deficiency, thalassemia, pyridoxine-responsive anemia, hemoglobinopathies]).

erythrocyte sedimentation rate (ESR). *Normal Values:* *Wintrobe Method:* males: 1–13 mm/hour; females: 0–20 mm/hour. *Westergren Method:* males: 0–13 mm/hour; females: 0–20 mm/hour.

Increase Rate: *Thyroid* (hyperthyroidism, hypothyroidism); *genital* (pelvic inflammation, ruptured ectopic pregnancy, normal pregnancy from 3rd month to termination plus 3 weeks postpartum, menstruation); *blood* (hyperglobulinemia, hypoalbuminemia, dextran or polyvinyl plasma substitutes; *infections* (many, but especially tuberculosis, necrosis); *collagen disease* (rheumatoid arthritis); neoplasm: *poison* (as in lead).

Not Increased Rate: *Bone and joints* (osteoarthritis); *heart* (angina pectoris); *stomach* (peptic ulcer); *genital* (unruptured ectopic pregnancy, early pregnancy); *blood* (polycythemia vera, sickle-cell anemia); *certain infections* (typhoid fever, undulant fever, malaria, infectious mononucleosis); acute appendicitis (first 24 hours), acute allergic disorders.

leukocytes, total count. *Normal Concentration:* 4300–10,800/μL (or mm^3).

—neutrophil counts. *Normal Concentration:* 1830–7250/μL (or mm^3) (34–71% of total).

Increased Concentration (leukocytosis): *skin and muscle* (exercise, seizures, burns, inflammation, gangrene, necrosis); *heart* (myocardial infarction); *genital* (eclampsia); *blood* (acute hemorrhage, acute hemolysis, myeloproliferative diseases [polycythemia vera, chronic myelocytic leukemia, myelofibrosis, idiopathic thrombocythemia]); *neoplasms* (malignant); *infections; chemical imbalances* (uremia, diabetic acidosis, gout); *drugs* (epinephrine, corticosteroids, lithium carbonate, parenteral foreign proteins, vaccines); *poisons* (venoms, mercury, black widow spider venom).

Decreased Concentration (leukopenia or neutropenia): *Bone marrow* (failure); *kidneys* (severe renal injury); *spleen* (hypersplenism, Felty's syndrome); *liver* (cirrhosis, portal obstruction); *blood* (pernicious anemia, folate deficiency, aleukemic leukemia, aplastic anemia, acute myeloblastic leukemia, cyclic neutropenia, autoimmune neutropenia); *congenital* (Gaucher's disease); infections (viral [infectious mononucleosis, hepatitis, HIV, influenza, rubeola rubella, psittacosis], bacterial [streptococcal, staphylococcal diseases, sepsis, tularemia, brucellosis, tuberculosis], *rickettsial diseases* [scrub typhus, sandfly fever]. *protozoal* [malaria, kala-azar]; *intake/output* (cachexia); *drugs and therapy* (cancer chemotherapy, sulfonamides, antibiotics, analgesics, antidepressants, arsenicals, antithyroid drugs, x-radiation); *poisons:* (benzene); *collagen disease* (systemic lupus erythematosus).

—eosinophil counts. *Normal Concentration:* 0–700/μL (or mm^3) (0–7.8% of WBC).

Increased Concentration (eosinophilia): *Skin* (pemphigus, dermatitis herpetiformis); *bone* (metastatic carcinoma to bone); *heart* (Loeffler parietal fibroplastic endocarditis); *gastrointestinal* (eosinophilic gastroenteritis, ulcerative colitis, regional enteritis); *spleen* (postsplenectomy); *blood* (pernicious anemia, hypereosinophilic syndrome), chronic myelocytic leukemia, polycythemia vera, Hodgkin's disease); *allergic disorders* (asthma, hay fever, urticaria, drug reactions); *infections* (scarlet fever, erythema multiforme); *parasitic infestations* (trichinosis, ecchynococcosis); *genital* (ovarian tumors); *miscellaneous* (polyarteritis nodosa, sarcoidosis); *irradiation; poisons* (phosphorus, black widow spider bite).

Decreased Concentration (eosinopenia): bone marrow failure; hypoadrenalism.

—basophil counts. *Normal Concentration:* 0–150/μL (or mm^3) (0–1.8% of WBC).

Increased Concentration (basophilia): *Thyroid* (myxedema); *spleen* (postsplenectomy); *kidneys* (nephrosis); *infections* (varicella, variola); *blood* (chronic myelocytic leukemia, polycythemia vera, myeloid metaplasia, Hodgkin's disease, chronic hemolytic anemias).

Decreased Concentration: *Thyroid* (hyperthyroidism); *genital* (pregnancy); *irradiation; blood* (bone marrow failure); *drugs* (chemotherapy, glucocorticoids).

lymphocyte counts. *Normal Concentration:* 1,500–4,000/μL (or mm^3) (19–52% of WBC).

Increased Concentration (lymphocytosis): *Lungs* (tuberculosis, viral pneumonia); *liver* (infectious hepatitis); *bowel* (cholera); *blood* (infectious lymphocytosis, infectious mononucleosis, lymphocytic leukemia, malignant lymphoma); *general infections* (rubella, brucellosis, systemic syphilis, toxoplasmosis, pertussis).

Decreased Concentration (lymphopenia): *acute infections; neoplasm* (carcinoma, lymphoma); *irradiation; drugs* (corticosteroids, cancer chemotherapy); idiopathic.

monocyte counts. *Normal Concentration:* 200–950/µL (or mm^3) (2.4–11.8% of WBC).

Increased Concentration (monocytosis): *bowel* (ulcerative colitis, regional enteritis); *blood* (monocytic leukemia, myeloid metaplasia, recovery from agranulocytosis); *congenital* (Gaucher's disease); *neoplasm; infections; protozoal* (malaria, kala-azar, trypanosomiasis); *rickettsial* (Rocky Mountain spotted fever, typhus); bacterial (subacute bacterial endocarditis, tuberculosis, brucellosis); *miscellaneous and multiple system* (systemic lupus erythematosus, sarcoidosis, syphilis).

platelet counts (thrombocytes). *Normal Concentration:* 150,000–400,000/µL (or mm^3).

Increased Concentration (thrombocytosis or thrombocythemia): *bone* (rheumatoid arthritis); *muscles* (exercise, bleeding, burns); *heart* (acute heart disease); *liver* (cirrhosis); *spleen* (postsplenectomy); *pancreas* (pancreatitis); *blood* (myeloproliferative diseases [polycythemia vera, myelocytic leukemia]; iron-deficiency anemia); *malignancy; acute infections, collagen disorders.*

Decreased Concentration (thrombocytopenia): *spleen* (hypersplenism [congestive splenomegaly, splenectomy, sarcoidosis, splenomegaly, Felty's syndrome]); *blood* (anemias [aplastic, myelophthisic, pernicious anemia, acquired hemolytic anemia, folate deficiency, contact with foreign substances in heart-lung machine during cardiac surgery]; polycythemia vera, myelocytic leukemia, thrombocytopenic purpura, primary hemorrhagic thrombocytopenia, massive blood transfusions, May-Hegglin anomaly, surgical operation in general); *infections* (subacute bacterial endocarditis, sepsis, AIDS, typhus); *congenital* (Gaucher's disease, Kasabach-Merritt syndrome); irradiation, *drugs* (marrow suppressants, nitrogen mustard, cancer chemotherapy, chloramphenicol, tranquilizers, antipyretics, heavy metals); *chemical imbalance* (azotemia, heatstroke); *poisons* (benzol, insect bites).

all cellular elements of the blood (erythrocytes, leukocytes, platelets). *Increased Concentration* (pancytosis): dehydration, polycythemia vera, the myeloproliferative syndromes.

Decreased Concentration (pancytopenia): *Bones* (marrow failure, multiple myeloma, carcinomatous invasion); *bacterial infections* (tuberculosis); *viral infections* (hepatitis); *blood* (multiple myeloma, lymphoma, pernicious anemia or folate deficiency, myeloblastic leukemia, paroxysmal hemoglobinuria, myelofibrosis); *collagen disease* systemic lupus erythematosus); *irradiation; drugs* (cancer chemotherapy, chloramphenicol); *poisons* (benzene).

coagulation factors.

Prothrombin Time (PT). *Normal:* 11–15 seconds. *Prolonged Time:* deficiencies in any of clotting factors I, II, V, VII, or X; liver disease; disseminated intravascular coagulation; vitamin K deficiency; steatorrhea; idiopathic; Coumadin administration; greatly decreased or abnormal fibrinogen.

Partial Thromboplastin Time (PTT). *Normal:* 22–37 seconds (activated. *Prolonged Time:* deficiency of *any of* clotting factors I, II, V, VIII, IX, X, XI, XII; disseminated intravascular coagulation; therapeutic doses of heparin; *drugs,* lupus erythematosus, and other antibody-mediated inhibitors of clotting factor activity.

Fibrinogen. *Normal:* 150–350 mg/dL. *Increased Concentration:* during menstruation; pregnancy, infections; hyperthyroidism. *Decreased Concentration:* congenital afibrinogenemia; disseminated intravascular coagulation; circulating anticoagulants; fibrinolysis.

Urinalysis

So much information about the patient's health can be rapidly obtained from examination of the urine that many physicians insist on personally performing this simple analysis in the small laboratories of an outclinic, hospital nursing unit, or office. Optimally, urine is collected as a midstream specimen from the first voiding in the morning and examined within one half hour. This practice tests renal concentrating ability and permits identification of casts before they disintegrate.

color. *Pathophysiology:* Either clear or cloudy (from precipitated normally excreted urates, phosphates, or sulfates) the urine is usually yellow to amber from urochrome pigments. Other colors provide clues to the presence of abnormal substances for which chemical tests should be applied: *dark yellow* *to green* (bile or bilirubin); *red to black* (erythrocytes, hemoglobin, myoglobin, homogentisic acid [plus sodium hydroxide]); *purple to brown* on standing in the sunlight from porphyrins.

acidity. Normal range of pH is from 4.6 to 8.0. Monitoring urinary pH helps physicians attempting to alkalinize or acidify the urine to enhance the solubility and excretion of certain substances and drugs.

specific gravity. *Pathophysiology:* An index of weight per unit volume, the specific gravity measures the kidney's ability to dilute or concentrate urine in response to the secretion of antidiuretic hormone (ADH). Fasting during 8 hours of sleep should produce a first morning specimen with a specific gravity exceeding 1.018.

Normal Range: 1.003–1.030 achieved with forced water drinking and fasting, respectively.

Increased Specific Gravity: fasting and dehydration, glycosuria, proteinuria, radiographic contrast media.

Decreased Specific Gravity: compulsive water drinking, diabetes insipidus.

Fixed Specific Gravity (isosthenuria = 1.010): severe renal parenchymal damage from many causes (gout, prolonged potassium deficiency, hypercalcemia, myeloma kidney, sickle cell disease).

proteinuria. *Pathophysiology:* Normally an adult excretes undetectable concentrations of protein (5–15 mg/dL). Tubular and glomerular disease may produce measurable proteinuria.

Low Concentrations: pyelonephritis, fever, benign orthostatic proteinuria, idiopathic focal glomerulonephritis.

High Concentrations: glomerulonephritis, diabetes mellitus, systemic lupus erythematosus, renal vein thrombosis, amyloidosis, and other causes of the nephrotic syndrome.

glucose. *Pathophysiology:* A function of the plasma glucose concentration, the glomerular filtration and tubular reabsorption of glucose, normal levels of glucose in randomly collected fresh urine specimens are undetectable at less than 25 mg/dL; less than 100 mg/dL during a glucose tolerance test. Dip sticks, impregnated with glucose oxidase and an indicator color, provide a convenient, rapid, and semiquantitative estimate for the patient and physician. Progressively diminished glucose utilization in a patient with uncontrolled diabetes mellitus leads to lypolysis with increasing plasma and urinary concentrations of acetoacetic acid, beta-hydroxybutyric acid, and ketones, which should be sought with other tests.

Normal Range: 3–25 mg/dL.

Increased Concentrations: hyperglycemia in diabetes mellitus; infrequently with renal abnormalities, including acute tubular damage, hereditary renal glycosuria and proximal tubular dysfunction as in the Fanconi syndromes.

urinary sediment. *Pathophysiology:* Normally excreted erythrocytes, leukocytes, hyaline casts, and crystals (urate, phosphate, oxalate) are found in the sediment of a fresh specimen collected after a night's fast. Centrifuge 10 mL of urine in a conical tube for 5 minutes, decant the supernatant, flick the tube to disperse formed elements in the remaining drop, and place it on a slide under a coverslip to examine with the high power objective of a microscope (hpf). Abnormal numbers of cells and casts or any bacteria reveal the presence of disease.

Erythrocytes: Normally, 0–5 RBC/hpf can be observed in concentrated specimens. *Microscopic hematuria* may occur with fever and exercise and many lesions of the urinary tract from glomerulus to urethra. Causes of *gross hematuria* include: coagulation defects, renal papillary necrosis, renal infarction, sickle cell disease, glomerulonephritis, Goodpasture's syndrome, stone or carcinoma of the kidney, hemorrhagic cystitis, stone or carcinoma of the bladder, and prostatitis.

Leukocytes: Normally, 0–10 WBC/hpf can be seen in concentrated specimens. In addition to neutrophils excreted into the urine from the same anatomic sites as erythrocytes, leukocytes from vaginal exudates frequently contaminate routine specimens collected from women. When pyuria exceeding 10 WBC/hpf is present in an uncontaminated specimen, a site of infection in the urinary tract should be sought.

Casts: Occasional *hyalin casts,* arising from the normal renal tubular secretion of mucoproteins, are seen in fresh concentrated specimens. Finding many broad fine or coarse *granular casts* (composed of serum proteins like albumin, IgG, transferrin, haptoglobin) in urine containing excessive protein, however, indicates renal parenchymal disease, especially when accompanied by red cell casts. The urine of patients with the nephrotic syndrome, who exhibit glomerular proteinuria and hyperlipoproteinuria, contains *fatty casts,* casts with *doubly refractile fat bodies,* and *maltese crosses* when examined in polarized light. *Red cell casts,* containing 10–50 distinct erythrocytes and doubly refractile fat bodies, indicate glomerular disease (glomerulonephritis). *White cell casts* are found in the urinary sediment of patients with pyelonephritis, polyarteritis, exudative glomerulonephritis, and renal infarction. *Bacteria* accompanying white cell casts indicate urinary tract infection. Broad orange or brown *hematin casts* occur in acute tubular injury and chronic renal failure.

Part III: Disease Patterns

(Chap. 12)

This section is devoted to the patterns of diagnostic clues for diseases and syndromes. In the search for clues with the other two modes, the examiner may encounter the names of diseases for which knowledge of more diagnostic clues is desired. The appropriate summaries are set forth here.

The boldface catchwords are the names of diseases and syndromes, followed by synonyms, brief descriptions, and chief diagnostic features. The basic material and terminology were derived from A. J. Finkel, B. L. Gordon, M. R. Baker, and C. M. Fanta: *Current Medical Information and Terminology,* 5th ed. American Medical Association, Chicago, 1981.

12

Diagnostic Clues of Diseases

This chapter contains short summaries of the diagnostic findings in various diseases mentioned but briefly in the text; consult the regular index to find the more detailed textual descriptions. The purpose of this chapter is to furnish a brief definition of a disease, with reminders of further symptoms and signs to seek and laboratory tests to obtain. The reader will wish to consult the textbooks for more details, after a beginning has been made with these clues.

In any index, the reader is frustrated in finding terms with multiple words. Which catchword was used to determine the alphabetic location? Here the term is stated in its usual sequence, except when one word refers to an anatomic region. When the term includes reference to an anatomic structure, the anatomic term comes first, whether it be adjective or noun. But when the adjective and noun for an anatomic region have different initials, the noun form is indexed. Whenever possible, the name for a disease coincides with the preference recommended in A. J. Finkel, B. L. Gordon, M. R. Baker, and C. M. Fanta: *Current Medical Information and Terminology*, 5th ed. American Medical Association, Chicago, 1981.

achondroplasia. Hereditary dominant disease of cartilage and endochondral bone growth. *Signs:* congenital dwarfism with recessed nasal bridge, large brachycephalic head, normal trunk, dorsal kyphosis, backward-tilting sacrum, slightly distended abdomen, short muscular limbs, stubby hands with thick fingers. *X-ray:* short bowed wide bones of increased density and expanded ends, characteristic cupping of metaphyses, incomplete glenoid fossa and acetabulum, wide joint spaces.

***acquired immunodeficiency syndrome* (*AIDS*).** An immunosuppressive syndrome predisposing to life-threatening opportunistic infections, Kaposi's sarcoma, and other malignancies was recognized in the United States in 1981. A retrovirus infection with a human T-cell lymphotrophic virus or human immunodeficiency virus (HIV), spread in the United States by sexual contact of semen and saliva, or by blood and blood products, progressed to an epidemic by the mid-1980s. Homosexual and bisexual males, intravenous drug users, Haitians, and hemophilic patients are the groups most frequently affected; however, transmission to spouses and children of affected persons has occurred. Opportunistic infections include: *parasites* (*Pneumocystis carinii* pneumonia, toxoplasmosis encephalitis, cryptosporidia enteritis), *viruses* (cytomegalovirus, Epstein-Barr virus, herpes simplex, herpes zoster), *fungi* (candidiasis, cryptococcosis, coccidioidomycosis, histoplasmosis, aspergillosis), *bacteria* (salmonellosis, mycobacteria, listeriosis, nocardiosis). *Symptoms:* chronic fever, dyspnea, diarrhea, weight loss, dementia. *Signs:* generalized lymphadenopathy, signs of opportunistic infections, disseminated pigmented skin nodules of Kaposi's sarcoma. *Lab.:* anemia, leukopenia, thrombocytopenia or pancytopenia; diminished concentration of T-helper lymphocytes and reversed ratio of T-helper/T-suppressor lymphocytes; antibody seropositivity to HIV. *Other tests:* cutaneous anergy to skin tests of candida, mumps, trichophyton, and purified protein derivative [W. J. Urba and D. L. Longo: Clinical Spectrum of Human Retroviral-induced Diseases, *Cancer Res.* (*Suppl.*), **45:**4637s–43s, 1985.].

acrocyanosis. Vasospasm of integumentary arterioles with secondary dilatation of capillary beds and subpapillary venous plexuses associated with anxiety, asthenia, and endocrinopathies. *Symptoms:* cold extremities. *Signs:* symmetric cyanosis of limbs with persistent blue or red mottling of wrists, ankles, and digits; cold sweat on digits; cold accentuates, warm relieves. *Tests:* intradermal injection of histamine produces exaggerated wheal and red flare.

acromegaly. Hypersection of growth hormone by eosinophilic adenoma or hyperplastic pituitary *after* closure of epiphyses. *Symptoms:* headache, visual loss, muscular weakness, backache, pain in limbs, sweating, amenorrhea, polydipsia, polyuria. *Signs:* exaggerated supraorbital ridges, exophthalmos, enlargement of hands, feet, mandible (separation of teeth), nose, lips, tongue; bitemporal hemianopsia to blindness; hepatomegaly and cardiomegaly; hypertrichosis; hypertension; goiter with signs of thyrotoxicosis; diabetes insipidus. *X-ray:* overgrowth of cancellous bone; enlarged sella turcica; osteoporosis; tufted phalangeal tips; osteoarthritic signs. *Lab.:* in active stage, elevated plasma growth hormone; increased urinary 17-ketosteroids; high serum inorganic P; elevated alkaline phosphatase; sometimes hyperglycemia and glycosuria.

actinomycosis. Chronic local or systemic granulomatous disease from *Actinomyces bovis* or *israeli,* often producing multiple draining sinuses. *Symptoms:* weight loss, weakness, fever; pain depending on tissue involved. *Signs:* vary depending on location; multiple draining sinuses suggestive; pus contains sulfur granules. *Lab.:* typical gram-positive fungi seen in microscopic examination of sulfur granules and grown in anaerobic cultures.

Addison's disease (adrenal cortical insufficiency). See alternative term.

adrenal cortical insufficiency, primary (Addison's disease). Primary failure of adrenal glands from idiopathic hypoplasia or destruction by tuberculosis, fungi, or other granulomatous processes, amyloidosis, hemochromatosis, or tumor. *Symptoms:* weakness, increased fatigability, lethargy, nausea and vomiting, diarrhea, weight loss, abdominal pain, craving for salt. *Signs:* mottled skin pigmentation; pigment in buccal mucosa (in Caucasians), lips, vagina, rectum; reduced growth of hair; arterial hypotension; signs of dehydration. *Lab.:* normochromic normocytic anemia, eosinophilia; low serum Na and Cl, high serum K; low urinary 17-ketosteroids and 17-hydroxysteroids. *Test:* decreased adrenocortical response to corticotropin administration. *X-ray:* rarely, calcification of adrenals.

adrenal cortical insufficiency, secondary. From pituitary insufficiency. *Symptoms:* less than in primary. *Signs:* less than in primary; pigmentation slight or absent. *Lab.:* usually increased adrenocortical response to corticotropin, but in long-standing adrenal suppression, negative tests should be repeated after daily injections of ACTH.

alkaptonuria (ochronosis). See alternative term.

alopecia areata. Sudden loss of hair associated with emotional disturbances or infections. *Signs:* painless loss of hair in patches, or complete denudation of body. No visible affection of the skin.

Alzheimer's disease (presenile dementia). Progressive dementia beginning before senility. *Signs:* progressive mental deterioration beginning insidiously with emotional disturbances of depression, anxiety, suspicion and later amnesia, agnosia, aphasia, shuffling gait, and rigidity. *Lab.:* normal CSF and blood counts. *CT or MRI scans:* diffuse atrophy of the cerebral cortex with symmetrical enlargement of the lateral and 3rd ventricles.

amaurosis fugax. monocular blindness of less than 10 minutes. This is a symptom of reduced cerebral circulation.

amaurotic familial idiocy, infantile (Tay-Sachs disease). Recessive trait occurring mainly among Jews of eastern European origin associated with abnormal metabolism of neuronal lipids and leading to cerebral atrophy. *Signs:* insidious onset at about 6 months in apparently healthy infants of decreased motor activity, flaccidity, apathy, and inattentiveness, followed by spasticity, clonus, Babinski sign, convulsions, increasing dementia, and finally blindness, idiocy, and death in about 3 to 4 years. Macular cherry red spot of retinal degeneration.

amebiasis. Infection with *Entamoeba histolytica,* after ingestion of contaminated water, leading to ulcerations of the colon and terminal ilium and liver abscess. *Symptoms: acute*—fulminant onset with cramping abdominal pain, bloody diarrhea, and tenesmus; *chronic*—episodes of milder abdominal cramps, diarrheal stools containing mucus or blood, alternating with intervals of normal function. *Signs: acute*—fever, diffuse abdominal tenderness, dehydration, and weight loss; *chronic*—fever, tenderness of cecum and ascending colon during cramping; liver tenderness and friction rub with liver abscess. *Lab.:* motile or encysted organisms in fresh stool specimens; ulcers of variable depth with raised edges, discrete small hemorrhages, and hyperemia on sigmoidoscopy. *X-ray:* rarely, irregular distribution of barium in cecum and ascending colon; sometimes positive liver scan reveals abscess.

amyloidosis. Disturbance of endogenous protein metabolism, either primary or as a result of chronic suppuration or tissue breakdown; deposition of amyloid either generally or locally, causing organ dysfunction. *Symptoms:* asthenia, weight loss, paresthesias, and symptoms depending on organs involved. *Signs:* depend on involved organs; macroglossia, hypertension, lymphadenopathy, hepatomegaly, splenomegaly, purpura, nephrotic syndrome, edema, joint and muscle pain, fluid in serous cavities. *Lab.:* biopsy specimen of gingiva, rectum, or other tissue produces green birefringence in polarized light when stained with Congo red or thioflavine-T; sometimes altered serum immunoglobulins.

amyotrophic lateral sclerosis. Hereditary disease of motor neurons. *Symptoms:* muscle aches and cramps; weakness of distal upper limbs, spreading downward, dysarthria, dysphagia, drooling. *Signs:* muscle fibrillation and atrophy, especially in upper limbs; hyperreflexia; spasticity of lower limbs; diminished superficial reflexes. *Tests:* EMG shows muscle fibrillation on mechanical stimulation; increased duration and amplitude of action potentials.

anaphyllactic shock. Antigen-antibody reaction following bee sting or injection of antisera, iron dextran, or drugs like penicillin. *Signs:* sudden vascular collapse preceded or accompanied by malaise, pruritus, palor, cyanosis, syncope, vomiting, diarrhea, tachypnea, tachycardia, and distant heart sounds.

aneurysm, dissecting. Rupture of the arterial intima permits blood from the lumen to extravasate between layers of the vessel wall, separating them. This often occludes the lumen. Extravasation may extend the entire length of the vessel below the point of rupture.

aneurysm, mycotic. Localized dilatation of an artery where the wall is weakened by the growth of microorganisms, as in subacute bacterial endocarditis.

angina pectoris. Myocardial ischemia secondary to reduced blood flow through partially obstructed coronary arteries. *Symptoms:* steady precordial pressure or pain, induced by effort, emotion, or eating, radiating to the jaw or left shoulder and arm; lasts for 1–20 minutes producing fear, perspiration, or nausea relieved by rest or nitroglycerin. *Signs:* occasionally there is a palpable precordial apical bulge that vanishes as pain disappears. *ECG:* occasional T-wave and ST-segment depression during pain.

angioneurotic edema. Sudden temporary edema in a localized area of skin or mucosa, from allergy, neurotic, or unknown causes. *Symptoms:* nausea, vomiting, diarrhea. *Signs:* single or multiple pruritic nonpitting swellings appear on the face, tongue, larynx, hands, feet, genitalia, and subside with or without treatment. *Lab.:* deficiency of C′ 1-esterase in hereditary form.

anorexia nervosa. Emotional disorder of young women who become emaciated as a result of refusing to eat. *Symptoms:* underlying maternal-patient conflict, retention of strength and unconcern for emaciation, spontaneous or self-induced vomiting, amenorrhea. *Signs:* loss of as much as 50% of body weight; low blood pressure and loss of breast tissue, no loss of axillary or pubic hair, no change in pigmentation, and no edema. *Lab.:* low BMR, anemia, and reduced cholesterol, gonadotropins, and 17-ketosteroid levels. Normal tests of thyroid hormone.

anthrax. Infection with *Bacillus anthracis* transmitted from infected wild or domestic animals by contact with hides or by ingestion or inhalation of the spores. *Symptoms:* malaise and painless pruritic pustule on the skin; dyspnea and hemoptysis during dissemination. *Signs:* "malignant pustule" begins on exposed surface as an erythematous papule and then vesiculates, ulcerates, and is surrounded by characteristic nontender brawny edema; a black eschar may form; occasional regional lymphadenopathy is present. *Lab.:* lesion or blood may yield gram-positive bacilli on culture; normal leukocyte count usually, but neutrophilic leukocytosis in severe cases.

aorta, aneurysm of. Dilation of a segment of the aorta caused by weakening of the wall by atherosclerosis, syphilis, or trauma. *Signs:* depend on location. *Tests:* frequently positive ultrasound findings in abdomen. *X-ray:* CT scan or angiography frequently positive.

aorta, coarctation of. Constriction of the aorta, near its isthmus, from congenital malformation or atherosclerosis, thrombosis, aneurysm, or compression. *Symptoms:* none, or epistaxis, intermittent claudication, dizziness, headaches, tinnitus. *Signs:* arterial hypertension, diminished femoral pulses, palpable pulsating arteries about the scapula and axilla. *X-ray:* notching of the lower rib borders, displacement of the esophageal shadow rightward. *ECG:* left ventricular hypertrophy.

aortic regurgitation. Insufficiency of the aortic valve may result from rheumatic fever, syphilis, localized bacterial endocarditis, Marfan's syndrome, dissecting aorta, aneurysm of Valsalva's sinus. *Symptoms:* none, or exertional dyspnea, orthopnea, weakness, anginal pain. *Signs:* accentuated precordial thrust at the apex, high-pitched blowing early diastolic murmur in right 2nd interspace and 3rd left interspace, accentuated A_2, collapsing pulse, high pulse pressure, pistolshot sound, Duroziez's sign, Mayne's sign. *X-ray:* enlarged left ventricle, aortic dilatation.

aortic stenosis. Narrowing of the aortic valve orifice by rheumatic fever, atherosclerosis, subacute bacterial endocarditis, subaortic narrowing from congenital malformation, or fusion of valve cusps. *Symptoms:* none, or exertional dyspnea, faintness, exertional syncope, cardiac pain. *Signs:* harsh crescendo-diminuendo medium-pitched systolic murmur at right upper sternum, sometimes at apex, transmitted to carotid arteries; systolic thrill at base; diminished A_2; decreased systolic pressure in arteries; occasionally, plateau pulse; accentuated precordial thrust at apex. *X-ray:* calcification of aortic valve ring; enlargement of left ventricle; prominent ascending aorta. *ECG:* high R waves; depressed T waves in I and precordial leads.

appendicitis. Inflammation of the appendix associated with luminal obstruction due to edema, lymphoid hyperplasia, fecaliths, foreign bodies, intestinal parasites, etc. *Symptoms:* generalized midabdominal discomfort or pain for several hours eventually localizing in the right lower abdominal quadrant, nausea, vomiting, frequently atypical pain or asymptomatic. *Signs:* occasionally tachycardia and fever, involuntary abdominal guarding, point tenderness in the right lower abdominal quadrant, rebound tenderness, tenderness on rectal or pelvic examination in lower right abdomen or upper pelvis. *Lab.:* neutrophilic leukocytosis in majority of but not all patients.

arachnodactyly (Marfan's syndrome). See alternative term.

argyria. Deposition of silver salts in the skin from excessive oral intake. *Symptoms:* none. *Signs:* permanent blue to bronze discoloration of skin and mucosa, darker in regions exposed to light.

arsenic poisoning. Accidental or homicidal ingestion of arsenical salts, often in form of insect poisons. *Symptoms:* nausea, vomiting, abdominal pain, diarrhea, headache, vertigo, increased fatigability, paresthesias, paralysis, mental impairment. *Signs:* mottled brown pigmentation of skin, hyperkeratoses on palms and soles, edema of cutis, transverse striate leukonychia, perforation of nasal septum, edema of eyelids, coryza, paralysis of limbs with impaired deep reflexes. *Lab.:* oliguria, hematuria, hemoglobinuria, macrocytic anemia; arsenic in urine, nails, and hair.

arterial thrombosis due to infection (Takayasu's pulseless disease). Cause often unknown. *Signs:* usually in females 5 to 15 years of age; diminished brachial and cervical pulses; hypertension in legs; arterial bruits; trophic changes in eyes.

arteritis, cranial (arteritis, temporal). A chronic granulomatous panarteritis of unknown cause principally involving temporal, ophthalmic, and retinal vessels. *Symptoms:* anorexia, malaise, and sweating precede boring unilateral headache with pain in face, teeth, jaws, eyes, and scalp; later photophobia, diplopia, and blindness may accompany systemic symptoms of joint pains, confusion, and delirium. *Signs:* very tender temporal arteries that are prominent, with painful, red edematous skin overlying them. *Lab.:* biopsy of the artery shows chronic inflammation; leukocytosis, increased erythrocyte sedimentation rate, and anemia characterize the peripheral blood.

arthritis, rheumatoid. Generalized disease of unknown cause. *Symptoms:* gradual onset with morning stiffness; joints become swollen, tender, with erythematous warm skin. *Signs:* sometimes fever; usually symmetric fusiform swelling of proximal phalangeal joints, wrists, elbows, feet, ankles, knees; temporomandibular joints occasionally involved; juxtaarticular nodes; muscle atrophy. *Lab.:* increased erythrocyte sedimentation rate; positive blood tests with bentonite or latex fixation; rheumatoid factor present. *X-ray:* normal early; later, narrowing of intraarticular spaces and bony fusion of articular surfaces.

arthritis, juvenile rheumatoid (Still's disease). This is rheumatoid disease in children. In contrast with the adult type, fever is more intense; nodules are rare; cardiac involvement with pericarditis and valvulitis is more common; frequently lymphadenopathy and hepatosplenomegaly. The arthritis interferes with bone growth, as in underdevelopment of the mandible.

aspergillosis. Infection by aspergillus fungi in patients with debilitating disease or in those receiving antibiotics, corticosteroids, or irradiation. *Symptoms:* dyspnea, cough, hemoptysis in pulmonary form; dissemination associated with fever, skin eruptions, arthralgias, and finally coma. *Signs:* fever and purulent sputum in pulmonary form; skin eruptions, infection of ears, eyes, sinuses, and fever during dissemination. *Lab.:* cultures from mouth and sputum. *X-ray:* pulmonary aspergillomas are unique with a crescentic radiolucency surrounding a circular shadow.

asthma. Paroxysms of peculiar dyspnea in those with hereditary predisposition to bronchospasm; initiated by allergic reactions, infections, irritation of bronchial mucosa, or emotional disturbances. Asthma may also be associated with necrotizing vasculitis. *Symptoms:* paroxysmal dyspnea with wheezing, coughing, and tightness in the chest. *Signs:* none between attacks; during attack, cyanosis, prolonged expiratory phase, sonorous and sibilant rales, hyperresonant thorax. *Lab.:* thick mucoid sputum with Curschmann's spirals and Charcot-Leyden crystals. *Test:* attack relieved by epinephrine inhaled or taken subcutaneously.

atrial septal defect from persistent ostium primum. Congenital opening in septum near AV valves, often with cleft mitral valve leaflet. *Symptoms:* dyspnea. *Signs:* rounded chest, rarely with precordial bulge; no cyanosis or clubbing of fingers; accentuated precordial apical thrust; accentuated P_2 with fixed splitting during inspiration and expiration; systolic thrill near sternal border; harsh systolic murmur at left sternal border; apical systolic murmur transmitted to axilla from mitral regurgitation; sometimes apical middiastolic murmur. *X-ray:* enlarged right and left ventricles and pulmonary artery. *ECG:* incomplete right bundle branch block.

atrial septal defect, persistent ostium secundum. Congenital defect at the fossa ovalis. *Symptoms:* dyspnea. *Signs:* accentuation of right ventricular precordial thrust; systolic ejection murmur in 2nd and 3rd left interspaces; wide splitting of P_2; short diastolic murmur along left sternal border. *X-ray:* enlargement of right atrium, right ventricle, and pulmonary artery. *ECG:* right-axis deviation and late R′ in right-sided leads.

Behçet's syndrome. A vasculitis of unknown cause, but related to isoimmunity, is characterized by the triad of *relapsing iridocyclitis, ulcerations in the mouth,* and *ulcers on the genitalia.* The great majority of cases has come from Greece, Cyprus, Turkey, the Middle East, and Japan, but an increasing number of U. S. natives are being found to have the disease. The disease is associated with a high incidence of erythema nodosa and arthritis. Almost one third of the patients have had thrombophlebitis, neurologic disorders, or intestinal involvement. The disease lasts for many years with relapses and remissions, but it can often be suppressed by corticosteroids.

beriberi. A nutritional disease resulting from thiamine deficiency. *Symptoms:* weakness, irritability, burning feet, pruritus, nausea and vomiting. *Signs:* tremor, diminished reflexes in lower limbs, muscle atrophy, edema, serous effusions. *Lab.:* anemia, lowered blood thiamine, decreased erythrocyte transketolase, high blood pyruvic acid. *Test:* no urinary excretion of thiamine after test dose given. *X-ray:* enlarged heart.

bezoar. Mass of hair, fibers, and other material in the stomach or intestines from swallowing indigestible substances for many months or years. *Symptoms:* nausea and vomiting with alternating constipation and diarrhea, epigastric discomfort, and bloating. *Signs:* palpable upper abdominal mass. *Lab.:* gastroscopy reveals a mass of hair, fibers of vegetables or fruits, seeds, and other material. *X-ray:* gastrointestinal series may demonstrate displacement of barium by a mass or radiopaque materials.

bilharziasis (schistosomiasis). See alternative term.

blackwater fever (hemoglobinuria, malarial). See alternative term.

blastomycosis, North American. A chronic disease caused by infection with *Blastomyces dermatiditis.* *Symptoms:* sweating, cough, nocturnal pains in joints. *Signs:* fever; involvement of skin, nervous system, bone, lungs, liver, spleen, and kidneys. Subcutaneous nodules and abscesses that discharge pus through sinuses. *Lab.:* organisms in the pus can be cultured; in systemic disease, fungi in bone marrow and sputum, positive complement fixation and skin test.

Bornholm disease (pleurodynia, epidemic). See alternative term.

botulism. An acute deadly disease caused by ingestion of *Clostridium botulinum* or its toxin. *Symptoms:* sudden weakness, headache, dizziness, dysphagia, abdominal pain, nausea and vomiting, diarrhea, diplopia. *Signs:* mydriasis, nystagmus, ptosis, irregular respiration; swollen tongue; hyporeflexia; incoordination. *Lab.:* injection of suspected food into mice kills them.

break-bone fever (dengue). See alternative term.

bronchiectasis. A chronic infectious process that results in multiple dilatations of the smaller bronchi, exuding a purulent discharge. *Symptoms:* cough and purulent sputum; occasionally hemoptysis or pneumonia. *Signs:* productive cough with copious purulent sputum; coarse rales at the lung bases; clubbing of the fingers. *Lab.:* sputum contains mixture of organisms, but not definitive: sputum forms layers on standing. *X-ray:* patches of increased density at lung bases; even advanced disease may give normal appearance, so bronchograms with opaque medium may be required. *Test:* postural drainage yields copious sputum. Bronchoscopic examination may assist in localization.

bronchitis. Caused by acute or chronic infections, allergy, and chemical irritants. *Symptoms:* cough with little or no sputum, laryngitis. *Signs:* may be fever; sibilant, sonorous, or moist rales; no areas of dullness or bronchial breathing. *Lab.:* leukocytosis. *X-ray:* chest films usually negative.

broncholithiasis. Perforation of a calcified tuberculous or fungal lymph node from the hilar region into the bronchial tree. *Symptoms:* sudden cough and sometimes massive hemoptysis. *Signs:* massive hemoptysis may contain fragments of calcium carbonate or phosphate, coarse rhonchi, fever; retinal hemorrhages may also be found. Bronchoscopy may locate broncholith or site of perforation. *X-ray:* calcified fragment in distal bronchus, calcification of hilar or paratracheal nodes.

bronchopleural fistula. A communication between bronchus and pleural cavity, usually caused by empyema draining through a bronchus or lung abscess invading pleural cavity. *Symptoms:* chronic cough with large volume of purulent sputum. *Signs:* dullness and absent breath sounds in lower hemithorax with resonant region above, the whole devoid of breath sounds; succussion splash; coin sound. *Test:* injection of methylene blue into pleural cavity results in dye appearing in sputum. *X-ray:* signs of hydropneumothorax.

brucellosis. Systemic infection with *Brucella abortus, suis,* or *melitensis.* *Symptoms:* lassitude, weight loss, recurrent fever and sweating; pain in joints. *Signs:* fever, splenomegaly, lymphadenopathy, tender bones or joints. *Lab.:* blood cultures, positive complement fixation test, anemia, leukocytosis, granulomas in bone marrow biopsy.

Budd-Chiari syndrome (hepatic vein thrombosis). See alternative term.

Buerger's disease (thromboangiitis obliterans). See alternative term.

bulbar paralysis, progressive (Duchenne's syndrome). Atrophy and glial overgrowth of motor nuclei of 5th, 7th, 9th, 10th, and 12th cranial nerves with subcortical involvement of corticobulbar tracts leading to death in 1 to 3 years from respiratory arrest or aspiration pneumonia. *Symptoms:* drooling, difficulty chewing, dysphagia, dysarthria, and nasal regurgitation. *Signs:* spasticity of arms and legs, hyperactive reflexes, ophthalmoplegia, fasciculation of muscles in tongue and lips, and emotional lability developing in the 5th and 6th decade.

Burnett's syndrome (milk-alkali syndrome). See alternative term.

candidiasis, disseminated. Occurs most frequently in immunosuppressed patients. *Symptoms:* fever, malaise. *Signs:* severe muscle tenderness, papuloerythematous rash. *Lab.:* abscesses contain mycelia resembling yeast, serum antigen titers are elevated.

carbon monoxide poisoning. Disease with excessive amounts of carboxyhemoglobin from inhalation of carbon monoxide. *Symptoms:* headache, dizziness, nausea and vomiting, mental confusion, visual disturbances. *Signs:* cherry-red skin and mucosa, bounding pulse, hypertension, muscular twitchings, stertorous breathing, dilated pupils, convulsions, coma. *Lab.:* blood grossly abnormally red, contains excessive carboxyhemoglobin in spectrographic examination; leukocytosis.

carcinoid, malignant. Metastases from carcinoid tumor of the gastrointestinal tract produces excessive amounts of serotonin. *Symptoms:* intermittent flushing of skin, recurrent diarrhea, nausea and vomiting; abdominal pain. *Signs:* intermittent migratory flushing of face and neck with rapid color changes between red, white, and violet. Right-sided heart failure may develop. *Lab.:* excessive 24-hour urinary excretion of 5-hydroxyindoleacetic acid (5-HIAA), but sprue and ingestion of bananas must be excluded for the test.

cardiospasm (esophageal achalasia). Deficient cholinergic innervation of the distal esophagus of unknown cause results in incoordinate contractions and tonic contraction of the lower esophageal sphincter. *Symptoms:* dysphagia and regurgitation of food, saliva, and esophageal secretions. *Signs:* weight loss. *X-ray:* esophageal dilatation with beaklike narrowing of distal segment, spasm of lower esophageal sphincter.

carotenemia. Deposition of carotene from excessive ingestion of pigmented vegetables or from failure of liver to metabolize in myxedema. *Symptoms:* none. *Signs:* yellow color in nasolabial folds, forehead, palms, and soles. No pigment in sclerae or buccal mucosa. *Lab.:* elevated plasma lipochromes and blood carotene.

carpal tunnel syndrome (median neuropathy). Compression of the median nerve by encroachment on the carpal tunnel by fibrosis of the tendon sheaths, trauma, arthritis, or soft-tissue swelling. *Symptoms:* numbness and tingling progressing to weakness of the first four fingers. *Signs:* anesthesia and weakness of the first four fingers with atrophy of the thenar eminence; increased paresthesia and pain with flexion of wrist, relieved by extension. *Lab.:* prolonged conduction of median nerve measured by electromyography.

cataplexy. Possibly hereditary episodic loss of motor and postural control precipitated by laughter or strong emotion of unknown etiology. *Signs:* momentary loss of voluntary motor power including speech, without loss of consciousness.

cataract. Opacification of the lens of the eye associated with aging, diabetes mellitus, genetic abnormalities, and trauma. *Symptoms:* diminished vision in one or both eyes. *Signs:* lenticular opacities of various shapes and degree noted with ophthalmoscopy and slit-lamp examination depending upon cause.

cat-scratch fever. Probably viral disease from the cat. *Symptoms:* malaise, headache. *Signs:* fever; scratch embellished by papule or vesicle; regional painful lymphadenopathy with overlying reddened skin; lymph nodes fluctuant but sterile. *Lab.:* skin test with antigen.

chancroid (soft chancre). Veneral infection with *Haemophilus ducreyi*. *Symptoms:* malaise, headache, anorexia. *Signs:* lesions begin on genitalia or adjacent skin as small red papules that suppurate, producing soft painful ulcers with undermined edges, regional lymphadenitis (bubo) in one third of patients, fever. *Lab.: ducreyi* bacilli identified in smear or culture.

Charcot-Marie-Tooth disease (peroneal muscular atrophy). See alternative term.

Charcot's joint (neurogenic arthropathy). Degeneration of joint from loss of proprioceptive sensation in tabes, syringomyelia, and diabetes mellitus. *Symptoms:* relatively painless in contrast to severe deformity. *Signs:* loss of joint contour with great instability and hypermobility. *X-ray:* severe degeneration.

Chiari-Frommel syndrome (Frommel's disease). Persistent amenorrhea and galactorrhea after delivery, probably secondary to excessive prolactin secretion. *Symptoms:* postpartum amenorrhea during lactation. *Signs:* persistent galactorrhea, small uterus. *Lab.:* low or absent urinary gonadotropins.

chickenpox (varicella). A contagious exanthematous disease from infection with varicella-zoster virus. *Symptoms:* fever, anorexia, malaise, headache, myalgia. Incubation period 11 to 21 days. *Signs:* crops of small red papules become clear umbilicated vesicles, spreading from trunk to face, little on limbs; generalized lymphadenopathy. *Lab.:* slight leukocytosis. Vesicular fluid contains multinucleated giant cells, epithelial cells with eosinophilic inclusion bodies, and virus.

cholangitis. Inflammation of the bile ducts, often associated with obstruction by gallstones. *Symptoms:* chills, colicky abdominal pain, nausea and vomiting. *Signs:* fever, jaundice; enlarged tender liver; sometimes palpable spleen. *Lab.:* leukocytosis; bilirubin in urine and plasma; high serum alkaline phosphatase; abnormal liver function tests.

cholecystitis. Inflammation of gallbladder by gram-negative bacteria. *Symptoms:* intermittent pain in epigastrium or RUQ referred to right shoulder or scapula; vomiting; intolerance to fat. *Signs:* fever; tenderness and rigidity in RUQ; rebound tenderness; percussion tenderness over liver; Murphy's inspiratory arrest sign; palpable gallbladder. *Lab.:* leukocytosis, increased ESR; increased bilirubin in plasma and urine. *X-ray:* nonvisualization on cholecystogram.

cholelithiasis. Gallstones in the gallbladder. *Symptoms:* often none; attacks of RUQ pain with residual soreness; intolerance to fat; nausea, flatulence. *Lab.:* sometimes increased bilirubin in plasma and urine. *X-ray:* calculi may be demonstrated with plain films or after giving opaque medium.

cholera. Acute infectious disease caused by *Vibrio cholerae.* *Symptoms:* sudden severe diarrhea, vomiting with abdominal cramps, thirst, oliguria. Incubation period 1–5 days. *Signs:* signs of severe dehydration with shriveled skin, dry mucosa; pinched features; cold skin; hypotension and tachycardia from shock. *Lab.:* watery mucoid stools; smears and culture from stools contain organisms. Agglutinin tests positive. Concentrated plasma proteins; serum electrolytes low; azotemia. Leukocytosis.

cholesteatoma, ear. A benign squamous metaplasia of epithelium in the middle ear producing a gradually expanding mass containing cholesterol crystals and keratinous debris, of unknown cause or associated with chronic otitis media. *Symptoms:* fullness in ear, pain, headache, hearing loss. *Signs:* chronic suppurative discharge from middle ear through perforated tympanic membrane, middle ear deafness, pearly gray mass visible with otoscope. *X-ray:* erosion of bones with enlargement of middle ear, opacification of air cells in mastoid process.

chordae tendineae, rupture of. In bacterial endocarditis, ulceration may result in rupture of a chorda tendinea. *Symptoms:* none or dyspnea, chest pain. *Signs:* sudden occurrence of loud raucous systolic sound in the heart.

chorea (Sydenham's chorea). Usually associated with infection, especially rheumatic fever. *Symptoms:* gradual onset of irritability, anxiety, poor memory, occasional involuntary movements. *Signs:* choreiform movements with hyperextended joints, inaccurate voluntary motions, hypotonia, diminished deep reflexes; sometimes speech impairment. *spinal Fluid:* increased pressure, sugar, and cell count.

chorea, progressive hereditary (Huntington's chorea). An autosomal dominant inherited disease appearing in middle life. *Symptoms:* gradual onset of failing memory, restlessness, lack of initiative. *Signs:* choreiform movements, shuffling gait, mental deterioration; deep reflexes normal or increased.

Christmas disease (factor IX deficiency). See alternative term.

circulatory overload. Acute heart failure from increase in blood volume. *Symptoms:* during or soon after intravenous infusion of blood, colloidal, or electrolyte solutions, the patient suddenly becomes dyspneic. *Signs:* intense cyanosis, orthopnea; loud sonorous and sibilant rales in chest; engorgement of peripheral veins; symptoms and signs promptly subside with emergency application of tourniquets to all four limbs and phlebotomy; otherwise, the patient may die suddenly.

coccidioidomycosis. Infection with the fungus *Coccidioides immitis.* *Symptoms:* chills, weight loss, productive cough, chest pain; pains in joints. *Signs:* fever; cervical adenopathy; skin lesions resembling erythema nodosum; pleural effusion, friction rub, rales in chest. *Lab.:* fungi in sputum; positive blood complement-fixing antibodies. *Tests:* positive skin test with coccidiomycin.

colitis, ulcerative. Chronic disease of unknown cause. *Symptoms:* diarrhea with passage of bloody mucus, anorexia, and weight loss; debility. *Signs:* fever; cachexia, hypotonus of muscles. *Lab.:* stools negative for pathogenic bacteria; anemia, leukocytosis, hypoproteinemia. *Sigmoidoscopic Examination:* friable mucosa with superficial bleeding ulcers. *X-ray:* late disease shows narrowing of colon, loss of haustral markings, indistinct outline of mucosa.

colonic diverticulitis. Inflammation of colonic diverticula. *Symptoms:* recurring pain in LLQ; vomiting, chills, diarrhea. *Signs:* fever, tenderness over descending colon most often, or other parts of the colon rarely. *X-ray:* shows diverticula and colonic spasm.

conjunctivitis, vernal. Allergic response to light or heat. *Symptoms:* lacrimation, photophobia, pruritus. *Signs:* recurrence in warm weather; conjunctival injection with mucoid secretion; sometimes hard flattened papillae with furrows on palpebral conjunctiva.

coryza (rhinitis). See alternative term.

costochondritis (Tietze's syndrome). A chronic inflammation that affects the costochondral joints; cause unknown. *Symptoms:* pain in chest, accentuated by respiratory movements. *Signs:* tenderness and swelling at the costochondral joints, especially of the 2nd and 3rd ribs.

cough fracture. A fatigue fracture of lower ribs from repeated coughing. *Symptoms:* pain in the chest, accentuated by respiratory movements; pressure on a remote segment of the rib causes pain in the fracture site. *X-ray:* films do not always reveal a fresh rib fracture.

cretinism (hypothyroidism, infantile). See alternative term.

cricoarytenoid joint, arthritis of. Ankylosis of this joint in rheumatoid arthritis. *Symptoms:* possible hoarseness; chronic shortness of breath. *Signs:* possibly stridor, respiratory acidosis; sudden coma.

crush syndrome. Shock and renal failure following extensive soft-tissue trauma and frequently leading to death. *Symptoms:* somnolence, thirst, nausea, and pain. *Signs:* external injury, shock, and oliguria. *Lab.:* elevated blood urea nitrogen, myoglobinuria, hyperpotassemia, and hyponatremia.

Cruveilhier-Baumgarten syndrome. This is characterized by liver cirrhosis with portal hypertension, and associated with congenital patency of umbilical or paraumbilical veins. *Signs:* hematemesis, ascites, splenomegaly, hypersplenism, esophageal varices, caput medusae, large tortuous veins in the abdominal wall. A *venous hum* can often be heard near the xiphoid process, often accompanied by a *thrill.* The hum may be augmented or diminished by Valsalva's maneuver.

Cushing's syndrome. Effects of hypercortisolism from adenoma or adenocarcinoma of the adrenal cortex, from stimulation by excess ACTH from a pituitary adenoma, or therapy with corticosteroids. *Symptoms:* weakness, weight gain, amenorrhea, back pain. *Signs:* moon face, acne, thoracic kyphosis, supraclavicular fat pad development, hypertrichosis, purplish striae on abdomen and thighs, peripheral edema, arterial hypertension. *Lab.:* increased plasma cortisol with failure of dexamethasone to suppress; increased urinary excretion of 17-ketosteroids and 17-hydroxysteroids. *X-ray:* occasionally shows enlarged sella turcica or adrenal tumor.

cystic fibrosis (mucoviscidosis, fibrocystic disease of pancreas). An autosomal recessive trait mostly found in children; but some escape attention and attain adulthood before recognition. This is primarily a disorder of the exocrine glands producing mucus blockage of the fine tubules in various organs. *Symptoms and Signs:* chronic cough, wheezing, with the production of very tenacious sputum. The patient has a voracious appetite, bulky malodorous stools. *Complications:* fecal impactions, intussusception, volvulus, bronchitis, cardiomegaly, clubbing of the fingers, excessive sweating that results in salt depletion and prostration. These patients are especially susceptible to upper respiratory infections and to diabetes mellitus. *Lab.:* The sweat contains more than 60 mEq/L of Cl^-. Agar (silver) plate hand test shows white palmar imprint from Cl^- in sweat. Pancreatic insufficiency is indicated by the starch tolerance test. The adult shows salt deficiency in sweat even after deprivation. Absence of pancreatic enzymes in duodenal aspirate of contents. Serum Cl^- and Na^+ are normal. *X-ray:* dilated loops of small intestine.

cystitis. Inflammation of the urinary bladder from infection, irradiation, or chemotherapy. *Symptoms:* in *acute cystitis*—urgency, frequency, dysuria, suprapubic pain, occasionally gross hematuria; in *chronic cystitis*—milder symptoms but also perineal or lower abdominal pain. *Signs:* tenderness of bladder and urethra. *Lab.:* pyuria, bacteriuria, positive culture, hematuria; cystoscopy (deferred until symptoms decrease), edema and injection of mucosal tissue and vasculature with ulceration, and patches of submucosal hemorrhage, chronically.

Dabney grip (pleurodynia, epidemic). See alternative term.

dacryocystitis. Inflammatory or neoplastic obstruction of the nasolacrimal duct. *Symptoms:* pain and epiphora increased by irritants such as wind, dust, or smoke. *Signs: acute*—pain, tenderness, swelling, and redness of the medial portion of the lower lid with a purulent discharge over the conjunctiva; *chronic*—fluid can be expressed with pressure on the puncta, conjunctivitis, blepharitis. *Lab.:* identification of bacteria by smear and/or culture of exudate.

dandy fever (dengue). See alternative term.

dementia paralytica (paresis, syphilitic). Syphilitic involvement of the central nervous system. *Symptoms:* slow mental deterioration, headaches, irresponsibility. *Signs:* tremor of the lips, tongue and hands; Argyll Robertson pupils; epileptiform seizures; memory loss; impaired judgment. *Spinal Fluid:* pleocytosis, increased protein; positive VDRL.

dengue (break-bone fever, dandy fever, Duengero fever, seven-day fever). Mosquito-transmitted arbor virus infection. *Symptoms:* abrupt onset of chills, fever, headache, arthralgias, and bone pain after 3–15 days' incubation. *Signs:* fever falls after 3–4 days, but rises 1–3 days later with recurrence of symptoms; red morbilliform or punctate rash starts on dorsa of hands and feet and spreads centripetally to trunk. *Lab.:* early viremia; after first week complement-fixing and neutralizing antibodies present, leukopenia.

dermatitis herpetiformis. Skin disease of unknown cause. *Symptoms:* intense pruritus and burning of skin. *Signs:* polymorphous lesions of urticarial wheals, vesicles, bullae, erythema; symmetric distribution on limbs and trunk. *Lab.:* eosinophilia.

dermatitis, stasis. Scarring, atrophy, and pigmentation of skin from venous stasis; especially on the legs and dorsa of feet.

dermatomyositis. Atrophy, edema, or fibrosis of the skin and nonsuppurative inflammation of striated muscle of unknown cause. *Symptoms:* malaise, weight loss, muscle stiffness, dysphagia. *Signs:* heliotrope discoloration of bridge of the nose, erythematous rashes or exfoliative dermatitis, Raynaud's phenomenon, proximal muscle weakness and stiffness, synovial and tendon friction rubs, lymphadenopathy, and splenomegaly. *Lab.:* creatinuria, hyperglobulinemia, anemia, and myoglobinuria, elevated ESR. *X-ray:* esophageal weakness.

Devil's grip (pleurodynia, epidemic). See alternative term.

dextrocardia. Congenital development with viscera reversed so the heart is on the right side, the mirror image of normal. *Symptoms:* none. *Signs:* apical impulse on the right; right border of the heart in the right midclavicular line; left border behind the sternum. *ECG:* inverted P and T; QRS negative in I; II resembles normal III and vice versa. *X-ray:* cardiac shadow reversed.

diabetes insipidus. Excessive constant water diuresis from lesion in hypothalamoneurohypophyseal tract. *Symptoms:* unquenchable thirst, polydipsia, tremendous polyuria. *Lab.:* urinary specific gravity seldom exceeds 1.008; water restriction fails to result in increased urinary concentration. *Tests:* Hare-Hickey test positive with the injection of hypertonic saline.

diabetes mellitus. Absolute deficit or dysfunction of insulin, cause unknown. *Symptoms:* polydipsia, polyuria, polyphagia; weight loss, weakness, amenorrhea, impotence. *Signs:* dryness of skin, pruritus, acetone on breath. *Lab.:* glycosuria, hyperglycemia. *Tests:* glucose tolerance test shows diminished sugar utilization.

diabetic acidosis. History of uncontrolled diabetes mellitus or overwhelming infection; rapid onset of weakness, vomiting, lethargy. *Signs:* mental clouding; Kussmaul breathing; acetone on breath; dry skin and mucosa, loss of skin turgor, soft eyeballs; subnormal temperature. *Lab.:* blood and urinary sugar depends upon immediately previous treatment. Blood CO_2 depressed; serum Na and Cl low; blood acetone high.

diaphragmatic hernia. Herniation of portion of stomach through esophageal hiatus of diaphragm. *Symptoms:* pain in epigastrium or lower chest, especially on reclining, relieved on standing. Pain may be retrosternal with radiation down left arm, as in angina pectoris. Hematemesis. *Signs:* usually none, but large herniation produces dullness in left lung base, with absent breath sounds; peristaltic sounds may be heard in this area. *X-ray:* barium swallow demonstrates stomach above diaphragm.

digitalis intoxication. *Symptoms:* anorexia, nausea and vomiting, somnolence, muscle weakness, diarrhea, yellow vision (xanthopsia). *Signs:* premature beats, bigeminy, atrial tachycardia with block, atrial fibrillation, nodal rhythm, ventricular tachycardia. *Lab.:* serum digoxin 2 ng/mL, digitoxin 30 ng/mL. *ECG:* in addition to the dysrhythmias, inversion of T waves, depression of S-T segment, increase of P-R interval are usual effects.

diphtheria. Pharyngitis and intoxication from *Corynebacterium diphtheriae*. *Symptoms:* sore throat, dysphagia, weakness. *Signs:* fever, pharyngeal redness, gray membrane in tonsillar regions, cervical lymphadenopathy. *Lab.:* leukocytosis. Organisms grown in throat culture.

Duchenne's syndrome. (bulbar paralysis, progressive). See alternative term.

ductus arteriosus, patent. Failure after birth of the obliteration of the ductus arteriosus between aorta and pulmonary artery. *Symptoms:* none, or retarded growth, exertional dyspnea. *Signs:* machinery-murmur throughout cardiac cycle with late systolic accentuation in left 2nd interspace and in left back; if large shunt, collapsing pulse and high pulse pressure. *X-ray:* accentuated pulmonary conus, prominent pulsating lung markings, pulmonary artery opacification on aortogram.

Duengero fever (dengue). See alternative term.

dumping syndrome (postgastrectomy syndrome). See alternative term.

dyschondroplasia. Cause unknown. *Signs:* unilateral joint deformity with knobby fingers or genu valgum. *X-ray:* bones shortened, rarefied shaft with streaks, dilated cortex, translucent metaphysis.

dysentery, amebic. Enterocolitis caused by *Entamoeba histolytica*. *Symptoms:* abdominal cramps, recurrent diarrhea, nausea and vomiting, arthralgia. *Signs:* abdominal tenderness, dehydration. *Sigmoidoscopy:* scattered shallow ulcers with raised edges and mucus or blood. *Lab.:* watery stools with mucus or blood; microscopic examination shows motile or encysted amebae.

dysentery, bacillary. Acute gastrointestinal infection with *Shigella* organisms. *Symptoms:* sudden diarrhea, tenesmus, abdominal cramps, nausea and vomiting, lassitude. *Signs:* fever, dehydration, tenderness in lower abdomen. *Sigmoidoscopic:* hyperemia, mural edema, purulent exudate. *Lab.:* mucus and pus in stools; leukocytosis or leukopenia; blood agglutinins against organisms; electrolyte imbalance from dehydration.

dysphagia, sideropenic (Plummer-Vinson syndrome). See alternative term.

echinococcosis (hydatid disease). Infection with *Echinococcus granulosis* or *E. multilocularis* larvae produces expanding cysts in liver or lungs. *Symptoms:* depend on the size and location of the cyst and the amount of tissue destroyed. *Signs:* anaphylactic reaction may result from rupture of cyst fluid into pleural or peritoneal cavities. *Lab.:* eosinophilia seldom present; skin tests (Casoni's antigen) and serologic tests are helpful. *X-ray:* radiograph, liver scan, CT or MRI scans may demonstrate cysts.

Eisenmenger's complex. Congenital defect in interventricular septum with overriding aorta. *Symptoms:* dyspnea, hemoptysis. *Signs:* cyanosis, systolic murmur in 4th left interspace, accentuated P_2, clubbing of fingers, accentuated precordial thrust of right ventricle. *ECG:* right-axis deviation or hypertrophy. *X-ray:* enlarged pulmonary arteries, vascular pulsations in lung fields.

encephalitis, St. Louis. Viral agent transmitted by mosquito or chicken mite. *Symptoms:* incubation period 4–21 days; sudden high fever, severe headache, stiff neck, lethargy, mental confusion, dysarthria, nausea and vomiting. *Signs:* tremor of tongue, lips, hands; ataxia, spastic paralysis; exaggerated deep reflexes, absent abdominal reflexes. *Lab.:* relative lymphocytosis with slightly increased total leukocyte count; virus demonstrated by animal inoculation; positive tests for complement fixation and neutralizing antibodies. *Spinal Fluid:* increased pressure; increased globulin and lymphocytes.

endocarditis, subacute bacterial. Inflammation of the endocardium, particularly the heart valves, caused by bacteria of low virulence that stimulate the formation of vegetations, serving as sources of bacterial emboli. *Symptoms:* chills, sweats, weight loss, anorexia, joint pains. *Signs:* fever, pallor, petechiae, splinter hemorrhages under nails, Osler's nodes, retinal hemorrhages with central pallor (Roth's spots), cerebral emboli with focal signs, systolic murmur from a heart valve. *Lab.:* leukocytosis, microscopic hematuria. Blood cultures positive for bacteria. Vegetations on heart valves detected with echocardiography.

endometriosis. Disseminated implants of endometrial tissue. *Symptoms:* lower abdominal pain and backache accentuated with menstruation, menorrhagia, dysmenorrhea, sterility. *Signs:* palpable tender masses in pelvis; nodular thickening of uterosacral ligament; fixed uterus; enlarged ovaries.

endometritis. Bacterial infection of endometrium. *Symptoms:* lower abdominal cramps, vaginal discharge, nausea and vomiting, prostration. *Signs:* fever, tenderness and muscle spasm in lower abdomen, vaginal discharge. *Lab.:* leukocytosis, smear and culture of discharge.

epidemic myalgia (pleurodynia, epidemic). See alternative term.

epilepsy, grand mal (major motor seizures). May occur in patients with congenital cerebral lesions, posttraumatic cerebral scars, brain tumor, or without structural abnormality or known cause. *Symptoms:* aura may include irritability, apathy, giddiness, headache, scintillating scotomata, nausea, choking sensation, paresthesias and myalgia. *Signs:* loss of postural tone, unconsciousness; muscular rigidity with opisthotonos, adduction and flexion of arms, extension of legs; tonic movements followed by clonic jerking of limbs and jaw; apnea, cyanosis; flaccidity and loss of tendon reflexes, gasping, incontinence on awakening. *Lab.:* postictal leukocytosis in the peripheral blood. *EEG:* paroxysmal diffuse outbursts of high voltage, many spikes in fast rhythm.

epilepsy, petit mal (absence or minor seizures). Either inherited without associated disease or acquired with vascular, infectious, neoplastic, or toxic brain disease. *Symptoms:* fleeting unconsciousness, amnesia, no aura. *Signs:* a vacant or dazed facial expression with rhythmic eyelid or head movements, pallor, incontinence, loss of postural control, picking at clothes or pursing lips after seizure; no convulsion. *EEG:* synchronous, 3-per-second, wave-spike dysrhythmia over frontal lobes.

ergotism. Excessive ingestion of ergot drugs or rye or wheat infected with the fungus *Claviceps purpurea.* *Symptoms:* colic, diarrhea, cramps of limbs, paresthesias, pruritus, convulsions, headache, drowsiness, nausea and vomiting. *Signs:* gangrene of tips of nose, ears, fingers, and toes.

erysipelas. A streptococcus infection of the skin. *Symptoms:* sudden chills, pain in the skin, feeling of tightness and warmth. *Signs:* fever, sharply demarcated red area of skin with elevated borders, local edema, and vesicles or bullae. *Lab.:* leukocytosis; streptococci in the vesicular fluid.

erysipeloid. Infection of the skin with *Erysipelothrix rhusiopathiae* from handling raw fish or animal hides. *Symptoms:* pain, pruritus. *Signs:* local tender violaceous swelling with elevated margins; rarely chills and fever; eruption brief and followed by brown pigmentation.

erythema ab igne. Erythema and subsequent mottled pigmentation of skin from exposure to radiant heat, such as an open fire.

erythema multiforme. Self-limited mucocutaneous reaction to systemic infection, herpes simplex, drug sensitivity, pregnancy, food allergy, deep x-ray, cancer. *Symptoms:* muscle and joint pains, mucosal erosion, itching, and malaise. *Signs:* sudden appearance of symmetrically distributed and sharply demarcated pruritic erythematous plaques on skin or mucous membranes; typical "target" lesion results from papule or vesicle formation in the center of the plaque, resolution without scarring; slight fever, pharyngitis.

erythema nodosum. A skin eruption occurring in association with generalized infection or allergic reaction. *Symptoms:* malaise, nausea and vomiting, abdominal cramps. *Signs:* crops of transient, symmetrically distributed, tender, painful, erythematous nodules under the skin; usually limited sharply to the legs and knees, seldom above. Lesions do not suppurate or ulcerate, although many have been incised because they were thought to contain pus. After involution, the lesions leave areas of pigmentation.

erythroblastosis fetalis. Best described by its British term of hemolytic disease of the newborn; the hemolytic anemia is caused in the fetus by antibodies in the mother's blood acting on the erythrocytes of the fetus; the mother lacks the blood cell antigens of the fetus and develops antibodies from contact with the red cells of the fetus or by transfusion from another person. *Signs in the Fetus:* large placenta, yellow vernix caseosa, jaundice, purpura, cyanosis, hepatomegaly, splenomegaly, ascites, edema, cerebral signs of kernicterus. *Lab.:* cytologic picture of hemolytic anemia; positive direct Coombs test on the infant's red cells; antibodies in the mother's blood specific for antigens in the child's erythrocytes.

erythromelalgia. Episodic bilateral vasodilatation with hyperemia of unknown cause but associated with local warmth, warm temperatures, exercise, or dependency of an arm or leg in patients with pseudopolycythemia, hypertension, hemiplegia, multiple sclerosis, and syphilis of the brain or cord. *Symptoms:* localized burning of skin on the palms and soles exacerbated by warmth but ameliorated by cool temperatures. *Signs:* engorgement of vasculature with warmth, perspiration, and swelling of involved area.

esophageal achalasia (cardiospasm). See alternative term.

esophageal laceration (Mallory-Weiss syndrome). Laceration near the esophagogastric junction following severe retching and vomiting. *Symptoms:* hematemesis after retching and vomiting. *Signs:* melena and shock; mucosal tear visualized on esophagogastroscopy.

esophageal perforation (Boerhaave's syndrome). Perforation of the esophagus secondary to carcinoma, foreign body, chemical burns, instrumentation, or from severe retching and vomiting in alcoholics or patients with esophagitis. *Symptoms:* retrosternal pain radiating to the back or epigastrium associated with hematemesis and melena after retching. *Signs:* hematemesis, melena, shock, fever, tachycardia, prostration. *Lab.:* leukocytosis, laceration of esophagus identified with esophagoscopy. *X-ray:* anterior displacement of trachea, pleural effusion, pneumothorax, sometimes mediastinal emphysema.

eunuchism. Testicular failure, congenital or acquired. *Signs:* when prepubertal, hypoplastic penis and testes; thin smooth skin; failure of voice to deepen; female escutcheon of pubic hair and absence of beard; poor muscles; long limbs, broad hips, gynecomastia. Postpubertal testicular atrophy; pallor. *Lab.:* normal or low androgens and 17-ketosteroids in urine; high urinary gonadotropin. *X-ray:* in prepubertal, delayed closure of epiphyses.

factor VIII deficiency (hemophilia). See alternative term.

factor IX deficiency (Christmas disease, hemophilia B, plasma thromboplastin component deficiency). Inherited sex-linked trait clinically indistinguishable from factor VIII deficiency. *Symptoms:* history of spontaneous bleeding or excessive hemorrhage following dental extractions and surgery since childhood. *Signs:* joint deformities and contractures. *Lab.:* prolonged partial thromboplastin time corrected by factor IX or normal serum.

familial periodic paralysis. Inherited as an autosomal dominant. *Symptoms:* headaches, thirst, lethargy. *Signs:* onset before 20 years of age; slow progressive weakness; intermittent muscular paralysis of shoulder and pelvic girdles; later, other regions involved; absent deep reflexes; no muscle weakness between attacks. *Lab.:* low serum K.

Fanconi's syndrome. A condition of various causes; there is a deficiency in renal tubular excretion, producing aminoaciduria, glycosuria, and hypophosphatemia. *Symptoms:* in children, polydipsia, malnutrition, increased susceptibility to infection. In adults, pain in weight-bearing joints, dehydration. *Signs:* retardation in growth and development; bony deformities similar to rickets; waddling gait; pathologic fractures. *Lab.:* aminoaciduria, cystinuria, glycosuria, phosphaturia. *X-ray:* pseudofractures.

favism. Acute hemolytic anemia results when Caucasians of Mediterranean ancestry with glucose-6-phosphate dehydrogenase deficiency inhale the pollen of or eat the whole fava bean. *Symptoms:* back pain, tiredness. *Signs:* mild fever, jaundice, pallor, tachycardia, dark red urine. *Lab.:* normochromic normocytic anemia, reticulocytosis, hyperbilirubinemia, hemoglobinuria, screening tests or enzyme assays show diminished erythrocyte glucose-6-phosphate dehydrogenase activity.

Felty's syndrome. A form of rheumatoid arthritis accompanied by splenomegaly and leukopenia.

filariasis (wuchereriasis). Mosquito-borne infection of lymphatic system with larvae of *W. bancrofti* or *W. malayi* producing inflammation and later scarring, obstruction, and lymphedema. *Symptoms:* headache, photophobia, vertigo, fatigue, low-grade fever, and myalgia. *Signs:* conjunctivitis, orchitis, lymphangitis, and lymphadenopathy acutely; later obstruction of lymphatic and venous drainage with edema, hydrocele, elephantiasis of breasts, scrotum, vulva, or legs.

Lab.: microfilariae appear in stained blood film, complement-fixation test sometimes positive, and eosinophilia.

fluoride toxicity (fluorosis). Ingestion of 2 g of sodium fluoride, an ingredient of insect poisons, is lethal. Hydrofluoric acid, formed in the stomachs of survivors of smaller doses, combines with calcium causing tetany. Fluoride inhibits carbohydrate metabolism. Chronic ingestion of small quantities mottles dental enamel. *Symptoms:* nausea and vomiting of corrosive gastric contents, abdominal pain, and diarrhea. *Signs:* hypertension, muscular irritability progresses to Chvostek's sign, tetany, and convulsions. *Lab.:* vomitus etches glass; hyperglycemia, prolonged blood clotting time. *X-ray:* osteosclerosis.

fragilitas ossium (osteogenesis imperfecta). See alternative term.

galactosemia. Autosomal recessive deficiency of galactose-1-phosphate uridyl transferase with failure to convert galactose to glucose and subsequent development of fatty cirrhotic liver. *Symptoms:* affects newborn. *Signs:* vomiting, diarrhea, and dehydration follow ingestion of milk after several days to weeks, failure to thrive and grow, jaundice, hepatosplenomegaly, cataracts, mental retardation. *Lab.:* diminished erythrocyte galactose-1-phosphate uridyl transferase activity, increased galactosemia and galactosuria, aminoaciduria, albuminuria.

gallbladder, hydrops. Obstruction of the cystic duct, usually by stone, with enlargement and tense thin edematous wall that occasionally ruptures. *Symptoms:* asymptomatic or accompanied by epigastric pain, nausea, and vomiting. *Signs:* RUQ abdominal tenderness or palpable tender mass, fever. *X-ray:* nonvisualization of the gallbladder on cholecystogram; cholelithiasis.

gas gangrene (anaerobic cellulitis). Tissue infection with gas-producing anaerobic bacteria, such as *Clostridium welchii, novyi, septicum, sordellii,* and *histolyticum.* *Symptoms:* history of deep contaminated wound; sudden pain in affected muscles; increasing prostration. *Signs:* fever, tachycardia, hypotension, pallor, apathy, and stupor; foul discharge from wound; the surrounding skin may be discolored; crepitus may be palpated in subcutaneous or muscular layers. *Lab.:*

leukocytosis; stained smears from wound show gram-positive encapsulated bacilli. *X-ray:* shows air in fascial planes.

gastritis, acute. Inflammation of the stomach associated with food poisoning, ingested irritants, alcohol, allergy, or uremia leading to erosions of papillae and hemorrhage. *Symptoms:* epigastric burning, anorexia, nausea, vomiting, fever, weakness. *Signs:* dehydration, epigastric tenderness, pallor, shock. *Lab.:* mucosal inflammation, engorgement, erosions, and hemorrhages seen with gastroscopy and biopsy. *X-ray:* thickened rugae.

Gaucher's disease. Familial disorder with disturbed cerebroside metabolism. *Symptoms:* heavy feeling in abdomen; painful sites of bone lesions. *Signs:* progressive abdominal distention with splenomegaly and hepatomegaly; brown pigmentation of conjunctiva; brown to yellow skin. *Lab.:* anemia, leukopenia, thrombocytopenia. *Bone Marrow:* Gaucher cells. *X-ray:* localized thinning of bony cortex; erosion and compression of femoral head.

gigantism. Excessive secretion of growth hormone from eosinophilic adenoma of pituitary, *before* epiphyseal closure. *Symptoms:* rapid excessive growth, weakness. *Signs:* excessive lengthening of long bones before epiphyseal closure; body proportions relatively normal; increased intracranial pressure; hyperplasia of all organs. *X-ray:* widening of sella turcica; enlarged frontal sinuses; tufting of distal phalanges; metacarpal and vertebral broadening; hyperplasia of mandible.

glanders. Infection of *Malleomyces mallei,* occasionally contracted by men who care for infected horses, mules, or asses, resulting in a fulminant febrile illness or in disseminated granulomatous lesions and abscesses in skin and respiratory tract. *Symptoms:* abrupt development of high fever, chills, prostration, myalgia, and vomiting. *Signs:* lymphadenopathy, local swelling, and the development of miliary lesions along lymphatics and subcutaneous tissues. *Lab.:* positive intradermal tests, complement fixation, and cultures of exudates, sputum, and blood are positive; leukocytosis.

glaucoma, narrow angle. Obstruction to drainage of aqueous from anterior chamber with narrowing of chamber angle and probable increased production of aqueous. *Symptoms:*

acute—there may be extreme ocular pain with loss of vision, nausea and vomiting; *chronic*—halos around lights, tunnel vision, ocular pain, and headache. *Signs:* chemosis, corneal edema, ciliary flush, fixed dilated pupil. *Tests:* narrow angles seen with gonioscopy, increased intraocular pressure (25–50 mm) with tonometry, cupping of disk.

glucoma, open angle. Increased secretion of aqueous with obstruction to outflow and normal chamber angles. *Symptoms:* most common type of glaucoma, occurs in older persons who may see colored halos around lights and experience insidious painless blindness. *Signs:* increased intraocular pressure, dilation of pupils, cupping of the disks. *Tests:* elevated intraocular pressure, loss of nasal and later peripheral visual fields, and eventually total blindness.

glomerulonephritis, acute (nephritis, acute glomular). An inflammatory reaction to infection with nephritogenic strain of hemolytic streptococci. *Symptoms:* several weeks after onset of streptococcal pharyngitis, acute onset of hematuria, facial edema, headache, anorexia, backache, vomiting. *Signs:* fever, facial edema, often generalized edema, arterial hypertension, tachycardia; sometimes rales in chest; increased venous pressure. *Lab.:* hematuria, cylindruria, azotemia, secondary anemia.

glomerulonephritis, chronic (nephritis, chronic glomerular). Reaction to infection with hemolytic streptococci; only a few cases develop from acute nephritis. *Symptoms:* gradual onset of dependent edema, weakness, lassitude, weight loss, blurred vision. *Signs:* pallor, edema, arterial hypertension; papilledema and retinal edema, retinal exudates and hemorrhages. *Lab.:* smoky urine containing erythrocytes, protein, and casts; anemia, azotemia, hypoalbuminemia, hypocalcemia, hyperphosphatemia; isosthenuria.

glycosuria, alimentary (glycosuria, digestive). Normal glycosuria preceded by the ingestion of sugar.

goiter. Enlargement of the thyroid gland or unknown cause (simple goiter) or secondary to iodine deficiency (endemic goiter) or the ingestion of goitrogens in genetically predisposed persons. *Symptoms:* usually asymptomatic but occasionally pressure-sensitive, dyspnea, dysphagia, or cough with large glands. *Signs: endemic goiter*—diffuse enlargement before puberty with progression unless treated with iodine or thyroid hormone, which produces regression; *simple goiter*—enlargement beginning in adolescent girls or pregnant lactating or menopausal women and regressing with thyroid hormone therapy. **Lab.:** *endemic goiter*—reduced PBI, increased plasma clearance and uptake of radioactive iodine; *simple goiter*—normal PBI, radioiodine kinetics, and cholesterol.

gonadal dysgenesis (Turner's syndrome, ovarian agenesis). Congenitally fibrotic ovarian anlagen associated with negative (male pattern) sex chromatin of buccal mucosal cells and neutrophils, and XO sex chromosome karyotype, with no Y and a diploid number of 45 in 80% of the cases. *Symptoms:* primary amenorrhea. *Signs:* short stature, webbed neck, shieldlike chest, infantile female genitalia and breasts, delayed growth of axillary and pubic hair, cubitus valgus, short metacarpals, and lymphedema of extremities. *Lab.:* elevated urinary gonadotropins. *X-ray:* osteoporosis, coarctation of aorta.

gonorrhea. Infection with the gonococcus. *Symptoms:* burning, frequency, and urgency of urination. *Signs in Male:* green, yellow, or sanguineous urethral discharge; meatal lips swollen and red; chordee; swelling, redness, and pain in anterior urethra. *Signs in Female:* purulent urethral discharge with urethral inflammation; swelling and tenderness in Skene's or Bartholin's glands. Either sex may have accompanying conjunctivitis or arthritis. *Lab.:* stained smears of pus contain gram-negative biscuit-shaped diplococci within leukocytes.

Goodpasture's syndrome. Intra-alveolar hemorrhage in the lungs and glomerulonephritis from antibody damage to alveolar and renal basement membranes progressing to death in several months or years. *Symptoms:* hemoptysis, cough, and exertional dyspnea. *Signs:* rales, rhonchi, and signs of uremia. *Lab.:* normochromic anemia; bloody sputum or gastric aspirates containing siderophages; hematuria. *X-ray:* bilateral perihilar patchy infiltrates.

gout. Inborn error of metabolism with uric acid overproduction, or acquired by excessive intake of purines or tissue breakdown. *Symptoms:* acute attacks of painful swelling of joints, often the great toe, with chills and fever; after many years, chronic stage with chronic arthritis, tophi, and ulceration. *Lab.:* increased blood uric acid and serum biurate crystals in joint aspirate. *X-ray:* late destructive joint changes with punched-out rarefactions, not diagnostic.

granuloma, midline (lethal midline or facial granuloma). Chronic inflammatory disease with thrombosis of small blood vessels and focal necrosis leading to destruction of nasal septum, palate, paranasal sinuses, and midfacial structures of unknown etiology. *Symptoms:* sneezing, nasal stuffiness, obstruction, and pain. *Signs:* more frequent in women beginning with rhinorrhea, nasal congestion, and paranasal sinusitis; progressing to inflammation and ulcerations of the nasal septum, palate, and nasal ali; followed by perforations and destruction of midfacial structures including pharynx, mouth, sinuses, eyes, with death from cachexia, pneumonia, meningitis, or hemorrhage. *Lab.:* leukopenia.

granulomatosis, Wegener's. A syndrome of necrotizing granulomas, arteritis, and glomerulonephritis leading to death. Cause unknown. *Symptoms:* rhinorrhea, epistaxis, cough, hemoptysis, malaise, and weight loss. *Signs:* ulceration of nasal cartilage and gingivae, conjunctivitis, uveitis, retinitis, chemosis, exophthalmos, signs of pleurisy or pneumonia, rashes, and polyarthritis. *Lab.:* anemia, leukocytosis, eosinophilia, hematuria, proteinuria, cylindruria, elevated blood urea nitrogen, and hyperglobulinemia. *Chest x-ray:* bronchopneumonic patches or multiple nodular densities.

Guillain-Barré syndrome (polyneuritis, acute idiopathic). See alternative term.

Haff disease. Poisoning of fisherman of the Koenigsberg Haff from arsine in waste water from the cellulose factories. Sudden seizure with severe pain in the extremities, great weakness, and myoglobinuria.

Hand-Schüller-Christian syndrome (lipoid histiocytosis). *Symptoms:* sore mouth, aural discharge, skin eruptions. *Signs:* swelling and necrosis of gums with extrusion of teeth; papular, seborrheic, or petechial rash; minute xanthomatous nodules; raised yellow to brown lesions in axillae or neck; retarded growth and sexual development; exophthalmos; diabetes insipidus. *Lab.:* anemia; fat and cholesterol in lesions. *X-ray:* sharply demarcated bony defects; pulmonary fibrosis.

hay fever. Rhinitis from pollen allergy. *Symptoms:* seasonal sneezing, itching of eyes, nose, and pharynx; irritability. *Signs:* lacrimation, photophobia, watery nasal discharge, injected conjunctiva; pale boggy edematous nasal mucosa. *Lab.:* increased eosinophils in nasal secretion. *Skin Tests:* positive reactions to causative pollens.

heart, tamponade of. Compression of the heart by pericardial effusion or hemopericardium. *Symptoms:* dyspnea, orthopnea, chest pain, syncope. *Signs:* cold clammy skin, tachycardia, distended neck veins, falling arterial pressure, paradoxical pulse, cyanosis, faint heart sounds, friction rub, increase in area of cardiac dullness. *X-ray:* widening of vascular and cardiac shadows. *ECG:* low voltage complexes.

heart failure, congestive. Precipitated by myocardial infarction, pneumonia, pulmonary embolism, anemia, dysrrhythmias, salt and water retention. *Symptoms:* exertional dyspnea, paroxysmal nocturnal dyspnea, nocturia, cough, weakness, pain in liver. *Signs:* orthopnea, cyanosis, engorgement of jugular veins from increased venous pressure, coarse rales, Cheyne-Stokes respiration, hydrothorax, ascites, dependent edema, hepatojugular reflux, hepatomegaly, diastolic gallop rhythm. *Lab.:* oliguria, proteinuria, hyalin casts, high urinary specific gravity. *X-ray:* enlarged cardiac shadow and increased vascular markings.

heart valve leaflet, rupture of. Rarely in the course of bacterial endocarditis a valve leaflet may rupture from erosion. This is indicated by the sudden appearance of a regurgitant murmur, usually loud, often raucous, with rapid progressive congestive cardiac failure.

heat exhaustion (heat prostration). Associated with cardiac output and vasomotor control insufficient for skin, muscles, and brain after exertion in hot environment. *Symptoms:* deficient salt intake may precede palpitation, faintness, lassitude, headache, vertigo, nausea, vomiting, and cramps. *Signs:* tachycardia, diaphoresis, ashen cold moist skin, dilated pupils, diminished blood pressure. *Lab.:* decreased plasma levels of sodium and chloride.

hematoma, subdural. A hemorrhage from a tear of the veins between the dura and the surface of the brain, usually secondary to cranial trauma. *Symptoms: acute*—headache, irritability, and association with severe bleeding; *chronic*—manifestations including intermittent headache and variable levels of consciousness that may occur hours, weeks, or months after trauma. *Signs: acute*—fluctuating levels of consciousness, with rapid progression of dilated pupils, hemiplegia, hyperreflexia, Babinski's sign, and convulsions; *chronic*—a more insidious onset with progressively impaired intellect, agitation, impulsive behavior, hemiparesis, stupor, and lucidity alternating to produce variable levels of consciousness. *Tests:* increased CSF pressure and protein with bloody or xanthochromic fluid, localized EEG disturbance, positive brain scan. *X-ray:* cranial fracture, shifted calcified pineal gland, avascular mass displacing cerebral and cranial vessels on angiography, positive CT and MRI scans.

hemiplegia. This is the result of cerebral artery thrombosis, embolism, or occlusion from other causes. *Symptoms:* sudden weakness and loss of function of arm and leg on the same side of the body. *Signs from Lesion in Cerebral or Internal Capsular Corticospinal Tract:* paralysis of arm and leg on opposite side; facial weakness on the same side. *Cortical or Subcortical:* convulsive seizures, dysphasia; cortical type of sensory loss. *Low Pontine Lesion:* paralysis of face on same side as involved limbs; paralysis of lateral gaze. *Lesion Low in Brain but above Decussation:* ipsilateral paralysis of palate or tongue; contralateral paralysis of arm and leg.

hemochromatosis. Excessive storage of iron in body from increased absorption or many blood transfusions. *Symptoms:* lassitude, weight loss, darkening of skin, abdominal pain. *Signs:* brown pigmentation of skin, hepatomegaly, loss of body hair, edema, ascites, peripheral neuritis, testicular atrophy. *Lab.:* high serum iron and decreased unsaturated iron binding capacity; sometimes glycosuria and hyperglycemia; biopsies of liver, bone marrow, or skin show excessive hemosiderin.

hemoglobinuria, cold. Hemolysis from autoantibodies activated by cold. *Symptoms:* exposure to cold followed by headache, pain in back and legs, abdominal cramps, vomiting, diarrhea, chills and fever. *Signs:* splenomegaly, hepatomegaly; possibly transient jaundice; pale fingers, toes, tip of nose. *Lab.:* hemoglobin in fresh urine with no red cells. Spectroscopy shows hemoglobin and methemoglobin in urine. *Test:* hemoglobinuria after immersion of hands or feet in ice water. Cold hemolysis in test tube. Donath-Landsteiner test may show hemolysis activated by cold but hemolyzing only when rewarmed.

hemoglobinuria, malarial (blackwater fever). A complication of falciparum malaria, cause unknown. *Symptoms:* sudden onset of chills and irregular fever, pain in liver and spleen, vomiting, headache. *Signs:* enlarged tender liver; splenomegaly; retinal hemorrhages, jaundice, shock. *Lab.:* hemoglobinuria, malarial parasites in blood smears.

hemoglobinuria, paroxysmal nocturnal. Increased sensitivity of RBC and other cells to complement. *Symptoms:* chronic anemia; abdominal, retrosternal, or lumbar pain. Superficial migratory thrombophlebitis, hemoglobinuria at night. *Lab.:* anemia, leukopenia; hemosiderin in leukocytes and urine, increased hemolysis in acid solution (Ham's test).

hemoglobinuria, paroxysmal, due to exertion (march hemoglobinuria). *Symptoms:* severe exertion causes pain in back and thighs, dark urine. *Signs:* red urine following mechanical trauma to RBC in microvasculature during strenous exercise. *Lab.:* spectroscopy shows hemoglobin in urine.

hemolysis, transfusion. Caused by transfusion of incompatible blood. *Symptoms:* sudden onset with anxiety, chills and fever, nausea, pains in back and thighs. *Signs:* flushed face, tachycardia, arterial hypotension. *Lab.:* urine contains hemoglobin without erythrocytes, hemoglobin casts. *Test:* fresh, centrifuged blood specimen shows gross hemoglobin in plasma.

hemophilia (factor VIII deficiency, hemophilia A). X-linked recessive mendelian trait transmitted through the usually unaffected mother to her male offspring. *Signs:* excessive bleeding from slight trauma including dental extractions and surgery; visceral bleeding; hemarthroses leading to contractures and degenerative arthritis. *Lab.:* prolonged partial thromboplastin time corrected by normal plasma or factor VIII, but not by hemophiliac plasma.

hemophilia A (hemophilia). See alternative term.

hemophilia B (factor IX deficiency). See alternative term.

hepatic vein thrombosis (Budd-Chiari syndrome). *Symptoms:* sudden epigastric pain and vomiting, or gradual onset with intermittent mild abdominal pain. *Signs:* large liver, tender initially; ascites and edema of the ankles, engorged venous collaterals in the epigastrium and lower thorax; splenomegaly; occasionally jaundice, shock, coma, and death. *X-ray:* obstruction visualized with angiography.

hepatitis, acute anicteric. Caused by virus. *Symptoms:* diarrhea, or otherwise asymptomatic. *Signs:* percussion tenderness over the liver. *Lab.:* elevated SGOT, SGPT.

hepatitis, fulminant. Caused by virus or toxic agents. *Symptoms:* severe nausea, vomiting, anorexia, chills and fever, abdominal pain. *Signs:* deep jaundice; rapidly shrinking liver, gastrointestinal hemorrhage; ascites, purpura; muscular twitching; oliguria, shock, death. *Lab.:* hyperbilirubinemia, lactic acidosis, leukocytosis.

hepatitis, viral. In *epidemic* type, A virus transmitted from gastrointestinal tract with incubation period 2–6 weeks; in *serum* type, B virus transmitted by blood of carriers with incubation period 6 weeks to 6 months. *Symptoms:* anorexia, fever, vomiting, weakness, diarrhea, jaundice. *Signs:* fever, jaundice, large tender liver with antedating percussion tenderness, dark urine, postcervical adenopathy. *Lab.:* Leukopenia, high ESR, bilirubinemia, bilirubinuria, high serum alkaline phosphatase, high SGOT, positive tests for HB_c Ag or HB_sAg indicate acute or chronic infections; anti-HB_s suggests previous infection.

hepatolenticular degeneration (Wilson's disease). Familial disorder of copper metabolism. *Signs:* jaundice, ascites, peripheral edema, vascular spiders, smoky brown ring on outer corneal margin (Kayser-Fleischer ring), brown skin, splenomegaly, choreiform movements, pill-rolling tremor, dystonia, masklike stare, dysarthria. *Lab.:* biopsy of liver shows cirrhosis and copper deposits; serum copper and ceruloplasmin decreased.

hereditary hemorrhagic telangiectasia (Osler's disease). Simple hereditary dominant profusion of telangiectases throughout body. *Symptoms:* profuse hemorrhages; often epistaxis. *Signs:* bright red elevated telangiectases that blanch with pressure; numbers increase with age. *X-ray:* sometimes visualizes arteriovenous fistulas. *Lab:* normal blood or posthemorrhagic anemia. No clotting disorder.

herpes simplex. Infection with herpes simplex virus. *Signs:* recurrent circumscribed grouped vesicles surrounded by erythema, forming crusts on rupture.

herpes zoster (shingles). Infections with Herpes zoster virus related to chickenpox. *Symptoms:* severe pain; sometimes chills and fever, malaise, meningismus. *Signs:* crops of clear vesicles along course of a cutaneous nerve; tender regional lymph nodes.

histiocytosis (Gaucher's disease, Hand-Schüller-Christian syndrome, Niemann-Pick disease). See alternative terms.

histoplasmosis. Disease caused by fungus *Histoplasma capsulatum.* *Symptoms:* asyptomatic or cough, malaise, dyspnea, weight loss, abdominal cramps, diarrhea, melena. *Signs:* fever, rales, ulcers in tongue, lips, lymphadenopathy; splenomegaly, hepatomegaly. *X-ray:* shows pneumonitis; later, calcified lesions. *Lab.:* cultures of organisms from blood, sputum, mouth, marrow and lesions; rising complement fixation titer. *Skin Test:* conversion from negative to positive reaction.

Hodgkin's disease. A malignant disease of lymphoid tissue, cause unknown. *Symptoms:* pruritus; painless enlargement of lymph nodes, abdominal pain; periodic or continuous fever, cachexia. *Signs:* firm, discrete, nontender, nonsuppurating lymph nodes; hepatomegaly, splenomegaly. *Lab.:* normocytic normochromic anemia, leukocytosis with lymphopenia. *X-ray:* anterior mediastinal or hilar lymphadenopathy; osteosclerotic or osteoporotic lesions. *Node Biopsy:* necessary for diagnosis; tissue contains Reed-Sternberg cells.

homocystinuria. Hereditary deficiency of cystathionine synthetase and abnormal methionine metabolism associated with intimal fibrosis, destruction of arterial elastic fibers and zonular fibers of the lens, fatty liver, and gliosis and focal necrosis of the midbrain. *Signs:* mental retardation and convulsions, cataracts and lenticular subluxation, sparse hair; older patients may have arachnodactyly, pectus excavatum, long thin trunk, arms, and legs; thromboembolic episodes. *Lab.:* increased levels of homocystine and methionine in cerebrospinal fluid, plasma, and urine.

hordeolum, external (external sty). Bacterial infection of sebaceous gland in the eyelid. *Symptoms:* painful foreign body sensation, lacrimation. *Signs:* erythematous tender indurated area that later supports a pustule on the lid margin.

hordeolum, internal (chalazion). Staphylococcal infection of meibomian gland. *Symptoms:* distressing pain on inner eyelid with lacrimation and photophobia. *Signs:* tender pustule under conjunctiva of inner eyelid.

Horner's syndrome. From destructive lesion of superior cervical ganglion. *Signs:* miosis, palpebral ptosis, absence of sweating on face and neck, all on the same side of the body.

hydatid disease (echinococcosis). See alternative term.

hydrarthrosis, intermittent. Cause unknown. *Symptoms:* usually unilateral, knees most often affected; joint becomes swollen, but painful only with weight-bearing; swelling lasts 3–5 days with normal intervals of 7–11 days. *Signs:* joint has classic signs of effusion without inflammatory changes. *Lab.:* leukocytosis in synovial fluid; villous synovitis on biopsy.

hydrocele, tunica vaginalis. Serous fluid accumulation in the cavity on the tunica vaginalis from trauma or infection. *Symptoms:* large amounts of fluid may produce a dragging sensation or interference with intercourse, smaller volumes are asymptomatic. *Signs:* nontender resilient scrotal swelling anterior to the testis and spermatic cord that is translucent. *Lab.:* fluid is like plasma unless infection produces an exudate.

hydrocephalus, communicating or obstructive. Congenital or acquired obstruction of circulation of cerebrospinal fluid. *Symptoms:* headache, vomiting, weakness of limbs, incoordination. *Signs:* enlargement of head, thinning of scalp, papilledema, eyes displaced downward, fontanels bulging. *Tests:* combined puncture of lateral ventricle and lumbar space with pressure measurements and determination of protein concentration in fluid. *X-ray:* thinning of cranial bones with dilated ventricles on CT or MRI scans.

hydronephrosis. Obstruction of urinary tract producing dilatation of renal pelvis, congenital or acquired. *Symptoms:* attacks of dull or colicky pain in abdomen or loin. *Signs:* kidney may be palpable. *Lab.:* pyuria, hematuria. *X-ray:* pyelography shows dilated renal pelvis with evidence of impaired kidney function.

hypercalcemia. From excessive vitamin D, or hyperparathyroidism, or nephritis, multiple myeloma, or carcinoma. *Symptoms:* nausea, headache, diarrhea, anorexia, lassitude. *X-ray:* calcified soft tissues. *Lab.:* urine and blood Ca high. ECG changes.

hypercalcemic syndrome, acute. A potentially fatal medical emergency caused by parathyroid intoxication, milk-alkali syndrome, vitamin D intoxication, or metastatic carcinoma. *Symptoms:* weakness, lethargy, nausea, intractable vomiting, and coma. *Signs:* hypotonia and muscular weakness. *Lab.:* hypercalcemia, hypercalciuria. *ECG:* shortened Q-T interval.

hyperinsulinism. From overdoses of insulin or excessive secretion from hyperplasia or adenoma of pancreatic islets. *Symptoms:* weakness, hunger, dyspnea, tachycardia, syncope, convulsive seizures, coma, all relieved by glucose administration. *Lab.:* hypoglycemia during an attack.

hypernephroma (carcinoma of the kidney). *Symptoms:* costovertebral angle tenderness, malaise, weight loss, fever. *Signs:* possibly palpable renal tumor. *Lab.:* often hematuria, anemia. *X-ray:* pyelography shows irregular pelvis and enlarged kidney; mass on CT or MRI scans; metastases to bones sometimes characteristic.

hyperparathyroidism, primary. Adenoma, hyperplasia, or neoplasia of the parathyroid gland with excessive secretion of parathyroid hormone causing bone resorption and inhibition of the renal tubular reabsorption of phosphate. The triad of complications that often suggests the diagnosis: peptic ulcer, urinary calculi, and pancreatitis. *Symptoms:* muscle weakness; loss of appetite, nausea, constipation; polyuria, polydipsia; weight loss, deafness, paresthesias, bone pain, and renal colic later. *Signs:* prolonged course, most common in middle-aged women; band (calcific) keratitis, hypotonia and weakness, tumor masses, fractures and skeletal deformities. *Lab.:* hypercalcemia, hypophosphatemia, hypercalciuria, hyperphosphaturia, elevated serum alkaline phosphatase. *X-ray:* skeletal deformities, generalized decreased density of bone on CT scan; cysts, tumors, and fractures. *ECG:* shortened Q-T interval.

hypertension, essential. Cause unknown. *Symptoms:* only produced by complications. *Signs:* diastolic pressure constantly above 90 mm Hg, accentuated A_2, forceful precordial apical thrust, spasm of retinal vessels, arteriovenous nicking of retinal vessels with widened arterial stripe; flame-shaped retinal hemorrhages, papilledema with malignant hypertension.

Lab.: serum cholesterol and lipids frequently elevated. *ECG:* left-axis deviation and increased voltage in the left precordial leads.

hypertension, paroxysmal (pheochromocytoma). Excess production of epinephrine by pheochromocytoma, a neoplasm frequently near the kidney. *Symptoms:* attacks of palpitation, diaphoresis, tremulousness, headache, vomiting, abdominal pain, syncope. *Signs:* during attack, high systolic and diastolic pressure, pallor, trembling, sometimes flushing of neck. Hypertension may be paroxysmal or sustained. *X-ray:* CT or MRI scans may reveal a mass near or in the adrenal. *Tests:* between attacks, paroxysm may be provoked by histamine intravenously; during hypertension, phentolamine (Regitine) intravenously lowers the pressure. Increased excretion of catecholamines in the urine.

hypertension, pulmonary (cor pulmonale). From primary pulmonary hypertension, mitral stenosis, left-to-right cardiac shunts, pulmonary emphysema, pneumoconiosis, pulmonary fibrosis, scleroderma, and others. *Symptoms:* retrosternal pain, cough, dyspnea. *Signs:* accentuated precordial thrust of the right ventricle, accentuated P_2, cyanosis, clubbed fingers. *Lab.:* erythrocytosis. *ECG:* right ventricular hypertrophy. *X-ray:* enlarged pulmonary artery and dilated right ventricle.

hyperthyroidism (thyrotoxicosis). Idiopathic hyperplasia of the thyroid gland with increased secretion of thyroid hormone. *Symptoms:* alertness, emotional lability, irritability, muscular weakness; palpitation; voracious appetite and weight loss, diarrhea; heat intolerance. *Signs:* hyperkinesia, rapid speech, quadriceps weakness, fine tremor; fine abundant hair, fine moist skin, onycholysis; lid lag, stare, chemosis, periorbital edema, proptosis; accentuated first heart sound, tachycardia, atrial fibrillation, wide pulse pressure, poor response to digitalis, dyspnea; frequent defecation, diarrhea. *Lab.:* increased basal metabolic rate, uptake of radioiodine by thyroid gland, T_3 uptake, total T_4 and free T_4. The TSH is suppressed.

hyperventilation. From emotional disturbances, pulmonary emphysema with anoxia, hypercapnea, respiratory acidosis. *Symptoms:* associated with dyspnea in anoxia or hypercapnea; in emotional disturbances, nervousness, restlessness, anxiety, fear, dizziness, faintness, ataxia, palpitation, paresthesias. *Signs:* tachycardia, hyperpnea, weak pulse, vasomotor collapse, tetany, convulsions, unconsciousness. *Lab.:* increased blood O_2 tension, decreased blood CO_2, low serum Na and K, increased Cl. Urine K, Na, and bicarbonate increased; Cl decreased.

hypocalcemia. Inadequate intake of Ca and vitamin D, hypoparathyroidism, poor intestinal absorption. *Symptoms:* vomiting, diarrhea. *Signs:* tetany with carpopedal spasm, Chvostek's and Trousseau's signs. *Lab.:* excess Ca in urine; low blood Ca and high blood P; possibly high BUN.

hypokalemia. Hypopotassemia from depletion of K, alkalosis, aldosteronism, or diuretics. *Symptoms:* apathy, muscle weakness. *Signs:* arterial hypotension, atonia, cardiac arrhythmias, impaired resiratory movements. *Lab.:* low plasma K, high urine K. *ECG:* prolonged Q-T interval, depressed S-T segment, flat or inverted T.

hypomagnesemia. Excessive loss of serum magnesium by dehydration, starvation, dialysis, alcoholism, or renal disease causes neuromuscular irritability like hypocalcemia, so that patients may have convulsive seizures, tetany, Chvostek's sign. In addition, weakness and vertigo are common. Dysphagia and vertical nystagmus may be found. The serum level of Mg is lowered.

hyponatremia. Low serum sodium from dilution, loss of Na in urine from diuresis or Addison's disease, excessive vomiting or diarrhea. *Symptoms:* cerebral depression, anorexia, asthenia, abdominal cramps. *Lab.:* low plasma Na; scanty Na and Cl in urine, except in Addison's disease.

hypoparathyroidism. From operative removal of parathyroid glands associated with thyroidectomy. *Symptoms:* nervousness, weakness, paresthesias, muscle stiffness and cramps, headaches, abdominal pain. *Signs:* tetany with carpopedal spasm, positive Chvostek's and Trousseau's signs, loss of hair, cataracts, papilledema. *Lab.:* low serum Ca and high P.

hypopituitarism syndrome (Simmonds' disease). See alternative term.

hypoprothrombinemia. From excessive bishydroxycoumarin, vitamin K deficiency from failure of absorption in obstructive jaundice or liver insufficiency. *Symptoms:* epistaxis, bleeding from gums, easy bruising, hematuria, melena, menorrhagia. *Signs:* ecchymoses. *Lab.:* prolonged prothrombin time. Administration of vitamin K_1 oxide decreases prothrombin time in coumarin poisoning or K deficiency from malabsorption, but not from deficit resulting from liver failure.

hypothyroidism, adult (myxedema). Decreased secretion of thyroid hormone of unknown cause or secondary to surgical ablation, irradiation, inflammation, or failure of anterior pituitary from ingestion of thyroid-suppressant substances (iodide, cyanates, or lithium), or secondary to thyroiditis, or carcinomatous replacement of thyroid tissue. *Symptoms:* dry skin and hair loss, broken nails; weight gain with diminished food intake, cold intolerance, constipation; menorrhagia, diminished libido; slow thinking. *Signs:* round puffy face, slow speech, hoarseness; hypokinesia, generalized muscle weakness, delayed relaxation of knee or ankle jerk; cold, dry, thick, scaling skin, dry coarse brittle hair, dry longitudinally ridged nails; periorbital edema; normal or faint cardiac impulse, indistinct heart tones, cardiac enlargement, bradycardia; ascites, ankle edema, pericardial effusion. *Lab.:* refractory macrocytic anemia; diminished thyroid uptake of radioiodine, decreased T_3 uptake, total T_4 and free T_4. The TSH is elevated; elevated serum cholesterol. *ECG:* low voltage of QRS complex.

hypothyroidism, infantile (cretinism). Congenital hypothyroidism, usually from an enzymatic defect, or iodine deficiency. *Symptoms:* none. *Signs:* dwarfism, yellow dry thick skin, overweight, thick lips and tongue; short hands with thick fingers; delayed deciduous dentition, retarded mental and sexual development; slow movements. *Lab.:* high TSH, decreased T_3 uptake, total T_4 and free T_4; decreased thyroidal uptake of ^{131}I. *X-ray:* retarded bone growth.

ichthyosis. Congenital or hereditary skin disease. *Symptoms:* dryness of skin, failure to sweat, worse in winter. *Signs:* skin dry, brittle, thickened, scaling; no sweating or oil excretion.

ileitis, regional Cause unknown. *Symptoms:* cramping pains near umbilicus; episodes of fever debility. *Signs:* tender immobile mass in lower abdomen, abdominal distention. *Lab.:* anemia, occult blood in feces; possibly hypoproteinemia. *X-ray:* granular or polypoid filling defects in blunted fused mucosal folds of small intestine, especially ileum; lumen narrowed or irregular.

ileus, paralytic. Inhibition of peristalsis in intestinal obstruction, peritonitis, mesenteric vessel thrombosis, pneumonia, hypokalemia, or other infections. *Symptoms:* generalized or localized abdominal pain; regurgitant vomiting. *Signs:* abdominal distention and tenderness; diminished or absent bowel sounds.

impetigo contagiosa. A streptococcal or staphylococcal infection of the skin. *Signs:* lesions distributed over head and limbs; may be vesicles, bullae, or pustules in various stages; crusting occurs when lesions rupture.

infectious mononucleosis. Infection with Epstein-Barr virus (EBV). *Symptoms:* sore throat with slight fever, malaise, cough, pain in the orbits. *Signs:* tender enlarged lymph nodes; pharynx red with edema, petechiae on palate and uvula; occasional morbilliform rash; conjunctivitis; splenomegaly; occasionally jaundice with tender enlarged liver. *Lab.:* leukopenia early, later leukocytosis with atypical large lymphocytes; rising titer of heterophil antibodies; may have positive monospot test and elevated titer of EBV antibody.

inferior vena cava, obstruction of. Caused by thrombosis, neoplasm in the vessel, or development anomalies. *Symptoms:* vomiting. *Signs:* edema of lower limbs, possible ascites; enlarged superficial veins in thighs, abdomen, and chest; jaundice; possible impaired renal or hepatic function.

influenza. Acute infectious disease from virus of type A, B, or C. *Symptoms:* chills and fever, dry throat, rhinitis, prostration, myalgia, headache, cough. *Signs:* dull red throat with hyperplastic lymphoid islands in pharynx; mucoid sputum, few rales in lungs. *Lab.:* leukopenia or slight leukocytosis with relative lymphopenia in either case; rising titer of hemagglutinin-inhibition antibodies.

insulinoma (pancreas, islet-cell tumor of). See alternative term.

intertrigo. Superficial dermatitis in skin folds secondary to abrasion of warm, moist skin and infection with bacteria or monilia. *Symptoms:* itching and burning. *Signs:* moist erythematous skin in folds of neck, breasts, groin, or buttocks. Diaper dermatitis may progress from redness to nodular, vesicular, or pustular lesions.

intervertebral disk, rupture of (nucleus pulposus, herniated). Stress on degenerated nucleus pulposus or annulus fibrosus from lifting, straining, or trauma leads to protrusion of the disk. *Symptoms:* cervical disk rupture may cause neck pain radiating to shoulder and arm with muscle weakness and paresthesias in the fingers; lumbar disk rupture results in low back pain with radiation into buttock and along sciatic nerve with muscle weakness, limping and paresthesias. *Signs:* unilateral impairment of biceps or triceps reflex or central cervical herniation resulting in pressure on cord with miosis and Brown-Sequard syndrome; lumbar herniation may result in pain with straight leg-raising and dorsiflexion of foot, diminished knee or ankle jerk, failure to walk on toes with disk protrusion at L-4–L-5 and failure to walk on heels with lesion at L-5–S-1. *X-ray:* tipping of vertebrae with narrowing of intervertebral space; filling defect on myelogram.

intestinal polyposis (Peutz-Jegher's syndrome). Inherited autosomal dominant. *Symptoms:* vague abdominal discomfort; gastrointestinal hemorrhages. *Signs:* pigmented brown oval or round spots on mucosa of lips and mouth, skin or face and hands. *Lab.:* anemia from hemorrhage; blood in feces. X-ray and sigmoidoscopic examination reveals polyps.

intestine, blind loop of. Surgical anastomosis performed for many reasons may lead to stasis and overgrowth of bacteria that compete with the host for vitamin B_{12} or folic acid. *Symptoms:* easy fatigue and exertional dyspnea. *Signs:* pallor and signs of pernicious anemia. *Lab.:* macrocytic anemia, hypersegmented neutrophils, decreased serum B_{12} level, deficient absorption of radioactive vitamin B_{12} not corrected with intrinsic factor. *X-ray:* "blind loop" of small bowel noted in fluoroscopy after ingestion of barium.

iodine poisoning. May produce acneiform eruption, papular or bullous rash. In acute overdosage, metallic taste in mouth; collapse, oliguria. The concentration in nasal secretions and saliva may produce corrosive effect on the skin and mucosa.

kala-azar. Visceral infection with the protozoon *Leishmania donovani* transmitted by the sandfly. *Symptoms:* irregular recurrent fever, weakness, sweating, cough, nausea and vomiting. *Signs:* pale macules, erythematous nodules, verrucae; splenomegaly, hepatomegaly, lymphadenopathy. *Lab.:* anemia, leukopenia; organisms cultured from bone marrow and lymph node fluid.

Kaposi's sarcoma (multiple idiopathic hemorrhagic sarcoma). An indolent sarcoma of multifocal origin involving skin and other organs with multiple vascular nodules, afflicting middle-aged to elderly white males. In the more aggressive form seen in young black males in Africa or in patients with AIDS, visceral involvement and lymphadenopathy occur much more frequently. *Symptoms:* painful burning or itching lesions. *Signs:* beginning as red-blue or bluish-brown plaques and nodules, some of the lesions become spongy or compressible tumors moving centripetally from the extremities; lymphadenopathy; lymphedema. *Lab.:* occasionally anemia or pancytopenia; diagnosis confirmed with biopsy.

keloid. Occurs in some families (Caucasian) and in some races (Blacks). It is a hyperplasia occurring in scars from any cause. *Symptoms:* tenderness and pain. *Signs:* fibrocellular elevation of a scar; dense and somewhat tender.

keratoconjunctivitis sicca syndrome (Sjögren's syndrome). This is an autoimmune disorder with the classical manifestations of keratoconjunctivitis, xerostomia, and rheumatoid arthritis. Similar manifestations have been reported in: Felty's syndrome, pulmonary fibrosis, systemic lupus erythematosus, progressive systemic sclerosis, dermatomyositis, polyarteritis nodosa, some myocardopathies, and a spectrum ranging from benign lymphoid hyperplasia to malignant lymphoproliferation (malignant lymphocytic and histiocytic lymphoma). *Lab.:* anemia, leukopenia, accelerated erythrocyte sedimentation rate, and the presence of antinuclear antibody. *Other Tests:* a labial biopsy frequently shows the typical heavy lymphocytic infiltration of salivary glands.

kidney, polycystic disease of. Congenital maturation defect of kidney tissue, probably inherited as an autosomal dominant, manifested in adults. *Symptoms:* headache, nausea, malaise, renal colic, and back pain. *Signs:* hypertension and bilateral enlargement of the kidneys. *Lab.:* hematuria, pyuria, and albuminuria, and rarely erythrocytosis or leukocytosis, cysts may be detected with ultrasonography. *X-ray:* pyelogram reveals blunted calices with oval and crescentic compression of kidney tissue and CT scans may reveal the cysts.

Laennec's cirrhosis (portal cirrhosis of liver). Scarring of the hepatic periportal regions from alcoholism, malnutrition, malaria, poisons. *Symptoms:* anorexia, weakness, increased fatigability, weight loss, abdominal pain. *Signs:* firm nontender liver, moderately enlarged, but may be small and impalpable; splenomegaly; late jaundice with engorged superficial veins of upper abdomen and lower thorax, ascites, edema of the legs, spider nevi, testicular atrophy, gynecomastia, palmar erythema, loss of axillary and pubic hair. *Lab.:* anemia, hypoalbuminemia, bilirubinemia, increased alkaline phosphatase. *X-ray:* esophageal varices with barium swallow. *Biopsy of Liver:* specimen obtained with needle biopsy may be diagnostic.

Laurence-Moon-Biedl syndrome. A recessive genetic disease. *Symptoms:* loss of central vision. *Signs:* retinitis pigmentosa, cataracts, nystagmus, strabismus, mental retardation, obesity, infantile genitalia; occasional dwarfism, mongolian facies, oxycephaly, syndactyly, deafness.

lead poisoning. *Symptoms:* anorexia, abdominal pain, weakness, headache, nausea and vomiting, constipation. *Signs:* lead line in gums, papilledema, ocular palsies, wrist drop, changes in reflexes, convulsions, delirium, coma. *Lab.:* stippled erythrocytes, anemia, leukocytosis; high concentration of lead in blood and urine; coproporphrynuria. *X-ray:* epiphyseal lead line. *Renal biopsy:* demonstrates pathognomonic acid-fast inclusion bodies in the tubular nuclei; these may also occur in the urinary sediment.

Legg-Calvé-Perthes' disease (osteochondrosis). See alternative term.

Legionnaires' disease. Caused by the Gram-negative bacterium *Legionella pneumophilia,* it was probably previously classed as *primary atypical pneumonia.* In some epidemics the agent has been airborne by the air-conditioning systems and in others, it has been waterborne. The *incubation period* has ranged from 2 to 10 days, but in one epidemic the time seemed to be 36 hours. The *prodrome* is *malaise, myalgia,* and *headache,* followed in 12 to 48 hours by sudden *sustained fever* (40 to 40.5° C), with chills and prostration. Nausea, vomiting, and diarrhea may occur. Two or 3 days later, a cough with little or no sputum develops; slight blood-tinged sputum may finally appear. *Chest pain* is common. The fever persists for 8 to 10 days; erythromycin seems to shorten the duration in the U. S. A mortality of 15% was reported in one epidemic; but this seems too high for the average experience. ***Signs:*** appearance of severe distress, with sweating and rapid respirations. There is relative bradycardia, considering the high temperature. The patient is often confused and disoriented, leading to the inference of encephalitis (M. N. Swartz: Clinical Aspects of Legionnaires' Disease. *Ann. Intern. Med.*, **90:**492–95, 1979). ***X-ray:*** initially chest films show unilateral lesions. The shadows are round and "fluffy" opacities that enlarge and spread to the other lobes progressing to dense consolidation. Pleural effusions are small. ***Lab.:*** moderate leukocytosis or a frank leukopenia; Gram-stained sputum contains few leukocytes and a paucity of bacteria usually causing pneumonia. *L. pneumophilia* is cultured from the sputum using special media; serologic changes may provide a diagnosis in retrospect.

leishmaniasis (kala-azar). See alternative term.

leprosy. Chronic granulomatous disease caused by *Mycobacterium leprae.* ***Symptoms:*** nasal discharge, dysphagia, hoarseness, skin anesthesia. ***Signs:*** nodules, papules, and macules symmetrically distributed on forehead, cheeks, and ears, generalized lymphadenopathy; persistent neuropathy; ulcerations and deformities. ***Lab.:*** organisms in blood and nasal secretions; false-positive VDRL reaction, anemia.

Leriche's syndrome. Occlusion at the bifurcation of the abdominal aorta, usually from atherosclerosis. ***Symptoms:*** pain or coldness in legs, intermittent claudication, impotence. ***Signs:*** absence of pulses in common iliac, femoral, popliteal, and pedal arteries.

Letterer-Siwe disease. Cause unknown; proliferation of the reticuloendothelial cells. ***Signs:*** febrile disease of young children with generalized lymphadenopathy, hepatomegaly, splenomegaly, maculopapular eruption, ulcerating gums. ***Lab.:*** leukocytosis, hypochromic anemia, thrombocytopenia. ***X-ray:*** destructive lesions in cranial bones.

leukemia, chronic lymphocytic. ***Symptoms:*** weakness, increased fatigability, anorexia, pruritus. ***Signs:*** hepatomegaly, splenomegaly, enlarged lymph nodes, fever. ***Lab.:*** normocytic anemia; leukocytes 10,000 to 500,000 with 80–90% mature lymphocytes; decreased platelets. *X-ray:* enlarged mediastinal nodes. *Bone Marrow:* increased lymphocytes.

leukemia, chronic myelocytic. *Symptoms:* weakness, loss of weight, pain in bones. *Signs:* splenomegaly, hepatomegaly, lymphadenopathy. *Lab.:* increased leukocyte count with increased granulocytes, monocytes; anemia; platelets may be increased. *Bone Marrow:* hypercellularity with myelocytic hyperplasia.

lichen planus. Cutaneous eruption of unknown cause. *Symptoms:* intense pruritus. *Signs:* violaceous papules, small and flat with angular bases; distributed symmetrically on flexural surfaces of forearms, wrists; inner aspects of thighs and knees; lower back; male genitalia. Lesions in mouth.

lipochondrodystrophy. Congenital disorder of lipid metabolism. *Symptoms:* stiff joints. *Signs:* grotesque deformities of head, trunk, and limbs; dwarfism, funnel breast, and corneal opacities; splenomegaly and hepatomegaly; mental retardation. *X-ray:* widened bone shafts; convex vertebrae.

liver, abscess of. Causes: staphylococcus, streptococcus, *Treponema pallidum*, gonococcus, colon bacillus, clostridia, amebas; secondary to cholecystitis, appendicitis, pylephlebitis, empyema thoracis, perforation of peptic ulcer. *Symptoms:* chills and fever, sweating, malaise, anorexia, diarrhea, RUQ pain radiating to shoulder. *Signs:* percussion tenderness over the liver, hepatomegaly, occasionally jaundice. *Lab.:* leukocytosis, possible positive blood culture, SGOT sometimes elevated. *X-ray:* elevated right diaphragm; positive CT scan.

liver, cirrhosis of (Laennec's cirrhosis). See alternative term.

liver, ecchinococcus cyst of (hydatid cyst). *Symptoms:* gradual onset of pain in RUQ, cough, hemoptysis. *Signs:* mass in liver; rarely, hydatid thrill on percussion of mass. *Lab.:* eosinophilia irregularly; scolices in sputum or urine. *X-ray:* cysts visible when walls calcified; positive CT scan.

liver, failure of. *Symptoms:* weakness, lethargy, anorexia. *Signs:* debility, mental blurring to coma; muscle twitching; purpura and hemorrhages, flapping tremor of hands and feet. *Lab.:* azotemia, anemia, hypoprothrombinemia uncorrected by giving vitamin K, procoagulant deficiency, high blood NH_3.

liver, fatty. Fatty infiltration from chronic alcoholism, malnutrition, obesity, chemical poisons. *Symptoms:* anorexia. *Signs:* hepatomegaly, jaundice, collapse, coma. *Lab.:* elevated SGOT, SGPT with necrosis.

liver, primary carcinoma (hepatoma). Frequently arising in a cirrhotic liver. *Signs:* hard nodular localized mass in liver with centrifugal extension; sometimes, overlying peritoneal friction rub. A bruit may be heard in the liver with cancer and alcoholic hepatitis. *Biopsy of Liver:* required for diagnosis. *X-ray:* positive CT scan.

lung, abscess of. Either from primary infection or from infarction or foreign body. *Symptoms:* cough, foul sputum, hemoptysis, chills and fever, night sweats, anorexia, weight loss. *Signs:* localized dullness in lung accompanied by bronchial breathing or absent breath sounds; foul purulent sputum forming layers on standing; clubbing of fingers. *Bronchoscopy:* may visualize foreign body, bronchial stenosis, or neoplasm. *X-ray:* visualizes pulmonary cavity with fluid level and surrounding pneumonitis. *Lab.:* sputum layers on standing; leukocytosis; sputum cultures uninformative.

lung, atelectasis of. Compression of a lung or a more localized region. *Symptoms:* dyspnea, pain in chest, fever. *Signs:* diminished respiratory movements on affected side when entire lobe involved; diminished breath sounds, dullness; tracheal displacement toward affected side if lobe involved. *Lab.:* leukocytosis. *X-ray:* density in lung; shifted mediastinum to affected side; elevated diaphragm on affected side.

lung, emphysema of. Result of long-standing coughing, asthma, or pulmonary fibrosis. *Symptoms:* exertional dyspnea and symptoms of underlying pulmonary disease. *Signs:* barrel chest, hyperresonance, diminished or absent breath sounds and heart sounds; cyanosis; clubbing of fingers. *Lab.:* reduced vital capacity unrelieved by administration of parenteral epinephrine; CO_2 retention in blood; polycythemia. *X-ray:* increased aeration of lungs in advanced cases, although physical signs appear earlier; occasionally emphysematous blebs or bullae; flattened diaphragms.

lungs, fibrosis of. Cause frequently unknown. *Symptoms:* increased fatigability, exertional dyspnea. *Signs:* slight pulmonary hyperresonance with few rales, accentuated P_2, clubbing of fingers. *Lab.:* slight sputum; reduced O_2 diffusion. *X-ray:* interstitial striations in lungs.

lung, infarction of. From pulmonary artery embolism or thrombosis. *Symptoms:* pain in chest, weakness, nausea, sweating, dyspnea. *Signs:* sometimes hemoptysis; area of pulmonary dullness with absent breath sounds; rales; pleural friction rub, cyanosis, mild jaundice. *Lab.:* leukocytosis. *X-ray:* usually an area of increased pulmonary density but only occasionally is it wedge-shaped to be identified as an infarct. *ECG:* changes of pulmonary embolism.

lupus erythematosus, systemic or disseminated. Cause unknown. *Symptoms:* irregular fever, migratory or rheumatoid type arthralgia; pleuritic or abdominal pain. *Signs:* may have butterfly eruption on cheeks of scaling nonpruritic erythematous papules; photosensitivity of skin. *Lab.:* hypochromic anemia; LE cells in blood; positive ANA; hyperglobulinemia; false-positive VDRL reaction; hypocomplimentemia during active disease.

Lyme disease. An immune-mediated inflammatory disease following transmission of a spirochete, *Borrelia burgdorferi,* by the tick *Ioxdes dammini* and involving nerve, heart, and joint tissues weeks to months later. *Symptoms and Signs:* a red macular skin lesion expanding to 20–30 cm with central clearing and induration (*erythema chronicum migrans*) days to weeks after a tick bite may be accompanied by chills, fever, headache, myalgias, stiff neck, malaise. Weeks later, Bell's palsy, pericarditis, arthralgias, lymphadenopathy, and splenomegaly are noted. Months to years later, attacks of arthritis of the knees and other joints lasting for a week may recur for up to 3 years. *Lab.: B. burgdorferi* spirochetes isolated from skin lesion, blood, and CSF; rising antibody titers to *Borrelia;* elevated ESR, leukocytosis, and anemia; negative ANA and rheumatoid factor.

lymphogranuloma venereum. Venereal disease caused by virus of psittacosis-lymphogranuloma group. *Symptoms:* headache, malaise, fever, joint pains. *Signs:* swollen matted adherent regional lymph nodes; bubo near the inguinal ligament; draining fistulas; proctitis; lymphatic obstruction of genitalia. *Lab.:* positive skin test with Frei antigen; complement-fixation test with same antigen.

macroglobulinemia. Proliferation and infiltration of bone marrow, spleen, and liver of plasmacytoid lymphocytes producing excessive quantities of macroglobulins, which in turn lead to increased viscosity of the blood. **Symptoms:** anorexia, malaise, and weakness with nasal, gingival bleeding, exertional dyspnea, and symptoms of heart failure. **Signs:** pallor, petechiae, ecchymoses, retinal hemorrhages, lymphadenopathy, hepatosplenomegaly, edema, and signs of heart failure. **Lab.:** anemia or pancytopenia, rouleau formation, increased sedimentation rate, prolonged bleeding time, plasmacytoid lymphocytes in bone marrow, positive Sia water test, increased plasma IgM on immunoelectrophoresis and ultracentrifugation.

Maffucci's syndrome. Mesodermal dysplasia of unknown cause. **Symptoms:** deformities of hands and feet. **Signs:** purple soft tender tumors in subcutaneous tissue, lips, and palate; pathologic fractures; poorly developed muscles. **X-ray:** cystlike areas in bones of hands and feet, occasionally in long bones, ribs, and vertebrae.

malaria. Disease transmitted by the bite of anopheline mosquitoes infected with *Plasmodium vivax, P. ovale, P. falciparum,* of *P. malariae.* **Symptoms:** abrupt onset of chills and fever, and sweating, preceded by headache and malaise, accompanied or followed by drowsiness and lethargy. **Signs:** fever lasts 1–8 hours; recurrence in 48 hours (*P. vivax*), 72 hours (*P. malariae*), irregularly (*P. falciparum*). During paroxysms the spleen is enlarged and tender. **Lab.:** blood smears taken during paroxysms contain protozoa; often anemia, urobilinuria.

Marchiafava-Micheli syndrome (hemoglobinuria, paroxysmal nocturnal). See alternative term.

Marfan's syndrome (arachnodactyly). Inherited as autosomal dominant. **Signs:** tall, extremely slender build, arm span exceeds height, with spider fingers, pigeon breast or funnel breast, hyperextensibility of joints and ligaments, kyphoscoliosis, hammer toes, long narrow skull, high palate, lenticular subluxations, myopia, cataracts; frequently death from dissecting aortic aneurysm. **Lab.:** homocystinuria; echocardiography demonstrates enlargement of aortic root. **X-ray:** deformities of aorta and pulmonary artery.

Marie-Bamberger syndrome (osteoarthropathy, hypertrophic). See alternative term.

mastoiditis. Pyogenic infection of mastoid process from a transmission of streptococcus or pneumococcus through eustachian tube or from otitis media. *Symptoms:* pain in mastoid, occipital, parietal regions, or in the ear from associated otitis media. *Signs:* swelling and tenderness of tissues behind ear and at the tip of the mastoid process; signs of otitis media by otoscopy. *Lab.:* leukocytosis. *X-ray:* loss of mastoid air cells.

McArdle's disease. Inherited absence of phosphorylase resulting in defective glycogenolysis in muscle. *Symptoms:* muscular cramps induced by lifting, climbing stairs, or running. *Signs:* intermittent myoglobinuria after painful attack. *Lab.:* electromyography reveals absent electrical activity of muscle during cramp; decreased lactate production with exercise. *Biopsy:* excessive muscle glycogen.

measles (rubeola, morbilli). A contagious exanthematous disease caused by the virus *Briareus morbillorum.* *Symptoms:* incubation period about 11 days; then prodrome with fever, malaise, myalgia, photophobia, lacrimation, sneezing, cough. *Signs:* during prodrome: Koplik's white spots on buccal mucosa opposite upper 1st and 2nd molars appearing 48 hours before rash; then blotchy erythematous eruption on face and neck spreading to trunk and limbs; discrete red-brown macules blanching with pressure; fever, cough; sneezing. *Lab.:* lymphocytosis; complement-fixation and neutralization tests may be employed.

measles, German (rubella). See alternative term.

Meig's syndrome. The occurrence of a benign ovarian fibroma may stimulate the production of ascites and pleural effusion. Removal of the tumor causes disappearance of the fluid.

Ménière's disease (labyrinthine hydrops). Swelling of endolymphatic labyrinthine spaces with degeneration of the organ of Corti of unknown cause but frequency of attacks is increased by stress or emotional disturbances in some patients. *Symptoms:* acute attack sometimes preceded by headaches, episodic vertigo, and uneasiness, followed by tinnitus, deafness on one or both sides, nausea, vomiting. *Signs:* nystagmus disappears with vertigo, nerve deafness for low tones early; later, all tones.

meningitis. Caused by viruses or many varieties of bacteria. *Signs:* fever, stiff neck; Kernig's sign, Brudzinski's sign.

Spinal Fluid: increased cell count, high globulin; culture reveals causative organism.

methemoglobinemia. Excessive intake of drugs with amino or nitro groups converts oxyhemoglobin of erythrocytes to methemoglobin that does not carry oxygen. *Symptoms:* headaches, dizziness, and weakness. *Signs:* cyanosis, tachycardia. *Lab.:* blood grossly chocolate-colored; spectroscopy identifies the methemoglobin.

migraine. A vascular disorder of the cerebral vessels, cause unknown. *Symptoms:* unilateral onset of severe headache, later may be bilateral; preceded by short period of depression, irritability, restlessness, voracious appetite; during attack, vomiting, scintillating scotomas, diplopia, and other signs of CNS involvement. *Signs:* facial flushing or pallor; prominence of scalp arteries; appearance of acute illness.

Mikulicz's syndrome. Bilateral painless enlargement of salivary and lacrimal glands, dryness of mouth, decreased lacrimation. Often unexplained, it may be a complication of tuberculosis, leukemia, lymphoma, or sarcoidosis. *X-ray:* sialography may demonstrate dilated salivary ducts.

milk-alkali syndrome (Burnett's syndrome). Hypercalcemia and renal failure developing a few days to several weeks in some patients ingesting large amounts of milk, cream, and calcium carbonate as therapy for peptic ulcer. *Symptoms:* anorexia, nausea, vomiting, irritability, headache, dizziness, and depression. *Signs:* confusion, band (calcific) keratitis, periarticular calcinosis. *Lab.:* hypercalcemia, normal to increased serum phosphate, normal alkaline phosphatase, normal to decreased urinary calcium, mild alkalosis, elevated BUN. *ECG:* shortened Q-T interval.

mitral regurgitation. From rheumatic endocarditis, subacute bacterial endocarditis, or cardiac dilatation and failure from any cause. *Symptoms:* dyspnea, increased fatigability, weakness, cough. *Signs:* harsh medium-pitched pansystolic murmur at apex often obliterating M_1; increased P_2, S_3 frequent; accentuated precordial apical thrust from left ventricular hypertrophy, systolic thrill. *X-ray:* enlarged left atrium and ventricle; definite systolic pulsation in left atrium; regurgitation on cineangiogram. *ECG:* left ventricular hypertrophy, left-axis deviation.

mitral stenosis. From rheumatic endocarditis or congenital anomaly. *Symptoms:* dyspnea, cough, hemoptysis. *Signs:* accentuated precordial thrust of right ventricle; apical low-pitched rumbling middiastolic murmur with presystolic crescendo; the murmur is sharply localized to a small area near the apex; opening snap of mitral valve from a flexible cusp, heard best in 3rd or 4th left interspace close to sternum; accentuated P_2; accentuated M_1, diminished M_2; diastolic thrill often felt; suffused face and lips; loss of crescendo component of diastolic murmur when atrial fibrillation occurs. *X-ray:* left atrial dilatation, straight left ventricular border, esophagus displaced posteriorly; occasionally, calcification of mitral ring. *ECG:* signs of left atrial and right ventricular hypertrophy.

mole, hydatidiform (hydatid mole). Benign proliferation of poorly vascularized chorionic villi in the absence of a fetus. Transformation to choriocarcinoma in 2–10%. *Symptoms:* uterine bleeding during the third or fourth month of pregnancy, hyperemesis, lack of fetal movement. *Signs:* excessive uterine enlargement, no fetal heart tones, ovarian enlargement, abortion. *Lab.:* levels of chorionic gonadotropin greater than in true pregnancy; positive biologic urine pregnancy test.

molluscum contagiosum. Viral infection of the skin. *Signs:* small lobular bodies with slightly umbilicated surfaces of the mucosa of lips and eyelids.

mongolism. (Down syndrome). Congenital disease. *Signs:* moderate to severe mental retardation; small anteroposterior cranial dimension; persistent epicanthus in Caucasians; short flat nose, protruding tongue, broad short neck, protuberant abdomen; short fingers with curved little finger, absent palmar creases. *Lab.:* pathognomonic karyotype, 47 chromosomes with trisomy 21. *X-ray:* small orbits, broad ilia, decreased acetabular angle.

moniliasis. Infection with *Candida albicans*. *Signs:* pruritic eroded areas in mouth, vagina, axillae, inguinal folds, and interdigital surfaces; scaling and crusting. *Lab.:* culture of surface yields *C. albicans*.

mouth, trench (stomatitis gangrenosa). See alternative term.

mucocutaneous lymph node syndrome. This is one of the necrotizing arteritides that is found in infants and children. It is unresponsive to antibiotics. It is accompanied by a *nonsuppu-*

rative lymphadenitis and an *erythema* involving lips, pharynx, and palms; the fingertips desquamate. A congestive *conjunctivitis* is common. Usually the disease is self-limited but 1 to 2% of the cases develop myocarditis, pericarditis, myocardial infarction, and cardiomegaly. About 1% die of coronary arteritis.

mucoviscidosis (pancreas, cystic fibrosis). See alternative term.

multiple myeloma. Cause unknown. *Symptoms:* pains in muscles and bones, weakness, weight loss, pallor. *Signs:* pallor, occasional palpable swellings on accessible bones; pathologic fractures. *Lab.:* normocytic or macrocytic anemia, Bence Jones proteinuria, monoclonal gammopathy; myeloma cells in peripheral blood and marrow; excessive rouleaux of red cells with high ESR. *X-ray:* punched-out lesions of bone, especially in skull; diagnosis sometimes suspected by encountering incidental bone lesions in x-ray examination.

multiple sclerosis. Scattered demyelinization of nervous system, cause unknown. *Symptoms:* visual disturbances, incoordination, myasthenia, paresthesias, loss of sphincter control. *Signs:* personality changes, ataxia, dysarthria, intention tremor, ocular palsies, retrobulbar neuritis; hyperactive deep reflexes, diminished abdominal reflexes, trophic changes in skin. Charcot's triad of signs is intention tremor, nystagmus, and scanning speech (INS). *Spinal Fluid:* increased protein, gamma globulin, mononuclear cells; *Other tests:* prolonged latency after visual evoked response; hypodense plaques of demyelinization on MRI. Visual signs exacerbated by a hot bath (Hot Bath Test).

mumps. A contagious disease caused by a myxovirus. *Symptoms:* incubation period 17–21 days; fever, chills, malaise, anorexia; pain in cheeks with chewing or swallowing, especially sour foods. *Signs:* tenderness at mandibular angle; tender swelling of parotid, submaxillary, and sublingual salivary glands; inflamed ducts, reddened mouth of parotid duct seen in buccal mucosa; orchitis frequent after puberty. *Lab.:* leukocytosis; elevated serum amylase; positive complement fixation.

Münchausen's syndrome. The name is applied to patients who rove from one hospital to another giving fantastically detailed and convincing histories of complicated serious diseases; hence they are submitted to serious diagnostic tests and surgical operations, only to be proved normal. Their motives seem inadequate and are not understood; they leave psychiatrists speechless. Unlike Baron Münchausen, their stories do not seem implausible.

muscular atrophy, progressive. Cause unknown. *Symptoms:* gradual weakness of hand muscles, extending to the arms and legs, unaccompanied by pain or paresthesias. *Signs:* muscular atrophy and fasciculations; absent deep reflexes.

muscular dystrophy, progressive. Hereditary and predominantly in males. *Symptoms:* weakness. *Signs:* gradual onset with waddling gait; lordosis; muscular atrophy around shoulder girdle, pelvis, thighs, and spinal extensors; pseudohypertrophy of calves; muscle wasting; reflexes normal or diminished. *Lab.:* high creatine in serum and urine, elevated SGOT, aldolase.

myasthenia gravis. Autoantibody binding of acetylcholine receptor at neuromuscular junction. *Symptoms:* increased fatigability; transient muscle weakness, diplopia, ptosis; easy fatigue with chewing and talking; regurgitation; dysphagia. *Signs:* lack of facial expression; abnormal speech, aphonia; cranial nerves frequently affected; sometimes cannot lift head from pillow without hand support; ptosis, eventually muscle atrophy. *Test:* weakness temporarily relieved by injection of neostigmine. *X-ray:* thymoma on CT scan in 15%.

myelofibrosis with myeloid metaplasia. Fibrosis or osteosclerosis of bone marrow and extramedullary hematopoiesis, cause unknown. *Symptoms:* weakness, increased fatigability, weight loss, pallor, fullness in LUQ. *Signs:* splenomegaly and hepatomegaly, dependent edema, bone pain, fever. *Lab.:* polycythemia or normochromic anemia with poikilocytosis and anisocytosis; normocytes in peripheral blood; leukocytosis with some myelocytes; thrombocytosis; increased staining of the polymorphs for alkaline phosphatase. *Bone Marrow:* fibrosis in biopsy, dry aspirate. *Liver Biopsy:* islands of extramedullary hematopoiesis. *X-ray:* mottled bone density.

myocardial infarction. Usually caused by acute coronary artery insufficiency in a vessel narrowed by atherosclerosis and followed by thrombosis; rarely arterial embolism is the cause of obstruction. *Symptoms:* sudden prolonged retrosternal pain often radiating to left arm, but also to right arm, neck, or epigastrium; pain not relieved by nitroglycerin; dyspnea, weakness; nausea and vomiting. *Signs:* pallor and sweating; shallow respiration; weakness; fever; often arterial hypotension, cardiac arrhythmias; muted heart sounds with diminished M_1; rales in lungs. *Lab.:* leukocytosis; elevated ESR and CPK. *ECG:* serial tracings show development of elevated S-T segments (injury current), inverted T wave; persisting Q or QS wave; depressed S-T segments.

myoglobinuria. From crushing injuries or severe exercise. *Symptoms:* sweating, weakened limb. *Signs:* hard swollen muscles in limb; recurrent attacks. *Lab.:* myoglobin in urine 8–12 hours after injury, demonstrated by spectroscopy.

myoglobinuria, march (march gangrene). Red urine occurs after long or forced march from trauma to muscles and release of myoglobin. *Lab.:* positive benzidine test of urine with demonstration of absorption band at 581μ with spectroscopic analysis.

myositis. Inflammation of muscle from trauma, or cause unknown. *Symptoms:* muscle pain, chill and fever. *Signs:* weakness, tender edematous muscle; later, shortening and fibrosis, with resulting contracture.

myositis ossificans, progressive. Inherited metabolic disorder. *Symptoms:* limited motion and pain. *Signs:* only voluntary muscles affected; first, the neck and back; swelling and edema; hemorrhage into fibrous tissue; fever. *X-ray:* bony deposits in muscle.

myositis ossificans, traumatic. Bony deposit in traumatized muscles. *Sign:* hard mass in muscle. *X-ray:* shows bony deposit.

myxedema. (hypothyroidism, adult). See alternative term.

narcolepsy. Idiopathic or secondary to head trauma, encephalitis, tumor, cerebrovascular insufficiency. Sudden episodes of somnolence during daytime. Idiopathic form usually occurs in young men and may be associated with cataplexy, sleep paralysis, visual or auditory hallucinations. *Symptoms:* unexpected, inappropriate, and irresistible short spells of sleep. *Signs:* several attacks per day of brief somnolent periods with no deterioration of mentation. *Lab.:* EEG is normal during an attack; rapid eye movements occur at onset of sleep.

nephritis, acute glomerular (glomerulonephritis, acute). See alternative term.

nephritis, chronic glomerular (glomerulonephritis, chronic). See alternative term.

nephritis, salt-losing. An uncommon type of chronic nephritis in which excessive amounts of Na and Cl are excreted in the urine. *Symptoms:* profound asthenia, malaise, anorexia, weight loss, polyuria. *Signs:* dehydration, arterial hypotension, uremic odor on breath. *Lab.:* anemia, urine specific gravity low, albuminuria, hyponatremia, hypochloremia.

nephrotic syndrome. A stage in chronic nephritis, or with unknown cause. *Symptoms:* anorexia, lassitude, vomiting, diarrhea. *Signs:* pallor, peripheral edema usually dependent, normal blood pressure. *Lab.:* proteinuria and cylindruria; hypercholesterolemia, hypoalbuminemia.

neurofibromatosis (Recklinghausen's disease). Congenital or hereditary. *Symptoms:* sometimes radicular pain. *Signs:* multiple soft sessile or pedunculated fleshy tumors distributed along nerve trunks; café-au-lait pigmented macules; occasionally, mental retardation and endocrine disorders. *X-ray:* occasionally, cavitation of bone.

neuropathy, diabetic. Often the result of poor control of diabetes mellitus. *Symptoms:* paresthesias, weakness, pain in limbs. *Signs:* diminished deep reflexes, diminished vibratory sense in the ankles, tender muscles and nerves, postural hypotension. *Lab.:* glycosuria.

neuropathy, median (carpal tunnel syndrome). See alternative term.

Niemann-Pick's disease. Familial deficiency in lipophosphatide metabolism. *Symptoms:* abdominal distention and vomiting in infants. *Signs:* hepatomegaly and splenomegaly, brown skin pigmentation, lymphadenopathy; macular degeneration with cherry spot; black pigmentation of mouth; deafness. *Lab.:* vacuolated monocytes and lymphocytes in peripheral blood; elevated serum lipids. *X-ray:* snowstorm shadows in lungs.

nucleus pulposus, herniated (intervertebral disk, rupture of). See alternative term.

ochronosis (alkaptonuria). Inability to oxidize completely tyrosine and phenylalanine, caused by inheritance of dominant genetic factor with incomplete penetrance. *Signs:* blue color to ears and sclerae, brown or black urine, osteoarthritis. *Lab.:* urine turns black with alkali or on standing; adding ferric chloride turns color deep blue; homogentisic acid present.

orchitis. Inflammation of the testis usually secondary to bacterial infection from urinary tract or from Coxsackie or mumps virus. *Symptoms:* sudden pain in testis radiating to inguinal canal and producing chills, nausea, and vomiting. *Signs:* swollen, tender testis with scrotal edema, hydrocele, and fever.

Osgood-Schlatter's disease (tibial tubercle, osteochondritis of). See alternative term.

Osler's disease (hereditary hemorrhagic telangiectasia). See alternative term.

Osteitis deformans (Paget's disease of bone). Cause unknown. *Symptoms:* bone pain, muscle cramps, impaired hearing, loss of stature. *Signs:* bowing of weight-bearing long bones, kyphosis, shortened spine, enlarged cranium, angioid streaks in retinae. *Lab.:* high serum alkaline phosphatase; normal serum Ca; normal or high serum P. *X-ray:* lessened bone density, thickened skull, patches of dense sclerotic bone.

osteitis fibrosa cystica generalisata (Recklinghausen's disease of bone). Bone changes from excessive parathyroid hormone produced by adenoma, or secondary to acidosis from chronic nephritis. *Symptoms:* anorexia, nausea and vomiting, constipation, asthenia, bone pain. *Signs:* pathologic fractures, bowing of long bones, deformities of spine and sternum. *Lab.:* in hyperparathyroidism, high serum Ca and alkaline phosphatase, low serum P, in acidosis, serum Ca normal or low, high serum P and BUN; CO_2 content low. *X-ray:* general or local decalcification of bone with deformities, sometimes cysts in primary type.

osteoarthritis. Degenerative disease of joints from trauma, wear and tear, and unknown causes. *Symptoms:* joint and muscle pains after rest, relieved by exercise. *Signs:* thickened bone ends, Heberden's nodes, joint crepitus, effusions into joint cavities. *X-ray:* narrowed joint spaces, lipped and spurred margins of articular surfaces and ligaments.

osteoarthropathy, hypertrophic (Marie-Bamberger syndrome). Inflammation of the periosteum, synovial membrane, articular capsule, and subcutaneous tissue produces clubbing of the fingers and toes, chronic periostitis, and arthritis. Cause unknown. Associated with bronchogenic carcinoma, pleural tumors, chronic lung infections, emphysema, cyanotic heart disease, subacute bacterial endocarditis, biliary cirrhosis, ulcerative colitis, regional enteritis, steatorrhea, and myxedema. *Symptoms:* warmth and burning in fingertips, hyperhidrosis of hands and feet, various rheumatic complaints. *Signs:* bilateral clubbing of the nails includes floating nails and loss of the unguophalangeal angle; dusky red, warm skin covers tender swollen knees, ankles, elbows, wrists, metacarpophalangeal joints, or pretibial surface. *X-ray:* flaring of terminal phalanges; osteoporosis; periosteal elevation of long bones; thinning of the cortex.

osteochondrosis (Legg-Calvé-Perthes' disease). Aseptic necrosis of the femoral head during the period of growth. *Symptoms:* pain in bones, limited motion of limbs, limping. *Signs:* slight bone absorption at epiphyseal plate; sclerosis and fissuring of bone.

osteogenesis imperfecta (fragilitas ossium). Congenital and hereditary disease of bone. *Symptoms:* fractures with little pain. *Signs:* exophthalmos, blue sclerae; deformed skull, trunk, limbs; hypermobility of joints. *X-ray:* hypoplastic bone; fracture deformities.

osteomalacia. Inadequate calcification of bone matrix secondary to diminished intestinal absorption of calcium, hypercalciuria, steatorrhea, or renal acidosis. Occurs after epiphyseal closure. Increased osteoblasts. *Symptoms:* anorexia, weight loss, muscular weakness, bone pains. *Signs:* skeletal deformities including skull, spine, and pelvis. *Lab.:* low or normal serum calcium and phosphorus, hypercalciuria, elevated level of alkaline phosphatase. *X-ray:* radiolucency of bone.

osteomyelitis. Infection of haversian canals and subperiosteal space from hematogenous spread or local extension with formation of necrotic bone sequestra; caused by pyogenic organisms, including staphylococcus and streptococcus. *Symptoms:* malaise, bone pain, chills, and feverishness. *Signs:* point tenderness at lesion, redness, edema, warmth, swelling of the limb, fever. *Lab.:* neutrophilic leukocytosis, bacteria cultured from lesion or blood. *X-ray:* bony rarefaction, periosteal elevation, and new bone formation.

osteoporosis. Increased osteoclastic resorption of trabecular and cortical bone with diminished bone density and weakness associated with many conditions including immobilization, malnutrition, senescence, postmenopausal estrogen deficiency, and hypercortisonism. *Symptoms:* back pain, bone pain, and muscular weakness. *Signs:* manifestations of fractures. *Lab.:* normal serum levels of alkaline phosphatase, calcium, and phosphorus. *X-ray:* increased radiolucency of bones, compression fractures of vertebrae, bending of long bones, decreased bone density on CT scan.

otitis media. *Acute*—inflammation and fluid in the middle ear usually following transmission of bacteria through eustachian tube from upper respiratory infection. *Chronic*—perforated tympanic membrane and complications of chronic suppuration, cholesteatoma, mastoiditis, osteomyelitis. *Symptoms: acute*—fever, rhinorrhea, lymphadenopathy, with loss of tympanic membrane's light reflex and later bulging red drum in children; signs not so marked in adults; *chronic*—perforated tympanic membrane and pus with tenderness and swelling of mastoid with complication. *Lab.: acute*—leukocytosis and elevated erythrocyte sedimentation rate.

otosclerosis. Idiopathic ankylosis of stapes to periphery of round window. *Symptoms:* tinnitus and progressive deafness occurring before middle age. *Signs:* evidence of middle ear disease with normal tympanic membrane, patent eustachian tube, and prolonged bone conduction.

ovarian agenesis (gonadal dysgenesis). See alternative term.

ovarian syndrome, bilateral polycystic (Stein-Leventhal syndrome). See alternative term.

Paget's disease of bone (osteitis deformans). See alternative term.

Paget's disease of breast. This is a malignant neoplasm beginning in the nipple. *Symptoms:* slowly progressive burning and pruritus of the nipple. *Signs:* enlargement of the nipple, fissuring, oozing, and ulceration.

Pancoast's syndrome (superior pulmonary sulcus syndrome). Tumor in apex of the lung or upper mediastinum invading brachial plexus and cervical sympathetic chain. *Symptoms:* severe pain in the shoulder and neuritic pain in the arm. *Signs:* weakness and atrophy of arm and hand muscles, Horner's syndrome. *X-ray:* apical lung mass, erosion of T-1 to T-3 ribs and vertebrae, and displaced trachea.

pancreas, cystic fibrosis (mucoviscidosis). Obstruction of pancreatic acini and ducts, cholangioles, and bronchial mucous glands by dried eosinophilic material; inherited as an autosomal recessive trait and associated with malabsorption, cirrhosis, chronic bronchitis, and increased sodium and chloride concentrations in the sweat of children and young adults. *Symptoms:* abdominal cramps and diarrhea yielding bulky foul-smelling stools, weight loss; dyspnea, productive cough; collapse in hot environment. *Signs:* retarded growth and cachexia; abdominal distention; viscid tenacious secretions. *Lab.:* increased sweat chloride estimated by noting degree of whiteness of palm print in an agar plate containing silver nitrate (patients have sweat chloride in excess of 60 mEq/L); decreased trypsin content causes stool to fail to dissolve gelatin on a piece of x-ray film. *X-ray:* obstructive emphysema and/or patchy atelectasis.

pancreas, islet-cell tumor of (insuloma). Episodic hypoglycemia precipitated by fasting or exercise. *Symptoms:* hunger, sweating, anxiety, headache, irritability, nausea, vertigo, syncope. *Signs:* pale, moist skin, tachycardia, speech impairment, hypothermia, incoordination. *Lab.:* persistent fasting blood sugar levels below 50 mg/100 mL, positive tolbutamide test, leucine sensitivity, elevated insulin levels, and flat oral glucose tolerance test curve.

pancreatitis, acute hemorrhagic. Parenchymatous extravasation of lytic pancreatic enzymes, cause unknown. *Symptom:* sudden excruciating epigastric pain referred to back or chest, with nausea and vomiting. *Signs:* abdominal distention, diminished or absent bowel sounds; jaundice; may be shock and death. *Lab.:* may be glycosuria and hyperglycemia; leukocytosis; high serum amylase during first day of attack.

pancreatitis, acute interstitial. Accompanying acute alcoholism, infections, and undefined disorders. *Symptoms:* vague epigastric discomfort or pain, bloating of the abdomen, nausea and vomiting, jaundice, prostration. *Signs:* abdominal distention, palpable firm mass under the pancreas. *Lab.:* leukocytosis; transiently elevated serum amylase; transient glycosuria.

pancreatitis, chronic. Chronic inflammation with pancreatic insufficiency, often associated with chronic cholecystitis. *Symptoms:* recurrent epigastric pain, nausea and vomiting, weight loss, diarrhea. *Signs:* abdominal distention, jaundice. *Lab.:* increased serum amylase, lipase, blood sugar; stools have foul odor and float in water. *Test:* administration of secretin may not stimulate pancreatic secretion into the duodenum.

paralysis agitans (Parkinson's disease). Lesion in the basal ganglion often from atherosclerosis or unknown cause. *Signs:* stooped posture, masklike facies, monotonous tone in speech; rest tremor of hands (pill rolling), arms, lips, eyelids; propulsive gait (festination), cogwheel rigidity of limbs.

paresis, syphilitic (dementia paralytica). See alternative term.

Parkinson's disease (paralysis agitans). See alternative term.

pellagra. Deficiency of nicotinic acid. *Symptoms:* anorexia, weight loss, weakness, burning tongue, diarrhea, mental depression. *Signs:* red-brown erythematous scaling dermatitis of glove and stocking distribution; erythematous oral mucosa; fiery red tongue; later bullous skin eruption with pigmentation; tremors, paralyses, psychosis. *Lab.:* normocytic or macrocytic anemia. *Test:* striking amelioration of symptoms and signs within 24 hours after administration of nicotinic acid.

pemphigus vulgaris. Cause unknown. *Symptoms:* skin blisters, pruritus, malaise. *Signs:* generalized bullous eruption on the skin with erythematous base; depression; death.

peptic ulcer. Ulcer of the stomach or duodenum, cause unknown. *Symptoms:* epigastric pain when stomach is empty, relieved by food or alkalis. *Signs:* usually point tenderness somewhere in the midline of the epigastrium. *Lab.* increased concentration of HCl in gastric contents; feces may contain occult blood. *Gastroscopy:* gastric ulcers usually visualized. *X-ray:* with barium meal, an ulcer niche, sometimes a crater, may be seen; spastic or deformed duodenal bulb; delayed gastric emptying.

periarteritis nodosa (polyarteritis nodosa). See alternative term.

pericarditis, acute. Caused by rheumatic fever; infections with pneumococcus, streptococcus, staphylococcus; uremia; myocardial infarction; trauma. *Symptoms:* sharp or dull precordial pain radiating to neck, shoulders, arms, or epigastrium accentuated by swallowing; dyspnea. *Signs:* fever, pericardial friction rub obliterated by effusion; effusion causes increased area of cardiac dullness, muffled heart sounds, cyanosis, paradoxic pulse. *Lab.:* leukocytosis, effusion demonstrated with ultrasonography. *ECG:* elevated S-T segments in all leads except for reciprocal depression in aV_r; T-wave flattened; diminished voltages of QRS.

pericarditis, constrictive. Cause frequently unknown. *Symptoms:* exertional dyspnea. *Signs:* engorged jugular veins, hepatomegaly, ascites, edema of the legs, pleural effusion, cyanosis, paradoxical pulse, low arterial pressure. *Tests:* prolonged circulation time; high venous pressure; low vital capacity. *ECG:* low voltage in QRS, flattened or inverted T-waves in I and II, notched P waves. *X-ray:* normal or enlarged cardiac shadow; calcium in pericardium; diminished pulsations; distinguished from effusion by ultrasound examination.

pernicious anemia. Anemia caused by atrophy of gastric mucosa and lack of Castle intrinsic factor. *Symptoms:* weakness, numbness and tingling of digits, sore tongue and mouth, constipation or diarrhea, anorexia. *Signs:* pallor, lemon-yellow color to skin, reddened tongue with smoothing caused by papillary atrophy, hepatosplenomegaly, pallanesthesia in legs, possibly peripheral neuritis, positive Romberg's sign, positive Babinski reflex, deep reflexes accentuated or diminished. *Lab.:* macrocytic anemia with poikilocytes and anisocytes, hyperchromia, granulopenia with increased lobulation of polymorphonuclear cells; high mean corpuscular hemoglobin; no reticulocytosis, without treatment; indirect hyperbilirubinemia. *Tests:* achlorhydria after histamine stimulation; Schilling's test shows diminished absorption of B_{12} labeled with ^{60}Co. Reticulocytosis 4–5 days after injection of B_{12}.

peroneal muscular atrophy (Charcot-Marie-Tooth disease). A hereditary disease of unknown cause. *Symptoms:* foot drop, pain, weakness, numbness, paresthesias of lower limbs. *Signs:* slowly progressive; clawfoot and foot drop, from weak Peronei, Tibialis anterior, Extensor longus digitorum; absent deep reflexes; cutaneous hypesthesia; slapping gait, forearm may be affected.

pertussis (whooping cough). Contagious respiratory disease caused by *Bordetella pertussis*. *Symptoms:* incubation period

7–14 days; gradual onset with rhinitis, sneezing, lacrimation. *Signs:* cough, gradually becoming more severe and developing characteristic inspiratory whoop, often followed by vomiting; cyanosis; fine rales in lungs; slight fever. *Lab.:* lymphocytosis; organism grown on culture plates exposed to patient's cough.

Peutz-Jehger's syndrome (intestinal polyposis). See alternative term.

pheochromocytoma (hypertension, paroxysmal). See alternative term.

pica. Unusual craving or appetite leading to the ingestion of unnatural foods such as clay, chips of old paint, plaster, laundry starch, etc. *Symptoms:* depend on substance eaten; ingestion of paint may cause lead poisoning; ingestion of laundry starch may cause obesity and hypochromic anemia.

pityriasis rosea. A skin eruption probably caused by a virus. *Symptoms:* skin rash, pruritus, lasting about 6–10 weeks. *Signs:* initial lesion on trunk; 4–10 days later, salmon-colored lesions with raised border and fine scale appear on trunk and limbs; occasionally papules or wheals.

placenta, abruptio. Premature separation of the placenta secondary to trauma, toxemia, or unknown cause. *Symptoms:* sudden onset of severe abdominal pain succeeded by a dull ache, vaginal bleeding, increased fetal activity, after the middle of gestation. *Signs:* firm tender enlarged uterine mass, diminished or irregular fetal heart tones, pale, cold, moist extremities, tachycardia, and shock. *Lab.:* anemia, hypofibrinogenemia from disseminated intravascular coagulation.

plasma thromboplastin component deficiency (factor IX deficiency). See alternative term.

pleurisy, fibrinous. Pleural irritation from pneumonia, pulmonary infarction, neoplasm, tuberculosis, fungi, or other causes. *Symptoms:* dull to sharp pain in one hemithorax, accentuated by respiratory movements or cough; diaphragmatic pleurisy produces pain in shoulder or abdomen; often fever and malaise. *Signs:* often none; sometimes pleural friction rub that can be heard and felt. *Lab.:* no distinguishing features. *X-ray:* no signs except diminished respiratory movements on affected side.

pleurodynia, epidemic (Bornholm disease, epidemic myalgia, Devil's grip, Dabney grip). Acute infection with Coxsackie

B virus. *Symptoms:* sudden seizure of sharp epigastric and rib pain accentuated by movement, after 2–14 days' incubation. Severe headache may accompany morning and evening fevers. *Signs:* pleural friction rub occurs in 25% of patients; mild pharyngeal infection, nonproductive cough, and transitory erythematous rashes occur in some. *Lab.:* virus isolated from throat and feces, positive complement fixation, and rising specific neutralizing antibodies.

Plummer-Vinson syndrome (sideropenic dysphagia). Postcricoid esophageal web sometimes present in women with severe iron deficiency. *Symptoms:* dysphagia, sore tongue, and dry mouth. *Signs:* cheilitis, erythematous buccal mucosa and tongue, spoon-shaped nails, and splenomegaly. *X-ray:* anterior displacement of barium by weblike stricture in upper esophagus.

pneumonia. Bacterial or viral infection causing consolidation of lung. *Symptoms:* chills, fever, cough, rust-colored sputum; pain in chest. *Signs:* appearance of serious acute illness; tachypnea or labored breathing; region of dullness in lung with early suppressed breath sounds, later bronchial breathing and crepitant rales; cyanosis. *Lab.:* leukocytosis. *X-ray:* increased density of parenchyma, often with lobar distribution.

pneumoperitoneum. Air in the peritoneal cavity from perforation of a viscus or therapeutic instillation. *Signs:* tympanitic abdomen with absent bowel sounds. *X-ray:* shows air between viscera.

pneumothroax. Air in the pleural cavity from rib fracture, rupture of an emphysematous bleb, bronchopleural fistula, or thoracentesis. *Symptoms:* when spontaneous, sudden onset with pain in affected side radiating to neck; often severe dyspnea and cyanosis. *Signs:* resonant hemithorax with absent breath sounds and tactile fremitus; if much air, trachea and heart shifted to unaffected side. *X-ray:* films of chest are diagnostic.

poliomyelitis, acute. Infection of gray matter of the spinal cord by poliomyelitis virus, types I, II, or III. *Symptoms:* headache, sore throat, stiff neck, pain in the back and limbs, inability to move one or more muscle groups. *Signs:* varying deep reflexes; hyperesthesia, paresthesia; lymphadenopathy; Kernig's and Brudzinski's signs present. *Lab.:* leukocytosis;

tissue cultures of virus from oropharynx, feces, or blood; neutralizing and complement-fixing antibodies in serum. *Spinal Fluid:* no specific findings; pleocytosis; increased protein.

polyarteritis nodosa (periarteritis nodosa). A chronic disease of vascular walls; cause unknown. *Symptoms:* anorexia, weight loss, abdominal pain, migratory or chronic arthritis, muscle pains, increased fatigability. *Signs:* fever; nodular swellings (palpable purpura) on arteries; peripheral neuritis; arterial hypertension. *Lab.:* leukocytosis, sometimes eosinophilia, hematuria, proteinuria. Biopsy of arterial segment confirms the diagnosis.

polycythemia vera. Cause unknown. *Symptoms:* headache, weakness, paresthesias, pruritus after bathing. *Signs:* flushed face, cyanotic mucosa, splenomegaly, hepatomegaly; engorgement of retinal veins. *Lab.:* increased hematocrit; increased leukocyte and platelet counts; increased blood volume and erythrocyte mass; hypercellular bone marrow; elevated leukocyte alkaline phosphatase; normal arterial oxygen saturation.

polyneuritis. Involvement of multiple peripheral nerves from action of alcohol, lead, arsenic, carbon monoxide, infections, bacterial toxins; occurs also in gout, diabetes mellitus, vitamin deficiencies. *Symptoms:* burning pain, hyperesthesia, anesthesia, paresthesia, muscle weakness, muscle cramps. *Signs:* loss of function of various motor and sensory nerves; tenderness of nerves accessible to palpation, flaccid paralysis; diminished or absent deep reflexes; trophic changes in the skin.

polyneuritis, acute idiopathic (Guillain-Barré syndrome). Cause unknown, probably autoimmune. *Symptoms:* ascending motor weakness with pain in back and limbs; headache, numbness and tingling, nausea and vomiting. *Signs:* slight fever; ascending flaccid paralysis; diminished deep and superficial reflexes; involvement of cranial nerves with dysphasia, dysphagia, dysarthria. *Spinal Fluid:* increased protein; normal cell count.

porphyria. The types are acute, intermittent, congenital, and cutanea tarda (consult textbooks for distinction). *Symptoms:* nausea and vomiting; abdominal pain; muscle spasm. *Signs:* peripheral neuritis, photosensitization of skin, skin pigmentation. *Urine:* contains either porphobilinogen, uroporphyrin I and III, or coproporphyrin I and III.

postgastrectomy syndrome ("dumping syndrome"). Postprandial jejunal distention with consequent reflex activity, hypermotility, and vasodilation. *Symptoms:* profound weakness, giddiness, warmth, sweating, palpitation, pallor, epigastric distress, nausea, and diarrhea occur at the end of a meal. *Signs:* flushing or pallor, sweating, and occasionally syncope. *Lab.:* reproduction of symptoms when hypertonic solutions are given by gastric tube; rapid gastric emptying on fluoroscopy.

Pott's disease (spine, tuberculosis of). See alternative term.

preeclampsia. Toxemia of pregnancy of unknown cause occurring during the end of gestation. *Symptoms:* headache, sudden weight gain, and visual disturbances developing during the last trimester of pregnancy. *Signs:* hypertension, spasm of retinal arterioles, and edema of eyelids, ankles, and hands. *Lab.:* proteinuria.

pregnancy, tubal or ectopic. *Symptoms:* unilateral or generalized abdominal pain. *Signs:* softened cervix uteri; tender palpable mass in region of ovarian tube. Uterine curettage yields decidual cells, but no chorionic villi.

proctalgia fugax. A neuralgia characterized by episodic sudden sharp pains high in the rectum.

prostate, carcinoma. Adenocarcinoma commonly involving posterior lobe and commonly associated with benign hyperplasia, of unknown etiology. *Symptoms:* asymptomatic until late when dysuria, frequency, urinary retention and suprapublic fullness, perineal pain, bone pain, and weight loss may supervene. *Signs:* small hard nodule on posterior lobe by rectal examination, later, rock-hard asymmetric fixed gland. *Lab.:* cytology or biopsy positive, increased serum acid phosphatase with metastasis, increased residual urine and BUN with urethral obstruction. *X-ray:* osteoblastic metastases to lumbar vertebrae, pelvic bones, femoral heads.

prostatitis. Pyogenic or other infection of the prostate from gonorrhea (less frequently), instrumentation, or hematogenous spread from remote abscess. *Symptoms: acute*—urgency, frequency, dysuria, chills, and perineal pain; *chronic*—fatigue, irritability, backache, gross hematuria and decreased sexual potency. *Signs: acute*—enlarged, tender, boggy prostate, fever, urethral discharge and/or urinary retention; *chronic*—prostate may become indurated. **Lab.:** pyuria, bacteriuria, hematuria, mucus shreds in terminal specimen of three-glass urine test.

pseudopancreatic cyst (pancreatic cyst, false). An accumulation of fluid in the lesser peritoneal cavity resulting from pancreatitis and the lytic action of the enzymes. *Symptoms:* epigastric pain, backache, nausea. *Signs:* rounded mass in the epigastrium; fever; weight loss. *Lab.:* demonstrated with ultrasonography, fat in the feces. *X-ray:* stomach and duodenum displaced anteriorly by a posterior mass; may be calcium in the cyst wall; positive CT scan.

pseudoxanthoma elasticum. Hereditary disease of unknown cause with degeneration of collagen and elastic fibers. *Symptoms:* intermittent claudication, increased fatigability, diminished vision. *Signs:* loose skin without resiliency; drooping ears; flat yellow plaques in the skin of the neck, axillae, and thighs; angioid streaks in the retina. *X-ray:* calcified arteries.

psoriasis. Chronic skin disease of unknown cause. *Symptoms:* mild pruritus. *Signs:* brown papules and plaques with silvery scales covering a bright red surface dotted with bleeding points.

pulmonary sulcus syndrome, superior (Pancoast's syndrome). See alternative term.

pulseless disease of Takayasu (arterial thrombosis due to infection). See alternative term.

purpura, autoimmune thrombocytopenic (purpura hemorrhagica). Bleeding into the skin and other tissues from deficiency of blood platelets. *Symptoms:* easy bruising; menorrhagia; excessive bleeding from trauma. *Signs:* petechiae and ecchymoses in the skin, especially over the legs. *Lab.:* low platelet counts, prolonged bleeding time; megakaryocytosis in bone marrow; increased platelet IgG.

purpura, capillary (Henoch-Schoenlein's purpura). An allergic response. *Symptoms:* headache, anorexia, vomiting, abdominal pain, arthralgia. *Signs:* irregular fever; rash resembling erythema multiforme. *Lab.:* increased capillary fragility (Rumpel-Leede test), eosinophilia.

pyelonephritis. Bacterial infection of the kidney predisposed by ureteral obstruction. *Symptoms:* sudden chills, fever, abdominal pain, backache, nausea and vomiting; pain with urination. *Signs:* fever, costovertebral angle tenderness; enlarged tender kidney; abdominal muscle spasm. *Lab.:* urine contains pus, erythrocytes, and bacteria. *X-ray:* dilatation of ureter and calyces; irregular narrowing of renal pelves, sometimes ureteral obstruction.

pyloric obstruction. Often from scarring of duodenal ulcer. *Symptoms:* vomiting of undigested food taken many hours before; weight loss; gastric discomfort. *Signs:* increased area of dullness in LUQ, succussion splash in stomach; sometimes epigastric mass; visible epigastric peristaltic wave. *X-ray:* gastric dilatation; delayed emptying time of stomach; narrowing of pylorus.

quartan fever. Chills and fever every third day from paroxysms caused by infection with *Plasmodium malariae.*

quotidian fever. Daily malarial paroxysms of chills and fever from infection with two strains of *Plasmodium vivax* maturing on alternate days.

rabies. Caused by neurotropic virus transmitted by the bite of infected mammals. *Symptoms:* local radiating dysthesia, malaise, nausea, sore throat; later restlessness and hallucinations. *Signs:* inflammation of wound with hyperesthesia; later dysarthria, dysphagia for fluids, convulsions, delirium, opisthotonos stimulated by lights or noises; shallow irregular breathing; hoarseness, aphonia; hyperactive deep reflexes; nuchal rigidity; Babinski's sign; flaccid paralysis, and death. *Lab.:* Saliva contains virus but diagnosis more quickly made by observing captured live animal that caused the wound, or microscopic examination of brain and spinal cord of the dead animal.

rat-bite fever, spirillary (sodoku). Acute infection of *Spirillum minus* transmitted by rat bite. *Symptoms:* pain at the site of the bite, malaise, chills, and relapsing fever of 2 to 4 days' duration occur 1 to 6 weeks after a rat bite. *Signs:* regional lymphadenitis, arthritis, fever, and asymmetric skin eruption are reported. *Lab.: Spirillum minus* seldom found in blood or tissue with dark-field examination but may be demonstrated after incubation in mice following administration of infected blood intraperitoneally. Leukocytes are normal or elevated and normochromic anemia may develop. Biologic false-positive tests for syphilis occur frequently.

Raynaud's disease and phenomenon. Cold fingers and hands after exposure to cold, of unknown cause (disease) or associated with cryoproteinemia, systemic lupus erythematosus, migraine, scleroderma, obliterative arterial disease, carpal tunnel syndrome, cervical arthritis, trauma from use of crutches or jack hammer, or lead poisoning (phenomenon). *Symptoms:* numb, cold, tingling, aching fingers after exposure to cold. *Signs:* begins in young adults with involvement of tips of fingers, later moving proximally to affect hands; attack starts with pallor and sweating and progresses to cyanosis with pain and then redness associated with tingling, throbbing, and edema over a 15- or 60-minute period; rarely, gangrene of the fingers supervenes.

Recklinghausen's disease (neurofibromatosis). See alternative term.

Reiter's syndrome. Triad of arthritis, conjunctivitis, and urethritis; cause unknown. *Symptoms:* fever, pain and swelling of joints, burning on urination, lacrimation and burning of the conjunctiva. *Signs:* arthritis of fingers, knees, ankles, and feet with vesicles and hyperkeratoses over affected joints; transient urethritis with seropurulent discharge; conjunctivitis. *Lab.:* leukocytosis, hematuria, or proteinuria.

relapsing fever. Infection with the spirochete *Borrelia recurrentis* or related types, transmitted by the bite of ticks or lice. *Symptoms:* initial attack from 2 to 8 days of sustained high fever beginning with chills; involution by crisis, then remission of 3 to 10 days, with relapse of various lengths; occasionally more relapses; headache, muscle and joint pains, nausea and vomiting; abdominal pain. *Signs:* profuse sweating; erythematous rash; petechiae; splenomegaly; hepatomegaly; jaundice; epistaxis. *Lab.:* large spirochetes seen with light microscope in wet blood preparation.

renal amyloidosis. One cause of the nephrotic syndrome consisting of proteinuria, cylindruria, hypoproteinemia, peripheral edema, and ascites; hypercholesterolemia. A specific cause can be diagnosed only by establishing the existence of systemic amyloidosis.

renal artery stenosis. Usually from atherosclerosis, the diminished renal circulation may cause arterial hypertension. The stenotic artery may produce a bruit to the left and above the umbilicus; this should lead to arteriography and demonstration of the stenosis; sometimes surgical repair and cure of the hypertension are possible.

Rendu-Osler-Weber syndrome (telangiectasia, hereditary hemorrhagic). See alternative term.

rheumatic fever. Cause unknown. *Symptoms:* migratory pains in joints and muscles; malaise, anorexia, weight loss, sweats, nosebleeds, precordial or abdominal pain. *Signs:* red, hot, swollen, tender large joints, with migration of inflammation from one to another, erythema marginatum, choreiform movements, subcutaneous nodules over bony prominences, pericardial friction rub, apical systolic murmur radiating to the axilla. Symptoms and signs show marked amelioration from administration of salicylates. *Lab.:* leukocytosis, elevated ESR; ASO titer; high serum C-reactive protein; beta-hemolytic streptococci in nose and throat cultures. *ECG:* prolongation of P-R interval.

rhinitis (coryza). Inflammation of nasal mucosa. *Symptoms:* dryness of nasal mucosa, conjunctivae, and soft palate followed by sneezing, nasal discharge, nasal obstruction, and concluding with purulent nasal discharge. *Signs:* erythematous nasal mucosa with discharge.

rickets (infantile osteomalacia). Vitamin D deficiency occurring before epiphyseal closure. *Symptoms:* restlessness, frequent crying, sweating. *Signs:* muscular atony and weakness, pot belly, scoliosis, craniotabes, Parrot's bosses, rachitic rosary, Harrison's grooves, contracted pelvis, genu valgum or varus, delayed and defective dentition. *Lab.:* subnormal serum calcium and phosphorus, increased serum alkaline phosphatase. *X-ray:* osteoporosis, cupping of diaphyses of long bones, lateral spurs and hollowed ends, late.

right subclavian artery, aberrant. Anomalous development with right subclavian artery formed on left side of aortic arch and crossing midline to right arm behind or in front of the esophagus. This produces difficulty in swallowing, *dysphagia lusoria,* that prompts an esophagram showing the indentation of the esophagus made by the transverse aberrant artery.

right-to-left shunt in the heart. Blood flow through a defect in the interatrial or interventricular septum through which blood goes from the right to the left side.

right ventricular wall aneurysm. A bulging of the right ventricular wall caused by thinning from an infarction or trauma. Palpation over the precordium often yields a palpable impulse in the area of right ventricular projection on the chest wall. Lateral or oblique x-ray projections may show the bulge.

Rocky Mountain spotted fever. Infection caused by *Rickettsia rickettsii* from the bite of the wood tick. *Symptoms:* chills, anorexia, malaise, headache; sudden pains in the limbs. *Signs:* fever, red or hemorrhagic maculopapules on wrists and ankles, spreading generally; cyanosis, splenomegaly. *Lab.:* leukopenia; complement-fixing antibodies; Felix-Weil reaction with Proteus OX-19.

rubella (measles, German). A contagious exanthematous viral disease. *Symptoms:* incubation period 14–21 days; fever, malaise, headache, myalgia, joint pains, coryza. *Signs:* abrupt fever with tender palpable postauricular and postoccipital lymph nodes; faint macular rash on face, extending to trunk and limbs, quite evanescent. *Lab.:* leukopenia, lymphocytosis.

rubeola (measles). See alternative term.

salicylate poisoning. *Symptoms:* headache, dizziness, tinnitus, hearing loss, mental confusion, sweating, nausea and vomiting, upper abdominal discomfort. *Signs:* fever, sweating, hyperpnea, tetany, convulsions, delirium, coma. *Lab.:* low serum CO_2 content, high serum pH, hyperglycemia. Urinary salicylates demonstrated by adding ferric chloride that produces purple color persisting after boiling (acetone gives similar color that disappears with boiling).

salivary duct calculi (sialolithiasis). *Symptoms:* dry mouth, recurrent sudden swelling of salivary gland while eating; pain. *Signs:* palpable stones in the ducts. *X-ray:* calculi may be demonstrated on plain films or after injection of opaque medium into the ducts.

salpingitis, acute. Usually caused by the gonococcus, it may also occur from streptococci, staphylococci, or tubercle bacilli. *Symptoms:* fever and lower abdominal pain. *Signs:* swollen tender ovarian tube with purulent exudate from the cervix. *Lab.:* organisms may be found in the cervical discharge by direct staining of smears or by culture.

sarcoidosis. A granulomatous disease of unknown cause. *Symptoms:* may be asymptomatic; weight loss, malaise, night sweats. *Signs:* may be fever; swelling of lymph nodes; uveitis and noncaseating granuloma of the conjunctiva; and involvement of, salivary glands, lungs, liver, kidneys, spleen, bones. *Lab.:* leukopenia, eosinophilia, monocytosis; microcytic hypochromic anemia; hypergammaglobulinemia; high serum alkaline phosphatase; hypercalcemia with normal serum P. Biopsy needed. *X-ray:* Great hilar lymphadenopathy bilaterally; translucent lesions in bones.

scarlet fever. Pharyngitis from beta-hemolytic streptococci with toxin production. *Symptoms:* excruciating sore throat, vomiting, malaise. *Signs:* brilliant red edematous pharynx with gray or white exudate or membrane; cervical adenopathy; tongue becomes denuded and beefy red; maculopapular erythematous blanching eruption on neck, axillae, groin, later generalized. After the rash, desquamation begins around the nails. *Lab.:* leukocytosis, proteinuria. *Throat Cultures:* beta-hemolytic streptococci.

Schamberg's disease (progressive pigmentary dermatosis). A benign chronic disorder, cause unknown, with repeated crops of petechiae on feet and legs that leave pigment spots of hemosiderin.

schistosomiasis. Infestation with *Schistosoma haematobium* as blood flukes, or *S. japonicum* and *S. mansoni* in intestinal venules; *S. haematobium* is found in plexuses of the bladder and pelvis; eggs migrate into liver, lung, and CNS. *Symptoms:* painful urination, malaise, lassitude. *Signs:* fever, urticaria, fibrous nodules in perineum; pedunculated papillomas in urethral orifice. *Cystoscopic Examination:* papillomas at trigone; reduced bladder capacity; calculi in ureters, renal pelves, bladder; rectovesical fistulas. *Lab.:* leukocytosis, eosinophilia, hematuria; ova in stools, occasionally in urine.

scleroderma. Collagen disease of unknown cause. *Symptoms:* gradual onset with anorexia, dyspnea, dysphagia, reduced sweating, arthralgias. *Signs:* slight fever, contracted skin with immobility and deformity in symmetric distribution; muscular weakness; limited chest expansion and opening of jaws. *Lab.:* no distinguishing finding.

scurvy. Deficiency in vitamin C (ascorbic acid). *Symptoms:* lassitude, irritability, anorexia, tenderness in gums, bone pains. *Signs:* rough, pigmented skin; hyperkeratotic follicles on lower limbs; perifollicular erythema and hemorrhages; swollen bleeding gums; tender shins. *Lab.:* diminished leukocyte and plasma concentration of vitamin C, anemia, reticulocytosis, increased capillary fragility with the Rumpel-Leede test. *X-ray:* ground-glass cortex in growing bone; white line on shaft ends; subperiosteal elevation from hemorrhages.

seizures, major motor (epilepsy, grand mal). See alternative term.

seizures, minor or absence (epilepsy, petit mal). See alternative term.

septicemia. Persistent growth of bacteria in the bloodstream. *Symptoms:* chills and fever; malaise. *Signs:* petechiae, purpura, metastatic abscesses, splenomegaly. *Lab.:* proteinuria, hematuria; blood cultures yield the infecting organism.

serum sickness. Allergic manifestation several days after injection of foreign protein or sensitizing drugs. *Symptoms:* pruritus, fever, malaise, nausea, vomiting, abdominal pain, arthralgia. *Signs:* fever, urticaria, erythematous rash, lymphadenopathy; swollen tender joints.

seven-day fever (dengue). See alternative term.

Sheehan's syndrome. Hypopituitarism secondary to pituitary necrosis because of hemorrhage and shock during delivery. *Symptoms:* failure of lactation, amenorrhea, lethargy, sensitivity to cold, diminished sweating. *Signs:* fine wrinkling of the skin, hair loss, depigmentation of the skin and areolae, mammary and genital atrophy. *Lab.:* diminished levels of pituitary and end-organ hormones, anemia, hypoglycemia, decreased urinary 17-ketosteroids and corticosteroids.

sialolithiasis (salivary duct calculi). See alternative term.

sick sinus syndrome. This includes a group of cardiac dysrhythmias having dysfunction of the sinoatrial node (NA: *sinuatrialis*) in common. Initially the list of disorders included bradycardias (sinus bradycardia, sinoatrial block, sinus arrest) with or without the tachycardias (tachycardia-bradycardia syndrome), to which has been added: severe sinus bradycardia, sinus arrest of varying intervals followed by atrial or junctional escape rhythms or cardiac arrest; generally there is an accompanying slow ventricular rate not due to digitalis; inability to resume sinus rhythm after conversion from atrial fibrillation; sinoatrial block not drug-induced. *Symptoms:* Adams-Stokes attacks, dizziness, and cerebrovascular accidents. *Signs:* the cardiovascular signs of one or more of the dysrhythmias of the aforementioned group (it is important to realize that the rhythm with which the patient presented may change to another in the group at any time); a minimal response of the heart rate to isometric exercise in bed; gentle carotid artery massage causes abrupt sinus arrest of 3 seconds; small increase in heart rate to Valsalva maneuver and small blood pressure overshoot afterward.

sickle-cell anemia. Inheritance of abnormal hemoglobin S. *Symptoms:* asymptomatic; or fever, malaise, headache, epistaxis, pains in legs and abdomen. *Signs:* tower skull, short trunk, thoracic kyphosis, abdominal and bone tenderness; pallor; yellow-green sclerae, cardiomegaly, hepatomegaly, splenomegaly; ulcers on shins. *Lab.:* anemia with immature circulating erythrocytes; sickling of anoxic erythrocytes; Howell-Jolly bodies in red cells; decreased osmotic fragility of red cells. *X-ray:* ground-glass appearance to skull; thickening and radial structure of diploë; cortical thickening; patchy medullary bone formation.

silicosis. Pulmonary fibrosis and inflammation from crystalline silica. *Symptoms:* exertional dyspnea, cough, sputum. *Signs:* barrel chest, hyperresonant lungs, diminished breath sounds; possibly a few rales. *Lab.:* discrete nodules in lungs, coalescence, fibrosis, and cavitation.

Simmonds' disease (hypopituitarism syndrome). Destruction of pituitary gland by tumor, injury, or granuloma, leading to progressive pituitary insufficiency and atrophy of thyroid, adrenal cortex, and gonads. *Symptoms:* cold intolerance; weakness, nausea and vomiting; impotence and amenorrhea. *Signs:* hypothermia, bradycardia, hypotension, atrophy of skin, pallor, hypotonia, areolar depigmentation, loss of axillary and pubic hair, atrophy of sex organs. *Lab.:* tests indicative of thyroid hypofunction, including decrease in circulating thyroid hormone and uptake of radioactive iodine; hypoglycemia, flat glucose tolerance curve, reduced ability to excrete a water load, positive response to ACTH, decreased excretion of urinary corticosteroids, anemia. *X-ray:* erosion of clinoid processes, calcified craniopharyngioma, enlarged sella turcica on radiograph or CT scan.

sinusitis. Bacterial, viral, or allergic inflammation of sinus mucosa with impaired drainage due to edema. *Symptoms:* aching over affected sinus accentuated by coughing or straining. More severe symptoms include pain over sinus, toothache, anorexia, photophobia, and malaise; chronic involvement may produce recurrent headache and pain over maxillary, frontal, retro-orbital, nasal, occipital, or nuchal regions. *Signs:* tenderness over sinuses, fever, and periorbital edema. *Tests:* leukocytosis, absent or diminished transillumination of sinus. *X-ray:* diminished radiolucency of sinus, fluid level.

Sjögren's syndrome (keratoconjunctivitis sicca syndrome). See alternative term.

smallpox (variola). A contagious exanthematous disease caused by a virus; declared eradicated 8 May 1980. *Symptoms:* incubation period 10–14 days; sudden onset with headache, chills, prostration. *Signs:* transient erythematous or petechial macular rash on face, scalp, thighs, and abdomen; mucosal ulcers with areolae appear in mouth; generalized tender papules surmounted by multilocular umbilicated vesicles; gradual desquamation; local hemorrhage into vesicles; lymphadenopathy, hepatomegaly, splenomegaly. *Lab.:* leukopenia; virus identification with electron microscope and isolation by growth in chicken embryo; rising titer of precipitating antibodies.

sodoku (rat-bite fever). See alternative term.

spine, tuberculosis of (Pott's disease). Infection of vertebrae with *Mycobacterium tuberculosis* from hematogenous route or invasion from contiguous lymph nodes leading to destruction of disks and compression of spinal cord. *Symptoms:* gradual onset of back pain and weight loss. *Signs:* gibbus, shortening of spine, muscle spasm and immobility, change of gait, paralysis. *Lab.:* positive tuberculin skin test. *X-ray:* wedge-shaped vertebrae, thinning of the intervertebral disk, spinal deformity, pulmonary tuberculosis.

spirillary rat-bite fever (rat-bite fever). See alternative term.

spondylitis, ankylosing (Marie-Strümpell-Bechterew disease). Rheumatoid arthritis of the spine, cause unknown. *Symptoms:* pain and stiffness in the back; low fever, weight loss. *Signs:* the painful sites progress upward in the spine, with local muscle spasm and limited motion; kyphosis; spinal ankylosis. *Lab.:* slight anemia, elevated C-reactive protein, elevated ESR. *X-ray:* irregular blurred sacroiliac joints; dense paravertebral ligaments; obliteration of intervertebral joint spaces, progressing cephalad.

spondylolisthesis. Forward slippage of vertebra and the spine it supports secondary to loss of the neural arch. *Symptoms:* pain in lower back and legs precipitated and/or aggravated by bending or lifting. *Signs:* shelflike depression above prominent spinous process of (usually) the 5th lumbar vertebra, horizontal pelvis, vertical sacrum, and flat buttocks. *X-ray:* anterior displacement of affected vertebra.

sporotrichosis. Infection with *Sporotrichum schenckii.* *Signs:* disseminated hard spherical nodules, turning pink, purple, and black, to ulcerate; ulcerating nodules along lymphatic vessels, felt as thick cords; polymorphous skin and mouth lesions. *Lab.:* smear and culture of discharges reveal fungi; complement-fixing antibodies appear.

sprue. A disease of unknown cause, characterized by impairment of intestinal absorption. *Symptoms:* diarrhea, anorexia, sore tongue. *Signs:* abdominal distention; malnutrition; follicular hyperkeratoses on the face; sometimes tetany. *Lab.:* megaloblastic anemia with normal gastric acid; excessive fat in feces; decreased serum carotene. *X-ray:* clumping or puddling of barium in small intestine. Biopsy of intestinal mucosa may confirm diagnosis.

Stein-Leventhal syndrome (bilateral polycystic ovarian syndrome). Enlarged cystic ovaries covered with a thickened tunica albuginea in a sterile young woman. May respond to wedge resection of ovarian cortex. Cause is unknown but may be associated with excess pituitary gonadotropic hormone secretion. *Symptoms:* sterility, periods of amenorrhea sometimes followed by menorrhagia. *Signs:* palpably enlarged cystic ovaries, hirsutism, underdeveloped breasts, obesity. *Lab.:* normal or elevated urinary 17-ketosteroids and luteinizing hormone, increased blood testosterone levels.

Still's disease (arthritis, juvenile rheumatoid). See alternative term.

stomatitis gangrenosa (Vincent's stomatitis, trench mouth). Infection with fusospirochetal organisms following nutritional deficiency, severe infections, or debilitating systemic diseases. *Symptoms:* tender ulcerated and/or bleeding gums. Signs: oral mucous membrane ulcer with gangrenous base. *Lab.:* culture of infected tissue yields fusospirochetal organisms.

stomatitis, Vincent's (stomatitis gangrenosa). See alternative term.

strabismus, comitant (nonparalytic squint). Abnormal fusional reflexes leading to inadequate simultaneous fixation of both eyes. *Symptoms:* difficulty in reading and loss of vision in nondominant eye, no diplopia. *Signs:* failure of simultaneous fixation on penlight, uncovered eye moves to fix on light in cover test.

strabismus, noncomitant (paralytic squint). Paralysis of extraocular muscles at birth or acquired. *Symptoms:* diplopia when affected eye fails to follow normal eye because of muscle palsy. *Signs:* squint occurs when affected eye is moved in direction of action of paralyzed muscle.

syphilis (lues). Infection with spirochete *Treponema pallidum* from sexual contact and presenting various clinicopathologic pictures depending upon tissues involved and the stage of the disease. *Symptoms: primary*—chancre or asymptomatic; *secondary*—headache, sore throat, myalgia, malaise, itching; *tertiary*—depends upon organ system involved. *Signs: primary*—a single, firm, painless, punched-out ulcer on or near the genitalia, and uncommonly on the lips, mouth or woman's breast, regional lymphadenopathy; *secondary*—maculopapular rash on the soles, palms, extremities appearing 6 weeks after a chancre; lymphadenopathy, fever, and alopecia; *tertiary*—aortic insufficiency, tabes dorsalis, general paresis, or gumma formation depending upon involvement. *Lab.:* treponema in dark-field examination of scrapings from chancre, or by positive serologic tests, positive *Treponema pallidum* immobilization, agglutination, antibody tests later in the disease.

syringomyelia. Abnormal fluid-filled cavities in the substance of the spinal cord from congenital malformation, trauma, or neoplasm. *Symptoms:* weakness of hands or feet, analgesia, shooting pains in limbs. *Signs:* depend on cord level involved; may have both upper and lower neuron lesions. *X-ray:* erosion of spinal canal; widening of interpedicular spaces; irregularity of articular surfaces and subchondral bone.

tabes dorsalis. Syphilis of the spinal cord. *Symptoms:* lightning-like pains in trunk and lower limbs; tabetic crises with abdominal pain and vomiting but relaxed belly wall; failing vision; paresthesias; urinary incontinence, impotence. *Signs:* Argyll Robertson pupils, ocular palsies, Romberg's sign, lost vibratory sense; absent deep reflexes; ataxia accentuated in the dark; Charcot's joints. *Blood:* VDRL positive; elevated serum globulin. *Spinal Fluid:* elevated pressure; positive VDRL test.

Takayasu's pulseless disease (arterial thrombosis due to infection). See alternative term.

telangiectasia, hereditary hemorrhagic (Rendu-Osler-Weber syndrome). A disease of multiple dilatations of venules and capillaries of skin and mucosa. Although it is a congenital vascular anomaly inherited as a simple dominant, bleeding occurs in adults and increases with aging. *Symptoms:* epistaxis, easy bruising, and prolonged bleeding from trivial trauma, hemoptysis, hematemesis, melena and hematuria. *Signs:* bright-red, 1–3-mm dilated vessels on oral or nasal mucosa, face or hands, that blanch with pressure. *Lab.:* normal tourniquet test, bleeding time, and tests of procoagulants. *X-ray:* pulmonary arteriovenous fistula is occasionally present.

temporal arteritis. Cause unknown. *Symptoms:* boring headache, weakness, weight loss, night sweats, arthralgia; pain in face, scalp, teeth, jaws, and eyes; photophobia; diplopia; mental confusion; hemiparesis. *Signs:* prominent tender temporal artery with painful nodular swelling and redness of overlying skin; oculomotor paresis, ptosis, papilledema.

tertian fever. Malarial paroxysms occurring on alternate days from a single inoculation strain of *Plasmodium vivax.*

tetanus (lockjaw). Caused by deep wound infection with *Clostridium tetani* that produces a neurotropic toxin. *Symptoms:* incubation period from 3 days to 4 weeks; restlessness, irritability, trismus, headache, chills, progressive muscular stiffness of face, neck, and limbs. *Signs:* fever; muscle spasm at wound site; later rigidity of neck, back, abdomen; risus sardonicus; tonic spasms with opisthotonos and sweating. *Spinal Fluid:* increased pressure.

tetany. Symptom complex produced by lowered serum Ca or elevated serum P in rickets, alkalosis, hypoparathyroidism, nephritis; hyperventilation causes it by changed pH of serum. *Signs:* carpopedal spasm, Chvostek's sign, Trousseau's sign, laryngospasm, stridor, nausea and vomiting, convulsions. *Lab.:* increased serum pH, increased P, lowered Ca. *Spinal Fluid:* increased pressure.

tetralogy of Fallot. Four malformations: pulmonary artery stenosis, interventricular septal defect, right ventricular hypertrophy, overriding aorta. *Signs:* cyanosis, clubbed fingers, accentuated right ventricular precordial thrust, systolic thrill at left midsternal border, systolic murmur in 5th left interspace near sternum. *ECG:* right-axis deviation, RS-T depression, inverted T in II and III, spiked P in II and III. *X-ray:* boot-shaped heart; small or absent pulmonary artery segment; diminished pulmonary vessel shadows.

thalassemia major (Cooley's anemia). Homozygous inheritance of defect of hemoglobin A synthesis with increased production of hemoglobin F and A_2. *Signs:* mongoloid facies, prominent frontal bosses, hepatomegaly, splenomegaly, pallor, cardiac dilatation, failure to grow normally. *Lab.:* hypochromic microcytic anemia; erythroblastic hyperplasia in the bone marrow; decreased osmotic fragility of erythrocytes; increased reticulocyte target cells; stippled cells; elevated serum iron; slightly increased serum bilirubin; high proportion of increased hemoglobin F and A_2. *X-ray:* increased trabeculation of bone; thin cortex in long bones; thickened cranial diploë.

thalassemia minor (Cooley's trait). Inherited heterozygous defect of thalassemia. *Symptoms:* increased fatigability. *Signs:* moderate splenomegaly. *Lab.:* moderate hypochromic microcytic anemia, poikilocytosis, stippled cells; high hemoglobin A_2, slightly increased HbF, some target cells.

thoracic empyema. From pulmonary infections or subphrenic abscess. *Symptoms:* pain in chest, fever, night sweats, weight loss. *Signs:* limited thoracic movements on affected side; dull area extending upward from base; absent breath sounds and tactile fremitus, or distant bronchial breathing. *Lab.:* leukocytosis. *Thoracentesis:* yields pus. *X-ray:* increased density with distribution of pleural fluid; mediastinal displacement away from affected side.

thromboangiitis obliterans (Buerger's disease). Inflammatory disease of arteries, cause unknown. *Symptoms:* coldness of limbs, tingling, burning, numbness. *Signs:* diminished or absent arterial pulsations in affected limb; arterial insufficiency of limb as evidenced by pallor on elevation, cyanosis on dependency; tender segments of veins; trophic changes in nails and digits. Distinguished from arteriosclerosis by being in younger age group and showing evidence of arterial spasm.

thrombosis, cavernous sinus. Thrombosis with occlusion and encephalitis around the cavernous sinus from bacterial infection of the upper lip, eyes, or face. *Symptoms:* pain in the eye and forehead with chills, fever, impaired vision. *Signs:* chemosis, edema of the eyelids, exophthalmos, hyperemia, papilledema, orbital tenderness, cranial nerve palsies of III, IV, VI; later leptomeningitis, blindness, intracerebral abscess, septicemia, and death. *Lab.:* peripheral leukocytosis or normal, increased cerebrospinal fluid turbidity and pressure.

thymoma. Neoplasm of the thymus gland sometimes associated with myasthenia gravis and pure red cell aplasia. *Symptoms:* cough, dyspnea, weakness. *Signs:* fever, pallor, widened area of retromanubrial dullness; evidence of tracheal compression. *Lab.:* hemolytic anemia, pancytopenia. *X-ray:* mass in anterior mediastinum demonstrated on lateral radiograph or CT scan.

thyrotoxicosis (hyperthyroidism). See alternative term.

tibial tubercle, osteochondritis of (Osgood-Schlatter's disease). From strain on the patellar ligament in growing bones. *Symptoms:* swelling and pain in the knee. *Signs:* localized swelling, tenderness, and heat over the tibial tubercle; often accompanied by an inflamed bursa. *X-ray:* irregular ossification of the tibial tubercle.

tic douloureux (trigeminal neuralgia). See alternative term.

Tietze's syndrome (costochondritis). See alternative term.

Toxic shock syndrome. A response to toxin elaborated by *Staphylococcus aureus* from contaminated vaginal tampons or, less frequently, from surgical wounds containing infected foreign bodies (sutures). *Symptoms and Signs:* The patient, who is usually unaware of the site of infection, suddenly experiences high fever, myalgia, nausea, vomiting, and diarrhea. Within a few days, a diffuse erythematous rash (like sunburn) appears, followed by altered mentation, adult respiratory distress syndrome (ARDS), hypotension and shock. *Lab.:* hypoalbuminemia, hypocalcemia, thrombocytopenia, azotemia, and elevated liver and muscle enzymes.

toxoplasmosis. Infection with the protozoan *Toxoplasma gondii.* *Symptoms:* malaise, myalgia, arthralgia, weakness. *Signs:* fever, lymphadenopathy, transient maculopapular rash, headache with mental confusion, signs of pneumonitis; occasional hepatomegaly or splenomegaly. *Cultures:* organisms in urine, spinal fluid, lymph node fluid. *Lab.:* rising serum antibody titer. *X-ray:* calcified area in brain in congenital form.

trichinosis. Infection with *Trichinella spiralis* from ingestion of incompletely cooked infected pork. *Symptoms:* 1–4 days after eating pork: nausea and vomiting, diarrhea, abdominal pain; 10 days later: fever, dyspnea, anorexia, myalgia and asthenia. *Signs:* periorbital edema, scarlatiniform rash, splinter hemorrhages under nails, tremors, involuntary movements. *Lab.:* eosinophilia with some leukocytosis; larva in blood early; later, larva in muscle biopsy; complement-fixing antibodies.

tricuspid regurgitation. Associated with right heart failure from any cause. *Signs:* prominent jugular pulses; pulsating liver; medium-pitched pansystolic murmur at left lower sternal margin accentuated during inspiration.

tricuspid stenosis. The result of rheumatic endocarditis, the lesion is usually associated with both mitral and aortic disease. *Signs:* accentuated precordial thrust of the right ventricle; diastolic thrill at the lower left sternal border; presystolic or middiastolic low-pitched rumbling murmur at left sternal border in 5th interspace; accentuation of murmur during inspiration; opening snap of tricuspid valve at right sternal border; pulsating liver; pronounced "a" wave in jugular pulse preceding the carotid artery pulse.

trigeminal neuralgia (tic douloureux). Cause unknown. *Symptoms:* paroxysms of excruciating pain along the course of a branch of the 5th cranial nerve, triggered by cold air on the face, shaving, chewing, or other movements. *Signs:* muscle spasms, flushing of the face, lacrimation, salivation, all during an attack.

trypanosomiasis, African (sleeping sickness). Infection with *Trypanosoma gambiense* from the bite of the tsetse fly. *Symptoms:* irregular fever, headache, insomnia, generalized pain, deep hyperesthesia; late lethargy, somnolence. *Signs:* erythema and swelling at inoculation site; erythematous patchy pruritic rash; generalized lymphadenopathy, hepatomegaly, splenomegaly, edema of the limbs; cachexia; tremors, convulsions, coma, and death. *Lab.:* trypanosomes in blood, lymph node fluid, spinal fluid.

trypanosomiasis, South American (Chagas' disease). Infection with *Trypanosoma cruzi* from the bite of reduviidae insects. *Signs:* swollen inoculation site with regional lymphadenitis; 2 weeks later, red macular rash on chest; later, unilateral conjunctivitis, facial edema, dyspnea, syncope, and precordial pain. *Lab.:* trypanosomes in blood, lymph node fluid, and spinal fluid.

tuberculosis. Transmissible infection of the lungs or other organ systems with *Mycobacterium tuberculosis.* *Symptoms:* asymptomatic or insidious onset of malaise, fevers, night sweats, weight loss, and, in cavitary pulmonary infections, hemoptysis. *Signs:* none or fevers, apical posttussive rales, amphoric, bronchial breath sounds, and signs of pleural effusion with advanced disease. *Lab.:* leukocytosis, increased sedimentation rate, positive tuberculin skin test, positive smear or culture of sputum or morning gastric aspirate. *X-ray:* apical infiltrates, mediastinal lymphadenopathy and cavities.

tularemia (rabbit fever). Infection with *Pasteurella tularensis* usually from handling meat or hides from infected dead animals. *Symptoms:* incubation 1–10 days; lassitude, headache, chill, nausea and vomiting, myalgia. *Signs of Ulceroglandular Type:* high fever, indolent ulcer on hand with painful regional lymphadenitis, splenomegaly. *Signs of Oculoglandular Type:* lacrimation, photophobia, edema of lids, lymphadenitis of cervical and facial drainage region. *Signs of Gastrointestinal Type:* hematemesis, melena, lymphadenitis. *Signs of Typhoidal Type:* severe fever, no lymphadenitis or ulceration. *Signs of Pleuropneumonic Type:* patchy pneumonia. *Lab.:* gram-negative bacilli in ulcers, lymph nodes, sputum, or blood. Later, development of agglutinins in blood serum.

Turner's syndrome (gonadal dysgenesis). See alternative term.

typhoid fever. Infection with *Salmonella typhosa.* *Symptoms:* incubation 10–12 days; chills and fever, prostration, cough, epistaxis, constipation or diarrhea. *Signs:* slowly progressing lassitude, abdominal distention and tenderness, splenomegaly, rose spots, delirium. *Lab.:* leukopenia, occult blood in feces; organisms cultured from blood early; later, cultures from stools and urine more frequent. Rising agglutinin titer in blood; positive Widal test.

typhus fever, epidemic. Infection with *Rickettsia prowazeki* from the bite of *Pediculus humanis corporis*. *Symptoms:* incubation 7–10 days; sudden onset of chills and fever, severe headaches, cough, gastrointestinal disturbances. *Signs:* generalized red macular rash, except on palms, soles, and face; flushing; red conjunctivae; in severe cases, confluent purpura, delirium. CNS involvement. *Lab.:* azotemia; rising antibody titer; positive Felix-Weil agglutination of Proteus OX-19.

typhus scrub. Infection with *Rickettsia tsutsugamushi* from mites. *Symptoms:* incubation 10–12 days; malaise, chills and fever; headache. *Signs:* erythematous inoculation site forming an ulcer; red macular rash on trunk; fever; rales; splenomegaly; lymphadenopathy. *Lab.:* positive Felix-Weil agglutination of Proteus OX-19.

uremia. A clinical picture associated with renal failure; it includes azotemia, although the symptoms do not necessarily parallel the degree of azotemia. *Symptoms:* increased fatigability, headache, anorexia, nausea and vomiting, diarrhea, hiccup, restlessness, depression. *Signs:* epistaxis, melena, dyspnea, Cheyne-Stokes breathing fetid breath, dehydration, muscle twitching, convulsions, delirium, coma. *Lab.:* azotemia, acidosis, high serum K and P, low Ca and CO_2; anemia; isosthenuria. The uremic breath contains many toxic metabolites, among which are dimethylamine and trimethylamine, which account for the fishy odor.

urinary bladder, rupture of. *Symptoms:* abdominal pain and muscle spasm, desire to urinate without being successful; passage of small amount of bloody urine. *Signs:* abdominal distention and muscle rigidity; mass in pelvic cul-de-sac; catheterization demonstrates urethral patency. *Lab.:* hematuria.

varicella (chickenpox). See alternative term.

variola (smallpox). See alternative term.

ventricular septal defect. A congenital anomaly or the result of infarction. *Signs:* accentuation of apical precordial thrust; medium-pitched pansystolic murmur at left sternal border in 4th or 5th interspace, often accompanied by a thrill in same region; murmur not influenced by inspiration, in contrast to the murmur of tricuspid regurgitation.

Whipple's disease (intestinal lipodystrophy). Invasion of intestinal mucosa and lamina propria with foamy macrophages filled with glycoprotein and producing lymphatic obstruction and malabsorption, of unknown cause. *Symptoms:* diffuse abdominal cramping and episodic diarrhea of fatty foul-smelling stools, weight loss, malaise and weakness, migratory polyarthralgias, cough, dyspnea. *Signs:* intermittent fever, hypotension, edema, lymphadenopathy, emaciation. *Lab.:* anemia, elevated ESR, increased excretion of fat in stools, hypocholesterolemia, hypoalbuminemia, biopsy of node or intestinal mucosa may reveal histiocytes containing PAS-positive material. *X-ray:* small-bowel x-ray may show flocculation and segmentation of barium as seen in malabsorption.

whooping cough (pertussis). See alternative term.

Wilson's disease (hepatolenticular degeneration). See alternative term.

Wolff-Parkinson-White syndrome. Congenital accessory conduction pathway in the heart, producing frequent dysrhythmia and distorted ECG. *Symptoms:* chest pain during the dysrhythmia. *Signs During Attack:* frequent attacks of paroxysmal tachycardia with fast regular ventricular beats without vagus slowing. *ECG Between Attacks:* shortened P-R interval; slightly widened QRS complex.

wuchereriasis (filariasis). See alternative term.

xanthelasma of eyelid. Localized deposits in the eyelids usually associated with hypercholesterolemia. *Signs:* soft, elevated beige-colored plaques on the eyelids, usually symmetric, often coalescent. *Lab.:* lipemia, hypercholesterolemia.

xanthoma disseminatum. Generalized skin deposits associated with hypercholesterolemia. *Signs:* small, closely packed red-to-brown papules and petechiae on scalp, face, trunk, axillae, and flexor surfaces of limbs. *Lab.:* hyperlipemia.

xanthoma, juvenile. Systemic deposits associated with familial type of disordered fat metabolism. *Signs:* relatively large red, brown, or yellow plaques on scalp, face, trunk, and extensor surfaces of limbs. In another familial type, nodules are palpable along the tendons and ligaments. *Lab.:* hypercholesterolemia, hyperlipemia.

xeroderma pigmentosum. A congenital disease of the skin with extreme sensitivity to light. *Symptoms:* slight light exposure causes skin inflammation; photophobia. *Signs:* light stimulates many freckles, keratoses, telangiectases; white spots of atrophy, superficial ulceration; verrucous malignant neoplasms.

yaws (frambesia). An endemic granulomatous disease of the tropics caused by *Treponema pertenue* and transmitted by close personal contact. *Symptoms:* irregular fever, headache, malaise, anorexia, arthralgia. *Signs:* primary lesion at point of implantation 2–8 weeks after contact; large red ulcerating granuloma with regional lymphadenopathy; secondary lesions in 6–10 weeks; macules and papules with adenopathy and desquamation; swellings over bones; tertiary lesions: one to many years later; deep granulomatous ulceration and bone lesions. *Lab.:* treponemes in exudates; positive VDRL, other serologies and treponema immobilization tests. *X-ray:* periosteal proliferation; rarefaction of long bone shafts.

yellow fever. A viral disease transmitted from man to man or from monkey to man by the bite of mosquitoes of genus Haemogogus or Aedes. *Symptoms:* incubation 3–6 days; nausea and vomiting; chills, headache; restlessness; prostration; pains in leg muscles. *Signs:* irregular fever; slowing pulse; jaundice, purpura and mucosal hemorrhages; hematemesis, melena; delirium, convulsions, coma. *Lab.:* leukopenia, diminished granulocytes, hypoglycemia, hyperbilirubinemia; proteinuria, oliguria, retention of Cl, blood in stools. Positive neutralization tests; virus isolated from blood.

Zollinger-Ellison syndrome. Pancreatic gastrinomas or adenomatous hyperplasia of non-Beta islet cells produce excess gastrin that stimulates high HCl in stomach and ulcers in esophagus, duodenum, and jejunum. *Symptoms:* recurrent attacks of epigastric pain, nausea and vomiting, diarrhea. *Lab.:* high basal and stimulated acid secretion; hypergastrinemia; positive secretin test. *X-ray:* multiple peptic ulcers in esophagus, duodenum, and jejunum; CT scan may reveal pancreatic gastrinoma.

References

Allergy and Immunology

Middleton, Elliott, Jr., Reed, Charles E., and Ellis, Elliott F., editors: *Allergy: Principles and Practice,* 2d ed., C. V. Mosby Co., St. Louis, 1983.

Patterson, Roy: *Allergic Diseases,* 3d. ed., J. B. Lippincott Co., Philadelphia, 1985.

Lachmann, P. J., and Peters, D. J., editors: *Clinical Aspects of Immunology,* 4th ed., C. V. Mosby Co., St. Louis, 1982.

Anatomy

Basmajian, J. V.: *Grant's Method of Anatomy,* 10th ed., The Williams & Wilkins Co., Baltimore, 1980.

Clemente, Carmine D., editor: *Gray's Anatomy of the Human Body,* 30th ed., Lea & Febiger, Philadelphia, 1984.

Pansky, Ben: *Review of Gross Anatomy,* 5th ed., Macmillan Publishing Co., New York, 1984.

Romanos, G. J., editor: *Cunningham's Manual of Practical Anatomy. Vol. 1, Upper & Lower Limbs; Vol. 2, Thorax & Abdomen; Vol. 3, Head, Neck & Brain;* 14th ed., Oxford University Press, Oxford, 1976–1979.

Woodburne, Russell T.: *Essentials of Human Anatomy,* 7th ed., Oxford University Press, New York, 1983.

Cardiology

Braunwald, Eugene, editor: *Heart Disease: A Textbook of Cardiovascular Medicine,* 2nd ed., W. B. Saunders Co., Philadelphia, 1984.

Hurst, J. Willis, Logue, R. Bruce, Schlant, Robert C., Sonnenblick, Edmund H., Wallace, Andus G., and Wenger, Nanette K., editors: *The Heart,* 6th ed., McGraw-Hill Book Co., New York, 1986.

Silber, Earl N.: *Heart Disease,* 2d ed. Macmillan Publishing Co., New York, 1987.

Dermatology

Fitzpatrick, Thomas B., Eisen, Arthur Z., Wolff, Klaus, Freedberg, Irwin B., and Austen, K. Frank, editors: *Dermatology in General Medicine,* 2d ed., McGraw-Hill Book Co., New York, 1979.

Diagnostic Imaging

Juhl, John H.: *Paul and Juhl's Essentials of Roentgen Interpretation,* 4th ed., Harper and Row Publishers, Inc., Hagerstown, Maryland, 1981.

Moss, Albert A., Gamsu, Gordon, and Genant, Harry K, editors: *Computed Tomography of the Body,* W. B. Saunders Co., Philadelphia, 1983.

Partain, C. Leon, James, A. Everette, Jr., Rollo, F. David, and Price, Ronald R., editors: *Nuclear Magnetic Resonance (NMR) Imaging,* W. B. Saunders Co., Philadelphia, 1983.

Diagnostic Reasoning

Cutler, Paul: *Problem Solving in Clinical Medicine: From Data to Diagnosis,* The Williams & Wilkins Co., Baltimore, 1985.

Elstein, A. S., Shulman, L. S., Sprafka, S. A., et al.: *Medical Problem Solving: An Analysis of Clinical Reasoning,* Harvard University Press, Cambridge, 1978.

Feinstein, Alvan R.: *Clinical Judgment,* The Williams & Wilkins Co., Baltimore, 1967.

Wulff, Henrik R.: *Rational Diagnosis and Treatment: An Introduction to Clinical Decision Making,* 2d ed., C. V. Mosby Co., St. Louis, 1981.

Diagnostic Tests

Henry, John B., editor: *Todd-Sanford-Davidsohn Clinical Diagnosis and Management by Laboratory Methods,* 17th ed., W. B. Saunders Co., Philadelphia, 1984.

Wallach, Jacques: *Interpretation of Diagnostic Tests: A Handbook Synopsis of Laboratory Medicine,* 3d ed., Little, Brown and Co., Boston, 1978.

Diagnostics

Hart, F. Dudley, editor: *French's Index of Differential Diagnosis,* 12th ed., PSG Publishing Co., Inc., Littleton, Massachusetts, 1985.

Endocrinology and Metabolism

Felig, Philip, Baxter, John D., Broadus, Arthur E., and Frohman, Lawrence C., editors: *Endocrinology and Metabolism,* McGraw-Hill Book Co., New York, 1981.

Wilson, Jean B., and Foster, Daniel W., editors: *William's Textbook of Endocrinology,* 7th ed., W. B. Saunders Co., Philadelphia, 1985.

Gastroenterology

Sleisenger, Marvin H., and Fordtran, John S.: *Gastrointestinal Disease: Pathophysiology, Diagnosis, Management,* 3d ed., W. B. Saunders Co., Philadelphia, 1983.

Spiro, Howard M.: *Clinical Gastroenterology,* 3d ed., Macmillan Publishing Co., New York, 1983.

Hematology

Williams, William J., et al.: *Hematology,* 3d ed., McGraw-Hill Book Co., New York, 1983.

Wintrobe, Maxwell M., et al.: *Clinical Hematology,* 8th ed., Lea & Febiger, Philadelphia, 1981.

Infectious Diseases

Braude, Abraham I.: *Infectious Diseases and Medical Microbiology,* 2d ed., Vol. 2, *The International Textbook of Medicine,* W. B. Saunders Co., Philadelphia, 1985.

Hoeprich, Paul D., editor: *Infectious Disease,* 3d ed., Harper Medical Publishers, Inc., New York, 1983.

Mandell, Gerald L., Douglas, R. Gordon, Jr., and Bennett, John E., editors: *Principles and Practice of Infectious Diseases,* 2d ed., John Wiley & Sons, Inc., New York, 1985.

Wehrle, Paul F., and Top, Franklin H., Sr.: *Communicable and Infectious Diseases,* 9th ed., The C. V. Mosby Co., St. Louis, 1981.

Internal Medicine

Wyngaarden, James B., and Smith, Floyd H., editors: *Cecil Textbook of Medicine,* 17th ed., W. B. Saunders Co., Philadelphia, 1985.

Petersdorf, R. G., Adams, R. D., Braunwald, E., Isselbacher, K. J., Martin, J. B., and Wilson, J. D., editors: *Harrison's Principles of Internal Medicine,* 10th ed., McGraw-Hill Book Co., New York, 1983.

Rubenstein, Edward, and Federman, Daniel D., editors: *Scientific American Medicine,* updated monthly, Scientific American, Inc., New York, 1984.

Nephrology

Brenner, Barry M., and Rector, Floyd C., editors: *The Kidney,* 2 Vols., 3d ed., W. B. Saunders Co., New York, 1985.

Massry, Shaul G., and Glassock, Richard J., editors: *Textbook of Nephrology,* 2 Vols., Williams and Wilkins, Baltimore, 1983.

Rose, Burton D.: *Pathophysiology of Renal Disease,* McGraw-Hill Book Co., New York, 1981.

Neurology

Adams, Raymond D., and Victor, Maurice: *Principles of Neurology*, 3d ed, McGraw-Hill Book Co., New York, 1985.

Rowland, Lewis P., editor: *Merritt's Textbook of Neurology*, 7th ed., Lea & Febiger, Philadelphia, 1984.

Van Allen, Maurice W.: *Pictorial Manual of Neurologic Tests*, Year Book Medical Publishers, Chicago, 1980.

Obstetrics and Gynecology

Danforth, David N., Dignam, William J., Hendricks, Charles H., and Maeck, John Van S., editors: *Obstetrics and Gynecology*, 4th ed., Harper and Row Publishers, Inc., Philadelphia, 1982.

Glass, Robert H.: *Office Gynecology*, 2d ed., Williams and Wilkins, Baltimore, 1981.

Pritchard, Jack A., and MacDonald, Paul C.: *Williams Obstetrics*, 17th ed., Appleton-Century-Crofts, Norwalk, Connecticut, 1984.

Oncology

Calabresi, Paul, Schein, Philip S., and Rosenberg, Saul A., editors: *Medical Oncology: Basic Principles and Clinical Management of Cancer*, Macmillan Publishing Co., New York, 1984.

DeVita, Vincent T., Hellman, Samuel, and Rosenberg, Steven A., editors: *Cancer: Principles and Practice of Oncology*, 2d ed., J. B. Lippincott Co., Philadelphia, 1985.

Holland, James F., and Frei, Emil, III, editors: *Cancer Medicine*, 2d ed., Lea & Febiger, Philadelphia, 1982.

Ophthalmology

Newell, Frank W.: *Ophthalmology Principles and Concepts*, 5th ed., The C. V. Mosby Co., St. Louis, 1982.

Vaughn, Daniel, and Asbury, Taylor: *General Ophthalmology*, 10th ed., Lange Medical Publications, Los Altos, California, 1983.

Orthopaedics

Edmonson, A. S., and Crenshaw, A. H., editors: *Campbell's Operative Orthopaedics*, 6th ed., The C. V. Mosby Co., St. Louis, 1980.

Evarts, C. McCollister, editor: *Surgery of the Musculoskeletal System*. Churchill Livingstone, New York, 1983.

Salter, Robert B.: *Textbook of the Disorders and Injuries of the Musculoskeletal System*, 2d ed., The Williams & Wilkins Co., Baltimore, 1983.

Turek, Samuel L.: *Orthopaedics: Principles and Their Application*, 4th ed., J. B. Lippincott Co., Philadelphia, 1983.

Otolaryngology

De Weese, David D., and Saunders, William H., editors: *Textbook of Otolaryngology,* 6th ed., The C. V. Mosby Co., St. Louis, 1982.

Pharmacology

Gilman, Alfred Goodman, Goodman, Louis S., Rall, Theodore W., and Murad, Ferid, editors: *Goodman and Gilman's The Pharmacological Basis of Therapeutics,* 7th ed., Macmillan Publishing Co., New York, 1985.

Spector, Reynold: *The Scientific Basis of Clinical Pharmacology: Principles and Examples,* Little, Brown and Co., Boston, 1986.

Physical Diagnosis (Medical)

Bates, Barbara: *A Guide to Physical Examination,* 4th ed., J. B. Lippincott Co., Philadelphia, 1983.

Delp, Mahlon H., and Manning, Robert T.: *Major's Physical Diagnosis,* 9th ed., W. B. Saunders Co., Philadelphia, 1981.

Judge, Richard D., Zuidema, George D., and Fitzgerald, Faith T., editors: *Clinical Diagnosis: A Physiologic Approach,* 4th ed., Little Brown and Co., Boston, 1982.

Prior, John A., and Silberstein, Jack S.: *Physical Diagnosis: The History and Examination of the Patient,* 6th ed., The C. V. Mosby Co., St. Louis, 1981.

Physical Diagnosis (Surgical)

Clain, Allan, editor: *Hamilton Bailey's Demonstrations of Physical Signs in Clinical Surgery,* 16th ed., PSG, Baltimore, 1980.

Silen, William, editor: *Cope's Early Diagnosis of the Acute Abdomen,* 16th ed., Oxford University Press, New York, 1983.

Physiology/Pathophysiology

Berne, Robert M., and Levy, Mathew N., editors: *Physiology,* C. V. Mosby Co., St. Louis, 1983.

Guyton, Arthur C., editor: *Textbook of Medical Physiology,* 7th ed., W. B. Saunders Co., Philadelphia, 1986.

Wright, Samson: *Samson Wright's Applied Physiology,* 13th ed., Oxford University Press, New York, 1982.

Psychiatry

Abram, Harry S., editor: *Basic Psychiatry for the Primary Care Physician,* Little, Brown and Co., Boston, 1979.

Kaplan, Harold I., and Sadock, Benjamin J., editors: *Comprehensive Textbook of Psychiatry IV,* 4th ed., The Williams & Wilkins Co., Baltimore, 1984.

Pulmonary Disease

Baum, Gerald L., and Wolinsky, E., editors: *Textbook of Pulmonary Diseases,* 3d ed., Little Brown and Co., Boston, 1983.

Cherniack, Reuben M., et al: *Respiration in Health and Disease,* 3d ed., W. B. Saunders Co., Philadelphia, 1983.

Guenter, Clarence H., and Welch, Martin H., editors: *Pulmonary Medicine,* 2d ed., J. B. Lippincott Co., Philadelphia, 1982.

Poe, Robert H., and Israel, Robert H., editors: *Problems in Pulmonary Medicine for the Primary Physician,* Lea & Febiger, Philadelphia, 1982.

Rheumatology

Kelley, William N., Harris, Edward Day, Jr., Ruddy, Shaun, and Sledge, Clement B., editors: *Textbook of Rheumatology,* 2d ed., W. B. Saunders Co., Philadelphia, 1985.

McCarty, Daniel J., Jr., editor: *Arthritis and Allied Conditions: A Textbook of Rheumatology,* 11th ed., Lea & Febiger, Philadelphia, 1985.

Terminology

Blakiston's Gould Medical Dictionary, 4th ed., McGraw-Hill Book Co., New York, 1979.

Dorland's Illustrated Medical Dictionary, 26th ed., W. B. Saunders Co., Philadelphia, 1981.

Stedman's Medical Dictionary, 24th ed., The Williams & Wilkins Co., Baltimore, 1981.

Ultrasonic Examination

Brown, Ross E.: *Ultrasonography: Basic Principles and Clinical Applications,* 2d ed., Warren H. Green, Inc., St. Louis, 1979.

Goldberg, Barry, and Wells, Peter N.: *Ultrasonics in Clinical Diagnosis,* 3d ed., Churchill Livingstone, New York, 1983.

Kremkau, Frederick W.: *Diagnostic Ultrasound: Principles, Instrumentation, and Exercises,* 2d ed., Grune and Stratton, Orlando, Florida, 1984.

Urology

Smith, Donald R.: *General Urology,* 11th ed., Lange Medical Publications, Los Altos, California, 1984.

Walsh, Patrick C., Perlmutter, Alan D., Gittes, Rubin F., and Stamey, Thomas A.: *Campbell's Urology,* 5th ed., W. B. Saunders Co., Philadelphia, 1985.

Procedures in Examination

Discussions of the following topics occur within the text in **boldface** type.

Index

Pages whose numbers are marked with asterisks bear figures pertinent to the subject.

Index

Index

Index

Index

Index

Index

Index

Index

Index

Index

Index

Index

Index

Index

Index